PHARMACOLOGY FOR NURSES
CANADIAN EDITION

A PATHOPHYSIOLOGICAL APPROACH

PHARMACOLOGY FOR NURSES
CANADIAN EDITION

A PATHOPHYSIOLOGICAL APPROACH

MICHAEL PATRICK ADAMS, PhD, RT(R)
Dean of Health Occupations
Pasco-Hernando Community College

LELAND NORMAN HOLLAND, Jr., PhD
Associate Academic Dean
Dean, College of Arts and Sciences
Southeastern University

PAULA MANUEL BOSTWICK, RN, MSN
Nursing Department Chair
Ivy Tech Community College

SHIRLEY LINDA KING, RN, BN, MN, PhD
Fellow, Canadian College of Neuropsychopharmacology
Instructor, Mount Royal School of Nursing
Mount Royal College

Pearson Canada
Toronto

Library and Archives Canada Cataloguing in Publication

Pharmacology for nurses : a pathophysiological approach / Michael Patrick Adams ... [et al.].—Canadian ed.

Includes bibliographical references and index.
ISBN 978-0-13-173123-3

1. Pharmacology. 2. Nurses. I. Adams, Michael, 1951–

RM301.P4565 2009   615'.1   C2008-907346-0

Original edition published by Pearson Education, Inc., Upper Saddle River, New Jersey, USA. Copyright © 2008, 2005. Pearson Education, Inc. This edition is authorized for sale only in Canada.

ISBN-13: 978-0-13-173123-3
ISBN-10: 0-13-173123-8

Vice-President, Editorial Director: Gary Bennett
Executive Editor: Michelle Sartor
Senior Marketing Manager: Colleen Gauthier
Senior Developmental Editor: Paul Donnelly
Production Editor: Avivah Wargon
Copy Editor: Kelly Davis
Proofreader: Kelly Coleman
Production Coordinator: Lynn O'Rourke
Compositor: Hermia Chung
Art Director: Julia Hall
Cover Designer: Anthony Leung
Interior Designer: Anthony Leung
Cover Image: Veer Inc.

Care has been taken to confirm the accuracy of information presented in this book. The authors, editors, and the publisher, however, cannot accept any responsibility for errors or omissions or for consequences from the application of the information in this book and make no warranty, expressed or implied, with respect to its contents.

The authors and publisher have exerted every effort to ensure that drug selections and dosages set forth in this text are in accord with current recommendations and practice at the time of publication. However, in view of ongoing research, changes in government regulations, and the constant flow of information relating to drug therapy and drug reactions, the reader is urged to check the package inserts of all drugs for any change in indications of dosage and for added warnings and precautions. This is particularly important when the recommended agent is a new or infrequently employed drug.

3 4 5   13 12 11

Printed and bound in the United States of America.

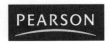

I dedicate this book to nursing educators, who contribute every day to making the world a better and more caring place.

—MPA

I would like to acknowledge the willful encouragement of Farrell and Norma Jean Stalcup. I dedicate this book to my beloved wife, Karen, and my three wonderful children, Alexandria Noelle, my double-deuce daughter, Caleb Jaymes, my number-one son, and Joshua Nathaniel, my number three "O."

—LNH

I dedicate the book to my husband Charles, the love of my life, my son C.J., and my daughter Bailey. Thank you for all of your love, support, and encouragement. I am so blessed to share my life with each of you.

—PMB

I dedicate this book to my nursing students, who inspire me always and who encouraged the authoring of this book. With your inquisitive minds, courageous spirits, and warm hearts, you have brought much joy to my life and work.

—SLK

BRIEF CONTENTS

CONTENTS

SPECIAL FEATURES

PHARMFACTS

PROTOTYPE DRUG

SPECIAL CONSIDERATIONS

LIFESPAN CONSIDERATIONS

PREFACE

When students are asked which subject in their nursing program is the most challenging, pharmacology always appears near the top of the list. The study of pharmacology demands that students apply knowledge from a wide variety of the natural and applied sciences. The successful prediction of drug action requires a thorough knowledge of anatomy, physiology, chemistry, and pathology, as well as the social sciences of psychology and sociology. Lack of proper application of pharmacology can result in immediate and direct harm to the client; thus, the stakes in learning the subject are high.

Pharmacology can be made more understandable if the proper connections are made to knowledge learned in other disciplines. The vast majority of drugs in clinical practice are prescribed for specific diseases, yet many pharmacology textbooks fail to recognize the complex interrelationships between pharmacology and pathophysiology. When drugs are learned in isolation from their associated diseases or conditions, students have difficulty connecting pharmacotherapy to therapeutic goals and client wellness. The pathophysiology approach of this textbook gives the student a clearer picture of the importance of pharmacology to disease, and ultimately to client care. The approach and rationale of this textbook focus on a holistic perspective to client care, which clearly shows the benefits and limitations of pharmacotherapy in curing or preventing illness. Although challenging, the study of pharmacology is truly a fascinating, lifelong journey.

Organization—A Body System and Disease Approach

Pharmacology for Nurses: A Pathophysiological Approach, Canadian Edition, is organized according to body systems (units) and diseases (chapters). Each chapter provides complete information on the drug classifications used to treat the disease(s). Specially designed headings cue students to each classification discussion.

The pathophysiology approach clearly places the drugs in context with how they are used therapeutically. The student is able to easily locate all relevant anatomy, physiology, pathology, and pharmacology in the same chapter in which the drugs are discussed. This approach provides the student with a clear view of the connection between pharmacology, pathophysiology, and the nursing care learned in other clinical courses. **PharmFacts** features present pertinent facts and statistics related to the disease and its treatment, providing a social and economic perspective.

PROTOTYPE APPROACH TO LEARNING DRUGS

The vast number of drugs available in clinical practice is staggering. To facilitate learning, we use prototypes where the one or two most representative drugs in each classifica-tion are introduced in detail in each chapter. Students are less intimidated when they can focus their learning on one representative drug in each class. **Prototype Drug** boxes clearly describe these important medications. Within these boxes, the **actions and uses** of the drug are succinctly presented, including **administration alerts,** which highlight vital information related to the administration of that drug and treatment of overdose and antidotes when known. **Pharmacokinetics** information regarding the absorption, distribution, metabolism, excretion, and half-life of drugs is included when known. **Adverse effects** and **drug-drug**, **herb-drug,** and **food-drug interactions** are also included.

FOCUSED COVERAGE OF THE NURSING PROCESS

This textbook features a focused approach to the Nursing Process, which allows students to quickly find the content that is essential for safe, effective drug therapy. **Nursing Considerations** sections appear within each drug class discussion. These sections discuss the major needs of the client, including general assessments, interventions, and client teaching for the classification. Client education discussions provide students with the essential information that they need to convey to their clients. **Integrated rationales** for nursing actions help students to learn the reasoning that is key to the development of critical thinking skills.

Nursing Process Focus charts provide a succinct, easy-to-read view of the most commonly prescribed drug classes for the disease. Need-to-know nursing actions are presented in a format that reflects the "flow" of the Nursing Process: nursing assessment, pattern identification and potential nursing diagnoses, planning, interventions, client education and discharge planning, and evaluation. Rationales for interventions are included in parentheses. The Nursing Process Focus charts identify clearly what nursing actions are most important. Some prototype drugs have important nursing actions that are specific to that drug; in these instances, we provide a Nursing Process Focus chart in the text devoted solely to the prototype drug. Nursing Process Focus charts for many of the prototype drugs can be found on the Companion Website (http://www.pearsoned.ca/adams-king). The 🌐 icon is provided at the bottom of each Prototype Drug box to remind the student that this content can be found on the Companion Website.

Holistic Pharmacology

Pharmacology for Nurses: A Pathophysiological Approach, Canadian Edition, examines pharmacology from a holistic perspective. The **Special Considerations** and **Lifespan Considerations** features present pharmacology and nursing issues related to **cultural, ethnic, age, gender,** and **psychoso-cial** aspects. These features remind students that a drug's efficacy is affected as much by its pharmacokinetics as by the uniqueness of the client. In addition, **pediatric** and **geriatric** considerations are integrated throughout the textbook.

Natural Therapies features present a popular herbal or dietary supplement that may be considered along with conventional drugs. Although the authors do not recommend the use of these alternative treatments in lieu of conventional medicines, many clients use complementary and alternative therapies and the nurse must become familiar with how they affect client health. **Herb-drug interactions** are also included within the Prototype Drug boxes. Non-pharmacological methods for controlling many diseases are also integrated into the chapters, and include **lifestyle and dietary modifications**.

Learning Pharmacology through Visuals

For nearly all students, learning is a highly visual process. This textbook incorporates generous use of artwork to illustrate and summarize key concepts. At the beginning of each unit, vivid and colourful illustrations help students recall important concepts of anatomy and physiology for that body system. Pharmacotherapy illustrations provide students with a visual overview of a drug therapy process, showing specifically how the drug acts to counteract the effects of disease on the body.

Pharmacology for Nurses: A Pathophysiological Approach, Canadian Edition, is the first nursing pharmacology textbook to incorporate **Mechanism in Action** animations, which use computer simulations to clearly demonstrate drug action at the molecular, tissue, and system levels. The MediaLink banner at the end of each chapter directs the student to full-colour animations, including audio narrations that describe each step of the mechanism, on the MediaLink DVD-ROM included with this book. Additional animations, which illustrate important pharmacological concepts such as agonists and antagonists, can also be found on the DVD-ROM.

The chapters on **Medication Incidents and Risk Reduction** and **Toxicology and Emergency Preparedness** include important content on the promotion of client safety, management of medication incidents, and the role of the nurse in situations involving toxicity and biochemical emergencies.

A NOTE ABOUT TERMINOLOGY

The term "healthcare provider" is used to denote the physician, nurse practitioner, and any other health professional that is legally authorized to prescribe drugs.

Student Resources

The following resources have been developed in support of the textbook to help students in their learning of pharmacology.

 MEDIALINK DVD-ROM

Packaged with every copy of the textbook, this dynamic DVD-ROM includes:

- **Audio Glossary** with pronunciations and definitions of every key term in the textbook
- **Drug Prototype Audio Pronunciations** of the most commonly used prototypes
- **Drug Dosage Calculator** to help you with conversions and calculations
- **Nursing in Action** video case studies for medication administration
- **CRNE (Canadian Registered Nurse Examination) Review** questions that emphasize the application of care and client education related to drug administration
- **Mechanism of Action** drug animation tutorials for prototype drugs, showing how drug action occurs at the tissue, organ, and system levels

 COMPANION WEBSITE

Serving students as an online review of the textbook, this Companion Website includes:

- Additional **CRNE Review** questions with comprehensive rationales
- Pharmacology review activities that test your understanding of the drugs from each chapter, such as **Classification Reviews, Drug Reviews,** and **Case Studies.**
- **Dosage Calculation** exercises that provide practice for drugs in the chapter
- **Nursing Process Focus** charts for drug prototypes
- **Preventing Medication Errors** review module and activities
- **Student Success** module with advice and activities to help you be a successful nursing student
- And much more!

STUDENT WORKBOOK

The workbook contains a large number and variety of practice questions and learning activities, including fill-ins, matching, multiple choice, case studies, and dosage calculations.

Instructor Resources

To aid in teaching your pharmacology course, the following resources have been designed to support the textbook.

INSTRUCTOR'S RESOURCE MANUAL

Designed to help faculty plan and manage the pharmacology course, this manual includes:

- Detailed lecture notes with correlations to PowerPoint slides, organized by learning objectives

- Suggestions for classroom and clinical activities
- Comprehensive test questions with rationales, mapped to learning objectives

It also includes a **Strategies for Instructor Success** module for faculty that explains learning theories, planning for instructions, how to use effective pedagogies, assessing learning, and more!

INSTRUCTOR'S RESOURCE DVD-ROM

This DVD-ROM includes all the textbook resources instructors need to teach pharmacology:

- Comprehensive **PowerPoint Presentation** that integrates lecture slides, images, animations, videos, and other resources
- Complete **Image Gallery** in PowerPoint
- Additional **Media Resources**, such as videos and animations, to enhance your classroom presentations
- **TestGen** with questions mapped to the chapter learning objectives

Acknowledgments

Authoring the first Canadian edition of this textbook has been a major undertaking made possible through the contributions of many individuals. First, I would like to acknowledge the efforts of the authors of the U.S. editions. Their work provided an excellent foundation for this textbook.

I thank the dedicated and talented team at Pearson Education Canada: acquisitions editor Michelle Sartor; marketing manager Colleen Gauthier; developmental editor Paul Donnelly; production editor Avivah Wargon; designer Anthony Leung; and production coordinators Patricia Ciardullo and Lynn O'Rourke. Thanks also go to copy editor Kelly Davis and proofreader Kelly Coleman.

I also want to thank the reviewers for their invaluable feedback on the drafts of this book:

Virginia Birnie, Camosun College
Marlene Del Pino, Red River College
Catherine Dunlop, Fanshawe College
Hope Graham, St. Francis Xavier University
Margaret Hadley, Grant MacEwan College
Trudy Hahn, University of New Brunswick
Lynne Hardwood-Lunn, York University
Jane Mackie, Trent University
Christa MacLean, SIAST
Cathy Michalenko, Red Deer College
Jane Mighton, Langara College
Mandi Newton, University of Alberta
Joe Noon, University of Alberta
Harry Plummer, University of Calgary
Jason Powell, Humber College
Jackie Santiago, Red River College
Margie Warren, Conestoga College
Catherine Wilkes, St. Lawrence College

I extend my enduring appreciation to my husband and children for their interest and encouragement.

Finally, very special thanks go to my students, who inspired and encouraged me to author a pharmacology textbook for Canadian nurses, and to whom this book is dedicated.

Shirley King

The vast majority of drugs are prescribed for specific diseases, yet many pharmacology textbooks fail to recognize the complex interrelationships between pharmacology and disease. Learning drugs in the context of their associated diseases will make it easier for you to connect pharmacotherapy to therapeutic goals and client wellness. The pathophysiology approach of this textbook gives you a clearer picture of the importance of pharmacology to disease, and, ultimately to nursing care.

ANGINA PECTORIS

23.3 Pathogenesis of Angina Pectoris

Angina pectoris is acute chest pain caused by insufficient oxygen reaching a portion of the myocardium. About 2% of Canadians have angina pectoris, with over 47,000 new cases each year. It is more prevalent in those over 55 years of age.

◀ Disease and Body System Approach

The organization by body systems (units) and diseases (chapters) clearly places the drugs in context with how they are used therapeutically. You can easily locate all relevant anatomy, physiology, pathophysiology, and pharmacology in the same chapter in which we present complete information for the drug classifications used to treat the disease(s) in each chapter. This organization builds the connection between pharmacology, pathophysiology, and the nursing care you learn in your clinical nursing courses.

Drugs at a Glance presents a quick way for you to see the classifications and prototypes that are covered in the chapter, organized by disorder drug class.

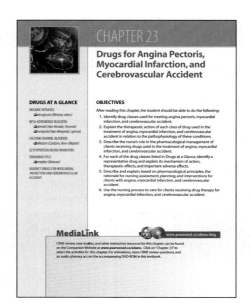

PharmFacts presents pertinent facts and statistics related to the disease, providing you with a social and economic perspective of the disease.

PHARMFACTS

Clients with Depressive Symptoms
- Major depression, manic depression, and situational depression are some of the most common mental health challenges worldwide.
- Clinical depression affects more than 6% of Canadians each year.
- Although depression can occur in anyone and at any age, the incidence is greater in females, Aboriginal Peoples, and older adults.
- Fewer than half of those suffering from depression actually seek medical treatment.
- Many clients consider depression a weakness rather than an illness.
- Depressed clients may self-treat with alcohol or street drugs.
- With antidepressants, about 40% recover fully and another 25% experience improvement in symptoms.
- Social support, psychotherapy, and culturally appropriate care are important components of depression treatment.

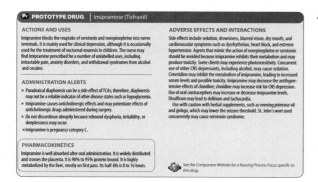

◀ Prototype Approach and Prototype Drug Boxes

The vast number of drugs available in clinical practice is staggering. To help you learn them, we use a prototype approach in which we introduce the one or two most representative drugs in each classification in detail. It can be less intimidating to focus your learning on one representative drug in each class. **Prototype Drug** boxes clearly summarize these important medications, presenting:
- Actions and Uses
- Administration Alerts
- Pharmacokinetics, including onset of action, duration, half-life, and peak effect, when known
- Adverse Effects and Interactions (with drugs, herbs, and food)

Providing a Nursing Focus

Once you understand how a drug works on the body—i.e., its actions, therapeutic effects, potential side effects and interactions, and more—you begin to understand the "why" of the interventions you will take as a nurse. Each chapter guides you to the content that is essential for you to provide safe, effective drug therapy.

NURSING CONSIDERATIONS

The role of the nurse in SSRI therapy involves careful monitoring of the client's condition and providing education as it relates to the prescribed drug regimen. The nurse should assess the client's need for antidepressant drugs, including intensity and duration of symptoms. The assessment should include identification of factors that led to the depression, such as life events or health changes. The nurse should obtain a careful drug history, including the use of CNS depressants, alcohol, and other antidepressants, especially MAO inhibitor therapy, as these may interact with SSRIs. The nurse should assess for hypersensitivity to SSRIs. The nurse should assess suicide ideation because the drugs may take several weeks before full therapeutic benefit is obtained. The medical history should include any disorders of sexual function since these drugs have a high incidence of side effects of this nature.

to reach their maximum therapeutic effectiveness. Following are other important points to include when teaching clients about SSRIs:

- Do not take any prescription or OTC drugs or herbal products without first consulting the healthcare provider.
- Maintain follow-up appointments with healthcare provider.
- Report side effects to healthcare provider as they occur.
- Do not drive or engage in hazardous activities until sedative effect is known; the SSRI may be taken at bedtime if sedation occurs.
- Do not discontinue drug abruptly after long-term use.
- Exercise and monitor caloric intake to avoid weight gain.

◀ **Nursing Considerations** appear within each drug class section and discuss the major needs of the client, including:

- General Assessments
- Interventions
- Lifespan Considerations
- Client education for all the drugs in that classification, when applicable

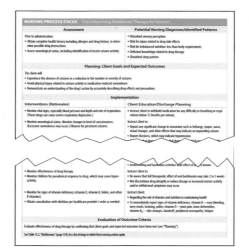

◀ **Nursing Process Focus** charts present need-to-know nursing actions in the nursing process—assessment, nursing diagnoses, planning, implementation with interventions and rationales, evaluation—and include client teaching and discharge planning. Additional **Nursing Process Focus** charts are available on the Companion Website.

Holistic Pharmacology

SPECIAL CONSIDERATIONS

Ethnic Groups and Smoking

Although smoking rates continue to decline in Canada, 22% of men and 17% of women are smokers. In the past 5 years, smoking rates for youth have declined from 28% to 18%. The incidence of tobacco use varies among racial and ethnic groups. Smoking prevalence is lower among foreign-born (16%) than native-born (25%) Canadians. The highest smoking rates are among Canadian Aboriginal Peoples (59%). The lowest rates are among Asian Canadians (11%). Each year, 42% of Canadian smokers attempt to quit. Smoking and tobacco use contribute to the leading causes of death—heart disease, cancer, and stroke. Clients who smoke should be informed about their increased risk of disease and the strategies and resources available to support smoking cessation.

◀ **Special Considerations** boxes present a variety of special issues related to ethnicity, gender, and psychosocial concerns that nurses must consider during drug therapy.

LIFESPAN CONSIDERATIONS

Dietary Supplements and the Older Adult

Can dietary supplements improve the health of older adults? A growing body of evidence is showing that the use of supplements can positively influence seniors' health. Dietary supplements have been successfully used to enhance their immune systems, reduce short-term memory loss, lessen the risks of Alzheimer's disease, and improve overall health. Nutritional deficiencies greatly increase with age, and supplements help to prevent or eliminate these deficiencies in older adults. In addition, some research has shown that older adults who have low levels of folate and vitamin B_{12} have an increased risk of developing Alzheimer's disease. The nurse should assess the need for such supplements in all older adults. The nurse should, however, be aware that herbal and dietary supplements can be expensive; thus, they should not automatically be included in treatment plans. In addition, older adults should be educated as to the risks of megavitamin therapy.

◀ **Lifespan Considerations** boxes specifically address client-care issues across the lifespan.

NATURAL THERAPIES

St. John's Wort for Depression

St. John's wort (*Hypericum perforatum*) is an herb found throughout Britain, Asia, Europe, and North America that is commonly used as an antidepressant. It gets its name from a legend that red spots once appeared on its leaves on the anniversary of St. John's beheading. The word *wort* is a British term for "plant." Researchers once claimed that it produced its effects the same way MAO inhibitors do, by increasing the levels of serotonin, norepinephrine, and dopamine in the brain. More recent evidence suggests that it may inhibit serotonin reuptake. Some claim that it is just as effective as fluoxetine (Prozac), paroxetine (Paxil), and sertraline (Zoloft) for mild to moderate depression and with milder side effects. It may also be used as an anti-infective agent for conditions such as *Staphylococcus* and *Streptococcus* infections, for nerve pain such as neuralgia and sciatica, and for mental burnout. St. John's wort should not be taken concurrently with antidepressant medications.

An active ingredient in St. John's wort is a photoactive compound that, when exposed to light, produces substances that can damage myelin. Clients have reported feeling stinging pain on the hands after sun exposure while taking this herbal remedy. Advise clients who take this herb to apply sunscreen or to wear protective clothing when outdoors.

◀ **Natural Therapies** boxes present popular herbal or dietary supplements clients may use along with conventional drugs. As a nurse, you need to assess clients to see if they are using any natural remedies that may have interactions with medications they are taking.

CULTURAL CONSIDERATIONS

Cultural Influences on Pain Expression and Perception

How a person responds to pain and the type of pain management chosen may be culturally determined. Establishment of a therapeutic relationship is of the utmost importance in helping a client attain pain relief. Respect the client's attitudes and beliefs about pain as well as the preferred treatment. An assessment of the client's needs, beliefs, and customs by listening, showing respect, and allowing the client to help develop and choose treatment options to attain pain relief is the most culturally sensitive approach.

When assessing pain, the nurse must remember that some clients may openly express their feelings and need for pain relief while others believe that the expression of pain symptoms, such as crying, is a sign of weakness. Pain management also varies according to cultural and religious beliefs. Traditional pain medications may or may not be the preferred method for pain control. For example, some Aboriginal Peoples and some Asian Canadians may prefer to use alternative therapies such as herbs, thermal therapies, acupuncture, massage, and meditation. Prayer plays an important role within some Canadian cultural groups, including some African Canadians.

◀ **Cultural Considerations** boxes explore issues specifically related to clients' cultural backgrounds, which may affect their responses to illness and their attitudes to drug therapy.

Teaching Through Visuals

For nearly all students, learning is a highly visual process. Thus, we use numerous visuals to help you review the anatomy and physiology of the body system as well as understand the principles of drug action on the body.

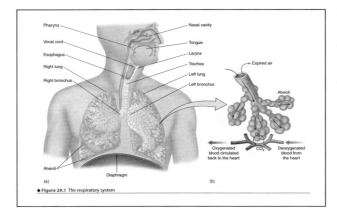

● Figure 29.1 The respiratory system

◀ **Vivid and Colorful Illustrations** help you review specific anatomy, physiology, and pathophysiology for a body system to help you better understand the impact of disease on that system.

Mechanism of Action Illustrations visually illustrate the drug therapy process and its impact on the disease, showing you specifically how the drug acts to counteract the effects of disease on the body.

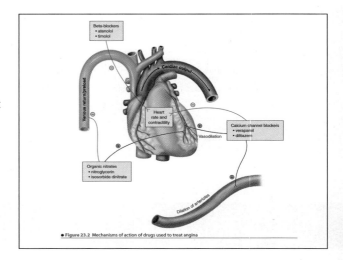

● Figure 23.2 Mechanisms of action of drugs used to treat angina

Mechanism of Action animated tutorials on your **Prentice Hall MediaLink DVD-ROM** clearly show drug action at the molecular, tissue, organ, and system levels. These interactive animations correlate to the **Prototype Drug** boxes in your book.
▼

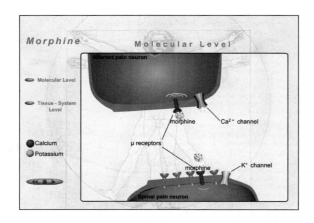

Putting It All Together

The tools at the end of each chapter and on the accompanying media resources help you test your understanding of the drugs and nursing care presented in that chapter. Using these tools will help you succeed in your pharmacology course, in the clinical setting, on the CRNE, and ultimately in professional nursing practice.

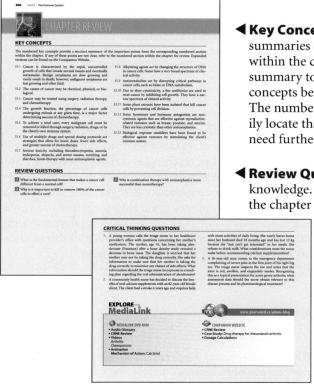

◀ **Key Concept Summary** provides expanded summaries of concepts that correlate to sections within the chapter. You can use this succinct summary to ensure that you understand the concepts before moving on to the next chapter. The numbering of these concepts helps you easily locate that section within the chapter if you need further review.

◀ **Review Questions** allow you to test your knowledge. You can easily scan through the chapter to check your answers.

◀ **Critical Thinking Questions** help you apply the essential components of nursing care through case-based scenarios. The Appendix provides answers.

◀ **Explore MediaLink** directs you to resources for that chapter on the **MediaLink DVD-ROM** and **Companion Website** that accompany your textbook.

MEDIALINK DVD-ROM

Packaged with every copy of the textbook, this dynamic DVD-ROM includes:

- **Audio Glossary** with pronunciations and definitions of every key term in the textbook
- **Drug Prototype Audio Pronunciations** of the most commonly used prototypes
- **Drug Dosage Calculator** to help you with conversions and calculations
- **Nursing in Action** video case studies for medication administration
- **CRNE (Canadian Registered Nurse Examination) Review** questions that emphasize the application of care and client education related to drug administration
- **Mechanism of Action** drug animation tutorials for prototype drugs, showing how drug action occurs at the tissue, organ, and system levels

COMPANION WEBSITE

Serving students as an online review of the textbook, this Companion Website includes:

- Additional **CRNE Review** questions with comprehensive rationales
- Pharmacology review activities that test your understanding of the drugs from each chapter, such as **Classification Reviews, Drug Reviews,** and **Case Studies**
- **Dosage Calculation** exercises that provide practice for drugs in the chapter
- **Nursing Process Focus** charts for drug prototypes
- **Preventing Medication Errors** review module and activities
- **Student Success** module with advice and activities to help you be a successful nursing student
- And much more!

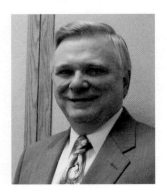

Michael Patrick Adams, PhD, RT(R), is the Dean of Health Occupations at Pasco-Hernando Community College. He is an accomplished and national speaker. The National Institute for Staff and Organizational Development in Austin, Texas, named Dr. Adams a Master Teacher. He has been registered by the American Registry of Radiologic Technologists for over 30 years. Dr. Adams obtained his Masters degree in Pharmacology from Michigan State University and his Doctorate in Education at the University of South Florida.

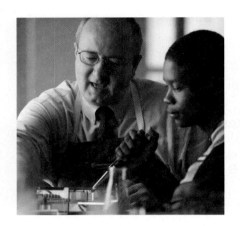

Leland Norman Holland, Jr., PhD (Norm) is the Associate Academic Dean and Dean of the College of Arts and Sciences at Southeastern University in Lakeland, Florida. He is actively involved in teaching and helping students prepare for service in medicine, nursing, dentistry, and allied health. He has taught pharmacology for 15 years at both the undergraduate and graduate levels. He is very much dedicated to the success of students preparing for work-life readiness. He comes to the teaching profession after spending several years doing basic science research at the VA Hospital in Augusta, Georgia, and the Medical College of Georgia, where he received his PhD in Pharmacology.

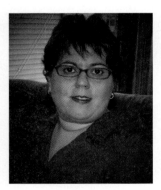

Paula Manuel Bostwick, RN, MSN is the Nursing Department Chair at Ivy Tech Community College in Fort Wayne, Indiana. She has been involved in nursing education for more than 15 years. She has clinical experience in medical-surgical and critical care nursing. Paula received her Masters of Science in Nursing from Ball State University.

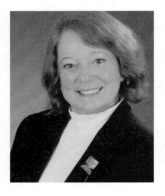

Shirley Linda King, RN, BN, MN, PhD, is a recipient of distinguished teaching and teaching excellence awards and teaches pharmacology in the Bachelor of Nursing program at Mount Royal School of Nursing. She has clinical experience in critical care and medical-surgical nursing. She is a member of several professional organizations, including the Canadian College of Neuropsychopharmacology. Shirley's research and publications focus on the neuroendocrine and psychological effects of traumatic stress and factors that influence the subsequent development of posttraumatic stress disorder (PTSD) and depression. She has received major fellowship, research, and academic awards for her work. She is an early adopter, leader, researcher, and enthusiastic mentor in the innovative use of technology for teaching and learning and a recipient of PanCanadian Technology Awards.

CONTRIBUTORS

This textbook is a culmination of writing provided by many writers. The authors wish to extend their special thanks to the many nurse contributors who provided their unique knowledge and wisdom to the original U.S. edition. Their willingness to make such sacrifices to meet deadlines is very much appreciated. Their dedication to quality nursing education is very evident in this text.

Text Contributors

Marti Burton, RN, BS
Canadian Valley Technology Center
El Reno, Oklahoma
Chapter 15: Drugs for Seizures
Chapter 17: Drugs for Psychoses
Chapter 22: Drugs for Lipid Disorders
Chapter 23: Drugs for Hypertension

Margaret Gingrich, RN, MSN
Harrisburg Area Community College
Harrisburg, Pennsylvania
Chapter 35: Drugs for Fungal, Protozoal,
*   and Helminthic Infections*

Corinne C. Harmon, RN, MS, EdD, AOCN
Clemson University
Clemson, South Carolina
Chapter 18: Drugs for the Control of Pain
Chapter 26: Drugs for Dysrhythmias
Chapter 29: Drugs for Shock
Chapter 31: Drugs for Fluid Balance, Electrolyte, and Acid–Base
*   Disorders*
Chapter 34: Drugs for Bacterial Infections
Chapter 37: Drugs for Neoplasia

Helen W. Jones, RN, PhD, APN-C
Raritan Valley Community College
Somerville, New Jersey
Chapter 8: Drug Administration Throughout the Lifespan
Chapter 9: Medication Errors and Risk Reduction
Chapter 14: Drugs for Anxiety and Insomnia
Chapter 16: Drugs for Emotional and Mood Disorders

Darcus Kottwitz, RN, MSN
Fort Scott Community College
Fort Scott, Kansas
Chapter 19: Drugs for Local and General Anesthesia
Chapter 21: Drugs for Neuromuscular Disorders
Chapter 24: Drugs for Heart Failure
Chapter 27: Drugs for Coagulation Disorders
Chapter 41: Drugs for Bowel Disorders and Other
*   Gastrointestinal Conditions*
Chapter 44: Drugs for Diabetes Mellitus
Chapter 49: Drugs for Eye and Ear Disorders

Claudia R. Stoffel, RN, MSN
West Kentucky Community and Technical College
Paducah, Kentucky
Chapter 8: Drug Administration Throughout the Lifespan
Chapter 20: Drugs for Degenerative Diseases of the Nervous
*   System*
Chapter 36: Drugs for Viral Infections
Chapter 38: Drugs for Allergic Rhinitis and the Common Cold
Chapter 40: Drugs for Peptic Ulcer Disease
Chapter 42: Drugs for Nutritional Disorders
Chapter 46: Drugs for Disorders and Conditions of the Male
*   Reproductive System*

Frances M. Warrick, RN, MS
El Centro College
Dallas, Texas
Chapter 28: Drugs for Hematopoietic Disorders
Chapter 32: Drugs for Immune System Modulation
Chapter 45: Drugs for Disorders and Conditions of the Female
*   Reproductive System*

Jan Weust, RN, MSN
Ivy Tech Community College
Terre Haute, Indiana
Chapter 25: Drugs for Angina Pectoris and
*   Myocardial Infarction*
Chapter 43: Drugs for Pituitary, Thyroid, and
*   Adrenal Disorders*
Chapter 47: Drugs for Bone and Joint Disorders
Chapter 48: Drugs for Skin Disorders

Julie Will, RN, MSN
Ivy Tech Community College
Terre Haute, Indiana
Chapter 30: Diuretic Therapy and Drugs for Renal Failure
Chapter 33: Drugs for Inflammation and Fever
Chapter 39: Drugs for Asthma and Other Pulmonary Disorders

PRENTICE HALL MEDIALINK DVD-ROM

Peggy Pryzbycien, RN, MSN
Onondaga Community College
Syracuse, New York

Margaret Gingrich, RN, MSN
Harrisburg Area Community College
Harrisburg, Pennsylvania

Patricia Teasley, RN, MSN, APRN, BC
Central Texas College
Killeen, Texas

(cont'd)

PRENTICE HALL MEDIALINK DVD-ROM
(continued)

Rachel Adema-Hannes, RN, MSc

Elaine Magowan, BPE, CPhT

Harry E. Peery, MS, PhD

Marcella Veenman-Mulder, RN, BScN

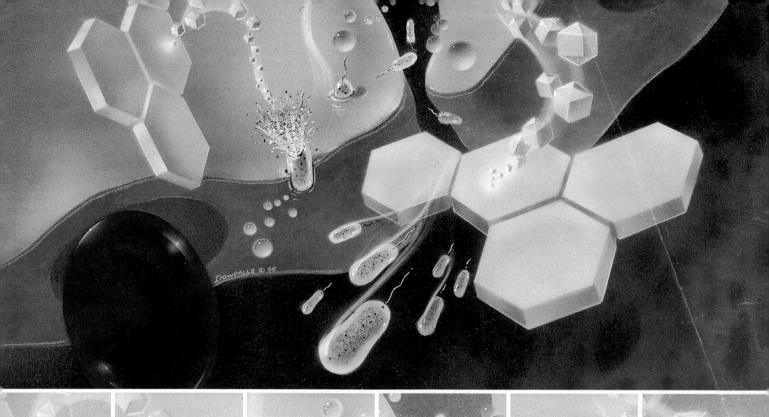

Unit 1 | Core Concepts in Pharmacology

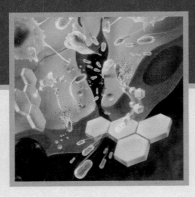

CHAPTER 1

Introduction to Pharmacology: Drug Regulation and Approval

OBJECTIVES

After reading this chapter, the student should be able to do the following:

1. Identify key events in the history of pharmacology.
2. Discuss the interdisciplinary nature of pharmacology.
3. Compare and contrast therapeutics and pharmacology.
4. Compare and contrast conventional drugs, biologics, and natural health products.
5. Identify the advantages and disadvantages of prescription and over-the-counter (OTC) drugs.
6. Identify key Canadian drug regulations that help to ensure the safety and efficacy of medications.
7. Discuss the role of Health Canada and the Health Products and Food Branch (HPFB) of Health Canada and its Therapeutic Products Directorate in the drug approval process.
8. Describe the stages of approval for therapeutic and biologic drugs in Canada.

MediaLink

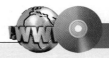

www.pearsoned.ca/adams-king

CRNE review, case studies, and other interactive resources for this chapter can be found on the Companion Website at **www.pearsoned.ca/adams-king**. Click on "Chapter 1" to select the activities for this chapter. For animations, more CRNE review questions, and an audio glossary, access the accompanying MediaLink DVD-ROM in this textbook.

More drugs are being prescribed to co
400 million prescriptions are dispensed ea
filled an average of 12 prescriptions in 2
purpose of this chapter is to introduce the subjt
emphasize the role of government in ensuring tha
natural alternatives are safe and effective for public use

1.1 History of Pharmacology

The story of pharmacology is rich and exciting, filled with a
and landmark events. Its history likely began when a huma
to relieve symptoms of disease. One of the oldest forms of
medicine has been practised in virtually every culture dating ba

The first recorded reference to the word *pharmacology* was i
entitled *Pharmacologia seu Manuductio ad Materiam Medicam,* by
in 1693. Although the exact starting date is obscure, modern phar.
thought to have begun in the early 1800s. At that time, chemists were
remarkable progress in isolating specific substances from complex mixture.
enabled chemists to isolate the active agents morphine, colchicine, cu
cocaine, and other early pharmacological agents from their natural produc.
Pharmacologists could then more precisely study the effects of these agents in
animals, using standardized amounts. Indeed, some early researchers used themselves as test subjects. Friedrich Serturner, who first isolated morphine from
opium in 1805, injected himself and three friends with a huge dose (100 mg) of
his new product. He and his cohorts suffered acute morphine intoxication for
several days afterward.

In the 20th century, the pace of change in all areas of medicine became exponential. Pharmacologists no longer needed to rely upon the slow, laborious
process of isolating active agents from scarce natural products; they could synthesize drugs in the laboratory. Hundreds of new drugs could be synthesized and
tested in a relatively short time. More importantly, it became possible to understand how drugs produced their effects, down to their molecular mechanism of
action.

The current practice of pharmacology is extremely complex and far advanced
compared with its early, primitive history. Whether a substance is extracted from
the Pacific yew tree, isolated from a fungus, or created completely in a laboratory,
the central purpose of pharmacology is to relieve suffering and improve quality
of life.

1.2 Pharmacology: The Study of Medicines

The word **pharmacology** is derived from two Greek words, *pharmakon,* which
means "medicine, drug," and *logos,* which means "study." Thus, pharmacology is
most simply defined as the study of medicines.

Pharmacology is an expansive subject ranging from understanding how drugs
are administered, to where they travel in the body, to the actual responses produced. To learn the discipline well, nursing students need a firm understanding
of concepts from various foundation areas such as anatomy and physiology,
chemistry, microbiology, and pathophysiology.

Over 10,000 brand name, generic, and combination agents are currently available. Each has its own characteristic set of therapeutic applications, interactions,
side effects, and mechanisms of action. Many drugs are prescribed for more than
one disease, and most produce multiple effects on the body. Further complicating
the study of pharmacology is the fact that drugs may elicit different responses
depending on individual client factors such as age, sex, body mass, health status,
and genetics. Indeed, learning the applications of existing medications and staying

drugs introduced every year is an enor-
for the nurse. The task, however, is a critical
he client and the healthcare practitioner. If
rly, drugs can dramatically improve the qual-
applied improperly, the consequences can be

harmacology and Therapeutics

ugh study of pharmacology is important to health-
roviders who prescribe or administer drugs. Although
al and provincial laws sometimes limit the kinds of
gs marketed and the methods used to dispense them, *all*
rses are directly involved with client care and are active in
ucating, managing, and monitoring the proper use of
rugs. This applies not only for nurses in clinics, hospitals,
and home healthcare settings, but also for nurses who teach
and for new students entering the nursing profession. In all
of these cases, a thorough knowledge of pharmacology is
necessary for them to perform their duties. As nursing students progress toward their chosen specialty, pharmacology
is at the core of client care and is integrated into every step
of the nursing process. As new drugs and research findings
emerge, nurses are challenged to evaluate the information
and incorporate relevant knowledge into evidence-based
practice.

Another important area of study for the nurse, sometimes difficult to distinguish from pharmacology, is the
study of therapeutics. Therapeutics is slightly different from
the field of pharmacology, although the disciplines are
closely connected. **Therapeutics** is the branch of medicine
concerned with the prevention of disease and treatment of
suffering. **Pharmacotherapy**, or **pharmacotherapeutics**, is
the administration of drugs for the purpose of disease prevention or treatment and relief of suffering. Drugs are just
one of many therapies available to the nurse for preventing
or alleviating human suffering.

1.4 Classification of Therapeutic Agents as Drugs, Biologics, or Natural Health Products

Substances applied for therapeutic purposes fall into one of
the following three general categories:

- Drugs or medications
- Biologics
- Natural health products

A **drug** is a chemical agent capable of producing biological responses within the body. These responses may be
desirable (therapeutic) or undesirable (adverse). A drug
that is considered medically therapeutic is commonly
referred to as a **medication**. Because drugs are defined so
broadly, it is necessary to separate them from other substances that can alter the body's biological activities, such as
foods, household products, and cosmetics. Agents such as
antiperspirants, sunscreens, toothpastes, and shampoos

might alter the body's biological activities, but they are not
considered to be drugs or medications. Sometimes it is not
clear whether a substance is a medication. For example,
alcohol (beer, red wine) may be considered medically therapeutic when used in small amounts for cardiovascular
effects or occasionally as a sleep aid, yet not be therapeutic
when used in excess.

While most modern drugs are synthesized in a laboratory,
biologics are agents naturally produced in animal cells, by
microorganisms, or by the body itself. Examples of biologics include hormones, monoclonal antibodies, natural
blood products and components, interferon, and vaccines.
Biologics are used to treat a wide variety of illnesses and
conditions.

Other therapeutic approaches include **natural health
products (NHPs)** and complementary and alternative
therapies. NHPs may include natural plant extracts, herbals,
vitamins, minerals, and dietary supplements. NHPs are discussed in detail in Chapter 11. **Complementary and alternative therapies** include therapies such as acupuncture,
hypnosis, biofeedback, and massage. Because of their growing popularity, herbal and alternative therapies are featured
throughout this text.

1.5 Prescription and Over-the-Counter Drugs

Legal drugs are obtained either by a prescription or over the
counter (OTC). There are major differences between the
two dispensing methods. To obtain prescription drugs, a
qualified healthcare provider must give an order authorizing
the client to receive the drug. The advantages to requiring
an authorization are numerous. The healthcare provider
has an opportunity to examine the client and determine a
specific diagnosis. The practitioner can maximize therapy
by ordering the proper drug for the client's condition and
controlling the amount and frequency of drug to be dispensed. In addition, the healthcare provider has an opportunity to teach the client the proper use of the drug and
what side effects to expect. In a few instances, a high margin
of safety observed over many years can prompt a change in
the status of a drug from prescription to OTC.

In contrast to prescription drugs, OTC drugs do not
require a prescription. In most cases, individuals may treat
themselves safely if they carefully follow instructions
included with the medication. If they do not follow these
guidelines, OTC drugs can have serious adverse effects.

Individuals prefer to take OTC drugs for many reasons.
They may be obtained more easily than prescription drugs.
No appointment with a physician is required, thus saving
time and money. Without the assistance of a healthcare
provider, however, choosing the proper drug for a specific
problem can be challenging for an individual. OTC drugs
may react with foods, herbal products, prescription medications, or other OTC drugs. Individuals may not be aware
that some drugs can impair their ability to function safely.
Self-treatment is sometimes ineffective, and the potential
for harm may increase if the disease is allowed to progress.

Consumer Spending on Prescription Drugs in Canada

About 22,000 drug products are on the market.

About 400 million prescriptions are filled annually.

Total pharmaceutical expenditures in Canada increased from $9.84 billion in 2000 to $16.57 billion in 2005.

- Spending on prescription drugs accounts for about 18% of total health-care costs in Canada.
- The average number of prescriptions per year increased from 9.5 prescriptions per person in 2000 to 12 prescriptions per person in 2005.
- Between 1990 and 2000, prescription drug expenditures increased by more than 200%.
- The two most commonly prescribed drug classes are cardiovascular drugs and psychotherapeutics.
- The average cost of a prescription increased from $35.48 in 2000 to $46.00 in 2005.
- In 2005, the average cost of a prescription was $63.79 for a brand name drug and $25.02 for a generic drug. Of all prescriptions filled, 43% were for generic drugs.

Source: IMS Health Canada, 2006; Canadian Pharmacists Association, 2007.

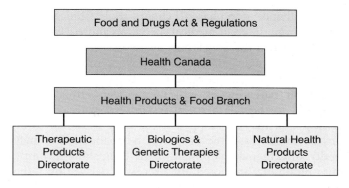

● **Figure 1.1** The governance structure for therapeutic products in Canada

1.6 Drug Regulations and Standards

Until the 19th century, there were few standards or guidelines to protect the public from drug misuse. The archives of drug regulatory agencies are filled with examples of early medicines, including rattlesnake oil for rheumatism; epilepsy treatment for spasms, hysteria, and alcoholism; and fat reducers for a slender, healthy figure. Many of these early concoctions proved ineffective, though harmless. At their worst, some contained hazardous levels of dangerous or addictive substances. It became quite clear that drug regulations were needed to protect the public.

1.7 Federal Drug Legislation

The Health Products and Food Branch (HPFB) of **Health Canada** is responsible for ensuring that health products and foods approved for sale to Canadians are safe and of high quality. The HPFB regulates the use of therapeutic products through directorates, as shown in Figure 1.1. The Therapeutic Products Directorate (TPD) authorizes marketing of a pharmaceutical drug or medical device once a manufacturer presents sufficient scientific evidence of the product's safety, efficacy, and quality as required by the Food and Drugs Act and Regulations. The Biologics and Genetic Therapies Directorate (BGTD) regulates biologic drugs (drugs derived from living sources) and radiopharmaceuticals. Products regulated by the BGTD include blood products, vaccines, tissues, organs, and gene therapy products. The Natural Health Products Directorate (NHPD) is the regulating authority for natural health products for sale in Canada. Natural health products and their regulation are presented in Chapter 11.

1.8 Approval Process for Prescription Drugs

Preclinical investigation involves extensive laboratory research. Over a 3- to 5-year period, scientists perform many tests on human and microbial cells cultured in the laboratory. Studies are performed in different species of animals to examine the drug's effectiveness at different doses and to look for adverse effects. Extensive testing on cultured cells and in animals is essential because it allows the scientist to predict whether the drug will cause harm to humans. Because laboratory tests do not always reflect the way a human responds, preclinical investigation results are always inconclusive. Animal testing may overestimate or underestimate the actual risk to humans.

If the drug has a desirable effect and is safe for animals, a Clinical Trial Application (CTA) is made to Health Canada, requesting permission to start clinical trials. The CTA includes detailed information about the drug's ingredients and proposed mechanism of action, the results of animal testing, and the proposed methodology for the clinical trials. An average of 1400 CTAs are made to Health Canada each year.

The manufacturer of a newly developed drug applies for **patent protection** that gives the manufacturer the right to sell the drug without competition for 20 years. When a patent has expired, competing pharmaceutical companies are permitted to manufacture and sell generic (chemically identical) versions of the drug.

Clinical trials, the second stage of drug testing, take place in three phases. Clinical trials are the longest part of the drug approval process. In phase I, clinical investigators perform tests on 20 to 100 healthy volunteers to determine dosage and to assess how the drug is absorbed, metabolized, and excreted by the body. In phase II, 100 to 300 clients with the particular disease the drug is intended to treat are given the medication to determine proper dosage and side effects. In phase III, 1000 to 3000 clients with the disease are given the medication. To eliminate bias, a double-blind study is generally used in which clients and investigators do not know whether the treatment the client is receiving is the drug or a placebo. Only about 10% of investigational drugs tested will make it to phase III clinical trials. Clinical investigators from different medical specialties address concerns such as whether the drug is effective, worsens other medical conditions, interacts unsafely with existing medications, or affects one type of client more than others.

Clinical trials are an essential component of drug evaluations due to the variability of responses among clients. A clinical trial may be stopped if the drug is shown to be unsafe. In this case, the drug may be abandoned or may undergo further development. If the drug shows promise but precautions are noted, the process is delayed until the pharmaceutical company addresses the concerns. If a drug appears to have dramatic benefits and be without serious side effects, it may be fast-tracked through the Health Canada approval process. A Priority Review Process is in place that may permit a drug to be used even sooner in special cases, with careful monitoring.

A **New Drug Submission (NDS)** must be submitted before a new drug is allowed to proceed to the next stage of the approval process. Health Canada receives about 80 NDSs for new drugs each year and approves about 10%. Health Canada reviews the submitted information and evaluates the drug's safety, efficacy, and quality. If Health Canada authorizes the drug to be marketed in Canada, a **Notice of Compliance (NOC)** and a **Drug Identification Number (DIN)** are issued to indicate official approval. The DIN must be displayed on the label of all prescription drugs, as shown in Figure 1.2. If there is insufficient evidence to support the safety, efficacy, or quality claims, authorization to market the drug will not be granted and a Notice of Deficiency or Notice of Non-Compliance is issued. Drug companies can then submit further information to support their claims and can appeal the decision not to authorize the drug.

Once drugs are marketed, the Marketed Health Products Directorate (MHPD) provides post-approval surveillance and regulation. Since clinical trials involve a limited number of individuals during a limited time period, they may detect only frequent or common adverse drug reactions (ADRs). It has been estimated that serious side effects may not be detected during clinical trials for as many as half of approved drugs. Under the Food and Drugs Act, manufacturers are required to continue to monitor the drug's safety and effects and report undesirable effects to the MHPD. MHPD activities include reviewing product safety data, investigating complaints, monitoring product advertising, and communicating product-related risks to healthcare professionals and consumers. Nurses can subscribe to MedEffect, an online service provided by Health Canada to quickly alert healthcare professionals about health product safety concerns. The Canadian Adverse Drug Reaction Information System (CADRIS) is a database of suspected adverse reactions to pharmaceuticals, biologics, and natural health products reported to Health Canada's Canadian Adverse Drug Reaction Monitoring Program (CADRMP). ADR reports are submitted voluntarily by health professionals or consumers. Only a small percentage of ADRs that occur are thought to be reported. Nurses play an important role in reporting ADRs and contributing to this database.

There are many sources of information about drugs marketed in Canada. Health Canada maintains an online **Drug Product Database** that is searchable by company, product name, active ingredient, DIN, or active ingredient group number. It is the most authoritative source of drugs marketed in Canada and contains listings for all human and veterinary drug products that have been assigned a DIN. The *Compendium of Pharmaceuticals and Specialties* (CPS) is a compilation of drug product monographs that are submitted by pharmaceutical manufacturers. Copies of the CPS are commonly available on nursing units, in pharmacies, and in physicians' offices. The contents are selected by the manufacturer and approved by Health Canada and frequently include information about product testing. Drug guides for nurses are published specifically to meet the need of nurses and their clients for accurate and concise information regarding drug action, desired and undesired effects, application of the nursing process, client teaching, and other aspects of drug therapy.

The drug approval process in Canada is outlined in Table 1.1. Many similarities exist between how drugs are regulated in Canada and the United States. These include the fact that both governments have realized a need to monitor natural products, dietary supplements and herbs, and newly developed drug therapies.

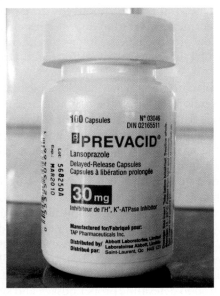

● **Figure 1.2** Example of a drug product labelled according to Canadian requirements: the generic drug name, Drug Identification Number (DIN), lot number, expiry date, and ingredients must be displayed

Source: Shirley King.

1.9 Pricing and Access to Prescription Drugs across Canada

Access to new drugs may be further delayed and may vary among the provinces. Once Health Canada has approved drugs for marketing in Canada, each province and territory

TABLE 1.1	Steps of Approval for Drugs Marketed in Canada
Step 1	Preclinical experiments in cultured cells, living tissue, and small animals are performed.
Step 2	A Clinical Trial Application (CTA) is submitted to Health Canada, followed by extensive clinical trials. Clinical trials are done in three phases: • phase I: small group of healthy humans • phase II: small group of humans with the target disorder • phase III: large group of humans with the target disorder
Step 3	The pharmaceutical company completes a New Drug Submission (NDS) to Health Canada. This report details important safety and efficacy information including testing data, how the drug product will be produced and packaged, expected therapeutic benefits, and adverse reactions.
Step 4	A committee of drug experts, including medical and drug scientists, reviews the NDS to identify potential drug benefits and risks.
Step 5	Health Canada reviews information about the drug product and passes on important details to healthcare practitioners and consumers.
Step 6	Health Canada issues a Notice of Compliance (NOC) and Drug Identification Number (DIN). Both are required for the manufacturer to market the drug product.
Step 7	Health Canada monitors the efficacy of the drug and any safety concerns after it has been marketed. This is done by regular inspection, notices, newsletters, and feedback from consumers and healthcare professionals.

must decide which drugs to list on the provincial formulary and to reimburse under the provincial drug plan. A **formulary** is a list of drugs available for prescribing or dispensing. Although each province and territory must make the final decision, the Common Drug Review (CDR) Directorate was established in 2002 to coordinate the jurisdictional review of new drugs and provide a listing recommendation. The CDR may require up to 6 months to make a recommendation. Generic and existing drugs are reviewed independently of the CDR by individual provinces, territories, and private insurers. Pharmacies, hospitals, and other health agencies make decisions about which drugs from the provincial formulary to include in their own formularies.

The cost of drugs influences access. Public and private insurers have budgets and thus consider the cost of drugs in making decisions about whether to list patented medicines as well as other medicines in their formularies. The Patented Medicine Prices Review Board (PMPRB) is a quasi-judicial body that operates under the Patent Act and is independent of Health Canada. The PMPRB regulates the prices charged by manufacturers for patented medicines to ensure they are not excessive in comparison to other countries. The PMPRB does not regulate non-patented drugs. Generic drugs that are bioequivalent to the brand drug may be marketed once patents expire and the NOC is received. Generic drugs cost, on average, about 45% less than their brand name equivalents. Insurance coverage for approved drugs is a federal responsibility for a few special populations, such as veterans, Aboriginal Peoples, and members of the Royal Canadian Mounted Police and the Canadian Armed Forces. For all other Canadians, the provincial governments and private insurers determine which drugs will be covered under their drug benefit plans and what level of coverage will be provided.

Advertising is another factor influencing drug product awareness and access.

Health Canada is the regulatory authority for drug advertising. Advertising Standards Canada (ASC) and the Pharmaceutical Advertising Advisory Board (PAAB) are responsible for ensuring that advertisements comply with rules set by Health Canada under the Food and Drugs Act and Regulations. Advertising in journals for healthcare providers may contain detailed drug information; however, unlike the United States, Canada limits direct-to-consumer advertising of prescription medications. Direct-to-consumer advertising is not allowed for prescription drugs and drugs that treat or cure serious diseases.

Through a **Special Access Program (SAP)**, Health Canada provides access to drugs not currently approved in Canada for treatment of clients with serious or life-threatening conditions for whom conventional therapies are ineffective, unavailable, or unsuitable. Health Canada reviews the Special Access Request Form. If approved, Health Canada sends a Letter of Authorization to the drug manufacturer and the client's physician. Pharmaceutical companies have the right to decide whether, and under what conditions, to provide the drug to the client.

LIFESPAN CONSIDERATIONS

How Prescription Drug Costs Affect Senior Citizens

Canadians over age 65 are only 13% of the population but account for about 34% of all prescriptions dispensed and 40% of all OTC medications purchased. Over 80% of all seniors take at least one prescribed medication each day. The average older person is taking more than four prescription medications at once, plus two OTC medications. Many of these medicines, such as those for hypertension and heart disease, are taken on a permanent basis.

Because seniors are usually retired, they are less likely than younger people to have insurance that substantially reimburses the cost of prescription medications. Every province offers coverage for low-income seniors, but the terms of coverage for non-low-income seniors vary considerably across provinces. One province requires that seniors not eligible for the publicly funded drug plan either have a private drug plan or pay out of pocket. Other provinces offer subsidized drug plans that require seniors to pay a portion of the cost. These portions may either be a percentage of the prescription cost or be capped at a fixed amount. For example, one province has a subsidized plan for seniors that covers 30%, to a maximum of $25.00 per prescription. As a result, some seniors may choose not to fill prescriptions.

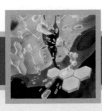

CHAPTER REVIEW

KEY CONCEPTS

The numbered key concepts provide a succinct summary of the important points from the corresponding numbered section within the chapter. If any of these points are not clear, refer to the numbered section within the chapter for review. Expanded versions can be found on the Companion Website.

1.1 The history of pharmacology began thousands of years ago with the use of plant products to treat disease.

1.2 Pharmacology is the study of medicines. It includes how drugs are administered and how the body responds.

1.3 The fields of pharmacology and therapeutics are closely connected. Pharmacotherapy is the application of drugs to prevent disease and ease suffering.

1.4 Therapeutic agents may be classified as traditional drugs, biologics, or natural health products (NHPs).

1.5 Drugs are available by prescription or over the counter (OTC). Prescription drugs require an order from a health-care provider.

1.6 Drug regulations were created to protect the public from drug misuse and to assume continuous evaluation of safety and effectiveness.

1.7 The regulatory agency responsible for ensuring that drugs are safe and effective is the Therapeutic Products Directorate of the Health Products and Food Branch of Health Canada.

1.8 Four levels of testing are required for therapeutic drugs and biologics. These progress from cellular and animal testing to use of the experimental drug in clients with the disease.

1.9 Once criticized for being too slow, Heath Canada has streamlined the process to get new drugs to market more quickly.

REVIEW QUESTIONS

1 Explain how the use of drugs has evolved since ancient times.

2 Explain why a client might seek treatment from an OTC drug instead of a more effective prescription drug.

3 What process does Health Canada use to ensure the safety and effectiveness of drugs?

4 Describe the role of the Health Products and Food Branch of Health Canada after initial drug approval.

EXPLORE MediaLink

MEDIALINK DVD-ROM
- Audio Glossary
- CRNE Review

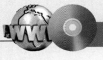

www.pearsoned.ca/adams-king

COMPANION WEBSITE
- CRNE Review
- **Case Study:** Client with psoriasis
- Expanded Key Concepts
- Challenge Your Knowledge

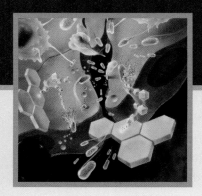

CHAPTER 2

Drug Classes and Schedules

OBJECTIVES

After reading this chapter, the student should be able to do the following:

1. Explain the basis for placing drugs into therapeutic and pharmacological classes.
2. Discuss the prototype approach to drug classification.
3. Describe what is meant by a drug's mechanism of action.
4. Distinguish between a drug's chemical name, generic name, and trade name.
5. Explain why the use of generic names is preferred to trade names when referring to drugs.
6. Discuss why drugs are sometimes placed on a restrictive list, and the controversy surrounding this issue.
7. Explain the meaning of a controlled substance.
8. Explain the Controlled Drugs and Substances Act (CDSA) of 1997 and the role of the Drug Strategy and Controlled Substances Programme (DSCSP) in controlling drug abuse and misuse.
9. Explain how drugs are scheduled according to the Canadian Food and Drugs Act, Controlled Drugs and Substances Act (CDSA), and the Narcotic Control Regulations (NCR).
10. Identify the drug schedules and give examples of drugs at each level.

MediaLink

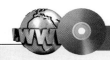

www.pearsoned.ca/adams-king

CRNE review, case studies, and other interactive resources for this chapter can be found on the Companion Website at **www.pearsoned.ca/adams-king**. Click on "Chapter 2" to select the activities for this chapter. For animations, more CRNE review questions, and an audio glossary, access the accompanying MediaLink DVD-ROM in this textbook.

The student beginning the study of pharmacology is quickly confronted with hundreds of drugs having specific dosages, side effects, and mechanisms of action. Without a means of grouping or organizing this information, most students would be overwhelmed by the vast amounts of new data. Drugs can be classified by a number of different methods that provide logical systems for identifying drugs and determining the limitations of their use. This chapter presents methods of grouping drugs by therapeutic or pharmacological classification and by drug schedules.

2.1 Therapeutic and Pharmacological Classification of Drugs

One useful method of organizing drugs is based on their therapeutic usefulness in treating particular diseases. This is referred to as **therapeutic classification**. Drugs may also be organized by **pharmacological classification**. A drug's pharmacological classification refers to the way the drug works at the molecular, tissue, and body system level. Both types of classification are widely used in categorizing the thousands of available drugs.

Table 2.1 shows the method of therapeutic classification, using cardiac care as an example. Many different types of drugs affect cardiovascular function. Some drugs influence blood clotting while others lower blood cholesterol or prevent the onset of stroke. Drugs may be used to treat elevated blood pressure, heart failure, abnormal rhythm, chest pain, heart attack, or circulatory shock. Thus, drugs that treat cardiac disorders may be placed in several types of therapeutic classes, for example, anticoagulants, antihyperlipidemics, and antihypertensives.

A therapeutic classification need not be complicated. For example, it is appropriate to simply classify a medication as a "drug used for stroke" or a "drug used for shock." The key to therapeutic classification is to clearly state what a particular drug does clinically. Other examples of therapeutic classifications include antidepressants, antipsychotics, drugs for erectile dysfunction, and antineoplastics.

The pharmacological classification addresses a drug's **mechanism of action**, or *how* a drug produces its effect in the body. Table 2.2 shows a variety of pharmacological classifications using hypertension as an example. A diuretic treats hypertension by lowering plasma volume. Calcium channel blockers treat this disorder by decreasing cardiac contractility. Other drugs block intermediates of the renin-angiotensin pathway. Notice that each example describes *how* hypertension might be controlled. A drug's pharmacological classification is more specific than a therapeutic classification and requires an understanding of biochemistry and physiology. In addition, pharmacological classifications may be described with varying degrees of complexity, sometimes taking into account drugs' chemical names.

When classifying drugs, it is common practice to select a single drug from a class and compare all other medications to this representative drug. A **prototype drug**

TABLE 2.1   Organizing Drug Information by Therapeutic Classification

Therapeutic Focus: Cardiac Care / Drugs Affecting Cardiovascular Function		
Therapeutic Usefulness	**Therapeutic Classification**	
inhibiting blood clotting	anticoagulants	
lowering blood cholesterol	antihyperlipidemics	
lowering blood pressure	antihypertensives	
restoring normal cardiac rhythm	antidysrhythmics	
treating angina	antianginals	

TABLE 2.2   Organizing Drug Information by Pharmacological Classification

Focus on How a Therapy Is Applied: Pharmacotherapy for Hypertension

Mechanism of Action	Pharmacological Classification
lowering plasma volume	diuretic
blocking heart calcium channels	calcium channel blocker
blocking hormonal activity	angiotensin-converting enzyme inhibitor
blocking stress-related activity	adrenergic antagonist
dilating peripheral blood vessels	vasodilator

is the well-understood drug model with which other drugs in a pharmacological class are compared. By learning the prototype drug, students may predict the actions and adverse effects of other drugs in the same class. For example, by knowing the effects of penicillin V, students can extend this knowledge to the other drugs in the penicillin class of antibiotics. The original drug prototype is not always the most widely used drug in its class. Newer drugs in the same class may be more effective, have a more favourable safety profile, or have a longer duration of action. These factors may sway healthcare providers from using the original prototype drug. In addition, healthcare providers and pharmacology textbooks sometimes differ as to which drug should be the prototype. In any case, becoming familiar with the drug prototypes and keeping up with newer and more popular drugs is an essential part of mastering drugs and drug classes.

2.2 Chemical, Generic, and Trade Names of Drugs

A major challenge in studying pharmacology is learning thousands of drug names. Adding to this difficulty is the fact that most drugs have multiple names. The three basic types of drug name are chemical, generic, and trade.

Chemical names are assigned using standard nomenclature established by the International Union of Pure and Applied Chemistry (IUPAC). A drug has only one chemical name, which is sometimes helpful in predicting its physical and chemical properties. Although chemical names convey a clear and concise meaning about the nature of a drug, they are often complicated and difficult to remember or pronounce. For example, few nurses know the chemical name for diazepam: 7-chloro-1,3-dihydro-1-methyl-5-phenyl-2H-1,4-benzodiazepin-2-one. In only a few cases, usually when the name is brief and easily remembered, will nurses use chemical names. Examples of useful chemical names include lithium carbonate, calcium gluconate, and sodium chloride.

More practically, drugs are sometimes classified by a *portion* of their chemical structure, known as the chemical group name. Examples are antibiotics such as fluoroquinolones and cephalosporins. Other common examples include phenothiazines, thiazides, and benzodiazepines. Although they may seem complicated when first encountered, knowledge of chemical group names will become

invaluable as the nursing student begins to learn and understand major drug classes and actions.

The **generic name**, or non-proprietary name, describes the chemical substance or pharmacological property of a drug. A generic name is the proper name of the drug ingredient or the common name if the ingredient has no proper name. An International Nonproprietary Name (INN) identifies a generic name as unique. An INN is the only internationally accepted generic name. Drugs that do not have a defined chemical composition or structure or that cannot adequately be described due to mixtures of substances cannot be assigned an INN. In Canada, INNs are used exclusively when they exist. Because there is only one generic name for each drug, healthcare providers often use this name, and students generally must memorize it. Importantly, the use of generic names increases safety since they are unique, while trade names may look and sound alike.

A drug's **trade (proprietary) name** is assigned by the company marketing the drug. The name is usually selected to be short and easy to remember. The trade name is sometimes called the product or brand name. The term *proprietary* suggests ownership. In Canada, a drug developer is given exclusive rights to name and market a drug for 20 years after a new drug application is submitted to Health Canada. Because it takes several years for a drug to be approved, the amount of time spent in approval is usually subtracted from the 20 years. For example, if it takes 7 years for a drug to be approved, competing companies will not be allowed to market a generic equivalent drug for another 13 years. The rationale is that the developing company should be allowed sufficient time to recoup the millions of dollars in research and development costs in designing the new drug. After 20 years, competing companies may sell a generic equivalent drug, sometimes using a different trade name, which Health Canada must approve.

Trade names may be a challenge for students to learn because of the dozens of products with different names but containing similar ingredients. In addition, **combination drugs** contain more than one active generic ingredient. This poses a problem in trying to match one generic name with one trade name. As an example, refer to Table 2.3 and consider the drug diphenhydramine (generic name), also called Benadryl (one of many trade names). Diphenhydramine is an antihistamine. Low doses of diphenhydramine may be purchased OTC; higher doses require a prescription. When

TABLE 2.3	Examples of Trade Name Products Containing Popular Generic Substances		
Generic Substance	**Trade Names**
acetylsalicylic acid (ASA)	Acuprin, Anacin, Aspergum, Aspirin, Bayer, Bufferin, Ecotrin, Empirin, Excedrin, Maprin, Norgesic, Salatin, Salocol, Salsprin, Supac, Talwin, Triaphen-10, Vanquish, Verin, ZORprin
diphenhydramine	Allerdryl, Benadryl, Benahist, Bendylate, Caladryl, Compoz, Diahist, Diphenadril, Eldadryl, Fenylhist, Fynex, Hydramine, Hydril, Insomnal, Noradryl, Nordryl, Nytol, Tusstat, Wehdryl
ibuprofen	Advil, Amersol, Apsifen, Brufen, Haltran, Medipren, Midol 200, Motrin, Neuvil, Novoprofen, Nuprin, Pamprin-IB, Rufen, Trendar

looking for diphenhydramine, the nurse may find it listed under many trade names, such as Allerdryl and Insomnal, provided alone or in combination with other active ingredients. Ibuprofen and aspirin are also examples of drugs with many different trade names. The rule of thumb is that the active ingredients in a drug are described by their generic name. When referring to a drug, the generic name is usually written in lowercase, whereas the trade name is capitalized. As stated in the Food and Drug Regulations, a drug is identified on its inner and outer label by the trade name (if there is one) followed by the generic name.

2.3 Differences between Brand Name Drugs and Their Generic Equivalents

During its 20 years of exclusive rights to a new drug, the pharmaceutical company determines the price of the medication. Because there is no competition, the price is generally quite high. The developing company sometimes uses legal tactics to extend its exclusive rights since this can bring in hundreds of millions of dollars per year in profits for a popular medicine. Once the exclusive rights end, competing companies market the generic drug for less money, and consumer savings may be considerable. In some jurisdictions, pharmacists may routinely substitute a generic drug when the prescription calls for a brand name. In other jurisdictions, the pharmacist must dispense drugs exactly as written by the healthcare provider or obtain approval before providing a generic substitute.

The companies marketing brand name drugs often lobby aggressively against laws that might restrict the routine use of their brand name products. The lobbyists claim that significant differences exist between a trade name drug and its generic equivalent and that switching to the generic drug may be harmful for the client. Consumer advocates, on the other hand, argue that generic substitutions should always be permitted because of the cost savings to clients.

Are there really differences between a brand name drug and its generic equivalent? The answer is unclear. Despite the fact that the dosages may be identical, drug formulations are not always the same. The two drugs may have different inert or added ingredients. For example, if in tablet form, the active ingredients may be more tightly compressed in one of the preparations.

The key to comparing brand name drugs and their generic equivalents lies in measuring the bioavailability of the two preparations. **Bioavailability** is the amount of drug that is absorbed into systemic circulation and therefore is physiologically available to reach its target cells and produce its effect. Bioavailability may indeed be affected by inert or added ingredients and tablet compression. Anything that affects absorption of a drug, or its distribution to the target cells, can certainly affect drug action. Measuring peak drug concentration in plasma and how long a drug takes to exert its effect gives a crude measure of bioavailability. For example, if a client is in circulatory shock and it takes the generic equivalent drug 5 minutes longer to produce its effect, that is significant; however, if a generic medication for arthritis pain relief takes 45 minutes to act, compared with the brand name drug which takes 40 minutes, it probably does not matter which drug is prescribed.

2.4 Drug Schedules

Throughout Canada, both prescription and non-prescription drugs must meet specific criteria for public distribution and use. Health Canada has established that all drugs used for medicinal purposes be grouped into the schedules as summarized in Table 2.4. Drugs that require a prescription are listed in Schedule F of the Food and Drug Regulations (FDR). In Canada, all Schedule F drugs must display "Pr" on the outside label of the product. Non-prescription drugs are provided according to guidelines and acts established by the respective Canadian provinces and territories. Pharmacies must monitor those drugs used specifically to treat self-limiting discomforts such as cold, flu, and mild gastrointestinal symptoms. Other non-prescription drugs may be sold without monitoring.

Canadian provinces and territories (except Quebec) use a national drug scheduling system to ensure consistent conditions of availability and sale among the provinces. Scheduling recommendations are made to provincial regulatory authorities by the National Drug Scheduling Advisory Committee (NDSAC). A set of factors are used to determine the schedule under which a drug can be sold. These factors include potential for dependency and abuse, adverse reactions, and interaction with other drugs. As illustrated in Table 2.4, Canada uses four categories (three schedules) for the sale of drugs.

Prescribers must follow standards of practice and legislation as set by national and provincial/territorial regulatory authorities. These authorities set out prescribing restrictions and the level of professional intervention and advice necessary for the safe and effective use of drugs by con-

TABLE 2.4	Schedule System for Drugs Sold in Canada
Schedule	**Description**
Schedule I	available only by prescription and provided by a pharmacist; includes the following: • all prescription drugs • drugs with no potential for abuse: Schedule F • controlled drugs: Schedule G • narcotic drugs
Schedule II	available only from a pharmacist; must be retained in an area with no public access
Schedule III	available via open access in a pharmacy or pharmacy area (OTC)
Unscheduled	can be sold in any store without professional supervision

sumers. Nurse prescribers must obtain special permits from their provincial nursing associations. Nurses can visit the website of their provincial nursing association to assess current licensing requirements.

2.5 Controlled Drugs and Substances

Some drugs and substances are frequently abused or have a high potential for addiction. Technically, addiction refers to the overwhelming feeling that drives someone to use a drug repeatedly. **Dependence** is a related term, often defined as a physiological or psychological need for a substance. Physical dependence refers to an altered physical condition caused by the nervous system adapting to repeated drug use. In this case, when the drug is no longer available, the individual experiences and shows physical signs of discomfort known as **withdrawal**. In contrast, when an individual is psychologically dependent, there are few signs of physical discomfort when the drug is withdrawn; however, the individual feels an intense compelling desire to continue drug use. These concepts are discussed in detail in Chapter 12.

Canada's Drug Strategy and Controlled Substances Programme (DSCSP) manages the 1997 Controlled Drugs and Substances Act (CDSA) and the Narcotic Control Regulations (NCR). Regulating drugs under the CDSA and the NCR protects the health and safety of Canadians by reducing the availability of substances on the illicit market that can alter mental processes and may produce harm to the health of an individual or to society when diverted or misused. These regulations control the import, production, export, distribution, and possession of narcotics and controlled substances. As a signatory to United Nations drug control conventions, Canada has an obligation to meet international requirements. Health Canada's Office of Controlled Substances (OCS) works to ensure that drugs and controlled substances are not diverted for illegal use.

The NCR governs the activities of manufacturers, pharmacies, hospitals, and healthcare professionals related to narcotic drugs. Licensed hospitals and other agencies must provide the required physical security measures for controlled substances in their possession and maintain records of all movements of controlled substances into and out of their inventory. Monitoring of compliance with the NCR is the responsibility of Health Canada. Offences under the CDSA and NCR are subject to criminal prosecution.

In Canada, **controlled substances** are those drugs outlined in the CDSA Schedules. A healthcare provider may only dispense these medications to clients suffering from specific diseases or illnesses. Controlled drugs must be labelled clearly with the letter *C* on the outside of the container. Narcotic drugs must be labelled clearly with the letter *N* on the outside of the container. The CDSA Schedules include restricted drugs such as amphetamines, barbiturates, anabolic steroids, morphine, and cannabis. Hallucinogens that are not intended for human use, such as LSD (lysergic acid diethylamide) and MDMA (3,4-methylenedioxy-N-methylamphetamine), better known as Ecstasy, are also listed in the CDSA Schedules. Examples of drugs listed by CDSA Schedule are presented in Table 2.5.

MediaLink ▶ Canadian Law and Drug Classification

TABLE 2.5	Controlled Drugs and Substance Act (CDSA) Drug Schedules
Drug Schedule	**Examples**
I	opium, codeine, hydrocodone, morphine, oxycodone, methamphetamine, dextromethorphan, naloxone, ketamine, fentanyl
II	cannabis, cannabis resin
III	amphetamines (except methamphetamine)
IV	barbiturates, phenobarbital, thiopental, meprobamate, benzodiazepines, clozapine, diazepam, lorazepam, anabolic steroids, testosterone, zolpidem
V	phenylpropanolamine
VI	ephedrine, ergotamine, lysergic acid diethylamide (LSD), pseudoephedrine
VII	cannabis, cannabis resin
VIII	cannabis, cannabis resin

2.6 United States Regulations Restricting Drugs of Abuse

In the United States, controlled substances are drugs whose use is restricted by the Controlled Substances Act of 1970 and later revisions. The Controlled Substances Act is also called the Comprehensive Drug Abuse Prevention and Control Act. Hospitals and pharmacies must register with the Drug Enforcement Administration (DEA) and then use their assigned registration numbers to purchase scheduled drugs. They must maintain complete records of all quantities purchased and sold. Drugs with higher abuse potential have more restrictions. For example, a special order form must be used to obtain Schedule II drugs, and orders must be written and signed by the healthcare provider. Telephone orders to a pharmacy are not permitted. Refills for Schedule II drugs are not permitted; clients must visit their healthcare provider first. Those convicted of unlawful manufacturing, distributing, or dispensing of controlled substances face severe penalties.

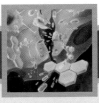

CHAPTER REVIEW

KEY CONCEPTS

The numbered key concepts provide a succinct summary of the important points from the corresponding numbered section within the chapter. If any of these points are not clear, refer to the numbered section within the chapter for review. Expanded versions can be found on the Companion Website.

2.1 Drugs may be organized by their therapeutic or pharmacological classification.

2.2 Drugs have chemical, generic, and trade names. A drug has only one chemical or generic name but may have multiple trade names.

2.3 Generic drugs are less expensive than brand name drugs, but they may differ in their bioavailability, which is the ability of the drug to reach its target tissue and produce its effect.

2.4 Drugs with potential for abuse are restricted by the Controlled Drugs and Substances Act (CDSA) and the Narcotic Control Regulations (NCR).

2.5 Canadian regulations restrict drugs with potential for abuse and label them as C (controlled) or N (narcotic).

2.6 In the United States, controlled substances are drugs whose use is restricted by the Controlled Substances Act.

REVIEW QUESTIONS

1 What is the difference between therapeutic and pharmacological classifications? Identify the following classifications as therapeutic or pharmacological: beta-adrenergic blocker, oral contraceptive, laxative, folic acid antagonist, antianginal agent.

2 What is a prototype drug, and how does it differ from other drugs in the same class?

3 A hospital pharmacist decides to switch from a trade name drug that was ordered by the physician to a generic equivalent. What advantages does this have for the client? What disadvantages might be caused by the switch?

4 Why are certain drugs placed in schedules? What extra precautions are required of healthcare providers when prescribing and administering scheduled drugs?

EXPLORE MediaLink
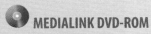

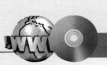

www.pearsoned.ca/adams-king

MEDIALINK DVD-ROM
- Audio Glossary
- CRNE Review

COMPANION WEBSITE
- CRNE Review
- Case Study: Generic drugs

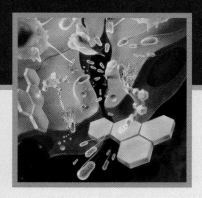

CHAPTER 3

Toxicology and Emergency Preparedness

OBJECTIVES

After reading this chapter, the student should be able to do the following:

1. Explain why drugs are important in the context of toxicity and emergency preparedness.
2. Describe common causes of toxicity and the meaning of exposure.
3. Discuss the role of the nurse in the prevention and management of poisoning.
4. Discuss the role of the nurse in preparing for and responding to a bioterrorist act.
5. Identify the purpose and components of the National Emergency Stockpile System (NESS).
6. Explain the threat of anthrax contamination and how anthrax is transmitted.
7. Discuss the clinical manifestations and treatment of anthrax exposure.
8. Identify specific viruses that would most likely be used in a bioterrorist act.
9. Explain the advantages and disadvantages of vaccination as a means of preventing illness due to bioterrorist acts.
10. Provide examples of chemical agents that might be used in a bioterrorism act, and their treatments.
11. Describe the symptoms of acute radiation exposure and the role of potassium iodide (KI) in preventing thyroid cancer.

MediaLink

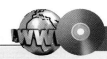 www.pearsoned.ca/adams-king

CRNE review, case studies, and other interactive resources for this chapter can be found on the Companion Website at **www.pearsoned.ca/adams-king**. Click on "Chapter 3" to select the activities for this chapter. For animations, more CRNE review questions, and an audio glossary, access the accompanying MediaLink DVD-ROM in this textbook.

It is important that nursing students are aware that some naturally occurring and manufactured substances can produce harmful effects on human health and that special services and drugs are available to help counter these effects. Drugs are the most powerful tools available for counteracting toxicity and for preventing or controlling global disease outbreaks and the effects of bioterrorist acts. If medical personnel could not identify, isolate, or treat the causes of global diseases, a major incident could easily overwhelm healthcare resources and produce a catastrophic loss of life. Drugs are a major component of emergency preparedness plans. This chapter discusses the role of pharmacology in the prevention and treatment of toxicity and diseases or conditions that might develop in the context of a biological, chemical, or nuclear attack.

PREVENTING AND CONTROLLING TOXICITY

Poisoning ranks, next to falls and motor vehicle collisions, as the third most frequent type of injury leading to hospitalization in Canada. Sources of toxicity or poisoning are numerous and include plants, household and industrial chemicals, drugs, and agents that may be used for bioterrorism. Nurses play key roles in preventing and minimizing harm from toxicity.

3.1 Toxicology

The Canadian Network of Toxicology Centres (CNTC) defines **toxicology** as the study of the harmful effects of naturally occurring and human-made substances on living organisms. Any substance can be toxic. **Exposure** occurs when a harmful substance enters the body through the skin, lungs, or gastrointestinal tract. Substances that are poorly absorbed reduce exposure. Substances that are stored in tissues prolong exposure. In general, the higher the dose and the longer the exposure to a potentially toxic substance, the greater the chance of an adverse effect. Carbon monoxide, arsenic, rattlesnake venom, botulinum toxin, and pesticides are some familiar sources of toxicity (poisoning). Yet many foods, beverages, drugs, and nutritional supplements have ingredients that can be toxic in large quantities. For example, vitamin A is an essential nutrient, but it can cause birth defects when taken at high doses during pregnancy. Health Canada is responsible for maintaining an adequate and safe food supply for Canadians and controlling exposure to toxins. Health Canada regulates the use of additives to prolong the shelf-life of foods, use of fertilizers and pesticides to protect crops, and use of growth stimulants and antibiotics to promote health and efficient growth in animals. Foods labels must indicate ingredients and additives. Drug labels must include directions for use. Products that may be hazardous must have clear warning labels.

Toxicity may be classified as acute or chronic. **Acute toxicity** refers to the rapid development of symptoms following short-term exposure (less than 24 hours) to a harmful substance. An example is nausea and vomiting following inhalation of bleach fumes. **Chronic toxicity** occurs following long-term repeated exposure to a harmful substance, with cumulative effects. A substance may produce both acute and chronic toxicity. Mechanisms of toxicity include disruption of nerve impulses, disruption of the body's ability to transport or use oxygen, damage to the immune system, and impairment of organ function. These effects may include reversible or irreversible physiological injury, disease, cancer, genetic damage or mutation, birth defects, or death. Individuals may differ in terms of their resistance (or susceptibility) to toxins. Nutrition, age, body mass, immune function, respiratory function, genetics, and other factors may affect susceptibility in humans. For example, clients with asthma may be more susceptible to toxins that affect respiration. Infants have less well developed immune systems and may be more susceptible to toxins from infectious agents. Developing fetuses are susceptible to environmental toxins such as drugs or alcohol taken during pregnancy. The Canadian Congenital Anomalies Surveillance Network (CCASN) was established in 2002 to monitor rates of birth defects across Canada.

Antidotes refer to substances used to reduce the effects of toxins. It is often difficult to identify a particular causative substance because individuals may be exposed to multiple substances that interact in different ways. Substances that when combined are less toxic than either would be individually are referred to as having antagonistic effects. Antagonistic substances may be used as antidotes for one another. When no specific antidote is available, activated charcoal may be used to bind drugs and poisons within the gastrointestinal tract so that they are expelled in the feces. Examples of some common sources of toxicity and their antidotes are presented in Table 3.1.

The **Canadian Association of Poison Control Centres (CAPCC)** was established in 1982 to provide a centralized forum for information exchange among Canadian poison control centres. Provinces/territories and regional jurisdictions have poison control and drug information centres that can be accessed by phone 24 hours a day. Centres are often staffed primarily with specially educated nurses and pharmacists who consult as needed with pharmaceutical companies, toxicologists, and physicians with expertise in toxicology and overdose management. The centres guide both laypersons and healthcare professionals in the event of chemical, herbal, or drug toxicity. The centres provide current, evidence-based advice about poisons and drugs specific to the caller's situation (either the layperson or the healthcare provider). About 70% of poison exposures can be safely and cost-effectively managed at home. Surveillance data are collected. Nurses should be knowledgeable about their local poison advisory centres. The CAPCC website maintains links to poison centres in Canada.

Priorities for treatment of poisoned clients are maintenance of airway, breathing, and circulation. The next priorities are to reduce absorption and action of the toxic substance by administering an antidote or activated charcoal. The use of syrup of ipecac to induce vomiting is often not recommended as significant quantities of the ingested substance may not be vomited or may already have passed through the stomach. There is an added risk that the client may lose consciousness and aspirate vomit during ipecac therapy.

The role of the nurse includes prevention of harm from toxins. This includes implementing the nursing process for clients receiving medications, as presented in Chapter 7. Nurses should know the antidotes that are available for each medication the client receives. The antidotes should be readily available in case toxicity occurs. Clients should be informed about proper use and safe storage of medicines, household cleaners, and other substances. Following are important points to include when teaching clients and families about prevention of toxicity:

- Immediately report known or suspected exposure to toxins to the local poison control centre for guidance and referral.
- Immediately report confusion, shortness of breath, chest congestion, heart palpitations, or other signs of adverse reaction.
- Store medications in their original containers and out of reach of children.
- Select products in containers with child-resistant safety caps.
- Read warning labels and follow directions when using medicines and household or industrial products.
- Ensure that contact information for the local poison and drug advisory centre is readily accessible.

TABLE 3.1	Common Toxins and Treatments
Toxin	**Antidote**
acetaminophen	acetylcysteine
anticholinergics (e.g., atropine)	physostigmine
beta-blockers	glucagon
benzodiazepines	flumazenil
botulinum toxin	botulinum antitoxin
carbon monoxide	oxygen (high concentration)
digitalis (foxglove)	digoxin immune Fab (digoxin antigen-binding fragments)
opioids	naloxone
organophosphate pesticides, nerve gas	atropine, pralidoxime
salicylates and various other substances	activated charcoal

PHARMFACTS

Poisoning

- Poisoning is the third most frequent type of injury leading to hospitalization in Canada.
- Medications are the most common substances in all poisonings.
- Except for children under 10 and adults 65 and over, most poisonings are intentionally self-inflicted.
- The highest incidence of self-inflicted poisoning is among women in their 20s to 40s who use tranquillizers, analgesics, antidepressants, and other psychotropic medications.
- Many poisonings occur in children under 6 years. Acetaminophen is one of the most common sources of poisoning in this age group.
- Adults can be poisoned by taking the wrong dose of medication, confusing different medications, or accidentally splashing a poison on the skin or in the eyes.
- Senior citizens are at increased risk of accidental poisonings when drugs are kept at the bedside.
- Poisoning can be prevented through education and awareness.

Source: Canadian Institute for Health Information (CIHI); Calgary's Poison and Drug Information System (PADIS).

MediaLink — Canadian Association of Poison Control Centres (CAPCC)

MediaLink — SafeCanada

EMERGENCY PREPAREDNESS

Bioterrorist activities and threats and the emergence of new infectious diseases such as severe acute respiratory syndrome (SARS) have led to widespread changes in emergency preparedness planning. Nurses play key roles in planning for such incidents.

3.2 The Nature of Bioterrorism

Prior to the September 11, 2001, terrorist attacks on the United States, the attention of healthcare providers regarding disease outbreaks was mainly focused on the spread of traditional infectious diseases. These included possible epidemics caused by influenza, tuberculosis, cholera, and HIV. Table 3.2 shows the 10 most dangerous infectious diseases ranked according to which caused the most deaths worldwide in the year 2000. Other diseases such as food poisoning and sexually transmitted infections were also common, though considered less important because they produced fewer fatalities.

The aftermath of the September 11, 2001, attacks prompted the healthcare community to expand its awareness of outbreaks and treatments to include bioterrorism and the health effects of biological and chemical weapons. **Bioterrorism** may be defined as the intentional use of infectious biological agents, chemical substances, or radiation to cause widespread harm or illness. The public has become more aware of the threat of bioterrorism because such agencies as the World Health Organization (WHO), Centre for Emergency Preparedness and Response (CEPR) of the Public Health Agency of Canada, and Centers for Disease Control and Prevention (CDC) in the United States have stepped up efforts to inform, educate, and prepare the public for disease outbreaks of a less traditional nature.

The goals of a bioterrorist are to create widespread public panic and cause as many casualties as possible. There is no shortage of agents that can be used for this purpose. Indeed, some of these agents are easily obtainable and require little or no specialized knowledge to disseminate. Areas of greatest concern include acutely infectious diseases such as anthrax, smallpox, plague, and hemorrhagic viruses; incapacitating chemicals such as nerve gas, cyanide, and chlorinated agents; and physical threats such as nuclear bombs and radiation. Biological threats have been categorized based on their potential impact on public health, as shown in Table 3.3.

3.3 Role of the Nurse in Emergency Preparedness

Emergency preparedness includes all activities, such as plans, procedures, contact lists, and exercises, undertaken in anticipation of a likely emergency. The goal of these preparedness activities is to make sure that the Public Health Agency of Canada, with the support of Health Canada, is ready and able to respond quickly and effectively in the event of an emergency. Emergency preparedness is not a new concept. For over 40 years, accredited hospitals have been required to develop disaster plans and to conduct periodic emergency drills to determine readiness. Originally, disaster plans and training focused on natural disasters such as tornados, hurricanes, and floods or on accidents such as explosions that could cause multiple casualties. More recently, bioterrorism and virulent infectious organisms have been included as possible scenarios in disaster preparedness. In the past few decades, infectious diseases have re-emerged as a growing threat to global health security. Both newer diseases, such as severe acute respiratory syndrome (SARS) and bovine spongiform encephalopathy (BSE), and older ones, such as tuberculosis and influenza, have had serious impacts on Canada and the world. Increases in antimicrobial resistance, in diseases transmitted from animals to humans, and in international trade and travel all compound the public health threat posed by infectious diseases. The WHO establishes the International Health Regulations (IHR) and leads international cooperation to ensure maximum security against the international spread of infectious diseases.

TABLE 3.2	The 10 Most Dangerous Infectious Diseases in the World, 2000		
Disease	**Cause**	**Target**	**Deaths per Year (millions)**
influenza	*Haemophilus influenzae*	respiratory system	3.7
tuberculosis	*Mycobacterium tuberculosis*	lungs	2.9
cholera	*Vibrio cholerae*	digestive tract	2.5
AIDS	human immunodeficiency virus	immune system	2.3
malaria	*Plasmodium falciparum*	blood	1.5
measles	rubeola virus	lungs and meninges	0.96
hepatitis B	hepatitis B virus (HBV)	liver	0.605
whooping cough	*Bordetella pertussis*	respiratory system	0.41
tetanus	*Clostridium tetani*	entire body (infections)	0.275
dengue fever	flavivirus	entire body (fever)	0.14

Source: World Health Organization data, www.ac-reunion.fr/pedagogie/anglaislp/OurFood/General_bacteriology.html.

Table 3.3	Categories of Infectious Agents	
Category	**Description**	**Examples**
A	agents that can be easily disseminated or transmitted person to person; cause high mortality, with potential for major public health impact; might cause public panic and social disruption; require special action for public health preparedness	*Bacillus anthracis* (anthrax) *Clostridium botulinum* toxin (botulism) *Francisella tularensis* (tularemia) variola major (smallpox) viral hemorrhagic fevers such as Marburg and Ebola *Yersinia pestis* (plague)
B	moderately easy to disseminate; cause moderate morbidity and low mortality; require specific enhancements of CDC's diagnostic capacity and enhanced disease surveillance	*Brucella species* (brucellosis) *Burkholderia mallei* (glanders) *Burkholderia pseudomallei* (melioidosis) *Chlamydia psittaci* (psittacosis) *Coxiella burnetii* (Q fever) epsilon toxin of *Clostridium perfringens* food safety threats such as *Salmonella* and *Escherichia coli* ricin toxin from *Ricinus communis* *Staphylococcus* enterotoxin B viral encephalitis water safety threats such as *Vibrio cholerae* and *Cryptosporidium parvum*
C	emerging pathogens that could be engineered for mass dissemination in the future because of their availability, ease of production and dissemination, and potential for high morbidity and mortality rates and major health impacts	hantaviruses multidrug-resistant tuberculosis Nipah virus (NiV) tick-borne encephalitis viruses yellow fever

Source: Centers for Disease Control and Prevention, www.bt.cdc.gov/Agent/agentlist.asp.

Emergency preparedness includes more than responding to the immediate casualties caused by a disaster: It also considers how an agency's healthcare delivery system will shift during a crisis and how it will return to normal operations following the incident. The expanded focus also includes how the individual healthcare agency will coordinate its efforts with community resources, such as other hospitals and public health agencies. National, provincial/territorial, and local agencies have revised their emergency preparedness guidelines in an attempt to more rationally plan for possible bioterrorist acts.

Planning for bioterrorist acts requires close cooperation among all the different healthcare professionals. Nurses are central to the effort. Because a bioterrorist incident may occur in any community without advance warning, nurses must be prepared to immediately respond. The Canadian Nurses Association (CNA) works with the Public Health Agency of Canada's Centre for Emergency Preparedness to combine expertise for a more effective response to emergency situations and to define nurses' role in a national emergency response plan. The CNA is a member of the International Council of Nurses (ICN), which published a position statement, "Nurses and Disaster Preparedness" (2001), providing information pertinent to global nursing issues such as coping with terrorism and disaster preparedness. The following elements underscore the key roles of nurses in meeting the challenges of a potential bioterrorist event:

- Education: Nurses must maintain a current knowledge and understanding of emergency management relating to bioterrorist activities.

- Resources: Nurses must maintain a current listing of health and law enforcement contacts and resources in their local community that would assist in the event of bioterrorist activity.

- Diagnosis and treatment: Nurses must be aware of the early signs and symptoms of chemical and biological agents, and their immediate treatment.

- Planning: Nurses should be involved in developing emergency management plans.

3.4 Emergency Stockpile System

Should a chemical or biological attack occur, it would likely be rapid and unexpected and produce multiple casualties. Although planning for such an event is an important part of emergency preparedness, individual healthcare agencies and local communities could easily be overwhelmed by such a crisis. Shortages of needed drugs, medical equipment, and supplies would be expected.

The Public Health Agency of Canada maintains a $300 million **National Emergency Stockpile System (NESS)** to quickly provide emergency supplies to provinces and territories when requested. The system consists of a central depot in Ottawa, as well as eight other warehouses and 1300 pre-positioned supply centres (under the combined management of the provinces and federal government) strategically located across Canada. It includes 165 mobile hospitals, with 200 beds in each, ready to be set up in buildings such as schools and community centres. The NESS contains everything that you would expect to find in a hospital, from blankets to a

MediaLink WHO: Epidemic and Pandemic Alert and Response (EPR)

MediaLink CNA: Emergencies, Disease Outbreaks and Disasters

MediaLink ICN: Nurses and Disaster Preparedness

supply of pharmaceuticals and a range of antibiotics. A 24-hour response capability is maintained. The Agency assesses and refurbishes stockpile units and distributes medical and pharmaceutical supplies at the request of provinces. The NESS has been used to support a number of emergencies, both in Canada and internationally.

The stockpiling of antibiotics and vaccines by local hospitals, clinics, or individuals for the purpose of preparing for a bioterrorist act is not recommended. Pharmaceuticals have a finite lifespan, and keeping large stores of drugs can be costly. Furthermore, stockpiling could cause drug shortages and prevent the delivery of these pharmaceuticals to communities where they may be needed most.

AGENTS USED IN BIOTERRORISM

Bioterrorists could potentially use any biological, chemical, or physical agent to cause widespread panic and serious illness. Knowing which agents are most likely to be used in an incident helps nurses to plan and implement emergency preparedness policies.

3.5 Anthrax

One of the first threats following the terrorist attacks on the World Trade Center was **anthrax**. In fall 2001, five people died as a result of exposure to anthrax, presumably due to purposeful, bioterrorist actions. At least 13 US citizens were infected, several governmental employees were threatened, and the US Postal Service was interrupted for several weeks. There was initial concern that anthrax outbreaks might disrupt many other essential operations throughout the country.

Anthrax is caused by the bacterium *Bacillus anthracis*, which normally affects domestic and wild animals. A wide variety of hoofed animals are affected by the disease, including cattle, sheep, goats, horses, donkeys, pigs, bison, antelopes, elephants, and lions. If transmitted to humans by exposure to an open wound, through contaminated food, or by inhalation, *B. anthracis* can cause serious damage to body tissues. Symptoms of anthrax infection usually appear 1 to 6 days after exposure. Depending on how the bacterium

is transmitted, specific types of anthrax "poisoning" may be observed, each characterized by hallmark symptoms. Clinical manifestations of anthrax are summarized in Table 3.4.

B. anthracis causes disease by the emission of two types of toxin, edema toxin and lethal toxin. These toxins cause necrosis and accumulation of exudate, which produces pain, swelling, and restriction of activity, the general symptoms associated with almost every form of anthrax. Another component, the anthrax binding receptor, allows the bacterium to bind to human cells and act as a "doorway" for both types of toxins to enter.

Further ensuring its chance to spread, *B. anthracis* is spore-forming. Anthrax spores can remain viable in soil for hundreds, and perhaps thousands, of years. Anthrax spores are resistant to drying, heat, and some harsh chemicals. These spores are the main cause for public health concern because they are responsible for producing inhalation anthrax, the most dangerous form of the disease. After entry into the lungs, *B. anthracis* spores are ingested by macrophages and carried to lymphoid tissue resulting in tissue necrosis, swelling, and hemorrhage. One of the main body areas affected is the mediastinum, which is a potential site for tissue injury and fluid accumulation. Meningitis is also a common pathology. If treatment is delayed, inhalation anthrax is lethal in almost every case.

B. anthracis is found in contaminated animal products such as wool, hair, dander, and bonemeal, but it can also be packaged in other forms making it transmissible through the air or by direct contact. Terrorists have delivered it in the form of a fine powder, making it less obvious to detect. The powder can be inconspicuously spread on virtually any surface, making it a serious concern for public safety.

The antibiotic ciprofloxacin has traditionally been used for anthrax prophylaxis and treatment. For prophylaxis, the usual dosage is 500 mg by mouth (PO, *per os*) every 12 hours for 60 days. If exposure has been confirmed, ciprofloxacin should be immediately administered by intravenous (IV) at a usual dose of 400 mg, every 12 hours. Other antibiotics are also effective against anthrax, including penicillin, vancomycin, ampicillin, erythromycin, tetracycline, and doxycycline. In the case of inhalation anthrax, the FDA has approved the use of ciprofloxacin and doxycycline in combination for treatment.

TABLE 3.4	Clinical Manifestations of Anthrax	
Type	**Description**	**Symptoms**
cutaneous anthrax	most common but least complicated form of anthrax; almost always curable if treated within the first few weeks of exposure; results from direct contact of contaminated products with an open wound or cut	small skin lesions develop and turn into black scabs; inoculation takes less than 1 week; cannot be spread by person-to-person contact
gastrointestinal anthrax	rare form of anthrax; without treatment, can be lethal in up to 50% of cases; results from eating anthrax-contaminated food, usually meat	sore throat, difficulty swallowing, cramping, diarrhea, and abdominal swelling
inhalation anthrax	least common, but most dangerous form of anthrax; can be successfully treated if identified within the first few days after exposure; results from inhaling anthrax spores	initially fatigue and fever for several days, followed by persistent cough and shortness of breath; without treatment, death can result within 4–6 days

Many members of the public have become intensely concerned about bioterrorism threats and have asked their healthcare provider to provide them with ciprofloxacin. The public should be discouraged from seeking the prophylactic use of antibiotics in cases when anthrax exposure has not been confirmed. Indiscriminate, unnecessary use of antibiotics can be expensive, cause significant side effects, and promote the appearance of resistant bacterial strains. Refer to Chapter 32 to review the precautions and guidelines regarding the appropriate use of antibiotics.

Although anthrax immunization (vaccination) has been in use for 30 years, it has not been widely used because of the extremely low incidence of this disease. The vaccine has been prepared from proteins from the anthrax bacterium, dubbed "protective antigens." Anthrax vaccine works the same way as other vaccines—by causing the body to make protective antibodies and thus preventing the onset of disease and symptoms. Immunization for anthrax consists of three subcutaneous (SC) injections given 2 weeks apart, followed by three additional SC injections given at 6, 12, and 18 months. Annual booster injections of the vaccine are recommended. At this time, vaccination is recommended only for select populations: laboratory personnel who work with anthrax, military personnel deployed to high-risk areas, and those who deal with animal products imported from areas with a high incidence of the disease.

There is an ongoing controversy regarding the safety of the anthrax vaccine and whether it is truly effective in preventing the disease. Until these issues are resolved, the use of anthrax immunization will likely remain limited to select groups. Vaccines and the immune response are discussed in more detail in Chapter 30.

3.6 Viruses

In 2002, the public was astounded as researchers in the United States announced that they had "built" a poliovirus, a threat considered essentially eradicated from the Western Hemisphere in 1994. Polio still persists among infants and children in areas with contaminated drinking water or food, mainly in underdeveloped regions of India, Pakistan, Afghanistan, western and central Africa, and the Dominican Republic. International travel can expose Canadians to infectious diseases, like polio, that are not frequently seen in North America.

The current concern regarding polio is that bioterrorists will culture the poliovirus and release it into regions where people have not been vaccinated. An even more dangerous threat is that a mutated strain, for which there is no effective vaccine, might be developed. Because the genetic code of the poliovirus is small (around 7500 base pairs), it can be manufactured in a relatively simple laboratory. Once the virus is isolated, hundreds of different mutant strains could be produced in a very short time.

In addition to polio, smallpox is considered a potential bioterrorism hazard. Smallpox was eradicated from the planet in the 1970s, but the variola virus that causes this disease is harboured in research labs in different countries.

Much of its genetic code (200,000 base pairs) has been sequenced and is public information. The disease is spread person to person as an aerosol or droplets or by contact with contaminated objects such as clothing or bedding. Only a few viral particles are needed to cause infection. If released into an unvaccinated population, as many as one in three could die from the virus.

There are no effective therapies for treating people infected by most types of viruses that could be used in a bioterrorist attack. For some viruses, however, it is possible to create a vaccine. The WHO does not recommend systematic vaccination against smallpox because the disease has already been eradicated. However, the WHO and many countries, including Canada, are stockpiling smallpox vaccine with which to combat new epidemics resulting from bioterrorist activity, if necessary. The variola vaccine provides a high level of protection if given prior to exposure or up to 3 days afterward. Re-vaccination may extend immunity for 10 to 20 years or more. Since mass vaccination in Canada ended in 1972, most people in Canada have little or no immunity to the virus that causes smallpox. As a result, people at high risk of infection in a bioterrorist attack—certain healthcare workers, public health personnel, and members of the military—are being vaccinated. Contraindications to receiving the smallpox vaccine include atopic dermatitis or eczema, altered immune states (e.g., HIV, AIDS, leukemia, lymphoma, taking immunosuppressive drugs), pregnancy, breastfeeding, and allergy to any component of the vaccine.

One suggestion has been that multiple vaccines be created, mass produced, and stockpiled to meet the challenges of a terrorist attack. Another suggestion has called for mass vaccination of the public, or at least those healthcare providers and law enforcement employees who might be exposed to infected members of the public; however, vaccines have side effects, some of which are quite serious. In addition, terrorists with some knowledge of genetic structure could create a modified strain of the virus that renders existing vaccines totally ineffective. It appears, then, that mass vaccination is not an appropriate solution until research can produce safer and more effective vaccines.

3.7 Toxic Chemicals

Although chemical warfare agents have been available since World War I, medicine has produced few drug antidotes. Many treatments provide minimal help, other than to relieve some symptoms and provide comfort following exposure. Most chemical agents used in warfare were created to cause mass casualties; others were designed to cause so much discomfort that soldiers would be too weak to continue fighting. Potential chemicals that could be used in a terrorist act include nerve gases, blood agents, choking and vomiting agents, and those that cause severe blistering. Table 3.5 provides a summary of selected chemical agents and known antidotes and first-aid treatments.

The category of main pharmacological significance is **nerve agents**. Exposure to these acutely toxic chemicals can

MediaLink Anthrax Vaccine Immunization Program (AVIP)

MediaLink Other Biological Threats

MediaLink Smallpox Vaccine

TABLE 3.5	Chemical Warfare Agents and Treatments		
Category	*Signs of Exposure*	*Antidotes/First Aid*	
Nerve Agents			
tabun or GA (liquid) sarin or GB (gaseous liquid) soman or GD (liquid) VX (gaseous liquid)	Depending on the nerve agent, symptoms may be slow to appear and cumulative depending on exposure time: miosis, runny nose, difficulty breathing, excessive salivation, nausea, vomiting, cramping, involuntary urination and defecation, twitching and jerking of muscles, headaches, confusion, convulsion, coma, death.	Nerve agent antidote and Mark I injector kits with atropine are available. Flush eyes immediately with water. Apply sodium bicarbonate or 5% liquid bleach solution to the skin. Vomiting should not be induced.	
Blood Agents			
hydrogen cyanide (liquid)	Red eyes, flushing of the skin, nausea, headaches, weakness, hypoxic convulsions, death	Flush eyes and wash skin with water. For inhalation of mist, oxygen and amyl nitrate may be given. For ingestion of cyanide liquid, 1% sodium thiosulfate may be given to induce vomiting.	
cyanogen chloride (gas)	Loss of appetite, irritation of the respiratory tract, pulmonary edema, death	Oxygen and amyl nitrate may be given. Give patient milk or water. Do not induce vomiting.	
Choking/Vomiting Agents			
phosgene (gas)	Dizziness, burning eyes, thirst, throat irritation, chills, respiratory and circulatory failure, cyanosis, frostbite-type lesions	Provide fresh air. Administer oxygen. Flush eyes with normal saline or water. Keep patient warm and calm.	
Adamsite or DM (crystalline compound dispensed in aerosol)	Irritating to the eyes and respiratory tract, tightness of the chest, nausea, and vomiting	Rinse nose and throat with saline, water, or 10% solution of sodium bicarbonate. Treat the skin with borated talcum powder.	
Blister/Vesicant Agents			
phosgene oxime (crystalline compound or liquid)	Destruction of mucous membranes, eye tissue, and skin (subcutaneous edema), followed by scab formation	Flush affected area with copious amounts of water. If ingested, do not induce vomiting.	
mustard-lewisite mixture or HL nitrogen mustard: HN-1, HN-2, HN-3 sulfur mustard agents	Irritating to the eyes, nasal membranes, and lungs; nausea and vomiting; formation of blisters on the skin; cytotoxic reactions in hematopoietic tissues including bone marrow, lymph nodes, spleen, and endocrine glands	Flush affected area with water. Treat the skin with 5% solution of sodium hypochlorite or household bleach. Give milk to drink. Do not induce vomiting. Skin contact with lewisite may be treated with 10% solution of sodium carbonate.	

Source: Chemical Fact Sheets, U.S. Army Center for Health Promotion and Preventative Medicine,
http://chemistry.about.com/gi/dynamic/offsite.htm?site=http%3A%2F%2Fchppm-www.apgea.army.mil%2Fdts%2Fdtchemfs.htm.

cause convulsions and loss of consciousness within seconds and respiratory failure within minutes. Almost all signs of exposure to nerve gas agents relate to overstimulation of the neurotransmitter acetylcholine (Ach) at both central and peripheral sites throughout the body.

Acetylcholine is normally degraded in the synaptic space by the enzyme acetylcholinesterase (AchE). Nerve agents block AchE, increasing the action of acetylcholine in the synaptic space; therefore, all symptoms of nerve gas exposure, such as salivation, increased sweating, muscle twitching, involuntary urination and defecation, confusion, convulsions, and death, are the direct result of Ach overstimulation. To remedy this condition, Mark I injector kits that contain the anticholinergic drug atropine and a related antidote are available in cases when nerve agent release is expected. Atropine blocks the attachment of Ach to recep-

tor sites and prevents the overstimulation caused by the nerve agent. Neurotransmitters, synapses, and autonomic receptors are discussed in detail in Chapter 13.

3.8 Ionizing Radiation

In addition to biological and chemical weapons, it is possible that bioterrorists could develop nuclear bombs capable of mass destruction. In such a scenario, the greatest number of casualties would occur due to the physical blast itself. Survivors, however, could be exposed to high levels of **ionizing radiation** from hundreds of different radioisotopes created by the nuclear explosion. Some of these radioisotopes emit large amounts of radiation and persist in the environment for years. As was the case in the 1986 Chernobyl nuclear accident in Ukraine, the resulting radioisotopes could travel by wind currents to land thousands of kilometres away from the initial explosion. Smaller scale radiation exposure could occur through terrorist attacks on nuclear power plants or by the release of solid or liquid radioactive materials into public areas.

The acute effects of ionizing radiation have been well documented and depend primarily on the dose of radiation received. **Acute radiation syndrome**, sometimes called radiation sickness, can occur within hours or days after extreme doses. Immediate symptoms are nausea, vomiting, and diarrhea. Later symptoms include weight loss, anorexia, fatigue, and bone marrow suppression. Clients who survive the acute exposure are at high risk of developing various cancers, particularly leukemia.

Symptoms of nuclear and radiation exposure remain some of the most difficult to treat pharmacologically. Apart from the symptomatic treatment of radiation sickness, taking potassium iodide (KI) tablets after an incident is the only recognized therapy specifically designed for radiation exposure. Following a nuclear explosion, one of the resultant radioisotopes is iodine-131 (I-131). Because iodine naturally concentrates in the thyroid gland, I-131 will immediately enter the thyroid and damage thyroid cells. For example, following the Chernobyl nuclear disaster, the incidence of thyroid cancer in Ukraine jumped from 4 to 6 cases per million people to 45 cases per million. If taken prior to, or immediately following, a nuclear incident, KI can prevent up to 100% of the radioactive iodine from entering the thyroid gland. It is effective even if taken 3 to 4 hours after radiation exposure. Generally, a single 130 mg dose is necessary.

MediaLink Potassium Iodide (KI)

PHARMFACTS

Potential Chemical and Biological Agents for Bioterrorism

- Robert Stevens, the 63-year-old employee of American Media who died in Florida on October 5, 2001, was the first person to die from anthrax in North America in 25 years.
- In 1979, accidental release of anthrax from a research lab in the former Soviet Union killed 68 people. The problem was traced to a faulty air filter.
- The Ebola virus causes death by hemorrhagic fever in up to 90% of the people who show clinical symptoms of infection.
- Ebola viruses are found in central Africa. Although the source of the viruses in nature remains unknown, monkeys appear to be susceptible to infection and serve as sources of virus if infected.
- Widespread public smallpox vaccinations ceased in Canada in 1972.
- Most of the nerve agents were originally produced in a search for insecticides, but because of their toxicity, they were evaluated for military use.
- Chemicals used in bioterrorist acts need not be sophisticated or difficult to obtain: Toxic industrial chemicals such as chlorine, phosgene, and hydrogen cyanide are used in commercial manufacturing and are readily available.

Unfortunately, KI only protects the thyroid gland from I-131. It has no protective effects on other body tissues, and it offers no protection against the dozens of other harmful radioisotopes generated by a nuclear blast. Like vaccines and antibiotics, the stockpiling of KI by local healthcare agencies or individuals is not recommended. Interestingly, I-131 is also a medication used to shrink the size of overactive thyroid glands. Thyroid medications are presented in Chapter 39.

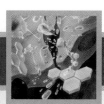

CHAPTER REVIEW

KEY CONCEPTS

The numbered key concepts provide a succinct summary of the important points from the corresponding numbered section within the chapter. If any of these points are not clear, refer to the numbered section within the chapter for review. Expanded versions can be found on the Companion Website.

3.1 Poisoning is the third most frequent type of injury leading to hospitalization in Canada. Drugs are the most common cause in all poisonings.

3.2 Bioterrorism is the deliberate use of a biological, chemical, or physical agent to cause panic and mass casualties. The health aspects of biological and chemical agents have become important public issues.

3.3 Nurses play key roles in emergency preparedness, including providing education, resources, diagnosis and treatment, and planning.

3.4 The National Emergency Stockpile System (NESS) is used to rapidly deploy medical necessities to communities experiencing a chemical or biological attack.

3.5 Anthrax can enter the body through ingestion, inhalation, or by the cutaneous route. Antibiotic therapy can be successful if given prophylactically or within a short time after exposure.

3.6 Viruses such as polio, smallpox, and the hemorrhagic fever viruses are potential biological weapons. If available, vaccines are the best treatments.

3.7 Chemicals and neurotoxins are potential bioterrorist threats for which specific antidotes are not always available.

3.8 Potassium iodide (KI) may be used to block the effects of acute radiation exposure on the thyroid gland, but it is not effective for protecting other organs.

REVIEW QUESTIONS

1 Explain the role of the nurse in the prevention and reduction of harm from poisoning.

2 Why is the medical community opposed to the mass vaccination of the general public for potential bioterrorist threats such as anthrax and smallpox?

3 Why does the protective effect of KI not extend to body tissues other than the thyroid gland?

4 Why do nurses play such a central role in emergency preparedness?

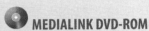

EXPLORE

MediaLink

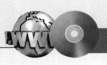

 www.pearsoned.ca/adams-king

MEDIALINK DVD-ROM
- Audio Glossary
- CRNE Review

COMPANION WEBSITE
- CRNE Review
- Case Study: Bioterrorism

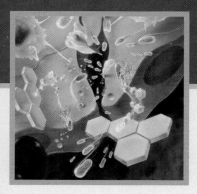

CHAPTER 4

Pharmacokinetics

OBJECTIVES

After reading this chapter, the student should be able to do the following:

1. Explain the applications of pharmacokinetics to clinical practice.
2. Identify the four components of pharmacokinetics.
3. Explain how substances travel across plasma membranes.
4. Discuss factors affecting drug absorption.
5. Explain the metabolism of drugs and its applications to pharmacotherapy.
6. Discuss how drugs are distributed throughout the body.
7. Describe how plasma proteins affect drug distribution.
8. Identify major processes by which drugs are excreted.
9. Explain how enterohepatic recirculation might affect drug activity.
10. Explain the applications of a drug's plasma half-life ($t_{1/2}$) to pharmacotherapy.
11. Explain how a drug reaches and maintains its therapeutic range in the plasma.
12. Differentiate between loading and maintenance doses.

MediaLink

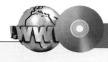

www.pearsoned.ca/adams-king

CRNE review, case studies, and other interactive resources for this chapter can be found on the Companion Website at **www.pearsoned.ca/adams-king**. Click on "Chapter 4" to select the activities for this chapter. For animations, more CRNE review questions, and an audio glossary, access the accompanying MediaLink DVD-ROM in this textbook.

Medications are given to achieve a desirable effect. To produce this therapeutic effect, the drug must reach its target cells and then be removed from the body, the process of pharmacokinetics. Drugs are exposed to many barriers and destructive processes after they enter the body. Care that the nurse provides may influence biochemical and psychological responses in a client that affect how drugs move through the body and achieve their effects. For example, providing a warm blanket can affect endogenous stress hormone levels and influence blood flow and other bodily processes that affect drug responses. The purpose of this chapter is to examine principles of pharmacokinetics and ways that the nurse can influence pharmacokinetics through purposeful use of dietary modifications and other supportive therapies.

4.1 Pharmacokinetics: How the Body Handles Medications

The term **pharmacokinetics** is derived from the root words *pharmaco*, which means "medicines," and *kinetics*, which means "movement or motion." Pharmacokinetics is thus the study of drug movement throughout the body. In practical terms, it describes how the body handles medications. Pharmacokinetics is a core subject in pharmacology, and a firm grasp of this topic allows nurses to better understand and predict the actions and side effects of medications.

Drugs face numerous obstacles in reaching their target cells. For most medications, the greatest barrier is crossing the many membranes that separate the drug from its target cells. A drug taken by mouth, for example, must cross the plasma membrane of the mucosal cells of the gastrointestinal tract and that of the capillary endothelial cells to enter the bloodstream. To leave the bloodstream, it must again cross capillary cells, travel through interstitial fluid, and enter target cells by passing through their plasma membrane. Depending on the mechanism of action, the drug may also need to enter cellular organelles such as the nucleus, which are surrounded by additional membranes. These are just some of the membranes and barriers that a drug must successfully penetrate before it can elicit a response.

While seeking their target cells and attempting to pass through the various membranes, drugs are subjected to numerous physiological processes. For medications given by the enteral route, stomach acid and digestive enzymes often act to break down the drug molecules. Enzymes in the liver and other organs may chemically change the drug molecule to make it less active. If seen as foreign by the body, phagocytes may attempt to remove the drug, or an immune response may be triggered. The kidneys, large intestine, and other organs attempt to excrete the medication from the body.

These examples illustrate pharmacokinetic processes: how the body handles medications. The many processes of pharmacokinetics are grouped into four categories: absorption, distribution, metabolism, and excretion, as illustrated in Figure 4.1.

4.2 The Passage of Drugs through Plasma Membranes

Pharmacokinetic variables depend on the ability of a drug to cross plasma membranes. With few exceptions, drugs must penetrate these membranes to produce their effects. Like other chemicals, drugs primarily use two processes to cross body membranes: (1) **diffusion**, a type of **passive transport**, is the movement of a substance from an area of higher concentration to an area of lower concentration, and (2) **active transport** is the movement of a substance

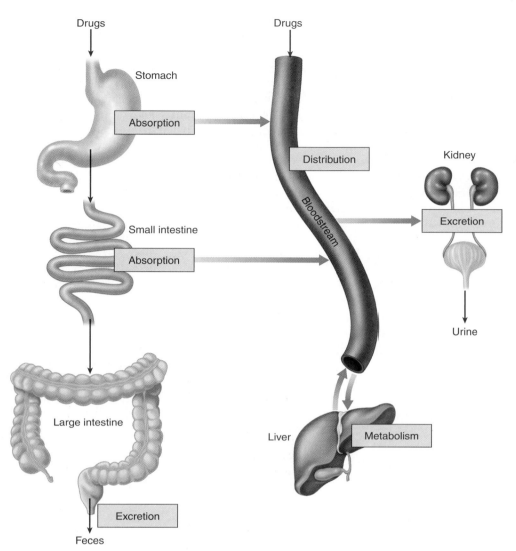

● **Figure 4.1** The four processes of pharmacokinetics: absorption, distribution, metabolism, and excretion

against a concentration or electrochemical gradient, which requires energy.

Plasma membranes consist of a lipid bilayer, with proteins and other molecules interspersed in the membrane. This lipophilic membrane is relatively impermeable to large molecules, ions, and polar molecules. These physical characteristics have direct application to pharmacokinetics. For example, drug molecules that are small, nonionized, and lipid soluble will usually pass through plasma membranes by simple diffusion and more easily reach their target cells. Small water-soluble agents such as urea, alcohol, and water can enter through pores in the plasma membrane. Large molecules, ionized drugs, and water-soluble agents, however, will have more difficulty crossing plasma membranes. These agents may use other means to gain entry, such as carrier proteins or active transport. In some cases, the drug may not need to enter the cell to produce its effects: once bound to the plasma membrane, some drugs activate a second messenger within the cell, which produces the physiological change (see Chapter 5).

4.3 Absorption of Medications

Absorption is a process involving the movement of a substance from its site of administration, across body membranes, to circulating fluids. Absorption may occur across the skin and associated mucous membranes or across membranes that line the gastrointestinal or respiratory tract. Most drugs, with the exception of a few topical medications, intestinal anti-infectives, and some radiological contrast agents, must be absorbed to produce an effect.

Absorption is the primary pharmacokinetic factor determining the length of time it takes a drug to produce its effect. In general, the more rapid the absorption, the faster the onset of drug action. Drugs that are used in critical care are designed to be absorbed within seconds or minutes. At the other extreme are drugs such as some hormones that may be injected deep into tissue in order to absorb slowly over a few weeks or months.

Absorption is conditional on many factors. Drugs administered by IV have the most rapid onset of action.

Drugs in elixir or syrup formulations are absorbed faster than tablets or capsules. Drugs administered in high doses are generally absorbed faster and have a more rapid onset of action than those given in low concentrations. Digestive motility, exposure to enzymes in the digestive tract, and blood flow to the site of drug administration also affect absorption.

The degree of ionization of a drug affects its absorption. A drug's ability to become ionized depends on the surrounding pH, which is a measure of the acidity or basicity of a solution. Acetylsalicylic acid (ASA) provides an excellent example of the effects of ionization on absorption, as depicted in Figure 4.2. In the acid environment of the stomach, ASA is in its nonionized form and is thus readily absorbed and distributed by the bloodstream. As ASA enters the alkaline environment of the small intestine, however, it becomes ionized. In its ionized form, ASA is not as likely to be absorbed and distributed to target cells. Unlike acidic drugs, medications that are weakly basic are in their nonionized form in an alkaline environment; therefore, basic drugs are absorbed and distributed better in alkaline environments such as in the small intestine. The pH of the

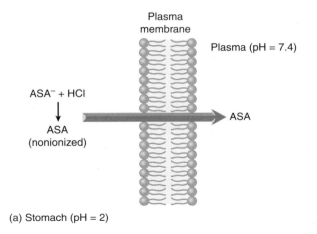

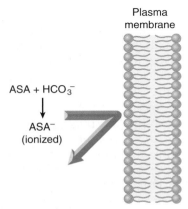

(a) Stomach (pH = 2)

(b) Small intestine (pH = 8)

● **Figure 4.2** Effect of pH on drug absorption: (a) a weak acid such as acetylsalicylic acid (ASA) is in a nonionized form in an acidic environment, and absorption occurs; (b) in a basic environment, ASA is mostly in an ionized form and absorption is prevented

local environment directly influences drug absorption through ionization of the drug. In simplest terms, it may help the student to remember that acids are absorbed in acids, and bases are absorbed in bases.

Drug manufacturers deliberately alter the forms of some drugs to mange these factors, as depicted in the examples in Figure 4.3. Drug products for oral use may be in regular, buffered, or enteric-coated forms. Enteric-coated products are intended to absorb in the alkaline environment of the small intestine. Regular (uncoated) acidic products dissolve and absorb in the stomach. Buffered products contain ions that decrease gastric acidity and slow absorption of acidic drugs.

Drug-drug or food-drug interactions may influence absorption. Many examples of these interactions have been discovered. For example, administering tetracyclines with food or drugs containing calcium, iron, or magnesium can significantly delay absorption of the antibiotic. High-fat meals can slow stomach motility significantly and delay the absorption of oral medications taken with the meal. The absorption of acidic drugs may be hastened by drinking citrus fruit juices that increase gastric acidity. Consuming alkaline substances with enteric-coated drugs may cause the coating to begin to breakdown prematurely before it reaches the intended alkaline environment of the small intestine. Dietary supplements may also affect absorption. Common ingredients in herbal weight-loss products such as aloe leaf, guar gum, senna, and yellow dock exert a laxative effect that may decrease intestinal transit time and reduce drug absorption (Scott & Elmer, 2002). Grapefruit juice but not orange juice inhibits the activity of an enzyme (cytochrome P450 3A4) in the intestinal wall. Even when taken in small quantities, grapefruit juice can significantly increase the absorption of some drugs such as nifedipine. The nurse must be aware of drug interactions and advise clients to avoid known combinations of foods and medications that significantly impact drug absorption and action.

4.4 Distribution of Medications

Distribution involves how pharmacological agents are transported throughout the body. The simplest factor determining distribution is the amount of blood flow to body tissues. The heart, liver, kidneys, and brain receive the most blood supply. Skin, bone, and adipose tissue receive a lower blood flow; therefore, it is more difficult to deliver high concentrations of drugs to these areas.

The physical properties of the drug greatly influence how it moves throughout the body after administration. Lipid solubility is an important characteristic because it determines how quickly a drug is absorbed, mixes within the bloodstream, crosses membranes, and becomes localized in body tissues. Lipid-soluble agents are not limited by the barriers that normally stop water-soluble drugs; thus, they are more completely distributed to body tissues.

Some tissues have the ability to accumulate and store drugs after absorption. The bone marrow, teeth, eyes, and adipose tissue have an especially high **affinity**, or attraction,

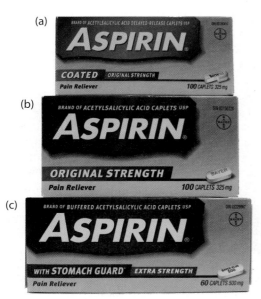

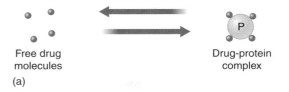

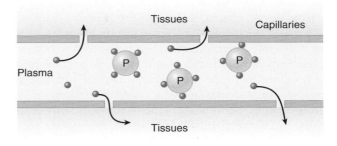

● **Figure 4.3** Drug products for oral use: (a) enteric-coated products are intended to absorb in the alkaline environment of the small intestine; (b) regular products dissolve and begin to absorb in the stomach; (c) buffered products contain ions that decrease gastric acidity and slow absorption
Source: Shirley King.

● **Figure 4.4** Plasma protein binding and drug availability: (a) drug exists in a free state or bound to plasma protein; (b) drug-protein complexes are too large to cross membranes

for certain medications. Examples of agents that are attracted to adipose tissue are thiopental, diazepam, and lipid-soluble vitamins. Tetracycline binds to calcium salts and accumulates in the bones and teeth. Once stored in tissues, drugs may remain in the body for many months.

Not all drug molecules in the plasma will reach their target cells because many drugs bind reversibly to plasma proteins, particularly albumin, to form **drug-protein complexes**. Drug-protein complexes are too large to cross capillary membranes; thus, the drug is not available for distribution to body tissues. Drugs bound to proteins circulate in the plasma until they are released or displaced from the drug-protein complex. Only unbound (free) drugs can reach their target cells. This concept is illustrated in Figure 4.4. Some drugs such as the anticoagulant warfarin are highly bound; 99% of the drug in the plasma exists in drug-protein complexes and is unavailable to reach target cells.

Drugs and other chemicals compete with each other for plasma protein binding sites, and some agents have a greater affinity for these binding sites than others. Drug-drug and drug-food interactions may occur when one agent displaces another from plasma proteins. The displaced medication can immediately reach high levels in the blood and produce adverse effects. An example is the drug warfarin. After administration, 99% of the warfarin molecules are bound to plasma proteins. Drugs such as ASA or cimetidine displace warfarin from the drug-protein complex, thus raising blood levels of free warfarin and dramatically enhancing the risk of hemorrhage. Most drug guides give the percentage of medication bound to plasma proteins; when giving multiple drugs that are highly bound, the nurse should monitor the client closely for adverse effects.

The brain and placenta possess special anatomical barriers that inhibit many chemicals and medications from entering. These barriers are referred to as the **blood-brain barrier** and **fetal-placental barrier**, respectively. Some medications such as sedatives, antianxiety agents, and anticonvulsants readily cross the blood-brain barrier to produce their actions on the central nervous system (CNS). On the other hand, most antitumour medications cannot cross this barrier, making brain cancers difficult to treat with chemotherapy.

The fetal-placental barrier serves an important protective function because it prevents potentially harmful substances from passing from the mother's bloodstream to the fetus. Substances such as alcohol, cocaine, caffeine, and certain prescription medications, however, easily cross the placental barrier and could potentially harm the fetus. Because of this, no prescription medication, OTC drug, or herbal therapy should be taken by a client who is pregnant without first consulting a healthcare provider. The healthcare provider should always question female clients in the childbearing years regarding their pregnancy status before prescribing a drug. Chapter 6 presents a list of drug pregnancy categories to assess fetal risk.

4.5 Metabolism of Medications

Metabolism, also called **biotransformation**, is the process of chemically converting a drug to a form that is usually more easily removed from the body. Metabolism involves a study of the complex biochemical pathways and reactions that alter drugs, nutrients, vitamins, and minerals. The liver is the primary site of drug metabolism, although the kidneys and cells of the intestinal tract also have high metabolic rates.

Many types of biochemical reactions occur to medications during phase I metabolism as they pass through the liver, including hydrolysis, oxidation, and reduction. Some drugs undergo phase II metabolism, during which the addition of side chains, known as **conjugates**, makes drugs more water-soluble and more easily excreted by the kidneys.

Most metabolism in the liver is accomplished by the **hepatic microsomal enzyme system**. This enzyme complex is sometimes called the P450 system, named after cytochrome P450, which is a key component of the system. As it relates to pharmacotherapy, the primary actions of the hepatic microsomal enzymes are to inactivate drugs and accelerate their excretion. In some cases, however, metabolism can produce a chemical alteration that makes the resulting molecule *more* active than the original. For example, the narcotic analgesic codeine undergoes bio-transformation to morphine, which has significantly greater ability to relieve pain. In fact, some agents, known as **prodrugs**, have no pharmacological activity unless they are first metabolized to their active form by the body. Examples of prodrugs include benazepril and losartan.

Changes in the function of the hepatic microsomal enzymes can significantly affect drug metabolism. A few drugs have the ability to increase metabolic activity in the liver, a process called **enzyme induction**. For example, phenobarbital causes the liver to synthesize more microsomal enzymes. By doing so, phenobarbital will increase the rate of its own metabolism, as well as that of other drugs metabolized in the liver. In these clients, higher doses of medication may be required to achieve therapeutic effect.

Certain clients have decreased hepatic metabolic activity, which may alter drug action. Hepatic enzyme activity is generally reduced in infants and elderly clients; therefore, pediatric and geriatric clients are more sensitive to drug therapy than middle-aged clients. Clients with severe liver damage, such as that caused by cirrhosis, will require reductions in drug dosage because of the decreased metabolic activity. Genetic polymorphisms among ethnically diverse populations may result in differences in metabolic function. Certain genetic disorders have been recognized in which clients lack specific metabolic enzymes. Drug dosages in these clients must be adjusted accordingly, or an alternate drug may be prescribed. The nurse should assess patterns in a client's responses to previous medications for evidence of possible altered metabolism and pay careful attention to laboratory values that may indicate liver disease so that doses may be adjusted accordingly.

Metabolism has a number of additional therapeutic consequences. As illustrated in Figure 4.5, drugs absorbed after oral administration cross directly from the small intestine into the hepatic portal circulation, which carries blood to the liver before it is distributed to other body tissues. As blood passes through the liver circulation, some drugs can be completely metabolized to an inactive form before they ever reach the general circulation. This **first-pass effect** is an important mechanism since a large number of oral drugs are rendered inactive by hepatic metabolic reactions. Alternate routes of delivery that bypass the first-pass effect (e.g., sublingual, rectal, or parenteral routes) may need to be considered for these drugs.

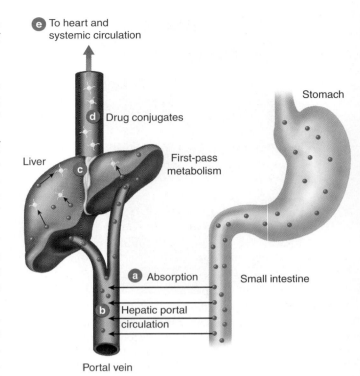

● **Figure 4.5** First-pass effect: (a) drug is absorbed; (b) drug enters hepatic portal circulation and goes directly to the liver; (c) hepatic microsomal enzymes metabolize drug to inactive forms; (d) drug conjugates leave liver; (e) distribution to general circulation

4.6 Excretion of Medications

Drugs are removed from the body by the process of **excretion**. The rate at which medications are excreted determines their concentration in the bloodstream and tissues. This is important because the concentration of drugs in the bloodstream determines their duration of action. Pathological states, such as liver disease or renal failure, often increase the duration of drug action in the body because they interfere with natural excretion mechanisms. Dosing regimens must be carefully adjusted in these clients.

Although drugs are removed from the body by numerous organs and tissues, the primary site of excretion is the kidney. In an average-sized person, approximately 180 L of blood are filtered by the kidneys each day. Free drugs, water-soluble agents, electrolytes, and small molecules are easily filtered by the glomerulus. Proteins, blood cells, conjugates, and drug-protein complexes are not filtered because of their large size.

Upon filtration, chemicals and drugs are subjected to the process of reabsorption in the renal tubule. Mechanisms of reabsorption are the same as absorption elsewhere in the body. Nonionized and lipid-soluble drugs cross renal tubular membranes easily and return to the circulation; ionized and water-soluble drugs generally remain in the filtrate for excretion.

Drug-protein complexes and substances too large to be filtered by the glomerulus are sometimes secreted into the distal tubule of the nephron. For example, only 10% of a dose of penicillin G is filtered by the glomerulus; 90% is secreted into the renal tubule. As with metabolic enzyme activity, secretion mechanisms are less active in infants and older adults.

Certain drugs may be excreted more quickly if the pH of the filtrate changes. Weak acids such as ASA are excreted faster when the filtrate is slightly alkaline because ASA is ionized in an alkaline environment and the drug will remain in the filtrate and be excreted in the urine. Weakly basic drugs such as diazepam are excreted faster with a slightly acidic filtrate because they are ionized in this environment. Nurses should be aware of common foods that alter the pH of urine since these may affect the excretion and duration of action of medications. Foods that acidify urine include cranberries, cheese, eggs, lentils, pasta, grains, plums, and prunes. Foods that alkalinize urine include milk, vegetables (except for corn), and fruits (except for cranberries, prunes, and plums). The relationship between pH and drug excretion can be especially important in critical care situations. To speed the renal excretion of acidic drugs such as ASA in an overdosed client, nurses can administer sodium bicarbonate. Sodium bicarbonate will make the urine more basic, which ionizes more ASA, causing it to be excreted more readily. The excretion of diazepam, on the other hand, can be enhanced by giving ammonium chloride, to acidify the filtrate.

Alteration of kidney function can dramatically affect pharmacokinetics. Clients with renal failure will have diminished ability to excrete medications and may retain drugs for an extended time. Doses for these clients must be reduced, to avoid drug toxicity. Because small to moderate changes in renal status can cause rapid increases in serum drug levels, the nurse must constantly monitor kidney function in clients receiving drugs that may be nephrotoxic or have a narrow margin of safety.

Other organs can serve as important sites of excretion. Drugs that can easily be changed into a gaseous form are especially suited for excretion by the respiratory system. The rate of respiratory excretion is dependent on factors that affect gas exchange, including diffusion, gas solubility, and pulmonary blood flow. The elimination of volatile anesthetics following surgery is primarily dependent on respiratory activity. The faster the breathing rate, the greater the excretion. Conversely, the respiratory removal of water-soluble agents such as alcohol is more dependent on blood flow to the lungs. The greater the blood flow into lung capillaries, the greater the excretion. In contrast to other methods of excretion, the lungs excrete most drugs in their original unmetabolized form.

Glandular activity is another elimination mechanism. Water-soluble drugs may be secreted into the saliva, sweat, or breast milk. The "funny taste" that clients sometimes experience when given IV drugs is due to the agent being secreted into the saliva. Another example of glandular excretion is the garlic smell that can be detected when standing next to a perspiring person who has recently eaten garlic. Excretion into breast milk is of considerable importance for basic drugs such as morphine and codeine as these

LIFESPAN CONSIDERATIONS

Adverse Drug Effects and the Elderly

Adverse drug effects are more commonly recorded in elderly clients than in young adults or middle-aged clients because the geriatric population takes more drugs simultaneously (an average of seven) than other age groups. In addition, chronic diseases that affect pharmacokinetics are present more often in the elderly. A recent study of over 2800 inpatients over age 70 found 500 adverse drug events at the time of admission (Doucet et al., 2002). Over 60% of the adverse drug events were caused by drug-drug interactions. Of these, over 46% were considered "preventable" because the drug-drug interaction was known. Excess doses were administered in almost 15% of the clients; prescribers often forgot to adjust doses for pharmacokinetic variables that change with aging.

can achieve high concentrations and potentially affect the nursing infant. Nursing mothers should always check with their healthcare provider before taking any prescription medication, OTC drug, or herbal supplement. Pharmacology for the pregnant or breastfeeding client is discussed in Chapter 6.

Some drugs are secreted in the bile, a process known as biliary excretion. In many cases, drugs secreted into bile will enter the duodenum and eventually leave the body in the feces. However, most bile is circulated back to the liver by **enterohepatic recirculation**, as illustrated in Figure 4.6. A percentage of the drug may be recirculated numerous times with the bile. Biliary reabsorption is extremely influential in prolonging the activity of cardiac glycosides, certain antibiotics, and phenothiazines. Recirculated drugs are ultimately metabolized by the liver and excreted by the kidneys. Recirculation and elimination of drugs through biliary excretion may continue for several weeks after therapy has been discontinued.

MediaLink Drugs and Breast Milk

4.7 Drug Plasma Concentration and Therapeutic Response

The therapeutic response of most drugs is directly related to their level in the plasma. Although the concentration of the medication at its *target tissue* is more predictive of drug action, this quantity is impossible to measure in most cases. For example, it is possible to conduct a laboratory test that measures the serum level of lithium, a bipolar disorder drug, by taking a blood sample; it is a far different matter to measure the quantity of this drug in neurons within the CNS. Indeed, it is common practice for nurses to monitor the plasma levels of certain drugs that have a low safety profile.

Several important pharmacokinetic principles can be illustrated by measuring the serum level of a drug following a single-dose administration. These pharmacokinetic values are shown graphically in Figure 4.7. This figure demonstrates two plasma drug levels. First is the **minimum effective concentration**, the amount of drug required to produce a therapeutic effect. Second is the **toxic concentration**, the level of drug that will result in serious adverse effects. The

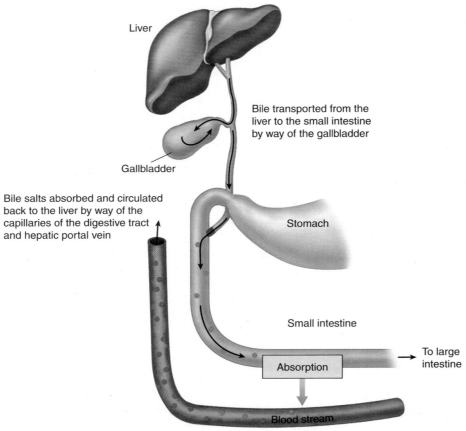

Liver

Bile transported from the
liver to the small intestine
by way of the gallbladder

Gallbladder

Bile salts absorbed and circulated
back to the liver by way of the
capillaries of the digestive tract
and hepatic portal vein

Stomach

Small intestine

To large
intestine

Absorption

Blood stream

● **Figure 4.6** Enterohepatic recirculation

plasma drug concentration between the minimum effective concentration and the toxic concentration is called the **therapeutic range** of the drug. These values have great

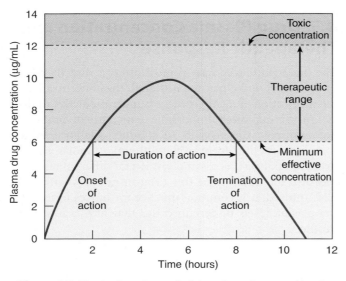

● **Figure 4.7** Single-dose drug administration: pharmacokinetic values for this drug are as follows: onset of action, 2 hours; duration of action, 6 hours; termination of action, 8 hours after administration; peak plasma concentration, 10 µg/mL; time to peak drug effect, 5 hours; $t_{1/2}$, 4 hours

clinical significance. For example, if the client has a severe headache and is given half of an ASA tablet, the plasma level will remain below the minimum effective concentration, and the client will not experience pain relief. Two or three tablets will increase the plasma level of ASA into the therapeutic range, and the pain will subside. Taking six or more tablets may result in adverse effects, such as gastrointestinal (GI) bleeding or tinnitus. For each drug administered, the nurse's goal is to keep its plasma concentration in the therapeutic range. For some drugs, this therapeutic range is quite wide; for other medications, the difference between a minimum effective dose and a toxic dose can be dangerously narrow.

4.8 Plasma Half-Life and Duration of Drug Action

The most common description of a drug's duration of action is its **plasma half-life ($t_{1/2}$)**, defined as the length of time required for a medication to decrease concentration in the plasma by one-half after administration. Some drugs have a half-life of only a few minutes, while others have a half-life of several hours or days. The greater the half-life, the longer it takes a medication to be excreted. For example, a drug with a $t_{1/2}$ of 10 hours would take longer to be excreted and thus produce a longer effect in the body than a drug with a $t_{1/2}$ of 5 hours.

The plasma half-life of a drug is an essential pharmacokinetic variable that has important clinical applications. Drugs with relatively short half-lives, such as ASA ($t_{1/2} = 15$ to 20 minutes), must be given every 3 to 4 hours. Drugs with longer half-lives, such as felodipine ($t_{1/2} = 10$ hours), need only be given once a day. If a client has extensive renal or hepatic disease, the plasma half-life of a drug will increase, and the drug concentration may reach toxic levels. In these clients, medications must be given less frequently, or the dosages must be reduced.

4.9 Loading Doses and Maintenance Doses

Few drugs are administered as a single dose. Repeated doses result in an accumulation of drug in the bloodstream, as shown in Figure 4.8. Eventually, a plateau will be reached where the level of drug in the plasma is maintained continuously within the therapeutic range. At this level, the amount of drug administered has reached equilibrium with the amount of drug being eliminated, resulting in a continuous therapeutic level of drug being distributed to body tissues. Theoretically, it takes approximately four half-lives to reach this equilibrium. If the medication is given as a continuous infusion, the plateau can be reached quickly and be maintained with little or no fluctuation in drug plasma levels.

The plateau may be reached faster by administration of loading doses followed by regular maintenance doses. A **loading dose** is a higher amount of drug, often given only once or twice, which is administered to "prime" the bloodstream with a level sufficient to quickly induce a therapeutic response. Before plasma levels can drop back toward zero, intermittent **maintenance doses** are given to keep the

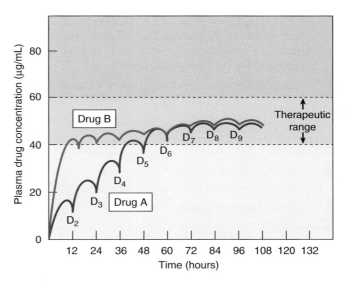

● **Figure 4.8** Multiple-dose drug administration: drug A and drug B are administered every 12 hours; drug B reaches the therapeutic range faster because the first dose is a loading dose

plasma drug concentration in the therapeutic range. Although blood levels of the drug fluctuate with this approach, the equilibrium state can be reached almost as rapidly as with a continuous infusion. Loading doses are particularly important for drugs with prolonged half-lives and for situations in which it is critical to raise drug plasma levels quickly, as might be the case when administering an antibiotic for a severe infection. In Figure 4.8, notice that it takes almost five doses (48 hours) before a therapeutic level is reached using a routine dosing schedule. With a loading dose, a therapeutic level is reached within 12 hours.

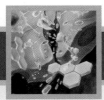

CHAPTER REVIEW

KEY CONCEPTS

The numbered key concepts provide a succinct summary of the important points from the corresponding numbered section within the chapter. If any of these points are not clear, refer to the numbered section within the chapter for review. Expanded versions can be found on the Companion Website.

4.1 Pharmacokinetics focuses on the movement of drugs throughout the body after they are administered.

4.2 The physiological properties of plasma membranes determine movement of drugs throughout the body. The four processes of pharmacokinetics are absorption, metabolism, distribution, and excretion.

4.3 Absorption is the process of moving a drug from the site of administration to the bloodstream. Absorption of a drug molecule depends on its size, lipid solubility, degree of ionization, and interactions with food or other medications.

4.4 Distribution represents how drugs are transported throughout the body. Distribution depends on the formation of drug-protein complexes and special barriers such as the placenta and blood-brain barrier.

4.5 Metabolism is a process that changes a drug's form and makes it more likely to be excreted. Changes in hepatic metabolism can significantly affect drug action.

4.6 Excretion processes remove drugs from the body. Drugs are primarily excreted by the kidneys but may be excreted by the lung or glands, or into bile.

4.7 The therapeutic response of most drugs depends on their concentration in the plasma. The difference between the minimum effective concentration and the toxic concentration is called the therapeutic range.

4.8 Plasma half-life represents the duration of action for most drugs.

4.9 Repeated dosing allows a plateau drug plasma level to be reached. Loading doses allow a therapeutic drug level to be reached rapidly.

REVIEW QUESTIONS

1 Describe the types of obstacles drugs face from the time they are administered until they reach their target cells.

2 Why is $t_{1/2}$ important to the nurse?

3 How does the ionization of a drug affect its distribution in the body?

4 Explain why drugs that are metabolized through the first-pass effect may need to be administered by the parenteral route.

5 Explain how onset of action, duration of action, and the time to peak effect can be estimated from a single-dose response curve.

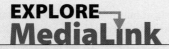

EXPLORE MediaLink

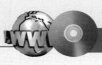

www.pearsoned.ca/adams-king

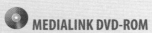

MEDIALINK DVD-ROM
- Audio Glossary
- CRNE Review

COMPANION WEBSITE
- CRNE Review
- **Case Study:** Client using herbal supplements

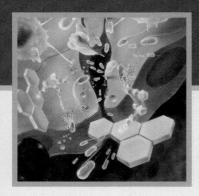

CHAPTER 5

Pharmacodynamics

OBJECTIVES

After reading this chapter, the student should be able to do the following:

1. Apply principles of pharmacodynamics to clinical practice.
2. Discuss how frequency response curves may be used to explain how clients respond differently to medications.
3. Explain the importance of the median effective dose (ED_{50}) to clinical practice.
4. Compare and contrast median lethal dose (LD_{50}) and median toxicity dose (TD_{50}).
5. Discuss how a drug's therapeutic index is related to its margin of safety.
6. Identify the significance of the graded dose-response relationship to clinical practice.
7. Compare and contrast the terms *potency* and *efficacy*.
8. Distinguish between an agonist, partial agonist, and antagonist.
9. Explain the relationship between receptors and drug action.
10. Explain possible future developments in the field of pharmacogenetics.

MediaLink

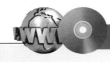

www.pearsoned.ca/adams-king

CRNE review, case studies, and other interactive resources for this chapter can be found on the Companion Website at **www.pearsoned.ca/adams-king**. Click on "Chapter 5" to select the activities for this chapter. For animations, more CRNE review questions, and an audio glossary, access the accompanying MediaLink DVD-ROM in this textbook.

In clinical practice, nurses quickly learn that medications do not affect all clients in the same way: a dose that produces a dramatic response in one client may have no effect on another. In some cases, the differences among clients are predictable, based on the pharmacokinetic principles discussed in Chapter 4. In other cases, the differences in response are not easily explained. Despite this client variability, healthcare providers must choose optimal doses while avoiding unnecessary adverse effects. This is not an easy task given the wide variation of client responses within a population. This chapter examines the mechanisms by which drugs affect clients and how the nurse can apply these principles to clinical practice.

5.1 Pharmacodynamics and Inter-Individual Variability

The term **pharmacodynamics** is composed of the root words *pharmaco*, which means "medicine," and *dynamics*, which means "change." In simplest terms, pharmacodynamics refers to how a drug *changes* the body. A more complete definition explains pharmacodynamics as the branch of pharmacology concerned with the mechanisms of drug action and the relationships between drug concentration and responses in the body.

Pharmacodynamics has important clinical applications. Healthcare providers must be able to predict whether a drug will produce a significant change in clients. Although clinicians usually begin therapy with average doses taken from a drug guide, intuitive experience often becomes the practical method for determining which doses of medications will be effective in a given client. Knowledge of therapeutic indexes, dose-response relationships, and drug-receptor interactions will help the nurse provide safe and effective treatment.

Inter-individual variability in responses to drugs can best be understood by examining a frequency distribution curve. A **frequency distribution curve**, shown in Figure 5.1, is a graphical representation of the number of individuals responding to a drug at different doses. Notice the wide range of doses that produced the responses shown in the curve. A few individuals responded to the drug at very low doses. As the dose was increased, more and more individuals responded. Some required very high doses to elicit the desired response. The peak of the curve indicates the largest number of individuals responding to the drug. The curve does not show the *magnitude* of response, only whether a measurable response occurred. As an example, think of the given response to an antihypertensive drug as being a reduction of 20 mm in systolic blood pressure. A few individuals experience the desired 20 mm reduction at a dose of only 10 mg of drug. A 50 mg dose produces the largest number of individuals with a 20 mm reduction in blood pressure; however, a few need as much as 90 mg of drug to produce the same 20 mm reduction.

The dose in the middle of the frequency distribution curve represents the drug's **median effective dose (ED$_{50}$)**. The ED$_{50}$ is the dose required to produce a specific therapeutic response in 50% of a group of clients. Drug guides sometimes report the ED$_{50}$ as the average or standard dose.

The inter-individual variability shown in Figure 5.1 has important clinical implications. First, the nurse should realize that the standard or average dose predicts a satisfactory therapeutic response for only *half* the population. In other words, many clients will require more or less than the average dose for optimum pharmacotherapy. Using the systolic blood pressure example, assume that a large group of clients is given the average dose of 50 mg. Some of these clients will experience toxicity at this level because they only needed 10 mg to achieve blood pressure reduction. Other clients in this group will probably have no reduction in

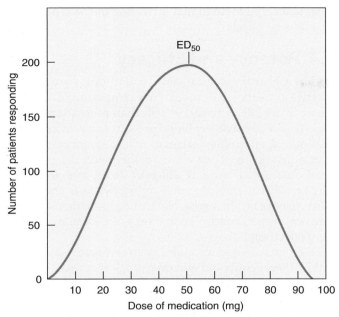

● **Figure 5.1** Frequency distribution curve: inter-individual variability in drug response

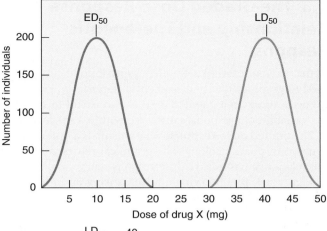

(a) Drug X : TI = $\dfrac{LD_{50}}{ED_{50}}$ = $\dfrac{40}{10}$ = 4

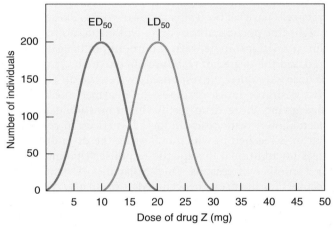

(b) Drug Z : TI = $\dfrac{LD_{50}}{ED_{50}}$ = $\dfrac{20}{10}$ = 2

● **Figure 5.2** Therapeutic index: (a) drug X has a therapeutic index (TI) of 4; (b) drug Z has a therapeutic index of 2

blood pressure. By observing the client, taking vital signs, and monitoring associated laboratory data, the skill of the nurse is critical in determining whether the average dose is effective for the client. It is not enough to simply memorize an average dose for a drug; the nurse must know when and how to adjust this dose to obtain the optimum therapeutic response.

5.2 Therapeutic Index and Drug Safety

Administering a dose that produces an optimum therapeutic response for each individual client is only one component of effective pharmacotherapy. The nurse must also be able to predict whether the dose being given is safe for the client.

Frequency distribution curves can also be used to represent the safety of a drug. For example, the **median lethal dose (LD$_{50}$)** is often determined in preclinical trials as part of the drug development process discussed in Chapter 1. The LD$_{50}$ is the dose of drug that will be lethal in 50% of a group of animals. As with ED$_{50}$, a group of animals will exhibit considerable variability in the lethal dose—what may be a non-toxic dose for one animal may be lethal for another.

To examine the safety of a particular drug, the LD$_{50}$ can be compared to the ED$_{50}$, as shown in Figure 5.2. In the top example, 10 mg of drug X is the average *effective* dose, and 40 mg is the average *lethal* dose. The ED$_{50}$ and LD$_{50}$ are used to calculate an important value in pharmacology, the **therapeutic index**, which is the ratio of a drug's LD$_{50}$ to its ED$_{50}$.

The larger the difference between the two doses, the greater the therapeutic index. In Figure 5.2a, the therapeutic index is 4 (40 mg ÷ 10 mg). Essentially, this means that it would

take an error in magnitude of *approximately* 4 times the average dose to be lethal to a client. Thus, the therapeutic index is a measure of a drug's safety margin—the higher the value, the safer the medication.

As another example, the therapeutic index of a second drug is shown in Figure 5.2b. Drug Z has the same ED$_{50}$ as drug X, but shows a different LD$_{50}$. The therapeutic index for drug Z is only 2 (20 mg ÷ 10 mg). The difference between an effective dose and a lethal dose is very small for drug Z; thus, the drug has a narrow safety margin. The therapeutic index offers the nurse practical information on the safety of a drug and a means to compare one drug to another.

Because the LD$_{50}$ cannot be experimentally determined in humans, the **median toxicity dose (TD$_{50}$)** is a more practical value in the clinical setting. The TD$_{50}$ is the dose that will produce a given toxicity in 50% of a group of clients. The TD$_{50}$ value may be extrapolated from animal data or based on adverse effects recorded in clinical trials.

5.3 The Graded Dose-Response Relationship and Therapeutic Response

In the previous examples, frequency distribution curves were used to graphically visualize client differences in responses to medications in a *population*. It is also useful to visualize the variability in responses observed within a *single client*.

The **graded dose-response** relationship is a fundamental concept in pharmacology. The graphical representation of this relationship is called a dose-response curve, as illustrated in Figure 5.3. By observing and measuring an individual's response at different doses of the drug, one can explain several important clinical relationships.

The three distinct phases of a dose-response curve indicate essential pharmacodynamic principles that have relevance to clinical practice. Phase 1 occurs at the lowest doses. The flatness of this portion of the curve indicates that few target cells have yet been affected by the drug. Phase 2 is the straight-line portion of the curve. This portion often shows a linear relationship between the amount of drug administered and the degree of response obtained. For example, if the dose is doubled, the response is twice as great. This is the most desirable range of doses for pharmacotherapeutics since giving more drug results in proportionately more effect; a lower drug dose produces less effect. In phase 3, a plateau is reached in which increasing the drug dose produces no additional therapeutic response. This may occur for a number of reasons. One explanation is that all the receptors for the drug are occupied. It could also mean that the drug has brought 100% relief, such as when a migraine headache has been terminated; giving higher doses produces no additional relief. In phase 3, although increasing the dose does not result in more therapeutic effect, the nurse should be mindful that increasing the dose may produce adverse effects.

5.4 Potency and Efficacy

Within a pharmacological class, not all drugs are equally effective at treating a disorder. For example, some antineoplastic drugs kill more cancer cells than others, some antihypertensive agents lower blood pressure to a greater degree than others, and some analgesics relieve severe pain better than others in the same class. Furthermore, drugs in the same class are effective at different doses; one antibiotic may be effective at a dose of 1 mg/kg, whereas another is most effective at 100 mg/kg. Nurses need a method to compare one drug to another so that they can administer treatment effectively.

There are two fundamental ways to compare medications within therapeutic and pharmacological classes. First is the concept of **potency**. A drug that is more potent will produce a therapeutic effect at a lower dose compared to another drug in the same class. Consider two agents, drug X and drug Y, which both produce a 20 mm drop in blood pressure. If drug X produced this effect at a dose of 10 mg, and drug Y at 60 mg, then drug X is said to be more potent. Thus, potency is a way to compare the doses of two independently administered drugs in terms of how much is needed to produce a particular response. A useful way to visualize the concept of potency is by examining dose-response curves. Compare the two drugs shown in Figure 5.4a. In this example, drug A is more potent because it requires a lower dose to produce the same response.

The second method used to compare drugs is **efficacy**, which is the magnitude of maximal response that can be produced from a particular drug. In the example in Figure 5.4b, drug A is more efficacious because it produces a higher maximal response.

Which is more important to the success of pharmacotherapy, potency or efficacy? Perhaps the best way to understand these concepts is to use the specific example of headache pain. Two common OTC analgesics are ibuprofen (200 mg) and acetylsalicylic acid (650 mg). The fact that ibuprofen relieves pain at a lower dose indicates that this agent is *more potent* than acetylsalicylic acid. At recommended doses, however, both are equally effective at relieving headache pain, thus, they have the *same efficacy*. But, if the client is experiencing severe pain, neither acetylsalicylic acid nor ibuprofen has sufficient efficacy to bring relief. Narcotic analgesics such as morphine have greater efficacy than acetylsalicylic acid and ibuprofen and could effectively treat this type of pain. From a pharmacotherapeutic perspective, efficacy is almost always more important than potency. In the previous example, the average dose is unimportant to the client, but headache relief is essential. As another comparison, the client with cancer is much more concerned about how many cancer cells have been killed (efficacy) than what dose the nurse administered (potency). Although the nurse will often hear claims that one drug is more potent than another, a more compelling concern is which drug is more efficacious.

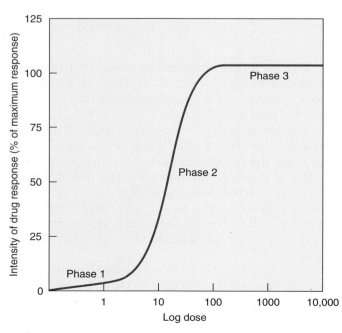

● **Figure 5.3** Dose-response relationship

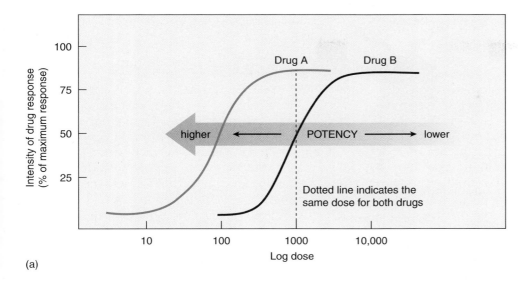

(a)

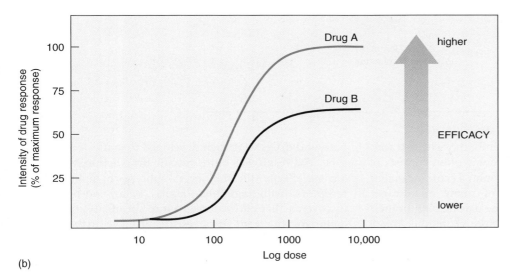

(b)

● **Figure 5.4** Potency and efficacy: (a) drug A has greater potency than drug B; (b) drug A has greater efficacy than drug B

5.5 Cellular Receptors and Drug Action

Cell signalling is part of a complex system of communication that enables cells to perceive and correctly respond to their environment and carry out basic cellular activities. Errors in cellular information processing are responsible for diseases such as diabetes, cancer, and autoimmune disorders. Cells receive information from their environment through a class of molecules known as **receptors**. A receptor is a molecule to which a medication binds to initiate its effect. While many receptors are cell surface proteins, some are found inside cells. Molecules that activate (or, in some cases, inhibit) receptors are called receptor **ligands**. These ligands can be classified as hormones, neurotransmitters, cytokines, or growth factors. The information that cells receive is then processed through signalling pathways. Activation of specific target proteins causes a particular cell response. Different types of cells may have the same receptor and receive the same signal but have different target proteins that produce different responses when activated.

Drugs act by modulating or changing existing physiological and biochemical processes. To effect such changes requires that the drug interact with specific molecules and chemicals normally found in the body. The concept of a drug binding to a receptor to cause a change in body chemistry or physiology is a fundamental theory in pharmacology. Receptor theory explains the mechanisms by which most drugs produce their effects. It is important to understand, however, that these receptors do not exist in the body solely to bind drugs. Their normal function is to bind endogenous molecules such as hormones, neurotransmitters, and growth factors.

Although a drug receptor can be any type of macromolecule, the vast majority are proteins. As shown in Figure 5.5, a receptor may be depicted as a three-dimensional protein

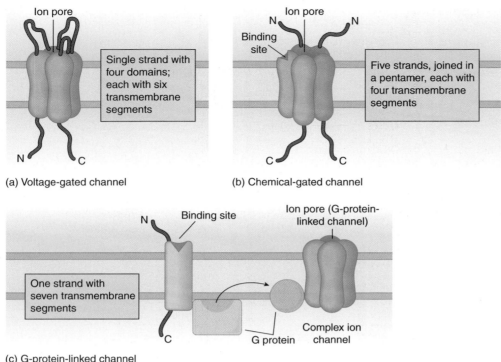

(a) Voltage-gated channel

Ion pore

Single strand with four domains; each with six transmembrane segments

(b) Chemical-gated channel

Ion pore

Binding site

Five strands, joined in a pentamer, each with four transmembrane segments

(c) G-protein-linked channel

Binding site

Ion pore (G-protein-linked channel)

One strand with seven transmembrane segments

G protein

Complex ion channel

● **Figure 5.5** Cellular receptors

associated with a cellular plasma membrane. The extracellular structural component of a receptor often consists of several protein subunits arranged around a central canal or channel. Other receptors consist of many membrane-spanning segments inserted across the plasma membrane.

A drug attaches to its receptor in a specific manner, much like a lock and key. Small changes to the structure of a drug, or its receptor, may weaken or even eliminate binding between the two molecules. Once bound, drugs may trigger a series of **second messenger** events within the cell, such as the conversion of adenosine triphosphate (ATP) to cyclic adenosine monophosphate (cyclic AMP), the release of intracellular calcium, or the activation of specific G proteins and associated enzymes. These biochemical cascades initiate the drug's action by either stimulating or inhibiting a normal activity of the cell.

Not all receptors are bound to plasma membranes; some are intracellular molecules such as DNA or enzymes in the cytoplasm. By interacting with these types of receptors, medications are able to inhibit protein synthesis or regulate events such as cell replication and metabolism. Examples of agents that bind intracellular components include steroid medications, vitamins, and hormones.

Receptors and their associated drug mechanisms are extremely important in therapeutics. Receptor subtypes are being discovered and new medications are being developed at a faster rate than at any other time in history. These subtypes permit the "fine-tuning" of pharmacology. For example, the first medications affecting the autonomic nervous system affected all autonomic receptors. It was discovered that two basic receptor types existed in the body, alpha and

beta, and drugs were then developed that affected only one type. The result was more specific drug action, with fewer adverse effects. Still later, several subtypes of alpha and beta receptors, including alpha$_1$, alpha$_2$, beta$_1$, and beta$_2$, were discovered that allowed even more specificity in pharmacotherapy. In recent years, researchers have further divided and refined these subtypes and discovered other receptors such as beta$_3$. It is likely that receptor research will continue to result in the development of new medications that activate very specific receptors and thus direct drug action that avoids unnecessary adverse effects.

Some drugs act independently of cellular receptors. These agents are associated with other mechanisms, such as changing the permeability of cellular membranes, depressing membrane excitability, or altering the activity of cellular pumps. Actions such as these are often described as **nonspecific cellular responses**. Ethyl alcohol, general anesthetics, and osmotic diuretics are examples of agents that act by non-specific mechanisms.

5.6 Types of Drug-Receptor Interactions

When a drug binds to a receptor, several therapeutic consequences can result. In simplest terms, a specific activity of the cell is either enhanced or inhibited. The actual biochemical mechanism underlying the therapeutic effect, however, may be extremely complex. In some cases, the mechanism of action is not known.

When a drug binds to its receptor, it may produce a response that *mimics* the effect of the endogenous regulatory molecule. For example, when the drug bethanechol is administered, it binds to acetylcholine receptors in the autonomic nervous system and produces the same actions as acetylcholine. A drug that produces the same type of response as the endogenous substance is called an **agonist**. Agonists sometimes produce a greater maximal response than the endogenous chemical. The term **partial agonist** describes a medication that produces a weaker, or less efficacious, response than an agonist.

A second possibility is that a drug will occupy a receptor and *prevent* the endogenous chemical from acting. This drug is called an **antagonist**. Antagonists often compete with agonists for the receptor binding sites. For example, the drug atropine competes with acetylcholine for specific receptors in the autonomic nervous system. If the dose is high enough, atropine will inhibit the effects of acetylcholine because acetylcholine cannot bind to its receptors.

Not all antagonism is associated with receptors. *Functional* antagonists inhibit the effects of an agonist, not by competing for a receptor, but by changing pharmacokinetic factors. For example, antagonists may slow the absorption of a drug. By speeding up metabolism or excretion, an antagonist can enhance the removal of a drug from the body. The relationships that occur between agonists and antagonists explain many of the drug-drug and drug-food interactions that occur in the body.

5.7 Pharmacology of the Future: Customizing Drug Therapy

Until recently, it was thought that single drugs should provide safe and effective treatment to every client in the same way. Unfortunately, a significant portion of the population either develops unacceptable side effects to certain drugs or is unresponsive to them. Many scientists and clinicians are now discarding the one-size-fits-all approach to drug therapy, which was designed to treat an entire population without addressing important inter-individual variation.

SPECIAL CONSIDERATIONS

Enzyme Deficiency in Certain Ethnic Populations

Pharmacogenetics has identified a number of people who are deficient in the enzyme glucose-6-phosphate dehydrogenase (G6PD). This enzyme is essential in carbohydrate metabolism. Males of Mediterranean and African descent are more likely to express this deficiency. It is estimated to affect 400 million people worldwide. The disorder is caused by mutations in the DNA that encode for G6PD, resulting in one or more amino acid changes in the protein molecule. Following administration of certain drugs, such as primaquine, sulphonamides, and nitrofurantoin, an acute hemolysis of red blood cells occurs due to the breaking of chemical bonds in the hemoglobin molecule. Up to 50% of the circulating red blood cells may be destroyed. Genetic typing does not always predict toxicity; thus, the nurse must observe clients carefully following the administration of these medications. Fortunately, there are good alternative choices for these medications.

With the advent of the Human Genome Project and other advances in medicine, researchers are hopeful that future drugs can be customized for clients with specific genetic similarities. In the past, unpredictable and unexplained drug reactions have been labelled **idiosyncratic responses**. It is hoped that by performing a DNA test before administering a drug, these idiosyncratic side effects can someday be avoided.

Pharmacogenetics is the area of pharmacology that examines the role of heredity in drug response. The greatest advances in pharmacogenetics have been the identification of subtle genetic differences in drug-metabolizing enzymes. Genetic differences in these enzymes are responsible for a significant portion of drug-induced toxicity. It is hoped that the use of pharmacogenetic information may someday allow for customized drug therapy. Although therapies based on a client's genetically based response may not be cost effective at this time, pharmacogenetics may radically change the way pharmacotherapy will be practised in the future.

MediaLink Animation: Agonist

MediaLink National Human Genome Research Institute

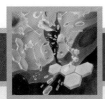

CHAPTER REVIEW

KEY CONCEPTS

The numbered key concepts provide a succinct summary of the important points from the corresponding numbered section within the chapter. If any of these points are not clear, refer to the numbered section within the chapter for review. Expanded versions can be found on the Companion Website.

5.1 Pharmacodynamics is the area of pharmacology concerned with how drugs produce *change* in clients and the differences in client responses to medications.

5.2 The therapeutic index, expressed mathematically as $TD_{50} \div ED_{50}$, is a value representing the margin of safety of a drug. The higher the therapeutic index, the safer the drug.

5.3 The graded dose-response relationship describes how the therapeutic response to a drug changes as the medication dose is increased.

5.4 Potency, the dose of medication required to produce a particular response, and efficacy, the magnitude of maximal response to a drug, are means of comparing medications.

5.5 Drug receptor theory is used to explain the mechanism of action of many medications.

5.6 Agonists, partial agonists, and antagonists are substances that compete with drugs for receptor binding and can cause drug-drug and drug-food interactions.

5.7 In the future, pharmacotherapy will likely be customized to match the genetic makeup of each client.

REVIEW QUESTIONS

1 If the ED_{50} is the dose required to produce an effective response in 50% of a group of clients, what happens in the "other" 50% of the clients after a dose has been administered?

2 Explain why a drug with a high therapeutic index is safer than one with a low therapeutic index.

3 On a dose-response curve, compare two drugs, drug D and drug E. Illustrate drug D as being more potent, but drug E as being more efficacious.

4 Two drugs are competing for a receptor on a mast cell that will cause the release of histamine when activated. Compare the effects of an agonist on this receptor to an antagonist. Which would likely be called an antihistamine, the agonist or the antagonist?

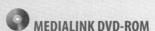
EXPLORE
MediaLink

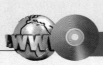 www.pearsoned.ca/adams-king

 MEDIALINK DVD-ROM
- **Audio Glossary**
- **CRNE Review**
- **Animation:** Antagonist

COMPANION WEBSITE
- **CRNE Review**
- **Case Study:** Potency and efficacy

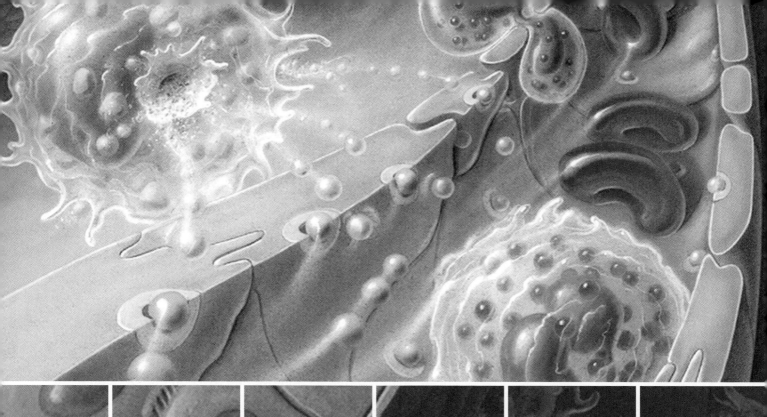

Unit 2 | Pharmacology and the Nurse–Client Relationship

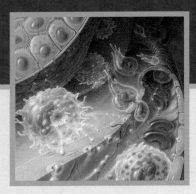

CHAPTER 6

Drug Administration throughout the Lifespan

OBJECTIVES

After reading this chapter, the student should be able to do the following:

1. Discuss the basic concepts of human growth and development in relation to pharmacotherapeutics.
2. Explain how physical, cognitive, and psychomotor development influence pharmacotherapeutics.
3. Match the five pregnancy categories with their definitions.
4. Identify the importance of teaching the breastfeeding mother about prescription and OTC drugs, as well as the use of herbal products.
5. Describe physiological and biochemical changes that occur in the older adult, and how these affect pharmacotherapy.
6. Discuss the nursing and pharmacologic implications associated with each of the following developmental age groups: prenatal, infancy, toddlerhood, preschool, school age, adolescence, young adulthood, middle adulthood, and older adulthood.

MediaLink

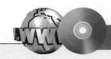

www.pearsoned.ca/adams-king

CRNE review, case studies, and other interactive resources for this chapter can be found on the Companion Website at **www.pearsoned.ca/adams-king**. Click on "Chapter 6" to select the activities for this chapter. For animations, more CRNE review questions, and an audio glossary, access the accompanying MediaLink DVD-ROM in this textbook.

Beginning with conception, and continuing throughout the lifespan, the organs and systems within the body undergo predictable physiological alterations that influence the absorption, metabolism, distribution, and elimination of medications. Nurses must have knowledge of such changes to ensure that drugs are delivered in a safe and effective manner to clients of all ages. The purpose of this chapter is to examine how principles of developmental physiology and lifespan psychology apply to pharmacotherapeutics.

6.1 Pharmacotherapy across the Lifespan

In order to collaborate effectively with the client, healthcare providers must consider the biophysical, psychosocial, ethnocultural, and spiritual characteristics that are unique to the client. To provide holistic and individualized care for the person receiving pharmacotherapy, nurses must understand *normal* growth and developmental patterns that occur throughout the lifespan. Growth characterizes the progressive increase in physical (body) size. Development refers to the functional evolution of the physical, psychomotor, and cognitive capabilities of a living being. It is from this benchmark that *deviations* from the norm can be recognized so that health pattern impairments can be appropriately addressed. The very nature of pharmacology requires that the specifics of age, growth, and development for each client be considered in relation to pharmacokinetics and pharmacodynamics.

PREGNANCY AND LACTATION

The decision to initiate pharmacotherapy during pregnancy and lactation is made in collaboration with the pregnant client with consideration of the risks and benefits for her and her fetus. Most drugs have not been tested in pregnant women and infants. When possible, drug therapy is postponed until after pregnancy and lactation, or safer alternatives are attempted. There are some conditions, however, that are severe enough to require pharmacotherapy in pregnant and lactating clients. These conditions include pre-existing illness, maternal illness unrelated to the pregnancy, and complications related to pregnancy. For example, if the client has epilepsy, hypertension, or a psychiatric disorder prior to the pregnancy, it could be unwise to discontinue therapy during pregnancy or lactation. Conditions such as gestational diabetes and gestational hypertension occur during pregnancy and must be treated for the safety of the growing fetus. In all cases, healthcare practitioners evaluate the therapeutic benefits of a given medication against its potential adverse effects and support the woman who may feel guilty for taking medically necessary drugs during pregnancy.

6.2 Pharmacotherapy during Pregnancy

The placenta is a semipermeable membrane through which some substances are passed to the fetus, and others are blocked. The fetal membranes contain enzymes that detoxify certain substances as they cross the membrane. For example, insulin from the mother is inactivated by placental enzymes during the early stages of pregnancy, preventing it from reaching the fetus. In general, drugs that are water soluble, ionized, or bound to plasma proteins are less likely to cross the placenta.

6.3 Pharmacokinetics during Pregnancy

During pregnancy, major physiological and anatomical changes occur in the endocrine, gastrointestinal (GI), cardiovascular, circulatory, and renal systems. Some of these changes alter the pharmacodynamics of drugs administered to the client and may affect the success of pharmacotherapy, as follows:

- Absorption: Hormonal changes as well as the pressure of the expanding uterus on the blood supply to abdominal organs affect the absorption of drugs. Gastric emptying is delayed, and transit time for food and drugs in the GI tract is slowed by progesterone, which allows a longer time for absorption of oral drugs. Gastric acidity is also decreased, which can affect the absorption of certain drugs. Changes in the respiratory system during pregnancy—increased tidal volume and pulmonary vasodilation—may cause inhaled drugs to be absorbed more quickly.

- Distribution and metabolism: Hemodynamic changes in the pregnant client increase cardiac output and plasma volume and change regional blood flow. The increased blood volume in the woman's body causes dilution of drugs and decreases plasma protein concentrations, affecting drug distribution. Blood flow to the uterus, kidneys, and skin is increased, whereas flow to the skeletal muscles is diminished. Alterations in lipid levels may alter drug transport and distribution, especially during the third trimester. Drug metabolism increases for certain drugs, most notably anticonvulsants such as carbamazepine, phenytoin, and valproic acid, which may require higher doses during pregnancy.

- Excretion: By the third trimester of pregnancy, blood flow through the kidneys increases 40% to 50%. This increase has a direct effect on renal plasma flow, glomerular filtration rate, and renal tubular absorption. Thus, drug excretion rates may be increased, affecting dosage timing and onset of action.

6.4 Gestational Age and Pharmacotherapy

The **prenatal** stage is the time span from conception to birth. This stage is subdivided into the embryonic period (conception to 8 weeks) and the fetal period (8 to 40 weeks or birth). In terms of pharmacotherapy, this is a strategic stage because the health and welfare of both the pregnant client and the baby in utero are taken into consideration (Fig. 6.1). Pharmacologically, the focus must be to eliminate potentially toxic agents that may harm the mother or unborn child. Agents that cause fetal malformations are termed **teratogens**. The baseline incidence of fetal malformations is approximately 3% of all pregnancies. Although causes of fetal malformations are difficult to confirm, Health Canada estimates that chemical and drug exposure, including alcohol and tobacco use, accounts for about 10% to 12% of these malformations.

During the first trimester (conception to 3 months) of pregnancy, when the skeleton and major organs begin to develop, the fetus is at greatest risk for developmental anomalies. If teratogenic drugs are used by the mother, major fetal malformations may occur, or the drug may even precipitate a spontaneous abortion. Unfortunately, acciden-

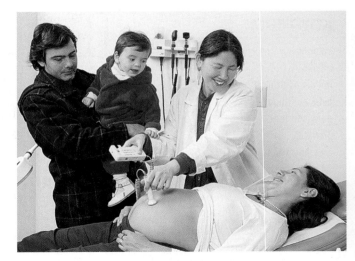

● **Figure 6.1** Pharmacotherapy of the pregnant client
Source: © Jenny Thomas Photography.

tal exposure may occur because the mother may take a medication before she knows she is pregnant. Whenever possible, drug therapy should be delayed until after the first trimester of pregnancy.

During the second trimester (4 to 6 months) of pregnancy, the development of the major organs has progressed considerably; however, exposure to certain substances taken by the mother can still cause considerable harm to the fetus. The nurse-client relationship is vital during this time, especially in terms of teaching. A woman who is pregnant can mistakenly believe that her unborn infant is safe from anything she consumes because the "infant is fully formed and just needs time to grow." During prenatal visits, the nurse must be vigilant in assessing and evaluating each client so that any mistaken beliefs can be clarified.

SPECIAL CONSIDERATIONS

Altered Pharmacokinetics during Pregnancy

- Increased progesterone levels can lead to delayed gastric emptying and decreased small intestinal motility, resulting in delayed or decreased drug *absorption*.

- Increased alveolar ventilation and cardiac output may lead to more rapid *absorption* of intramuscular and inhaled drugs.

- Nausea and vomiting may prevent drug *absorption*.

- Some hepatic enzymes are induced during pregnancy, resulting in increased *metabolism* of some drugs, while other hepatic enzymes are inhibited, resulting in decreased metabolism of other drugs.

- Renal blood flow is markedly increased, resulting in more rapid *excretion* of many drugs.

- Increased maternal blood volume may cause a decrease in serum concentration of the drug, thus decreasing *distribution*.

- Decreased serum albumin and protein levels may decrease plasma protein binding of some drugs, resulting in more free drug and increased drug *distribution*.

Source: Gibson, P. (2003). Baby safe: Which drugs are safe during pregnancy? Canadian Journal of CME, 15, 67–76.

During the third trimester (7 to 9 months) of pregnancy, blood flow to the placenta increases and placental vascular membranes become thinner. Such alterations allow the transfer of more substances from the maternal circulation to the fetal blood. As a result, the fetus will receive larger doses of medications and other substances taken by the mother. Because the fetus lacks mature metabolic enzymes and efficient excretion mechanisms, medications will have a prolonged duration of action in the unborn child.

6.5 Pregnancy Drug Categories

Health Canada uses the drug pregnancy categories developed by the United States Food and Drug Administration (FDA) to rate medications as to their risks during pregnancy. Table 6.1 shows the five pregnancy categories, which guide the healthcare team and the client in selecting drugs that are the least hazardous for the fetus. Nurses who routinely work with women who are pregnant must learn the drug pregnancy categories for medications commonly prescribed for their clients. Examples of category D or X drugs that have been associated with teratogenic effects include testosterone, estrogens, ergotamine, all angiotensin-converting enzyme (ACE) inhibitors, methotrexate, thalidomide, tetracycline, valproic acid, and warfarin. In addition, alcohol, nicotine, and illicit drugs such as cocaine also affect the unborn child.

It is impossible to experimentally test drugs for teratogenicity in human subjects during clinical trials. Although drugs are tested in pregnant laboratory animals, the structure of the human placenta is unique. Pregnancy drug categories are extrapolated from this animal data and may be crude approximations of the actual risk to a human fetus. The actual risk to a human fetus may be much less, or magnitudes greater, than that predicted from animal data. No prescription drug, OTC medication, or herbal product should be taken during pregnancy unless the physician verifies that the therapeutic benefits to the mother clearly outweigh the potential risks to the fetus.

The current A, B, C, D, and X pregnancy labelling system is simplistic and gives no specific clinical information to help guide nurses or their clients as to whether a medication is truly safe. The system does not indicate how the dose should be adjusted during pregnancy or lactation. Most drugs are category C, as very high doses often produce teratogenic effects in animals. The FDA is in the process of updating these categories to provide more descriptive information on the risks and benefits of taking each medication. The new labels are expected to include pharmacokinetic and pharmacodynamic information that will suggest optimum doses for the childbearing client. To gather this information, the FDA is encouraging all pregnant women who are taking medication to join a pregnancy registry that will survey drug effects on both the client and the fetus or newborn. Evaluation of a large number of pregnancies is needed to determine the effects of a medication on the fetus.

6.6 Pharmacotherapy during Lactation

Breastfeeding is highly recommended as a means of providing nutrition, emotional bonding, and immune protection to the neonate. Many drugs, however, are able to enter breast milk in small amounts, and a few have been shown to be harmful. As with the placenta, drugs that are ionized, water soluble, or bound to plasma proteins are less likely to enter breast milk. Central nervous system (CNS) medications are very lipid soluble and thus are more likely to be present in higher concentrations in milk and can be expected to have a greater effect on an infant. Although concentrations of CNS drugs in breast milk are found in higher amounts, they often remain at subclinical levels. Regarding the role of protein binding, drugs that remain in the maternal plasma bound to albumin are not able to penetrate the mother's milk supply. For example, warfarin is strongly bound to plasma proteins and thus has a low level in breast milk.

TABLE 6.1	FDA Pregnancy Categories
Category	**Definition**
A	Adequate, well-controlled studies in pregnant women have not shown an increased risk of fetal abnormalities.
B	Animal studies have revealed no evidence of harm to the fetus; however, there are no adequate, well-controlled studies in pregnant women. or Animal studies have shown an adverse effect, but adequate, well-controlled studies in pregnant women have failed to demonstrate a risk to the fetus.
C	Animal studies have shown an adverse effect and there are no adequate, well-controlled studies in pregnant women. or No animal studies have been conducted and there are no adequate, well-controlled studies in pregnant women.
D	Studies, adequate, well controlled, or observational, in pregnant women have demonstrated a risk to the fetus; however, the benefits of therapy may outweigh the potential risk.
X	Studies, adequate, well controlled, or observational, in animals or pregnant women have demonstrated positive evidence of fetal abnormalities. The use of the product is contraindicated in women who are or may become pregnant.

Source: U.S. Food and Drug Administration, 2001.

It is imperative, however, to teach the mother that many prescription medications, OTC drugs, and herbal products may be excreted in breast milk and have the potential to affect her child (Fig. 6.2). The same guidelines for drug use apply during the breastfeeding period as during pregnancy—drugs should only be taken if the benefits to the mother clearly outweigh the potential risks to the infant. The nurse should explore the possibility of postponing pharmacotherapy until the baby is weaned, or perhaps selecting a safer, non-pharmacological alternative therapy. If a drug is indicated, it is sometimes useful to administer it immediately after breastfeeding, or when the infant will be sleeping for an extended period, so that the longest possible time elapses before the next feeding. This will reduce the amount of active drug in the mother's milk when she does breastfeed her infant. The nurse can assist the mother in protecting the child's safety by teaching her to avoid illicit drugs, alcohol, and tobacco products during breastfeeding. Also, the mother should be advised to consult a healthcare provider before taking any OTC drugs or herbals.

When considering the effects of drugs on the breastfeeding infant, the amount of drug that actually reaches the infant's tissues must be considered. Some medications are destroyed in the infant's GI system, are unable to be absorbed through the wall of the GI tract, or are rapidly metabolized by the liver. Thus, although many drugs are found in breast milk, some are present in such small amounts that they cause no harm.

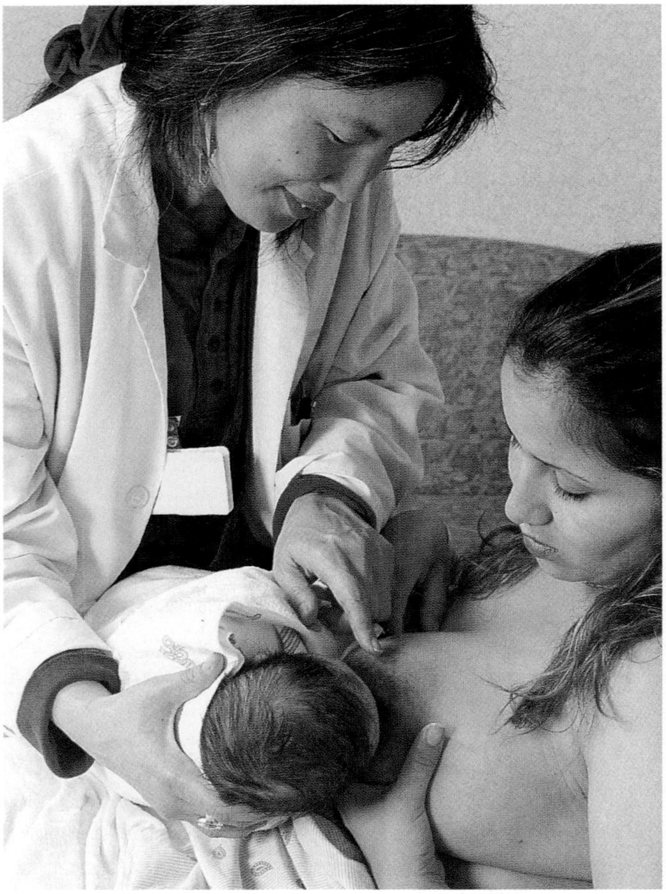

The last key factor in the effect of drugs on the infant relates to the infant's ability to metabolize small amounts of drugs. Premature, neonatal, and ill infants may be at greater risk for adverse effects because they lack drug metabolizing enzymes. Some recommendations regarding medications given during lactation are as follows (Hale, 2004):

- Drugs with a shorter half-life are preferable. They generally peak rapidly and then are eliminated from the maternal plasma, which reduces the amount of drug exposure to the infant. The mother should not breastfeed while the drug is at its peak level.

- Drugs that have long half-lives (or metabolites) should be avoided because they can accumulate in the infant's plasma. Examples include barbiturates, benzodiazepines, meperidine, and fluoxetine.

- Whenever possible, drugs with high protein-binding ability should be selected because they do not transfer as readily to the milk.

- Herbal products and dietary supplements should be avoided, unless specifically prescribed by the healthcare provider, because they may contain chemical ingredients that are harmful to the infant.

Health Canada's Food and Nutrition Branch provides guidance on which drugs should be avoided during breastfeeding to protect the infant's safety. Medications that pass into breast milk are indicated in drug guides. Nurses who work with women who are pregnant or breastfeeding should refer to this information. Table 6.2 shows select drugs that enter the breast milk and have been shown to produce adverse effects.

● **Figure 6.2** Pharmacotherapy of the breastfeeding client
Source: © Jenny Thomas Photography.

PharmFacts

Possible Fetal Effects Caused by Drug Use during Pregnancy

- Marijuana: low birth weight, increased risk of birth defects, increased risk of leukemia, increased behavioural problems, decreased attention span
- Cocaine: increased risk of miscarriage, premature delivery, malformations of fetal limbs and kidneys, later learning difficulties
- Heroin: increased risk of miscarriage, low birth weight, neonatal abstinence syndrome (diarrhea, fever, sneezing, yawning, tremors, seizures, irregular breathing, and irritability)
- Tobacco: increased risk of stillbirths, premature delivery, low birth weight, increased risk of sudden infant death syndrome (SIDS)
- Alcohol: alcohol-related birth defects, ranging from miscarriage and stillbirth to fetal alcohol syndrome (small stature, joint problems, and problems with attention, memory, intelligence, coordination, and problem solving)

Source: Data from Prevention Source, Vancouver, BC.

TABLE 6.2	Select Drugs Associated with Adverse Effects during Breastfeeding
Drug	**Reported Effect or Reason for Concern**
amphetamine	irritability, poor sleeping pattern
cocaine	cocaine intoxication: irritability, vomiting, diarrhea, tremulousness, seizures
heroin	tremors, restlessness, vomiting, poor feeding
phencyclidine	potent hallucinogen
acebutolol	hypotension, bradycardia, tachypnea
atenolol	cyanosis, bradycardia
bromocriptine	suppresses lactation; may be hazardous to the mother
acetylsalicylic acid (ASA)	metabolic acidosis
ergotamine	vomiting, diarrhea, convulsions (doses used in migraine medications)
lithium	one-third to one-half therapeutic blood concentration in infants
phenindione	increased prothrombin and partial thromboplastin time
phenobarbital	sedation, infantile spasms after weaning from milk containing phenobarbital, methemoglobinemia
primidone	sedation, feeding problems
sulfasalazine	bloody diarrhea

Source: American Academy of Pediatrics, Committee on Drugs. (2001). The transfer of drugs and other chemicals into human breast milk. Pediatrics, 108, 776–782. Reprinted by permission.

CHILDHOOD

6.7 Pharmacotherapy of Infants

Infancy is the period from birth to 12 months of age. During this time, nursing care and pharmacotherapy are directed toward safety of the infant, proper dosing of prescribed drugs, and teaching parents how to administer medications properly.

When an infant is ill, it is sometimes traumatic for the parents. By having knowledge of growth and development, the nurse can assist the parents in caring for the infant (Fig. 6.3). The nurse should assess the infant's normal routines at home and attempt to follow these routines as closely as possible while the infant is hospitalized. Parents should be kept informed of specific orders for the infant, such as fluid restrictions. Encourage the parents to participate in the care of the infant as much as they are able. Medications administered at home to infants are often given via droppers into the eyes, ears, nose, or mouth. Infants with well-developed sucking reflexes may be willing to ingest oral drugs with a pleasant taste through a bottle nipple. Infant drops are given by placing the drops in the buccal pouch for the infant to swallow. Oral medications should be administered slowly to avoid aspiration. If rectal suppositories are administered, the buttocks should be held together for 5 to 10 minutes to prevent expulsion of the drug before absorption has occurred.

Special considerations must be observed when administering intramuscular (IM) or intravenous (IV) injections to infants. Unlike adults, infants lack well-developed muscle masses, so the smallest needle appropriate for the drug preferably a 1 cm (3/8-inch) needle should be used. The vastus lateralis is the preferred site for IM injections because it has few nerves and is relatively well developed in infants. The gluteal site is usually contraindicated because of potential damage to the sciatic nerve, which may result in permanent disability. Because of the lack of choices for injection sites, the nurse must take care not to overuse a particular location as inflammation and excessive pain may result. For IV sites, the feet and scalp often provide good venous access. After gaining IV access, it is important that the IV remain secured so the infant does not dislodge it. It is also important to check the IV site frequently and assess for signs of inflammation or infiltration.

Medications for infants are often prescribed in milligrams per kilogram per day (mg/kg/24h) rather than according to the infant's age in weeks or months. An alternate method of calculating doses is to use the infant's body surface area (BSA). Because the liver and kidneys of infants are immature, drugs will have a greater impact due to their prolonged duration of action. For these reasons, it is important to consider age and size in determining safe dosages of medications for infants.

From early infancy, the natural immunity a child receives from the mother in utero slowly begins to decline. The child's developing immune system must then take over. Childhood diseases that were once damaging or fatal can now be controlled through routine immunizations. The nurse plays a key role in educating parents about the importance of keeping their child's immunizations current. Vaccinations are discussed in Chapter 30.

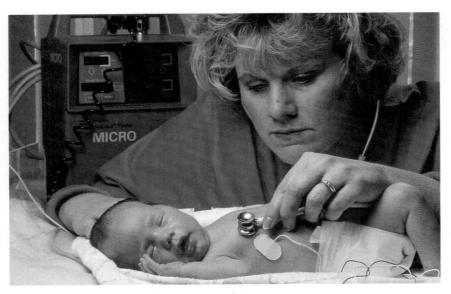

● **Figure 6.3** Pharmacotherapy of the infant
Source: PearsonEducation/PH College.

6.8 **Pharmacotherapy of Toddlers**

Toddlerhood is the age from 1 to 3 years. During this period, a toddler displays a tremendous sense of curiosity. The child begins to explore, wants to try new things, and tends to place everything in the mouth. This becomes a major concern for medication and household product safety. The nurse must be instrumental in teaching parents that poisons come in all shapes, sizes, and forms and include medicines, cosmetics, cleaning supplies, arts and crafts materials, plants, and food products that are improperly stored. Parents should be instructed to request child-resistant containers from the pharmacist and to store all medications in secure cabinets.

Toddlers can swallow liquids and may be able to chew solid medications. When prescription drugs are supplied as flavoured elixirs, it is important to stress that the child not be given access to the medication. Drugs must never be left at the bedside or within easy reach of the child. To a child who has access to a bottle of cherry-flavoured acetaminophen, the tasty liquid may produce a fatal overdose. About half of all poisonings reported to poison control centres occur in children less than 6 years old. Nurses should educate parents about the following means to protect their children from poisoning:

- Read and carefully follow directions on the label before using drugs and household products.
- Store all drugs and harmful agents out of the reach of children and in locked cabinets.
- Keep all household products and drugs in their original containers. Never put chemicals in empty food or drink containers.
- Always ask for medication to be placed in child-resistant containers.
- Never tell children that medicine is candy.

- Keep a bottle of syrup of ipecac in the home to induce vomiting. **Do not give this medication unless instructed to do so by a healthcare provider.**
- Keep the poison control centre number near the phones and call immediately on suspicion of a poisoning.
- Never leave medication unattended in a child's room or in areas where the child plays.

Administration of medications to toddlers can be challenging for the nurse. At this stage, the child is rapidly developing increased motor ability and learning to assert independence but has extremely limited ability to reason or understand the relationship of medicines to health. Giving long, detailed explanations to the toddler will prolong the procedure and create additional anxiety. Short, concrete explanations followed by immediate drug administration are best for this age group. Physical comfort in the form of touching, hugging, or verbal praise following drug administration is important.

Oral medications that taste bad should be mixed with a vehicle such as jam, syrup, or fruit puree, if possible. The medication may be followed with a carbonated beverage or mint-flavoured candy. Nurses should teach parents to avoid placing medicine in milk, orange juice, or cereals because the child may associate these healthy foods with bad-tasting medications. Pharmaceutical companies often formulate pediatric medicines in sweet syrups to increase the ease of drug administration.

IM injections for toddlers may be given into the vastus lateralis muscle. IV injections may use scalp or feet veins; additional peripheral site options become available in late toddlerhood. Suppositories may be difficult to administer due to the resistance of the child. For any of these invasive administration procedures, having a parent in close proximity will usually reduce the toddler's anxiety and increase cooperation. Ask the parent prior to the procedure if he or she would like to assist. The nurse should take at least one helper into the room for assistance in restraining the toddler, if necessary.

6.9 Pharmacotherapy of Preschoolers and School-Aged Children

The **preschool child** ranges in age from 3 to 5 years. During this period, the child begins to refine gross and fine motor skills and develop language abilities. The child initiates new activities and becomes more socially involved with other children.

Preschoolers can sometimes comprehend the difference between health and illness and that medications are administered to help them feel better. Nonetheless, medications and other potentially dangerous products must still be safely stowed out of the child's reach.

In general, principles of medication administration that pertain to the toddler also apply to this age group. Preschoolers cooperate in taking oral medications if they are crushed or mixed with food or flavoured beverages. After a child has been walking for about a year, the ventrogluteal site may be used for IM injections as it causes less pain than the vastus lateralis site. The scalp veins can no longer be used for IV access; peripheral veins are used for IV injections.

Like the toddler, preschoolers often physically resist medication administration and a long, detailed explanation of the procedure will promote additional anxiety. A brief explanation followed quickly by medication administration is usually the best method. Uncooperative children may need to be restrained, and clients over 4 years of age may require two adults to administer the medication. Before and after medication procedures, the child may benefit from opportunities to play-act troubling experiences with dolls. When the child plays the role of doctor or nurse by giving a "sick" doll a pill or injection, comforting the doll, and explaining that the doll will now feel better, the little actor feels safer and more in control of the situation.

SPECIAL CONSIDERATIONS

Pediatric Drug Research and Labelling

An estimated 75% of the medications prescribed for children contain no specific dosing information for pediatric clients. Without specific labelling information, healthcare providers have largely based their doses on the smaller weight of the child. Children, however, are not merely small adults; they have unique differences in physiology and biochemistry that may place them at risk to effects of drug therapy.

Inclusion of children in clinical trials is an expensive and potentially risky process. Large numbers of children in different age groups are needed for adequate drug testing. Manufacturers also face liability and malpractice issues associated with testing new medications in children. The US FDA provided financial incentives for pharmaceutical manufacturers to test drugs in children. As a result, over 28 drugs have been investigated in children, and 18 drug labels have been changed to incorporate the results of the research findings. Drugs that now have more specific pediatric labelling include ibuprofen, ranitidine, fluvoxamine, and midazolam.

The **school-aged child** is between 6 and 12 years of age. Some refer to this period as the middle childhood years. This is the time in a child's life when there is progression away from the family-centred environment to the larger peer relationship environment. Rapid physical, mental, and social development occur and early ethical-moral development begins to take shape. Thinking processes become progressively logical and more consistent.

During this time, most children remain relatively healthy, with immune system development well under way. Respiratory infections and gastrointestinal upsets are the most common complaints. Because the child feels well most of the time, there is little concept of illness or the risks involved with ingesting a harmful substance offered to the child by a peer or older person.

The nurse is usually able to gain considerable cooperation from school-aged children. Longer, more detailed explanations may be of value because the child has developed some reasoning ability and can understand the relationship between the medicine and feeling better. When children are old enough to welcome choices, they can be offered limited dosing alternatives to provide a sense of control and encourage cooperation. The option of taking one medication before another or the chance to choose which drink will follow a chewable tablet helps to distract children from the issue of whether they will take the medication at all. It also makes an otherwise strange or unpleasant experience a little more enjoyable. Making children feel that they are willing participants in medication administration, rather than victims, is an important foundation for compliance. Praise for cooperation is appropriate for any pediatric client and will set the stage for successful medication administration in the future.

School-aged children can take chewable tablets and may be able to swallow tablets or capsules. Many still resist injections; however, an experienced pediatric nurse can usually administer parenteral medications quickly and compassionately, without the need for restraining the child. The ventrogluteal site is preferred for IM injections, although the muscles of older children are developed enough for the nurse to use other sites.

6.10 Pharmacotherapy of Adolescents

Adolescence is the time between ages 13 and 18 years. A person in this age group is able to think in abstract terms and come to logical conclusions based on a given set of observations. Rapid physical growth and psychological maturation have a great impact on personality development. The adolescent relates strongly to peers, wanting and needing their support, approval, and presence. Physical appearance and conformity with peers in terms of behaviour, dress, and social interactions is important.

The most common needs for pharmacotherapy in this age group are skin problems, headaches, menstrual symptoms, and sports-related injuries. There is an increased need for contraceptive information and counselling about sexually related health problems. Since bulimia occurs in this population, the nurse should carefully question adolescents about their eating habits and their use of OTC appetite suppressants or laxatives. Tobacco use and illicit drug experimentation may be prevalent in this population. Teenage athletes may use amphetamines to delay the onset of fatigue, as well as anabolic steroids to increase muscle strength and endurance. The nurse assumes a key role in educating adolescent clients about the hazards of tobacco use and illicit drugs.

The adolescent has a need for privacy and control in drug administration. The nurse should seek complete cooperation and communicate with the teen more in the manner of an adult than a child. Teens usually appreciate thorough explanations of their treatment, and ample time should be allowed for them to ask questions. Adolescents are often reluctant to admit their lack of knowledge, so the nurse should carefully explain important information regarding their medications and expected side effects, even if the client claims to understand. Teens are easily embarrassed, and the nurse should be sensitive to their need for self-expression, privacy, and individuality, particularly when parents, siblings, or friends are present.

ADULTHOOD

When considering adult health, it is customary to divide this period of life into three stages: **young adulthood** (18 to 40 years), **middle adulthood** (40 to 65 years), and **older adulthood** (over 65 years). Within each of these divisions are similar biophysical, psychosocial, and spiritual characteristics that impact nursing and pharmacotherapy.

6.11 Pharmacotherapy of Young and Middle-Aged Adults

The health status of younger adults is generally good; absorption, metabolic, and excretion mechanisms are at their peak. There is minimal need for prescription drugs unless chronic diseases such as diabetes or immune-related conditions exist. The use of vitamins, minerals, and herbal remedies is prevalent in young adulthood. Prescription drugs are usually related to contraception or agents needed during pregnancy and delivery. Medication compliance is positive within this age range as there is clear comprehension of benefit in terms of longevity and feeling well.

Substance abuse is a cause for concern in the 18 to 24 age group, with alcohol, tobacco products, amphetamines, and illicit drugs (marijuana and cocaine) being a problem. For young adults who are sexually active with multiple partners, prescription medications for the treatment of herpes, gonorrhea, syphilis, and HIV infection may be necessary.

The physical status for the middle-aged adult is on par with the young adult until about 45 years of age. During this period of life, numerous transitions occur that often result in excessive stress. Middle-aged adults are sometimes

---

SPECIAL CONSIDERATIONS

Gender-Related Differences in Pharmacokinetics

- Oral contraceptives and sex hormone replacement therapies for women can affect hepatic *metabolism* and other metabolism of drugs.
- The *metabolism* of alcohol is slower in women.
- Renal function is greater in men, resulting in more efficient drug *excretion*.
- Hormonal fluctuations in women across the menstrual cycle and the lifespan may potentially affect all phases of pharmacokinetics; research is needed to assess the effects.
- Body size and surface area, which are usually greater in men, can affect drug *distribution*.
- Adipose tissue, which is usually greater in women, can affect drug storage.

---

referred to as the "sandwich generation" because they are often caring for aging parents as well as children and grandchildren. Because of the pressures of work and family, they often take medication to control health alterations that could best be treated with positive lifestyle modifications. The nurse must emphasize the importance of lifestyle choices to overall health, such as limiting lipid intake, maintaining optimum weight, and exercising.

Health impairments related to cardiovascular disease, hypertension, obesity, arthritis, cancer, and anxiety begin to surface in middle age. Gender-related differences in pharmacokinetics and disease comorbidity may influence pharmacotherapeutics. The use of drugs to treat hypertension, hyperlipidemia, digestive disorders, erectile dysfunction, and arthritis is becoming more common. Respiratory disorders related to lifelong tobacco use or exposure to second-hand smoke and environmental toxins may develop that require drug therapies. Adult onset diabetes mellitus often emerges during this time of life. The use of antidepressants and antianxiety agents is prominent in the over-50 population.

6.12 Pharmacotherapy of Older Adults

During the 20th century, an improved quality of life and the ability to effectively treat many diseases contributed to increased longevity. The risk of chronic health disorders is greater in older adults, and they are more likely to be prescribed drugs to treat them. The taking of multiple drugs concurrently, known as **polypharmacy**, has become commonplace among many older adults. Polypharmacy dramatically increases the risk of drug interactions and side effects.

Although predictable physiological and psychosocial changes occur with aging, significant variability exists among clients. Cognitive decline and memory loss may occur in older adults. However, many older adults are healthy and live independently. The nurse should avoid preconceived notions that elderly clients will have physical or cognitive impairment simply because they have reached a certain age. Careful assessment is always necessary (Fig. 6.4).

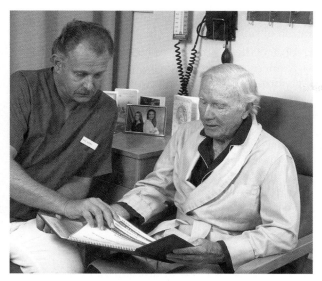

● **Figure 6.4** Pharmacotherapy of the older adult
Source: PearsonEducation/PH College.

When administering medications to older adults, offer the client the same degree of independence and dignity that would be afforded middle-aged adults, unless otherwise indicated. Like their younger counterparts, older clients have a need to understand why they are receiving a drug and what outcomes are expected. Accommodations must be made for older adults who have certain impairments. Visual and auditory changes make it important for the nurse to provide drug instructions in large type and to obtain client feedback to be certain that medication instructions have been understood. Elderly clients with cognitive decline and memory loss can benefit from aids such as alarmed pill containers, medicine management boxes, and clearly written instructions. During assessment, the nurse should determine if the client is capable of self-administering medications or whether the assistance of a caregiver will be required. As long as small children are not present in the household, older clients with arthritis should be encouraged to ask the pharmacist for medication bottles with caps specially designed for ease of opening.

Older clients experience more adverse effects from drug therapy than any other age group. Although some of these effects are due to polypharmacy, many of the adverse events are predictable, based on normal physiological and biochemical processes that may occur during aging. The principal complications of drug therapy in the older adult population are degeneration of organ systems, multiple and severe illnesses, multiple drug therapy, and unreliable compliance. By understanding these changes, the nurse can avoid many adverse drug effects in older clients. In older clients, the functioning of all major organ systems slowly declines. For this reason, all phases of pharmacokinetics are affected, and appropriate adjustments in therapy need to be implemented. Although most of the pharmacokinetic changes are due to reduced hepatic and renal drug elimination, other systems may also show a variety of changes. For

Special Considerations

Altered Pharmacokinetics during Older Adulthood

- Increased gastric pH, delayed gastric emptying, and decreased peristaltic rate may affect medication *absorption*. Often, when laxatives are used to compensate for slower peristalsis, medications may be rapidly *excreted* from the body before they can provide their full therapeutic benefit.
- The liver's production of enzymes decreases, thus decreasing hepatic drug metabolism and resulting in increased serum drug concentration; more drug is available for *distribution* and the effects of some drugs are prolonged.
- The aging liver produces less albumin, resulting in decreased plasma protein binding and increased levels of free drug in the bloodstream; *distribution*, drug effects, and the potential for drug-drug interactions are increased.
- The ratio of body fat to water increases, affecting *distribution* and storage of fat-soluble drugs and vitamins. The ratio of fat to muscle increases, slowing *metabolism*.
- The aging cardiovascular system causes decreased cardiac output and less efficient blood circulation, which slow drug *distribution*. This makes it important to initiate pharmacotherapy with smaller dosages and slowly increase the amount to a safe, effective level.
- The percentage of body water decreases, contributing to dehydration and changes in drug concentration and *distribution*. The risk of drug toxicity is increased by fluid deficit.
- Blood flow to the kidney decreases, resulting in a decrease in the amount of drug being delivered to the kidney for *excretion*.

example, immune system function diminishes with aging, so autoimmune diseases and infections occur more frequently in elderly clients. Thus, there is an increased need for influenza and pneumonia vaccinations. Normal physiological changes that affect pharmacotherapy of the older adult are summarized as follows:

- Absorption: In general, absorption of drugs is slower in the older adult owing to diminished gastric motility and decreased blood flow to digestive organs. Increased gastric pH can delay absorption of medications that require high acidity to dissolve.

- Distribution: Increased body fat in the older adult provides a larger storage compartment for lipid-soluble drugs and vitamins. Plasma levels are reduced, and the therapeutic response is diminished. Older adults have less body water, making the effects of dehydration more dramatic and increasing the risk for drug toxicity. For example, elderly clients who have reduced body fluid experience more orthostatic hypotension. The decline in lean body mass and total body water leads to an increased concentration of water-soluble drugs because the drug is distributed in a smaller volume of water. The aging liver produces less albumin, resulting in decreased plasma protein binding ability and increased levels of free drug in the bloodstream, thereby increasing the potential for drug-drug interactions. The aging cardiovascular system has decreased cardiac output and less efficient blood circulation, which slow drug distribution. This makes it important to initiate pharmacotherapy

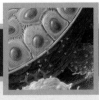

with smaller dosages and slowly increase the amount to a safe, effective level.

- Metabolism: The liver's production of enzymes decreases, liver mass decreases, and the visceral blood flow is diminished, resulting in reduced hepatic drug metabolism. This change leads to an increase in the half-life of many drugs, which prolongs and intensifies the drug response. The decline in hepatic function reduces first-pass metabolism. (Recall that first-pass metabolism relates to the amount of a drug that is metabolized during the first circulation through the liver after the drug has been absorbed by the intestinal tract.) Thus, plasma levels are elevated, and tissue concentrations are increased for the particular drug. This change alters the standard dosage, the interval between doses, and the duration of side effects.

- Excretion: Older adults have reductions in renal blood flow, glomerular filtration rate, active tubular secretion, and nephron function. This decreases excretion for drugs that are eliminated by the kidneys. When excretion is reduced, serum drug levels and the potential for toxicity markedly increase. Administration schedules and dosage amounts may need to be altered in many older adults owing to these changes in kidney function. Keep in mind that the most common etiology of adverse drug reactions in older adults is caused by the accumulation of toxic amounts of drugs secondary to impaired renal excretion.

CHAPTER REVIEW

KEY CONCEPTS

The numbered key concepts provide a succinct summary of the important points from the corresponding numbered section within the chapter. If any of these points are not clear, refer to the numbered section within the chapter for review. Expanded versions can be found on the Companion Website.

6.1 To contribute to safe and effective pharmacotherapy, it is essential for the nurse to comprehend and apply fundamental concepts of growth and development.

6.2 Pharmacotherapy during pregnancy should only be conducted when the benefits to the mother outweigh the potential risks to the unborn child.

6.3 During pregnancy, major physiological and anatomical changes occur that can alter the pharmacodynamics of administered drugs.

6.4 Gestational age must be considered when prescribing drugs to pregnant clients.

6.5 Pregnancy categories guide the healthcare provider in prescribing drugs for these clients.

6.6 Breastfeeding clients must be aware that drugs and other substances can appear in milk and affect the infant.

6.7 During infancy, pharmacotherapy is directed toward the safety of the child and teaching the parents how to properly administer medications and care for the infant.

6.8 Drug administration to toddlers can be challenging; short, concrete explanations followed by immediate drug administration are usually best for the toddler.

6.9 Preschool and younger school-aged children can begin to assist with medication administration.

6.10 Pharmacological compliance in the adolescent is dependent on an understanding and respect for the uniqueness of the person in this stage of growth and development.

6.11 Young adults comprise the healthiest age group and generally need few prescription medications. Middle-aged adults begin to suffer from lifestyle-related illnesses such as hypertension.

6.12 Older adults take more medications and experience more adverse drug events than any other age group. For drug therapy to be successful, the nurse must make accommodations for age-related changes in physiologic and biochemical functions.

REVIEW QUESTIONS

1 How is drug safety for the three trimesters of pregnancy determined?

2 What factors should be considered before administering medications to an infant, a toddler, a school-aged child, and an adolescent?

3 What physiological changes make it important to consider advanced age when prescribing or administering medication?

4 A client who is on several medications for psychiatric disorders has just delivered her infant and is about to begin breastfeeding. What information should she receive before she is discharged from the ward?

CRITICAL THINKING QUESTIONS

1. A 22-year-old pregnant client is diagnosed with pyelonephritis and an antibiotic is prescribed. What information does the nurse need to have to safely administer the drug?

2. An 86-year-old male client is confused and anxious. His daughter wonders if "a small dose" of diazepam (Valium) might help her father to be less anxious. Prior to responding to the daughter or consulting the prescribing authority, the nurse should consider age-related factors affecting pharmacotherapeutics. What are these? Discuss these with reference to the pharmacokinetics and effects of diazepam.

3. An 8-month-old child is prescribed acetaminophen (Tylenol) elixir for management of fever. The child is recovering from gastroenteritis and is still having several loose stools per day. She spits some of the elixir on her shirt. Should the nurse repeat the dose? What are the implications of this child's age and physical condition for oral drug administration?

EXPLORE
MediaLink

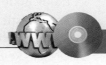 **www.pearsoned.ca/adams-king**

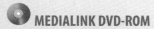 **MEDIALINK DVD-ROM**
- **Audio Glossary**
- **CRNE Review**

 COMPANION WEBSITE
- **CRNE Review**
- **Case Study:** Pharmacotherapy of toddlers

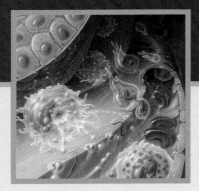

CHAPTER 7

The Nursing Process in Pharmacology

OBJECTIVES

After reading this chapter, the student should be able to do the following:

1. Explain the steps of the nursing process in relation to pharmacotherapeutics.
2. Identify assessment data to be gathered that is pertinent to medication administration.
3. Develop appropriate nursing diagnoses for clients receiving medications.
4. Set realistic goals and outcomes during the planning stage for clients receiving medications.
5. Discuss key intervention strategies to be carried out for clients receiving medications.
6. Evaluate the outcomes of medication administration.
7. Apply the nursing process when giving medications, using the Nursing Process Focus flowcharts found in Chapters 13 through 48.

MediaLink

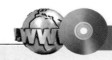 www.pearsoned.ca/adams-king

CRNE review, case studies, and other interactive resources for this chapter can be found on the Companion Website at **www.pearsoned.ca/adams-king**. Click on "Chapter 7" to select the activities for this chapter. For animations, more CRNE review questions, and an audio glossary, access the accompanying MediaLink DVD-ROM in this textbook.

The nursing process, a systematic method of problem solving, forms the foundation of all nursing practice. The use of the nursing process is particularly essential during medication administration. By using the steps of the nursing process, nurses can ensure that the interdisciplinary practice of pharmacology results in safe, effective, and individualized medication administration and outcomes for all clients under their care.

7.1 Review of the Nursing Process

Most nursing students enter a pharmacology course after taking a course on the fundamentals of nursing, during which the steps of the **nursing process** are discussed in detail. This section presents a brief review of those steps before discussing in detail how they can be applied to pharmacology. Students who are unfamiliar with the nursing process are encouraged to consult one of the many excellent fundamentals of nursing textbooks for a more detailed explanation.

Assessing, the first step in the nursing process, is an ongoing process that begins with the nurse's initial contact with the client and continues with every interaction thereafter. During the initial assessment, **baseline data** are gathered which will be used to compare to information obtained during later interactions. Assessing consists of gathering **subjective data**, which include what the client says or perceives, and **objective data**, which are gathered through physical assessment, laboratory tests, and other diagnostic sources.

Identifying patterns, or **diagnosing**, is the second step in the nursing process. This step begins once the initial assessment data are gathered. The nurse interprets, analyzes, and synthesizes data in order to identify patterns of problems, health and safety risks, related needs, and strengths. If gaps in the data are observed, the nurse collects the missing data. The judgments made by nurses in this step are commonly referred to as **nursing diagnoses** to differentiate them from medical diagnoses. Identifying patterns, or diagnosing, provides the basis for establishing goals and outcomes, planning interventions to meet those goals and outcomes, and evaluating the effectiveness of the care given.

Diagnosing is often the most challenging part of the nursing process. Sometimes the nurse identifies what is believed to be the client's problem, only to discover from further assessment that the planned goals, outcomes, and interventions have not "solved" the problem. Diagnosing is an ongoing reasoning process and focuses on the client's problems and needs. A nursing role in primary healthcare is to enable clients to become active participants in their own care. By verifying identified problems and their associated needs collaboratively with the client, the nurse encourages the client to take a more active role in resolving these problems.

Identifying patterns in health problems and needs is integral to the nursing process. Use of the term *diagnosing* to describe this activity is common to most nursing practice models. In this book, the terms *diagnosing* and *nursing diagnoses* are used generally and do not refer specifically to the structured list of nursing diagnoses approved by the North American Nursing Diagnosis Association (NANDA).

In **planning**, the third step of the nursing process, the nurse plans ways to assist the client to resolve problems and return to an optimum level of wellness. Short- or long-term **goals** are established that focus on what the client will be able to do or achieve, not what the nurse will do. **Outcomes** are the objective measures of those goals. They specifically define what the client will do, under what circumstances, and within what time frame. Goals and outcomes are also verified with the client or caregiver and are prioritized to address immediate needs first.

Planning links strategies, or interventions, to the established goals and outcomes. It is the formal written process that communicates with all members of the healthcare team what the nurse will do to assist the client in meeting those goals.

Each healthcare organization decides how this plan of care will be communicated, and it may be nurse-centred or interdisciplinary.

Implementing, the fourth step in the nursing process, occurs when the nurse caries out the planned nursing interventions. Interventions are designed to meet the client's needs and ensure safe, effective care. As the nurse provides care, reassessment is ongoing and new data are compared to the earlier data. The nurse compares the data to established nursing diagnoses, goals, and outcomes and begins the process of **evaluating**, the fifth step in the nursing process. Established needs are reviewed while taking into consideration the client's response to care. More assessment data are gathered as needed, and goals and outcomes are considered as to whether they were met, partially met, or not met at all. The process comes full circle as new or modified needs are identified and diagnosed, goals and outcomes redefined, and new interventions planned.

Nursing has not always relied on such an organized approach to nursing care but has always been concerned with delivering safe and effective care. The administration of medications requires the use of the nursing process to ensure the best possible outcomes for the client. These steps will now be applied specifically to drug administration.

7.2 Assessing the Client in Relation to Drug Administration

A health history and physical assessment are usually completed during the initial meeting between a nurse and client. Many pieces of data are gathered during this initial assessment, which have specific implications for the process of drug administration. Ongoing assessments after this time will provide additional data to help the nurse evaluate the outcomes of medication use. This section discusses pertinent assessment components and how they relate to drug administration.

The initial health history is tailored to the client's clinical condition. A complete history is the most detailed, but the appropriateness of this history must be considered given the client's condition. Often a problem-focused or "chief complaint" history is taken, focusing on the symptoms that led the client to seek care. In any history, key components must be assessed that may affect the successful outcome of drug administration. Essential questions to ask in the initial history relate to allergies; past medical history; medications used currently and in the recent past; responses to medications taken in the past; patterns of compliance with medications; personal and social history such as the use of alcohol, tobacco, or caffeine; health risks such as the use of street drugs or illicit substances; and reproductive health questions such as the pregnancy status of women of childbearing age. Table 7.1 provides pertinent questions that may be asked during an initial health history to provide baseline data before the administration of medications. The health history is tailored to the client's condition, so all questions may not be appropriate during the initial assessment. Keep in mind that what is *not* being said may be as important, or more,

than what *is* said. For instance, a client may deny or downplay any symptoms of pain while grimacing or guarding a certain area from being touched. Nurses must use their keen skills of observation during the history to gather such critical data.

Along with the health history, a physical assessment is completed to gather objective data on the client's condition. Vital signs, height and weight, a head-to-toe physical assessment, and lab specimens may be obtained. These values provide the baseline data to compare with future assessments and guide the healthcare provider in deciding which medications to prescribe. Many medications can affect the heart rate and blood pressure and these vitals signs should be noted. Baseline electrolyte values are important parameters to obtain because many medications affect electrolyte balance. Renal and hepatic function tests are essential for many clients, particularly older adults and those who are critically ill, as these will be used to determine the proper drug dosage.

In addition to assessing the client, the nurse must assess the prescribed medication. Is the order complete? Is the order current or has it expired? Are the drug, dose, route, and time of administration specified and appropriate for this client, considering factors such as the client's age, gender, weight, ethnicity, and medical diagnoses? Are there any contraindications to using this drug for this client? Does the drug require special assessments or client teaching?

Once pharmacotherapy is initiated, ongoing assessments are conducted to determine the effects of the medications. Assessment should first focus on determining whether the client is experiencing the expected therapeutic benefits from the medications. For example, if a drug is given for symptoms of pain, is the pain subsiding? If an antibiotic is given for an infection, are the signs of that infection—elevated temperature, redness or swelling, drainage from infected sites, etc.—improving over time? If a client is not experiencing the therapeutic effects of the medication, then further assessment must be done to determine the reason. Dosages and the scheduling of medications are reviewed, and serum drug levels may be obtained.

Assessment during pharmacotherapy also focuses on any side or adverse effects the client may be experiencing. Often these effects are manifested in dermatological, cardiovascular, gastrointestinal, or neurological symptoms. Here again, baseline data are compared with the current assessment to determine what changes have occurred since the initiation of pharmacotherapy. The Nursing Process Focus flowcharts provided in Chapters 13 through 48 illustrate key assessment data to be gathered associated with specific medications or classes of drugs.

Finally, an assessment of the ability of the client to assume responsibility for his or her own drug administration is necessary. Will the client require assistance obtaining or affording the prescribed medications, or with taking them safely? What kind of medication storage facilities exist and are they adequate to protect the client, others in the home, and the efficacy of the medication? Does the client understand the uses and effects of this medication and how it is

TABLE 7.1	Health History Assessment Questions Pertinent to Drug Administration
Health History Component	**Pertinent Questions**
chief complaint	• How do you feel? (Describe.) • Are you having any pain? (Describe.) • Are you experiencing other symptoms? (Especially pertinent to medications are nausea, vomiting, headache, itching, dizziness, shortness of breath, nervousness or anxiousness, palpitations or heart "fluttering," weakness, or fatigue.)
allergies	• Are you allergic to any medications? • Are you allergic to any foods, environmental substances (e.g., pollen or "seasonal" allergies), tape, soaps, or cleansers? • What specifically happens when you experience an allergy?
past medical history	• Do you have a history of diabetes, heart or vascular conditions, respiratory conditions, neurological conditions? • Do you have any dermatological conditions? • How have these been treated in the past? Currently?
family history	• Has anyone in your family experienced difficulties with any medications? (Describe.) • Does anyone in your family have any significant medical problems?
drug history	• What prescription medications are you currently taking? (List drug name, dosage, frequency of administration.) • What non-prescription/OTC medications are you taking? (List drug name, dosage, frequency.) • What drugs, prescription or OTC, have you taken within the past month or two? • Have you ever experienced any side effects or unusual symptoms with any medications? (Describe.) • What do you know, or have been taught, about these medications? • Do you use any herbal or homeopathic remedies? Any nutritional substances or vitamins?
health management	• When was the last time you saw a healthcare provider? • What is your normal diet? • Do you have any trouble sleeping?
reproductive history	• Is there any possibility you are pregnant? (Ask *every* woman of childbearing age.) • Are you breastfeeding?
personal-social history	• Do you smoke? • What is your normal alcohol intake? • What is your normal caffeine intake? • Do you have any religious or cultural beliefs or practices concerning medications or your health that we should know about? • What is your occupation? What hours do you work? • Do you have any concerns regarding insurance or the ability to afford medications?
health risk history	• Do you have any history of depression or other mental illness? • Do you use any street drugs or illicit substances?

properly taken? Would assessment data suggest that the use of this medication might present a problem, such as difficulty swallowing large capsules or an inability to administer medication when home anticoagulant therapy has been ordered parenterally?

7.3 Diagnosing for the Client Receiving Medications

Assessment data are analyzed in order to identify patterns of problems, health and safety risks, related needs, and strengths. This process is referred to as diagnosing. The identified patterns are summarized in a list of nursing diagnoses. The nursing diagnoses are verified and prioritized in collaboration with the client. They are then used to set goals and plan care. This section discusses common

nursing diagnoses related to medication administration, and the development of appropriate nursing diagnosis statements.

Diagnosing that focuses on drug administration is the same as for other client condition-specific responses. Nursing diagnoses may address actual problems, such as the treatment of pain; focus on potential problems, such as a risk for fluid volume imbalance; or concentrate on maintaining the client's current level of wellness. There are many problems and needs common to clients receiving medications. The nurse can manage some problems independently, whereas other problems are multidisciplinary and require collaboration with other members of the healthcare team. For any of the medications given to a client, there are often combinations of nursing-independent and collaborative diagnoses that can be established.

Two of the most common nursing diagnoses in medication administration are inadequate knowledge and non-adherence. Inadequate knowledge may be that the client has been given a new prescription and has no previous experience with the medication. It may also be applicable when a client has not received adequate education about the drugs used in the treatment of his or her condition. When obtaining a medication history, the nurse should assess the client's knowledge regarding the drugs currently being taken and evaluate whether the drug education has been adequate. Sometimes a client refuses to take a drug that has been prescribed or refuses to follow the directions correctly. Non-adherence assumes that the client has been properly educated about the medication and has made an informed decision not to take it. Because labelling a client's response as non-compliant may have a negative impact on the nurse-client relationship, it is vital that the nurse assess all possible factors leading to the non-adherence *before* establishing this diagnosis. Does the client understand why the medication has been prescribed? Has dosing and scheduling information been explained? Are side effects causing the client to refuse the medication? Do social issues or cultural, religious, or health beliefs have an impact on taking the medication? Is the non-adherence related to inadequate resources, either financial or social? A thorough assessment of possible causes should be conducted before labelling the client's response as non-compliant.

Nursing diagnoses applicable to drug administration are often collaborative problems that require communication with other healthcare providers. For example, fluid volume deficit related to diuretic drugs may require additional interventions such as medical orders by the physician to ensure that electrolytes and intravascular fluid volume remain within normal limits. Nurses may, independent of medical orders, assist the client with ambulation if weakness or postural hypotension occurs as a result of this fluid volume deficit.

7.4 Setting Goals and Outcomes for Drug Administration

After the nurse has gathered client assessment data, identified patterns and needs, and established priorities, the goals and outcomes are developed to assist the nurse in planning care, carrying out interventions, and evaluating the effectiveness of that care. Before administering and monitoring the effects of medications, nurses should establish clear goals and outcomes so that planned interventions ensure safe and effective use of these agents.

Goals are somewhat different than outcomes. Goals focus on what the client should be able to achieve and do, based on the nursing diagnosis established from the assessment data. Outcomes provide the specific, measurable criteria that will be used to evaluate the degree to which the goal was met. For example, a goal may be that the client will learn to self-inject insulin. One outcome related to this goal may be that the client will demonstrate the correct technique for withdrawing insulin from a vial into a syringe without prompting. Both goals and outcomes are focused on what the client will achieve or do, are realistic, and are verified with the client or caregiver. Priorities are established based on the assessment data and nursing diagnoses, with high-priority needs addressed before low-priority items. Safe and effective administration of medications, with the best therapeutic outcome possible, is the overall goal of any nursing plan of care.

Goals may be focused on the short term or long term, depending on the setting and situation. In the acute care or ambulatory setting, short-term goals may be most appropriate, whereas in the rehabilitation setting, long-term goals may be more commonly identified. For a client with a thrombus in the lower extremity who has been placed on anticoagulant therapy, a short-term goal may be that the client will not experience an increase in clot size as evidenced by improving circulation to the lower extremity distal to the clot. A long-term goal might focus on teaching the client to effectively administer parenteral anticoagulant therapy at home. Like assessment data, goals should focus first on the therapeutic outcomes of medications, then on the limitation or treatment of side effects. For the client on pain medication, relief of pain is a priority established before treating the nausea, vomiting, or dizziness caused by the medication. The Nursing Process Focus flowcharts provided in Chapters 13 through 48 outline some of the common goals that might be developed with the client.

Outcomes are the specific criteria used to measure attainment of the selected goals. They are written to include the subject (the client in most cases), the actions required by that subject, under what circumstances the actions are to be

SPECIAL CONSIDERATIONS

Clients with Speaking, Visual, or Hearing Impairments

Speaking impairments may make obtaining responses from the client difficult. Communication may be facilitated by having the client write, demonstrate, or draw responses. Clarify by paraphrasing the response back to the client. Use gestures, body language, and yes/no questions if writing or drawing is difficult. Allow adequate time for responses. Be especially aware of nonverbal clues, such as grimacing, when performing interventions that may cause discomfort or pain.

Provide adequate lighting for clients with visual impairments and be aware of the phrasing of verbal communication and how phrasing affects the message conveyed. Remember that the nonverbal cues involved in communication may be missed by the client. Paraphrase responses back to the client to be sure he or she understood the message in the absence of nonverbal cues. Explain interventions in detail before implementing procedures or activities with the client.

Clients with hearing impairments benefit from communication that is spoken clearly and slowly in a low-pitched voice. Sit near the client and avoid speaking loudly or shouting, especially if hearing devices are used. Limit the amount of background noise when possible. Write or draw to clarify verbal communication and use nonverbal gestures and body language to aid communication. Allow adequate time for communication and responses. Alert other members of the healthcare team that the client has a hearing impairment and may not hear a verbal answer to the nurse's call light given over an intercom system.

carried out, the expected performance, and the specific time frame in which the performance will be accomplished. In the example of the client who will be taught to self-administer anticoagulant therapy at home, an outcome may be written as follows: Client will demonstrate the injection of enoxaparin (Lovenox) using the preloaded syringe provided, given subcutaneously into the anterior abdominal areas, in 2 days (1 day prior to discharge). This outcome includes the subject (client), actions (demonstrate injection), circumstances (using a preloaded syringe), performance (SC injection into the abdomen), and time frame (2 days from now—1 day before discharge home). Writing specific outcomes also gives the nurse a concrete time frame to work toward to assist the client to meet the goals.

After goals and outcomes are identified based on the nursing diagnoses, a plan of care is written. Each agency determines whether this plan will be communicated as nursing-centred, interdisciplinary, or both. All plans should be client focused and verified with the client or caregiver. The goals and outcomes identified in the plan of care will assist the nurse, and other healthcare providers, in carrying out interventions and evaluating the effectiveness of that care.

7.5 Key Interventions for Drug Administration

After the plan of care has been written, explicitly stating any goals and outcomes based on established nursing diagnoses, the nurse implements this plan. Interventions are aimed at returning the client to an optimum level of wellness and limiting adverse effects related to the client's medical diagnosis or condition. The nurse plays a key role in promoting optimal responses to drugs and minimizing adverse effects. Chapter 8 discusses interventions specific to drug administration, such as the six rights and the techniques of administering medications. This section focuses on other key intervention strategies that the nurse completes for a client receiving medications.

A thorough knowledge of pharmacokinetics and pharmacodynamics is essential for the safe and effective care of clients receiving medications. Not only medications, but almost every intervention that the nurse provides may influence biochemical and psychological responses in a client. For example, providing a warm blanket can affect endogenous stress hormone levels differently than administering an intramuscular injection. This, in turn, can influence blood flow and other bodily processes that affect drug responses. Ways that the nurse can influence pharmacokinetics through purposeful use of dietary modifications and other supportive therapies are presented in Chapter 4.

Monitoring drug effects is a primary intervention that nurses perform. A thorough knowledge of the actions of each medication is necessary to carry out this monitoring process. The nurse should first monitor for the identified therapeutic effect. A lack of sufficient therapeutic effect suggests the need to reassess pharmacotherapy and related interventions. Monitoring may require a reassessment of the client's physical condition, vital signs, body weight, lab values, and/or serum drug levels. The client's statements about pain relief, as well as objective data, such as a change in blood pressure, are used to monitor the therapeutic outcomes of pharmacotherapy. The nurse also monitors for side and adverse effects and attempts to prevent or limit these effects when possible. Some side effects may be managed by the nurse independently of medical orders, whereas others require collaboration with physicians to alleviate client symptoms. For example, a client with nausea and vomiting after receiving a narcotic pain reliever may be comforted by the nurse who provides small frequent meals, sips of carbonated beverages, or changes of linen. However, the physician may need to prescribe an antiemetic drug to control the side effect of intense nausea.

Documentation of both therapeutic and adverse effects is completed during the intervention phase. This includes appropriate documentation of the administration of the medication as well as the effects observed. Additional objective assessment data, such as vital signs, may be included in the documentation to provide more details about the specific drug effects. A client's statements can provide subjective detail to the documentation. Each healthcare facility determines where, when, and how to document the administration of medications and any follow-up assessment data that have been gathered. The nurse's role in reporting adverse drug reactions is presented in Chapter 9.

Client teaching is a vital component of the nurse's interventions for a client receiving medications. Knowledge deficit and even non-adherence are directly related to the type and quality of medication education that a client has received. Nurse practice standards and regulating bodies such as professional nursing associations consider teaching to be a primary role for nurses, giving it the weight of law and key importance in accreditation standards. Because the goal of pharmacotherapy is the safe administration of medications, with the best therapeutic outcomes possible, teaching is aimed at providing the client with the information necessary to ensure this occurs. Every nurse-client interaction can present an opportunity for teaching. Small portions of education given over time are often more effective than large amounts of information given on only one occasion. Discussing medications each time they are administered is an effective way to increase the amount of education accomplished. Providing written material also assists the client to retain the information and review it later. Some medications come with a self-contained teaching program that includes videotapes. A word of caution on the use of audio and print material is necessary, however. The client must be able to read and understand the material provided. Pharmacies may dispense client education pamphlets that detail all of the effects of a medication and the monitoring required, but they are ineffective if the reading level is above what the client can understand or is in a language unfamiliar to the client. Having the client "teach" the nurse, or summarize key points after the teaching has been provided, is a safety check that may be used to verify that the client understands the information.

Elderly and pediatric clients often present special challenges to client teaching. Age-appropriate print or video materials, and teaching that is repeated slowly and provided in small increments, may assist the nurse in teaching these clients. It is often necessary to co-teach the client's caregiver.

Table 7.2 summarizes key areas of teaching and provides sample questions the nurse might ask, or observations that can be made, to verify that teaching has been effective. The Nursing Process Focus flowcharts in Chapters 13 through 48 also supply information on specific drugs and drug classes that is important to include in client teaching.

7.6 Evaluating the Effects of Drug Administration

Evaluation is the final step of the nursing process. It considers the effectiveness of the interventions in meeting established goals and outcomes. The process comes full circle as the nurse reassesses the client, reviews the nursing diagnoses, makes necessary changes, reviews and rewrites goals and outcomes, and carries out further interventions to meet the goals and outcomes. When evaluating the effectiveness of drug administration, the nurse assesses for therapeutic effects and a minimal occurrence of side or adverse effects. The nurse also evaluates the effectiveness of teaching provided and notes areas where further drug education is needed. Evaluation is not the end of the process, but the beginning of another cycle as the nurse continues to work to ensure safe and effective medication use and active client involvement in his or her care. It is a checkpoint where the

CULTURAL CONSIDERATIONS

Non-English-Speaking and Culturally Diverse Clients

Nurses should know in advance what translation services and interpreters are available in their healthcare facility to assist with communication. The nurse should use an interpreter's services when available, validating with the interpreter that he or she is able to understand the client. Many dialects are similar but not the same, and knowing another language is not the same as understanding the culture. Can the interpreter understand the client's language and cultural expressions or nuances well enough for effective communication to occur? If a family member is interpreting, especially if a child is interpreting for a parent or relative, be sure that the interpreter first understands and repeats the information back to the nurse before explaining it to the client in the client's own language. This is especially important if the interpretation is a summary of what has been said rather than a line-by-line interpretation. Before an interpreter is available, or if one is unavailable, use pictures, simple drawings, nonverbal cues, and body language to communicate with the client.

In some cultures, time may not be important and compliance with dosage schedules may require greater emphasis. Be aware of culturally based nonverbal communication behaviours (e.g., use of personal space, eye contact, or lack of eye contact). Gender sensitivities related to culture (e.g., male nurse or physician for female clients) and the use of touch are often important issues. In Western cultures, an informal and personal style is often the norm. When working with older clients and clients of other cultures, adopting a more formal style may be more appropriate.

nurse considers the overall goal of safe and effective administration of medications, with the best therapeutic outcome possible, and takes the steps necessary to ensure success. The nursing process acts as the overall framework to work toward this success.

TABLE 7.2	Important Areas of Teaching for Clients Receiving Medications
Area of Teaching	**Important Questions and Observations**
therapeutic use and outcomes	• Can you tell me the name of your medicine and what the medicine is used for? • What will you look for to know that the medication is effective? (How will you know that the medicine is working?)
monitoring side and adverse effects	• Which side effects can you handle by yourself? (e.g., simple nausea, diarrhea) • Which side effects should you report to your healthcare provider? (e.g., extreme cases of nausea or vomiting, extreme dizziness, bleeding)
medication administration	• Can you tell me how much of the medication you are to take? (mg, number of tablets, mL of liquid, etc.) • Can you tell me how often you are to take it? • What special requirements are necessary when you take this medication? (e.g., take with a full glass of water, take on an empty stomach and remain upright for 30 minutes) • Is there a specific order in which you are to take your medications? (e.g., bronchodilator before corticosteroid inhaler) • Can you show me how you will give yourself the medication? (e.g., eye drops, subcutaneous injections) • What special monitoring is required before you take this medication? (e.g., pulse rate) Can you demonstrate this for me? Based on that monitoring, when should you NOT take the medication? • Do you know how, or where, to store this medication? • What should you do if you miss a dose?
other monitoring and special requirements	• Are there any special tests you are to have related to this medication? (e.g., fingerstick glucose levels, therapeutic drug levels) • How often should these tests be done? • What other medications should you NOT take with this medication? • Are there any foods or beverages you must not have while taking this medication?

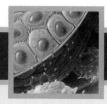

CHAPTER REVIEW

KEY CONCEPTS

The numbered key concepts provide a succinct summary of the important points from the corresponding numbered section within the chapter. If any of these points are not clear, refer to the numbered section within the chapter for review. Expanded versions can be found on the Companion Website.

7.1 The nursing process is a systematic method of problem solving and consists of clearly defined steps: assessing; diagnosing client problems, strengths, and needs; planning care through the formulation of goals and outcomes; implementing interventions; and evaluating the care provided.

7.2 Assessing the client receiving medications includes obtaining health history information, physical assessment data, lab values, and other measurable data and assessing medication effects, both therapeutic and side effects. It also includes assessment of the medication ordered in relation to the client's medical condition, culture, ethnicity, gender, age, and other factors.

7.3 Diagnosing occurs after an analysis of the assessment data and identifies the client's problems and needs in relation to drug administration. Nursing diagnoses are verified with the client or caregiver.

7.4 In planning, goals and outcomes are established from the nursing diagnoses. Goals focus on what the client should be able to achieve, and outcomes provide the specific, measurable criteria that will be used to measure goal attainment. Interventions are planned to meet the goals.

7.5 Interventions are implemented in order to return the client to an optimum level of wellness. These include the safe and effective administration of medications. Key interventions required of the nurse include monitoring drug effects, documenting medications, promoting optimal responses to medications, preventing or limiting adverse effects, and client teaching.

7.6 Evaluating whether the medication is producing desired effects is an important nursing responsibility. Evaluation begins a new cycle as new assessment data are gathered and analyzed, nursing diagnoses are reviewed, goals and outcomes are refined, and new interventions are carried out.

REVIEW QUESTIONS

1 A client visits an outpatient clinic for treatment of a sore throat that is diagnosed as being caused by *Streptococcus* bacteria and is given a prescription for an antibiotic. What pertinent medical history information would the nurse gather, given the short duration of this client's visit, that would ensure optimum outcomes from this prescription?

2 Develop two possible nursing diagnoses for the client in question 1 related to the use or administration of the medication.

3 Write a pertinent goal for this client related to antibiotic use. Write an outcome statement.

4 What essential areas should be covered when teaching this client before discharge from the clinic?

5 This client returns to the clinic in 3 days for a problem unrelated to the previous infection. What would the nurse evaluate at this time in relation to the antibiotic prescription to demonstrate success or areas that still need to be addressed?

CRITICAL THINKING QUESTIONS

1. A 13-year-old client who is a cheerleader from a rural community has been diagnosed with type 1 diabetes. She is supported by a single mother who is frustrated with her daughter's eating habits. The client has lost weight since beginning her insulin regimen. The nurse notes that the client and her mother, who is very well dressed, are both extremely thin. Identify additional data that the nurse would need to obtain before making the nursing diagnosis of non-adherence.

2. Regarding the client in question 1, her drug regimen is evaluated and the healthcare provider suggests a subcutaneous insulin pump to help control the client's fluctuating blood glucose levels. Identify three client needs related to this new therapy.

3. A nursing student is assigned to a licensed preceptor who is administering oral medications. The student notes that the preceptor administers the drugs safely but routinely fails to offer the client information about the drug being administered. Discuss this action in relation to the concept of safe drug administration.

EXPLORE
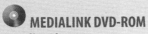
MediaLink

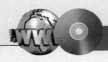 www.pearsoned.ca/adams-king

MEDIALINK DVD-ROM
- **Audio Glossary**
- **CRNE Review**

COMPANION WEBSITE
- **CRNE Review**
- **Case Study:** Safe medication administration

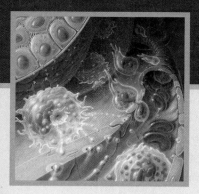

CHAPTER 8

Principles of Drug Administration

OBJECTIVES

After reading this chapter, the student should be able to do the following:

1. Discuss drug administration as a component of safe, effective nursing care, utilizing the nursing process.
2. Describe the roles and responsibilities of the nurse regarding drug administration.
3. Explain how the seven rights of drug administration impact client safety.
4. Give specific examples of how the nurse can increase client adherence in taking medications.
5. Interpret drug orders that contain abbreviations.
6. Compare and contrast the three systems of measurement used in pharmacology.
7. Explain the proper methods to administer enteral, topical, and parenteral drugs.
8. Compare and contrast the advantages and disadvantages of each route of drug administration.

MediaLink

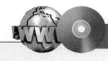

www.pearsoned.ca/adams-king

CRNE review, case studies, and other interactive resources for this chapter can be found on the Companion Website at **www.pearsoned.ca/adams-king**. Click on "Chapter 8" to select the activities for this chapter. For animations, more CRNE review questions, and an audio glossary, access the accompanying MediaLink DVD-ROM in this textbook.

The primary role of the nurse in drug administration is to ensure that prescribed medications are delivered in a safe manner. Drug administration is an important component of providing comprehensive nursing care that incorporates all aspects of the nursing process. In the course of drug administration, nurses collaborate closely with physicians, pharmacists, and, of course, their clients. The purpose of this chapter is to introduce the roles and responsibilities of the nurse in delivering medications safely and effectively.

NURSING MANAGEMENT OF DRUG ADMINISTRATION

8.1 Medication Knowledge, Understanding, and Responsibilities of the Nurse

Whether administering drugs or supervising drug use, the nurse is expected to understand the pharmacotherapeutic principles for all medications received by each client. Given the large number of different drugs and the potential consequences of medication errors, this is indeed an enormous task. The nurse's responsibilities include knowledge and understanding of the following:

- What drug is ordered
- Drug name (generic and trade) and classification
- Intended or proposed use
- Effects on the body
- Contraindications
- Special considerations (i.e., how age, gender, weight, body fat distribution, diet, genetics, and individual pathophysiological states affect pharmacokinetics, pharmacodynamics, and overall pharmacotherapeutic response)
- Side effects
- Why the medication has been prescribed for this particular client
- How the medication is to be administered, including dosage ranges
- What nursing process considerations related to the medication apply to this client

Before any drug is administered, the nurse must obtain and process pertinent information regarding the client's medical history, physical assessment, disease processes, and learning needs and capabilities. Growth and developmental factors must always be considered. It is important to remember that a large number of variables influence a client's response to medications. Having a firm understanding of these variables can increase the success of pharmacotherapy.

A major role of the nurse in pharmacotherapy is to promote optimal responses to the medication and to prevent or limit the number and severity of adverse drug events. Many adverse drug reactions (ADRs) are preventable. Professional nurses can routinely prevent many serious adverse drug reactions in their clients by applying their experience and knowledge of pharmacotherapeutics to clinical practice. Some ADRs, however, are not preventable. It is vital that the nurse be prepared to recognize and respond to potential adverse effects of medications. Professional responsibilities in reporting adverse drug reactions are presented in Chapter 9.

Allergic and anaphylactic reactions are particularly serious ADRs that must be carefully monitored and prevented, when possible. An **allergic reaction** is an acquired hyperresponse of body defences to a foreign substance (allergen). Signs of allergic reactions vary in severity and include skin rash with or without itching, edema, nausea, diarrhea, runny nose, and reddened eyes with tearing. Upon discovering that the client is allergic to a product, it is the nurse's responsibility to alert all personnel by documenting the allergy in the medical record and by applying labels to the chart and **medication administration record (MAR)**. An appropriate, agency-approved bracelet should be placed on the client next to the identification bracelet to alert all caregivers of the specific drug allergy. It is good practice to verify allergy information on the bracelet with the client. Stress at the time of hospitalization may cause the client to forget to mention a significant allergy. Information related to drug allergy must be communicated to the physician and pharmacist so the medication regimen can be evaluated for cross-sensitivity between various pharmacological products.

Anaphylaxis is a severe type of allergic reaction that involves the massive, systemic release of histamine and other chemical mediators of inflammation that can lead to life-threatening shock. Symptoms such as acute dyspnea and the sudden appearance of hypotension or tachycardia following drug administration are indicative of anaphylaxis, which must be treated immediately. The pharmacotherapy of anaphylaxis and allergic reactions is covered in Chapters 27 and 31, respectively.

8.2 The Rights of Drug Administration

The **seven rights of drug administration** form the operational basis for the safe delivery of medications. The seven rights offer simple and practical guidance for the nurse to use during drug preparation, delivery, administration, and documentation. If followed consistently, the chance of a medication error is greatly reduced. The seven rights are as follows:

1. Right client
2. Right medication
3. Right dose
4. Right route of administration
5. Right time of delivery
6. Right documentation
7. Right reason

The seven rights require that the nurse complete the assessment of the client and research the prescribed drug, as presented in Chapter 7. Once the nurse determines that the drug as prescribed is appropriate and safe for this client at this time, the drug is prepared adhering to the "rights" and administered in accordance with the guidelines for safe drug administration presented in Table 8.1.

Additional rights have been added over the years, depending on particular academic curricula or agency policies. Additions to the original five rights include the now standard sixth right, right documentation, and seventh right,

right reason. Other considerations include the right to refuse medication, the right to receive drug education, the right assessment, and the right preparation.

The **three checks of drug administration** that nurses use in conjunction with the seven rights help to ascertain client safety and drug effectiveness. Traditionally, these checks incorporate checking the drug with the MAR or the medication information system at the following times:

1. When removing the drug from the medication drawer, refrigerator, or controlled substance locker
2. When preparing the drug, pouring it, taking it out of the unit dose container, or connecting the IV tubing to the bag
3. Immediately before administering the drug to the client

Despite all attempts to provide safe drug delivery, errors continue to occur, some of which are fatal. Although the nurse is held accountable for preparing and administering medications, safe drug practices are a result of multidisciplinary endeavours. Responsibility for accurate drug administration lies with multiple individuals, including physicians, pharmacists, and other healthcare professionals. Factors contributing to medication errors and strategies to prevent medication errors are presented in Chapter 9. The student should review the guidelines for safe drug administration in Table 8.1 before proceeding to subsequent sections.

PHARMFACTS

Potentially Fatal Drug Reactions

Toxic Epidermal Necrolysis (TEN)

- Severe and potentially fatal drug-induced reaction
- Characterized by widespread epidermal sloughing caused by massive disintegration of keratinocytes
- Severe epidermal detachment involving the top layer of the skin and mucous membranes
- Multisystem organ involvement and death if the reaction is not recognized and diagnosed
- Occurs when the liver fails to properly break down a drug, which then cannot be excreted normally
- Associated with the use of some anticonvulsants such as phenytoin and carbamazepine, the antibiotic trimethoprim/sulfamethoxazole, and other drugs, but can occur with the use of any prescription or OTC preparation, including ibuprofen
- Risk of death decreased if the offending drug is quickly withdrawn and supportive care is maintained
- Skin sloughing of 30% or more of the body

Stevens-Johnson Syndrome (SJS)

- Usually prompted by the same or similar drugs as for TEN
- Begins within 1 to 14 days of pharmacotherapy
- Non-specific upper respiratory infection with chills, fever, and malaise usually signals the start of SJS
- Generalized blister-like lesions within a few days
- Skin sloughing of 10% of the body

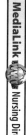

MediaLink · Nursing Directories for Drug Information

TABLE 8.1	Guidelines for Safe Drug Administration

Certain protocols and techniques are common to all methods of drug administration:

- Know and apply the medication policies of the hospital or agency.
- Review the medication order and check for drug allergies.
- Wash hands and apply gloves, if indicated.
- Use aseptic technique when preparing and administering parenteral medications.
- Identify the client by asking the person to state his or her full name (or by asking the parent or guardian), checking the identification band, and comparing this information with the MAR.
- Ask the client about known allergies.
- Inform the client of the drug name, intended effect, and method of administration.
- Position the client for the appropriate route of administration.
- For enteral drugs, assist the client to a sitting position.
- If the drug is pre-packaged (unit dose), remove it from its packaging at the bedside, when possible. This enables the nurse to check the package label directly, provides a safe way to preserve the medication if the client is unable to receive the drug at the last moment (e.g., vomits), and provides an opportunity for the nurse to demonstrate checking the label for the "right drug" for able clients.
- Unless specifically instructed to do so in the orders, do not leave drugs at the bedside. Remain with the client until all medication has been swallowed.
- When giving more than one medication to a client, the following chronological order is recommended: Give tablets and capsules followed by water or other liquid; then give liquids diluted with water as required. Cough medicine is given undiluted and is not followed by liquids. Sublingual and buccal tablets are given last.
- Document the medication administration and any pertinent client responses on the MAR. Documenting immediately after administration decreases the chance that another dose of the drug is given by another caregiver.

8.3 Client Adherence and Successful Pharmacotherapy

Adherence is a major factor affecting pharmacotherapeutic success. As it relates to pharmacology, **adherence** is taking a medication in the manner prescribed by the practitioner or, in the case of OTC drugs, following the instructions on the label. Client non-adherence ranges from not taking the medication at all, to taking it at the wrong time or in the wrong manner.

Although the nurse may be extremely conscientious in applying all the principles of effective drug administration, these strategies are of little value unless the client agrees that the prescribed drug regimen is personally worthwhile. Before administering the drug, the nurse should use the nursing process to formulate a personalized care plan that will best enable the client to become an active participant in his or her care (see Chapter 7). This allows the client to accept or reject the pharmacological therapy based on accurate information that is presented in a manner that addresses individual learning styles. It is imperative to remember that a responsible, well-informed adult always has the legal option of refusing to take any medication.

In the plan of care, it is important to address essential information that the client must know regarding the prescribed medications. This includes factors such as the name of the drug, why it has been ordered, expected drug actions, associated side effects, and potential interactions with other medications, foods, herbal supplements, or alcohol. Clients need to be reminded that they share an active role in ensuring their own medication effectiveness and safety.

SPECIAL CONSIDERATIONS

The Challenges of Pediatric Drug Administration

Administering medication to infants and young children requires special knowledge and techniques.

- Weight must be assessed; drug dosages are commonly determined by the child's weight.
- The nurse must have knowledge of growth and developmental patterns and modify interventions accordingly.
- A caregiver may be asked to verify a young child's name when checking the bracelet for the "right client."
- When possible, give the child a choice regarding the use of a spoon, dropper, or syringe. Present a matter-of-fact attitude in giving a child medication; using threats or dishonesty is unacceptable.
- Oral medications that must be crushed for the child to swallow can be mixed with honey, flavoured syrup, jelly, or fruit puree to avoid unpleasant tastes. Iced products such as popsicles can dull bitter taste. Medications should not be mixed with certain foods, such as potatoes, milk, or fruit juices, to mask the taste because the child may develop an unpleasant association with these items and refuse to consume them in the future.
- To prevent nausea, medications can be preceded and followed with sips of a carbonated beverage that is poured over crushed ice.
- The nurse may have to rely on nonverbal cues and objective data when assessing and evaluating the effects of drugs such as pain medications.

Many factors can influence whether clients comply with pharmacotherapy. The drug may be too expensive or not approved by the client's health insurance plan. Clients sometimes forget doses of medications, especially when they must be taken three or four times per day. Clients often

Grapefruit Juice and Drug Interactions

- Grapefruit juice may not be safe for people who take certain medications.
- Chemicals (most likely flavonoids) in grapefruit juice lower the activity of specific enzymes in the intestinal tract that normally break down medications. This allows a larger amount of medication to reach the bloodstream, resulting in increased drug activity.
- Drugs that may be affected by grapefruit juice include midazolam, cyclosporine, erythromycin, antihyperlipidemics such as lovastatin and simvastatin, certain antihistamines such as astemizole (Hismanal), and certain antifungals such as itraconazole, ketoconazole, and mibefradil.
- Grapefruit juice should be consumed at least 2 hours before or 5 hours after taking a medication that may interact with it.
- Some drinks that are flavoured with fruit juice could contain grapefruit juice, even if grapefruit is not part of the name of the drink. Check the ingredients label.

discontinue the use of drugs that have annoying side effects or those that impair major lifestyle choices. Adverse effects that often prompt non-adherence are headache, dizziness, nausea, diarrhea, and impotence.

Clients often take medications in an unexpected manner, sometimes self-adjusting their doses. Some clients believe that if one tablet is good, two must be better. Others believe they will become dependent on the medication if it is taken as prescribed; thus, they take only half the required dose. Clients are usually reluctant to admit or report non-adherence to the nurse for fear of being reprimanded or feeling embarrassed. Because the reasons for non-adherence are many and varied, the nurse must be vigilant in questioning clients about their medications. When pharmacotherapy

fails to produce the expected outcomes, non-adherence should be considered a possible explanation.

8.4 Drug Orders and Time Schedules

Healthcare providers use accepted abbreviations to communicate the directions and times for drug administration. Table 8.2 lists common abbreviations.

A **STAT order** refers to any medication that is needed immediately and is to be given only once. It is often associated with emergency medications that are needed for life-threatening situations. The term *STAT* comes from *statim*, the Latin word meaning "immediately." The physician normally notifies the nurse of any STAT order, so it can be obtained from the pharmacy and administered immediately. The time frame between writing the order and administering the drug should be 5 minutes or less. Although not as urgent, an **ASAP order** (as soon as possible order) should be available for administration to the client within 30 minutes of the written order.

The **single order** is for a drug that is to be given only once and at a specific time, such as a preoperative order. A **PRN order**, from the Latin *pro re nata*, is administered *as required* by the client's condition. The nurse makes the judgment, based on client assessment, as to when such a medication is to be administered. A **continuing order** is for a drug that is to be given on an ongoing basis for a specific number of doses or days. An example is "ampicillin 250 mg PO qid for 5 days." Continuing orders usually are initiated within 2 hours of the time the order is written by the physician. Sometimes a **standing order** is written in advance of a routine situation and is to be carried out under specific circumstances. An example is a set of postoperative PRN

TABLE 8.2	Drug Administration Abbreviations		
Abbreviation	**Meaning**	**Abbreviation**	**Meaning**
ac	before meals	qd	every day*
ad lib	as desired/directed	qh	every hour
AM	morning	qhs	bedtime (every night)*
bid	twice per day	qid	four times per day
cap	capsule	qod	every other day*
/d	per day	q2h	every 2 hours (even)
gtt	drop	q4h	every 4 hours (even)
h or hr	hour	q6h	every 6 hours (even)
hs	hour of sleep/bedtime	q8h	every 8 hours (even)
no	number	q12h	every 12 hours
pc	after meals; after eating	Rx	take
PM	afternoon	STAT	immediately; at once
PO	by mouth; orally	tab	tablet
PRN or prn	when needed/necessary	tid	three times per day
q	every		

*The Institute for Safe Medical Practices recommends the following changes to avoid medication errors: for qd, use "daily" or "every day"; for qhs, use "nightly"; for qod, use "every other day."

prescriptions that are written for all clients who have undergone a specific surgical procedure. "Acetaminophen elixir 325 mg PO q4h PRN sore throat" may be ordered for all clients who have undergone a tonsillectomy. The nurse must then assess the safety of implementing the order for a particular client. Because of the legal implications of putting all clients into a single treatment category, such orders are not permitted in some facilities. It is important to be aware that agencies differ in the way that they define the terms *continuing order* and *standing order* and to clarify how the term is defined in a particular agency.

Agency policies dictate that drug orders be reviewed by the attending physician within specific time frames, usually at least every 7 days. Prescriptions for narcotics and other scheduled drugs are often automatically discontinued after 72 hours, unless specifically re-ordered by the physician. Automatic stop orders do not generally apply when the number of doses, or an exact period of time, is specified.

Some medications must be taken at specific times. If a drug causes stomach upset, it is usually administered with meals to prevent epigastric pain, nausea, and vomiting. Other medications should be administered between meals because food interferes with absorption. Some CNS drugs and antihypertensives are best administered at bedtime because they may cause drowsiness. Sildenafil (Viagra) is unique in that it should be taken 30 to 60 minutes prior to expected sexual intercourse to achieve an effective erection. The nurse must pay careful attention to educating clients about the timing of their medications to enhance adherence and to increase the potential for therapeutic success.

Once medications are administered, the nurse must correctly document that they have been given to the client. It is necessary to include the drug name, dosage, time administered, any assessments, and the nurse's signature. If a medication is refused or omitted, this fact must be recorded on the appropriate form within the medical record. It is customary to document the reason, when possible. Should the client voice any concerns or complaints about the medication, these are also included.

8.5 Systems of Measurement

Dosages are labelled and dispensed according to their weight, quantity, or volume. Three systems of measurement are used in pharmacology: metric, apothecary, and household.

The **International System of Units (SI)**, the modern **metric system**, is the most common system of drug measurement. The volume of a drug is expressed in terms of the litre (L) or millilitre (mL). The cubic centimetre (cc) is a common measurement of volume that is equivalent to 1 mL of fluid. The metric weight of a drug is stated in terms of kilograms (kg), grams (g), milligrams (mg), or micrograms (mcg or μg). A **unit (U)** is a particular quantity. Insulin is an example of a drug that is prescribed in units.

The **apothecary system** and **household system of measurement** are older systems of measurement. Although most physicians and pharmacies use the metric system, these older systems are still encountered. Approximate equivalents between metric, apothecary, and household units of volume and weight are listed in Table 8.3.

Because Canadians are very familiar with the teaspoon, tablespoon, and cup, it is important for the nurse to be able to convert between the household and metric systems of measurement. In the hospital, a glass of fluid is measured in millilitres or cubic centimetres—an 8 ounce glass of water is recorded as 240 mL. If a client being discharged is ordered to drink 2400 mL of fluid per day, the nurse may instruct the client to drink ten 8 ounce glasses, or 10 cups, of fluid per day. Likewise, when a child is to be given a drug that is administered in elixir form, the nurse should explain that

TABLE 8.3	Approximate Metric, Apothecary, and Household Measurement Equivalents	
Metric	**Apothecary**	**Household**
1 mL	15 minims	15 drops
5 mL	1 fluidram	1 teaspoon or 75 drops
15 mL	4 fluidrams	1 tablespoon or 3 teaspoons
30 mL	8 fluidrams or 1 fluid ounce	2 tablespoons
240–250 mL	8 fluid ounces (1/2 pint)	1 glass or cup
500 mL	1 pint	2 glasses or 2 cups
1 L	32 fluid ounces or 1 quart	4 glasses or 4 cups or 1 quart
1 mg	1/60 grain	—
60–64 mg	1 grain	—
300–325 mg	5 grains	—
1 g	15–16 grains	—
1 kg	—	2.2 pounds

To convert grains to grams: Divide grains by 15 or 16.
To convert grams to grains: Multiply grams by 15 or 16.
To convert minims to millilitres: Divide minims by 15.

5 mL of the drug is the same as 1 teaspoon. The nurse should encourage the use of accurate medical dosing devices at home, such as oral dosing syringes, oral droppers, cylindrical spoons, and medication cups. These are preferred over the traditional household measuring spoon because they are more accurate. Eating utensils that are commonly referred to as teaspoons or tablespoons often do not hold the volume that their names imply.

ROUTES OF DRUG ADMINISTRATION

The three broad categories of routes of drug administration are enteral, topical, and parenteral, with subsets within each. Each route has both advantages and disadvantages. While some drugs are formulated to be given by several routes, others are specific to only one route. Pharmacokinetic considerations, such as how the route of administration affects drug absorption and distribution, are discussed in Chapter 4.

8.6 Enteral Drug Administration

The **enteral route** of drug administration includes drugs given orally and those administered through nasogastric or gastrostomy tubes. Oral drug administration is the most common, most convenient, and usually the least costly of all routes. It is also considered the safest route because the skin barrier is not compromised, and, in cases of overdose or error, medications remaining in the stomach can be retrieved. Oral preparations are available in tablet, capsule, and liquid forms. Medications administered by the enteral route take advantage of the vast absorptive surfaces of the oral mucosa, stomach, or small intestine.

Tablets and Capsules Tablets and capsules are the most common forms of drugs. Clients prefer tablets or capsules over other routes and forms because of their ease of use. In some cases, tablets may be scored for more individualized dosing. Clients should be instructed to take tablets and capsules with a full glass of water and then to sit up for 15 minutes.

Some clients, particularly children, have difficulty swallowing tablets and capsules. Although crushing tablets or opening capsules and sprinkling the drug over food or mixing it with juice could make it more palatable and easier to swallow, this should be avoided in many situations. Do *not* crush tablets or open capsules unless the manufacturer specifically states that this is permissible. Some drugs are inactivated by crushing or opening, while others severely irritate the stomach mucosa and cause nausea or vomiting. Occasionally, drugs should not be crushed because they irritate the oral mucosa, are extremely bitter, or contain dyes that stain the teeth. Most drug guides provide lists of drugs that may not be crushed. Another reason not to mix medicine with food is that children may become less willing to eat the food. Guidelines for administering tablets and capsules are given in Table 8.4.

The strongly acidic contents within the stomach can present a destructive obstacle to the absorption of some medications. To overcome this barrier, tablets may have a hard, waxy coating that enables them to resist the acidity. These **enteric-coated** tablets are designed to dissolve in the alkaline environment of the small intestine. It is important that the nurse not crush enteric-coated tablets as the medication would then be directly exposed to the stomach environment.

Studies have clearly demonstrated that adherence declines as the number of doses per day increases. With this in mind, pharmacologists have attempted to design new drugs so that they may be administered only once or twice daily. **Sustained-release** tablets or capsules are designed to dissolve very slowly. This releases the medication over an extended time and results in a longer duration of action for the medication. Also called extended-release (XR), long-acting (LA), or slow-release (SR) medications, these forms allow for the convenience of once- or twice-daily dosing. Extended-release medications must not be crushed or opened.

Giving medications by the oral route has certain disadvantages. The client must be conscious and able to swallow properly. Certain types of drugs, including proteins, are inactivated by digestive enzymes in the stomach and small intestine. Medications absorbed from the stomach and small intestine first travel to the liver, where they may be inactivated before they ever reach their target organs. This process, called first-pass metabolism, is discussed in Chapter 4. The significant variation in the motility of the GI tract and in its ability to absorb medications can create differences in bioavailability. In addition, children and some adults have an aversion to swallowing large tablets and capsules or to taking oral medications that are distasteful.

Sublingual and Buccal Drug Administration For sublingual and buccal administration, the tablet is not swallowed, but kept in the mouth. The mucosa of the oral cavity contains a rich blood supply that provides an excellent absorptive surface for certain drugs. Medications given by this route are not subjected to destructive digestive enzymes and do not undergo hepatic first-pass metabolism.

For the **sublingual (SL)** route, the medication is placed under the tongue and allowed to dissolve slowly, as shown in Figure 8.1a on page 73. Because of the rich blood supply in this region, the sublingual route results in a rapid onset of action. Sublingual dosage forms are most often formulated as rapidly disintegrating tablets or as soft gelatin capsules filled with liquid drug.

When multiple drugs have been ordered, the sublingual preparations should be administered after oral medications have been swallowed. The client should be instructed not to move the drug with the tongue and not to eat or drink anything until the medication has completely dissolved. The sublingual mucosa is not suitable for extended-release formulations because it is a relatively small area and is constantly being bathed by a substantial amount of saliva. Table 8.4 presents important points regarding sublingual drug administration.

TABLE 8.4	Enteral Drug Administration
Drug Form	**Administration Guidelines**
tablet, capsule, and liquid	1. Assess that client is alert and has ability to swallow. 2. Place tablets or capsules into medication cup. (A tablet in a single dose packet may be torn at the top, ready to hand to the client.) 3. If liquid, shake the bottle to mix the agent, if it is a suspension, and measure the dose into the cup at eye level. 4. Hand the client the medication cup. 5. Offer a glass of water to facilitate swallowing the medication. Milk or juice may be offered if not contraindicated. 6. Remain with client until all medication is swallowed.
sublingual	1. Assess that client is alert and has ability to hold medication under tongue. 2. Place sublingual tablet under tongue. 3. Instruct client not to chew or swallow the tablet or move the tablet around with tongue. 4. Instruct client to allow tablet to dissolve completely before swallowing saliva. 5. Remain with client to determine that all of the medication has dissolved. 6. Offer a glass of water, if client desires.
buccal	1. Assess that client is alert and has ability to hold medication between the gums and the cheek. 2. Place buccal tablet between the gum line and the cheek. 3. Instruct client not to chew or swallow the tablet or move the tablet around with tongue. 4. Instruct client to allow tablet to dissolve completely before swallowing saliva. 5. Remain with client to determine that all of the medication has dissolved. 6. Offer a glass of water, if client desires.
nasogastric and gastrostomy	1. Administer liquid forms when possible to avoid clogging the tube. 2. If solid, crush finely into powder and mix thoroughly with at least 30 mL of warm water until dissolved. 3. Assess and verify tube placement. 4. Turn off feeding, if applicable to client. 5. Aspirate stomach contents and measure the residual volume. If greater than 100 mL for an adult, check agency policy. 6. Return residual via gravity and flush with water. 7. Pour medication into syringe barrel and allow to flow into the tube by gravity. Give each medication separately, flushing between with water. 8. Keep head of bed elevated for 1 hour to prevent aspiration. 9. Re-establish continual feeding, as scheduled. Keep head of bed elevated 45 degrees to prevent aspiration.

To administer by the **buccal route**, the tablet or capsule is placed in the oral cavity between the gum and the cheek, as shown in Figure 8.1b. The client must be instructed not to manipulate the medication with the tongue, otherwise it could get displaced to the sublingual area where it would be more rapidly absorbed, or to the back of the throat where it could be swallowed. The buccal mucosa is less permeable to most medications than the sublingual area, providing for slower absorption. The buccal route is preferred over the sublingual route for sustained-release delivery because of its greater mucosal surface area. Drugs formulated for buccal administration generally do not cause irritation and are small enough to not cause discomfort to the client. Like the sublingual route, the buccal route avoids first-pass metabolism by the liver and the enzymatic processes of the stomach and small intestine. Table 8.4 provides important guidelines for buccal drug administration.

Elixirs, Syrups, and Suspensions Liquids come in three forms. Elixirs contain drugs that are in a solution of water and alcohol. Cough medicines are often available as elixirs.

A syrup contains the drug in a sugary, sticky solution. Acetaminophen is available as a syrup, for example. A suspension contains finely divided drug particles dispersed in a liquid. A suspension must always be shaken to ensure the drug is dispersed evenly throughout the liquid before it is poured. Failure to shake the bottle every time it is used allows the drug to settle to the bottom, so the last dose poured would contain the largest dose of drug. Some antibiotics are available in suspensions.

Nasogastric and Gastrostomy Drug Administration
Clients with a nasogastric tube or enteral feeding mechanism such as a gastrostomy tube may have their medications administered through these devices. A nasogastric (NG) tube is a soft, flexible tube inserted by way of the nasopharynx with the tip lying in the stomach. A gastrostomy (G) tube is surgically placed directly into the client's stomach. Generally, the NG tube is used for short-term treatment, whereas the G tube is inserted for clients requiring long-term care. Drugs administered through these tubes are usually in liquid form. Although solid drugs can be crushed or dissolved,

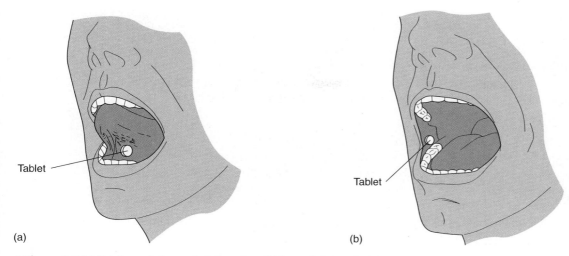

Tablet

(a)

Tablet

(b)

● **Figure 8.1** (a) Sublingual drug administration; (b) buccal drug administration

they tend to cause clogging of the tubes. Sustained-release drugs should not be crushed and administered through NG or G tubes. Drugs administered by this route are exposed to the same physiological processes as those given orally. Table 8.4 lists important guidelines for administering drugs through NG and G tubes.

8.7 Topical Drug Administration

Topical drugs are those applied locally to the skin or the membranous linings of the eye, ear, nose, respiratory tract, urinary tract, vagina, and rectum. These applications include the following:

- Dermatological preparations: Drugs are applied to the skin; this is the topical route most commonly used. Formulations include creams, lotions, gels, powders, and sprays.

- Instillations and irrigations: Drugs are applied into body cavities or orifices. These include the eyes, ears, nose, urinary bladder, rectum, and vagina.

- Inhalations: Drugs are applied to the respiratory tract by inhalers, nebulizers, or positive-pressure breathing apparatuses. The most common indication for inhaled drugs is bronchoconstriction due to bronchitis or asthma; however, a number of illegal, abused drugs are taken by this route because it provides a very rapid onset of drug action (see Chapter 12). Additional details on inhalation drug administration can be found in Chapter 29.

Many drugs are applied topically to produce a *local* effect. For example, antibiotics may be applied to the skin to treat skin infections. Antineoplastic agents may be instilled into the urinary bladder via a catheter to treat tumours of the bladder mucosa. Corticosteroids are sprayed into the nostrils to reduce inflammation of the nasal mucosa due to allergic rhinitis. Local, topical delivery produces fewer side effects compared with the same drug given orally or parenterally. This is because, when given topically, these drugs are absorbed very slowly and the amounts reaching the general circulation are minimal.

Some drugs are given topically to provide for slow release and absorption of the drug to the general circulation. These agents are given for their *systemic* effects. For example, a nitroglycerin patch is not applied to the skin to treat a local skin condition, but to treat a systemic condition—coronary artery disease. Likewise, prochlorperazine suppositories are inserted rectally not to treat a disease of the rectum, but to alleviate nausea.

The distinction between topical drugs given for local effects and those given for systemic effects is an important one for the nurse. In the case of local drugs, absorption is undesirable and may cause side effects. For systemic drugs, absorption is essential for the therapeutic action of the drug. With either type of topical agent, drugs should not be applied to abraded or denuded skin, unless directed to do so.

Transdermal Delivery System The use of transdermal patches provides an effective means of delivering certain medications. Examples include nitroglycerin for angina pectoris and scopolamine for motion sickness. Although transdermal patches contain a specific amount of drug, the rate of delivery and the actual dose received may be variable. Patches are changed on a regular basis, using a site rotation routine, which should be documented in the MAR. Before applying a transdermal patch, the nurse should verify that the previous patch has been removed and disposed of appropriately. Drugs to be administered by this route avoid the first-pass effect in the liver and bypass digestive enzymes. Table 8.5 and Figure 8.2 explain the major points of transdermal drug delivery.

Ophthalmic Administration The ophthalmic route is used to treat local conditions of the eye and surrounding structures. Common indications include excessive dryness, infections, glaucoma, and dilation of the pupil during eye examinations. Ophthalmic drugs are available in the form of eye irrigations, drops, ointments, and medicated disks. Table 8.5 and Figure 8.3 on page 75 give guidelines for adult administration. Although the procedure is the same with a

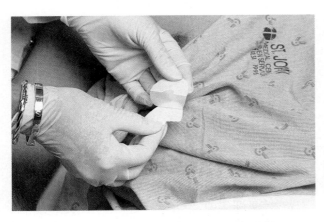 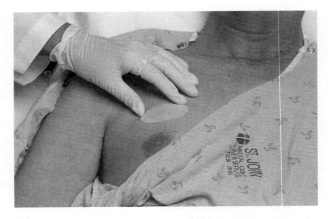

● **Figure 8.2** Transdermal patch administration: (a) protective coating removed from patch; (b) patch immediately applied to clean, dry, hairless skin and labelled with date, time, and initials
Source: Pearson Education/PH College.

child, it is advisable to enlist the help of an adult caregiver. In some cases, the infant or toddler may need to be immobilized with arms wrapped to prevent accidental injury to the eye during administration. For the young child, demonstrating the procedure using a doll facilitates cooperation and decreases anxiety.

TABLE 8.5	Topical Drug Administration
Drug Form	**Administration Guidelines**
transdermal	1. Obtain transdermal patch and read manufacturer's guidelines. Application site and frequency of changing differ according to medication. 2. Apply gloves before handling to avoid absorption of the agent by the nurse. 3. Remove previous medication or patch and cleanse area. 4. If using a transdermal ointment, apply the ordered amount of medication in an even line directly on the pre-measured paper that accompanies the medication tube. 5. Press patch or apply medicated paper to clean, dry, and hairless skin. 6. Rotate sites to prevent skin irritation. 7. Label patch with date, time, and initials.
ophthalmic	1. Instruct client to lie supine or to sit with head slightly tilted back. 2. With non-dominant hand, pull lower lid down gently to expose the conjunctival sac, creating a pocket. 3. Ask client to look upward. 4. Hold eyedropper 0.5 cm above the conjunctival sac. Do not hold dropper over eye as this may stimulate the blink reflex. 5. Instill prescribed number of drops into the centre of the pocket. Avoid touching eye or conjunctival sac with tip of eyedropper. 6. If applying ointment, apply a thin line of ointment evenly along inner edge of lower lid margin, from inner to outer canthus. 7. Instruct the client to close eye gently. Apply gentle pressure with finger to the nasolacrimal duct at the inner canthus for 1–2 minutes to avoid overflow drainage into nose and throat, thus minimizing risk of absorption into the systemic circulation. 8. With tissue, remove excess medication around eye. 9. Replace dropper. Do not rinse eyedropper.
otic	1. Instruct client to lie on side or to sit with head tilted so that affected ear is facing up. 2. If necessary, clean the pinna of the ear and the meatus with a clean washcloth to prevent any discharge from being washed into the ear canal during the instillation of the drops. 3. Position the pinna backward and upward for an adult (see Fig. 8.4, p. 76). Position the pinna backward and slightly downward for a child (see Fig. 8.5, p. 76). This straightens the ear canal. 4. Hold dropper 0.5 cm above ear canal and instill prescribed number of drops into the side of the ear canal, allowing the drops to flow downward. Avoid placing drops directly on the tympanic membrane. 5. Gently apply intermittent pressure to the tragus of the ear three or four times. 6. Instruct client to remain on side for up to 10 minutes to prevent loss of medication. 7. If cotton ball is ordered, pre-soak with medication and insert it into the outermost part of ear canal. 8. Wipe any solution that may have dripped from the ear canal with a tissue.

TABLE 8.5	Topical Drug Administration *(Continued)*
Drug Form	**Administration Guidelines**
nasal drops	1. Ask the client to blow the nose to clear nasal passages.
	2. Instruct client to lie or sit with head tilted back and slightly toward the side of the target nostril/sinus (head tilted slightly to the left for the left nostril/sinus; head tilted slightly to the right for the right nostril/sinus).
	3. Draw up the correct volume of drug into dropper.
	4. Instruct the client to open and breathe through the mouth.
	5. Hold the tip of the dropper just above the nostril and, without touching the nose with the dropper, direct the solution laterally toward the midline of the superior concha of the ethmoid bone—not the base of the nasal cavity, where it will run down the throat and into the eustachian tube.
	6. Ask the client to remain in position for 5 minutes.
	7. Discard any remaining solution that is in the dropper.
vaginal	1. Instruct the client to assume a supine position with knees bent and separated.
	2. Place water-soluble lubricant into medicine cup.
	3. Apply gloves; open suppository and lubricate the rounded end.
	4. Expose the vaginal orifice by separating the labia with non-dominant hand.
	5. Insert the rounded end of the suppository about 8–10 cm along the posterior wall of the vagina, or as far as it will pass.
	6. If using a cream, jelly, or foam, gently insert applicator 5 cm along the posterior vaginal wall and slowly push the plunger until empty. Remove the applicator and place on a paper towel.
	7. Ask the client to lower legs and remain lying in the supine or side-lying position for 5–10 minutes following insertion.
rectal suppositories	1. Instruct the client to lie on left side (Sims' position).
	2. Apply gloves; open suppository and lubricate the rounded end.
	3. Lubricate the gloved forefinger of the dominant hand with water-soluble lubricant.
	4. Inform the client when the suppository is to be inserted; instruct the client to take slow, deep breaths and deeply exhale during insertion to relax the anal sphincter.
	5. Gently insert the lubricated end of suppository into the rectum, beyond the anal-rectal ridge to ensure retention.
	6. Instruct the client to remain in the Sims' position or to lie supine to prevent expulsion of the suppository.
	7. Instruct the client to retain the suppository for at least 30 minutes to allow absorption to occur, unless the suppository is administered to stimulate defecation.

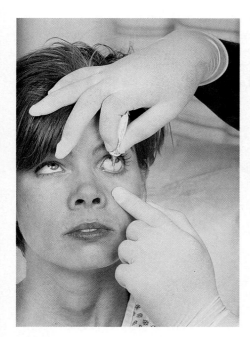 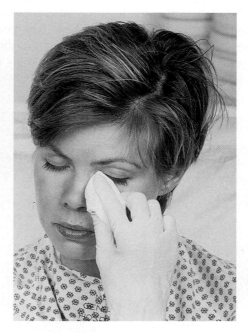

● **Figure 8.3** Ophthalmic administration: (a) instilling an eye ointment into the lower conjunctival sac; (b) pressing on the nasolacrimal duct

Source: © Jenny Thomas Photography.

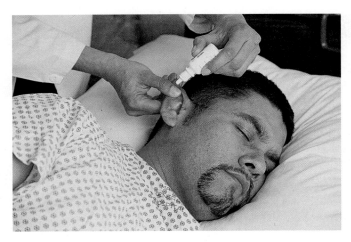

● **Figure 8.4** Position pinna backward and upward when instilling eardrops in adults

Source: © Elena Dorfman.

Otic Administration

The otic route is used to treat local conditions of the ear, including infections and soft blockages of the auditory canal. Otic medications include eardrops and irrigations, which are usually ordered for cleaning purposes. Figure 8.4 illustrates the procedure for otic administration in adults. Administration to infants and young children must be performed carefully to avoid injury to sensitive structures of the ear, as shown in Figure 8.5. Table 8.5 presents key points in administering otic medications.

Nasal Administration

The nasal route is used for both local and systemic drug administration. The nasal mucosa provides an excellent absorptive surface for certain medications. Advantages of this route include ease of use and avoidance of the first-pass effect and digestive enzymes. Nasal spray formulations of corticosteroids have revolutionized the treatment of allergic rhinitis due to their high safety margin when administered by this route.

Although the nasal mucosa provides an excellent surface for drug delivery, there is the potential for damage to the cilia within the nasal cavity, and mucosal irritation is common. In addition, unpredictable mucus secretion among some individuals may affect drug absorption from this site.

Drops or sprays are often used for their local **astringent effect**, which is to shrink swollen mucous membranes or to loosen secretions and facilitate drainage. This brings immediate relief from the nasal congestion caused by the common cold. The nose also provides the route to reach the nasal sinuses and the eustachian tube. Proper positioning of the client prior to instilling nose drops for sinus disorders depends on which sinuses are being treated. The same holds true for treatment of the eustachian tube. Table 8.5 and Figure 8.6 illustrate important points related to nasal drug administration.

Vaginal Administration

The vaginal route is used to deliver medications for treating local infections and to relieve vaginal pain and itching. Vaginal medications are inserted as suppositories, creams, jellies, or foams. It is important that the nurse explain the purpose of treatment and provide for privacy and client dignity. Before inserting vaginal drugs, the nurse should instruct the client to empty her bladder to lessen both the discomfort during treatment and the possibility of irritating or injuring the vaginal lining. The client should be offered a perineal pad following administration. Figure 8.7 illustrates administration of a vaginal suppository and cream. Table 8.5 provides guidelines regarding vaginal drug administration.

Rectal Administration

The rectal route may be used for either local or systemic drug administration. It is a safe and effective means of delivering drugs to clients who are comatose or who are experiencing nausea and vomiting. Rectal drugs are normally in suppository form, although a few laxatives and diagnostic agents are given via enema.

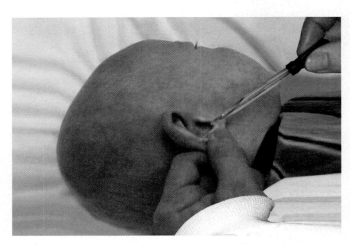

● **Figure 8.5** Position pinna backward and slightly downward when instilling eardrops in children

Source: Shirley King.

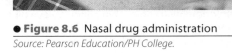

● **Figure 8.6** Nasal drug administration

Source: Pearson Education/PH College.

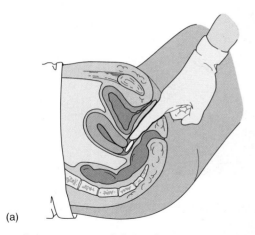 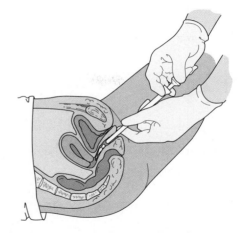

(a)   (b)

● **Figure 8.7** Vaginal drug administration: (a) instilling a vaginal suppository; (b) using an applicator to instill a vaginal cream
Source: Pearson Education/PH College.

Although absorption is slower than by other routes, it is steady and reliable provided the medication can be retained by the client. Venous blood from the lower rectum is not transported by way of the liver; thus, the first-pass effect is avoided, as are the digestive enzymes of the upper GI tract. Table 8.5 gives details regarding rectal suppository administration.

8.8 Parenteral Drug Administration

Parenteral administration refers to the dispensing of medications by routes other than oral or topical. The **parenteral route** delivers drugs via a needle into the skin layers, subcutaneous tissue, muscles, or veins. More advanced parenteral delivery includes administration into arteries, body cavities (such as intrathecal), and organs (such as intracardiac). Parenteral drug administration is much more invasive than topical or enteral. Because of the potential for introducing pathogenic microbes directly into the blood or body tissues, aseptic techniques must be strictly applied. The nurse is expected to identify and use appropriate materials for parenteral drug delivery, including specialized equipment and techniques involved in the preparation and administration of injectable products. The nurse must know the correct anatomical locations for parenteral administration and the safety procedures regarding hazardous equipment disposal.

Intradermal and Subcutaneous Administration

Injection into the skin delivers drugs to the blood vessels that supply the various layers of the skin. Drugs may be injected either intradermally or subcutaneously. The major difference between these methods is the depth of injection. An advantage of both methods is that they offer a means of administering drugs to clients who are unable to take them orally. Drugs administered by these routes avoid the hepatic first-pass effect and digestive enzymes. Disadvantages are that only small volumes can be administered, and injections can cause pain and swelling at the injection site.

An **intradermal (ID)** injection is administered into the dermis layer of the skin, as illustrated in Figure 8.8 on page 78. Because the dermis contains more blood vessels than the deeper subcutaneous layer, drugs are more easily absorbed. This method is usually employed for allergy and disease screening or for local anesthetic delivery prior to venous cannulation. Intradermal injections are limited to very small volumes of drug, usually only 0.1 to 0.2 mL. The usual sites for ID injections are the non-hairy skin surfaces of the upper back, over the scapulae, the high upper chest, and the inner forearm. Guidelines for intradermal injections are provided in Table 8.6 on page 79.

A **subcutaneous (SC)** injection is delivered to the subcutaneous (fatty) tissue. Insulin, heparin, vitamins, some vaccines, and other medications are given in this tissue because it is easily accessible and contains no large blood vessels. Body sites that are ideal for SC injections include the following:

- Outer aspect of the upper arms, in the area above the triceps muscle
- Middle two-thirds of the anterior thigh area
- Subscapular areas of the upper back
- Upper dorsogluteal and ventrogluteal areas
- Abdominal areas, above the iliac crest and below the diaphragm, 4 to 5 cm out from the umbilicus

Subcutaneous doses are small in volume, usually ranging from 0.5 to 1 mL. The needle size varies with the client's quantity of body fat. The length is usually one-half the size of a pinched/bunched skin fold that can be grasped between the thumb and forefinger. It is important to rotate injection sites in an orderly and documented manner to promote absorption, minimize tissue damage, and alleviate discomfort. For insulin, however, rotation should be within an anatomical area to promote reliable absorption and maintain consistent blood glucose levels. Movement from one anatomical area to another should occur in a systematic order in accordance with agency and regional policies. Movement to a new anatomical area will allow previous areas time to rejuvenate.

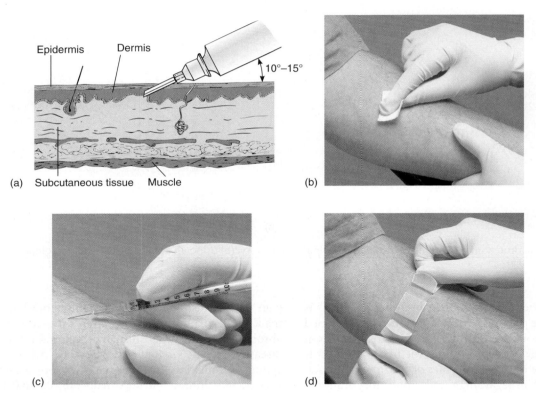

● **Figure 8.8** Intradermal drug administration: (a) cross-section of skin showing depth of needle insertion; (b) the administration site is prepped; (c) the needle is inserted, bevel up, at a 10–15 degree angle; (d) the needle is removed and the puncture site is covered with an adhesive bandage

Source: Pearson Education/PH College.

TABLE 8.6	Parenteral Drug Administration	
Drug Form	**Administration Guidelines**	
intradermal (ID)	1. Prepare medication in a tuberculin or 1 mL syringe, using a 25–27 gauge, 1.0–1.6 cm (3/8–5/8 inch) needle.	
	2. Apply gloves and cleanse injection site with antiseptic swab in a circular motion. Allow to air dry.	
	3. With thumb and index finger of non-dominant hand, spread skin taut.	
	4. Insert needle, with bevel facing upward, at angle of 10–15 degrees.	
	5. Advance needle until entire bevel is under skin; do not aspirate.	
	6. Slowly inject medication to form small wheal or bleb.	
	7. Withdraw needle quickly, and pat site gently with sterile 2 × 2 gauze pad. Do not massage area.	
	8. Instruct the client not to rub or scratch the area.	
subcutaneous route (SC)	1. Prepare medication in a 1–3 mL syringe using a 23–25 gauge, 1.3–1.6 cm (1/2–5/8 inch) needle. For heparin and insulin, the recommended needle is 1 cm (3/8 inch) and 25–27 gauge. Insulin syringes are marked in units and usually have needles already attached.	
	2. Choose site, avoiding areas of bony prominence, major nerves, and blood vessels. For heparin, check with agency policy for the preferred injection sites.	
	3. Check previous rotation sites and select a new area for injection. (Selection of sites for insulin is discussed in Chapter 40.)	
	4. Apply gloves and cleanse injection site with antiseptic swab in a circular motion. Allow to air dry.	
	5. Bunch the skin between thumb and index finger of non-dominant hand or spread taut if there is substantial subcutaneous tissue.	
	6. Insert needle at 45 or 90 degree angle depending on body size and depth of subcutaneous tissue: 90 degrees if obese or average; 45 degrees if underweight. If the client is very thin, gather skin at area of needle insertion and administer at 90 degree angle.	
	7. Aspiration is usually not required for SC injections. If agency policy requires aspiration for non-heparin injections, aspirate by pulling back on plunger. If blood appears, withdraw the needle, discard the syringe, and prepare a new injection. For heparin, do not aspirate as this can damage surrounding tissues and cause bruising.	
	8. Inject medication slowly.	
	9. Remove needle quickly, and gently pat site with antiseptic swab or gauze. For heparin, do not massage the site, as this may cause bruising or bleeding.	

TABLE 8.6	**Parenteral Drug Administration** *(Continued)*
Drug Form	**Administration Guideline**
intramuscular (IM): ventrogluteal site	1. Prepare medication using a 20–23 gauge, 3.8 cm (1.5 inch) needle. 2. Apply gloves and cleanse ventrogluteal injection site with antiseptic swab in a circular motion. Allow to air dry. 3. Locate site by placing the hand with heel on the greater trochanter and thumb toward umbilicus. Point to the anterior iliac spine with the index finger, spreading the middle finger to point toward the iliac crest (forming a V). Injection of medication is given within the V-shaped area of the index and third finger. 4. Insert needle with smooth, dart-like movement at a 90 degree angle within V-shaped area. 5. Aspirate, and observe for blood. If blood appears, withdraw the needle, discard the syringe, and prepare a new injection. 6. Inject medication slowly with smooth, even pressure on the plunger. 7. Remove needle quickly. 8. Apply pressure to site with a dry, sterile 2 × 2 gauze and massage vigorously to create warmth and promote absorption of the medication into the muscle.

intravenous (IV)	1. To add drug to an IV fluid container:
	   a. Verify order and compatibility of drug with IV fluid.
	   b. Prepare medication in a 5–20 mL syringe using a 2.5–3.8 cm (1–1.5 inch), 19–21 gauge needle.
	   c. Locate medication port on IV fluid container and cleanse with antiseptic swab.
	   d. Carefully insert needle or access device into port and inject medication.
	   e. Withdraw needle and mix solution by rotating container end to end.
	   f. Apply gloves and assess injection site for signs and symptoms of inflammation or extravasation.
	   g. Hang container and check infusion rate.
	 2. To add drug to an IV bolus (IV push) using existing IV line or IV lock (reseal):
	   a. Verify order and compatibility of drug with IV fluid.
	   b. Determine the correct rate of infusion.
	   c. Determine if IV fluids are infusing at proper rate (IV line) and that IV site is adequate.
	   d. Prepare drug in a syringe with 25–26 gauge needle.
	   e. Apply gloves and assess injection site for signs and symptoms of inflammation or extravasation.
	   f. Select injection port, on tubing, closest to insertion site (IV line).
	   g. Cleanse tubing or lock port with antiseptic swab and insert needle into port.
	   h. If administering medication through an existing IV line, occlude tubing by pinching just above the injection port.
	   i. Slowly inject medication over designated time, not usually faster than 1 mL/min, unless specified.
	   j. Withdraw syringe. Release tubing and ensure proper IV infusion if using an existing IV line.
	   k. If using an IV lock, check agency policy for use of saline flush before and after injecting medications.

Site preparation should be in accordance with agency policies. Alcohol preparation may be preferred for hygienic reasons in some situations. However, alcohol swabs can be drying and toxic to cells with repeated application, and some clients prefer to cleanse the site with soapy water and rinse with plain water prior to injection. Soap and water and proper site rotation may help to reduce **lipoatrophy**, the damage and scarring of subcutaneous tissue, in diabetic clients. When performing SC injections, it is not necessary to aspirate prior to the injection. Note that tuberculin syringes and insulin syringes are not interchangeable, so the nurse should not substitute one for the other. Table 8.6 and Figure 8.9 provide important information regarding SC drug administration.

Intramuscular Administration

An **intramuscular (IM)** injection delivers medication into specific muscles. Because muscle tissue has a rich blood supply, medication moves quickly into blood vessels to produce a more rapid onset of action than with oral, ID, or SC administration. The anatomical structure of muscle permits this tissue to receive a larger volume of medication than the subcutaneous region. An adult with well-developed muscles can safely tolerate up to 5 mL of medication in a large muscle, although only 2 to 3 mL is recommended. The deltoid and triceps muscles should receive a maximum of 1 mL.

A major consideration for the nurse regarding IM drug administration is the selection of an appropriate injection site. Injection sites must be located away from bone, large blood vessels, and nerves. The size and length of needle are determined by body size and muscle mass, the type of drug to be administered, the amount of adipose tissue overlying the muscle, and the age of the client. Information regarding IM injections is given in Table 8.6 and Figure 8.10. The

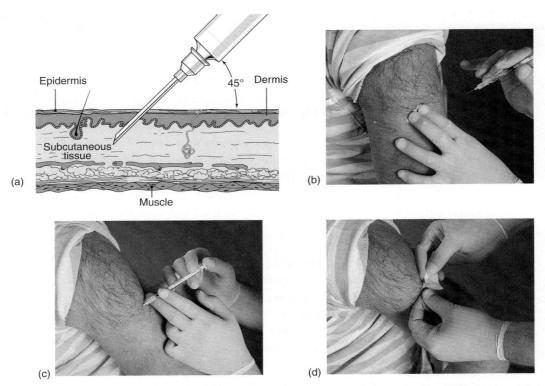

● **Figure 8.9** Subcutaneous drug administration: (a) cross-section of skin showing depth of needle insertion; (b) the administration site is prepped; (c) the needle is inserted, bevel up, at a 45 degree angle; (d) the needle is removed and the puncture site is covered with an adhesive bandage

Source: Pearson Education/PH College.

four common sites for intramuscular injections are as follows:

- Ventrogluteal: This is the preferred site for IM injections. This area provides the greatest thickness of gluteal muscles, contains no large blood vessels or nerves, is sealed off by bone, and contains less fat than the buttock area, thus eliminating the need to determine the depth of subcutaneous fat. It is a suitable site for children and infants over 7 months of age.

- Deltoid: This site is used in adults and well-developed teens for volumes of medication not to exceed 1 mL. Because the radial nerve lies in close proximity, the deltoid is not generally used except for small-volume vaccines, such as hepatitis B in adults.

- Dorsogluteal: This site is used for adults and for children who have been walking for at least 6 months. The site is safe as long as the nurse appropriately locates the injection landmarks to avoid puncture or irritation of the sciatic nerve and blood vessels.

- Vastus lateralis: Usually thick and well developed in both adults and children, the middle third of the muscle is the site for IM injections.

Intravenous Administration Intravenous (IV) medications and fluids are administered directly into the blood-

stream and are immediately available for use by the body. The IV route is used when a very rapid onset of action is desired. Like other parenteral routes, IV medications bypass the enzymatic process of the digestive system and the first-pass effect of the liver. The three basic types of IV administration are as follows:

- Large-volume infusion: This is used for fluid maintenance, replacement, or supplementation. Compatible drugs may be mixed into a large-volume IV container with fluids such as normal saline or Ringer's lactate. Table 8.6 and Figure 8.11 describe and illustrate this technique. Do not add a drug to an IV bag that is already connected to the client and infusing, because concentrated drug may be drawn into the infusion line before being distributed in the solution bag. An IV drug should be added to a full bag of solution, rotated to promote even distribution, and then connected to the client.

- Intermittent infusion: This is a small amount of IV solution that is arranged tandem or piggy-backed to the primary large-volume infusion. It is used to instill adjunct medications, such as antibiotics or analgesics, over a short time period. This is illustrated in Figure 8.12 on page 82.

- IV bolus (push): A concentrated dose is delivered directly to the circulation via syringe. This is used to administer single-dose medications. Bolus injections

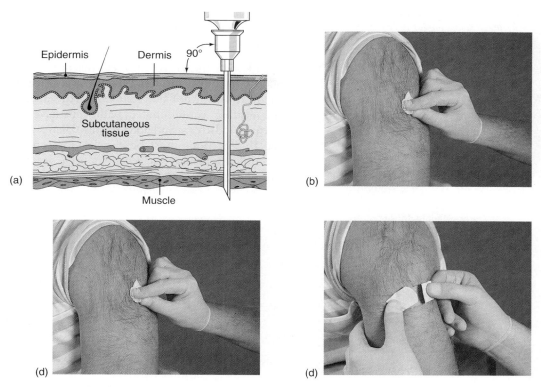

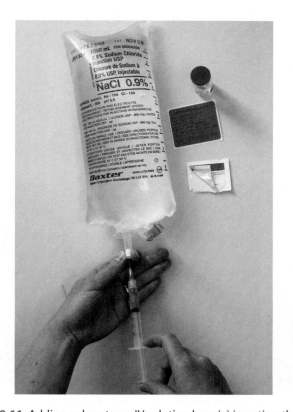

Figure 8.10 Intramuscular drug administration: (a) cross-section of skin showing depth of needle insertion; (b) the administration site is prepped; (c) the needle is inserted at a 90 degree angle; (d) the needle is removed and the puncture site is covered with an adhesive bandage

Source: Pearson Education/PH College.

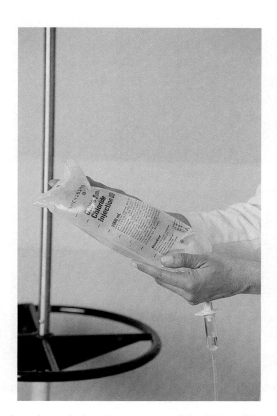

Figure 8.11 Adding a drug to an IV solution bag: (a) inserting the drug through the injection port of the IV bag; (b) rotating the IV bag to distribute the drug

Sources: (left) Shirley L. King; (right) © Elena Dorfman.

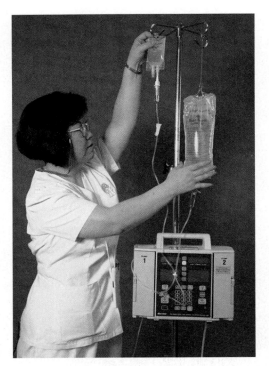

● **Figure 8.12** An intermittent IV infusion given piggy-back to the primary infusion

Source: Pearson Education/PH College.

may be given through an intermittent injection port or by direct IV push. Details on the bolus administration technique are given in Table 8.6 and Figure 8.13.

Although the IV route offers the fastest onset of drug action, it is also the most dangerous. Once injected, the medication cannot be retrieved. If the drug solution or the needle is contaminated, pathogens have a direct route to the bloodstream and body tissues. Clients who are receiving IV injections must be closely monitored for adverse reactions. Some adverse reactions occur immediately after injection; others may take hours or days to appear. Antidotes for drugs that can cause potentially dangerous or fatal reactions must always be readily available.

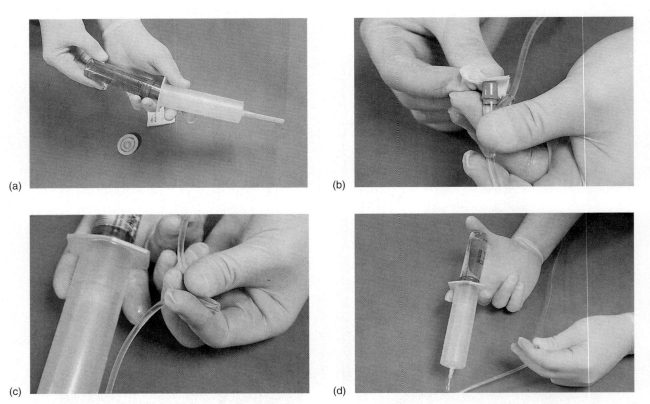

(a) (b) (c) (d)

● **Figure 8.13** Intravenous bolus administration: (a) drug is prepared; (b) administration port is cleaned; (c) line is pinched; (d) drug is administered

Source: Pearson Education/PH College.

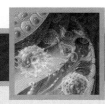

CHAPTER REVIEW

KEY CONCEPTS

The numbered key concepts provide a succinct summary of the important points from the corresponding numbered section within the chapter. If any of these points are not clear, refer to the numbered section within the chapter for review. Expanded versions can be found on the Companion Website.

8.1 The nurse must have comprehensive knowledge of the actions and side effects of drugs before they are administered to limit the number and severity of adverse drugs reactions.

8.2 The seven rights and three checks are guidelines to safe drug administration, which is a collaborative effort among nurses, physicians, and other healthcare professionals.

8.3 For pharmacological adherence, the client must understand and personally accept the value associated with the prescribed drug regimen. Understanding the reasons for non-adherence can help the nurse increase the success of pharmacotherapy.

8.4 There are established orders and time schedules by which medications are routinely administered. Documentation of drug administration and reported side effects are important responsibilities of the nurse.

8.5 Systems of measurement used in pharmacology include the metric, apothecary, and household systems. Although the metric system is most commonly used, the nurse must be able to convert dosages among the three systems of measurement.

8.6 The enteral route includes drugs given orally and those administered through nasogastric or gastrostomy tubes. This is the most common route of drug administration.

8.7 Topical drugs are applied locally to the skin or membranous linings of the eye, ear, nose, respiratory tract, urinary tract, vagina, and rectum.

8.8 Parenteral administration is the dispensing of medications via a needle, usually into the skin layers (ID), subcutaneous tissue (SC), muscles (IM), or veins (IV).

REVIEW QUESTIONS

1 Why is it that errors continue to occur in spite of the fact that the nurse follows the seven rights and three checks of drug administration?

2 What strategies can the nurse employ to promote drug adherence for a client who is refusing to take his or her medication?

3 Compare the oral, topical, IM, SC, and IV routes. Which has the fastest onset of drug action? Which routes avoid the hepatic first-pass effect? Which require strict aseptic technique?

EXPLORE

MediaLink

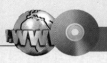

www.pearsoned.ca/adams-king

MEDIALINK DVD-ROM
- **Audio Glossary**
- **CRNE Review**
- **Video:** Epidural Placement
- **Nursing in Action Videos**
  Administering a Nasal Spray
  Administering a Z Track Medication
  Administering an IM Medication
  Administering Dermatologic Medications
  Administering Ear Drops
  Administering Eye Drops
  Administering Medications by Inhaler
  Administering Medications by IV Piggyback
  Administering Medications through a NG Tube
  Administering Medications by IV Push
  Administering Subcutaneous Q Meds
  Administering Subcutaneous Q Meds (Abdomen)

COMPANION WEBSITE
- **CRNE Review**
- **Case Study:** Client taking glyburide
- **Expanded Key Concepts**
- **Challenge Your Knowledge**

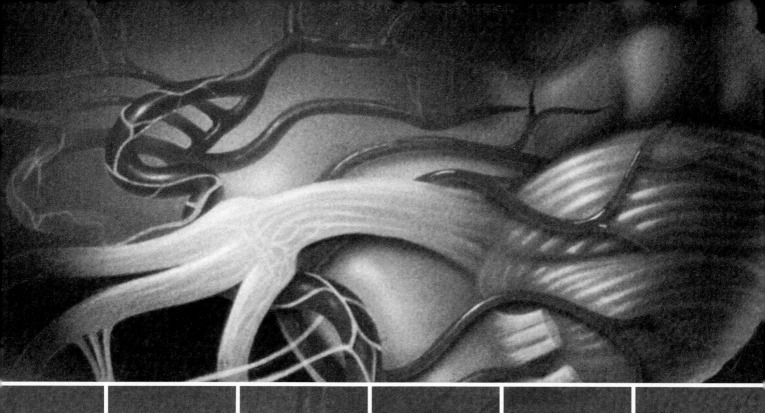

Unit 3 | Professional, Personal, and Cultural Influences in Pharmacotherapy

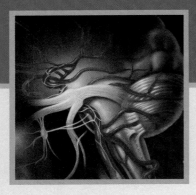

CHAPTER 9

Medication Incidents and Risk Reduction

OBJECTIVES

After reading this chapter, the student should be able to do the following:

1. Explain how the ethical principles contained in the "Code of Ethics for Registered Nurses" by the Canadian Nurses Association (CNA) are used to guide nurses in their practice.
2. Apply general moral principles to the effective administration of medications.
3. Discuss the standards of care in the application of the nursing process.
4. Explain the importance of documentation in the administration of medications.
5. Discuss factors contributing to medication incidents.
6. Identify the process in reporting and managing medication incidents.
7. Describe strategies that the nurse may implement to prevent medication incidents.
8. Describe the role of the nurse in reporting adverse drug reactions (ADRs).
9. Discuss client education that is important for safe medication usage.

MediaLink

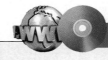

www.pearsoned.ca/adams-king

CRNE review, case studies, and other interactive resources for this chapter can be found on the Companion Website at **www.pearsoned.ca/adams-king**. Click on "Chapter 9" to select the activities for this chapter. For animations, more CRNE review questions, and an audio glossary, access the accompanying MediaLink DVD-ROM in this textbook.

KEY TERMS

adverse drug reaction (ADR)   page 87

beneficence   page 87

ethics   page 89

medication errors   page 87

non-maleficence   page 87

standards of care   page 89

standards of professional practice   page 89

In their clinical practice, nurses are sensitive to the complexities of medication administration and the potential for incidents involving medications to occur. Medication incidents that put clients at risk include medication errors and adverse drug reactions. Although nurses highly value proficiency and strive for 100% accuracy in giving medications, they may inadvertently be involved in an incident that places their client at risk for injury. Doing harm to a client is every nurse's greatest fear. "To do no harm" is the ethical principle of **non-maleficence**, and **beneficence** is the obligation to seek interventions that are beneficial for the client. These two principles guide nursing care in both theory and practice.

9.1 Medication Incidents

Medication incidents that put clients at risk include medication errors and adverse drug reactions. Medication incidents impede pharmacotherapeutic outcomes, increase hospitalization costs, and can result in serious illness or death. An **adverse drug reaction (ADR)** is an undesired and unexpected client response to an administered medication. ADRs can range from rashes to anaphylaxis and death. **Medication errors** are situations where the wrong drug or medication is prescribed or given, the medication is improperly administered, or an incorrect dosage or protocol is used. According to Health Canada, medication errors are the most common single preventable cause of client injury. Medication incidents may lead to litigation against the nurse, physician, pharmacist, or healthcare agency. Medication errors occur even among the most conscientious healthcare professionals.

9.2 National Programs for Monitoring Medication Incidents and Reducing Risk

Health Canada is concerned with medication incidents at the national level. The Canadian Medication Incident Reporting and Prevention System (CMIRPS), funded by Health Canada, is a new national medication incident reporting and prevention system. A number of healthcare and client safety organizations, including the Canadian Patient Safety Institute (CPSI), Institute for Safe Medication Practices Canada (ISMP Canada), Canadian Institute for Health Information (CIHI), Canadian Nurses Association (CNA), Canadian Medical Association (CMA), and Canadian Pharmacists Association (CPhA), helped to develop the system. CMIRPS is aimed at promoting an open, "blame-free," non-punitive system that encourages healthcare practitioners to voluntarily report medication incidents.

CMIRPS categorizes errors using the algorithm (step-by-step process) shown in Figure 9.1. This algorithm was developed by the United States' National Coordinating Council for Medication Error Reporting and Prevention (NCC MERP). Analysis focuses on the extent of harm that an error can cause, as shown in Figure 9.2, and is used to plan strategies to promote safe medication practices and prevent medication errors.

Health Canada's Marketed Health Products Directorate (MHPD) developed the MedEffect program to provide easy, centralized access to current, relevant, and reliable health product safety information. This includes access to Health Canada's advisories, warnings, and recalls; the Canadian Adverse Reaction Newsletter (CARN); and the Canadian Adverse Drug Reaction Monitoring Program (CADRMP).

The MedEffect program aims to increase awareness about the importance of reporting adverse drug reactions to Health Canada and to make it as simple as possible for health professionals and consumers to complete and file ADR reports

MediaLink   Canadian Medication Incident Reporting and Prevention System (CMIRPS)

MediaLink   Institute for Safe Medication Practices Canada (ISMP Canada)

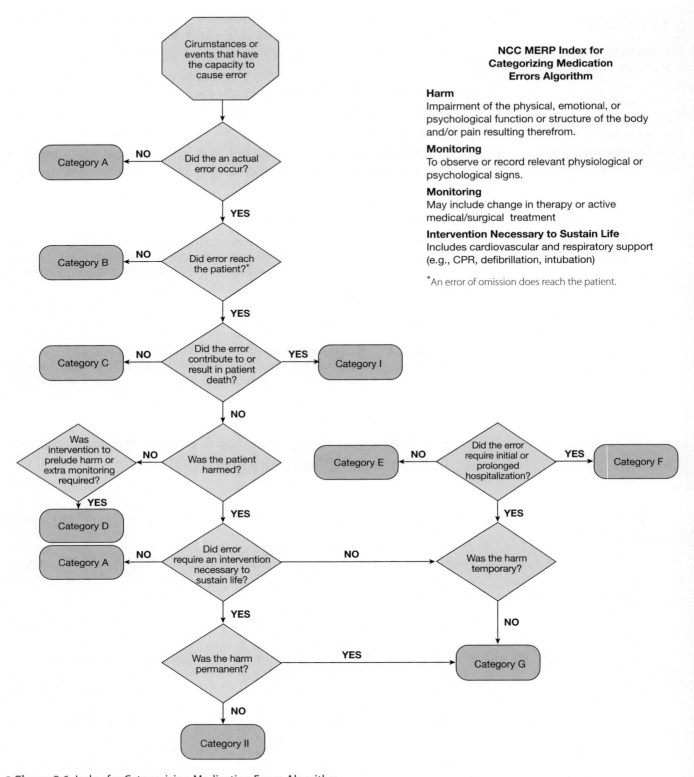

NCC MERP Index for Categorizing Medication Errors Algorithm

Harm
Impairment of the physical, emotional, or psychological function or structure of the body and/or pain resulting therefrom.

Monitoring
To observe or record relevant physiological or psychological signs.

Monitoring
May include change in therapy or active medical/surgical treatment

Intervention Necessary to Sustain Life
Includes cardiovascular and respiratory support (e.g., CPR, defibrillation, intubation)

*An error of omission does reach the patient.

● **Figure 9.1** Index for Categorizing Medication Errors Algorithm

via the Web, phone, fax, or mail. *It is the responsibility of the nurse to become familiar with this program and know how to file an ADR report in the event of an occurrence.* An ADR report should be filed whenever an ADR is suspected; con-firmation of the ADR is not required. The accuracy of available drug information on potentially harmful effects depends on reporting. Sometimes ADR reports result in drugs being removed from the market to protect client safety.

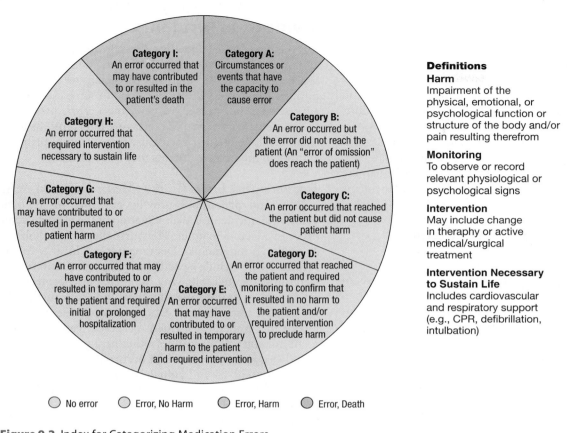

Category I:
An error occurred that may have contributed to or resulted in the patient's death

Category A:
Circumstances or events that have the capacity to cause error

Category H:
An error occurred that required intervention necessary to sustain life

Category B:
An error occurred but the error did not reach the patient (An "error of omission" does reach the patient)

Category G:
An error occurred that may have contributed to or resulted in permanent patient harm

Category C:
An error occurred that reached the patient but did not cause patient harm

Category F:
An error occurred that may have contributed to or resulted in temporary harm to the patient and required initial or prolonged hospitalization

Category E:
An error occurred that may have contributed to or resulted in temporary harm to the patient and required intervention

Category D:
An error occurred that reached the patient and required monitoring to confirm that it resulted in no harm to the patient and/or required intervention to preclude harm

Definitions
Harm
Impairment of the physical, emotional, or psychological function or structure of the body and/or pain resulting therefrom

Monitoring
To observe or record relevant physiological or psychological signs

Intervention
May include change in theraphy or active medical/surgical treatment

Intervention Necessary to Sustain Life
Includes cardiovascular and respiratory support (e.g., CPR, defibrillation, intulbation)

○ No error   ○ Error, No Harm   ○ Error, Harm   ○ Error, Death

● **Figure 9.2** Index for Categorizing Medication Errors

9.3 Ethics and Standards of Nursing Practice

Drug administration is one of the most important responsibilities of the nurse, and one that has obvious ethical and legal connections to nursing practice. Knowledge of applicable codes of **ethics** and standards of practice is essential to provide for client safety.

The Canadian Nurses Association (CNA) published the "Code of Ethics for Registered Nurses" to provide guidance for decision-making concerning ethical matters and a basis for evaluating ethical nursing practice. The code informs nurses, other healthcare professionals, and members of the public about the ethical responsibilities and moral commitments expected of nurses. Because the registered nurse and nursing student are required to practise and administer medications in accordance with the code, they should obtain a current copy of the complete code from the CNA website.

Standards of professional practice specify the skills and learning that are expected to be possessed by members of a profession. Standards of professional practice demonstrate to the public, government, and other stakeholders that a profession is dedicated to maintaining public trust and upholding the criteria of its legal scope of practice.

In nursing, standards of practice are defined and enforced by provincial or territorial regulatory bodies (professional nursing associations). The rule of reasonable and prudent action also defines **standards of care**. This rule defines the standard of care as the actions that a reasonable and prudent nurse with equivalent preparation would do under similar circumstances. The nurse's actions would be legally judged by whether he or she acted within the standards of practice and whether the actions were what a reasonable and prudent nurse would have done when faced with a similar dilemma.

Standards of nursing practice include definition of roles, responsibilities, and practices, part of which includes the safe delivery of medications. Each province and territory has a professional nursing association or regulatory body that establishes, monitors, and enforces standards of professional practice. The professional nurse must be qualified to administer medications as specified in the standards for the particular province or territory in which he or she is working.

Every nurse and student nurse is responsible for consulting their provincial/territorial practice standards prior to implementing care to clients. Nurses are also responsible for regularly reviewing their nursing practice standards for amendments and updates.

MediaLink — Health Canada: MedEffect Canada

MediaLink — Canadian Nurses Association (CNA)

Nurses who practise in clinical agencies need to understand and follow the policies and procedures governing medication administration of the organization in which they practise. These policies and procedures establish the standards of care for that particular hospital or organization, and it is important that nurses adhere to those established policies and procedures. Common errors relate to failing to administer a medication at the prescribed time. For example, an agency policy may identify that it is permissible to give a medication 30 minutes early or 30 minutes late for medications taken four times a day. The standards of care and the agency's policy manual are designed to help the nurse prevent medication incidents and maintain client safety.

9.4 The Impact of Medication Incidents

Medication incidents are the most common cause of morbidity and preventable death within hospitals. When a medication error occurs, the repercussions can be emotionally devastating for the nurse and extend beyond the particular nurse and client involved. A medication error can increase the client's length of stay in the hospital, which increases costs and the time that a client is separated from his or her family. The nurse making the medication error may suffer self-doubt and embarrassment. If a high error rate occurs within a particular unit, the nursing unit may develop a poor reputation within the facility. If frequent medication errors or serious errors are publicized, the reputation of the facility may suffer because it may be perceived as unsafe.

The goal of every healthcare organization should be to improve medication administration systems to prevent harm to clients due to medication incidents. All errors, whether or not they affect the client, should be investigated with the goal of identifying ways to improve the medication administration process to prevent future errors. The investigation should occur in a non-punitive manner that will encourage staff to report errors, thereby building a culture of safety within an organization. An error can alert nurses and healthcare administrators to the fact that a new policy or procedure needs to be implemented to reduce or eliminate medication incidents.

PHARMFACTS

Medication Safety Considerations

- About 30% of adults with health problems in Canada reported that they had experienced a medication error or medical error in the past 2 years. The majority of these people said the error caused serious health consequences.
- Preventable adverse drug events cause about 700 deaths in Canada per year.
- Most medication incidents are preventable.
- Strict adherence to the seven rights of drug administration greatly reduces the chance of error.

9.5 Documenting and Reporting Medication Incidents

It is the nurse's legal and ethical responsibility to document and report all incidents involving medications. The nurse in charge and, in most cases, the physician are immediately notified about a medication incident. In some cases, serious adverse reactions caused by medication errors may require the immediate initiation of life-saving interventions for the client. Following such incidents, intense monitoring and additional medical treatments may be required.

Documenting in the Client's Medical Record Agency policies and procedures provide guidance on reporting medication incidents. Documentation of the incident should occur in a factual manner: The nurse should avoid blaming or making judgments. Documentation in the medical record must include specific nursing interventions that were implemented following the incident to protect client safety, such as monitoring vital signs and assessing the client for possible complications. Documentation does not simply record that a medical incident occurred. Failure to document nursing actions implies either negligence or failure to acknowledge that the incident occurred. The nurse should also document all individuals who were notified of the incident. Incidents that involve a medication that was given in error or that was omitted should also be recorded on the medication administration record (MAR).

Completing a Written Incident Report In addition to documenting in the client's medical record, the nurse who made or discovered the incident should complete a written incident report. The specific details of the incident should be recorded in a factual and objective manner. The incident report provides the nurse an opportunity to identify factors that contributed to the incident. Agency policy specifies whether a copy of the incident report is to be included in the client's medical record.

Accurate documentation in the medical record and the incident report is essential for legal reasons. These documents verify that the client's safety was protected and serve as tools to improve medication administration processes. Legal situations may worsen if there is an attempt to hide a mistake or delay corrective action, or if the nurse forgets to document interventions in the client's chart.

Hospitals and agencies monitor medication incidents through quality improvement programs. The results of quality improvement programs alert staff and administrative personnel about trends within particular units. Through data analyses, specific strategies can be developed to prevent such incidents.

Reporting at the National Level Health Canada requests that nurses and other healthcare providers report medication incidents in order to build an up-to-date database that can be used to develop national strategies to improve medication safety. Medication errors, or situations that can lead to errors, may be reported in confidence directly to Health Canada through CMIRPS or ISMP Canada. Adverse drug reactions can be reported to Health Canada through MedEffect.

9.6 Factors Contributing to Medication Incidents

Safe medication administration involves collaboration between the nurse and the client and between the nurse and other members of the healthcare team. Factors contributing to medication incidents include, but are not limited to, the following:

- Omitting one of the seven rights of drug administration (see Chapter 8). Common errors include giving an incorrect dose, not giving an ordered dose, and giving an unordered drug.

- Failing to perform an agency system check. Both pharmacists and nurses must collaborate on checking the accuracy and appropriateness of drug orders prior to administering drugs to clients.

- Failing to account for client variables such as age, body size, and renal or hepatic function. Nurses should always review recent laboratory data and other information in the client's chart before administering medications, especially those drugs that have a narrow margin of safety.

- Giving medications based on verbal orders or phone orders, which may be misinterpreted or go undocumented. Nurses should remind the prescribing health-care practitioner that medication orders must be in writing before the drug can be administered.

- Giving medications based on an incomplete order or an illegible order, when the nurse is unsure of the correct drug, dosage, or administration method. Incomplete orders should be clarified with the healthcare provider before the medication is administered. Characteristics of orders that improve safety include avoidance of certain abbreviations (Table 9.1) and inclusion of the following:

  - A brief notation of purpose (e.g., for pain)
  - Metric system measurements, except for therapies that use standard units (e.g., insulin or vitamins)
  - Client age and, when appropriate, weight
  - Drug name, exact metric weight or concentration, and dosage form
  - A leading zero preceding a decimal number less than one (e.g., 0.5 mg)
  - Avoidance of abbreviations for drug names (e.g., MOM, HCTZ) and avoidance of Latin directions for use

- Practising under stressful work conditions. The rate of medication errors increases when nurses have high stress levels and when individual nurses are assigned to clients who are the most acutely ill.

Clients, or their home caregivers, may also contribute to medication incidents by doing the following:

- Taking drugs prescribed by several healthcare practitioners without informing those providers about all prescribed medications

TABLE 9.1	Abbreviations to Avoid in Medication Administration	
Abbreviation	**Intended Meaning**	**Common Error**
U	units	Mistaken as a zero or a four (4), resulting in overdose. Also mistaken for "cc" (cubic centimetres) when poorly written.
μg	micrograms	Mistaken for "mg" (milligrams), resulting in an overdose.
q.d.	Latin abbreviation for every day	The period after the "q" has sometimes been mistaken for an "I", and the drug has been given "qid" (four times daily) rather than daily.
q.o.d.	Latin abbreviation for every other day	Misinterpreted as "qd" (daily) or "qid" (four times daily). If the "O" is poorly written, it looks like a period or "I."
SC	subcutaneous	Mistaken as "SL" (sublingual) when poorly written.
t i w	three times a week	Misinterpreted as "three times a day" or "twice a week."
D/C	discharge; also discontinue	Medications have been prematurely discontinued when D/C (intended to mean "discharge") was misinterpreted as "discontinue," because it was followed by a list of drugs.
hs	half strength	Mistaken as the Latin abbreviation "hs" (hour of sleep).
cc	cubic centimetres	Mistaken as "U" (units) when poorly written.
AU, AS, AD	Latin abbreviation for both ears, left ear, right ear	Misinterpreted as the Latin abbreviation "OU" (both eyes), "OS" (left eye), "OD" (right eye).
IU	international unit	Mistaken as IV (intravenous) or 10 (ten).
MS, MS04, MgS04	confused for one another	Can mean morphine sulfate or magnesium sulfate.

Source: © 1998–2006 National Coordinating Council for Medication Error Reporting and Prevention. All Rights Reserved.

- Getting their prescriptions filled at more than one pharmacy
- Not filling or refilling their prescriptions
- Taking medications incorrectly
- Taking medications that may have been left over from a previous illness or prescribed for something else

9.7 Preventing Medication Incidents

What can the nurse do in the clinical setting to prevent medication incidents? The nurse can begin by using the four steps of the nursing process:

1. Assessment: Ask the client about allergies to food or medications, current health concerns, and use of OTC medications and herbal supplements. Ensure that the client is receiving the right dose, at the right time, and by the right route. Assess renal and liver function and check for impairments of other body systems that may affect pharmacotherapy. Identify areas of needed client education with regard to medications.

2. Planning: Minimize factors that contribute to medication errors. Avoid using abbreviations that can be misunderstood, question unclear orders, do not accept verbal orders, and follow specific facility policies and procedures related to medication administration. Have the client restate dosing directions, including the correct dose of medication and the right time to take it. Ask the client to demonstrate an understanding of the goals of therapy.

3. Implementation: Avoid distractions during medication administration if at all possible. When engaged in a medication-related task, focus entirely on the task. Noise, other events, and talking co-workers can distract the nurse's attention and result in a medication error. Practise the rights of medication administration: right client, right time and frequency of administration, right dose, right route of administration, right drug, and right documentation. Keep the following steps in mind as well:

   - Positively verify the identity of each client using two means (i.e., name and birthdate) before administering the medication, according to facility policy and procedures.
   - Use the correct procedures and techniques for all routes of administration. Use sterile materials and aseptic techniques when administering parenteral or eye medications.
   - Calculate medication doses correctly and measure liquid drugs carefully. Some medications, such as heparin, have a narrow safety margin for producing serious adverse effects. When giving these medications, ask a colleague to check the calculations to make certain the dosage is correct. Always double-check pediatric calculations prior to administration.
   - Open medications immediately prior to administering the medication and in the presence of the client.
   - Record the medication on the MAR immediately after administration.
   - Always confirm that the client has swallowed the medication. Never leave the medication at the bedside unless there is a specific order that medications may be left there.
   - Be alert for long-acting oral dosage forms with indicators such as LA, XL, and XR. These tablets or capsules must remain intact for the extended-release feature to be effective. Instruct the client not to crush, chew, or break the medication in half because doing so could cause an overdose.
   - Re-check any medications that the client states "look different" (e.g., different colour, larger pill).

4. Evaluation: Assess the client for expected outcomes and determine if any adverse effects have occurred.

Nurses must be zealous in keeping up-to-date on pharmacotherapeutics and should never administer a medication until they are familiar with its uses, contraindications, interactions, and side effects. There are many venues by which the nurse can obtain updated medication information. Each nursing unit should have current drug references available. Nurses can also call the pharmacy to obtain information about the drug or, if available, look it up on the Internet using reliable sources. Many nurses are now relying on personal digital assistants (PDAs) to provide current information. These devices can be updated daily or weekly by downloading information, so the information is always current. PDAs have the advantage of being portable for easy access right at the bedside or point of care. Nurses need to familiarize themselves with research on preventing medical errors to maintain evidence-based practice skills.

LIFESPAN CONSIDERATIONS

Issues in Medication Safety and Risk Reduction

Children

Children are vulnerable to medication incidents because they receive medication dosages based on weight (which increases the possibility of dosage miscalculations) and the therapeutic dosages are much smaller.

- Always double-check calculations for pediatric clients with another nurse.
- Medications may need to be crushed or administered in a liquid form.
- Medications can have idiosyncratic effects on pediatric clients.
- Keep medications out of reach and use child-safe tops on medication containers.

Older Adults

Almost half of fatal medication errors occur in clients older than 60 years. There is an increase in the risk for errors in older adults because they often take multiple medications, have numerous healthcare providers, and may have normal age-related changes in pharmacokinetics.

- Be alert for individual responses to pharmacotherapy and assess laboratory reports.
- Complete a thorough medication history on admission.
- Provide written and oral instructions on discharge.

Nurses have a collaborative role to play in improving systems for managing medications in their practice settings. For example, nurses may make recommendations for improving lighting in a medication preparation area or for stocking and storing medications. Modifications to policies and procedures may be recommended. Nurses may advocate for use of modern technologies that could improve client safety, such as the use of automated, computerized, locked cabinets for medication storage; in this system, each nurse on the unit has a code for accessing the cabinet and removing a medication dose. These automated systems maintain an inventory of drug supplies. Nurses may seek opportunities to become involved in committees that focus on examining and reducing risk of medication incidents.

9.8 Providing Client Education for Safe Medication Usage

An essential strategy for avoiding medication errors is to educate the client. Provide age-appropriate handouts and audiovisual teaching aids about the medication, and provide contact information about whom to notify in the event of an adverse reaction. Teach clients to do the following:

- Keep a lifetime record of all medications and natural health products taken.
- Carry a list of all medications they are currently taking, including prescribed drugs, OTC drugs, dietary supplements, and herbals.
- Know the names of all medications they are currently taking, their uses, when they should be taken, and the doses.
- Know what side effects need to be reported immediately.
- Read the label prior to each drug administration.
- Use the measuring device that comes with liquid medications rather than using household measuring spoons.
- Do not use expired medications.
- Wear a MedicAlert bracelet for allergies and health conditions.
- Use one pharmacy for all prescriptions because the pharmacist is able to identify interactions and provide information about scheduling doses.
- Keep contact information for the nearest poison control centre accessible.
- Ask questions. Healthcare providers want to be partners in maintaining client safety with respect to medications.

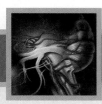

CHAPTER REVIEW

KEY CONCEPTS

The numbered key concepts provide a succinct summary of the important points from the corresponding numbered section within the chapter. If any of these points are not clear, refer to the numbered section within the chapter for review. Expanded versions can be found on the Companion Website.

9.1 Medication incidents that put clients at risk include medication errors and adverse drug reactions. Medication incidents impede pharmacotherapeutic outcomes, increase hospitalization costs, and can result in serious illness or death.

9.2 Health Canada has two programs aimed at monitoring and reducing risk of medication incidents. Medication errors should be reported to the Canadian Medication Incident Reporting and Prevention System (CMIRPS). Adverse drug reactions should be reported to MedEffect. Both programs provide easy online reporting.

9.3 Standards of nursing practice include definition of roles, responsibilities, and practices relating to the safe delivery of medications.

9.4 Medication errors affect client morbidity, mortality, and length of hospital stay. Nurses must be vigilant to prevent errors and protect clients.

9.5 Nurses are legally and ethically responsible for reporting medication errors—whether or not they cause harm to a client—to the physician and for documenting them in the client's medical record and the incident report.

9.6 Numerous factors contribute to medication errors, including failing to adhere to the seven rights of drug administration, failing to follow agency procedures or consider client variables, giving medications based on verbal orders, not confirming orders that are illegible or incomplete, and working under stressful conditions.

9.7 Nurses can reduce medication incidents by adhering to the steps of the nursing process, by knowing common types of medication errors and strategies for their prevention, and by keeping up-to-date on pharmacotherapeutics.

9.8 Client teaching includes providing age-appropriate medication handouts and encouraging clients to keep a list of all prescribed medications, OTC drugs, herbal therapies, and vitamins they are taking and to report them to all healthcare providers.

REVIEW QUESTIONS

1 What are standards of care? How do they relate to the regulation of nursing practice?

2 Discuss the CNA's Code of Ethics for Registered Nurses and its relationship to the administration of medications.

3 Explain the medical and legal responsibilities of the nurse in documenting medication incidents.

4 What strategies can the nurse use to prevent medication incidents?

CRITICAL THINKING QUESTIONS

1. A registered nurse is assigned a group of eight clients. Six of these clients have medications scheduled for once-a-day dosing at 10 AM. Explain how this nurse will be able to administer these drugs to the clients at the "right time."

2. A healthcare provider writes an order for Tylenol #3 PO q3–4 for mild pain. The nurse evaluates this order and is concerned that it is incomplete. Discuss the probable concern and describe what the nurse should do prior to administering this drug.

3. Advanced nurse practitioners have achieved prescriptive authority in several healthcare regions. Describe the process that would be required to obtain prescriptive authority in your province or territory.

4. A new nurse does not check an antibiotic dosage ordered by a healthcare provider on a pediatric unit. The nurse subsequently overdoses a 2-year-old client before an experienced nurse notices the error during the shift change. Who is responsible for the error? Who should report the incident? If you were the nurse responsible for the error, how would you respond when you became aware of it? Who could you consult to discuss your concerns and get advice about how to manage the situation?

EXPLORE
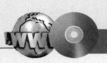
MediaLink

 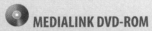 www.pearsoned.ca/adam-king

MEDIALINK DVD-ROM
- **Audio Glossary**
- **CRNE Review**

COMPANION WEBSITE
- **CRNE Review**
- **Case Study:** Documentation of medication administration

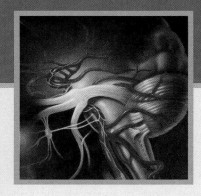

CHAPTER 10

Psychosocial and Cultural Influences on Pharmacotherapy

OBJECTIVES

After reading this chapter, the student should be able to do the following:

1. Describe fundamental concepts underlying a holistic approach to pharmacotherapy.
2. Describe the components of the human integration pyramid model.
3. Identify psychosocial and spiritual factors that can impact pharmacotherapeutics.
4. Explain how ethnicity can affect pharmacotherapeutic outcomes.
5. Identify examples of how cultural values and beliefs can influence pharmacotherapeutic outcomes.
6. Explain how community and environmental factors can affect pharmacotherapeutic outcomes.
7. Convey how genetic polymorphisms can influence pharmacotherapy.
8. Relate the implications of gender to the actions of certain drugs.

MediaLink

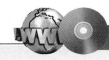

www.pearsoned.ca/adams-king

CRNE review, case studies, and other interactive resources for this chapter can be found on the Companion Website at **www.pearsoned.ca/adams-king**. Click on "Chapter 10" to select the activities for this chapter. For animations, more CRNE review questions, and an audio glossary, access the accompanying MediaLink DVD-ROM in this textbook.

MediaLink   Healthy People 2010

t is convenient for a nurse to learn an average drug dose, administer the medication, and expect all clients to achieve the same outcomes. Unfortunately, this is rarely the case. For pharmacotherapy to be successful, the needs of each individual client must be assessed and evaluated. In Chapter 4, variables such as absorption, metabolism, plasma protein binding, and excretion were examined in an attempt to explain how these modify client responses to drugs. In Chapter 5, variability among client responses was explained in terms of differences in drug-receptor interactions. Chapter 6 examined how these pharmacokinetic and pharmacodynamic factors change client responses to drugs throughout the lifespan. This chapter examines additional psychological, social, and biological variables that must be considered for optimum pharmacotherapy.

10.1 The Concept of Holistic Pharmacotherapy

To deliver the highest quality of care, the nurse must fully recognize the individuality and totality of the client. Each person must be viewed holistically as an integrated biological, psychosocial, cultural, spiritual, communicating whole, existing and functioning within the environment. This approach helps to better understand how risk factors such as age, genetics, biological characteristics, personal habits, lifestyle, and environment increase a person's likelihood of acquiring specific diseases and influence pharmacotherapeutic outcomes.

The human integration pyramid, shown in Figure 10.1, is a model of six categories that compartmentalize the functional environment in which human beings exist, while maintaining an interrelated connection between them. This representation provides a useful approach to addressing the nursing and pharmacological needs of clients within the collaborative practices of healthcare delivery. Where appropriate, concepts illustrated in the pyramid will be presented throughout this book as they relate to the various drug categories. All levels of the pyramid are important and connected: some are specific to certain drug classes and nursing activities, whereas others apply more diversely across the nursing-pharmacology spectrum.

By its very nature, modern (Western) medicine as it is practised in Canada is seemingly incompatible with **holistic** medicine. Western medicine focuses on specific diseases, their causes, and treatments. Disease is viewed as a malfunction of a specific organ or system. Sometimes, the disease is viewed even more specifically and is categorized as a change in DNA structure or a malfunction of one enzyme. Sophisticated technology is used to image and classify the specific structural or functional abnormality. Somehow, the total client is lost in this focus of categorizing disease. Too often, it does not matter how or why the client developed cancer, diabetes, or hypertension, or how they feel about it; the psychosocial and cultural dimensions are lost. Yet these dimensions can profoundly impact the success of pharmacotherapy. The nurse must consciously direct care toward a holistic treatment of each individual client, in his or her psychosocial, spiritual, and social context.

10.2 Psychosocial Influences on Pharmacotherapy

Whereas science and medicine are founded on objective, logical, critical deliberation, psychology and sociology are based more on intuitive and subjective considerations. **Psychology** is the science that deals with normal and abnormal mental processes and their impact on behaviour. **Sociology** studies human behaviour within the context of groups and societies. **Spirituality** incorporates the capacity to love, to convey compassion and empathy, to give and forgive, to enjoy life, and to find peace of mind and fulfillment in living. The spiritual life

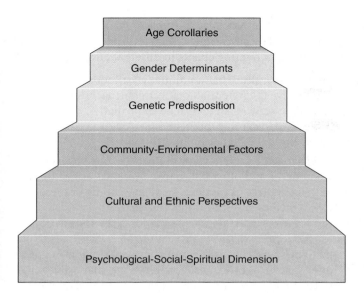

Age Corollaries

Gender Determinants

Genetic Predisposition

Community-Environmental Factors

Cultural and Ethnic Perspectives

Psychological-Social-Spiritual Dimension

● **Figure 10.1** The human integration pyramid care model

SPECIAL CONSIDERATIONS

Alcoholism: Cultural and Environmental Influences

Alcoholism is considered a disease with both social and biological components. It clearly has a genetic basis that sensitizes some individuals to the action of ethanol. It also is known to develop in individuals who are exposed, from an early age, to situations where drinking is considered socially acceptable. It is supported by cultural customs, poverty, traumatic experiences, and other environmental factors. The nurse is often the key healthcare professional who is trained to identify these factors during client assessment and to refer the client to the proper health or social agency for assistance. The condition must be considered and treated in a holistic and compassionate manner if the problem is to be controlled.

overlaps with components of the emotional, mental, physical, and social aspects of living.

From a healthcare perspective, every human being should be considered as an integrated psychological, social, and spiritual being. Health impairments related to an individual's psychosocial situation often require a blending of individualized nursing care and therapeutic drugs, in conjunction with psychotherapeutic counselling. The term *psycho-social-spiritual* is appearing more frequently in nursing literature. It is now acknowledged that when clients have strong spiritual or religious beliefs, these may greatly influence their perceptions of illness and their preferred modes of treatment. In many situations, these beliefs have a strong bearing on pharmacotherapy. When illness imposes threats to health, the client commonly presents with psychological, social, and spiritual issues along with physical symptoms. Clients face concerns related to ill health, suffering, loneliness, despair, and death and at the same time look for meaning, value, and hope in their situation. Such issues can have a great impact on wellness and preferred methods of medical treatment, nursing care, and pharmacotherapy.

The client's psychosocial history is an essential component of the initial client interview and assessment. This history delves into the personal life of the client, with inquiries directed toward lifestyle preferences, religious beliefs, sexual practices, alcohol intake, and tobacco and non-prescription drug use. The nurse must show extreme sensitivity when gathering the data. If a trusting nurse-client relationship is not quickly established, the client will be reluctant to share important personal data that could affect nursing care.

The psychological dimension can exert a strong influence on pharmacotherapy. Clients who are convinced that their treatment is important and beneficial to their well-being will demonstrate better compliance with drug therapy. The nurse must ascertain the client's goals in seeking treatment and determine whether drug therapy is compatible with those goals. Past experiences with healthcare may lead a client to distrust medications. Drugs may not be acceptable for the social environment of the client. For example, having to take drugs at school or in the workplace may cause embarrassment; clients may fear that they will be viewed as weak, unhealthy, or dependent.

Clients who display positive attitudes toward their personal health and have high expectations regarding the results of their pharmacotherapy are more likely to achieve positive outcomes. The nurse plays a pivotal role in encouraging the client's positive expectations. The nurse must always be forthright in explaining drug actions and potential side effects. Trivializing the limitations of pharmacotherapy or minimizing potential adverse effects can cause the client to have unrealistic expectations regarding treatment. The nurse-client relationship may be jeopardized, and the client may acquire an attitude of distrust.

10.3 Cultural and Ethnic Influences on Pharmacotherapy

Despite the apparent diverse cultural and ethnic differences among humans, we are, indeed, one species. It has been estimated that all humans share 99.8% of the same DNA sequences. The remaining 0.2% of the sequences that differ is shared among peoples with similar historic and geographic heritage.

SPECIAL CONSIDERATIONS

Religious Affiliation and Disease Incidence

Religious affiliation is correlated with a reduction in the incidence of some diseases such as cancer and coronary artery disease. Religious and spiritual factors often figure into important decisions for clients facing terminal illness and death, for example, the employment of advance directives such as the living will and the durable power of attorney for healthcare. Considerations of the meaning, purpose, and value of human life are used to make choices about the desirability of cardiopulmonary resuscitation (CPR) and aggressive life support and whether and when to forgo life support and accept death as appropriate and natural under the circumstances.

PHARMFACTS

Ethnic Considerations

- Canada is one of the most ethnically diverse nations in the world, with more than 200 different ethnic origins reported in the 2001 Census.
- In 2001, visible minorities (persons, other than Aboriginal Peoples, who are non-Caucasian in race or non-white in colour) accounted for 13% of the total population.
- In 2001, Aboriginal Peoples accounted for 3.4% of the total population. Of this total, 62% were North American Indian, 30% were Métis, and 5% were Inuit.

Source: Statistics Canada, 2001 Census of Population, www12.statcan.ca/.

An **ethnic** group is a community of people having a common history and similar genetic heritage. Members of an ethnic group share distinctive social and cultural traditions, which are maintained from generation to generation. These beliefs include a shared perception of health and illness.

Culture is a set of beliefs, values, religious rituals, and customs shared by a group of people. In some respects, culture and ethnicity are similar, and many people use the words interchangeably. Ethnicity more often is used to refer to biological and genetic similarities. For example, many African Canadians have adopted the cultural norms of European Canadians. Others have kept some of their African cultural traditions and beliefs that have been passed on from generation to generation. As a group, however, all African Canadians share genetic similarities to people living in Africa today and thus are considered as belonging to the same ethnic group.

Culture can be a dominant force influencing the relationship between the client and the nurse. The practitioner-client relationship is a cross-cultural encounter, with the client bringing religious and ideological beliefs that may challenge or conflict with what the healthcare provider believes to be in the best interests of the client. The client's definition of illness is, in fact, often based on cultural beliefs and values. It is also important to remember that diversity not only exists *between* different cultures but also *within* individual cultures. Examples include differences between age groups or between genders within a given culture.

Cultural sensitivity must be demonstrated by the nurse during the initial phase of the nursing process, when the nurse and client first meet and culturally specific information is obtained during the medical history. Cultural competence requires knowledge of the values, beliefs, and practices of various peoples, along with an attitude of awareness, openness, and sensitivity. Understanding and respecting the beliefs of the client are key to establishing and maintaining a positive therapeutic relationship that culminates in culturally sensitive nursing care. Therapeutic communication mandates that all healthcare providers bear in mind the cultural, racial, and social factors that make up each person and how these impact behaviour. Failure to take these beliefs seriously can undermine the client's ability to trust the nurse and may even persuade some clients to avoid seeking medical care when it is needed.

Culture and ethnicity can impact pharmacotherapy in many ways. The nurse must keep in mind the following variables when treating clients in different ethnic groups:

- Diet: Every culture has a unique set of foods and spices, which have the potential to affect pharmacotherapy. For example, some Asian diets tend to be high in carbohydrates and lower in protein and fat. African Canadian diets tend to be higher in lipid content.

- Alternative therapies: Many cultural groups believe in using herbs and other alternative therapies either along with or in place of modern medicines. Some of these folk remedies and traditional treatments have existed for thousands of years and helped to form the foundation for modern medical practice. Some Chinese clients may go to herbalists to treat their illnesses. Aboriginal Peoples often take great care in collecting, storing, and using herbs to treat and prevent disease. Certain cultures use spices and herbs to maintain a balance of hot and cold, which is thought to promote wellness. Therapeutic massage, heat, and tea infusions are used by many cultures. The nurse needs to interpret how these herbal and alternative therapies will impact the desired pharmacotherapeutic outcomes.

- Beliefs of health and disease: Each culture has distinct ways to view sickness and health. Some individuals seek the assistance of people in their community who they believe are blessed with healing powers. First Nations may seek help from a tribal medicine man. Some African Canadians may know of neighbours who have gifts of healing through the laying on of hands. Clients may place great trust in these alternative healers. Culturally sensitive care respects the local knowledge, values, and wisdom of ethnic minority peoples.

- Genetic differences: With the advent of DNA sequencing, hundreds of structural variants in metabolic enzymes have been discovered. Some of these appear more frequently in certain ethnic groups and have an impact on pharmacotherapeutics, as discussed in Section 10.5.

10.4 Community and Environmental Influences on Pharmacotherapy

A number of community and environmental factors have been identified that influence disease and its subsequent treatment. Population growth, complex technological advances, and evolving globalization patterns have all affected healthcare. Communities vary significantly with regard to urbanization, age distribution, socioeconomic status, occupational pattern, and industrial growth. All of these have the potential to affect health and access to pharmacotherapy.

Access to healthcare is perhaps the most obvious community-related influence on pharmacotherapy. There are many potential obstacles to obtaining appropriate healthcare. Without an adequate prescription drug plan, some people on limited incomes are reluctant to seek healthcare for fear the cost of prescription drugs may be too high. Older adults may fear losing their retirement savings or being placed in a nursing home for the remainder of their lives. Families living in rural areas may have to travel great distances to obtain necessary treatment. The nurse must be aware of these variables and have knowledge of agencies in the local community that can assist in improving healthcare access.

Literacy is another community-related variable that can affect healthcare. The 2003 Adult Literacy and Life Skills Survey (ALL Survey) measured the literacy skills of adults in seven countries, including Canada, and found that 4 in 10 Canadian adults lack the literacy skills that are desired for a knowledge-based economy. Canada's Aboriginal population has even lower literacy rates, and 22% of adult Canadians have serious problems dealing with printed materials. People who do not have access to computers also have significantly lower literacy skills than computer users. The functional illiteracy rate is higher in non-English-speaking individuals and older adults. The nurse must be aware that these clients may not be able to read drug labels, understand written treatment instructions, or read brochures describing their disease or therapy. Functional illiteracy can result in a lack of understanding about the importance of pharmacotherapy and lead to poor compliance. The nurse must attempt to identify clients with low literacy and provide them with brochures, instructions, and educational materials that can be understood. For non-English-speaking clients or those for whom English is their second language, the nurse should have proper materials in the client's primary language or should provide an interpreter who can help with accurate interpretation. The nurse should ask the client to repeat important instructions, to ensure comprehension. The use of more graphical materials is appropriate for certain therapies.

For many clients, belief in a higher spiritual being is important to wellness, and prayer may be an essential component of daily life. When serious illness occurs, or when death is imminent, clients may find comfort and support from religious rituals and artifacts. For these clients, the nurse should provide proper spiritual support. The nurse may want to provide information on local ministers, priests, or rabbis who visit the hospital on a regular basis. Spiritual guidance may provide clients with positive expectations regarding their health and may improve compliance.

10.5 Genetic Influences on Pharmacotherapy

Although humans are 99.8% alike in their DNA sequences, the remaining 0.2% may result in significant differences in clients' ability to metabolize medications. These differences are created when a mutation occurs in the gene (portion of DNA) responsible for encoding a certain metabolic enzyme. A single base mutation in DNA may result in an amino acid change in the enzyme, which changes its function. Hundreds of such mutations have been identified. These changes in enzyme structure and function are called **genetic polymorphisms**. The change may result in either increased or decreased drug metabolism depending on the exact type of genetic polymorphism. The study of these polymorphisms is called pharmacogenetics.

Genetic polymorphisms are most often identified in specific ethnic groups because people of an ethnic group have been located in the same geographic area and have married others within the same ethnic group for many generations. This allows the genetic polymorphism to be amplified within that population.

The relationship between genetic factors and drug response has been documented for decades. The first polymorphism was discovered in the enzyme acetyltransferase, which metabolizes isoniazid (INH). The metabolic process, known as acetylation, occurs slowly in certain Caucasians. The slow clearance can cause the drug to build up to toxic levels in these clients, who are known as slow acetylators. The opposite effect, fast acetylation, is found in many Japanese people.

In recent years, several other enzyme polymorphisms have been identified. People of Asian descent are less likely to be able to metabolically convert codeine to morphine due to an inherent absence of the enzyme debrisoquine hydroxylase, a defect that interferes with the analgesic properties of codeine. In another example, some persons of African descent receive decreased effects from beta-adrenergic antagonist drugs such as propranolol due to genetically influenced variances in plasma renin levels. A set of oxidation enzyme polymorphisms have been found that alter the response to warfarin, diazepam, and several other medications. Table 10.1 summarizes the three most common polymorphisms. Expanding knowledge about the physiological impact of heredity on pharmacological treatment may

TABLE 10.1   Enzyme Polymorphisms of Importance to Pharmacotherapy

Enzyme	Result of Polymorphism	Drugs Using This Metabolic Enzyme/Pathway
acetyltransferase	slow acetylation in Scandinavians, Jews, North African Caucasians fast acetylation in Japanese	isoniazid, chlordiazepam, hydralazine, procainamide, caffeine
debrisoquine hydroxylase	poor metabolization in Asians and Africans	imipramine, perphenazine, haloperidol, propranolol, metoprolol, codeine, morphine
mephenytoin hydroxylase	poor metabolization in Asians and Africans	diazepam, imipramine, barbiturates, warfarin

someday allow for personalization of the drug treatment process.

10.6 Gender Influences on Pharmacotherapy

A person's gender influences many aspects of health maintenance, promotion, and treatment, as well as drug response. It is a substantiated fact, for example, that women pay more attention to changes in health patterns and seek healthcare earlier than their male counterparts. Conversely, many women do not seek medical attention for potential cardiac problems because heart disease is considered to be a "man's disease." Alzheimer's disease affects both men and women, but studies in various populations have shown that between 1.5 and 3 times as many women as men suffer from the disease. Alzheimer's disease is becoming recognized as a major "women's health issue," comparable to osteoporosis, breast cancer, and fertility disorders.

Acceptance or rejection of the use of particular categories of medication may be gender based. Because of the side effects associated with certain medications, some clients do not take them appropriately—or take them at all. A common example is the use of certain antihypertensive agents in men. These may cause, as a common side effect, male impotence. In certain instances, male clients have suffered a stroke because they abruptly stopped taking the drug and did not communicate this fact to their healthcare provider.

With open communication, dilemmas regarding drug problems and side effects can be brought into the open so that alternative drug therapies can be considered. As with so many areas of healthcare, appropriate client teaching by the nurse is a key aspect in preventing or alleviating pharmacological-related health problems.

Local and systemic responses to some medications can differ between genders. These response differences may be based on differences in body composition such as the fat-to-muscle ratio. In addition, cerebral blood flow variances between males and females may alter the response to certain analgesics. Some of the benzodiazepines used for anxiety have slower elimination rates in women, and this difference becomes even more significant if the woman is concurrently taking oral contraceptives. There are numerous gender-related situations that the nurse must understand in order to monitor drug actions and effects appropriately.

Until recently, the vast majority of drug research studies were conducted using only male subjects. It was wrongly assumed that the conclusions of these studies applied in the same manner to females. In the late 1990s, Health Canada formalized policies that require the inclusion of subjects of both genders during development of drugs intended for use by both genders. This includes analyses of clinical data by gender, assessment of potential pharmacokinetic and pharmacodynamic differences between genders, and, where appropriate, conducting additional studies specific to women's health.

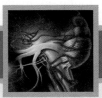

CHAPTER REVIEW

KEY CONCEPTS

The numbered key concepts provide a succinct summary of the important points from the corresponding numbered section within the chapter. If any of these points are not clear, refer to the numbered section within the chapter for review. Expanded versions can be found on the Companion Website.

10.1 To deliver holistic treatment, the nurse must consider the client's psychosocial and spiritual needs in a social context.

10.2 The psychosocial domain must be considered when taking client medical histories. Positive attitudes and high expectations toward therapeutic outcomes in the client may increase the success of pharmacotherapy.

10.3 Culture and ethnicity are two interconnected factors that can impact nursing care and pharmacotherapy. Differences in diet, use of alternative therapies, perceptions of wellness, and genetic makeup can influence client drug response.

10.4 Community and environmental factors affect health and impact the public's access to healthcare and pharmacotherapy. Inadequate access to healthcare resources and an inability to read or understand instructions may negatively impact treatment outcomes.

10.5 Genetic differences in metabolic enzymes that occur among different ethnic groups must be considered for effective pharmacotherapy. Small differences in the structure of enzymes can result in profound changes in drug metabolism.

10.6 Gender can influence many aspects of health maintenance, promotion, and treatment, as well as medication response.

REVIEW QUESTIONS

1 Give examples of how cultural beliefs can influence a client's symptoms.

2 What are three features of culturally sensitive care?

3 What influence can the nurse's own culture or cultural-ethnic background have on the attitudes toward the use of prescription drugs and alcohol?

4 Why is a particular enzyme polymorphism seen more frequently in one ethnic group versus another?

CRITICAL THINKING QUESTIONS

1. A 72-year-old African Canadian client, who has been treated for a heart condition and atrial flutter, is taking warfarin sodium (Coumadin) 2.5 mg PO once a day. He comes to the outpatient clinic for his routine international normalized ratio (INR), which is no longer in the therapeutic range. The client lives in a rural area and grows vegetables. What questions would a nurse need to ask in order to evaluate the cause of the decreased drug effectiveness?

2. An 82-year-old female client is admitted to the emergency department. She has been taking furosemide (Lasix) 40 mg PO daily as part of a regimen for congestive heart failure. She is confused and dehydrated. What gender-related considerations should the nurse be aware of when assessing this client?

3. A 19-year-old Inuit male presents to a northern nursing outpost clinic. He describes severe pain in his lower jaw. An assessment reveals two abscessed molars and other oral health problems. Discuss the probable reasons for this client's condition. Discuss cultural factors that should be considered in planning care and teaching for this client.

EXPLORE
MediaLink

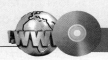 www.pearsoned.ca/adams-king

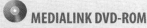 **MEDIALINK DVD-ROM**
- **Audio Glossary**
- **CRNE Review**

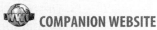 **COMPANION WEBSITE**
- **CRNE Review**
- **Case Study:** Cultural and ethnic influences

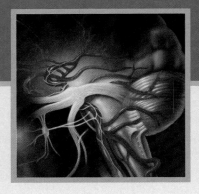

CHAPTER 11

Natural Health Products and Alternative Therapies

OBJECTIVES

After reading this chapter, the student should be able to do the following:

1. Explain the role of complementary and alternative medicine in client wellness.
2. Discuss reasons why herbal and dietary supplements have increased in popularity.
3. Identify the parts of an herb that may contain active ingredients and the types of formulations made from these parts.
4. Discuss the regulatory process for natural health products licensed for sale in Canada.
5. Describe some adverse effects that may be caused by herbal preparations.
6. Discuss the role of the nurse in teaching clients about complementary and alternative therapies.
7. Identify common drug-herbal interactions.

MediaLink

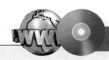

www.pearsoned.ca/adams-king

CRNE review, case studies, and other interactive resources for this chapter can be found on the Companion Website at **www.pearsoned.ca/adams-king**. Click on "Chapter 11" to select the activities for this chapter. For animations, more CRNE review questions, and an audio glossary, access the accompanying MediaLink DVD-ROM in this textbook.

Natural therapies, including herbal products, are increasingly used by Canadians. Despite the fact that these therapies have not been subjected to the same scientific scrutiny as prescription medications, consumers have turned to these treatments for a variety of reasons. Many people have the impression that natural substances have more healing power than synthetic medications. This impression and the ready availability of herbal products at a reasonable cost have convinced many consumers to try them. This chapter examines the role of complementary and alternative therapies in the prevention and treatment of disease.

11.1 Complementary and Alternative Therapies

Complementary and alternative medicine (CAM) comprises an extremely diverse set of therapies and healing systems that are considered to be outside mainstream healthcare. Although diverse, the major CAM systems have the following common characteristics:

- Focus on treating each person as an individual
- Consider the health of the whole person
- Integrate mind and body
- Promote disease prevention, self-care, and self-healing
- Acknowledge the role of spirituality in health and healing

Because of its popularity, considerable attention is now being focused on the effectiveness, or lack of effectiveness, of CAM. Although research into these alternative systems is beginning to appear worldwide, few CAM therapies have been subjected to rigorous clinical and scientific study. It is likely that some of these therapies will be found ineffective, while others will become mainstream treatments. The line between what is defined as an alternative therapy and what is considered mainstream is constantly changing. Increasing numbers of healthcare providers are now accepting CAM therapies and recommending them to their clients. Table 11.1 lists many of these therapies.

Nurses have long known the value of CAM therapies in preventing and treating disease. Prayer, meditation, massage, and yoga, for example, have been used to treat both body and mind for centuries. From a pharmacotherapeutic perspective, the value of CAM therapies lies in their ability to reduce the need for medications. For example, if a client can find anxiety relief through herbal products, massage, or biofeedback therapy, then the use of anxiolytic drugs may be reduced or eliminated. Reduction of traditional drug doses leads to fewer adverse effects.

The nurse should be sensitive to the client's need for alternative treatment and not be judgmental. Both advantages and limitations must be presented to clients so they may make rational and informed decisions on their treatment. Pharmacotherapy and alternative therapies can serve complementary and essential roles in the healing of the total client.

11.2 Brief History of Natural Health Products

An **herb** is technically a **botanical** without woody tissue such as stems or bark. Over time, the terms *botanical* and *herb* have come to be used interchangeably to refer to any plant product with some useful application either as a food enhancer, such as flavouring, or as a medicine.

The use of botanicals has been documented for thousands of years. One of the earliest recorded uses of plant products was a prescription for garlic in 3000 BCE. Eastern and Western medicine have recorded thousands of herbs and herb

TABLE 11.1 Complementary and Alternative Therapies

Healing Method	Examples
biological-based therapies	herbal therapies
	nutritional supplements
	special diets
alternate healthcare systems	naturopathy
	homeopathy
	chiropractic
	Aboriginal medicine (e.g., sweat lodges, medicine wheel)
	Chinese traditional medicine (e.g., acupuncture, Chinese herbs)
manual healing	massage
	pressure-point therapies
	hand-mediated biofield therapies
mind-body interventions	yoga
	meditation
	hypnotherapy
	guided imagery
	biofeedback
	movement-oriented therapies (e.g., music, dance)
spiritual	shamans
	faith and prayer
others	bioelectromagnetics
	detoxifying therapies
	animal-assisted therapy

TABLE 11.2 Best-Selling Herbal Supplements, in Rank Order

Herb	Medicinal Part	Primary Use(s)
ginkgo	leaves and seeds	improve memory, reduce dizziness
echinacea	entire plant	enhance immune system, anti-inflammatory
garlic	bulbs	reduce blood cholesterol, reduce blood pressure, anticoagulation
ginseng	root	relieve stress, enhance immune system, decrease fatigue
soy	beans	source of protein, vitamins, and minerals, relieve menopausal symptoms, prevent cardiovascular disease, anticancer
saw palmetto	ripe fruit/berries	relieve urinary problems related to prostate enlargement
St. John's wort	flowers, leaves, stems	reduce depression, reduce anxiety, anti-inflammatory
valerian	roots	relieve stress, promote sleep
cranberry	berries/juice	prevent urinary tract infection
black cohosh	roots	relieve menopausal symptoms
kava kava	rhizome	reduce stress, promote sleep
milk thistle	seeds	antitoxin, protect against liver disease
evening primrose	seeds/oil	source of essential fatty acids, relieve premenstrual or menopausal symptoms, relieve rheumatoid arthritis and other inflammatory symptoms
grape seed	seeds/oil	source of essential fatty acids, antioxidant, restore microcirculation to tissues
bilberry	berry/leaf	terminate diarrhea, improve and protect vision, antioxidant

Source: Data from Information Resources, Inc., Chicago.

combinations reputed to have therapeutic value. Some of the most popular herbal supplements and their primary uses are shown in Table 11.2.

With the birth of the pharmaceutical industry in the late 1800s, interest in herbal medicines began to wane. Synthetic drugs could be standardized and produced more cheaply than natural herbal products. Regulatory agencies required that products be safe and effective. The focus of healthcare was on diagnosing and treating specific diseases rather than promoting wellness and holistic care. Most alternative therapies were no longer taught in medical or nursing schools; these healing techniques were criticized as being unscientific relics of the past.

Beginning in the 1970s and continuing to the present, alternative therapies and herbal medicines have experienced a remarkable resurgence, such that the majority of adults in Canada are currently using CAM therapies. These therapies now represent a multibillion-dollar industry. This increase in popularity is due to factors such as increased availability of herbal products, aggressive marketing by the herbal industry, increased attention to natural alternatives, and a renewed interest in preventive medicine. The gradual aging of the population has led to more clients seeking therapeutic alternatives for chronic conditions such as pain, arthritis, menopausal symptoms, and prostate difficulties. In addition, longer waiting times for access to healthcare services have driven many clients to self-treat, despite the high cost of herbal medicines.

11.3 Regulation of Natural Health Products (NHPs)

Internationally, the regulation of natural products varies. Generally, they are regulated as drugs in the European Union. In Australia, many products are classified as "complementary medicines." In the United States, many products are regulated as "dietary supplements," a category that does not require pre-market review or proof of safety or efficacy.

In Canada, vitamins and minerals, herbal products, homeopathic medicines, and other such products with health claims are classified as **natural health products (NHPs)**. A recent survey shows that 71% of Canadians regularly take vitamins and minerals and other NHPs. Since 2004, NHPs, also referred to as complementary medicines or traditional remedies, are subject to the Natural Health Products Regulations of the Food and Drugs Act of Health Canada. The Natural Health Products Directorate (NHPD) is responsible for defining NHPs and determining licensing requirements, labelling standards, manufacturing practices, adverse event reporting, quality control, and more. Because the NHPD is a recent establishment, labels may differ among products. NHPs may display different numbering systems, as shown in Figure 11.1. Information about ingredients, indications, and cautions on the labels of NHPs may vary in completeness, as shown in Figure 11.2. To be licensed, an NHP must have at least some efficacy and be relatively safe at the recommended dosage. The NHPD establishes toler-

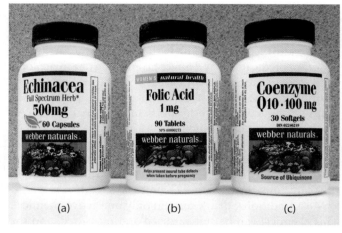

● **Figure 11.1** Natural health product labels may display different numbering systems: (a) no number, indicating that no health claims are made and the product has not been evaluated by Health Canada; (b) Natural Product Number (NPN), indicating that the product has been approved for sale by the NHPD of Health Canada; (c) Drug Identification Number (DIN), indicating that the product has been evaluated by the Therapeutic Products Directorate of Health Canada and approved for sale in Canada
Source: Shirley King.

ance levels for impurities in NHPs. Canadians want NHPs that are as free of contaminants as possible for a product that is natural. Potential contaminants include heavy metals, microorganisms, foreign matter, pesticides and herbicides, radioactive elements, and parts of other plants. The inclusion of unintended or undeclared botanicals in a product represents a serious problem as it is one of the most common causes of adverse effects. For most botanicals, the biologically active ingredients that produce the desired therapeutic effect have not been conclusively identified. The nurse should access Health Canada's MedEffect website to monitor product safety concerns and recalls.

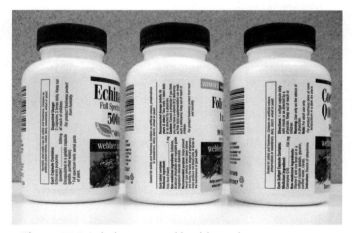

● **Figure 11.2** Labels on natural health products vary: some labels suggest a use for the product, some display warnings, but all recommend a dosage
Source: Shirley King.

MediaLink Health Canada: Natural Health Products

MediaLink Health Canada: MedEffect Canada

11.4 Herbal Product Formulations

Herbal products can interact with other drugs. Nurses need to have knowledge of products that can interact with prescription medications and affect health. The pharmacologically active chemicals in an herbal product may be present in only one specific part of the plant or in all parts. For example, the active chemicals in chamomile are in the above ground portion that includes the leaves, stems, and flowers. For other herbs, such as ginger, the underground rhizomes and roots are used for their healing properties. If collecting herbs for home use, it is essential to know which portion of the plant contains the active chemicals.

Most traditional drugs contain only one active chemical. This chemical can be standardized and measured, and the amount of drug received by the client is precisely known. It is a common misunderstanding that herbs also contain one active ingredient, which can be extracted and delivered to clients in precise doses, like drugs. Herbs may contain dozens of active chemicals, many of which have not yet been isolated, studied, or even identified. It is possible that some of these substances work together synergistically and may not have the same activity in isolation. Furthermore, the strength of an herbal preparation may vary depending on where the herb was grown and how it was collected and stored.

SPECIAL CONSIDERATIONS

Herbal Products

- Because an herbal product comes from plants and is labelled "natural," this does not mean it is safe. Many plants are poisonous and are harmful to human bodies.
- Herbals can act in the same way as drugs and can cause side effects and health problems if not used correctly or if taken in large amounts.
- The active ingredients in many herbs and herbal products are not known. There may be dozens of active compounds in one herbal product.
- Research is needed to identify the active ingredients in herbals and determine how they work in the body.
- Actual contents of herbal products may differ from batch to batch depending on growing conditions and manufacturing processes. "Standardization" may not guarantee uniformity.
- Some herbal products have been found to be contaminated with lead, pesticides, microorganisms, and other substances.
- Women who are pregnant or nursing and children should be especially cautious about using herbal products.
- Clients who are taking prescription medications should be advised to consult their healthcare provider before using an herbal product. Some herbals are known to interact with medications in ways that cause health problems.
- Advertisements should be evaluated for accuracy since some may provide information that is unclear or misleading.
- Adverse effects of herbal products should be reported as for prescription medicines (see Chapter 9).

Source: Natural Health Products Directorate (NHPD),www.hc-sc.gc.ca; National Center for Complementary and Alternative Medicine (NCCAM), http://nccam. nih.gov/.

LIFESPAN CONSIDERATIONS

Dietary Supplements and the Older Adult

Can dietary supplements improve the health of older adults? A growing body of evidence is showing that the use of supplements can positively influence seniors' health. Dietary supplements have been successfully used to enhance their immune systems, reduce short-term memory loss, lessen the risks of Alzheimer's disease, and improve overall health. Nutritional deficiencies greatly increase with age, and supplements help to prevent or eliminate these deficiencies in older adults. In addition, some research has shown that older adults who have low levels of folate and vitamin B_{12} have an increased risk of developing Alzheimer's disease. The nurse should assess the need for such supplements in all older adults. The nurse should, however, be aware that herbal and dietary supplements can be expensive; thus, they should not automatically be included in treatment plans. In addition, older adults should be educated as to the risks of megavitamin therapy.

Some attempts have been made to standardize herbal extracts using a marker substance such as the percent of flavones in ginkgo or the percent of lactones in kava kava. Some of these standardizations are shown in Table 11.3. Until science can better characterize these substances, however, it is best to conceptualize the active ingredient of an herb as being the herb itself.

The two basic formulations of herbal products are solid and liquid. Solid products include pills, tablets, and capsules made from the dried herbs (see Figure 11.1). Other solid products are salves and ointments that are administered topically. Liquid formulations are made by extracting the active chemicals from the plant using solvents such as water, alcohol, or glycerol. The liquids are then concentrated in various strengths and ingested. The various liquid formulations of herbal preparations are described in Table 11.4. Figure 11.3 illustrates formulations of the popular herbal *Ginkgo biloba*.

11.5 Specialty Supplements

Specialty supplements are non-herbal dietary products used to enhance a wide variety of body functions. These supplements form a diverse group of substances obtained from plant and animal sources. They are more specific in their action than herbal products and are generally targeted for one or a smaller number of conditions. The most popular specialty supplements are listed in Table 11.5.

In general, specialty supplements have a legitimate rationale for their use. For example, chondroitin and glucosamine are natural substances in the body necessary for cartilage growth and maintenance. Amino acids are natural building blocks of muscle protein. Flaxseed and fish oils contain omega fatty acids that have been shown to reduce the risk of heart disease in certain clients. As with herbal products, the link between most specialty supplements and their claimed benefits is unclear. In some cases, the body already has sufficient quantities of the substance and taking additional amounts may provide no benefit. In other cases, the supplement is marketed for conditions for which the

TABLE 11.3 Standardization of Select Herb Extracts

Herb	Standardization	Percent
black cohosh rhizome	triterpene glycosides	2.5
cascara sagrada bark	hydroxyanthracenic heterosides	20
Echinacea purpurea herb	phenolics	4
ginger rhizome	pungent compounds	> 10
ginkgo leaf	flavone glycosides	24–25
	lactones	6
ginseng root	ginsehosides	20–30
kava kava rhizome	kavalactones	40–45
milk thistle root	silymarin	80
St. John's wort herb	hypericins	0.3–0.5
	hyperforin	3–5
saw palmetto fruit	total fatty acids	80–90

TABLE 11.4 Liquid Formulations of Herbal Products

Product	Description
tea	fresh or dried herbs are soaked in hot water for 5–10 minutes before ingestion; convenient
infusion	fresh or dried herbs are soaked in hot water for long periods, at least 15 minutes; stronger than teas
decoction	fresh or dried herbs are boiled in water for 30–60 minutes until much of the liquid has boiled off; very concentrated
tincture	extraction of active ingredients by soaking the herb in alcohol; alcohol remains as part of the liquid
extract	extraction of active ingredients using organic solvents to form a highly concentrated liquid or solid form; solvent may be removed or be part of the final product

TABLE 11.5 Select Specialty Supplements

Product	Common Uses
acidophilus	maintain intestinal health
amino acids	build protein, muscle strength, and endurance
coenzyme Q10	prevent heart disease, provide antioxidant therapy
chondroitin	alleviate arthritis and other joint problems
dehydroepiandrosterone (DHEA)	boost immune and memory functions
elk velvet antler (EVA)	relieve symptoms of rheumatoid arthritis and muscle and joint pain
fish oil	reduce cholesterol levels, enhance brain function, increase visual acuity due to presence of the omega-3 fatty acids
flaxseed oil	reduce cholesterol levels, enhance brain function, increase visual acuity due to presence of the omega-3 fatty acids
glucosamine	alleviate arthritis and other joint problems
methyl sulfonyl methane (MSM)	reduce allergic reactions to pollen and foods, relieve pain and inflammation of arthritis and similar conditions
soy isoflavone	reduce the risk of certain types of cancer

supplement has no proved effect. The good news is that these substances are generally not harmful, unless taken in large amounts. The bad news, however, is that they can give clients false hope of an easy cure for chronic conditions such as heart disease or the pain of arthritis. As with herbal products, the healthcare professional should advise clients to be skeptical about the health claims regarding the use of these supplements until benefits and safety are shown through research. Studies are being conducted by nurse researchers and other scientists to assess the potential efficacy of some of the more popular products.

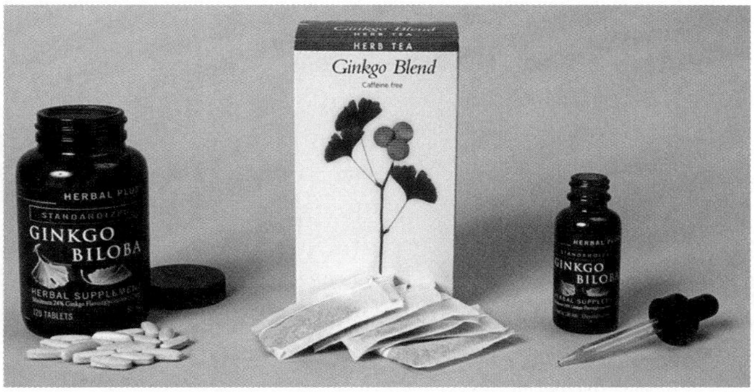

11.6 The Pharmacological Actions and Safety of Natural Products

A key concept to remember when dealing with alternative therapies is that "natural" is not synonymous with "better" or "safe." There is no question that some botanicals contain powerful active chemicals, perhaps more effective than

● **Figure 11.3** Three different ginkgo formulations: tablets, tea bags, and liquid extract

currently approved medications. Thousands of years of experience, combined with current scientific research, have shown that some herbal remedies have therapeutic actions. Because a substance comes from a natural product, however, does not make it safe or effective. For example, poison ivy is natural but it certainly is not safe or therapeutic. Natural products may not offer an improvement over conventional therapy in treating certain disorders and, indeed, may be of no value whatsoever. Furthermore, a client who substitutes an unproven alternative therapy for an established, effective medical treatment may delay healing and suffer irreparable harmful effects.

Some herbal products contain ingredients that may serve as agonists or antagonists to prescription drugs. When obtaining medical histories, nurses should include questions on dietary supplements. Clients taking medications with potentially serious drug-herbal interactions such as insulin, warfarin, or digoxin should be warned to never take any herbal product or dietary supplement without first discussing their needs with a physician. Drug interactions with selected herbs are shown in Table 11.6.

When using natural products, one must also beware of allergic reactions. Most herbal products contain a mixture of ingredients, many of which have not been identified. It is not unusual to find dozens of different chemicals in teas and infusions made from the flowers, leaves, or roots of a plant. Clients who have known allergies to food products or medicines should seek medical advice before taking a new herbal product. It is always wise to take the smallest amount possible when starting herbal therapy, even less than the recommended dose, to see if allergies or other adverse effects occur.

Nurses have an obligation to seek the latest medical information on herbal products since their clients may be using them to supplement traditional medicines. Clients should be advised to be skeptical of claims on the labels of dietary supplements and to seek health information from reputable sources. Nurses should never judge or condemn a client's use of alternative medicines, but instead should be supportive and seek to understand the client's goals for taking the supplements. They should also gather information about the benefits the clients report to experience. The healthcare provider will often need to educate clients on the role of CAM therapies in the treatment of their disorder and discuss which treatment or combination of treatments will best meet their health goals.

TABLE 11.6 Common Herb-Drug Interactions		
Common and Scientific Names	**Drugs of Interaction**	**Comments**
echinacea (*Echinacea purpurea*)	amiodarone	Possible increased hepatotoxicity
	anabolic steroids	Possible increased hepatotoxicity
	ketoconazole	Possible increased hepatotoxicity
	methotrexate	Possible increased hepatotoxicity
feverfew (*Tanacetum parthenium*)	ASA	Increased bleeding potential
	heparin	Increased bleeding potential
	NSAIDs	Increased bleeding potential
	warfarin	Increased bleeding potential
garlic (*Allium sativum*)	ASA	Increased bleeding potential
	insulin	Additive hypoglycemic effects
	NSAIDs	Increased bleeding potential
	oral hypoglycemic agents	Additive hypoglycemic effects
	warfarin	Increased bleeding potential
ginger (*Zingiber officinalis*)	ASA	Increased bleeding potential
	heparin	Increased bleeding potential
	NSAIDs	Increased bleeding potential
	warfarin	Increased bleeding potential
ginkgo (*Ginkgo biloba*)	anticonvulsants	May decrease anticonvulsant effectiveness
	ASA	Increased bleeding potential
	heparin	Increased bleeding potential
	NSAIDs	Increased bleeding potential
	tricyclic antidepressants	May decrease seizure threshold
	warfarin	Increased bleeding potential
ginseng (*Panax quinquefolius/ Eleutherococcus senticosus*)	CNS depressants	Potentiate sedation
	digoxin	Increased toxicity
	diuretics	May attenuate diuretic effects
	insulin	Increased hypoglycemic effects
	MAO inhibitors	Hypertension, manic symptoms, headaches, nervousness
	oral hypoglycemic agents	Increased hypoglycemic effects
	warfarin	Decreased anticoagulant effects

TABLE 11.6   Common Herb-Drug Interactions *(continued)*

Common and Scientific Names	Drugs of Interaction	Comments
goldenseal (*Hydrastis canadensis/ Eleuterococcus senticosus*)	diuretics	May attenuate diuretic effects
kava kava (*Piper methysticum*)	barbiturates	Potentiate sedation
	benzodiazepines	Potentiate sedation
	CNS depressants	Potentiate sedation
	levodopa/carbidopa	Worsening of Parkinson's symptoms
	phenothiazines	Increased risk and severity of dystonic reactions
St. John's wort (*Hypericum perforatum*)	CNS depressants	Potentiate sedation
	cyclosporine	May decrease cyclosporine levels
	efavirenz	Decreased antiretroviral activity
	MAO inhibitors	May cause hypertensive crisis
	opiate analgesics	Increased sedation
	protease inhibitors	Decreased antiretroviral activity of indinavir
	reserpine	Antagonize hypotensive effects
	selective serotonin reuptake inhibitors	May cause serotonin syndrome[*]
	theophylline	Decreased theophylline efficacy
	tricyclic antidepressants	May cause serotonin syndrome[*]
	warfarin	Decreased anticoagulant effects
valerian (*Valeriana officinalis*)	barbiturates	Potentiate sedation
	benzodiazepines	Potentiate sedation
	CNS depressants	Potentiate sedation

[*]Serotonin syndrome: headache, dizziness, sweating, agitation
Source: Data modified from www.prenhall.com/drugguides.

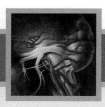

CHAPTER REVIEW

KEY CONCEPTS

The numbered key concepts provide a succinct summary of the important points from the corresponding numbered section within the chapter. If any of these points are not clear, refer to the numbered section within the chapter for review. Expanded versions can be found on the Companion Website.

11.1 Complementary and alternative medicine (CAM) is a set of diverse therapies and healing systems used by many people for disease prevention and self-healing.

11.2 Natural products obtained from plants have been used as medicines for thousands of years.

11.3 Natural health products are regulated by the Natural Health Products Regulations of the Food and Drugs Act.

11.4 Herbal products are available in a variety of formulations, some containing standardized extracts and others containing whole herbs.

11.5 Specialty supplements are non-herbal dietary products used to enhance a wide variety of body functions.

11.6 Natural health products may have pharmacological actions and result in adverse effects, including significant interactions with prescription medications.

REVIEW QUESTIONS

1 When obtaining a medical history, the nurse finds the client is taking St. John's wort. How might this affect the treatment plan for this client who has been diagnosed with clinical depression?

2 How does the federal regulation of drugs differ from that of dietary supplements?

3 Using specific examples, give the types of claims or statements that are *not* allowed on a dietary supplement label, according to the Natural Health Products Directorate of Health Canada.

4 An 80-year-old client is suffering from chronic back pain and has been unresponsive to non-narcotic medications. Name complementary therapies the client might consider to find pain relief.

CRITICAL THINKING QUESTIONS

1. A 44-year-old breast cancer survivor is placed on tamoxifen (Nolvadex) 20 mg PO daily. Since receiving chemotherapy, the client has not had a menstrual cycle. She is concerned about being menopausal and wonders about the possibility of using a soy-based product as a form of natural hormone replacement. How should the nurse advise the client?

2. A 62-year-old male client is recuperating from a myocardial infarction. He is on the anticoagulant warfarin sodium (Coumadin) and antidysrhythmic digitalis. He talks to his wife about starting garlic to help lower his blood lipid levels and ginseng because he has heard it helps coronary artery disease. Discuss the potential concerns about the use of garlic and ginseng by this client.

3. A 22-year-old female college student is brought to the emergency room. She has just experienced a seizure in her dormitory. Her apical pulse is 122 and blood pressure is 166/92 mm Hg. Her roommate states that she "has never done this before" and takes no prescribed medications. What should the nurse consider when conducting the assessment?

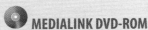 EXPLORE
MediaLink

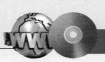

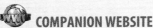 www.pearsoned.ca/adams-king

MEDIALINK DVD-ROM
- **Audio Glossary**
- **CRNE Review**

COMPANION WEBSITE
- **CRNE Review**
- **Case Study:** Alternative Therapies

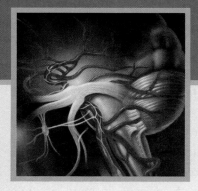

CHAPTER 12

Substances of Addiction

DRUGS AT A GLANCE:
Substances of Addiction

CNS DEPRESSANTS
Sedatives
  barbiturates
  benzodiazepines
Opioids
Ethyl alcohol

CANNABINOIDS
Marijuana

HALLUCINOGENS
LSD
Other hallucinogens

CNS STIMULANTS
Amphetamines and methylphenidate
Cocaine
Caffeine

NICOTINE

OBJECTIVES

After reading this chapter, the student should be able to do the following:

1. Describe underlying causes of addiction.
2. Differentiate psychological and physical dependence.
3. Compare withdrawal syndromes for the various addictive substance classes.
4. Describe signs of drug tolerance, drug dependence, and withdrawal.
5. Describe the major characteristics of addiction, dependence, and tolerance resulting from the following substances: alcohol, nicotine, marijuana, hallucinogens, CNS stimulants, sedatives, and opioids.
6. Describe the role of the nurse in delivering care to individuals with drug addictions.

MediaLink

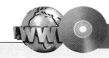 www.pearsoned.ca/adams-king

CRNE review, case studies, and other interactive resources for this chapter can be found on the Companion Website at **www.pearsoned.ca/adams-king**. Click on "Chapter 12" to select the activities for this chapter. For animations, more CRNE review questions, and an audio glossary, access the accompanying MediaLink DVD-ROM in this textbook.

Throughout history, individuals have self-administered both natural substances and prescription drugs to increase performance, assist with relaxation, alter psychological state, or to simply fit in with the crowd. **Substance abuse** is the self-administration of a drug in a manner that does not conform to the norms within one's given culture or society. Many of these substances are addictive. Substance addiction has a tremendous economic, social, and public health impact on society. Although the terms *drugs of addiction* and *substances of addiction* are sometimes used interchangeably, *substances of addiction* is more accurate because some abused agents are not considered drugs. For example, glue is not classified as a drug. The term *substance of addiction* may be preferable to *abused substance* since it shifts the focus to labelling the substance rather than the behaviour of the individual suffering from the stigma and despair of living with an addiction.

12.1 Overview of Substances of Addiction

Addictive substances belong to a number of diverse chemical classes. They have few structural similarities but have the common ability to affect the nervous system, particularly the brain. Some substances, such as opium, marijuana, cocaine, nicotine, caffeine, and alcohol, are obtained from natural sources. Others are synthetic or **designer drugs** created in illicit laboratories for the express purpose of making fortunes in illicit drug trafficking.

Although the public often associates substance addiction with illicit drugs, this is not necessarily the case: alcohol and nicotine are the two most common substances of addiction. Prescription medications such as methylphenidate (Ritalin) and meperidine (Demerol) are sometimes addictive. Substances used illicitly that are frequent sources of addiction include marijuana, volatile inhalants such as aerosols and paint thinners, cocaine, sedatives sold on the street, and hallucinogens such as lysergic acid diethylamide (LSD) and phencyclidine hydrochloride (PCP).

Several drugs once used therapeutically are now illicit due to their high potential for addiction. Cocaine was once widely used as a local anesthetic, but today nearly all the cocaine acquired by users is obtained illicitly. LSD is now illicit, although in the 1940s and 1950s, it was used in psychotherapy. Phencyclidine was popular in the early 1960s as an anesthetic but was withdrawn from the market in 1965 due to clients reporting hallucinations, delusions, and anxiety after recovering from anesthesia. Many amphetamines once used for bronchodilation were discontinued in the 1980s after psychotic episodes were reported.

PHARMFACTS

Substances of Addiction in Canada

- Caffeine is the most commonly used psychoactive substance.
- About 79.3% of Canadians aged 15 years or older consume alcohol; about 6.2% of these are heavy drinkers.
- Drinking rates peak between 18 and 24 years.
- Cannabis is the most commonly used illicit drug; about 44.5% of Canadians report using cannabis at least once in their lifetime.
- More than 30% of teenagers use cannabis.
- The use of addictive substances by Canadian Aboriginal Peoples is higher than the national average. Addictive substances are often acquired through prescriptions. Readily accessible solvents and glue may be used by youth.

12.2 Neurobiological and Psychosocial Components of Substance Addiction

Behaviours such as eating, drinking, and engaging in sexual activity that are necessary for survival of the species are reinforced through stimulation of "reward pathways" in the brain that provide pleasure. Thus, the brain naturally encourages behaviours that lead to pleasure. The addictive process is hypothesized to involve stimulation of these reward pathways by an addictive substance that mimics and even surpasses that of its naturally occurring chemical counterpart. With repeated self-administration of the addictive substance, tolerance develops and, with it, the perceived need to continue to use the substance in order to experience pleasure. **Addiction** is an overwhelming compulsion that drives someone to repetitive drug-taking behaviour despite serious health and social consequences. It is impossible to accurately predict whether a person will become addicted to a substance. Attempts to predict a person's addictive tendency using psychological profiles or genetic markers have largely been unsuccessful. Substance addiction depends on multiple complex, interacting variables. These variables focus on the following categories:

- Agent or drug factors: cost, availability, dose, mode of administration (e.g., oral, IV, inhalation), speed of onset/termination, length of drug use

- User factors: genetic factors (e.g., metabolic enzymes, innate tolerance), propensity for risk-taking behaviour, prior experiences with drugs, disease that may require a scheduled drug

- Environmental factors: social/community norms, role models, peer influences, educational opportunities

In the case of prescription drugs, addiction may begin with a legitimate need for pharmacotherapy. For example, narcotic analgesics may be indicated for pain relief or sedatives, for a sleep disorder. These drugs may result in a favourable experience, such as pain relief or sleep, and clients will want to repeat these positive experiences.

It is a common misunderstanding, even among some health professionals, that the therapeutic use of scheduled drugs creates large numbers of addicted clients. In fact, prescription drugs rarely cause addiction when used according to accepted medical protocols. The risk of addiction for prescription drugs is primarily a function of the dose and the length of therapy. Because of this, medications having the potential for addiction are usually prescribed at the lowest effective dose and for the shortest time necessary to treat the medical problem. Nurses should administer these medications as prescribed for the relief of client symptoms without undue fear of producing dependency. As mentioned in Chapters 1 and 2, numerous laws have been passed in an attempt to limit drug addiction.

12.3 Physical and Psychological Dependence

Whether a substance is addictive is related to how easily an individual can stop taking the substance on a repetitive basis. When a person has an overwhelming desire to take a drug and cannot stop, this is referred to as substance dependence. Substance dependence is classified by two categories, physical dependence and psychological dependence.

Physical dependence refers to an altered physical condition caused by the nervous system adapting to repeated substance use. Over time, the body's cells start to respond as though it is normal for the substance to be continually present. With physical dependence, uncomfortable symptoms known as withdrawal result when the agent is discontinued. Opioids, such as morphine and heroin, may produce physical dependence rather quickly with repeated doses, particularly when taken intravenously. Alcohol, sedatives, some stimulants, and nicotine are other examples of substances that may produce physical dependence easily with extended use.

In contrast, **psychological dependence** produces no signs of physical discomfort after the agent is discontinued. The user, however, has an overwhelming desire to continue using the substance despite obvious negative economic, physical, or social consequences. This intense craving may be associated with the client's home environment or social contacts. Strong psychological craving for a substance may continue for months or even years and is often responsible for relapses during substance addiction therapy and a return to drug-seeking behaviour. Psychological dependence usually requires relatively high doses for a prolonged time, such as with marijuana and antianxiety drugs; however, psychological dependence may develop quickly, perhaps after only one use, with crack—a potent, inexpensive form of cocaine.

12.4 Withdrawal Syndrome

Once a client becomes physically dependent and the substance is discontinued, a **withdrawal syndrome** will occur. Symptoms of withdrawal syndrome may be particularly severe for clients who are physically dependent on alcohol and sedatives. Because of the severity of the symptoms, the process of withdrawal from these agents is best accomplished in a substance addiction treatment facility. Examples of the types of withdrawal syndromes experienced with different addictive substances are shown in Table 12.1.

Prescription drugs may be used to reduce the severity of withdrawal symptoms. For example, alcohol withdrawal can be treated with a short-acting benzodiazepine such as oxazepam, and opioid withdrawal can be treated with methadone. Symptoms of nicotine withdrawal may be relieved by nicotine replacement therapy in the form of patches or chewing gum. No specific pharmacological intervention is indicated for withdrawal from CNS stimulants, hallucinogens, marijuana, or inhalants.

With chronic use of addictive substances, clients will often associate their conditions and surroundings, including social contacts with other users, with the taking of the drug. Users tend to revert back to drug-seeking behaviour when they return to the company of other users of addictive substances. Counsellors often encourage users to refrain from associating with past social contacts or engaging in relationships with other people with addictions to lessen the possibility of relapse. The formation of new social contacts as a result of association with self-help groups such as Alcoholics Anonymous helps some clients transition to a drug-free lifestyle.

12.5 Tolerance

Tolerance is a biological condition that occurs when the body adapts to a substance after repeated administration. Over time, higher doses of the agent are required to produce the same initial effect. For example, at the start of pharmacotherapy, a client may find that 2 mg of a sedative is effective at inducing sleep. After taking the medication for several months, the client notices that it takes 4 mg or perhaps 6 mg to fall asleep. Development of drug tolerance is

LIFESPAN CONSIDERATIONS

Pediatric Use of Volatile Inhalants

Many parents are concerned about their children smoking tobacco or marijuana or becoming addicted to crack or amphetamines. Yet few parents consider that the most common sources of addictive substances lie in their own homes. Inhaling volatile chemicals, known as huffing, is most prevalent in the 10- to 12-year-old age group and then declines with age; one in five children has tried huffing by the eighth grade. Virtually any organic compound can be huffed, including nail polish remover, spray paint, household glue, correction fluid, propane, gasoline, and even whipped cream propellants. These agents are readily available, inexpensive, and can be used anytime and anywhere. Children can die after a single exposure or suffer brain damage, which may be manifested as slurred or slow speech, tremor, memory loss, or personality changes. Nurses who work with pediatric clients should be aware of the widespread nature of this type of addiction and should advise parents to keep close watch on volatile substances.

common for substances that affect the nervous system. Tolerance should be thought of as a natural consequence of continued drug use and not be considered evidence of addiction.

Tolerance does not develop at the same rate for all actions of a drug. For example, clients usually develop tolerance to the nausea and vomiting produced by narcotic analgesics after only a few doses. Tolerance to the mood-altering effects of these drugs and to their ability to reduce pain develops more slowly but eventually may be complete. Tolerance to the drug's ability to constrict the pupils never develops. Clients will often endure annoying side effects of drugs, such as the sedation caused by antihistamines, if they know that tolerance will develop quickly to these effects.

Once tolerance to a substance develops, it often extends to closely related drugs. This phenomenon is known as **cross-tolerance**. For example, a heroin addict will be tolerant to the analgesic effects of other opioids such as morphine and meperidine. Clients who have developed tolerance to alcohol will show tolerance to other CNS depressants such as barbiturates, benzodiazepines, and some general anesthetics. This has important clinical implications for the nurse as doses of these related medications will have to be adjusted accordingly to obtain maximum therapeutic benefit.

The terms *immunity* and *resistance* are often confused with tolerance. These terms more correctly refer to the immune system and infections and should not be used interchangeably with tolerance. For example, microorganisms become resistant to the effects of an antibiotic—they do not become tolerant. Clients become tolerant to the effects of pain relievers—they do not become resistant.

12.6 CNS Depressants

CNS depressants form a group of drugs that cause clients to feel sedated or relaxed. Drugs in this group include barbiturates, non-barbiturate sedative-hypnotics, benzodiazepines, alcohol, and opioids. Although the majority of these are available by prescription, they are controlled under the Controlled Drugs and Substances Act (CDSA) due to their addictive potential.

TABLE 12.1	Withdrawal Symptoms of Select Substances of Addiction
Drug	**Symptoms**
opioids	excessive sweating, restlessness, dilated pupils, agitation, goosebumps, tremor, violent yawning, increased heart rate and blood pressure, nausea/vomiting, abdominal cramps and pain, muscle spasms with kicking movements, weight loss
barbiturates and similar sedative-hypnotics	insomnia, anxiety, weakness, abdominal cramps, tremor, anorexia, seizures, hallucinations, delirium
benzodiazepines	insomnia, restlessness, abdominal pain, nausea, sensitivity to light and sound, headache, fatigue, muscle twitches
alcohol	tremors, fatigue, anxiety, abdominal cramping, hallucinations, confusion, seizures, delirium
cocaine and amphetamines	mental depression, anxiety, extreme fatigue, hunger
nicotine	irritability, anxiety, restlessness, headaches, increased appetite, insomnia, inability to concentrate, decrease in heart rate and blood pressure
marijuana	irritability, restlessness, insomnia, tremor, chills, weight loss
hallucinogens	rarely observed; dependent on specific drug

Sedatives **Sedatives**, also known as tranquilizers, are primarily prescribed for sleep disorders and certain forms of epilepsy. The two primary classes of sedatives are the barbiturates and the non-barbiturate sedative-hypnotics. Their actions, indications, safety profiles, and addictive potential are roughly equivalent. Physical dependence, psychological dependence, and tolerance develop when these agents are taken for extended periods at high doses. Individuals sometimes obtain these drugs by faking prescriptions or by sharing medication with friends. They are commonly combined with other substances of addiction, such as CNS stimulants or alcohol. Addicted individuals often alternate between amphetamines, which keep them awake for several days, and barbiturates, which are needed to help them relax and fall sleep.

Many sedatives have a long duration of action: effects may last an entire day, depending on the specific drug. Clients may appear dull or apathetic. Higher doses resemble alcohol intoxication, with slurred speech and motor incoordination. Barbiturates commonly used in addiction include pentobarbital and secobarbital. The medical use of barbiturates and non-barbiturate sedative-hypnotics has declined markedly over the past 20 years. The use of barbiturates in treating sleep disorders is discussed in Chapter 14, and their use in epilepsy is presented in Chapter 15.

Overdoses of barbiturates and non-barbiturate sedative-hypnotics are extremely dangerous. The drugs suppress the respiratory centres in the brain, and the user may stop breathing or lapse into a coma. Death may result from barbiturate overdose. There is no specific antidote for barbiturates. Withdrawal symptoms from these drugs resemble those of alcohol withdrawal and may be life-threatening.

Benzodiazepines are another group of CNS depressants that have the potential for addiction. They are one of the most widely prescribed classes of drug and have largely replaced the barbiturates for certain disorders. Their primary indication is anxiety (Chapter 14), although they are also used to prevent seizures (Chapter 15) and treat muscle spasms (Chapter 45). Common benzodiazepines include alprazolam, diazepam, temazepam, triazolam, and midazolam.

Although benzodiazepines are the most frequently prescribed drug class, benzodiazepine abuse is not common. Individuals abusing benzodiazepines may appear carefree, detached, sleepy, or disoriented. Death due to overdose is rare, even with high doses. The antidote for benzodiazepines is flumazenil. Users may combine these agents with alcohol, cocaine, or heroin to augment their drug experience. If combined with these other agents, overdose may be lethal. The benzodiazepine withdrawal syndrome is less severe than that of barbiturates and alcohol.

Opioids **Opioids**, also known as narcotic analgesics, are prescribed for severe pain, persistent cough, and diarrhea. The opioid class includes natural substances obtained from the unripe seeds of the poppy plant, such as opium, morphine, and codeine, and synthetic drugs such as meperidine, oxycodone, fentanyl, methadone, and heroin. The thera-peutic effects of the opioids are discussed in detail in Chapter 19.

The effects of *oral* opioids begin within 30 minutes and may last over a day. *Parenteral* forms produce immediate effects, including the brief, intense rush of euphoria sought by heroin addicts. Individuals experience a range of CNS effects, from extreme pleasure to slowed body activities and profound sedation. Signs include constricted pupils, an increase in the pain threshold, and respiratory depression.

Addiction to opioids can occur rapidly, and withdrawal can produce intense symptoms. While extremely unpleasant, withdrawal from opioids is not life-threatening, compared to barbiturate withdrawal. Methadone is a narcotic sometimes used to treat opioid addiction. Although methadone has addictive properties of its own, it does not produce the same degree of euphoria as other opioids and its effects are longer lasting. Heroin addicts are switched to methadone to prevent unpleasant withdrawal symptoms. Since methadone is taken orally, clients are no longer exposed to serious risks associated with intravenous drug use, such as hepatitis and AIDS. Clients sometimes remain on methadone maintenance for a lifetime. Withdrawal from methadone is more prolonged than with heroin or morphine, but the symptoms are less intense.

Ethyl Alcohol Ethyl alcohol, commonly known as alcohol, is one of the most commonly abused drugs. Alcohol is readily available to adults as beer, wine, and liquor. The economic, social, and health consequences of alcohol abuse are staggering. Despite the enormous negative consequences associated with long-term use, small quantities of alcohol consumed on a daily basis have been found to reduce the risk of stroke and heart attack.

Alcohol is classified as a CNS depressant because it slows the region of the brain responsible for alertness and wakefulness. Alcohol easily crosses the blood-brain barrier, so its effects are observed within 5 to 30 minutes of consumption. Effects of alcohol are directly proportional to the amount consumed and include relaxation, sedation, memory impairment, loss of motor coordination, reduced judgment, and decreased inhibition. Alcohol also imparts a characteristic odour to the breath and increases blood flow in certain areas of the skin, causing a flushed face, pink cheeks, or red nose. Although flushing and lack of coordination are easily recognized, the nurse must be aware that other substances and disorders may cause similar symptoms. For example, many antianxiety agents, sedatives, and antidepressants can cause drowsiness, memory difficulties, and loss of motor coordination. Certain mouthwashes contain alcohol and cause the breath to smell alcoholic. During assessment, the skilled nurse must consider these factors before suspicion of alcohol use can be confirmed.

The presence of food in the stomach will slow the absorption of alcohol, thus delaying the onset of drug action. Metabolism, or detoxification, of alcohol by the liver occurs at a slow, constant rate, which is not affected by the presence of food. The average rate is about 15 mL per hour—the practical equivalent of one alcoholic beverage per hour. If consumed at a higher rate, alcohol will accumulate in the blood and produce greater effects on the brain. Acute overdoses of alcohol produce vomiting, severe hypotension, respiratory failure, and coma. Death due to alcohol poisoning is not uncommon. The nurse should teach clients to never combine alcohol with the use of other CNS depressants as their effects are cumulative and profound sedation or coma may result.

Chronic alcohol consumption produces both psychological and physiological dependence and results in a large number of adverse health effects. The organ most affected by chronic alcohol use is the liver. Alcoholism is a common cause of cirrhosis, a debilitating and often fatal failure of the liver to perform its vital functions. Liver failure results in abnormalities in blood clotting and nutritional deficiencies, and sensitizes the client to the effects of all medications metabolized by the liver. For alcoholic clients, the nurse should begin therapy with lower than normal doses until the adverse effects of the medication can be assessed.

The alcohol withdrawal syndrome is severe and may be life-threatening. The use of anticonvulsants in the treatment of alcohol withdrawal is discussed in Chapter 15. Long-term treatment for alcohol addiction includes behavioural counselling and self-help groups such as Alcoholics Anonymous. Disulfiram may be given to discourage relapses. Disulfiram inhibits acetaldehyde dehydrogenase, the enzyme that metabolizes alcohol. If alcohol is consumed while taking disulfiram, the client becomes violently ill within 5 to 10 minutes, with headache, shortness of breath, nausea/vomiting, and other unpleasant symptoms. Disulfiram is only effective in highly motivated clients since the success of pharmacotherapy is entirely dependent on client adherence. Alcohol sensitivity continues for up to 2 weeks after disulfiram has been discontinued. As a pregnancy category X drug, disulfiram should never be taken during pregnancy.

12.7 Cannabinoids

Cannabinoids are agents obtained from the hemp plant *Cannabis sativa,* which thrives in tropical climates. Cannabinoid agents are usually smoked and include marijuana, hashish, and hash oil. Although over 61 cannabinoid chemicals have been identified, the ingredient responsible for most of the psychoactive properties is delta-9-**tetrahydrocannabinol (THC).**

Marijuana Marijuana, also known as grass, pot, weed, reefer, or dope, is a natural product obtained from *C. sativa.* It is the most commonly used illicit drug in Canada. Use of marijuana slows motor activity, decreases coordination, and causes disconnected thoughts, feelings of paranoia, and euphoria. It increases thirst and craving for food, particularly chocolate and other candies. One hallmark symptom of marijuana use is red or bloodshot eyes, caused by dilation of blood vessels. THC accumulates in the gonads.

When inhaled, marijuana produces effects that occur within minutes and last up to 24 hours. Because marijuana smoke is inhaled more deeply and held within the lungs for a longer time than cigarette smoke, marijuana smoke introduces four times more particulates (tar) into the lungs than tobacco smoke. Smoking marijuana on a daily basis may increase the risk of lung cancer and other respiratory disorders. Chronic use is associated with a lack of motivation in achieving or pursuing life goals.

Unlike many addictive substances, marijuana produces little physical dependence and/or tolerance. Withdrawal symptoms are mild, if they are experienced at all. Metabolites of THC, however, remain in the body for months to years, allowing laboratory specialists to easily determine whether someone has used marijuana. For several days after use, THC can also be detected in the urine. Despite numerous attempts to demonstrate therapeutic applications for marijuana, results have been controversial and the medical value of the drug remains to be proven.

12.8 Hallucinogens

Hallucinogens consist of a diverse class of chemicals that have in common the ability to produce an altered, dream-like state of consciousness. Sometimes called **psychedelics,** the prototype substance for this class is lysergic acid diethylamide (LSD). All hallucinogens are Schedule I drugs—they have no medical use.

LSD For nearly all drugs of addiction, predictable symptoms occur in every user. Effects from hallucinogens, however, are highly variable and dependent on the mood and expectations of the user and the surrounding environment in which the substance is used. Two clients taking the same agent will report completely different symptoms, and the same client may report different symptoms with each use. Users who take LSD or psilocybin, also known as magic mushrooms or shrooms, may experience symptoms such as laughter, visions, religious revelations, and deep personal insights. The structures of these hallucinogens are shown in Figure 12.1. Common occurrences are hallucinations and after-images being projected onto people as they move. Users also report unusually bright lights and vivid colours. Some users hear voices; others report smells. Many experience a profound sense of truth and deep-directed thoughts. Unpleasant experiences can be terrifying and may include anxiety, panic attacks, confusion, severe depression, and paranoia.

LSD, also called acid, the beast, blotter acid, and California sunshine, is derived from a fungus that grows on rye and other grains. LSD is nearly always administered orally and can be manufactured in capsule, tablet, or liquid form. A common and inexpensive method of distributing LSD is to place drops of the drug on paper, often containing the images of cartoon characters or graphics related to the drug culture. After drying, the paper containing the LSD is ingested to produce the drug's effects.

LSD is distributed throughout the body immediately after use. Effects are experienced within an hour and may last from 6 to 12 hours. It affects the central and autonomic

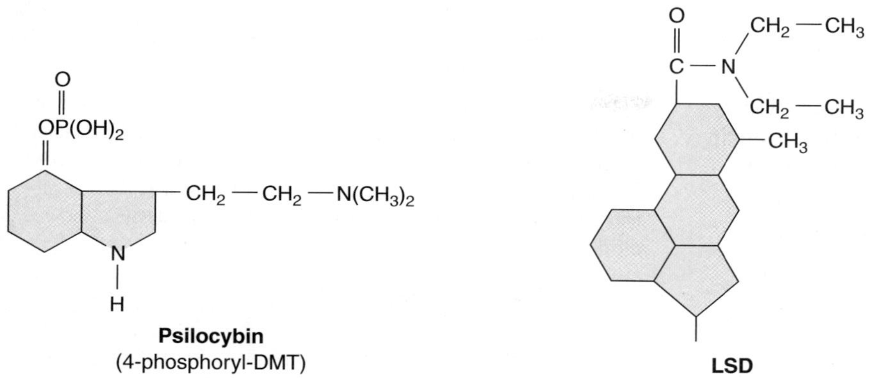

● **Figure 12.1** Comparison of the chemical structures of psilocybin (derived from a mushroom) and LSD (derived from a fungus)

Source: Pearson Education/PH College.

nervous systems, increasing blood pressure, elevating body temperature, dilating pupils, and increasing heart rate. Repeated use may cause impaired memory and inability to reason. In extreme cases, clients may develop psychoses. One unusual adverse effect is flashbacks, in which the user experiences the effects of the drug again, sometimes weeks, months, or years after the drug was initially taken. While tolerance is observed, little or no dependence occurs with the hallucinogens.

Other Hallucinogens   In addition to LSD, other hallucinogens that are abused include the following:

- Mescaline: found in the peyote cactus of Mexico and Central America (Figure 12.2)
- MDMA (3,4-methylenedioxymethamphetamine; XTC or Ecstasy): an amphetamine originally synthesized for research purposes that has since become extremely popular among teens and young adults
- DOM (2,5-dimethoxy-4-methylamphetamine; STP): a recreational drug often linked with rave parties
- MDA (3,4-methylenedioxyamphetamine): called the love drug due to a belief that it enhances sexual desire
- Phenylcyclohexylpiperidine (PCP; angel dust or phencyclidine): produces a trance-like state that may last for days and results in severe brain damage
- Ketamine (date rape drug or special K): produces unconsciousness and amnesia; primary approved use is as an anesthetic

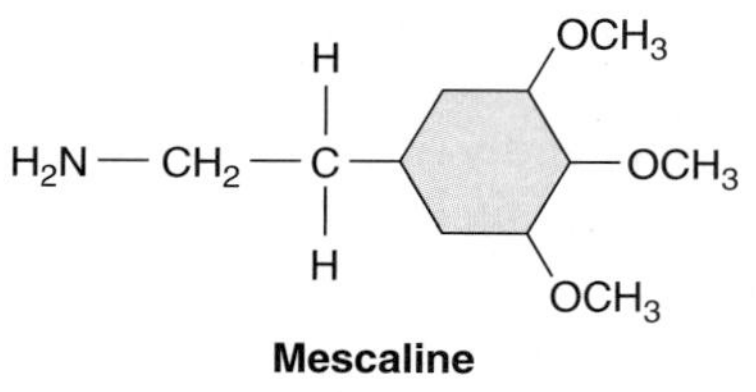

● **Figure 12.2** The chemical structure of mescaline (derived from the peyote cactus)

Source: Pearson Education/PH College.

12.9 CNS Stimulants

Stimulants include a diverse family of drugs known for their ability to increase the activity of the CNS. Some are available by prescription for the treatment of narcolepsy, obesity, and attention deficit disorder. As drugs of addiction, CNS stimulants are taken to produce a sense of exhilaration, improve mental and physical performance, reduce appetite, prolong wakefulness, or simply "get high." Stimulants include the amphetamines, methylphenidate, cocaine, and caffeine.

Amphetamines and Methylphenidate   CNS stimulants have effects similar to the neurotransmitter norepinephrine (see Chapter 13). Norepinephrine affects awareness and wakefulness by activating neurons in a part of the brain called the **reticular formation**. High doses of amphetamines give the user a feeling of self-confidence, euphoria, alertness, and empowerment; but just as short-term use induces favourable feelings, long-term use often results in feelings of restlessness, anxiety, and fits of rage, especially when the user is coming down from a high induced by the drug.

Most CNS stimulants affect cardiovascular and respiratory activity, resulting in increased blood pressure and increased respiration rate. Other symptoms include dilated pupils, sweating, and tremors. Overdoses of some stimulants lead to seizures and cardiac arrest.

Amphetamines and dextroamphetamines were once widely prescribed for depression, obesity, drowsiness, and congestion. In the 1960s it became recognized that the medical uses of amphetamines did not outweigh their risk of dependence. Due to the development of safer medications, the current therapeutic uses of these drugs are extremely limited. Illicit laboratories can easily produce amphetamines and sell them for tremendous profit.

Dextroamphetamine may be used for short-term weight loss, when all other attempts to reduce weight have been exhausted, and to treat narcolepsy. Methamphetamine, commonly called ice, is often used as a recreational drug for users who like the rush that it gives them. It usually is administered in powder or crystal form, but it may also be smoked. Most users obtain it from illicit methamphetamine laboratories. A structural analog of methamphetamine, methcathinone (street name, Cat) is made illicitly and is snorted, taken orally, or injected IV.

Methylphenidate (Ritalin) is a CNS stimulant widely prescribed for children diagnosed with **attention deficit disorder (ADD)**. Methylphenidate has a calming effect in children who are inattentive or hyperactive. It stimulates the alertness centre in the brain, and the child is able to focus on tasks for longer periods of time. This explains the paradoxical calming effects that this stimulant has on children, which is usually opposite to the effects on adults. The therapeutic applications of methylphenidate are discussed in Chapter 16.

Methylphenidate is a CDSA Schedule III drug that has many of the same effects as cocaine and amphetamines. It is sometimes abused by adolescents and adults seeking euphoria. Tablets are crushed and used intranasally or dissolved in liquid and injected IV. Methylphenidate is sometimes mixed with heroin, a combination called a speedball.

Cocaine   Cocaine is a natural substance obtained from leaves of the coca plant, which grows in the Andes Mountain region of South America. Documentation suggests that the plant has been used by Andean cultures since 2500 BCE. Natives in this region chew the coca leaves or make tea from the dried leaves. Because it is taken orally and is absorbed slowly, and because the leaves contain only 1% cocaine, users do not suffer the ill effects caused by chemically pure extracts from the plant. In the Andean culture, use of coca leaves is not considered substance abuse because it is part of the social norms of that society.

Cocaine is a CDSA Schedule I drug that produces actions similar to the amphetamines, although its effects are usually more rapid and intense. It is the second most commonly used illicit drug in Canada. Routes of administration include snorting, smoking, and injecting. In small doses, cocaine produces feelings of intense euphoria, a decrease in hunger, analgesia, illusions of physical strength, and increased sensory perception. Larger doses will magnify these effects and also cause rapid heartbeat, sweating, dilation of the pupils, and an elevated body temperature. After the feelings of euphoria diminish, the user is left with a sense of irritability, insomnia, depression, and extreme distrust. Some users report the sensation that insects are crawling under their skin. Users who snort cocaine develop a chronic runny nose, a crusty redness around the nostrils, and deterioration of the nasal cartilage. Overdose can result in dysrhythmias, convulsions, stroke, or death due to respiratory arrest. The withdrawal syndrome for amphetamines and cocaine is much less intense than that for alcohol and barbiturates.

Caffeine   Caffeine is a natural substance found in the seeds, leaves, or fruits of more than 63 plant species throughout the world. Significant amounts of caffeine are consumed in chocolate, coffee, tea, soft drinks, and ice cream. Caffeine is sometimes added to OTC pain relievers because it has been shown to increase the effectiveness of these medications. Caffeine travels to almost all parts of the body after ingestion,

NATURAL THERAPIES

Herbal Stimulants and Ephedra

Recovering from addiction may be a difficult experience. Individuals claim that discretionary use of some herbal stimulants may ease the symptoms associated with recovery. Examples are kola, damiana, Asiatic and Siberian ginseng, and gotu kola. These agents are thought to stimulate the CNS, providing just enough of an effect to reduce the tension and stresses associated with drug craving.

Ephedra is an herbal stimulant. In addition to its stimulant effects of increasing wakefulness and alertness, the herb affects the cardiovascular system to potentially cause increases in blood pressure and heart rate. Ephedra is an ingredient in a variety of products marketed as dietary supplements for weight loss, energy enhancement, and body-building purposes. It has been implicated in several deaths and serious adverse effects, such as heart attack and stroke, and may be removed from the market due to safety concerns. Nurses should advise their clients to never take this herbal stimulant until they have consulted with their physician.

and several hours are needed for the body to metabolize and eliminate the drug. Caffeine has a pronounced diuretic effect.

Caffeine is considered a CNS stimulant because it produces increased mental alertness, restlessness, nervousness, irritability, and insomnia. The physical effects of caffeine include bronchodilation, increased blood pressure, increased production of stomach acid, and changes in blood glucose levels. Repeated use of caffeine may result in physical dependence and tolerance. Withdrawal symptoms include headaches, fatigue, depression, and impaired performance of daily activities.

12.10 Nicotine

Nicotine is sometimes considered a CNS stimulant, and although it does increase alertness, its actions and long-term consequences place it into a class by itself. Nicotine is unique among addictive substances in that it is not illicit but is strongly addictive and highly carcinogenic. Furthermore, use of tobacco can cause harmful effects to those in the immediate area due to second-hand smoke.

Tobacco Use and Nicotine   The most common method by which nicotine enters the body is through the inhalation of cigarette, pipe, or cigar smoke. Tobacco smoke contains over 1000 chemicals, a significant number of which are carcinogens. The primary addictive substance present in cigarette smoke is nicotine. Effects of inhaled nicotine may last from 30 minutes to several hours.

Nicotine affects many body systems including the nervous, cardiovascular, and endocrine systems. Nicotine stimulates the CNS directly, causing increased alertness and ability to focus, feelings of relaxation, and light-headedness. Stimulation of dopamine release in the pleasure area of the brain may contribute to its addictive potential. The cardiovascular effects of nicotine include an accelerated heart rate and increased blood pressure caused by activation of nicotinic receptors located throughout the autonomic nervous system (see Chapter 13). These cardiovascular effects can be particularly serious in clients taking oral contraceptives: the risk of a fatal heart attack is five times greater in smokers than in non-smokers. Muscular tremors may occur with moderate doses of nicotine, and convulsions may result from very high doses. Nicotine affects the endocrine system by increasing the basal metabolic rate, leading to weight loss. Nicotine also reduces appetite. Chronic use leads to bronchitis, emphysema, and lung cancer.

Both psychological and physical dependence occur relatively quickly with nicotine. Once started on tobacco, clients tend to continue their drug use for many years despite overwhelming medical evidence that their quality of life will be adversely affected and their lifespan shortened. Discontinuation results in agitation, weight gain, anxiety, headache, and an extreme craving for the drug. Although nicotine replacement patches and gum assist clients in dealing with the unpleasant withdrawal symptoms, only 25% of clients who attempt to stop smoking remain tobacco-free a year later.

12.11 The Nurse's Role in Substance Addiction

The nurse serves a key role in the prevention, diagnosis, and treatment of substance addiction. A thorough medical history must include questions about the use of addictive substances. In the case of IV drug users, the nurse must consider the possibility of HIV infection, hepatitis, and associated diagnoses. Clients are often reluctant to report their drug use for fear of embarrassment or being arrested. The nurse must be knowledgeable about the signs of substance dependence and withdrawal symptoms and must develop a keen sense of perception during the assessment stage. A trusting nurse-client relationship is essential to helping clients deal with their dependence.

It is often difficult for a healthcare provider not to condemn or stigmatize a client for his or her substance addiction. Nurses are all too familiar with the devastating medical, economic, and social consequences of heroin and cocaine. Yet, compassion and encouragement may help motivate the client who uses illicit and addictive substances to receive treatment. A list of social agencies dealing with dependency should be readily available to provide to clients. When possible, the nurse should attempt to involve family members and other close social contacts in the treatment. Educating the client and family members about the long-term consequences of the use of substances of addiction is essential.

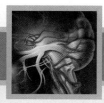

CHAPTER REVIEW

KEY CONCEPTS

The numbered key concepts provide a succinct summary of the important points from the corresponding numbered section within the chapter. If any of these points are not clear, refer to the numbered section within the chapter for review. Expanded versions can be found on the Companion Website.

12.1 A wide variety of addictive substances may be used by individuals, all of which share the common characteristic of altering brain physiology and/or perception.

12.2 Addiction is an overwhelming compulsion to continue repeated drug use that has both neurobiological and psychosocial components.

12.3 Certain substances can cause both physical and psychological dependence, which result in continued drug-seeking behaviour despite negative health and social consequences.

12.4 The withdrawal syndrome is a set of uncomfortable symptoms that occur when a substance to which an individual is addicted is no longer available. The severity of the withdrawal syndrome varies among the different drug classes.

12.5 Tolerance is a biological condition that occurs with repeated use of certain substances and results in higher doses being needed to achieve the same initial response. Cross-tolerance occurs between closely related drugs.

12.6 CNS depressants, which include sedatives, opioids, and ethyl alcohol, decrease the activity of the central nervous system.

12.7 Cannabinoids, which include marijuana, are the most frequently used class of addictive substances. They cause less physical dependence and tolerance than the CNS depressants.

12.8 Hallucinogens, including LSD, cause an altered state of thought and perception similar to that found in dreams. Their effects are extremely variable and unpredictable.

12.9 CNS stimulants, including amphetamines, methylphenidate, caffeine, and cocaine, increase the activity of the central nervous system and produce increased wakefulness.

12.10 Nicotine is a powerful and highly addictive cardiovascular and CNS stimulant that has serious adverse effects with chronic use.

12.11 The nurse serves an important role in educating clients about the consequences of substance addiction and in recommending appropriate treatment.

REVIEW QUESTIONS

1 What is the difference between physical dependence and psychological dependence? How does a client know when he or she is physically dependent on a substance?

2 Name three uncontrolled addictive substances that are used more commonly than illicit drugs. Are these natural or synthetic substances?

3 By examining and interviewing a client, how can a nurse distinguish whether the client is under the influence of marijuana or hallucinogens?

4 Name three classes of CNS stimulants and give examples for each class. Name three major systems in the body affected by stimulants.

CRITICAL THINKING QUESTIONS

1. A 16-year-old male is hospitalized in the ICU following ingestion of a high dose of MDMA (Ecstasy) at a street dance. His mother cannot understand why her son could have such serious renal and cardiovascular complications after "just one dose." The nurse is concerned that the mother lacks sufficient knowledge to be helpful. What teaching does the nurse conduct?

2. The wife of a 24-year-old professional football player is admitted to the ER after being beaten and verbally abused by her husband. She says that he is under a great deal of stress and has been working hard to maintain peak athletic

fitness. She says she has noticed that her husband easily becomes irritable. What assessments and interventions should the nurse perform?

3. A 44-year-old businessman travels weekly for his company and has had difficulty sleeping in "one hotel after another." He consulted his healthcare provider and has been taking secobarbital nightly to help him sleep. The client has called the nurse at his healthcare provider's office and said, "I have just got to have something stronger." What does the nurse consider as part of the assessment?

EXPLORE MediaLink

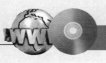   www.pearsoned.ca/adams-king

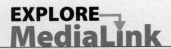 **MEDIALINK DVD-ROM**
- **Audio Glossary**
- **CRNE Review**
- **Animations:** Cirrhosis, Cocaine

 COMPANION WEBSITE
- **CRNE Review**
- **Case Study:** CNS depressants
- **Dosage Calculations**

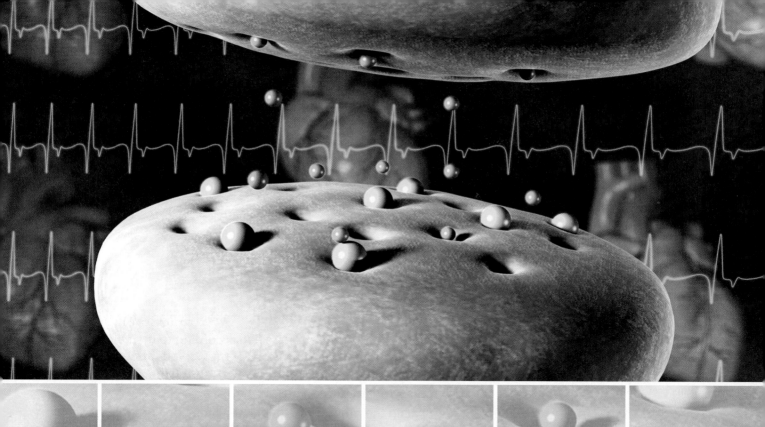

Unit 4 | The Nervous System

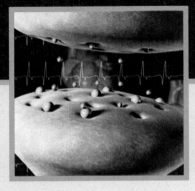

CHAPTER 13

Drugs Affecting the Autonomic Nervous System

DRUGS AT A GLANCE

CHOLINERGICS
- 🖸 *bethanechol (PMS-Bethanechol)*

ANTICHOLINERGICS
- 🖸 *atropine*

Other prototypes
- 🖸 *benztropine (Apo-Benztropine)*: Chapter 18
- 🖸 *ipratropium (Atrovent, others)*: Chapter 29

ADRENERGICS
- 🖸 *phenylephrine (Neo-Synephrine)*

Other prototypes
- 🖸 *norepinephrine (Levophed)*: Chapter 27
- 🖸 *dopamine (Dopastat, others)*: Chapter 27
- 🖸 *epinephrine (Adrenalin)*: Chapter 31

ANTIADRENERGICS
- 🖸 *prazosin (Minipress)*

Other prototypes
- 🖸 *atenolol (Apo-Atenolol, Tenormin)*: Chapter 23
- 🖸 *carvedilol (Coreg)*: Chapter 24
- 🖸 *doxazosin (Cardura)*: Chapter 21
- 🖸 *metoprolol (Apo-Metoprolol, Lopresor)*: Chapter 23
- 🖸 *propranolol (Inderal)*: Chapter 25
- 🖸 *timolol (Apo-Timop, others)*: Chapter 48

OBJECTIVES

After reading this chapter, the student should be able to do the following:

1. Discuss how drugs are classified according to their effects on each of the two fundamental divisions of the nervous system.
2. Compare and contrast the actions of the sympathetic and parasympathetic nervous systems.
3. Explain the process of synaptic transmission and the neurotransmitters important to the autonomic nervous system.
4. Discuss how drugs are used to modify functions of the autonomic nervous system.
5. Compare and contrast the types of responses that occur when a drug activates $alpha_1$-, $alpha_2$-, $beta_1$-, or $beta_2$-adrenergic receptors.
6. Describe the nurse's role in the pharmacological management of clients receiving drugs affecting the autonomic nervous system.
7. For each of the drug classes listed in Drugs at a Glance, explain the mechanism of drug action, primary actions, and important adverse effects.
8. Use the nursing process to care for clients receiving cholinergics, anticholinergics, adrenergics, and adrenergic blockers.

MediaLink

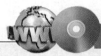

www.pearsoned.ca/adams-king

CRNE review, case studies, and other interactive resources for this chapter can be found on the Companion Website at **www.pearsoned.ca/adams-king**. Click on "Chapter 13" to select the activities for this chapter. For animations, more CRNE review questions, and an audio glossary, access the accompanying MediaLink DVD-ROM in this textbook.

KEY TERMS

Neuropharmacology represents one of the largest, most complicated, and least understood branches of pharmacology. Nervous system drugs are used to treat a large and diverse set of conditions, including pain, anxiety, depression, schizophrenia, insomnia, and convulsions. By their action on nerves, medications are used to treat disorders affecting many body systems. Examples include abnormalities in heart rate and rhythm, hypertension, glaucoma, asthma, and even a runny nose.

The study of nervous system pharmacology extends over the next eight chapters of this textbook. Traditionally, the study of neuropharmacology begins with the autonomic nervous system. A firm grasp of autonomic physiology is necessary to understand nervous, cardiovascular, and respiratory pharmacology. This chapter serves dual purposes. First, it is a comprehensive review of autonomic nervous system physiology, a subject that is often covered superficially in anatomy and physiology classes. Second, it introduces the four fundamental classes of autonomic drugs.

THE AUTONOMIC NERVOUS SYSTEM

13.1 The Peripheral Nervous System

The nervous system has two major divisions: the **central nervous system (CNS)** and the **peripheral nervous system**. The CNS consists of the brain and spinal cord. The peripheral nervous system consists of all nervous tissue outside the CNS, including sensory and motor neurons. The basic functions of the nervous system are as follows:

- Recognize changes in the internal and external environments
- Process and integrate the environmental changes that are perceived
- React to the environmental changes by producing an action or response

Figure 13.1 shows the functional divisions of the nervous system. In the peripheral nervous system, neurons either recognize changes to the environment (sensory division) or respond to these changes by moving muscles or secreting chemicals (motor division). The **somatic nervous system** consists of nerves that provide *voluntary* control over skeletal muscle. Nerves of the **autonomic nervous system (ANS)**, on the other hand, have *involuntary* control over the contraction of smooth muscle and cardiac muscle, and the secretion of glands. Organs and tissues regulated by neurons from the autonomic nervous system include the heart, digestive tract, respiratory tract, reproductive tracts, arteries, salivary glands, and portions of the eye. Whereas only a few medications directly affect the somatic nervous system, a large number affect autonomic nerves.

13.2 The Autonomic Nervous System: Sympathetic and Parasympathetic Branches

The autonomic nervous system has two divisions: the sympathetic and the parasympathetic nervous systems. With a few exceptions, organs and glands receive nerves from both branches of the autonomic nervous system. The ultimate action of the smooth muscle or gland depends on which branch is sending the most signals at a given time. The major actions of the two divisions are shown in Figure 13.2. It is essential that the student learn these actions early in the study of pharmacology because knowledge of autonomic effects is used to predict the actions and side effects of many drugs.

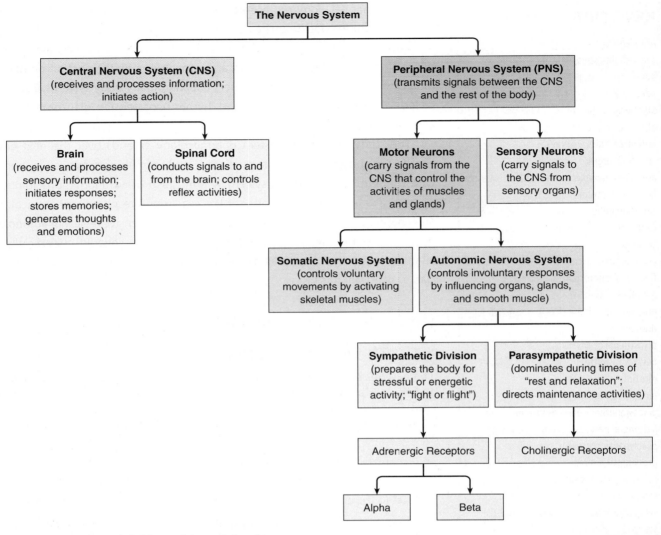

● **Figure 13.1** Functional divisions of the peripheral nervous system

The **sympathetic nervous system** is activated under conditions of stress and produces a set of actions called the **fight-or-flight response**. Activation of this system will ready the body for an immediate response to a potential threat. The heart rate and blood pressure increase, and more blood is shunted to skeletal muscles. The liver immediately produces more glucose for energy. The bronchi dilate to allow more air into the lungs, and the pupils dilate for better vision.

Conversely, the **parasympathetic nervous system** is activated under non-stressful conditions and produces symptoms called the **rest-and-digest response**. Digestive processes are promoted, and heart rate and blood pressure decline. Not as much air is needed, so the bronchi constrict. Most of the actions of the parasympathetic division are opposite to those of the sympathetic division.

A proper balance of the two autonomic branches is required for internal homeostasis. Under most circumstances, the two branches cooperate to achieve a balance of readiness and relaxation. Because they have mostly opposite effects, homeostasis may be achieved by changing one or

both branches. For example, heart rate can be increased by either *increasing* the firing of sympathetic nerves or *decreasing* the firing of parasympathetic nerves. This allows the body a means of fine-tuning its essential organ systems.

The sympathetic and parasympathetic divisions are not always opposite in their effects. For example, the constriction of arterioles is controlled entirely by the sympathetic branch. Sympathetic stimulation causes constriction of arterioles, whereas lack of stimulation causes vasodilation. Sweat glands are controlled only by sympathetic nerves. In the male reproductive system, the roles are complementary. Erection of the penis is a function of the parasympathetic division, and ejaculation is controlled by the sympathetic branch.

13.3 Structure and Function of Synapses

For information to be transmitted throughout the nervous system, neurons must communicate with each other and with muscles and glands. In the autonomic nervous system,

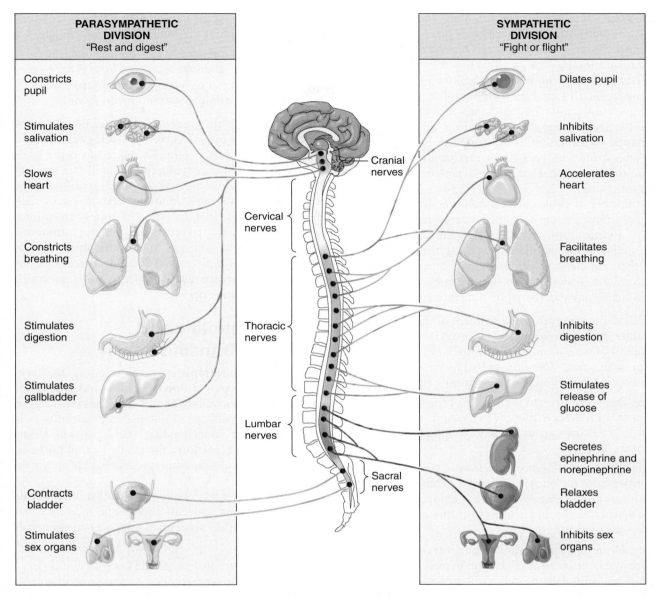

● **Figure 13.2** Effects of the sympathetic and parasympathetic nervous systems

Source: Krogh, D. (2002). Biology: A Guide to the Natural World (2nd ed., p. 558). Upper Saddle River, NJ: Prentice Hall. Reprinted by permission.

this involves the connection of two neurons in series. As an action potential travels along the first nerve, it encounters a structure at the end called a **synapse**. The synapse contains a physical space called the synaptic cleft, which must be bridged for the impulse to reach the next nerve. The nerve carrying the original impulse is called the **presynaptic neuron**. The nerve on the other side of the synapse, waiting to receive the impulse, is the **postsynaptic neuron**. If this

connection occurs outside the CNS, it is called a **ganglion**. The basic structure of a synapse is shown in Figure 13.3.

The physical space of the synaptic cleft is bridged by **neurotransmitters**, which are released into the synaptic cleft when a nerve impulse reaches the end of the presynaptic neuron. The neurotransmitter diffuses across the synaptic cleft to reach receptors on the postsynaptic neuron, which results in the impulse being regenerated. Outside the CNS,

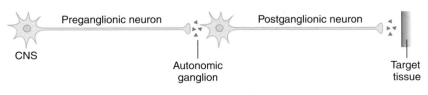

● **Figure 13.3** Basic structure of an autonomic pathway

the regenerated action potential travels along the postganglionic neuron until it reaches its target: a type of synapse called a neuroeffector junction, which is located on smooth muscle, cardiac muscle, or a gland. When released at the neuroeffector junction, the neurotransmitter induces the target tissue to elicit its characteristic response. Generally, the more neurotransmitter released into the synapse, the greater and longer lasting will be its effect. This process, called **synaptic transmission**, is illustrated in Figure 13.4. There are several different types of neurotransmitters located throughout the nervous system, and each is associated with particular functions.

A large number of drugs affect autonomic function by altering neurotransmitter activity. Some drugs are identical to endogenous neurotransmitters, or have a similar chemical structure, and are able to directly activate the gland or muscle. Others are used to block the activity of endogenous neurotransmitters. Following are the five general mechanisms by which drugs affect synaptic transmission:

1. Synthesis: Drugs may affect the *synthesis* of the neurotransmitter in the presynaptic nerve. Drugs that decrease the amount of neurotransmitter synthesis will inhibit autonomic function. Those drugs that increase neurotransmitter synthesis will have the opposite effect.

2. Storage: Drugs can prevent the *storage* of the neurotransmitter in vesicles within the presynaptic nerve. Prevention of neurotransmitter storage will inhibit autonomic function.

3. Release: Drugs can influence the *release* of the neurotransmitter from the presynaptic nerve. Promoting neurotransmitter release will stimulate autonomic function, whereas slowing neurotransmitter release will have the opposite effect.

4. Binding: Drugs can *bind* to the receptor site on the postsynaptic neuron. Drugs that bind to postsynaptic receptors and stimulate the nerve will increase autonomic function. Drugs that attach to the postsynaptic

neuron and prevent the natural neurotransmitter from reaching its receptors will inhibit autonomic function.

5. Reuptake: Drugs can *prevent the reuptake or normal destruction* of the neurotransmitter. Drugs that cause the neurotransmitter to remain in the synapse for a longer time will stimulate autonomic function.

It is important for the student to understand that autonomic drugs are not given to correct physiological defects in the autonomic nervous system. Compared to other body systems, the autonomic nervous system itself has remarkably little disease. Rather, drugs are used to stimulate or inhibit *target organs* of the autonomic nervous system, such as the heart, lungs, or digestive tract. With few exceptions, the disorder lies in the target organ, not the autonomic nervous system. Thus, when an "autonomic drug" such as norepinephrine is administered, it does not correct an autonomic disease—it corrects disorders of target organs through its effects on autonomic nerves.

13.4 Acetylcholine and Cholinergic Transmission

The two primary neurotransmitters of the autonomic nervous system are **norepinephrine (NE)**, also known as noradrenaline, and **acetylcholine (Ach)**. A detailed knowledge of the underlying physiology of these neurotransmitters is required for proper understanding of drug action. When reading the following sections, the student should refer to the sites of acetylcholine and norepinephrine action shown in Figure 13.5.

Nerves releasing acetylcholine are called **cholinergic** nerves. There are two types of cholinergic receptors that bind acetylcholine; they are named after certain chemicals that bind to them:

• Nicotinic receptors: postganglionic neurons ending in ganglia in both the sympathetic and parasympathetic nervous systems

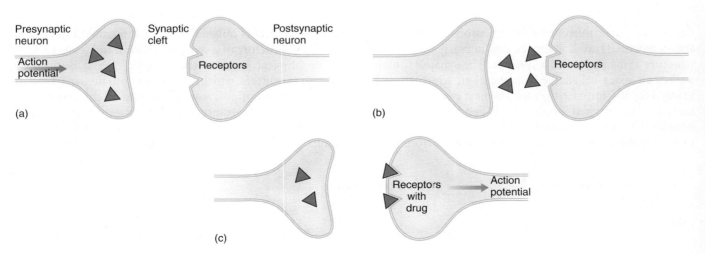

● **Figure 13.4** Synaptic transmission: (a) action potential reaches synapse; (b) neurotransmitter released into synaptic cleft; (c) neurotransmitter reaches receptors to regenerate action potential

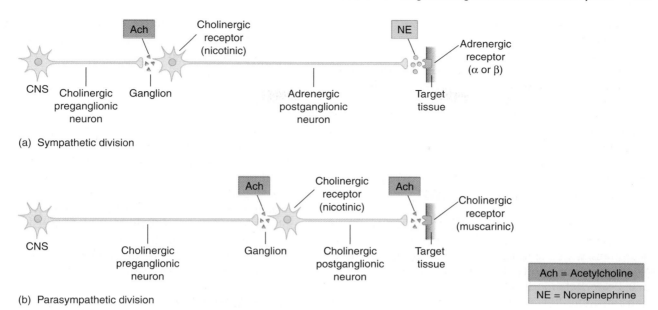

● **Figure 13.5** Receptors in the autonomic nervous system: (a) sympathetic division; (b) parasympathetic division

● Muscarinic receptors: postganglionic neurons ending in neuroeffector target tissues in the parasympathetic nervous system

Early research on laboratory animals found that the actions of acetylcholine at the *ganglia* resemble those of nicotine, the active agent found in tobacco. Because of this similarity, receptors for acetylcholine in the ganglia are called **nicotinic** receptors. Nicotinic receptors are also present in skeletal muscle, which is controlled by the somatic nervous system. Because these receptors are present in so many locations, drugs affecting nicotinic receptors produce profound effects on both the autonomic and somatic nervous systems. Activation of the nicotinic acetylcholine receptors causes tachycardia, hypertension, and increased tone and motility in the digestive tract. Although nicotinic receptor blockers were some of the first drugs used to treat hypertension, the only current therapeutic application of these agents, known as ganglionic blockers, is to produce muscle relaxation during surgical procedures (Chapter 20).

Activation of acetylcholine receptors at *postganglionic* nerve endings in the parasympathetic nervous system results in the classic symptoms of parasympathetic stimulation shown in Figure 13.2. Early research discovered that these actions closely resemble those produced when a client ingests the poisonous mushroom *Amanita muscaria*. Because of this similarity, these acetylcholine receptors were named **muscarinic** receptors. Unlike the nicotinic receptors that have few pharmacological applications, a number of medications affect muscarinic receptors, and these are discussed in subsequent sections of this chapter. The locations of nicotinic and muscarinic receptors are illustrated in Figure 13.5. Table 13.1 summarizes the actions produced by the two types of acetylcholine receptors.

The physiology of acetylcholine affords several mechanisms by which drugs may act. Acetylcholine is synthesized in the presynaptic nerve terminal from choline and acetyl coenzyme A. The enzyme that catalyzes this reaction is called **acetylcholinesterase (AchE)**, or simply cholinesterase. (Note the suffix -*erase* can be thought of as wiping out the

TABLE 13.1	Types of Autonomic Receptors		
Neurotransmitter	**Receptor**	**Primary Locations**	**Responses**
acetylcholine (cholinergic)	muscarinic	parasympathetic target: organs other than the heart	stimulation of smooth muscle and gland secretions
		heart	decreased heart rate and force of contraction
	nicotinic	postganglionic neurons and neuromuscular junctions of skeletal muscle	stimulation of smooth muscle and gland secretions
norepinephrine (adrenergic)	alpha₁	all sympathetic target organs except the heart	constricted blood vessels; dilated pupils
	alpha₂	presynaptic adrenergic nerve terminals	inhibited release of norepinephrine
	beta₁	heart and kidneys	increased heart rate and force of contraction; release of renin
	beta₂	all sympathetic target organs except the heart	inhibition of smooth muscle

Ach.) Once synthesized, acetylcholine is stored in vesicles in the presynaptic neuron. When an action potential reaches the nerve ending, acetylcholine is released into the synaptic cleft, where it diffuses across to find nicotinic or muscarinic receptors. Acetylcholine in the synaptic cleft is rapidly destroyed by acetylcholinesterase, and choline is reformed. The choline is taken up by the presynaptic neuron to make more acetylcholine, and the cycle is repeated. Drugs can affect the formation, release, receptor activation, or destruction of acetylcholine.

13.5 Norepinephrine and Adrenergic Transmission

In the sympathetic nervous system, norepinephrine is the neurotransmitter released at almost all postganglionic nerves. Norepinephrine belongs to a class of endogenous agents called **catecholamines**, all of which are involved in neurotransmission. Other catecholamines include epinephrine (adrenaline) and dopamine. The receptors at the ends of postganglionic sympathetic neurons are called **adrenergic**, which comes from the word *adrenaline*.

Adrenergic receptors are of two basic types: **alpha (α)-receptors** and **beta (β)-receptors**. These receptors are further divided into the subtypes alpha$_1$, alpha$_2$, and beta$_1$, beta$_2$, beta$_3$. Activation of each receptor subtype results in a characteristic set of physiological responses, which are summarized in Table 13.1.

The significance of these receptor subtypes to pharmacology cannot be overstated. Some drugs are selective and activate only one type of adrenergic receptor, whereas others affect all receptor subtypes. Furthermore, a drug may activate one type of receptor at low doses and begin to affect other receptor subtypes as the dose is increased. Committing the receptor types and their responses to memory is an essential step in learning autonomic pharmacology.

Norepinephrine is synthesized in the nerve terminal through a series of steps that require the amino acids phenylalanine and tyrosine. The final step of the synthesis involves the conversion of dopamine to norepinephrine. Norepinephrine is stored in vesicles until an action potential triggers its release into the synaptic cleft. It then diffuses across the cleft to alpha- or beta-receptors on the effector organ. The reuptake of norepinephrine back into the presynaptic neuron terminates its action. Once reuptake occurs, norepinephrine in the nerve terminal may be returned to vesicles for future use or destroyed enzymatically by **monoamine oxidase (MAO)**. The primary method for termination of norepinephrine action is through reuptake. Many drugs affect autonomic function by influencing the synthesis, storage, release, reuptake, or destruction of norepinephrine.

The adrenal medulla is a tissue closely associated with the sympathetic nervous system that has a much different anatomical and physiological arrangement than the rest of the sympathetic branch. The preganglionic neuron from the spinal cord terminates in the adrenal medulla and releases the neurotransmitter epinephrine directly into the blood.

Epinephrine travels to target organs, where it elicits the classic fight-or-flight symptoms. The action of epinephrine is terminated through hepatic metabolism rather than reuptake.

Other types of adrenergic receptors exist. Beta$_3$-receptors are located in the central and autonomic nervous systems and may play a role in lipolysis. Although dopamine was once thought to function only as a chemical precursor to norepinephrine, research has determined that dopamine serves a larger role as neurotransmitter. Five dopaminergic receptors (D$_1$ through D$_5$) have been discovered in the CNS. Dopaminergic receptors in the CNS are important to the action of certain antipsychotic medicines (Chapter 17) and in the treatment of Parkinson's disease (Chapter 18). Dopamine receptors in the peripheral nervous system are located in the arterioles of the kidney and other viscera. These receptors likely have a role in autonomic function.

AUTONOMIC DRUGS

13.6 Classification and Naming of Autonomic Drugs

Given the opposite actions of the sympathetic and parasympathetic nervous systems, autonomic drugs are classified based on one of four possible actions:

1. Stimulation of the sympathetic nervous system: These drugs are called **adrenergics**, sympathomimetics, or adrenergic agonists, and they produce the classic symptoms of the fight-or-flight response.

2. Stimulation of the parasympathetic nervous system: These drugs are called **cholinergics**, parasympathomimetics, or muscarinic agonists, and they produce the characteristic symptoms of the rest-and-digest response.

3. Inhibition of the sympathetic nervous system: These drugs are called **adrenergic antagonists, antiadrenergics**, or adrenergic blockers, and they produce actions *opposite* to those of the adrenergics.

4. Inhibition of the parasympathetic nervous system: These drugs are called **anticholinergics**, parasympatholytics, or muscarinic blockers, and they produce actions *opposite* to those of the cholinergics.

Students beginning their study of pharmacology often have difficulty understanding the terminology and actions of autonomic drugs. Upon examining the four drug classes, however, it is evident that only one group need be learned because the others are logical extensions of the first. If the fight-or-flight actions of the adrenergics are learned, the other three groups are either the same or opposite. For example, both the adrenergics and the anticholinergics increase heart rate and dilate the pupils. The other two groups, the cholinergics and the adrenergic antagonists, have the opposite effects of slowing heart rate and constricting the pupils. Although this is an oversimplification and exceptions do exist, it is a timesaving means of learning the basic actions and adverse effects of dozens of drugs affecting the autonomic nervous system. It should be emphasized again that mastering the actions and terminology of autonomic drugs early in the study of pharmacology will reap rewards later in the course when these drugs are applied to various systems.

CHOLINERGICS

Cholinergics (parasympathomimetics) are drugs that activate the parasympathetic nervous system. These drugs induce the rest-and-digest response. They are listed in Table 13.2.

13.7 Clinical Applications of Cholinergics

The classic cholinergic (parasympathomimetic) is acetylcholine, the endogenous neurotransmitter at cholinergic synapses in the autonomic nervous system. Acetylcholine, however, has almost no therapeutic use because it is rapidly destroyed after administration and it produces many side effects. Recall that acetylcholine is the neurotransmitter at the ganglia in both the parasympathetic and sympathetic divisions and at the neuroeffector junctions in the parasympathetic nervous system, as well as in skeletal muscle. It is not surprising then that administration of acetylcholine or drugs that mimic acetylcholine will have widespread and varied effects on the body.

Cholinergics are divided into two subclasses, direct acting and indirect acting, based on their mechanism of action. Direct-acting agents bind to cholinergic receptors to produce the rest-and-digest response and increase smooth muscle tone. For example, bethanechol causes the detrusor muscle in the bladder wall to contract and expel urine. Because they are relatively resistant to the enzyme acetylcholinesterase, they have a longer duration of action than acetylcholine. They are poorly absorbed across the GI tract and generally do not cross the blood-brain barrier. They have little effect on acetylcholine receptors in ganglia. Because they are moderately selective to muscarinic receptors when used at therapeutic doses, they are sometimes called muscarinic agonists.

The indirect-acting cholinergics, such as neostigmine, inhibit the action of acetylcholinesterase. This inhibition allows endogenous acetylcholine to avoid rapid destruction and remain on cholinergic receptors for a longer time, thus prolonging its action. These drugs are called cholinesterase inhibitors. Unlike the direct-acting agents, the cholinesterase inhibitors are non-selective and affect all acetylcholine sites: autonomic ganglia, muscarinic receptors, skeletal muscle, and acetylcholine sites in the CNS.

Physostigmine was one of the first indirect-acting cholinergics to be discovered. It was obtained from the dried ripe seeds of *Physostigma venenosum,* a plant found in West Africa. The bean of this plant was used in tribal rituals. During World War II, similar compounds were synthesized that produced potent neurological effects that could be used during chemical warfare. This class of agents now includes organophosphate insecticides, such as malathion and parathion, and toxic nerve gasses such as sarin. Nurses who work in agricultural areas may become quite familiar with the symptoms of acute poisoning with organophosphates. Poisoning results in intense stimulation of the parasympathetic nervous system, which may result in death if untreated.

Because of their high potential for serious adverse effects, few cholinergics are widely used in pharmacotherapy. Some have clinical applications in ophthalmology because they reduce intraocular pressure in clients with glaucoma (Chapter 48). Others are used for their stimulatory effects on the smooth muscle of the bowel or urinary tract.

Several drugs in this class are used for their effects on acetylcholine receptors in skeletal muscle or in the CNS, rather than for their parasympathetic action. **Myasthenia gravis** is a disease characterized by destruction of nicotinic receptors on skeletal muscle. Administration of neostigmine will stimulate skeletal muscle contraction and help to reverse the severe muscle weakness characteristic of this disease. Galantamine is used to treat Alzheimer's disease because of its ability to inhibit cholinesterase and thus increase the amount of acetylcholine at receptors in the CNS (Chapter 18).

NURSING CONSIDERATIONS

The role of the nurse in drug therapy with cholinergics involves careful monitoring of the client's condition and providing education as it relates to the prescribed drug treatment. Both direct- and indirect-acting cholinergics are contraindicated for clients with hypersensitivity. These drugs should not be used in clients with obstruction of the gastrointestinal and urinary systems because they increase muscular tone and contraction. Additionally, they should not be used in clients with active asthma, bradycardia, hypotension, or Parkinson's disease.

TABLE 13.2	Cholinergics	
Type	**Drug**	**Primary Use**
direct acting (muscarinic agonists)	bethanechol (PMS-Bethanechol)	increase urination
	pilocarpine (Salagen)	glaucoma
indirect acting (cholinesterase inhibitors)	edrophonium (Tensilon)	diagnosis of myasthenia gravis
	galantamine hydrobromide (Reminyl)	Alzheimer's disease
	neostigmine (Prostigmin)	myasthenia gravis, increase urination

Indirect-Acting Cholinergics Indirect-acting cholinergics are contraindicated for clients with mechanical obstruction of either the intestine or urinary tract due to their ability to intensify smooth muscle contractions. Smooth muscle contractions can also occur in the bronchi, so extreme caution must be exercised when treating clients with asthma or chronic obstructive pulmonary disease (COPD).

Due to the ability of these medications to inhibit acetylcholinesterase at many locations, acetylcholine will accumulate at the muscarinic receptors and neuromuscular junctions and cause side effects such as increased salivation, increased muscle tone, urinary frequency, bronchoconstriction, and bradycardia. Monitor the client for drug-induced insomnia. Also assess pregnancy and breastfeeding status, as these agents are contraindicated for both situations.

Cholinergic crisis occurs when acetylcholine increases to toxic levels. Cholinergic crisis is characterized by excessive parasympathetic activity, including excessive salivation and profound muscle weakness. Atropine, an anticholinergic, should be available to counteract the increased levels of acetylcholine by providing selective blockage of muscarinic cholinergic receptors.

For clients with myasthenia gravis, it is important to perform a baseline physical assessment of neuromuscular and respiratory function. In myasthenia gravis, the nicotinic receptors on skeletal muscle are destroyed. As a result, the muscles of the respiratory tract and other muscle groups used for chewing, swallowing, and speaking are weakened. Therefore, it is important to assess the client's swallowing ability prior to administering an oral drug.

See "Nursing Process Focus: Clients Receiving Cholinergic Therapy" for specific points to include when teaching clients about indirect-acting cholinergics.

Direct-Acting Cholinergics Due to the stimulation of the CNS by these agents, several additional nursing actions are required. These include assessment of past medical history for any of the following: angina pectoris, recent myocardial infarction, and dysrhythmias. Obtain history information on the possible use of lithium and adenosine because both drugs are contraindicated due to their interaction with nicotine. Lithium is a CNS agent that can produce significant muscarinic blockade to atropine. Adenosine is an antidysrhythmic agent, and its effect with nicotine can cause an increased risk of heart block. For mothers who are breastfeeding, monitor the infant's respiratory patterns and any CNS changes prior to and after feedings. Monitor elderly clients for episodes of dizziness and sleep disturbances caused by CNS stimulation from the parasympathomimetic.

See "Nursing Process Focus: Clients Receiving Cholinergic Therapy" for specific points to include when teaching clients about direct-acting cholinergics.

ANTICHOLINERGICS

Anticholinergics are drugs that inhibit parasympathetic impulses. By suppressing the parasympathetic division, symptoms of the fight-or-flight response are induced. The anticholinergics are listed in Table 13.3 on page 132.

Pr PROTOTYPE DRUG | Bethanechol (PMS-Bethanechol)

ACTIONS AND USES

Bethanechol is a direct-acting cholinergic that interacts with muscarinic receptors to cause actions typical of parasympathetic stimulation. Its effects are most noted in the digestive and urinary tracts, where it will stimulate smooth muscle contraction. These actions are useful in increasing smooth muscle tone and muscular contractions in the GI tract following general anesthesia. In addition, it is used to treat non-obstructive urinary retention in clients with atony of the bladder.

ADMINISTRATION ALERTS

- Never administer by IM or IV.
- Oral and SC doses are *not* interchangeable.
- Monitor blood pressure, pulse, and respirations before administration and for at least 1 hour after SC administration.
- Bethanechol is pregnancy category C.

PHARMACOKINETICS

Bethanechol is poorly absorbed from the GI tract, but it may still be administered orally. It can be given by SC injection. Peak effect is 30 minutes SC and 60 minutes PO.

ADVERSE EFFECTS AND INTERACTIONS

The side effects of bethanechol are predicted from its parasympathetic actions. It should be used with extreme caution in clients with disorders that could be aggravated by increased contractions of the digestive tract, such as suspected obstruction, active ulcer, or inflammatory disease. The same caution should be exercised in clients with suspected urinary obstruction or chronic obstructive pulmonary disease (COPD). Side effects include increased salivation, sweating, abdominal cramping, and hypotension that could lead to fainting. It should not be given to clients with asthma.

Drug interactions with bethanechol include increased effects from cholinesterase inhibitors and decreased effects from procainamide, quinidine, atropine, and epinephrine.

 See the Companion Website for a Nursing Process Focus specific to this drug.

NURSING PROCESS FOCUS   Clients Receiving Cholinergic Therapy

Assessment	Potential Nursing Diagnoses/Identified Patterns
Prior to administration: ■ Obtain complete health history including vital signs, allergies, and drug history for possible drug interactions. ■ Assess reason for drug administration. ■ Assess for contraindications of drug administration. ■ Assess for urinary retention, urinary patterns initially and throughout therapy (direct acting). ■ Assess muscle strength, neuromuscular status, ptosis, diplopia, and chewing.	■ Need for knowledge regarding drug therapy ■ Impaired physical mobility ■ Urinary incontinence ■ Risk for injury related to drug side effects

Planning: Client Goals and Expected Outcomes

The client will:
■ Exhibit increased bowel/bladder function and tone by regaining normal pattern of elimination (direct acting)
■ Exhibit a decrease in myasthenia gravis symptoms such as muscle weakness, ptosis, and diplopia (indirect acting)
■ Demonstrate understanding of the drug by accurately describing the drug's purpose, action, side effects, and precautions

Implementation

Interventions (Rationales)	Client Education/Discharge Planning
All Cholinergics	
■ Monitor for adverse effects such as abdominal cramping, diarrhea, excessive salivation, difficulty breathing, and muscle cramping. (These may indicate cholinergic crisis, which requires atropine.) ■ Monitor liver enzymes with initiation of therapy and weekly for 6 weeks (for possible hepatotoxicity). ■ Assess and monitor for appropriate self-care administration to prevent complications.	■ Instruct client to report nausea, vomiting, diarrhea, rash, jaundice, change in colour of stool, or any other adverse reactions to the drug. ■ Instruct client to adhere to laboratory testing schedule for serum blood level tests of liver enzymes as directed. Instruct client to: ■ Take drug as directed on regular schedule to maintain serum levels and control symptoms ■ Not chew or crush sustained-release tablets ■ Take oral cholinergics on an empty stomach to lessen incidence of nausea and vomiting and to increase absorption
Direct Acting	
■ Monitor intake and output ratio. Palpate abdomen for bladder distention. (These drugs have an onset of action of 60 minutes due to binding of the drug to cholinergic receptors on the smooth muscle of the bladder, which contracts the bladder to stimulate urination.) ■ Monitor for blurred vision (a cholinergic effect). ■ Monitor for orthostatic hypotension.	■ Advise client to be near bathroom facilities after taking drug. ■ Advise client that blurred vision is a possible side effect and to take appropriate precautions. ■ Instruct client not to drive or perform hazardous activities until effects of the drug are known. ■ Instruct client to avoid abrupt changes in position and prolonged standing in one place.
Indirect Acting (Cholinesterase Inhibitors)	
■ Monitor muscle strength, neuromuscular status, ptosis, diplopia, and chewing to determine if the therapeutic effect is achieved. ■ Schedule other medications around meal times unless contraindicated. (The indirect-acting cholinergic will aid in chewing and swallowing.) ■ Schedule activities to avoid fatigue.	■ Instruct client to report difficulty with vision or swallowing. ■ Instruct client to take indirect-acting cholinergic about 30 minutes before meal. ■ Instruct client to plan activities according to muscle strength and fatigue. ■ Instruct client to take frequent rest periods.

continued

NURSING PROCESS FOCUS   Clients Receiving Cholinergic Therapy   (*continued*)

Indirect Acting (Cholinesterase Inhibitors)

■ Monitor for muscle weakness. (This symptom, depending on time onset, indicates cholinergic crisis—overdose—OR myasthenic crisis—underdose.)	Instruct client to: ■ Report any severe muscle weakness that occurs 1 hour after administration of medication ■ Report any muscle weakness that occurs 3 or more hours after medication administration as this is a major symptom of myasthenic crisis ■ Not allow prescription to run out, especially if the medication is essential for breathing (respiratory muscle function)

Evaluation of Outcome Criteria

Evaluate effectiveness of drug therapy by confirming that client goals and expected outcomes have been met (see "Planning").

See Table 13.2 (page 129) for a list of drugs to which these nursing applications apply.

TABLE 13.3   Anticholinergics

Drug	Primary Use
atropine	increase heart rate, dilate pupils
benztropine (Apo-Benztropine)	Parkinson's disease
cyclopentolate (Cyclogyl)	dilate pupils
dicyclomine (Bentylol)	irritable bowel syndrome
glycopyrrolate	produce a dry field prior to anesthesia, peptic ulcers
ipratropium (Atrovent)	asthma
oxybutynin (Ditropan)	incontinence
propantheline (Pro-Banthine)	irritable bowel syndrome, peptic ulcer
scopolamine (Hyoscine)	motion sickness, irritable bowel syndrome, adjunct to anesthesia

SPECIAL CONSIDERATIONS

Impact of Anticholinergics on Male Sexual Function

A functioning autonomic nervous system is essential for normal male sexual health. The parasympathetic nervous system is necessary for erections, whereas the sympathetic division is responsible for the process of ejaculation. Anticholinergic drugs will block transmission of parasympathetic impulses and may interfere with normal erections. Adrenergic antagonists can interfere with the smooth muscle contractions in the seminal vesicles and penis, resulting in an inability to ejaculate.

For clients receiving autonomic medications, include questions about sexual activity during the assessment process. For male clients who are not sexually active, these side effects may be unimportant. For clients who are sexually active, however, drug-induced sexual dysfunction may be a major cause of non-adherence. The client should be informed to expect such side effects and to report them to their healthcare provider immediately. In most cases, alternative medications are available that do not affect sexual function. Inform the client that supportive counselling is available.

NATURAL THERAPIES

Valerian

Valerian root (*Valeriana officinalis*) is a perennial native to Europe and North America that is an herbal choice for nervous tension and anxiety. This natural product promotes rest without affecting rapid eye movement (REM) sleep and has a reputation for calming an individual without causing side effects or discomfort. Its name comes from the Latin *valere,* which means "to be well." One thing that is *not well,* however, is its pungent odour, though many users claim that the smell is well worth the benefits. Valerian also is purported to reduce pain and headaches without the worry of dependency. There is no drug hangover, as is sometimes experienced with tranquilizers and sedatives. It is available as a tincture (alcohol mixture), tea, or extract. Sometimes it is placed in juice and consumed immediately before taking a nap or going to bed.

13.8 Clinical Applications of Anticholinergics

Agents that block the action of acetylcholine are known by a number of names, including anticholinergics, cholinergic blockers, muscarinic antagonists, and parasympatholytics. Although the term *anticholinergic* is most commonly used, the most accurate term for this class of drug is *muscarinic antagonists* because at therapeutic doses, these drugs are selective for acetylcholine muscarinic receptors and thus have little effect on acetylcholine nicotinic receptors.

Anticholinergics act by competing with acetylcholine for binding of muscarinic receptors. When anticholinergics occupy these receptors, no response is generated at the neuroeffector organs. By suppressing the effects of acetylcholine, symptoms of sympathetic nervous system activation predominate. Most therapeutic uses of the anticholinergics are predictable extensions of their parasympathetic-blocking actions: dilation of the pupils, increase in heart rate, drying of secretions, and relaxation of the bronchi. Note that these are also symptoms of sympathetic activation (fight-or-flight response).

Therapeutic uses of anticholinergics include the following:

- GI disorders: Anticholinergics decrease the secretion of gastric acid in peptic ulcer disease (Chapter 36). They also slow intestinal motility and may be useful for reducing the cramping and diarrhea associated with irritable bowel syndrome (Chapter 37).

- Ophthalmic procedures: Anticholinergics may be used to cause mydriasis or cycloplegia during eye procedures (Chapter 48).

- Cardiac rhythm abnormalities: Anticholinergics can be used to accelerate the heart rate in clients experiencing bradycardia.

- Pre-anesthesia: Combined with other agents, anticholinergics can decrease excessive respiratory secretions and reverse the bradycardia caused by anesthetics (Chapter 20).

- Asthma: A few agents, such as ipratropium (Atrovent), are useful in treating asthma due to their ability to dilate the bronchi (Chapter 29).

The Prototype Drug, atropine, is used for several additional medical conditions due to its effective muscarinic receptor blockade. These applications include reversal of adverse muscarinic effects and treatment of muscarinic agonist poisoning, including that caused from overdose of bethanechol, cholinesterase inhibitors, or accidental ingestion of certain types of mushrooms or organophosphate pesticides.

Some of the anticholinergics are used for their effects on the CNS rather than their autonomic actions. Scopolamine is used for sedation and motion sickness (Chapter 37), and benztropine is prescribed to reduce the muscular tremor and rigidity associated with Parkinson's disease.

Anticholinergics exhibit a relatively high incidence of side effects. Important adverse effects that limit their usefulness include tachycardia, CNS stimulation, and the tendency to cause urinary retention in men with prostate disorders. Adverse effects such as dry mouth and dry eyes occur due to blockade of muscarinic receptors on salivary glands and lacrimal glands, respectively. Blockade of muscarinic receptors on sweat glands can inhibit sweating, which may lead to hyperthermia. Photophobia can occur due to the pupil being unable to constrict in response to bright light. Symptoms of overdose include fever, visual changes, difficulty swallowing, psychomotor agitation, and/or hallucinations. The development of safer, and sometimes more effective, drugs has greatly decreased the current use of anticholinergics. An exception is ipratropium, a relatively new anticholinergic used for clients with COPD. Because it is delivered via aerosol spray, this agent produces more localized action with fewer systemic side effects than atropine.

NURSING CONSIDERATIONS

The role of the nurse in anticholinergic therapy involves careful monitoring of the client's condition and providing education as it relates to the prescribed drug treatment. Perform a thorough medical history, including medications the client is currently taking that could cause drug-drug interactions. Antihistamines, in particular, can lead to excessive muscarinic blockade. Check for a history of taking herbal supplements; some have atropine-like actions that potentiate the effects of the medication and can be harmful to the client. For example, aloe, senna, buckthorn, and cascara sagrada may increase atropine's effect, particularly with chronic use of the herbs.

This classification of drugs should not be used if the client has a history of acute angle-closure glaucoma. Anticholinergics block muscarinic receptors in the eye, creating paralysis of the iris sphincter, which can increase intraocular pressure. Safety has not been established for pregnancy and lactation. Anticholinergics may produce fetal tachycardia.

Anticholinergics are contraindicated in clients with cardiopulmonary conditions such as COPD, asthma, heart disease, and hypertension because blockade of cardiac muscarinic receptors prevents the parasympathetic nervous system from slowing the heart. This can result in an acceleration of heart rate that may exacerbate these conditions. Clients with hyperthyroidism should not be given these medications because in hyperthyroidism, the heart rate is generally high and administration of anticholinergics can cause dysrhythmias due to norepinephrine release from sympathetic nerves that regulate heart rate.

The nurse should also assess for baseline bowel and bladder function. Renal conditions are contraindications to anticholinergic therapy because they impair the ability of the bladder to empty. Gastrointestinal conditions such as ulcerative colitis and ileus are contraindicated because blockade of muscarinic receptors in the intestine can decrease the tone and motility of intestinal smooth muscle, which can exacerbate intestinal conditions. Monitor clients with esophageal reflux and hiatal hernia because anticholinergics reduce GI motility. Clients with gastroesophageal reflux disease (GERD) and hiatal hernia experience decreased muscle tone in the lower esophageal sphincter and delayed stomach emptying. Anticholinergics exacerbate these symptoms, increasing the risk of esophageal injury and aspiration. Clients with Down syndrome may be more sensitive to the effects of atropine due to structural differences in the CNS caused by chromosomal abnormality (trisomy). Clients with Down syndrome also tend to have disorders such as GERD and heart disease, which may be adversely affected by anticholinergics.

See "Nursing Process Focus: Clients Receiving Anticholinergic Therapy" on page 135 for specific points to include when teaching clients about this class of drug.

Pr PROTOTYPE DRUG | Atropine

ACTIONS AND USES

By occupying muscarinic receptors, atropine blocks the parasympathetic actions of acetylcholine and induces symptoms of the fight-or-flight response. Most prominent are increased heart rate, bronchodilation, decreased motility in the GI tract, mydriasis, and decreased secretions from glands. At therapeutic doses, atropine has no effect on nicotinic receptors in ganglia or skeletal muscle.

Atropine is particularly important as an antidote to cholinergic toxicity. Atropine may also be used to suppress secretions during surgical procedures, to increase the heart rate in clients with bradycardia, and to dilate the pupil during eye examinations. Once widely used to cause bronchodilation in clients with asthma and to treat hypermotility diseases of the GI tract such as irritable bowel syndrome, atropine is now rarely prescribed for these disorders because of the development of drugs with less unpleasant side effects.

PHARMACOKINETICS

Atropine can be given IV, SC, IM, or PO. Atropine is well absorbed. It is widely distributed, crosses the blood-brain barrier and placenta, and enters breast milk. It is mostly metabolized by the liver. About 40% is excreted unchanged by the kidneys. Its half-life is 4 to 5 hours in adults.

ADMINISTRATION ALERTS

- Atropine may be given by direct IV (push) or by infusion.
- It may cause initial paradoxical bradycardia, lasting up to 2 minutes, especially at lower doses.
- The drug may induce ventricular fibrillation in cardiac clients.
- Atropine is pregnancy category C.

ADVERSE EFFECTS AND INTERACTIONS

The side effects of atropine limit its therapeutic usefulness and are predictable extensions of its autonomic actions. Expected side effects include dry mouth, constipation, urinary retention, and an increased heart rate. Initial CNS excitement may progress to delirium and even coma. Atropine is usually contraindicated in clients with glaucoma because the drug may increase pressure within the eye. Accidental poisoning has occurred in children who eat the colourful, purple berries of the deadly nightshade, mistaking them for cherries. Symptoms of poisoning are those of intense parasympathetic stimulation.

Drug interactions with atropine include an increased effect with antihistamines, tricyclic antidepressants, quinidine, and procainamide. Atropine decreases effects of levodopa. Use with caution with herbal supplements, such as aloe, senna, buckthorn, and cascara sagrada, which may increase atropine's effect, particularly with chronic use of these herbs.

 See the Companion Website for a Nursing Process Focus specific to this drug.

ADRENERGICS

Adrenergics (sympathomimetics) stimulate adrenergic receptors, thereby activating the sympathetic nervous system and inducing symptoms characteristic of the fight-or-flight response. These drugs have clinical applications in the treatment of shock and hypotension. They are listed in Table 13.4.

13.9 Clinical Applications of Adrenergics

The adrenergics, also known as adrenergic agonists and sympathomimetics, produce many of the same responses as the anticholinergics. However, because the sympathetic nervous system has both alpha- and beta-subreceptors, the

TABLE 13.4   Adrenergics

Drug	Primary Receptor Subtype	Primary Use
salbutamol (Ventolin)	beta$_2$	asthma
clonidine (Catapres)	alpha$_2$ in CNS	hypertension
dobutamine (Dobutrex)	beta$_1$	cardiac stimulant
dopamine (Intropin)	alpha$_1$ and beta$_1$	shock
epinephrine (Adrenalin)	alpha and beta	cardiac arrest, asthma
formoterol (Foradil)	beta$_2$	asthma, COPD
isoproterenol (Isuprel)	beta$_1$ and beta$_2$	asthma, dysrhythmias, heart failure
isoproterenol	beta$_2$	asthma
methyldopa	alpha$_2$ in CNS	hypertension
norepinephrine (Levophed)	alpha$_1$ and beta$_1$	shock
phenylephrine (Neo-Synephrine)	alpha	nasal congestion
pseudoephedrine	alpha and beta	nasal congestion

NURSING PROCESS FOCUS Clients Receiving Anticholinergic Therapy

Assessment	Potential Nursing Diagnoses/Identified Patterns
Prior to administration: ■ Obtain complete health history, including drug history to determine possible drug interactions and allergies. ■ Assess reason for drug administration. ■ Assess heart rate, blood pressure, temperature, and elimination patterns (initially and throughout therapy).	■ Need for knowledge regarding drug therapy ■ Decreased cardiac output ■ Changes in body temperature ■ Dry oral mucous membrane ■ Constipation ■ Urinary retention

Planning: Client Goals and Expected Outcomes

The client will:
■ Exhibit a decrease in symptoms for which the medication is prescribed
■ Demonstrate an understanding of the drug by accurately describing the drug's purpose, action, side effects, and precautions
■ Verbalize techniques to avoid hazardous side effects associated with anticholinergic therapy

Implementation

Interventions (Rationales)	Client Education/Discharge Planning
■ Monitor for signs of anticholinergic crisis resulting from overdosage: fever, tachycardia, difficulty swallowing, ataxia, reduced urine output, psychomotor agitation, confusion, hallucinations. ■ Report significant changes in heart rate, blood pressure, or the development of dysrhythmias. ■ Observe for side effects such as drowsiness, blurred vision, tachycardia, dry mouth, urinary hesitancy, and decreased sweating. ■ Provide comfort measures for dry mucous membranes, such as applying lubricant to moisten lips and oral mucosa, assisting in rinsing mouth, using artificial tears for dry eyes, as needed. ■ Minimize exposure to heat and cold and strenuous exercise. (Anticholinergics can inhibit sweat gland secretions due to direct blockade of the muscarinic receptors on the sweat glands. This can increase their risk for hyperthermia since sweating is necessary for clients to cool down) ■ Monitor intake and output ratio. Palpate abdomen for bladder distention. ■ Monitor client for abdominal distention and auscultate for bowel sounds.	■ Instruct clients to report side effects related to therapy such as shortness of breath, cough, dysphagia, syncope, fever, anxiety, right upper quadrant pain, extreme lethargy, or dizziness. ■ Instruct client to monitor vital signs, ensuring proper use of home equipment. Instruct client to: ■ Report side effects ■ Avoid driving and hazardous activities until effects of the drug are known ■ Wear sunglasses to decrease the sensitivity to bright light ■ Instruct client that oral rinses, sugarless gum or candy, and frequent oral hygiene may help relieve dry mouth. Avoid alcohol-containing mouthwashes that can further dry oral tissue. ■ Advise client to limit activity outside when the temperature is hot. Strenuous activity in a hot environment may cause heat stroke. ■ Instruct client to notify healthcare provider if difficulty in voiding occurs. ■ Advise client to increase fluid and add bulk to the diet if constipation becomes a problem.

Evaluation of Outcome Criteria

Evaluate effectiveness of drug therapy by confirming that client goals and expected outcomes have been met (see "Planning").

See Table 13.3 (page 132) for a list of drugs to which these nursing actions apply.

---

actions of many adrenergics are more specific and have wider therapeutic application (see Table 13.4).

Adrenergics may be classified as catecholamines or non-catecholamines. The catecholamines have a chemical structure similar to norepinephrine, a short duration of action, and must be administered parenterally. The non-catecholamines can be taken orally and have longer durations of action because they are not rapidly destroyed by monoamine oxidase.

Most adrenergics act by directly binding to and activating adrenergic receptors. Examples include the three endogenous catecholamines: epinephrine, norepinephrine, and dopamine. Other medications in this class act indirectly by causing the release of norepinephrine from its vesicles on the presynaptic neuron or by inhibiting its reuptake or destruction. Those that act by indirect mechanisms, such as amphetamine and cocaine, are used for their central effects on the brain rather than their autonomic effects. A few agents, such as ephedrine, act by both direct and indirect mechanisms.

Most effects of adrenergics are predictable based on their autonomic actions, depending on which adrenergic subreceptors are stimulated. Because the receptor responses are so different, the student will need to memorize the specific receptor subtypes activated by each adrenergic. Therapeutic applications of the different receptor subtype activations are as follows:

- Alpha$_1$-receptor agonists: treatment of nasal congestion or hypotension; induction of mydriasis during ophthalmic examinations
- Alpha$_2$-receptor agonists: treatment of hypertension through non-autonomic (central-acting) mechanism
- Beta$_1$-receptor agonists: treatment of cardiac arrest, heart failure, and shock
- Beta$_2$-receptor agonists: treatment of asthma and premature labour contractions

Some adrenergics are non-selective, stimulating more than one type of adrenergic receptor. For example, epinephrine stimulates all four types of adrenergic receptors and is used for cardiac arrest and asthma. Pseudoephedrine (Sudafed and others) stimulates both alpha$_1$- and beta$_2$-receptors and is used as a nasal decongestant. Isoproterenol (Isuprel) stimulates both beta$_1$- and beta$_2$-receptors and is used to increase the heart's rate and force of contraction and speed of electrical conduction, and occasionally to treat asthma. The non-selective drugs generally cause more autonomic-related side effects than the selective agents.

The side effects of the adrenergics are mostly extensions of their autonomic actions. Cardiovascular effects such as tachycardia, hypertension, and dysrhythmias are particularly troublesome and may limit therapy. Large doses can induce CNS excitement and seizures. Other adrenergic responses that may occur are dry mouth, nausea, and vomiting. Some of these agents cause anorexia, which has led to their historical use as appetite suppressants. Because of prominent cardiovascular side effects, adrenergics are now rarely used for this purpose.

Drugs in this class are presented as Prototype Drugs in many other chapters in this textbook: dopamine and norepinephrine in Chapter 27, oxymetazoline and epinephrine in Chapter 31, and salmeterol in Chapter 29.

NURSING CONSIDERATIONS

Since the purposes and indications of drugs within this class vary greatly, the Nursing Process Focus applies to all clients receiving adrenergic drugs. For specific nursing considerations, contraindications, and precautions, see Chapters 27, 29, and 31.

Pr PROTOTYPE DRUG | Phenylephrine (Neo-Synephrine)

ACTIONS AND USES

Phenylephrine is a selective alpha-adrenergic agonist that is available in several different formulations, including intranasal, ophthalmic, IM, SC, and IV. All of its actions and indications are extensions of its sympathetic stimulation. When applied intranasally by spray or drops, it reduces nasal congestion by constricting small blood vessels in the nasal mucosa. Applied topically to the eye during ophthalmic examinations, phenylephrine is used to dilate the pupil. The parenteral administration of phenylephrine can reverse acute hypotension caused by spinal anesthesia or vascular shock. Because it lacks beta-adrenergic agonist activity, it produces relatively few cardiac side effects at therapeutic doses. Its longer duration of activity and lack of significant cardiac effects give phenylephrine some advantages over epinephrine and norepinephrine in treating acute hypotension.

ADMINISTRATION ALERTS

- Do not use solution if it is brown or contains precipitate (particles).
- Parenteral administration can cause severe tissue injury with extravasation.
- Phenylephrine ophthalmic drops may damage soft contact lenses.
- Phenylephrine is pregnancy category C.

PHARMACOKINETICS

Phenylephrine is rapidly absorbed. It is metabolized in the liver and tissues by monoamine oxidase. Its half-life is unknown.

ADVERSE EFFECTS AND INTERACTIONS

When used topically or intranasally, side effects are uncommon. Intranasal use can cause burning of the mucosa and rebound congestion if used for prolonged periods (see Chapter 31). Ophthalmic preparations can cause narrow-angle glaucoma, secondary to their mydriatic effect. High doses can cause reflex bradycardia due to the elevation of blood pressure caused by stimulation of alpha$_1$-receptors. When used parenterally, the drug should be used with caution in clients with advanced coronary artery disease or hypertension. Anxiety, restlessness, and tremor may occur due to the drug's stimulation effect on the CNS. Clients with hyperthyroidism may experience a severe increase in basal metabolic rate, resulting in increased blood pressure and tachycardia. Drug interactions may occur with MAO inhibitors, causing a hypertensive crisis. Increased effects may also occur with tricyclic antidepressants. This drug is incompatible with iron preparations (ferric salts).

 See the Companion Website for a Nursing Process Focus specific to this drug.

NURSING PROCESS FOCUS Clients Receiving Adrenergic Therapy	
Assessment	**Potential Nursing Diagnoses/Identified Patterns**
Prior to administration: ■ Determine reason for drug administration. ■ Monitor vital signs, urinary output, and cardiac output (initially and throughout therapy). ■ For treatment of nasal congestion, assess the nasal mucosa for changes such as excoriation or bleeding. ■ Obtain complete health history including allergies, drug history, and possible drug interactions.	■ Need for knowledge regarding drug therapy ■ Adequate sleep ■ Nasal congestion ■ Risk for injury related to side effects of drug therapy ■ Decreased cardiac output ■ Risk for decreased tissue perfusion

Planning: Client Goals and Expected Outcomes
The client will: ■ Exhibit a decrease in the symptoms for which the drug is being given ■ Demonstrate understanding of the drug's action by accurately describing drug side effects and precautions ■ Demonstrate proper nasal/ophthalmic drug instillation technique

Implementation	
Interventions (Rationales)	**Client Education/Discharge Planning**
■ Closely monitor IV insertion sites for extravasation with IV administration. Use an infusion pump to deliver the medication. ■ Use a tuberculin syringe when administering SC doses that are extremely small. ■ For metered dose inhalation, shake container well and wait at least 2 minutes between medications. ■ Instill only the prescribed number of drops when using ophthalmic solutions.	Instruct client to: ■ Use the drug strictly as prescribed, and not "double up" on doses ■ Take medication early in day to avoid insomnia
■ Monitor the client for side effects. (Side effects of adrenergics may be serious and limit therapy.)	Instruct client to: ■ Immediately report shortness of breath, palpitations, dizziness, chest/arm pain or pressure, or other angina-like symptoms ■ Consult healthcare provider before attempting to use adrenergics to treat nasal congestion or eye irritation ■ Monitor blood pressure, pulse, and temperature to ensure proper use of home equipment
■ Monitor breathing patterns and observe for shortness of breath and/or audible wheezing.	■ Instruct client to immediately report any difficulty breathing. Instruct clients with a history of asthma to consult their healthcare provider before using OTC drugs to treat nasal congestion.
■ Observe the client's responsiveness to light. (Some adrenergics cause photosensitivity by affecting the pupillary light accommodation/response.) ■ Provide eye comfort by reducing exposure to bright light in the environment; shield the eyes with a rolled washcloth or eye bandages for severe photosensitivity.	■ Instruct clients using ophthalmic adrenergics that transient stinging and blurred vision upon instillation is normal. Headache and/or brow pain may also occur. ■ Instruct client to avoid driving and other activities requiring visual acuity until blurring subsides.
■ For clients receiving nasal adrenergics, observe the nasal cavity. Monitor for rhinorrhea and epistaxis.	Instruct client to: ■ Observe nasal cavity for signs of excoriation or bleeding before instilling nasal spray or drops; review procedure for safe instillation of nasal sprays or eye drops ■ Limit OTC usage of adrenergics; inform client about rebound nasal congestion

Evaluation of Outcome Criteria
Evaluate effectiveness of drug therapy by confirming that client goals and expected outcomes have been met (see "Planning").

See Table 13.4 (page 134) for a list of drugs to which these nursing actions apply.

ADRENERGIC ANTAGONISTS

Adrenergic antagonists inhibit the sympathetic nervous system and produce many of the same rest-and-digest symptoms as the cholinergics. They have wide therapeutic application in the treatment of hypertension. The adrenergic antagonists are listed in Table 13.5.

13.10 Clinical Applications of Adrenergic Antagonists

Adrenergic antagonists act by directly blocking adrenergic receptors. The actions of these agents are specific to either alpha or beta blockade. Medications in this class have great therapeutic application: they are the most widely prescribed class of autonomic drug.

Alpha-adrenergic antagonists, or simply alpha-blockers, are used for their effects on vascular smooth muscle. By relaxing vascular smooth muscle in small arteries, alpha$_1$-blockers such as doxazosin cause vasodilation, which results in decreased blood pressure. They may be used either alone or in combination with other agents in the treatment of hypertension (Chapter 21). A second use is in the treatment of benign prostatic hyperplasia, due to their ability to increase urine flow (Chapter 42). The most common adverse effect of alpha-blockers is orthostatic hypotension, which occurs when a client abruptly changes from a recumbent to an upright position. Reflex tachycardia, nasal congestion, and impotence are other important side effects that occur due to increased parasympathetic activity.

Beta-adrenergic antagonists may block beta$_1$-receptors, beta$_2$-receptors, or both. Regardless of their receptor specificity, the therapeutic applications of all beta-blockers relate to their effects on the cardiovascular system. Beta-blockers will decrease the rate and force of contraction of the heart and slow electrical conduction through the atrioventricular node. Drugs that selectively block beta$_1$-receptors, such as atenolol, are called cardioselective agents. Because they have little effect on non-cardiac tissue, they exert fewer side effects than non-selective agents such as propranolol.

The primary use of beta-blockers is in the treatment of hypertension. Although the exact mechanism by which beta-blockers reduce blood pressure is not completely understood, it is thought that the reduction may be due to the decreased cardiac output or suppression of renin release by the kidney. The student should refer to Chapter 21 for a more comprehensive description of the use of beta-blockers in hypertension management.

Beta-adrenergic antagonists have several other important therapeutic applications, discussions of which appear in many chapters in this textbook. By decreasing the cardiac workload, beta-blockers can ease the symptoms of angina pectoris (Chapter 23). By slowing electrical conduction across the myocardium, beta-blockers are able to treat certain types of dysrhythmias (Chapter 25). Other therapeutic uses include the treatment of heart failure (Chapter 24), myocardial infarction (Chapter 23), and narrow-angle glaucoma (Chapter 48).

NURSING CONSIDERATIONS

Because the purposes and indications of drugs within this class vary greatly, the Nursing Process Focus applies to all clients receiving adrenergic antagonist drugs. For specific nursing considerations, contraindications, and precautions, see Chapters 21, 23, and 48 for more information about alpha- and beta-adrenergic blockers.

TABLE 13.5	Adrenergic Antagonists	
Drug	**Primary Receptor Subtype**	**Primary Use**
acebutolol (Monitan)	beta$_1$	hypertension, dysrhythmias, angina
atenolol (Tenormin)	beta$_1$	hypertension, angina
carvedilol (Coreg)	alpha$_1$, beta$_1$, and beta$_2$	hypertension
doxazocin (Cardura)	alpha$_1$	hypertension
metoprolol (Lopresor)	beta$_1$	hypertension
nadolol (Corgard)	beta$_1$ and beta$_2$	hypertension
phentolamine	alpha	severe hypertension
prazosin (Minipress)	alpha$_1$	hypertension
propranolol (Inderal)	beta$_1$ and beta$_2$	hypertension, dysrhythmias, heart failure
sotalol (Apo-Sotalol)	beta$_1$ and beta$_2$	dysrhythmias
terazosin (Apo-Terazosin)	alpha$_1$	hypertension
timolol (Timoptic)	beta$_1$ and beta$_2$	hypertension, angina, glaucoma

Pr PROTOTYPE DRUG | Prazosin (Minipress)

ACTIONS AND USES

Prazosin is a selective alpha$_1$-adrenergic antagonist that competes with norepinephrine at its receptors on vascular smooth muscle in arterioles and veins. Its major action is a rapid decrease in peripheral resistance that reduces blood pressure. It has little effect on cardiac output or heart rate, and it causes less reflex tachycardia than some other drugs in this class. Tolerance to prazosin's antihypertensive effects may occur. Its most common use is in combination with other agents, such as beta-blockers or diuretics, in the pharmacotherapy of hypertension. Prazosin has a short half-life and is often taken two or three times per day.

PHARMACOKINETICS

Prazosin is 60% absorbed after oral administration. It is widely distributed and highly protein bound. It is extensively metabolized by the liver. Its half-life is 2 to 3 hours.

ADMINISTRATION ALERTS

- This drug increases urinary metabolites of vanillylmandelic acid (VMA) and norepinephrine, which are measured to screen for pheochromocytoma (adrenal tumour), so prazosin will cause false-positive results.
- Prazosin is pregnancy category C.

ADVERSE EFFECTS AND INTERACTIONS

Like other alpha-blockers, prazosin has a tendency to cause orthostatic hypotension due to alpha$_1$ inhibition in vascular smooth muscle. In rare cases, this hypotension can be so severe as to cause unconsciousness about 30 minutes after the first dose. This is called the *first-dose phenomenon*. To avoid this situation, the first dose should be very low and given at bedtime. Dizziness, drowsiness, or light-headedness may occur as a result of decreased blood flow to the brain due to the drug's hypotensive action. Reflex tachycardia may occur due to the rapid falls in blood pressure. The alpha blockade may also result in nasal congestion or inhibition of ejaculation.

Drug interactions include increased hypotensive effects with concurrent use of antihypertensives and diuretics.

 See the Companion Website for a Nursing Process Focus specific to this drug.

NURSING PROCESS FOCUS   Clients Receiving Adrenergic Antagonist Therapy

Assessment	Potential Nursing Diagnoses/Identified Patterns
Prior to administration: - Assess vital signs, urinary output, and cardiac output (initially and throughout therapy). - Assess reason for drug administration. - Obtain complete health history, including allergies, drug history, and possible drug interactions.	- Need for knowledge regarding drug therapy - Impaired sensory perception - Risk for injury related to dizziness, syncope - Urinary retention - Sexual dysfunction

Planning: Client Goals and Expected Outcomes

The client will:
- Exhibit a decrease in blood pressure with no adverse effects
- Report a decrease in urinary symptoms such as hesitancy and difficulty voiding
- Demonstrate an understanding of the drug by accurately describing the drug's purpose, action, side effects and precautions

Implementation

Interventions (Rationales)	Client Education/Discharge Planning
- For prostatic hypertrophy, monitor for urinary hesitancy/feeling of incomplete bladder emptying, interrupted urinary stream.	- Instruct client to report increased difficulty with urinary voiding to healthcare provider.
- Monitor for syncope. (Alpha-adrenergic antagonists produce first-dose syncope phenomenon and may cause loss of consciousness.)	Instruct client to: - Take this medication at bedtime, and to take the first dose *immediately* before getting into bed - Avoid abrupt changes in position Warn client about the first dose phenomenon; reassure that this effect diminishes with continued therapy.
- Monitor vital signs, level of consciousness, and mood. (Adrenergic antagonists can exacerbate existing mental depression.)	- Instruct client to immediately report any feelings of dysphoria. - Interview client regarding suicide potential; obtain a "no self-harm" verbal contract from the client.

continued

NURSING PROCESS FOCUS Clients Receiving Adrenergic Antagonist Therapy *(continued)*

Implementation

▪ Monitor carefully for dizziness, drowsiness, or light-headedness. (These are signs of decreased blood flow to the brain due to the drug's hypotensive action.)	Instruct client: ▪ To monitor vitals signs, especially blood pressure, ensuring proper use of home equipment ▪ Regarding the normotensive range of blood pressure; instruct client to consult the nurse regarding "reportable" blood pressure readings ▪ To report dizziness or syncope that persists beyond the first dose, as well as paresthesias and other neurological changes
▪ Observe for side effects, which may include blurred vision, tinnitus, epistaxis, and edema.	Instruct client: ▪ That nasal congestion may be a side effect ▪ To report any adverse reactions to the healthcare provider Warn client about the potential danger of concomitant use of OTC nasal decongestants.
▪ Monitor liver function (due to increased risk for liver toxicity).	Instruct client to: ▪ Adhere to a regular schedule of laboratory testing for liver function as ordered by the healthcare provider ▪ Report signs and symptoms of liver toxicity: nausea, vomiting, diarrhea, rash, jaundice, abdominal pain, tenderness or distention, or change in colour of stool Inform client of the importance of ongoing medication adherence and follow-up.

Evaluation of Outcome Criteria

Evaluate effectiveness of drug therapy by confirming that client goals and expected outcomes have been met (see "Planning").

See Table 13.5 (page 138) for a list of drugs to which these nursing actions apply.

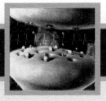

CHAPTER REVIEW

KEY CONCEPTS

The numbered key concepts provide a succinct summary of the important points from the corresponding numbered section within the chapter. If any of these points are not clear, refer to the numbered section within the chapter for review. Expanded versions can be found on the Companion Website.

13.1 The peripheral nervous system is divided into a somatic portion, which is under voluntary control, and an autonomic portion, which is involuntary and controls smooth muscle, cardiac muscle, and glandular secretion.

13.2 Stimulation of the sympathetic division of the autonomic nervous system causes symptoms of the fight-or-flight response, whereas stimulation of the parasympathetic branch induces rest-and-digest responses.

13.3 Drugs can affect nervous transmission across a synapse by preventing the storage or release of the neurotransmitter, binding receptors for the neurotransmitter, or preventing the destruction of the neurotransmitter.

13.4 Acetylcholine is the primary neurotransmitter released at cholinergic receptors (nicotinic and muscarinic) in both the sympathetic and parasympathetic nervous systems. It is also the neurotransmitter at nicotinic receptors in skeletal muscle.

13.5 Norepinephrine is the primary neurotransmitter released at adrenergic receptors, which are divided into alpha and beta subtypes.

13.6 Autonomic drugs are classified by which receptors they stimulate or block: adrenergics stimulate adrenergic receptors of sympathetic nerves, and cholinergics stimulate cholinergic receptors of parasympathetic nerves; adrenergic antagonists inhibit the sympathetic division, whereas anticholinergics inhibit the parasympathetic branch.

13.7 Cholinergics act directly by stimulating cholinergic receptors or indirectly by inhibiting acetylcholinesterase. They have few therapeutic uses because of their numerous side effects.

13.8 Anticholinergics act by blocking the effects of acetylcholine at muscarinic receptors and are used to dry secretions, treat asthma, and prevent motion sickness.

13.9 Adrenergics act directly by activating adrenergic receptors or indirectly by increasing the release of norepinephrine

from nerve terminals. They are primarily used for their effects on the heart, bronchial tree, and nasal passages.

13.10 Adrenergic antagonists are primarily used for hypertension and are the most widely prescribed class of autonomic drug.

REVIEW QUESTIONS

1 How are drugs affecting the autonomic nervous system classified?

2 Why do the adrenergic agonists produce many of the same symptoms as the anticholinergics?

3 Both cholinergics and adrenergic blockers produce similar actions. Why are the adrenergic blockers used to treat hypertension, but the cholinergics are not used for this purpose?

4 Atropine is used as an antidote for cholinergic toxicity. Why is it used for this purpose?

5 A new drug has been developed that is classified as an adrenergic-receptor antagonist. Why is it important to know which type of adrenergic receptor is blocked before administering this medication?

CRITICAL THINKING QUESTIONS

1. A 24-year-old female college student is diagnosed with Raynaud's disease, a disorder characterized by inadequate peripheral blood flow. She reports that her hands are constantly cold and dusky and that her fingers and toes become white with numbness and throbbing when exposed to cold. She is prescribed prazosin, an alpha-adrenergic blocker. What is the drug's therapeutic action? What side effects can be anticipated? How might this drug affect her studies? What evidence would indicate that the drug is effective?

2. A 74-year-old female client has undergone a retropubic urethral suspension. She required a Foley catheter for 4 days post-op and was unable to void after it was removed. She was re-catheterized and a bladder rehabilitation program was begun, which included bethanechol. What does the nurse need to know about this drug in order to plan

safe, effective care? What interventions may enhance the drug's effectiveness? What side effects may occur?

3. A 42-year-old male client has been diagnosed with having Parkinson's disease for 4 years. He is being treated with amantadine, an indirect-acting dopaminergic agent, and benztropine. The nurse identifies benztropine as an anticholinergic agent. Discuss the potential side effects of benztropine that the nurse should assess for in this client. What should the client be taught about this drug?

4. A 16-year-old male reports to the school nurse that his heart rate increases when he uses his isoproterenol inhaler for asthma. How is this drug classified? Is his increased heart rate likely to be due to the effects of this drug? What assessment is important for a client on this drug? What interventions would you plan to enhance the effectiveness and minimize the side effects of this drug?

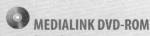
EXPLORE
MediaLink

 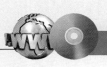
ww.pearsoned.ca/adams-king

MEDIALINK DVD-ROM
- **Audio Glossary**
- **CRNE Review**

COMPANION WEBSITE
- **CRNE Review**
- **Case Study:** Cholinergics
- **Dosage Calculation**
- **Nursing Process Focus Charts**

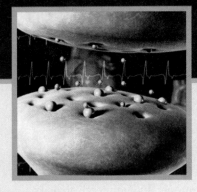

CHAPTER 14

Drugs for Anxiety and Insomnia

DRUGS AT A GLANCE

BENZODIAZEPINES
　　🔊 *lorazepam (Ativan)*

BARBITURATES

NON-BENZODIAZEPINE/NON-BARBITURATE CNS DEPRESSANTS
　　🔊 *zopiclone (Imovane)*

OBJECTIVES

After reading this chapter, the student should be able to do the following:

1. Discuss factors contributing to anxiety and insomnia and explain some non-pharmacological therapies used to manage each of these disorders.
2. Identify drug classes used for treating anxiety and sleep disorders.
3. Explain the therapeutic action of drugs used for treating anxiety disorders and insomnia.
4. Describe the nurse's role in the pharmacological management of clients with anxiety disorders and insomnia.
5. For each of the drug classes listed in Drugs at a Glance, identify a representative drug and explain its mechanism of action, therapeutic effects, and important adverse effects.
6. Describe and explain, based on pharmacological principles, the rationale for nursing assessment, planning, and interventions for clients with anxiety disorders and insomnia.
7. Use the nursing process to care for clients receiving drug therapy for anxiety and insomnia.

MediaLink

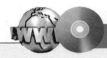 www.pearsoned.ca/adams-king

CRNE review, case studies, and other interactive resources for this chapter can be found on the Companion Website at **www.pearsoned.ca/adams-king**. Click on "Chapter 14" to select the activities for this chapter. For animations, more CRNE review questions, and an audio glossary, access the accompanying MediaLink DVD-ROM in this textbook.

People experience nervousness and tension more often than any other symptoms. Seeking relief from these symptoms, clients often turn to a variety of pharmacological and alternative therapies. Most healthcare providers agree that even though drugs do not cure the underlying problem, they can provide short-term help to clients who are experiencing acute anxiety or insomnia. This chapter deals with drugs that treat anxiety, cause sedation, or help clients sleep.

ANXIETY DISORDERS

According to the *International Classification of Diseases,* 10th edition (ICD-10), **anxiety** is a state of "apprehension, tension, or uneasiness that stems from the anticipation of danger, the source of which is largely unknown or unrecognized." Anxious individuals can often identify at least some factors that bring on their symptoms. Most state that their feelings of anxiety are disproportionate to any actual dangers.

14.1 Types of Anxiety Disorders

The anxiety experienced by people faced with a stressful environment is called **situational anxiety**. To a certain degree, situational anxiety is beneficial because it motivates people to accomplish tasks in a prompt manner—if for no other reason than to eliminate the source of nervousness. Situational stress may be intense, though clients often learn coping mechanisms to deal with the stress without seeking conventional medical intervention. From an early age, ego defence mechanisms begin to develop that serve as defences against anxiety.

Generalized anxiety disorder (GAD) is a difficult-to-control, excessive anxiety that lasts 6 months or more. It focuses on a variety of life events or activities and interferes with normal, day-to-day functions. It is by far the most common type of stress disorder, and the one most frequently encountered by the nurse. Symptoms include restlessness, fatigue, muscle tension, nervousness, inability to focus or concentrate, an overwhelming sense of dread, and sleep disturbances. Autonomic signs of sympathetic nervous system activation include blood pressure elevation, heart palpitations, varying degrees of respiratory change, dry mouth, and increased reflexes. Parasympathetic responses may consist of abdominal cramping, diarrhea, fatigue, urinary urgency, and numbness and tingling of the extremities. Females are slightly more likely to experience GAD, and its prevalence is highest in the 20 to 35 age group.

A second category of anxiety, called **panic disorder**, is characterized by intense feelings of immediate apprehension, fearfulness, terror, or impending doom that are accompanied by increased autonomic nervous system activity. Although panic attacks usually last less than 10 minutes, clients may describe them as seemingly endless. As much as 5% of the population will experience one or more panic attacks during their lifetime, with women being affected about twice as often as men.

Other categories of anxiety disorders include phobias, obsessive-compulsive disorder, and posttraumatic stress disorder. **Phobias** are fearful feelings attached to situations or objects. Common phobias include fear of snakes, spiders, crowds, or heights. Phobias compel a client to avoid the fearful stimulus. **Obsessive-compulsive disorder (OCD)** involves recurrent, intrusive thoughts or repetitive behaviours that interfere with normal activities or relationships. Common examples include fear of exposure to germs and repetitive handwashing. **Posttraumatic stress disorder (PTSD)** is a type of anxiety that develops in response to re-experiencing a previous life event. Traumatic life events such as war, physical or sexual abuse, natural disasters, or murder may lead to a sense of helplessness and re-experiencing of the traumatic event. In the aftermath of the terrorist attack of September 11, 2001, the incidence of PTSD increased considerably.

14.2 Regions of the Brain Responsible for Anxiety and Wakefulness

Neural systems associated with anxiety and restlessness include the limbic system and the reticular activating system. These are illustrated in Figure 14.1.

The **limbic system** is an area in the middle of the brain responsible for emotional expression, learning, and memory. Signals routed through the limbic system ultimately connect with the hypothalamus. Emotional states associated with this connection include anxiety, fear, anger, aggression, remorse, depression, sexual drive, and euphoria.

The hypothalamus is an important centre responsible for unconscious responses to extreme stress such as elevated blood pressure, elevated respiratory rate, and dilated pupils. These are responses associated with the fight-or-flight

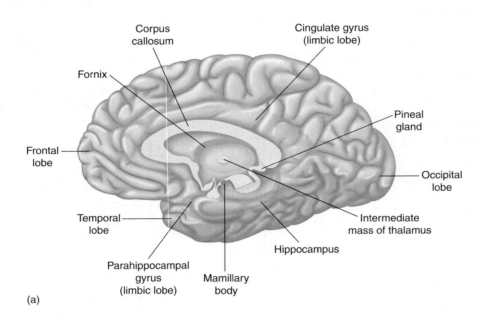

(a)

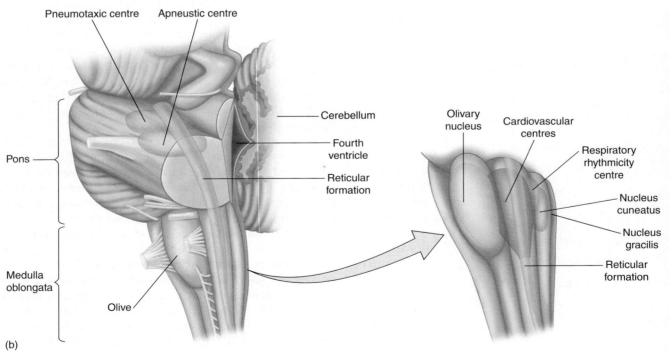

(b)

● **Figure 14.1** Brain regions strongly associated with anxiety, expressions of emotion, and a restless state: (a) the limbic system; (b) the reticular formation, a nucleus where nervous signals ascend to higher centres of the brain; this entire neural network is called the reticular activating system

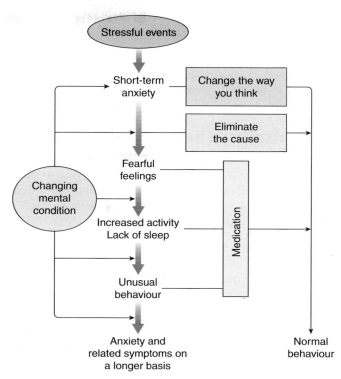

● **Figure 14.2** A model of anxiety in which stressful events or a changing mental condition can produce unfavourable symptoms, some of which may be controlled by medication

response of the autonomic nervous system, as presented in Chapter 13. The many endocrine functions of the hypothalamus are discussed in Chapter 39.

The hypothalamus also connects with the **reticular formation**, a network of neurons found along the entire length of the brainstem, as shown in Figure 14.1b. Stimulation of the reticular formation causes heightened alertness and arousal; inhibition causes general drowsiness and the induction of sleep.

The larger area in which the reticular formation is found is called the **reticular activating system (RAS)**. This structure projects from the brainstem to the thalamus. The RAS is responsible for sleeping and wakefulness and performs an alerting function for the cerebral cortex. It also helps a person to focus attention on individual tasks by transmitting information to higher brain centres.

If signals are prevented from passing through the RAS, no emotional signals are sent to the brain, resulting in a reduction in general brain activity. If signals coming from the hypothalamus are allowed to proceed, then those signals are further routed through the RAS and on to higher brain centres. This is the neural mechanism thought to be responsible for emotions such as anxiety and fear. It is also the mechanism associated with restlessness and an interrupted sleeping pattern.

14.3 Anxiety Management through Pharmacological and Non-Pharmacological Strategies

Although stress itself may be incapacitating, it is often only a symptom of an underlying disorder. It is considered more productive to uncover and address the cause of the anxiety rather than to merely treat the symptoms with medications. Clients should be encouraged to explore and develop non-pharmacological coping strategies to deal with the underlying causes. Such strategies may include behavioural therapy,

biofeedback techniques, meditation, and other complementary therapies. One model for stress management is shown in Figure 14.2.

When anxiety becomes severe enough to significantly interfere with daily activities of life, pharmacotherapy in addition to non-pharmacological strategies is indicated. In most types of stress, **anxiolytics**, which are drugs with the ability to relieve anxiety, are quite effective. Anxiolytics are usually meant to address generalized anxiety on a short-term basis. Longer-term pharmacotherapy for phobias and obsessive-compulsive and posttraumatic stress disorders may include mood disorder drugs (Chapter 16).

INSOMNIA

Insomnia is a condition characterized by a client's inability to fall asleep or remain asleep. Pharmacotherapy may be indicated if the sleeplessness interferes with normal daily activities.

14.4 Insomnia and Its Link to Anxiety

Why is it that we need sleep? During an average lifetime, about 33% of the time is spent sleeping, or trying to sleep. Although it is well established that sleep is essential for well-being, scientists are unsure of its function or how much is needed. Following are some theories:

- Inactivity during sleep gives the body time to repair itself.
- Sleep is a function that evolved as a protective mechanism. Throughout history, nighttime was the safest time of day.
- Sleep deals with "electrical" charging and discharging of the brain. The brain needs time for processing and filing new information collected throughout the day. When this is done without interference from the outside environment, these vast amounts of data can be retrieved through memory.

14.5 Insomnia and the Role of Melatonin

Melatonin is a natural hormone (N-acetyl-5 methoxytryptamine) produced in the pineal gland, especially at night. Its secretion is stimulated by darkness and inhibited by light. Tryptophan is converted to serotonin and finally to melatonin. As melatonin production rises, alertness decreases and body temperature starts to fall, both of which make sleep more inviting. Melatonin production is also related to age. Children manufacture more melatonin than elderly people; however, melatonin production begins to drop at puberty.

Supplemental melatonin, 0.5 to 3.0 mg at bedtime, is purported to decrease the time required to fall asleep and to produce a deep and restful sleep. Although melatonin is sold OTC without a prescription in several countries, the sale of melatonin in Canada is banned. There are several safety concerns about the use of melatonin. People with severe allergies, autoimmune diseases, and immune system cancers such as lymphoma and leukemia should not take melatonin because it could exacerbate such conditions by stimulating the immune system. Clients taking corticosteroids should not take melatonin because it may interfere with the efficacy of these hormones. Melatonin use in some children with seizure disorders may lead to increased seizure activity. Melatonin should not be given to healthy children as they already produce it in abundance. The safety of melatonin use by pregnant or nursing women has not been established. Large doses of melatonin may inhibit ovulation.

The acts of sleeping and waking are synchronized to many different bodily functions. Body temperature, blood pressure, hormone levels, and respiration all fluctuate on a cyclic basis throughout the 24-hour day. When this cycle becomes impaired, pharmacological or other interventions may be needed to readjust it. Increased levels of the neurotransmitter serotonin help initiate the various processes of sleep.

Insomnia, or sleeplessness, is a disorder sometimes associated with anxiety. There are several major types of insomnia. Short-term or behavioural insomnia may be attributed to stress caused by a hectic lifestyle or the inability to resolve day-to-day conflicts within the home environment or the workplace. Worries about work, marriage, children, and health are common reasons for short-term loss of sleep. When stress interrupts normal sleeping patterns, people cannot sleep because their minds are too active.

Foods or beverages containing stimulants such as caffeine may interrupt sleep. People may also find that the use of tobacco products makes them restless and edgy. Alcohol, while often enabling a person to fall asleep, may produce vivid dreams and frequent awakening that prevent restful sleep. Ingestion of a large meal, especially one high in protein and fat, close to bedtime can interfere with sleep due to the increased metabolic rate needed to digest the food. Certain medications cause CNS stimulation, and these should not be taken immediately before bedtime. Stressful conditions such as too much light, uncomfortable room temperature (especially one that is too warm), snoring, sleep apnea, and recurring nightmares also interfere with sleep. Long-term insomnia may be caused by depression, manic disorders, and chronic pain.

Non-pharmacological means should be attempted prior to initiating drug therapy for sleep disorders. Long-term use of sleep medications is likely to worsen insomnia and may cause physical or psychological dependence. Some clients experience a phenomenon referred to as **rebound insomnia.** This occurs when a sedative drug is discontinued abruptly or after it has been taken for a long time; sleeplessness and symptoms of anxiety then become markedly worse.

Older clients are more likely to experience medication-related sleep problems. Drugs may seem to help the insomnia of an elderly client for a night or two, only to produce gen-

PHARMFACTS

Insomnia and Insulin Resistance

- Chronic lack of sleep may make people more prone to developing type 2 diabetes mellitus.
- Chronic lack of sleep can provide the impetus for the body to acquire a reduced sensitivity to insulin.
- In one study, healthy adults who averaged little more than 5 hours of sleep per night over eight consecutive nights secreted 50% more insulin than those who averaged 8 hours of sleep per night for the same period. Those who slept less were 40% less sensitive to insulin than those who got more sleep.
- Sleep deprivation (6.5 hours or less per night) may explain why type 2 diabetes is becoming more prevalent.

eralized brain dysfunction as the medication accumulates in the system. The agitated client may then be mistakenly overdosed with further medication. Nurses, especially those who work in geriatric settings, are responsible for making accurate observations and reporting client responses to drugs so the healthcare provider can determine the lowest effective maintenance dose. The need for PRN medication for sleep requires individualized assessment by the nurse as well as follow-up evaluation and documentation of its effect on the client.

14.6 Use of the Electroencephalogram to Diagnose Sleep and Seizure Disorders

The **electroencephalogram (EEG)** is a tool for the diagnosis of sleep disorders, seizure activity, depression, and dementia. Four types of brain waves—alpha, beta, delta, and theta—are identified by their shape, frequencies, and height on a graph. Brain waves give the healthcare provider an idea of how brain activity changes during various stages of sleep and consciousness. For example, alpha waves indicate an awake but drowsy client. Beta waves indicate an alert client whose mind is active.

Two distinct types of sleep can be identified on the EEG: non-rapid eye movement (NREM) sleep and **rapid eye movement (REM) sleep**. There are four progressive stages that advance into REM sleep. After going through the four stages of NREM sleep, the sequence goes into reverse. Under normal circumstances, after returning from the depths of stage 4 back to stage 1 of NREM, a person will still not awaken. Sleep quality begins to change: it is not as deep, and hormone levels and body temperature begin to rise. At that point, REM sleep occurs. REM sleep is often called paradoxical sleep because this stage has a brain wave pattern similar to when persons are drowsy but awake. This is the stage when dreaming occurs. People with normal sleep patterns move from NREM to REM sleep about every 90 minutes.

Clients who are deprived of stage 4 NREM sleep experience depression and a feeling of apathy and fatigue. Stage 4 NREM sleep appears to be linked to repair and restoration of the physical body, while REM sleep is associated with learning, memory, and the capacity to adjust to changes in the environment. The body requires the dream state associated with REM sleep to keep the psyche functioning normally. When test subjects are deprived of REM sleep, they experience a **sleep debt** and become frightened, irritable, paranoid, and even emotionally disturbed. Judgment is impaired and reaction time is slowed. It is speculated that, to make up for their lack of dreaming, they experience far more daydreaming and fantasizing throughout the day. The stages of sleep are shown in Table 14.1.

CENTRAL NERVOUS SYSTEM DEPRESSANTS

CNS depressants are used to slow brain activity in clients experiencing anxiety or sleep disorders. These medications are grouped into three classes: benzodiazepines, barbiturates, and non-barbiturate/non-benzodiazepine CNS depressants.

14.7 Treating Anxiety and Insomnia with CNS Depressants

CNS depressants are drugs that slow neuronal activity in the brain. CNS depression should be viewed as a continuum ranging from relaxation, to sedation, to the induction of sleep and anesthesia. Coma and death are the end stages of CNS depression. Some drug classes are capable of producing the full range of CNS depression from calming to anesthesia, whereas others are less efficacious. CNS depressants used for anxiety and sleep disorders are categorized into two major classes, the benzodiazepines and the barbiturates. A third class consists of miscellaneous drugs that are chemically unrelated to the benzodiazepines or barbiturates but have similar therapeutic uses. Other CNS depressants include the opioids (Chapter 19) and ethyl alcohol (Chapter 12).

Medications that depress the CNS are sometimes called **sedatives** because of their ability to sedate or relax a client. At higher doses, some of these drugs are called **hypnotics** because of their ability to induce sleep. Thus, the term **sedative-hypnotic** is often used to describe a drug with the ability to produce a calming effect at lower doses while having the ability to induce sleep at higher doses. *Tranquilizer* is an older term sometimes used to describe a drug that produces a calm or tranquil feeling.

TABLE 14.1	Stages of Sleep
Stage	**Description**
NREM stage 1	At the onset of sleep, the person is in a stage of drowsiness for about 1 to 7 minutes. During this time, the person can be easily awakened. This stage lasts for about 4% to 5% of total sleep time.
NREM stage 2	The person can still be easily awakened. The stage comprises the greatest amount of total sleep time, 45% to 55%.
NREM stage 3	The person may move into or out of a deeper sleep. Heart rate and blood pressure fall; gastrointestinal activity rises. This stage lasts for about 4% to 6% of total sleep time.
NREM stage 4	The deepest stage of sleep; this stage lasts a little longer than stage 1 or stage 3, about 12% to 15%. This is the stage during which nightmares occur in children. Sleepwalking is also a common behaviour for this stage. Heart rate and blood pressure remain low; gastrointestinal activity remains high.
REM	This stage is characterized by eye movement and a loss of muscle tone. Eye movement occurs in bursts of activity. Dreaming takes place in this stage. The mind is very active and resembles a normal waking state.

Many CNS depressants can cause physical and psychological dependence, as discussed in Chapter 12. The withdrawal syndrome for some CNS depressants can cause life-threatening neurological reactions, including fever, psychosis, and seizures. Other withdrawal symptoms include increased heart rate and lowered blood pressure; loss of appetite; muscle cramps; impairment of memory, concentration, and orientation; abnormal sounds in the ears; blurred vision; and insomnia, agitation, anxiety, and panic. Obvious withdrawal symptoms typically last 2 to 4 weeks. Subtle ones can last months.

BENZODIAZEPINES

The benzodiazepines are one of the most widely prescribed drug classes. The root word *benzo* refers to an aromatic compound, one having a carbon ring structure attached to different atoms or another carbon ring. Two nitrogen atoms incorporated into the ring structure are the reason for the *diazepine* (*di* = two; *azepine* = nitrogen) portion of the name.

14.8 Treating Anxiety and Insomnia with Benzodiazepines

The benzodiazepines, listed in Table 14.2, are drugs of choice for various anxiety disorders and for insomnia. Since the introduction of the first benzodiazepines—chlordiazepoxide and diazepam—in the 1960s, the class has become one of the most widely prescribed in medicine. Although several benzodiazepines are available, all have the same actions and adverse effects and differ primarily in their onset and duration of action. The benzodiazepines are categorized as Controlled Drugs and Substances Act (CDSA) Schedule IV drugs, although they produce considerably less physical dependence and result in less tolerance than the barbiturates.

Benzodiazepines act by binding to the gamma-aminobutyric acid (GABA) receptor–chloride channel complex. These drugs intensify the effect of GABA, which is a natural inhibitory neurotransmitter found throughout the brain. Most are metabolized in the liver to active metabolites and are excreted primarily in urine. One major advantage of the benzodiazepines is that they do not produce life-threatening respiratory depression or coma if taken in excessive amounts. Death is unlikely unless the benzodiazepines are taken in large quantities in combination with other CNS depressants or the client suffers from sleep apnea.

Most benzodiazepines are given orally. Those that can be given parenterally, such as diazepam and lorazepam, should be used with caution due to their rapid onset of CNS effects and possible respiratory depression.

The benzodiazepines are drugs of choice for the short-term treatment of insomnia caused by anxiety, having replaced the barbiturates because of their greater margin of safety. Benzodiazepines shorten the length of time it takes to fall asleep and reduce the frequency of interrupted sleep. Although most benzodiazepines increase total sleep time, some reduce stage 4 sleep, and some affect REM sleep. In general, the benzodiazepines used to treat short-term insomnia are different from those used to treat generalized anxiety disorder.

Benzodiazepines have a number of other important indications. Diazepam is featured as a Prototype Drug in Chapter 15 for its use in treating seizure disorders. Other uses include treatment of alcohol withdrawal symptoms, central muscle relaxation (Chapter 45), and induction of general anesthesia (Chapter 20).

TABLE 14.2 Benzodiazepines for Anxiety and Insomnia	
Drug	*Route and Adult Dose*
Anxiety Therapy	
alprazolam (Xanax)	For anxiety: PO; 0.25–0.5 mg tid
	For panic attacks: PO; 1–2 mg tid
chlordiazepoxide (Librium)	Mild anxiety: PO; 5–10 mg tid or qid
	IM/IV; 50–100 mg 1 hr before a medical procedure
	Severe anxiety: PO; 20–25 mg tid or qid
	IM/IV; 50–100 mg followed by 25–50 mg tid or qid
clonazepam (Apo-Clonazepam)	PO; 1–2 mg/day in divided doses (max 4 mg/day)
clorazepate (Apo-Clorazepate)	PO; 15 mg/day at hs (max 60 mg/day in divided doses)
diazepam (Valium)	PO; 2–10 mg bid;
	IM/IV; 2–10 mg, repeat if needed in 3–4 hr
lorazepam (Ativan)	PO; 2–6 mg/day in divided doses (max 10 mg/day)
oxazepam (Apo-Oxazepam)	PO; 10–30 mg tid or qid
Insomnia Therapy	
flurazepam (Dalmane)	PO; 15–30 mg at hs
temazepam (Restoril)	PO; 7.5–30 mg at hs
triazolam (Halcion)	PO; 0.125–0.25 mg at hs (max 0.5 mg/day)

NURSING CONSIDERATIONS

The role of the nurse in benzodiazepine therapy involves careful monitoring of the client's condition and providing education as it relates to the prescribed drug regimen. Assess the client's need for antianxiety drugs, including intensity and duration of symptoms. The assessment should include identification of factors that precipitate anxiety or insomnia: physical symptoms, excessive CNS stimulation, excessive daytime sleep, or too little exercise or activity. Obtain a drug history, including hypersensitivity and the use of alcohol and other CNS depressants. Assess for the likelihood of drug abuse and dependence, and identify coping mechanisms used in managing previous episodes of stress, anxiety, and insomnia. These drugs should be used with caution in clients with suicidal tendency as the risk of suicide may be increased. Assess for the existence of a primary sleep disorder, such as sleep apnea, as benzodiazepines depress respiratory drive.

Alterations in neurotransmitter activity produce changes in intraocular pressure; therefore, benzodiazepines are contraindicated in narrow-angle glaucoma. The presence of any organic brain disease is contraindicated, as these drugs alter the level of consciousness. Liver and kidney function should be monitored in long-term use, and these drugs should be used cautiously in those clients with impaired renal or liver function. Because benzodiazepines cross the placenta and are excreted in breast milk, they are not recommended in pregnant or nursing women (pregnancy category D).

The risk of respiratory depression should be taken into consideration when administering IV doses and when administering to clients with impaired respiratory function or those taking other CNS depressants. Assess for common side effects related to CNS depression such as drowsiness and dizziness as these increase a client's risk of injury and may indicate a need for dose reduction. Should an overdose occur, flumazenil is a specific benzodiazepine receptor antagonist that can be administered to reverse CNS depression.

Benzodiazepines are used illicitly for recreation, most often by adolescents, young adults, and individuals addicted to opioids or cocaine. Nurses should help clients evaluate the social context of their environment and take any precautions necessary to safeguard the medication supply.

See "Nursing Process Focus: Clients Receiving Benzodiazepine and Non-Benzodiazepine Antianxiety Therapy" on page 151 for specific teaching points.

BARBITURATES

Barbiturates are drugs derived from barbituric acid. They are powerful CNS depressants prescribed for their sedative, hypnotic, and antiseizure effects that have been used in pharmacotherapy since the early 1900s.

14.9 Use of Barbiturates as Sedatives

Until the discovery of the benzodiazepines, barbiturates were the drugs of choice for treating anxiety and insomnia. While barbiturates are still indicated for several conditions, they are rarely, if ever, prescribed for treating anxiety or insomnia because of significant side effects and the availability of more effective medications. Table 14.3 provides a list of barbiturates. The risk of psychological and physical dependence is high—several are Schedule II drugs. The withdrawal syndrome from barbiturates is extremely severe and can be fatal. Overdose results in profound respiratory depression, hypotension, and shock. Barbiturates have been used to commit suicide, and death due to overdose is not uncommon.

Pr PROTOTYPE DRUG | Lorazepam (Ativan)

ACTIONS AND USES

Lorazepam is a benzodiazepine that acts by potentiating the effects of GABA, an inhibitory neurotransmitter, in the thalamic, hypothalamic, and limbic levels of the CNS. It is one of the most potent benzodiazepines. It has an extended half-life that allows for once- or twice-daily oral dosing. In addition to its use as an anxiolytic, lorazepam is used as a pre-anesthetic medication to provide sedation and for the management of status epilepticus.

ADMINISTRATION ALERTS

- When administering IV, monitor respirations every 5 to 15 minutes. Have airway and resuscitative equipment accessible.
- Lorazepam is pregnancy category D.

PHARMACOKINETICS

Lorazepam is well absorbed after oral administration. It is widely distributed, crosses the blood-brain barrier and placenta, and enters breast milk. It is almost completely metabolized by the liver. Its half-life is 10 to 16 hours.

ADVERSE EFFECTS AND INTERACTIONS

The most common side effects of lorazepam are drowsiness and sedation, which may decrease with time. When given in higher doses or by the IV route, more severe effects may be observed, such as amnesia, weakness, disorientation, ataxia, sleep disturbance, blood pressure changes, blurred vision, double vision, nausea, and vomiting.

Lorazepam interacts with multiple drugs. For example, concurrent use of CNS depressants, including alcohol, potentiates sedation effects and increases the risk of respiratory depression and death. Lorazepam may contribute to digoxin toxicity by increasing the serum digoxin level. Symptoms include visual changes, nausea, vomiting, dizziness, and confusion.

Use with caution with herbal supplements. For example, sedation-producing herbs such as kava, valerian, chamomile, or hops may have an additive effect with lorazepam. Stimulant herbs such as gotu kola and ma huang may reduce the drug's effectiveness.

 See the Companion Website for a Nursing Process Focus specific to this drug.

TABLE 14.3	Barbiturates for Sedation and Insomnia
Drug	**Route and Adult Dose**
Short Acting	
pentobarbital sodium (Nembutal)	Sedative: PO; 20–30 mg bid or qid
	Hypnotic: PO; 120–200 mg, IM; 150–200mg
secobarbital (Novo-Secobarb)	Sedative: PO; 100–300 mg/day in three divided doses
	Hypnotic: PO/IM; 100–200 mg
Long Acting	
mephobarbital (Mebaral)	Sedative: PO; 32–100 mg tid or qid
phenobarbital (PMS-Phenobarbital) (see page 160 for the Prototype Drug box)	Sedative: PO; 30–120 mg/day IV/IM; 100–200 mg/day

Barbiturates are capable of depressing CNS function at all levels. Like benzodiazepines, barbiturates act by binding to GABA receptor–chloride channel complexes, intensifying the effect of GABA throughout the brain. At low doses they reduce anxiety and cause drowsiness. At moderate doses they inhibit seizure activity (Chapter 15) and promote sleep, presumably by inhibiting brain impulses travelling through the limbic system and the reticular activating system. At higher doses, some barbiturates can induce anesthesia (Chapter 20).

When taken for prolonged periods, barbiturates stimulate the microsomal enzymes in the liver that metabolize medications. Thus, barbiturates can stimulate their own metabolism as well as that of hundreds of other drugs that use these enzymes for their breakdown. With repeated use, tolerance develops to the sedative effects of the drug; this includes cross-tolerance to other CNS depressants such as the opioids. Tolerance does not develop, however, to the respiratory depressant effects (see "Nursing Process Focus: Clients Receiving Barbiturate Therapy for Seizures" in Chapter 15, page 161).

14.10 Other CNS Depressants for Anxiety and Sleep Disorders

The final group of CNS depressants used for anxiety and sleep disorders consists of miscellaneous agents that are chemically unrelated to either benzodiazepines or barbiturates, as shown in Table 14.4. Some of the older drugs, such as paraldehyde and chloral hydrate, are now rarely prescribed. Several newer agents, such as buspirone and zopiclone, are commonly prescribed for their anxiolytic and hypnotic effects.

The mechanism of action for buspirone is unclear but appears to be related to dopamine D_2-receptors in the brain. The drug has agonist effects on presynaptic dopamine receptors and a high affinity for serotonin receptors. Buspirone is less likely than benzodiazepines to affect cognitive and motor performance and rarely interacts with other CNS depressants. Common side effects include dizziness, headache, and drowsiness. Dependence and withdrawal problems are less of a concern with buspirone. Therapy may take several weeks to achieve optimal results. Buspirone is pregnancy category B.

Zopiclone is a hypnotic agent with sedative, anxiolytic, anticonvulsant, and muscle relaxant properties. It exerts specific agonist action at central GABA(A) receptors. Zopiclone reduces time to onset of sleep and the frequency of nocturnal awakenings to increase duration of sleep. It decreases stage 1 and increases stage 2 NREM sleep while preserving or prolonging the deep stages (3 and 4) and REM sleep. Zopiclone may be used to treat short-term and chronic insomnia in adults (including difficulty falling asleep and nocturnal awakening). Regardless, the treatment period should be as

TABLE 14.4	Non-Benzodiazepine/Non-Barbiturate
Drug	**Route and Adult Dose**
buspirone (BuSpar)	PO; 7.5–15 mg in divided doses; may increase by 5 mg/day every 2–3 days if needed (max 60 mg/day)
chloral hydrate (PMS-Chloral Hydrate)	Sedative: PO or suppositories; 250 mg tid after meals
	Hypnotic: PO; 500 mg–1 g 15–30 min before hs
ethchlorvynol (Placidyl)	Sedative: PO; 200 mg bid or tid
	Hypnotic: PO; 500 mg–1 g at hs
paraldehyde (Paracetaldehyde)	Sedative: PO; 5–10 mL prn
	Hypnotic: PO; 10–30 mL prn
zopiclone (Imovane)	PO; 5–7.5 mg at hs

Pr PROTOTYPE DRUG | Zopiclone (Imovane)

ACTIONS AND USES

Zopiclone is a hypnotic agent with sedative, anxiolytic, anticonvulsant, and muscle relaxant properties. It exerts specific agonist action at central GABA(A) receptors. It reduces time to onset of sleep and the frequency of nocturnal awakenings, while preserving or prolonging deep sleep. Zopiclone may be used to treat short-term and chronic insomnia in adults.

PHARMACOKINETICS

Zopiclone is absorbed rapidly and peaks within 2 hours. Absorption is not affected by food. The risk of drug interactions is low due to weak plasma protein binding. Its elimination half-life is 5 hours (may be longer in older adults). There is no accumulation of zopiclone or its metabolites, even in older adults. It is excreted from the kidneys and lungs.

ADMINISTRATION ALERTS

- Give drug immediately before bedtime.
- Do not take drug with alcohol.
- Taper off if used long term.
- Zopiclone is pregnancy category C.

ADVERSE EFFECTS AND INTERACTIONS

The most common side effects include dizziness, headache, residual somnolence, dyspepsia, dry mouth, bitter taste, nausea, and anterograde amnesia.

 See the Companion Website for a Nursing Process Focus specific to this drug.

short as possible, and doses should be tapered if zopiclone is used for 3 weeks or longer. Side effects are usually mild and include bitter taste. Because of rapid absorption, it should be taken just prior to bedtime. Zopiclone is contraindicated in myasthenia gravis, respiratory failure, severe sleep apnea, and severe hepatic insufficiency.

As with other CNS depressants, these non-benzodiazepine/non-barbiturate agents should be used cautiously in clients with respiratory impairment, older adults, and those tak-

ing them concurrently with other CNS depressants. Lower dosage may be necessary.

Diphenhydramine (Benadryl) and hydroxyzine (Vistaril) are antihistamines that produce drowsiness and may be beneficial in calming clients. They offer the advantage of not causing dependence, although their use is often limited by anticholinergic side effects. Diphenhydramine is a common component of OTC sleep aids (see Prototype Drug box in Chapter 31, page 412).

NURSING PROCESS FOCUS   Clients Receiving Benzodiazepine and Non-Benzodiazepine Antianxiety Therapy

Assessment	Potential Nursing Diagnoses/Identified Patterns
Prior to administration: - Obtain complete health history (both physical and mental), including allergies and drug history for possible drug interactions. - Identify factors that precipitate anxiety or insomnia. - Assess likelihood of drug abuse and dependence. - Establish baseline vital signs and level of consciousness.	- Risk for injury - Anxiety - Need for knowledge regarding drug therapy - Disturbed sleep - Coping pattern

Planning: Client Goals and Expected Outcomes

The client will:
- Experience an increase in psychological comfort
- Report absence of physical and behavioural manifestations of anxiety
- Demonstrate an understanding of the drug's action by accurately describing drug side effects and precautions

Implementation

Interventions (Rationales)	Client Education/Discharge Planning
- Monitor vital signs. Observe respiratory patterns, especially during sleep, for evidence of apnea or shallow breathing. (Benzodiazepines can reduce the respiratory drive in susceptible patients.)	Instruct client: - To consult the healthcare provider before taking this drug if snoring is a problem. Snoring may indicate an obstruction in the upper respiratory tract resulting in hypoxia - Regarding methods to monitor vital signs at home, especially respirations
- Monitor neurological status, especially level of consciousness. (Confusion or lack of response may indicate overmedication.)	- Instruct client to report extreme lethargy, slurred speech, disorientation, or ataxia.

continued

NURSING PROCESS FOCUS Clients Receiving Benzodiazepine and Non-Benzodiazepine Antianxiety Therapy *(Continued)*	
Interventions (Rationales)	**Client Education/Discharge Planning**
■ Ensure client safety. (Drug may cause excessive drowsiness.)	Instruct client: ■ To not drive or perform hazardous activities until effects of drug are known ■ To request assistance when getting out of bed and ambulating until effect of medication is known
■ Monitor the client's intake of stimulants, including caffeine (in beverages such as coffee, tea, cola and other soft drinks, and in OTC analgesics such as Excedrin) and nicotine (from tobacco products and nicotine patches). (These products can reduce the drug's effectiveness.)	Instruct client to: ■ Avoid taking OTC sleep-inducing antihistamines, such as diphenhydramine ■ Consult the healthcare provider before self-medicating with any OTC preparation
■ Monitor affect and emotional status. (Drug may increase risk of mental depression, especially in patients with suicidal tendencies.)	Instruct client to: ■ Report significant mood changes, especially depression ■ Avoid consuming alcohol or taking other CNS depressants while on benzodiazepines because these increase depressant effect
■ Avoid abrupt discontinuation of therapy. (Withdrawal symptoms, including rebound anxiety and sleeplessness, are possible with abrupt discontinuation after long-term use.)	Instruct client: ■ To take drug exactly as prescribed ■ To keep all follow-up appointments as directed by healthcare provider to monitor response to medication ■ About non-pharmacological methods for re-establishing sleep regimen

Evaluation of Outcome Criteria

Evaluate effectiveness of drug therapy by confirming that client goals and expected outcomes have been met (see "Planning").

See Tables 14.2 (page 148) and 14.4 (page 150) for lists of drugs to which these nursing actions apply.

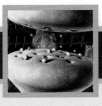

CHAPTER REVIEW

KEY CONCEPTS

The numbered key concepts provide a succinct summary of the important points from the corresponding numbered section within the chapter. If any of these points are not clear, refer to the numbered section within the chapter for review. Expanded versions can be found on the Companion Website.

14.1 Generalized anxiety disorder is the most common type of anxiety; phobias, obsessive-compulsive disorder, panic attacks, and posttraumatic stress disorder are other important categories.

14.2 The limbic system and the reticular activating system are specific regions of the brain responsible for anxiety and wakefulness.

14.3 Anxiety can be managed through pharmacological and non-pharmacological strategies.

14.4 Insomnia is a sleep disorder that may be caused by anxiety. Non-pharmacological means should be attempted prior to initiating pharmacotherapy.

14.5 The electroencephalogram records brain waves and is used to diagnose sleep and seizure disorders.

14.6 CNS depressants, including anxiolytics, sedatives, and hypnotics, are used to treat anxiety and insomnia.

14.7 Benzodiazepines are drugs of choice for generalized anxiety and insomnia.

14.8 Because of their side effects and high potential for dependency, barbiturates are rarely used to treat insomnia.

14.9 Some commonly prescribed CNS depressants used for anxiety and sleep disorders are not related to either benzodiazepines or barbiturates.

REVIEW QUESTIONS

1 Compare and contrast each of following terms in relation to anxiety and alertness: CNS depressants, sedatives, hypnotics, and anxiolytics.

2 What is the major drug class used to treat generalized anxiety disorder and panic disorder? Name common drugs within this class.

3 Why might a client not be able to enjoy normal sleep? Why is long-term pharmacotherapy for lack of sleep not recommended?

4 Identify the major drug classes used for daytime sedation and insomnia. Why are CNS depressants especially dangerous if administered in high doses?

5 How can the nurse best support a client who is suffering from anxiety and insomnia?

CRITICAL THINKING QUESTIONS

1. A 58-year-old male client had an emergency coronary artery bypass graft 5 days ago. He suffered respiratory complications while in the cardiac intensive care unit (ICU). He is still experiencing a high degree of pain and also states that he cannot fall asleep. The client has been ordered secobarbital (Novo-Secobarb) hs for sleep and also has a prescribed opioid analgesic. Should the nurse medicate the client with both agents? Why or why not?

2. A 42-year-old female client with ovarian cancer suffered profound nausea and vomiting after her first round of chemotherapy. The oncologist has added lorazepam (Ativan)

2 mg per IV piggyback with ondansetron (Zofran) as part of the pre-chemotherapy regimen. Consult a drug handbook and discuss the purpose for adding this benzodiazepine.

3. An 82-year-old female client complains that she "just can't get good rest and sleep anymore." She questions whether she should ask her doctor to prescribe something to help her sleep. What information can the nurse offer this client regarding the normal changes in sleep patterns associated with aging? What would you recommend for this client?

EXPLORE MediaLink

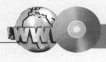

www.pearsoned.ca/adams-king

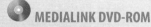 **MEDIALINK DVD-ROM**
- **Audio Glossary**
- **CRNE Review**
- **Videos**
  Obsessive-Compulsive Disorder 1
  Obsessive-Compulsive Disorder 2
  Obsessive-Compulsive Disorder 3
  Panic Disorder 1
  Panic Disorder 2
- **Animation**
  Mechanism of Action Escitalopram

 COMPANION WEBSITE
- **CRNE Review**
- **Case Study:** Client taking lorazepam and digoxin
- **Dosage Calculation**
- **Nursing Process Focus Charts**

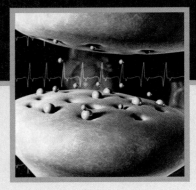

CHAPTER 15

Drugs for Seizures

DRUGS AT A GLANCE

DRUGS THAT POTENTIATE GABA ACTION

Barbiturates
- *phenobarbital (PMS-Phenobarbital)*

Miscellaneous GABA agents

Benzodiazepines
- *diazepam (Valium)*

HYDANTOINS AND PHENYTOIN-LIKE DRUGS

Hydantoins
- *phenytoin (Dilantin)*

Phenytoin-like drugs
- *valproic acid (Depakene)*

SUCCINIMIDES
- *ethosuximide (Zarontin)*

OBJECTIVES

After reading this chapter, the student should be able to do the following:

1. Identify drug classes used for treating epilepsy and seizures.
2. For each of the drug classes listed in Drugs at a Glance, identify a representative drug and explain its mechanism of action, primary actions, and important adverse effects.
3. Describe the nurse's role in the pharmacological management of clients with epilepsy.
4. Describe and explain, based on pharmacological principles, the rationale for nursing assessment, planning, and interventions for clients with epilepsy.
5. Explain the importance of client adherence in the pharmacotherapy of epilepsy.
6. Use the nursing process to care for clients receiving drug therapy for epilepsy.

MediaLink

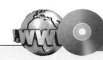 www.pearsoned.ca/adams-king

CRNE review, case studies, and other interactive resources for this chapter can be found on the Companion Website at **www.pearsoned.ca/adams-king**. Click on "Chapter 15" to select the activities for this chapter. For animations, more CRNE review questions, and an audio glossary, access the accompanying MediaLink DVD-ROM in this textbook.

Epilepsy is a common neurological disease. **Epilepsy** may be defined as any disorder characterized by recurrent seizures. The symptoms of epilepsy depend on the type of seizure and may include blackout, fainting spells, sensory disturbances, jerking body movements, and temporary loss of memory. Epilepsy affects approximately 0.6% of Canadians. This chapter will examine the pharmacotherapy used to treat the different types of seizures.

SEIZURES

A **seizure** is a disturbance of electrical activity in the brain that may affect consciousness, motor activity, and sensation. The symptoms of seizure are caused by abnormal or uncontrollable neuronal discharges within the brain. These abnormal discharges can be measured using an electroencephalogram (EEG), a valuable tool in diagnosing seizure disorders. Figure 15.1 compares normal and abnormal EEG recordings.

The terms *convulsion* and *seizure* are not synonymous. **Convulsions** specifically refer to involuntary, violent spasms of the large skeletal muscles of the face, neck, arms, and legs. While some types of seizures do indeed involve convulsions, other seizures do not. Thus, it may be stated that all convulsions are seizures, but not all seizures are convulsions. Because of this difference, agents used to treat epilepsy should correctly be called antiseizure medications, rather than anticonvulsants.

15.1 Causes of Seizures

A seizure is considered a symptom of an underlying disorder rather than a disease in itself. There are many different etiologies of seizure activity. Seizures can result from acute situations or occur on a chronic basis, as with epilepsy. In some cases, the exact etiology may not be identified. The following are known causes of seizures:

- Infectious diseases: Acute infections such as meningitis and encephalitis can cause inflammation in the brain.
- Trauma: Physical trauma such as direct blows to the skull may increase intracranial pressure; chemical trauma such as the presence of toxic substances or the ingestion of poisons may cause brain injury.

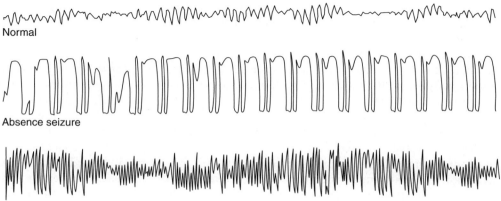

● **Figure 15.1** EEG recordings showing the differences between normal, absence seizure, and generalized tonic-clonic seizure tracings

- Metabolic disorders: Changes in fluid and electrolytes such as hypoglycemia, hyponatremia, and water intoxication may cause seizures by altering electrical impulse transmission at the cellular level.

- Vascular diseases: Changes in oxygenation, such as that caused by respiratory hypoxia and carbon monoxide poisoning, and changes in perfusion, such as that caused by hypotension, cerebral vascular accidents, shock, and cardiac dysrhythmias, may be causes.

- Pediatric disorders: Rapid increase in body temperature may result in a febrile seizure.

- Neoplastic disease: Tumours, especially rapidly growing ones, may occupy space, increase intracranial pressure, and damage brain tissue by disrupting blood flow.

Certain medications for mood disorders, psychoses, and local anesthesia when given in high doses may cause seizures because of increased levels of stimulatory neurotransmitters. Seizures may also occur from drug abuse, as with cocaine, or during withdrawal syndromes from alcohol or sedative-hypnotic drugs.

Pregnancy is a major concern for clients with epilepsy. Additional barrier methods of birth control should be practised to avoid unintended pregnancy as some antiseizure medications decrease the effectiveness of oral contraceptives. Most antiseizure drugs are pregnancy category D. Clients should consult with their healthcare provider prior to pregnancy to determine the most appropriate plan of action for seizure control, given their seizure history. As some antiseizure drugs may cause folate deficiency, a condition correlated with increased risk of neural tube defects, vitamin supplements may be necessary. Pregnant women may experience seizures with eclampsia, a pregnancy-induced hypertensive disorder.

In some cases, the etiology of the seizures cannot be found. Clients may have a lower tolerance to environmental triggers, and seizures may occur when the client is sleep deprived, exposed to strobe or flickering lights, or experiences small fluid and electrolyte imbalances. Seizures represent the most common serious neurological problem affecting children, with an overall incidence approaching 2% for febrile seizures and 1% for idiopathic epilepsy. Seizures that result from acute situations generally do not reoccur after the situation has been resolved. If a brain abnormality exists after the acute situation resolves, continuing seizures are likely.

Seizures can have a significant impact on quality of life. They may cause serious injury if they occur while a person is driving a vehicle or performing a dangerous activity. Without pharmacotherapy, epilepsy can severely limit participation in school, employment, and social activities and can affect self-esteem. Chronic depression may accompany poorly controlled seizures. Proper treatment, however, can eliminate seizures completely in many clients. Important considerations in nursing care include identifying clients at risk for seizures, documenting the pattern and type of seizure activity, and implementing safety precautions. In

MediaLink Epilepsy Canada

MediaLink Canadian Epilepsy Alliance

collaboration with the client, healthcare provider, and pharmacist, the nurse is instrumental in achieving positive therapeutic outcomes. Through a combination of pharmacotherapy, client-family support, and education, effective seizure control can be achieved by the majority of clients.

15.2 Types of Seizures

The differing presentation of seizures relates to the areas of the brain affected by the abnormal electrical activity. Symptoms of a seizure can range from sudden, violent shaking and total loss of consciousness (LOC) to muscle twitching or slight tremor of a limb. Staring into space, altered vision, and difficulty speaking are other symptoms a person may exhibit during a seizure. Determining the cause of recurrent seizures is important in order to plan appropriate treatment options.

Methods of classifying epilepsy have evolved over time. The terms *grand mal* and *petit mal* epilepsy have, for the most part, been replaced by more descriptive and detailed categorization. Epilepsies are typically identified, using the International Classification of Epileptic Seizures nomenclature, as partial (focal), generalized, or special epileptic syndromes. Types of partial or generalized seizures may be recognized based on symptoms observed during a seizure episode. Some symptoms are subtle and reflect the simple nature of neuronal misfiring in specific areas of the brain; others are more complex.

Partial Seizures **Partial (focal) seizures** involve a limited portion of the brain. They may start on one side and travel only a short distance before they stop. The area where the abnormal electrical activity starts is known as an abnormal focus (plural = *foci*).

Simple partial seizures have an onset that may begin as a small, limited focus and subsequently progress to a generalized seizure. Clients with simple partial seizures may feel for a brief moment that their precise location is vague, and they may hear and see things that are not there. Some clients smell and taste things that are not present or have an upset stomach. Others may become emotional and experience a sense of joy, sorrow, or grief. The arms, legs, or face may twitch.

Complex partial seizures (formerly known as psychomotor or temporal lobe seizures) show sensory, motor, or autonomic symptoms with some degree of altered or impaired consciousness. Total loss of consciousness may not occur during a complex partial seizure, but a brief period of somnolence or confusion may follow the seizure. Such seizures are often preceded by an aura that is often described as an unpleasant odour or taste. Seizures may start with a blank stare, and clients may begin to chew or swallow repetitively. Some clients fumble with clothing; others may try to take off their clothes. Most clients will not pay attention to verbal commands and act as if they are having a psychotic episode. After the seizure, clients do not remember the seizure incident.

Generalized Seizures
As the name suggests, **generalized seizures** are not localized to one area but travel throughout the entire brain on both sides. The seizure is thought to originate bilaterally and symmetrically within the brain.

Absence seizures (formerly known as petit mal seizures) most often occur in children and last only a few seconds. Absence seizures involve a loss or reduction of normal activity. Staring and transient loss of responsiveness are the most common signs, but there may be slight motor activity with eyelid fluttering or myoclonic jerks. Because these episodes are subtle and only last a few seconds, absence epilepsy may go unrecognized for a long time or be mistaken for daydreaming or attention deficit disorder.

Atonic seizures are sometimes called drop attacks because clients often stumble and fall for no apparent reason. Episodes are very short, lasting only a matter of seconds.

Tonic-clonic seizures are the most common type of seizure in all age groups. Seizures may be preceded by an aura, a warning that some clients describe as a spiritual feeling, a flash of light, or a special noise. Intense muscle contractions indicate the tonic phase. A hoarse cry may occur at the onset of the seizure due to air being forced out of the lungs, and clients may temporarily lose bladder or bowel control. Breathing may become shallow and even stop momentarily. The clonic phase is characterized by alternating contraction and relaxation of muscles. The seizure usually lasts 1 to 2 minutes, after which the client becomes drowsy, disoriented, and sleeps deeply (known as the postictal state).

Special Epileptic Syndromes
Special epileptic seizures include the febrile seizures of infancy, reflex epilepsies, and other forms of myoclonic epilepsies. Myoclonic epilepsies often go along with other neurological abnormalities or progressive symptoms.

Febrile seizures typically cause tonic-clonic motor activity lasting 1 or 2 minutes with rapid return of consciousness. They occur in conjunction with a rapid rise in body temperature and usually occur only once during any given illness. Febrile seizures are most likely to occur in the 3-month to 5-year age group, and as many as 5% of all children experience febrile seizures. Preventing the onset of high fever is the best way to control these seizures.

Myoclonic seizures are characterized by large, jerking body movements. Major muscle groups contract quickly, and clients appear unsteady and clumsy. They may fall from a sitting position or drop whatever they are holding. Infantile spasms exemplify a type of generalized, myoclonic seizure distinguished by short-lived muscle spasms involving the trunk and extremities. Such spasms are often not identified as seizures by parents or healthcare providers because the movements are much like the normal infantile Moro (startle) reflex.

Status epilepticus is a medical emergency that occurs when a seizure is repeated continuously. It could occur with any type of seizure, but usually generalized tonic-clonic seizures are exhibited. When generalized tonic-clonic seizures are prolonged or continuous, the time in which breathing is affected by muscle contraction is lengthened and hypoxia may develop. The continuous muscle contraction also can lead to hypoglycemia, acidosis, and hypothermia due to increased metabolic needs, lactic acid production, and heat loss during contraction. Carbon dioxide retention also leads to acidosis. If not treated, status epilepticus could lead to brain damage and death. Medical treatment involves the IV administration of antiseizure medications. Steps must also be taken to ensure that the airway remains open.

LIFESPAN CONSIDERATIONS

Epilepsy across the Lifespan
- Epilepsy affects 0.6% of the Canadian population.
- Epilepsy can occur at any age.
- About 30% of new cases begin in childhood, particularly in early childhood and around the time of adolescence.
- Another period of relatively high onset occurs over the age of 65 years.
- Drug dosages may require adjustment due to age-related changes in pharmacokinetics.
- Side effects may decrease drug adherence in all age groups.
- Older adults may experience more severe adverse effects.

Source: Epilepsy Canada, http://www.epilepsy.ca/eng/content/epidemio.html.

PHARMFACTS

Epilepsy
- The word *epilepsy* is derived from the Greek word *epilepsia,* meaning "to take hold of or to seize."
- Contrary to popular belief, it is impossible to swallow the tongue during a seizure, and one should never force an object into the mouth of someone who is having a seizure.
- Epilepsy is not a mental illness; children with epilepsy have equivalent IQ scores to children without the disorder.
- Famous people who had epilepsy include Julius Caesar, Alexander the Great, Napoleon, Vincent van Gogh, Charles Dickens, Joan of Arc, and Socrates.
- About 60% of adult alcoholics who go to the emergency department with withdrawal complaints have seizures within 6 hours after arriving.

15.3 General Concepts of Epilepsy Pharmacotherapy

The choice of drug for epilepsy pharmacotherapy depends on the type of seizure the client is experiencing, the client's previous medical history, diagnostic studies, and the pathological processes causing the seizures. Once a medication is selected, the client is placed on a low initial dose. The amount is gradually increased until seizure control is achieved or the side effects of the drug prevent additional increases in dose. Serum drug levels may be obtained to assist the healthcare provider in determining the most effective drug concentration. If seizure activity continues, a different medication is added in small dose increments while the dose of the first drug is slowly reduced. Because seizures are likely to occur with abrupt withdrawal, antiseizure medication is withdrawn over a period of 6 to 12 weeks.

In most cases, effective seizure management can be obtained using a single drug. In some clients, two antiseizure medications may be necessary to control seizure activity, although additional side effects may become evident. Some antiseizure drug combinations may actually increase the incidence of seizures. The nurse should consult current drug guides regarding compatibility before administering a second antiseizure agent.

Once seizures have been controlled, clients are continued indefinitely on the antiseizure drug. After several years of being seizure-free, clients may question the need for their medication. In general, withdrawal of antiseizure drugs should only be attempted after at least 3 years of being seizure-free, and only under the close direction of the healthcare provider. Doses of medications are reduced slowly, one at a time, over a period of several months. If seizures recur during the withdrawal process, pharmacotherapy is resumed, usually with the same drug. The nurse must strongly urge clients to maintain adherence with pharmacotherapy and not attempt to discontinue antiseizure drug use without professional guidance. Table 15.1 shows antiseizure drugs, based on the type of seizure.

Living a healthy, active lifestyle is good therapy for epilepsy, but only as an adjunct to a medically prescribed antiseizure drug, not instead of it. With a valid diagnosis of epilepsy, there is no substitute for effective antiseizure pharmacotherapy. There are situations, however, when the medicines cannot be tolerated. Sometimes another medical therapy, such as the ketogenic diet, is used, along with natural remedies.

Antiseizure pharmacotherapy is directed at controlling the movement of electrolytes across neuronal membranes or affecting neurotransmitter balance. In a resting state, neurons are normally surrounded by a higher concentration of sodium, calcium, and chloride ions. Potassium levels are higher inside the cell. An influx of sodium or calcium into the neuron *enhances* neuronal activity, whereas an influx of chloride *suppresses* neuronal activity.

The goal of antiseizure pharmacotherapy is to suppress neuronal activity just enough to prevent abnormal or repetitive firing. To this end, there are three general mechanisms by which antiseizure drugs act:

1. Stimulating an influx of chloride ions, an effect that potentiates the inhibitory neurotransmitter, gamma-aminobutyric acid (GABA)

2. Delaying an influx of sodium ions

3. Delaying an influx of calcium ions

DRUGS THAT POTENTIATE GABA

Several important antiseizure drugs act by changing the action of **gamma-aminobutyric acid (GABA)**, the primary inhibitory neurotransmitter in the brain. These agents mimic the effects of GABA by stimulating an influx of chloride ions that interact with the GABA receptor–chloride channel complex. A model of this receptor is shown in Figure 15.2. When the receptor is stimulated, chloride ions move into the cell, thus suppressing the ability of neurons to fire.

BARBITURATES AND MISCELLANEOUS GABA AGENTS

Barbiturates, benzodiazepines, and several miscellaneous drugs reduce seizure activity by intensifying GABA action. The major effect of enhancing GABA activity is CNS depression. These agents are shown in Table 15.2. The antiseizure properties of phenobarbital were discovered in

TABLE 15.1	Drugs for the Management of Specific Types of Seizure				
	Partial Seizures			*Generalized Seizures*	
	Simple , Complex	Absence		Atonic, Myoclonic	Tonic-Clonic, Status Epilepticus
Benzodiazepines					
diazepam (Valium)					✓
lorazepam (Ativan)					✓
Phenytoin-Like Agents					
phenytoin (Dilantin)	✓				✓
carbamazepine (Tegretol)	✓				✓
valproic acid (Depakene)	✓	✓		✓	✓
Succinimides					
ethosuximide (Zarontin)		✓		✓	

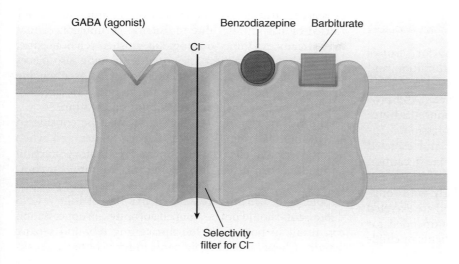

● **Figure 15.2** Model of the GABA receptor–chloride channel complex

1912, and the drug is still one of the most commonly prescribed for epilepsy.

15.4 Treating Seizures with Barbiturates and Miscellaneous GABA Agents

As a class, barbiturates have a low margin of safety, cause profound CNS depression, and have a high potential for dependence. Phenobarbital, however, is able to suppress abnormal neuronal discharges without causing sedation. It is inexpensive, long acting, and produces a low incidence of adverse effects. When given orally, several weeks may be necessary to achieve optimum antiseizure activity.

Other barbiturates are occasionally used for epilepsy. Mephobarbital is converted to phenobarbital in the liver and offers no significant advantages over phenobarbital. Amobarbital is an intermediate-acting barbiturate that is given IM or IV to terminate status epilepticus. Unlike phenobarbital, which is a Schedule IV drug, amobarbital is a Schedule II drug and has a higher risk for dependence; it is not given orally as an antiseizure drug.

Several non-benzodiazepine/non-barbiturate agents act by the GABA mechanism. An example of these newer drugs, first approved in the 1990s, is gabapentin.

TABLE 15.2	Antiseizure Drugs That Potentiate GABA Action
Drug	**Route and Adult Dose**
Barbiturates	
pentobarbital (Nembutal)	PO/IM; 150–200 mg in two divided doses IV; 100 mg, may increase to 500 mg if necessary
phenobarbital (PMS-Phenobarbital)	For seizures: PO; 100–300 mg day IV/IM; 200–600 mg up to 20 mg/kg For status epilepticus: IV; 15–18 mg/kg in single or divided doses (max 20 mg/kg)
Benzodiazepines	
clonazepam (Rivotril)	PO; 1.5 mg/day in three divided doses, increased by 0.5–1.0 mg every 3 days until seizures are controlled
clorazepate (Apo-Clorazepate)	PO; 7.5 mg tid
diazepam (Valium)	IM/IV; 5–10 mg (repeat as needed at 10–15 min intervals up to 30 mg; repeat again as needed every 2–4 hr) IV push; administer emulsion at 5 mg/min
lorazepam (Ativan) (see page 149 for the Prototype Drug box)	IV; 4 mg injected slowly at 2 mg/min; if inadequate response after 10 min, may repeat once
Miscellaneous Agents	
gabapentin (Neurontin)	For additional therapy: PO; start with 300 mg on day 1; 300 mg bid on day 2; 300 mg tid on day 3; continue to increase over 1 week to a dose of 1200 mg/day (400 mg tid); may increase to 1800–2400 mg/day
primidone (Apo-Primidone)	PO; 250 mg/day; increased by 250 mg/week up to max of 2 g in two to four divided doses
topiramate (Topamax)	PO; Start with 50 mg/day; increase by 50 mg/week to effectiveness (max 1600 mg/day)

NURSING CONSIDERATIONS

The role of the nurse in barbiturate therapy for seizures involves careful monitoring of the client's condition and providing education as it relates to the prescribed drug regimen. Of those drugs that mimic or enhance GABA production, barbiturates produce the most pronounced adverse effects, including sedation and respiratory depression.

Barbiturates are metabolized in the liver and excreted primarily in urine. These drugs should be used with caution in clients with impaired hepatic or renal capacity; liver and kidney function must be monitored regularly with long-term usage. Barbiturates cross the placenta and are excreted in breast milk; therefore, they are not recommended for pregnant or nursing women. Assess female clients of child-bearing age for pregnancy or intent to become pregnant. There is an increased risk of congenital malformations when the drug is taken during the first trimester (pregnancy category D). These drugs may also produce folic acid deficiency, which is associated with an increased risk of neural tube birth defects, including spina bifida and hydrocephalus. Barbiturates may also decrease the effectiveness of oral contraceptives.

Barbiturates produce biochemical changes at the cellular level that result in accelerated metabolism and subsequent depletion of nutrients such as vitamins D and K. Alterations in vitamin synthesis can result in reduced bone density (vitamin D deficiency) and impaired blood coagulability (vitamin K deficiency). Bleeding caused by vitamin K deficiency may present as simple bruising or petechiae or may manifest as a more serious adverse reaction, such as epistaxis, GI bleeding, menorrhagia, or hematuria. Older adults can be particularly at risk of significant vitamin deficiency caused by barbiturates due to nutritional imbalances that may already exist due to aging. Diminished renal, hepatic, and respiratory function associated with aging also places older adults at risk of CNS depression. GABA-enhancing drugs may produce an idiosyncratic response in children, resulting in restlessness and psychomotor agitation.

The risk of respiratory depression must be considered when administering IV doses of barbiturates and when administering to clients with impaired respiratory function and those taking other CNS depressants. Monitor for common side effects such as drowsiness, dizziness, and postural hypotension, which increase a client's risk of injury. CNS depressants should not be stopped abruptly; abrupt cessation can result in potentially life-threatening rebound seizure activity. Clients should avoid consuming alcohol while taking barbiturates. The use of the herb *Ginkgo biloba* may decrease the antiseizure effect of these drugs. Concurrent use of other antiseizure drugs may also decrease their antiseizure effect.

Clients taking gabapentin should be monitored for dizziness and drowsiness. Drugs with GABA-intensifying action are not recommended for pregnant or nursing women (pregnancy category C).

See "Nursing Process Focus: Clients Receiving Barbiturate Therapy for Seizures" for specific teaching points.

BENZODIAZEPINES

Like barbiturates, benzodiazepines intensify the effect of GABA in the brain. The benzodiazepines bind to the GABA receptor directly, suppressing abnormal neuronal foci. These agents are listed in Table 15.2.

Pr PROTOTYPE | Phenobarbital (PMS-Phenobarbital)

ACTIONS AND USES

Phenobarbital is a long-acting barbiturate used for the management of a variety of seizures. It is also used for insomnia. Phenobarbital should not be used for pain relief as it may increase a client's sensitivity to pain.

Phenobarbital acts biochemically in the brain by enhancing the action of the neurotransmitter GABA, which is responsible for suppressing abnormal neuronal discharges that can cause epilepsy.

PHARMACOKINETICS

Phenobarbital PO is slowly absorbed. Distribution is unknown. It is mostly metabolized by the liver. About 25% is excreted unchanged in urine. The half-life is 2 to 6 days in adults and 1.5 to 3 days in children.

ADMINISTRATION ALERTS

- Parenteral phenobarbital is a soft tissue irritant. IM injections may produce local inflammatory reaction. IV administration is rarely used because extravasation may produce tissue necrosis.
- Phenobarbital is pregnancy category D.

ADVERSE EFFECTS AND INTERACTIONS

Phenobarbital is a Schedule IV drug that may cause dependence. Common side effects include drowsiness, vitamin deficiencies (vitamin D, folate, and B_{12}), and laryngospasm. With overdose, phenobarbital may cause severe respiratory depression, CNS depression, coma, and death.

Phenobarbital interacts with many other drugs. For example, it should not be taken with alcohol or other CNS depressants. These substances potentiate the action of barbiturates, increasing the risk of life-threatening respiratory depression or cardiac arrest. Phenobarbital increases the metabolism of many other drugs, reducing their effectiveness.

 See the Companion Website for a Nursing Process Focus specific to this drug.

NURSING PROCESS FOCUS   Client Receiving Barbiturate Therapy for Seizures

Assessment	Potential Nursing Diagnoses/Identified Patterns
Prior to administration: ■ Obtain complete health history including allergies and drug history, to determine possible drug interactions. ■ Assess neurological status, including identification of recent seizure activity.	■ Disturbed sensory perception ■ Risk for injury related to drug side effects ■ Risk for imbalanced nutrition: less than body requirements ■ Deficient knowledge related to drug therapy ■ Disturbed sleep pattern

Planning: Client Goals and Expected Outcomes

The client will:

■ Experience the absence of seizures or a reduction in the number or severity of seizures
■ Avoid physical injury related to seizure activity or medication-induced somnolence
■ Demonstrate an understanding of the drug's action by accurately describing drug effects and precautions

Implementation

Interventions (Rationales)	Client Education/Discharge Planning
■ Monitor vital signs, especially blood pressure and depth and rate of respirations. (These drugs can cause severe respiratory depression.)	■ Instruct client to withhold medication for any difficulty in breathing or respirations below 12 breaths per minute.
■ Monitor neurological status. Monitor changes in level of consciousness. (Excessive somnolence may occur.) Observe for persistent seizures.	Instruct client to: ■ Report any significant change in sensorium such as lethargy, stupor, auras, visual changes, and other effects that may indicate an impending seizure ■ Report dizziness, which may indicate hypotension ■ Be aware that drug will cause initial drowsiness, which may diminish with continued therapy ■ Keep a seizure diary to chronicle symptoms
■ Monitor for signs of hepatic or renal toxicity. (Barbiturates are metabolized by the liver and excreted by the kidneys.)	Instruct client to: ■ Observe for signs of toxicity such as nausea; vomiting; diarrhea; rash; jaundice; abdominal pain, tenderness, or distention; change in colour of stool; flank pain; hematuria ■ Adhere to a regular schedule of laboratory testing for liver and kidney function as ordered by the healthcare provider
■ Ensure client safety. (Barbiturates can cause drowsiness and dizziness.)	Instruct client to: ■ Request assistance when getting out of bed and ambulating until effect of drug is known ■ Avoid driving and hazardous activities until effect of drug is known
■ Monitor effectiveness of drug therapy. ■ Monitor children for paradoxical response to drug, which may cause hyperactivity.	Instruct client to: ■ Be aware that full therapeutic effect of oral barbiturate may take 2 to 3 weeks ■ Not discontinue drug abruptly or reduce dosage as increased seizure activity and/or withdrawal symptoms may occur
■ Monitor for signs of vitamin deficiency (vitamin D, vitamin K, folate, and other B vitamins). ■ Obtain consultation with dietitian per healthcare provider's order as needed.	Instruct client: ■ Regarding the role of vitamins and nutrition in maintaining health ■ To immediately report signs of vitamin deficiency: vitamin K—easy bleeding, tarry stools, bruising, pallor; vitamin D—joint pain, bone deformities; vitamin B_6—skin changes, dandruff, peripheral neuropathy, fatigue

Evaluation of Outcome Criteria

Evaluate effectiveness of drug therapy by confirming that client goals and expected outcomes have been met (see "Planning").

See Table 15.2, "Barbiturates" (page 159), for a list of drugs to which these nursing actions apply.

15.5 Treating Seizures with Benzodiazepines

Benzodiazepines used in treating epilepsy include clonazepam, clorazepate, lorazepam, and diazepam. Indications include absence seizures and myoclonic seizures. Parenteral diazepam is used to terminate status epilepticus. Because tolerance may begin to develop after only a few months of therapy with benzodiazepines, seizures may recur unless the dose is periodically adjusted. These agents are generally not used alone in seizure pharmacotherapy, but instead serve as adjuncts to other antiseizure drugs for short-term seizure control.

The benzodiazepines are one of the most widely prescribed classes of drugs, used not only to control seizures but also for anxiety, skeletal muscle spasms, and alcohol withdrawal symptoms.

NURSING CONSIDERATIONS

The following content provides nursing considerations that apply to benzodiazepines when given to treat seizure disorders. For the complete nursing process applied to benzodiazepine therapy, see "Nursing Process Focus: Clients Receiving Benzodiazepine and Non-Benzodiazepine Antianxiety Therapy" in Chapter 14, page 151.

The role of the nurse in benzodiazepine therapy for seizures involves careful monitoring of the client's condition and providing education as it relates to the prescribed drug regimen. Assess the client's need for seizure medication. The assessment should include identification of factors associated with the seizures, such as frequency, symptoms, and previous therapies. A drug history should be obtained, including the use of CNS depressants and OTC drugs. Assess for the likelihood of drug abuse and dependence as benzodiazepines are Schedule IV drugs. Assess women of childbearing age for pregnancy, intent to become pregnant, and lactation status as these drugs are pregnancy category D and are secreted into breast milk. Benzodiazepines may also decrease the effectiveness of oral contraceptives.

Alterations in neurotransmitter activity produce changes in intraocular pressure; therefore, benzodiazepines are contraindicated in narrow-angle glaucoma. Liver and kidney function should be monitored in long-term use and these drugs should be used cautiously in those with impaired renal or liver function.

The risk of respiratory depression should be taken into consideration, especially when administering IV doses and when administering to clients with impaired respiratory function and those taking other CNS depressants. Assess for common side effects related to CNS depression such as drowsiness and dizziness. Should an overdose occur, flumazenil is a specific benzodiazepine receptor antagonist that can be administered to reverse CNS depression.

Intravenous benzodiazepines such as diazepam and lorazepam are used in the treatment of status epilepticus or continuous seizures. When administering these drugs IV, it is important to have supplemental oxygen and resuscitation equipment available. Monitor respiratory effort and oxygen saturation. Because the desired action is to terminate seizure activity, severe respiratory depression would be treated with intubation and ventilation rather than by reversing the benzodiazepine effects with flumazenil. Because IV administration may cause hypotension, tachycardia, and muscular weakness, monitoring of heart rhythm, heart rate, and blood pressure is necessary. These drugs have a tendency to

---

Pr **PROTOTYPE DRUG** | Diazepam (Valium)

ACTIONS AND USES

Diazepam binds to the GABA receptor–chloride channels throughout the CNS. It produces its effects by suppressing neuronal activity in the limbic system and subsequent impulses that might be transmitted to the reticular activating system. Effects of this drug are suppression of abnormal neuronal foci that may cause seizures, calming without strong sedation, and skeletal muscle relaxation. When used orally, maximum therapeutic effects may take from 1 to 2 weeks. Tolerance may develop after about 4 weeks. When given IV, effects occur in minutes and its anticonvulsant effects last about 20 minutes.

PHARMACOKINETICS

Diazepam PO is rapidly absorbed. It is widely distributed, crosses the blood-brain barrier and placenta, and enters breast milk. It is highly metabolized by the liver. Its half-life is 20 to 50 hours in adults.

ADMINISTRATION ALERTS

- When administering IV, monitor respirations every 5 to 15 minutes. Have airway and resuscitative equipment accessible.
- Diazepam is pregnancy category D.

ADVERSE EFFECTS AND INTERACTIONS

Diazepam should not be taken with alcohol or other CNS depressants because of combined sedation effects. Other drug interactions include cimetidine, oral contraceptives, valproic acid, and metoprolol, which potentiate diazepam's action; and levodopa and barbiturates, which decrease diazepam's action. Diazepam increases the levels of phenytoin in the bloodstream and may cause phenytoin toxicity. When given IV, hypotension, muscular weakness, tachycardia, and respiratory depression are common. Because of tolerance and dependency, use of diazepam is reserved for short-term seizure control or for status epilepticus.

Use with caution with herbal supplements, such as kava and chamomile, which may cause an increased effect.

 See the Companion Website for a Nursing Process Focus specific to this drug.

precipitate from solution and are irritating to veins. They should not be mixed with other drugs or IV fluid additives and should be given in a large vein if possible.

Client education as it relates to benzodiazepines should include goals, reasons for obtaining baseline data, and possible side effects. Following are points to include when teaching regarding benzodiazepines:

- Avoid alcohol and other CNS depressants, including herbal and OTC drugs, unless advised by the healthcare provider.
- Tobacco use (and nicotine patches) can decrease benzodiazepine effectiveness.
- Benzodiazepines can potentiate the action of digoxin, thus raising blood levels.
- Do not drive or perform hazardous activities until effects of the drug are known.
- Do not discontinue drug abruptly as this may result in rebound seizure activity.
- Take with food if GI upset occurs.
- Benzodiazepines are used illegally for recreation; clients should evaluate the social context of their environment and take any precautions necessary to safeguard their medication supply.

DRUGS THAT SUPPRESS SODIUM INFLUX

This class of drug dampens CNS activity by delaying an influx of sodium ions across neuronal membranes. Hydantoins and several other related antiseizure drugs act by this mechanism.

HYDANTOIN AND PHENYTOIN-LIKE DRUGS

Sodium channels guide the movement of sodium across neuronal membranes into the intracellular space. Sodium movement is the major factor that determines whether a neuron will undergo an action potential. If these channels are temporarily inactivated, neuronal activity will be suppressed. With hydantoin and phenytoin-like drugs, sodium channels are not blocked; they are just desensitized. If channels are blocked, neuronal activity completely stops, as occurs with local anesthetic drugs. These agents are shown in Table 15.3.

15.6 Treating Seizures with Hydantoins and Phenytoin-Like Drugs

The oldest and most commonly prescribed hydantoin is phenytoin. Approved in the 1930s, phenytoin is a broad-spectrum drug that is useful in treating all types of epilepsy except absence seizures. It is able to provide effective seizure suppression without the abuse potential or CNS depression associated with barbiturates. Clients vary significantly in their ability to metabolize phenytoin; therefore, dosages are highly individualized. Because of the very narrow range between a therapeutic dose and a toxic dose, clients must be carefully monitored. The other hydantoins are used much less frequently than phenytoin.

Several widely used drugs share a mechanism of action similar to the hydantoins, including carbamazepine and valproic acid, which is also available as valproate and divalproex sodium. Carbamazepine is a drug of choice for tonic-clonic and partial seizures because it produces fewer adverse effects than phenytoin or phenobarbital. Valproic acid is a drug of choice for absence seizures. Both carbamazepine and valproic acid are also used for bipolar disorder (Chapter 16). Newer antiseizure drugs, such as lamotrigine, have more limited uses.

NURSING CONSIDERATIONS

The role of the nurse in hydantoin and phenytoin-like drug therapy involves careful monitoring of the client's condition and providing education as it relates to the prescribed drug regimen. Some of these drugs are monitored via serum drug levels, so regular laboratory testing is required. When serum drug levels stray outside the normal range, dosage adjustments are made.

TABLE 15.3	**Hydantoins and Phenytoin-Like Drugs**
Drug	*Route and Adult Dose*
Hydantoins	
fosphenytoin (Cerebyx)	IV; Initial dose 15–20 mg PE/kg at 100–150 mg PE/min followed by 4–6 mg PE/kg/day (PE = phenytoin equivalents)
phenytoin (Dilantin)	PO; 15–18 mg/kg or 1 g initial dose; then 300 mg/day in one to three divided doses; may be gradually increased 100 mg/week
Phenytoin-Like Agents	
carbamazepine (Tegretol)	PO; 200 mg bid; gradually increased to 800–1200 mg/day in three to four divided doses
lamotrigine (Lamictal)	PO; 50 mg/day for 2 weeks, then 50 mg bid for 2 weeks; may increase gradually up to 300–500 mg/day in two divided doses (max 700 mg/day)
valproic acid (Depakene)*	PO/IV; 15 mg/kg/day in divided doses when total daily dose is greater than 250 mg; increase 5–10 mg every week until seizures are controlled (max 60 mg/kg/day)

*Other formulations of valproic acid include its salts, valproate, and divalproex sodium.

Common signs of hydantoin toxicity include dizziness, ataxia, diplopia, and lethargy. These drugs affect vitamin K metabolism; therefore, blood dyscrasias and bleeding may ensue. Because hydantoins may increase serum glucose levels, a complete blood count (CBC) and urinalysis should be obtained. Urinalysis is also important to identify the presence of hematuria; phenytoin may change urine colour to pink, red, or brown. These drugs should be used cautiously in clients with hepatic or renal disease.

There have been several cases of fatal hepatotoxicity in clients taking valproic acid. The risk is higher for clients taking multiple antiseizure drugs, those with existing liver disease, those with organic brain disease, and those under 2 years of age. Extreme caution must be taken when administering this drug to these clients.

Pregnancy tests must be conducted on all women of childbearing age before beginning therapy since drugs in this class are pregnancy class D (phenytoin, carbamazepine, and valproic acid) or class C (felbamate and lamotrigine). Hydantoins may also decrease the effectiveness of oral contraceptives. Additional contraindications include heart block and seizures due to hypoglycemia.

Client education as it relates to hydantoin and phenytoin-like drugs should include goals, reasons for obtaining baseline data, and possible side effects. See "Nursing Process Focus: Clients Receiving Antiseizure Drug Therapy" for specific teaching points.

DRUGS THAT SUPPRESS CALCIUM INFLUX

Succinimides are medications that suppress seizures by delaying calcium ion influx into neurons. They are generally only effective against absence seizures.

SUCCINIMIDES

15.7 Treating Seizures with Succinimides

Neurotransmitters, hormones, and some medications bind to neuronal membranes, stimulating the entry of calcium ions. Without calcium influx, neuronal transmission would not be possible. Succinimides delay entry of calcium into neurons by blocking calcium channels, increasing the electrical threshold, and reducing the likelihood that an action potential will be generated. By raising the seizure threshold, succinimides keep neurons from firing too quickly, thus suppressing abnormal foci. The succinimides are shown in Table 15.4 on page 166.

Pr PROTOTYPE | Phenytoin (Dilantin)

ACTIONS AND USES

Phenytoin acts by desensitizing sodium channels in the CNS responsible for neuronal responsivity. Desensitization prevents the spread of disruptive electrical charges in the brain that produce seizures. It is effective against most types of seizure except absence seizures. Phenytoin has antidysrhythmic activity similar to lidocaine (class IB). An unlabelled use is for digitalis-induced dysrhythmias.

ADMINISTRATION ALERTS

- When administering IV, mix with saline only and infuse at the maximum rate of 50 mg/min. Mixing it with other medications or dextrose solutions produces precipitate.
- Always prime or flush IV lines with saline before hanging phenytoin as a piggyback since traces of dextrose solution in an existing main IV or piggyback line can cause microscopic precipitate formation, which becomes emboli if infused. Use an IV line with filter when infusing this drug.
- Injectable phenytoin is a soft tissue irritant that causes local tissue damage following extravasation.
- To reduce the risk of soft tissue damage, do not give IM; inject into a large vein or via central venous catheter.
- Avoid using hand veins to prevent serious local vasoconstrictive response (purple glove syndrome).
- Phenytoin is pregnancy category D.

PHARMACOKINETICS

Phenytoin is slowly absorbed from the GI tract. It is widely distributed, crosses the placenta, and enters breast milk and cerebrospinal fluid (CSF). It is mostly metabolized by the liver. Its half-life is about 22 hours.

ADVERSE EFFECTS AND INTERACTIONS

Phenytoin may cause dysrhythmias, such as bradycardia or ventricular fibrillation, severe hypotension, and hyperglycemia. Severe CNS reactions include headache, nystagmus, ataxia, confusion and slurred speech, paradoxical nervousness, twitching, and insomnia. Peripheral neuropathy may occur with long-term use. Phenytoin can cause multiple blood dyscrasias, including agranulocytosis and aplastic anemia. It may cause severe skin reactions, such as rashes, including exfoliative dermatitis, and Stevens-Johnson syndrome. Connective tissue reactions include lupus erythematosa, hypertrichosis, hirsutism, and gingival hypertrophy.

Phenytoin interacts with many other drugs, including oral anticoagulants, glucocorticoids, H_2-receptor antagonists, antituberculin agents, and food supplements such as folic acid, calcium, and vitamin D. It impairs the efficacy of drugs such as digitoxin, doxycycline, furosemide, estrogens and oral contraceptives, and theophylline. Phenytoin can trigger seizures when combined with tricyclic antidepressants.

Use with caution with herbal supplements, such as herbal laxatives (buckthorn, cascara sagrada, and senna), which may increase potassium loss.

 See the Companion Website for a Nursing Process Focus specific to this drug.

Pr PROTOTYPE | Valproic Acid (Depakene)

ACTIONS AND USES

The mechanism of action of valproic acid is the same as phenytoin, although effects on GABA and calcium channels may cause some additional actions. It is useful for a wide range of seizure types, including absence seizures and mixed types of seizure. Other uses include prevention of migraine headaches and treatment of bipolar disorder.

ADMINISTRATION ALERTS

- Valproic acid is a GI irritant. Extended-release tablets must not be chewed, as mouth soreness will occur.
- Valproic acid syrup must not be mixed with carbonated beverages because they will trigger immediate release of the drug, which causes severe mouth and throat irritation.
- Capsules may be opened and sprinkled on soft foods.
- It is contraindicated in clients with liver disease.
- Valproic acid is pregnancy category D

PHARMACOKINETICS

Valproic acid is well-absorbed from the GI tract. It is widely distributed, crosses the blood-brain barrier and placenta, and enters breast milk. It is mostly metabolized by the liver. Its half-life is 8 to 17 hours in adults.

ADVERSE EFFECTS AND INTERACTIONS

Side effects include sedation, drowsiness, GI upset, and prolonged bleeding time. Other effects include visual disturbances, muscle weakness, tremor, psychomotor agitation, bone marrow suppression, weight gain, abdominal cramps, rash, alopecia, pruritus, photosensitivity, erythema multiforme, and fatal hepatotoxicity.

Valproic acid interacts with many drugs. For example, ASA, cimetidine, chlorpromazine, erythromycin, and felbamate may increase valproic acid toxicity. Concomitant warfarin, ASA, or alcohol use can cause severe bleeding. Alcohol, benzodiazepines, and other CNS depressants potentiate CNS depressant action. Lamotrigine, phenytoin, and rifampin lower valproic acid levels. Valproic acid increases serum phenobarbital and phenytoin levels. Use of clonazepam concurrently with valproic acid may induce absence seizures.

 See the Companion Website for a Nursing Process Focus specific to this drug.

NURSING PROCESS FOCUS   Clients Receiving Antiseizure Drug Therapy

Assessment	Potential Nursing Diagnoses/Identified Patterns
Prior to administration: - Obtain complete health history including allergies and drug history, to determine possible drug interactions. - Assess neurological status, including identification of recent seizure activity. - Assess growth and development.	- Risk for injury related to drug side effects - Deficient knowledge related to drug therapy - Non-adherence

Planning: Client Goals and Outcomes

The client will:
- Experience the absence of seizures or a reduction in the number or severity of seizures
- Avoid physical injury related to seizure activity or medication-induced sensory changes
- Demonstrate an understanding of the drug's action by accurately describing drug effects and precautions

Implementation

Interventions (Rationales)	Client Education/Discharge Planning
- Monitor neurological status, especially changes in level of consciousness and/or mental status. (Sedation may indicate impending toxicity.)	Instruct the client to: - Report any significant change in sensorium, such as slurred speech, confusion, hallucinations, or lethargy - Report any changes in seizure quality or unexpected involuntary muscle movement, such as twitching, tremor, or unusual eye movement
- Protect the client from injury during seizure events until therapeutic effects of drugs are achieved.	- Instruct client to avoid driving and other hazardous activities until effects of the drug are known.

continued

NURSING PROCESS FOCUS   Clients Receiving Antiseizure Drug Therapy   *(Continued)*

Interventions (Rationales)	Client Education/Discharge Planning
■ Monitor effectiveness of drug therapy. Observe for developmental changes, which may indicate a need for dose adjustment.	Instruct client to: ■ Keep a seizure diary to record symptoms during dosage adjustment phases and whenever seizures occur ■ Take the medication exactly as ordered, including the same manufacturer's drug each time the prescription is refilled (Switching brands may result in alterations in seizure control.) ■ Take a missed dose as soon as remembered, but not to take double doses (Doubling doses could result in toxic serum level.)
■ Monitor for adverse effects. Observe for hypersensitivity, nephrotoxicity, and hepatotoxicity.	■ Instruct client to report side effects specific to drug regimen.
■ Monitor oral health. Observe for signs of gingival hypertrophy, bleeding, or inflammation (phenytoin specific).	Instruct client to: ■ Use a soft toothbrush and oral rinses as prescribed by the dentist ■ Avoid mouthwashes containing alcohol ■ Report changes in oral health such as excessive bleeding or inflammation of the gums ■ Maintain a regular schedule of dental visits
■ Monitor gastrointestinal status. (Valproic acid is a GI irritant and anticoagulant.) ■ Conduct guaiac stool testing for occult blood. (Phenytoin's CNS depressant effects decrease GI motility, producing constipation.)	Instruct client to: ■ Take drug with food to reduce GI upset ■ Immediately report any severe or persistent heartburn, upper GI pain, nausea, or vomiting ■ Increase exercise, fluid and fibre intake to facilitate stool passage
■ Monitor nutritional status. (Phenytoin's action on electrolytes may cause decreased absorption of folic acid, vitamin D, magnesium, and calcium. Deficiencies in these vitamins and minerals lead to anemia and osteoporosis. Valproic acid may cause an increase in appetite and weight.)	■ Instruct client in dietary or drug administration techniques specific to prescribed medications. ■ Instruct client to report significant changes in appetite or weight gain.

Evaluation of Outcome Criteria

Evaluate effectiveness of drug therapy by confirming that client goals and expected outcomes have been met (see "Planning").

See Tables 15.3 (page 163) and 15.4 for lists of drugs to which these nursing actions apply.

Ethosuximide is the most commonly prescribed drug in this class. It remains a drug of choice for absence seizures, although valproic acid is also effective for these types of seizures. Some of the newer antiseizure agents, such as lamotrigine, are being investigated for their roles in treating absence seizures.

NURSING CONSIDERATIONS

The role of the nurse in succinimide therapy involves careful monitoring of the client's seizure activity and providing education as it relates to the prescribed drug regimen. Obtain a medical history confirming the baseline seizure activity. Baseline renal and hepatic function tests should be obtained because these drugs are metabolized by the liver and excreted by the kidneys. Succinimides should be used cautiously in clients with liver or renal insufficiency. Succinimides are pregnancy category C.

Review the client's current drug history to determine if any medications interact with succinimides. Succinimides may alter the effectiveness of other antiseizure drugs. Many drugs that alter CNS activity, such as phenothiazines and antidepressants, lower the seizure threshold and can decrease the effectiveness of succinimides.

The nurse should observe for common adverse reactions during therapy, including drowsiness, headache, fatigue, dizziness, depression or euphoria, nausea and vomiting,

TABLE 15.4   Succinimides

Drug	Route and Adult Dose
⏺ ethosuximide (Zarontin)	PO; 250 mg, bid, increased every 4–7 days (max 1.5 g/day)
methsuximide (Celontin)	PO; 300 mg/day; may increase every 4–7 days (max 1.2 g/day)

diarrhea, weight loss, and abdominal pain. Life-threatening adverse reactions include severe mental depression with overt suicidal intent, Stevens-Johnson syndrome, and blood dyscrasias such as agranulocytosis, pancytopenia, and leukopenia.

Seizure activity should be monitored during therapy to confirm the drug's efficacy. Symptoms of overdose include CNS depression, stupor, ataxia, and coma. These symptoms may occur when ethosuximide is given alone or in combination with other anticonvulsants. Combined usage must be monitored carefully, with regular testing for serum levels of each drug.

Client education as it relates to succinimides should include goals, reasons for obtaining baseline data, and possible side effects. Following are the points the nurse should include when teaching clients about succinimides:

- Immediately report changes in mood, mental depression, and suicidal urges.

- Do not drive or perform hazardous activities until effect of drug is known.

- Do not discontinue drug abruptly as this may result in rebound seizure activity.

- Take with food if GI upset occurs.

- Immediately report symptoms suggestive of infection (e.g., fever, sore throat, malaise).

- Report weight loss and anorexia.

NATURAL THERAPIES

The Ketogenic Diet

The ketogenic diet is used when seizures cannot be controlled through pharmacotherapy or there are unacceptable side effects of the medications. Before antiepileptic drugs were developed, this diet was a primary treatment for epilepsy. The ketogenic diet may be used for babies, children, or adults. With adults, however, it is harder to produce the ketones that are necessary for the therapeutic effect.

The ketogenic diet is a stringently calculated diet that is high in fat and low in carbohydrates and protein. It limits water intake to avoid ketone dilution and carefully controls caloric intake. Each meal has the same ketogenic ratio of 4 g of fat to 1 g of protein and carbohydrate. Extra fat is usually given in the form of cream. Research suggests that the diet produces success rates similar to the use of medication, with one-third of the children using it becoming seizure-free, one-third having their seizures reduced, and one-third not responding.

The diet appears to be equally effective for every seizure type, though drop attacks (atonic seizures) may be the most rapid responders. It also helps children with Lennox-Gastaut syndrome and shows promise in babies with infantile spasms. Side effects include hyperlipidemia, constipation, vitamin deficiencies, kidney stones, acidosis, and possibly slower growth rates. Those interested in trying the diet must consult with their healthcare provider; this is not a do-it-yourself diet and may be harmful if not carefully monitored by skilled professionals.

Pr PROTOTYPE DRUG | Ethosuximide (Zarontin)

ACTIONS AND USES

Ethosuximide is a drug of choice for absence (petit mal) seizures. It depresses the activity of neurons in the motor cortex by elevating the neuronal threshold. It is usually ineffective against psychomotor or tonic-clonic seizures; however, it may be given in combination with other medications, which better treat these conditions. It is available in tablet and flavoured syrup formulations.

ADMINISTRATION ALERTS

- Abrupt withdrawal of this medication may induce grand mal seizures.
- Ethosuximide is pregnancy category C.

PHARMACOKINETICS

Ethosuximide is rapidly absorbed. It is mostly metabolized by the liver. Its half-life is 60 hours in adults and 30 hours in children.

ADVERSE EFFECTS AND INTERACTIONS

Ethosuximide may impair mental and physical abilities. Psychosis or extreme mood swings, including depression with overt suicidal intent, can occur. Behavioural changes are more prominent in clients with a history of psychiatric illness. CNS effects include dizziness, headache, lethargy, fatigue, ataxia, sleep pattern disturbances, attention difficulty, and hiccups. Bone marrow suppression and blood dyscrasias are possible, as is systemic lupus erythematosa.

Other reactions include gingival hypertrophy and tongue swelling. Common side effects are abdominal distress and weight loss.

Drug interactions include phenytoin since ethosuximide increases phenytoin serum levels. Valproic acid causes ethosuximide serum levels to fluctuate (increase or decrease).

 See the Companion Website for a Nursing Process Focus specific to this drug.

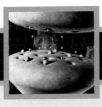

CHAPTER REVIEW

KEY CONCEPTS

The numbered key concepts provide a succinct summary of the important points from the corresponding numbered section within the chapter. If any of these points are not clear, refer to the numbered section within the chapter for review. Expanded versions can be found on the Companion Website.

15.1 Seizures are associated with many causes, including head trauma, brain infection, fluid and electrolyte imbalance, hypoxia, stroke, brain tumours, and high fever in children.

15.2 The three broad categories of seizure are partial seizures, generalized seizures, and special epileptic syndromes. Each seizure type has a characteristic set of signs, and different drugs are used for different types.

15.3 Antiseizure drugs act by distinct mechanisms: potentiation of GABA and delaying the influx of sodium or calcium ions into neurons. Pharmacotherapy may continue for many years, and withdrawal from these agents must be done gradually to avoid seizure recurrence.

15.4 Barbiturates act by potentiating the effects of GABA. Phenobarbital is used for tonic-clonic and febrile seizures.

15.5 Benzodiazepines reduce seizure activity by intensifying GABA action. Their use is limited to short-term adjuncts to other more effective agents.

15.6 Hydantoin and phenytoin-like drugs act by delaying sodium influx into neurons. Phenytoin is a broad-spectrum drug used for all types of epilepsy except absence seizures.

15.7 Succinimides act by delaying calcium influx into neurons. Ethosuximide is a drug of choice for absence seizures.

REVIEW QUESTIONS

1. While obtaining a medical history, a new client claims to have a history of epilepsy but cannot remember the type. What sort of questions should the nurse ask to determine the type of seizure this client has experienced?

2. Explain the importance of the neurotransmitter GABA in neuronal transmission.

3. A client has been seizure-free for 4 years and wants to be taken off phenytoin. Explain the process by which this withdrawal should be accomplished.

CRITICAL THINKING QUESTIONS

1. The nurse reviews the laboratory results on a 16-year-old male who presents to the clinic with fatigue and pallor. The client's hematocrit is 26%, and the nurse notes multiple small petechiae and bruises over his arms and legs. This client has a generalized tonic-clonic seizure disorder that has been managed well on carbamazepine (Tegretol). Relate the drug regimen to this client's presentation.

2. A 24-year-old woman is brought to the emergency room by her husband. He tells the triage nurse that his wife has been treated for seizure disorder secondary to a head injury she received in an automobile accident. She takes phenytoin (Dilantin) 100 mg q8 hours. He relates a history of increasing drowsiness and lethargy in his wife over the past 24 hours. A phenytoin level is performed and the nurse notes that the result is 89 µmol/L. What is the prob-

able cause of this client's CNS depression? What priority nursing interventions should be implemented?

3. The nurse is admitting a 17-year-old female client who has broken her leg in a car crash, in which she was the driver. The client has a history of seizure disorder. The client states that she hates having to take phenytoin (Dilantin) and that she stopped the drug because she couldn't drive and it was making her irritable. Instead of reassuring the client, the nurse first considers the possible side effects of long-term phenytoin therapy. Discuss these and how they might impact client adherence. Develop a nursing care plan for this client. Consider how this care plan could be modified to accommodate cultural beliefs and needs of clients with various ethnic backgrounds.

EXPLORE
MediaLink

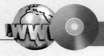 www.pearsoned.ca/adams-king

MEDIALINK DVD-ROM
- **Audio Glossary**
- **CRNE Review**
- **Videos**
  Complex Partial Seizure
  Epilepsy
  Extrapyramidal Side Effects: Torticollis
  Tonic-Clonic Seizure
- **Animations**
  Mechanism of Action: Diazepam
  Mechanism of Action: Valproic acid

COMPANION WEBSITE
- **CRNE Review**
- **Case Study:** Client with seizure
- **Care Plans**
- **Dosage Calculation**
- **Nursing Process Focus Charts**

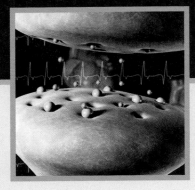

CHAPTER 16

Drugs for Emotional and Mood Disorders

DRUGS AT A GLANCE

ANTIDEPRESSANTS

Tricyclic antidepressants
- *imipramine (Tofranil)*

Selective serotonin reuptake inhibitors
- *fluoxetine (Prozac)*

Atypical antidepressants

MAO inhibitors
- *phenelzine (Nardil)*

DRUGS FOR BIPOLAR DISORDER: MOOD STABILIZERS
- *lithium (Carbolith)*

Miscellaneous drugs

DRUGS FOR ATTENTION DEFICIT–HYPERACTIVITY DISORDER (ADHD)

CNS stimulants
- *methylphenidate (Ritalin)*

Non-stimulant drugs for ADHD

OBJECTIVES

After reading this chapter, the student should be able to do the following:

1. Identify drug classes used for treating emotional and mood disorders.
2. Explain the therapeutic action of antidepressant drugs in relation to physiological aspects of neurotransmission.
3. For each of the drug classes listed in Drugs at a Glance, identify a representative drug and explain its mechanism of action, primary actions, and important adverse effects.
4. Explain the therapeutic action of drugs used for treating attention deficit–hyperactivity disorder.
5. Discuss the nurse's role in the pharmacological management of clients with depression, bipolar disorder, or attention deficit–hyperactivity disorder.
6. Describe and explain, based on pharmacological principles, the rationale for nursing assessment, planning, and interventions for clients with mood disorders.
7. Use the nursing process to care for clients receiving drug therapy for mood and emotional disorders.

MediaLink

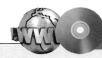

www.pearsoned.ca/adams-king

CRNE review, case studies, and other interactive resources for this chapter can be found on the Companion Website at **www.pearsoned.ca/adams-king**. Click on "Chapter 16" to select the activities for this chapter. For animations, more CRNE review questions, and an audio glossary, access the accompanying MediaLink DVD-ROM in this textbook.

KEY TERMS

attention deficit–hyperactivity disorder (ADHD)   page 184

atypical antidepressants   page 183

bipolar disorder (manic depression)   page 183

depression   page 171

electroconvulsive therapy (ECT)   page 172

major depressive episode   page 171

mania   page 183

monoamine oxidase (MAO) inhibitors   page 178

mood disorder   page 171

mood stabilizer   page 184

selective serotonin reuptake inhibitors (SSRIs)   page 176

serotonin syndrome (SES)   page 177

SSRI discontinuation syndrome   page 177

tricyclic antidepressants (TCAs)   page 173

tyramine   page 179

Mood disorders are common mental health disorders. A large percentage of all drug prescriptions filled in Canada are for mood disorders. Although mood changes are a normal part of life, when those changes become severe and result in impaired functioning within the family, work environment, or interpersonal relationships, an individual may be diagnosed as having a **mood disorder**. The two major categories of mood disorders are depression and bipolar disorder. A third emotional disorder, attention deficit–hyperactivity disorder, is also included in this chapter.

DEPRESSION

Depression is a disorder characterized by a sad or despondent mood. Many symptoms are associated with depression, including lack of energy, sleep disturbances, abnormal eating patterns, and feelings of despair, guilt, and misery.

16.1 Characteristics of Depression

Major depressive disorder is the most common mood disorder in Canada, affecting about 6% of adults. In order to meet the criteria for a diagnosis of **major depressive episode**, according to the *Diagnostic and Statistical Manual of Mental Disorders,* 4th Edition (DSM-IV), the client must experience at least five of the following symptoms for a minimum period of 2 weeks:

- Feeling depressed, sad, or empty or appearing tearful most of the day, nearly every day
- Markedly decreased interest or pleasure in most activities, most of the day, nearly every day
- Poor appetite or overeating nearly every day, or a loss or gain of 5% of body weight
- Feeling guilty, worthless, like a failure, or having let self or others down nearly every day
- Fatigue or having little energy nearly every day
- Difficulty falling or staying asleep, or sleeping too much nearly every day
- Difficulty concentrating on things, such as reading a newspaper or watching television, or making decisions nearly every day
- Moving or speaking so slowly that other people have noticed, or the opposite—being restless, fidgety, and moving around a lot more than usual, nearly every day
- Recurrent thoughts of being better off dead or harming oneself

The majority of depressed clients are not found in psychiatric hospitals, but in mainstream everyday settings. Many go undiagnosed. The recognition of depression, in order for proper diagnosis and treatment to occur, is a collaborative effort among healthcare providers. Because depressed clients are present in multiple settings and in all areas of practice, every nurse should possess proficiency in the assessment and nursing care of clients afflicted with this disorder. Nurses may recognize depression in clients admitted for reasons other than depression or in their family members. A drug history of self-medication with remedies to enhance mood or sleep may alert the nurse to the possibility of depression.

People suffer from depression for a variety of reasons. Depression may be biological, or organic, in origin, associated with dysfunction of neurological processes leading to an imbalance of neurotransmitters. Family history of depression

SPECIAL CONSIDERATIONS

Cultural Influences on Depression and Its Management

- Depression (and other mental illnesses) is often ignored in many Asian communities because of the tremendous amount of stigma attached to it. Emotions are largely suppressed. Asian clients tend to come to the attention of mental health workers late in the course of their illness and often come with a feeling of hopelessness.

- Close to one-quarter of elderly Chinese immigrants report symptoms of depression.

- The incidence of mental illness, including depression, and alcoholism is higher in many Aboriginal communities than in the general Canadian population. The rate of suicide in Aboriginal youth is five to six times higher. Depression may be viewed as an imbalance within the individual and between the individual and the environment that arose from not living life in a good way. Traditional healers or elders may use rituals, charms, and other practices to help restore the balance.

- Some people of European origin deny that mental illness exits and therefore believe that depression will subside on its own.

- The ability to metabolize drugs used for emotional and mood disorders may vary significantly among ethnic groups due to differences in the genes for cytochrome P450 enzymes. Asian clients may require lower doses of antidepressants, lithium, and some other drugs.

increases the risk for biological depression. In some cases, depression may be situational or reactive, meaning that it results from challenging circumstances, such as severe physical illness, loss of a job, death of a loved one, divorce, or financial difficulties, coupled with inadequate psychosocial support. Depression is the most common mental health disorder of older adults, encompassing a variety of physical, emotional, cognitive, and social considerations.

Some women experience intense mood shifts associated with hormonal changes during the menstrual cycle, pregnancy, childbirth, and menopause. For example, up to 80% of women experience depression 2 weeks to 6 months after the birth of a baby. Many women face additional stresses such as responsibilities both at work and home, single parenthood, and caring for children and aging parents. If mood is severely depressed and persists long enough, many women may benefit from medical treatment, including women with premenstrual distress disorder, postpartum depression, or menopausal distress.

During the dark winter months, some clients experience a type of depression known as seasonal affective disorder (SAD). This type of depression is associated with a reduced release of the brain neurohormone melatonin. Exposing clients on a regular basis to specific wavelengths of light may relieve SAD depression and prevent future episodes.

16.2 Assessment and Treatment of Depression

The first step in implementing appropriate treatment for depression is a complete health examination. Certain drugs, such as glucocorticoids and oral contraceptives, can cause the same symptoms as depression, and the healthcare provider should rule out this possibility. Depression may be mimicked by a variety of medical and neurological disorders, ranging from B vitamin deficiencies to thyroid gland problems to early Alzheimer's disease. If underlying causes for the depression are ruled out, a psychological evaluation is often performed by a psychiatrist or psychologist to confirm the diagnosis.

During health examinations, inquiries should be made about alcohol and drug use and whether the client has thoughts about death or suicide. Ask the client about a family history of depressive illness; if other family members have been treated, document the therapies received and whether they were effective. Assess for symptoms of depression. In general, severe depressive illness, particularly that which is recurrent, will require both medication and psychotherapy to achieve the best response. Counselling therapies help clients gain insight and resolve their problems through verbal "give-and-take" with the therapist. Behavioural therapies help clients learn how to obtain more satisfaction and rewards through their own actions and how to unlearn the behavioural patterns that contribute to or result from their depression.

Short-term psychotherapies that are helpful for some forms of depression are interpersonal and cognitive-behavioural therapies. Interpersonal therapy focuses on the client's disturbed personal relationships that both cause and exacerbate the depression. Cognitive-behavioural therapies help clients change the negative styles of thought and behaviour that are often associated with their depression.

Psychodynamic therapies focus on resolving the client's internal conflicts. These therapies are often postponed until the depressive symptoms are significantly improved.

In clients with serious and life-threatening mood disorders that are unresponsive to pharmacotherapy, **electroconvulsive therapy (ECT)** has been the traditional treatment. Although ECT has been found to be safe, there are still deaths (1 in 10,000 clients) and other serious complications related to the seizure activity and anesthesia (Janicak, 2002). Recent studies suggest that repetitive transcranial magnetic stimulation (rTMS) is an effective somatic treatment for major depression. In contrast to ECT, it has minimal effects on memory, does not require general anesthesia, and produces its effects without a generalized seizure.

Even with the best professional care, the client with depression may take a long time to recover. Many clients with major depression have multiple bouts of the illness over the course of a lifetime. This can take its toll on the client's family, friends, and other caregivers who may sometimes feel burned out, frustrated, or even depressed themselves. They may experience episodes of anger toward the depressed loved one, only to subsequently suffer reactions of guilt over being angry. Although such feelings are common, they can be distressing, and the caregiver may not know where to turn for help, support, or advice. It is often the nurse who is best able to assist the family members of a person suffering from emotional and mood disorders. Family members may need counselling themselves.

LIFESPAN CONSIDERATIONS

Depression across the Lifespan

- Depression can occur at any age, but it is more prevalent in older adults.
- Drug dosages may require adjustment due to age-related changes in pharmacokinetics.
- Elderly clients are at increased risk of falls, confusion, and other side effects due to the sedating effects of some antidepressants and altered pharmacokinetics.
- Depressed teens and older adults have an increased risk of suicide.
- A healthy lifestyle should be promoted in all age groups to help reduce depressive symptoms and enhance antidepressant effectiveness.

PHARMFACTS

Clients with Depressive Symptoms

- Major depression, manic depression, and situational depression are some of the most common mental health challenges worldwide.
- Clinical depression affects more than 6% of Canadians each year.
- Although depression can occur in anyone and at any age, the incidence is greater in females, Aboriginal Peoples, and older adults.
- Fewer than half of those suffering from depression actually seek medical treatment.
- Many clients consider depression a weakness rather than an illness.
- Depressed clients may self-treat with alcohol or street drugs.
- With antidepressants, about 40% recover fully and another 25% experience improvement in symptoms.
- Social support, psychotherapy, and culturally appropriate care are important components of depression treatment.

ANTIDEPRESSANTS

Drugs for depression are called antidepressants. Antidepressants treat major depression by enhancing mood.

16.3 Mechanism of Action of Antidepressants

Depression is associated with an imbalance of neurotransmitters in certain regions of the brain. Although medication does not completely restore these chemical imbalances, it does help to reduce depressive symptoms while the client develops effective means of coping. Antidepressants enhance the action of certain neurotransmitters in the brain, including norepinephrine and serotonin, which is also known by its chemical name, 5-hydroxytryptamine (5-HT). The two basic mechanisms of action are blocking the enzymatic breakdown of norepinephrine and slowing the reuptake of serotonin. The four primary classes of antidepressant drugs, also shown in Tables 16.1 and 16.2, are as follows:

1. Tricyclic antidepressants (TCAs)
2. Selective serotonin reuptake inhibitors (SSRIs)
3. Monoamine oxidase (MAO) inhibitors
4. Atypical antidepressants

TRICYCLIC ANTIDEPRESSANTS

Tricyclic antidepressants (TCAs) are drugs named for their three-ring chemical structure. They were the mainstay of

TABLE 16.1   Antidepressants: An Overview

	Typical			Atypical		
	Monoamine Oxidase Inhibitors	Tricyclic Antidepressants	Selective Serotonin Reuptake Inhibitors	Norepinephrine (NE) Reuptake Inhibitors	NE and Dopamine Reuptake Inhibitors	Serotonin and NE Reuptake Inhibitors
Generic Drugs	phenelzine tranylcypromine	imipramine clomipramine amitriptyline desipramine doxepin trimipramine	fluoxetine sertraline paroxetine fluvoxamine citalopram	reboxetine atomoxetine	bupropion	venlafaxine
Mechanism of Action	inhibit monoamine oxidase	inhibit NE, serotonin, and dopamine reuptake	inhibit serotonin reuptake	inhibit NE reuptake	inhibit NE and dopamine reuptake	inhibit serotonin and NE reuptake
Therapeutic Effect	↑ NE ↑ serotonin ↑ dopamine ↑ NE	↑ NE ↑ serotonin ↑ dopamine ↑ NE	↑ serotonin	↑ NE	↑ NE ↑ dopamine	↑ NE ↑ serotonin
Key Side Effects	orthostatic hypotension (hypertensive crisis with tyramine), headache, insomnia, diarrhea	anticholinergic effects: sweating, sedation, orthostatic hypotension	nervousness, insomnia, sexual dysfunction, weight gain	dry mouth, hypotension, decreased libido, constipation, increased heart rate	increased appetite	nausea, headache, nervousness, hypertension
Serious Interactions	tyramine, many OTC and prescriptiondrugs	MAO inhibitors	MAO inhibitors, warfarin	MAO inhibitors	MAO inhibitors	MAO inhibitors

TABLE 16.2 Antidepressants

Drug	Route and Adult Dose
Tricyclic Antidepressants (TCAs)	
amitriptyline (Elavil)	Adult: PO; 75–100 mg/day (may gradually increase to 150–300 mg/day) Geriatric: PO; 10–25 mg at hs (may gradually increase to 25–150 mg/day)
amoxapine (Asendin)	Adult: PO; begin with 100 mg/day, may increase on day 3 to 300 mg/day Geriatric: PO; 25 mg at hs; may increase every 3–7 days to 50–150 mg/day (max 300 mg/day)
desipramine (Apo-Desipramine)	Adult: PO; 75–100 mg day; may increase to 150–300 mg/day
doxepin (Sinequan)	PO; 30–150 mg/day at hs; may gradually increase to 300 mg/day
imipramine (Tofranil)	PO; 75–100 mg/day (max 300 mg/day)
trimipramine (Surmontil)	PO; 75–100 mg/day (max 300 mg/day)
Selective Serotonin Reuptake Inhibitors (SSRIs)	
citalopram (Celexa)	PO; Start at 20 mg/day (max 40 mg/day)
fluoxetine (Prozac)	PO; 20 mg/day in the AM (max 80 mg/day)
fluvoxamine (Luvox)	PO; Start with 50 mg/day (max 300 mg/day)
paroxetine (Paxil)	Depression: PO; 10–50 mg/day (max 80 mg/day) Obsessive-compulsive disorder: PO; 20–60 mg/day Panic attacks: PO; 40 mg/day
sertraline (Zoloft)	Adult: PO; start with 50 mg/day; gradually increase every few weeks to a range of 50–200 mg Geriatric: PO; start with 25 mg/day
MAO Inhibitors	
phenelzine (Nardil)	PO; 15 mg tid (max 90 mg/day)
tranylcypromine (Parnate)	PO; 30 mg/day (give 20 mg in AM and 10 mg in PM); may increase by 10 mg/day at 3-week intervals up to 60 mg/day
Atypical Antidepressants	
bupropion (Wellbutrin)	PO; 75–100 mg tid (greater than 450 mg/day increases risk for adverse reactions)
mirtazapine (Remeron)	PO; 15 mg/day in a single dose at hs; may increase every 1–2 weeks (max 45 mg/day)
trazodone (Desyrel)	PO; 150 mg/day; may increase by 50 mg/day every 3–4 days up to 400–600 mg/day
venlafaxine (Effexor)	PO; 25–125 mg tid

depression pharmacotherapy from the early 1960s until the 1980s and are still used today.

16.4 Treating Depression with Tricyclic Antidepressants

Tricyclic antidepressants act by inhibiting the reuptake of norepinephrine and serotonin, and, to a lesser extent, dopamine, into presynaptic nerve terminals, as shown in Figure 16.1. TCAs are used mainly for major depression and occasionally for milder situational depression. Clomipramine is approved for the treatment of obsessive-compulsive disorder, and other TCAs are sometimes used as unlabelled treatments for panic attacks. One use for TCAs, not related to psychopharmacology, is the treatment of childhood enuresis (bedwetting).

Shortly after their approval as antidepressants in the 1950s, it was found that the TCAs produced fewer side effects and were less dangerous than MAO inhibitors. However, TCAs have some unpleasant and serious side effects. The most common side effect is orthostatic hypotension, which occurs due to alpha₁ blockade on blood vessels. The most

serious adverse effect occurs when TCAs accumulate in cardiac tissue. Although rare, cardiac dysrhythmias can occur.

Sedation is a frequently reported complaint at the initiation of therapy, though clients may become tolerant to this effect after several weeks of treatment. Most TCAs have a long half-life, which increases the risk of side effects for clients with delayed excretion. Anticholinergic effects, such as dry mouth, constipation, urinary retention, blurred vision, and tachycardia, are common. These effects are less severe if the drug is gradually increased to the therapeutic dose over 2 to 3 weeks. Significant drug interactions can occur with CNS depressants, sympathomimetics, anticholinergics, and MAO inhibitors. With the availability of newer antidepressants that have fewer side effects, TCAs are less likely to be used as first-line drugs in the treatment of depression.

NURSING CONSIDERATIONS

The role of the nurse in TCA therapy involves careful monitoring of the client's condition and providing education as

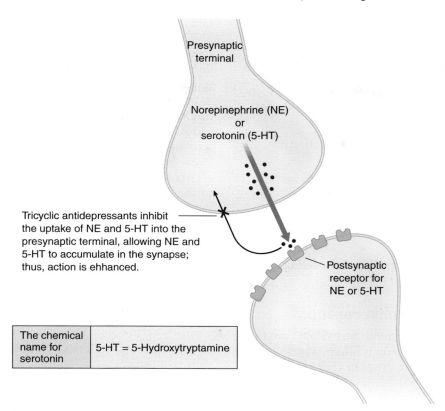

● **Figure 16.1** Tricyclic antidepressants produce their effects by inhibiting the reuptake of neurotransmitters, particularly norepinephrine and serotonin (5-HT), into presynaptic nerve terminals

it relates to the prescribed drug regimen. Clients should be advised that the therapeutic effects of TCAs may take 2 to 6 weeks to occur. Although the neurotransmitter deficiencies are corrected quickly, subsequent changes in the receptors for the neurotransmitters occur more slowly over a period of weeks, resulting in a delay in the onset of therapeutic effects. Individual responses to drug therapy may vary and require assessment. Responses may be affected by variations in serum albumin levels (since TCAs are more than 90% bound to plasma proteins), genetic differences in metabolizing enzymes, and differences in receptor changes.

Suicide potential increases as blood levels of a TCA increase but have not yet reached their peak therapeutic level. While in the depths of depression, clients may lack the energy for suicide. As clients begin to recover from depression, their energy level rises and with it their ability to plan and enact suicide. The nurse needs to monitor the client closely for symptoms of suicidal ideation throughout treatment.

TCAs are contraindicated in clients in the acute recovery phase of a myocardial infarction (MI) and in clients with heart block or a history of dysrhythmias because of their effects on cardiac tissue. Because TCAs lower the seizure threshold, clients with epilepsy must be carefully monitored. Clients with urinary retention, narrow-angle glaucoma, or prostatic hypertrophy may not be good candidates for TCAs because of anticholinergic side effects. Annoying

anticholinergic effects, coupled with the weight gain effect of TCAs, may lead to non-adherence. Tricyclics must be given with extreme caution to clients with asthma, cardiovascular disorders, gastrointestinal disorders, alcoholism, and other psychiatric disorders, including schizophrenia and bipolar disorder. Most TCAs are pregnancy category C or D, so they are only used during pregnancy and lactation when medically necessary. Should a client desire to become pregnant while taking a TCA, she should immediately discuss her depression medication with her healthcare provider. The TCAs should be withdrawn over several weeks and not discontinued abruptly.

Significant drug interactions may occur with TCAs. Oral contraceptives may decrease the efficacy of tricyclics. Cimetidine interferes with their metabolism and excretion. Tricyclics affect the efficacy of clonidine and guanethidine. Concurrent use of alcohol and other CNS depressants may result in excessive sedation and should be avoided.

Client education as it relates to TCAs should include goals, reasons for obtaining baseline data such as vital signs and tests for cardiac and renal disorders, and possible side effects. Following are other important points to include when teaching clients about TCAs:

- Be aware that it may take several weeks or more to achieve the full therapeutic effect of the drug.

- Maintain follow-up appointments with the healthcare provider.

- Sweating, along with other anticholinergic side effects, may occur.
- Take medication exactly as prescribed, and report side effects if they occur.
- Do not take any prescription drugs, OTC drugs, or herbal products without first consulting with the healthcare provider.
- Change position slowly, especially when sitting or standing from a lying position.
- Do not drive or engage in hazardous activities until sedative effect is known; drowsiness may be considerable in the first weeks.
- Note that the TCA may be taken at bedtime if sedation occurs.
- Older adults may be more prone to the sedating effects and have an increased risk of falls.

SELECTIVE SEROTONIN REUPTAKE INHIBITORS

Selective serotonin reuptake inhibitors (SSRIs) are drugs that slow the reuptake of serotonin into presynaptic nerve terminals. They have become drugs of choice in the treatment of depression.

16.5 Treating Depression with SSRIs

Serotonin is a natural neurotransmitter in the CNS, found in high concentrations in certain neurons in the hypothalamus, limbic system, medulla, and spinal cord. It is important to several body activities, including the cycling between NREM and REM sleep, pain perception, and emotional states. Lack of adequate serotonin in the CNS can lead to depression. Serotonin is metabolized to a less active substance by the enzyme monoamine oxidase (MAO).

In the 1970s, it became increasingly clear that serotonin had a more substantial role in depression than once thought. Clinicians knew that the TCAs altered the sensitivity of serotonin to certain receptors in the brain, but they did not know how this was connected with depression. Ongoing efforts to find antidepressants with fewer side effects led to the development of another category of medications, the SSRIs.

While the tricyclic class inhibits the reuptake of both norepinephrine and serotonin into presynaptic nerve terminals, the SSRIs are selective for serotonin. Increased levels of serotonin in the synaptic gap induce complex neurotransmitter changes in pre- and postsynaptic neurons in the brain. Presynaptic receptors become less sensitive, while postsynaptic receptors become more sensitive. This concept is illustrated in Figure 16.2.

SSRIs have approximately the same efficacy at relieving depression as the MAO inhibitors and the tricyclics. The major advantage of the SSRIs, and the one that makes them drugs of choice, is their greater safety. Sympathomimetic effects (increased heart rate and hypertension) and anticholinergic effects (dry mouth, blurred vision, urinary retention, and constipation) are less common with this drug class. Sedation is also experienced less frequently. Cardiac conduction changes are common with SSRIs. Babies

---

Pr PROTOTYPE DRUG | Imipramine (Tofranil)

ACTIONS AND USES

Imipramine blocks the reuptake of serotonin and norepinephrine into nerve terminals. It is mainly used for clinical depression, although it is occasionally used for the treatment of nocturnal enuresis in children. The nurse may find imipramine prescribed for a number of unlabelled uses, including intractable pain, anxiety disorders, and withdrawal syndromes from alcohol and cocaine.

ADMINISTRATION ALERTS

- Paradoxical diaphoresis can be a side effect of TCAs; therefore, diaphoresis may not be a reliable indicator of other disease states such as hypoglycemia.
- Imipramine causes anticholinergic effects and may potentiate effects of anticholinergic drugs administered during surgery.
- Do not discontinue abruptly because rebound dysphoria, irritability, or sleeplessness may occur.
- Imipramine is pregnancy category C.

PHARMACOKINETICS

Imipramine is well absorbed after oral administration. It is widely distributed and crosses the placenta. It is 90% to 95% protein bound. It is highly metabolized by the liver, mostly on first pass. Its half-life is 8 to 16 hours.

ADVERSE EFFECTS AND INTERACTIONS

Side effects include sedation, drowsiness, blurred vision, dry mouth, and cardiovascular symptoms such as dysrhythmias, heart block, and extreme hypertension. Agents that mimic the action of norepinephrine or serotonin should be avoided because imipramine inhibits their metabolism and may produce toxicity. Some clients may experience photosensitivity. Concurrent use of other CNS depressants, including alcohol, may cause sedation. Cimetidine may inhibit the metabolism of imipramine, leading to increased serum levels and possible toxicity. Imipramine may decrease the antihypertensive effects of clonidine; clonidine may increase risk for CNS depression. Use of oral contraceptives may increase or decrease imipramine levels. Disulfiram may lead to delirium and tachycardia.

Use with caution with herbal supplements, such as evening primrose oil and ginkgo, which may lower the seizure threshold. St. John's wort used concurrently may cause serotonin syndrome.

 See the Companion Website for a Nursing Process Focus specific to this drug.

born to women on SSRIs are at greater risk for lung and heart defects. Drugs in the SSRI class have similar efficacy in inhibiting serotonin reuptake and improving depression. However, they differ in some effects due to differences in interactions with receptors other than serotonin. For example, sertraline has dopamine reuptake inhibition properties that may improve attention and cognitive function as well as mood. Fluoxetine has norepinephrine reuptake inhibition action that may improve depression and also contribute to jitteriness, nervousness, and sleep problems that are common in early weeks of treatment. Fluoxetine may be associated with QT prolongation on the electrocardiogram (ECG). Clients who do not respond well to one SSRI may respond better to another.

The most common side effects of SSRIs relate to sexual dysfunction. Up to 70% of both men and women can experience decreased libido and lack of ability to reach orgasm. In men, delayed ejaculation and impotence may occur. For clients who are sexually active, these side effects may result in non-adherence with pharmacotherapy. Other common side effects of SSRIs include nausea, headache, anxiety, and insomnia.

Serotonin syndrome (SES) may occur when taking another medication that affects the metabolism, synthesis, or reuptake of serotonin, causing serotonin to accumulate in the body. Symptoms can begin as early as 2 hours after taking the first dose, or as late as several weeks after initiating pharmacotherapy. Symptoms of serotonin syndrome include mental status changes (confusion, anxiety, restlessness), hypertension, tremors, sweating, hyperpyrexia, and ataxia. Serotonin syndrome can be caused by the concurrent administration of an SSRI with an MAO inhibitor, a TCA, lithium, meperidine, or a number of other medications and herbals. Because deaths have been caused by administering meperidine and other drugs to clients receiving SSRIs, it is very important to always check for interactions. Early recognition of symptoms and early treatment can help prevent deaths from SES. Conservative treatment is to discontinue the SSRI and provide supportive care. In severe cases, mechanical ventilation and muscle relaxants may be necessary.

Some clients may experience **SSRI discontinuation syndrome** when SSRI therapy is discontinued. Symptoms include lowered mood, dizziness, lethargy, paresthesia, nausea, vivid dreams, irritability, electric shock sensations, and confusion. Symptoms are more frequent with shorter half-life SSRIs, such as fluvoxamine or paroxetine. Symptoms may persist for up to 21 days despite slowly tapered SSRI withdrawal. Symptoms may be relieved within 24 hours by restarting the medication.

NURSING CONSIDERATIONS

The role of the nurse in SSRI therapy involves careful monitoring of the client's condition and providing education as it relates to the prescribed drug regimen. The nurse should

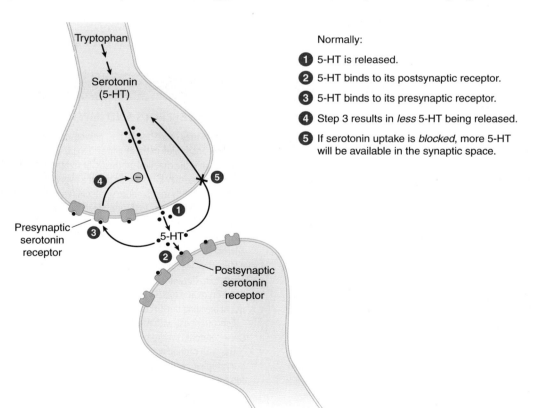

Normally:

1. 5-HT is released.
2. 5-HT binds to its postsynaptic receptor.
3. 5-HT binds to its presynaptic receptor.
4. Step 3 results in *less* 5-HT being released.
5. If serotonin uptake is *blocked*, more 5-HT will be available in the synaptic space.

● **Figure 16.2** SSRIs block the reuptake of serotonin into presynaptic nerve terminals: increased levels of serotonin induce complex changes in pre- and postsynaptic neurons of the brain; presynaptic receptors become less sensitive, while postsynaptic receptors become more sensitive

assess the client's need for antidepressant drugs, including intensity and duration of symptoms. The assessment should include identification of factors that led to the depression, such as life events or health changes. The nurse should obtain a careful drug history, including the use of CNS depressants, alcohol, and other antidepressants, especially MAO inhibitor therapy, as these may interact with SSRIs. The nurse should assess for hypersensitivity to SSRIs. The nurse should assess suicide ideation because the drugs may take several weeks before full therapeutic benefit is obtained. The medical history should include any disorders of sexual function since these drugs have a high incidence of side effects of this nature.

Although the SSRIs are safer than other antidepressants, serious adverse effects can still occur. Baseline liver function laboratory tests should be obtained because SSRIs are metabolized in the liver and hepatic disease can result in higher serum levels. A baseline body weight should be obtained as SSRIs can cause weight gain.

Client education as it relates to SSRIs should include goals, reasons for obtaining baseline data such as vital signs and concurrent medications, and possible side effects. The nurse should inform the client that SSRIs take up to 5 weeks to reach their maximum therapeutic effectiveness. Following are other important points to include when teaching clients about SSRIs:

- Do not take any prescription or OTC drugs or herbal products without first consulting the healthcare provider.
- Maintain follow-up appointments with healthcare provider.

- Report side effects to healthcare provider as they occur.
- Do not drive or engage in hazardous activities until sedative effect is known; the SSRI may be taken at bedtime if sedation occurs.
- Do not discontinue drug abruptly after long-term use.
- Exercise and monitor caloric intake to avoid weight gain.

MONOAMINE OXIDASE INHIBITORS

Monoamine oxidase (MAO) inhibitors inhibit monoamine oxidase, the enzyme that terminates the actions of neurotransmitters such as dopamine, norepinephrine, epinephrine, and serotonin. Because of their low safety margin, these drugs are reserved for clients who have not responded to TCAs or SSRIs.

16.6 Treating Depression with MAO Inhibitors

As discussed in Chapter 13, the action of norepinephrine at adrenergic synapses is terminated through two means: reuptake into the presynaptic nerve and enzymatic destruction by the enzyme monoamine oxidase.

MAO inhibitors inhibit the breakdown of norepinephrine, dopamine, and serotonin in CNS neurons. The higher levels of these neurotransmitters in the brain intensify neurotransmission and alleviate the symptoms of depression. MAO is located within presynaptic nerve terminals, as shown in Figure 16.3.

The MAO inhibitors were the first drugs approved to treat depression, in the 1950s. They are as effective as TCAs and

---

Pr PROTOTYPE DRUG | Fluoxetine (Prozac)

ACTIONS AND USES

Therapeutic actions of fluoxetine can be attributed to its ability to selectively inhibit serotonin reuptake into presynaptic nerve terminals. Its main use is clinical depression, although it may be prescribed for obsessive-compulsive disorder and eating disorders. Therapeutic actions include improved affect, mood enhancement, and increased appetite, with maximum effects observed after several days to weeks.

ADMINISTRATION ALERTS

- Fluoxetine is available in both daily and weekly dose oral formulations. Weekly dose capsules should be dispensed in small quantity or in the healthcare setting to reduce the risk of suicide by overdose.
- Fluoxetine is pregnancy category B.

PHARMACOKINETICS

Fluoxetine is well absorbed after oral administration. It is widely distributed and crosses the blood-brain barrier. It is 95% protein bound. Fluoxetine tends to be eliminated slowly and to accumulate in the body. Active metabolites may persist for weeks. This is of consequence when discontinuation of the drug is required and drugs that may interact with fluoxetine, or its metabolite norfluoxetine (also an antidepressant), are subsequently prescribed.

ADVERSE EFFECTS AND INTERACTIONS

Fluoxetine may cause headaches, nervousness, insomnia, nausea, and diarrhea. Foods high in the amino acid tryptophan should be avoided since tryptophan is the chemical precursor for serotonin synthesis. Concurrent use with selegiline may increase the risk of a hypertensive crisis. TCAs administered concurrently may produce serotonin syndrome. Symptoms of fluoxetine overdose include fever, confusion, shivering, sweating, and muscle spasms. Fluoxetine cannot be used if the client took an MAO inhibitor within the past 14 days. Concurrent use of benzodiazepines may cause increased adverse CNS effects. Concurrent use of beta-blockers can cause their decreased elimination, leading to hypotension or bradycardia. Concurrent use of phenytoin, clozapine, or theophylline may lead to decreased elimination of these drugs and toxicity. Concurrent use of warfarin may lead to increased risk of bleeding due to competitive protein binding.

Concurrent use with meperidine, fentanyl, or dextromethorphan may cause serotonin syndrome.

Use with caution with herbal supplements, such as St. John's wort and L-tryptophan, which may cause serotonin syndrome, and kava, which may increase the effects of fluoxetine.

 See the Companion Website for a Nursing Process Focus specific to this drug.

SSRIs in treating depression. However, because of drug-drug and food-drug interactions, hepatotoxicity, and the development of safer antidepressants, MAO inhibitors are now reserved for clients who are not responsive to other antidepressant classes.

Common side effects of the MAO inhibitors include orthostatic hypotension, headache, insomnia, and diarrhea. A primary concern is that these agents interact with a large number of foods and other medications, sometimes with serious effects. A hypertensive crisis can occur when an MAO inhibitor is used concurrently with other antidepressants or sympathomimetic drugs. Combining an MAO inhibitor with an SSRI can produce serotonin syndrome. If given with antihypertensives, the client can experience excessive hypotension. MAO inhibitors also potentiate the hypoglycemic effects of insulin and oral antidiabetic drugs. Hyperpyrexia is known to occur in clients taking MAO inhibitors with meperidine (Demerol), dextromethorphan, and TCAs.

A hypertensive crisis can also result from an interaction between MAO inhibitors and foods containing **tyramine**, a form of the amino acid tyrosine. In many respects, tyramine resembles norepinephrine. Tyramine is usually degraded by MAO in the intestines. If a client is taking MAO inhibitors, however, tyramine enters the bloodstream in high amounts and displaces norepinephrine in presynaptic nerve terminals. The result is a sudden increase in norepinephrine,

causing acute hypertension. Symptoms usually occur within minutes of ingesting the food and include occipital headache, stiff neck, flushing, palpitations, diaphoresis, and nausea. Calcium channel blockers may be given as an antidote. Examples of foods containing tyramine are shown in Table 16.3.

NURSING CONSIDERATIONS

The role of the nurse in MAO inhibitor therapy involves careful monitoring of the client's condition and providing education as it relates to the prescribed drug regimen. Assess the client's need for antidepressant drugs, including intensity and duration of symptoms. The assessment should include identification of factors that led to depression, such as life events or health changes. Assess suicide ideation because the drugs may take several weeks before full therapeutic benefit is obtained. Cardiovascular status should be assessed as these agents may affect blood pressure. Phenelzine is contraindicated in cardiovascular disease, heart failure, cerebrovascular accident, hepatic or renal dysfunction, and paranoid schizophrenia. A CBC should be obtained because MAO inhibitors can inhibit platelet function. Assess for the possibility of pregnancy; these agents are pregnancy category C and enter breast milk. A client taking an MAO inhibitor must refrain from foods that contain tyramine,

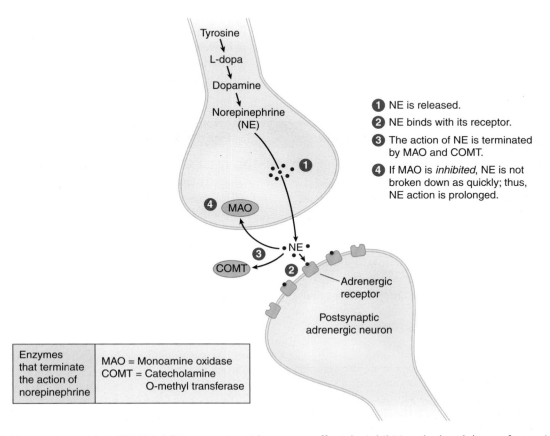

● **Figure 16.3** Monoamine oxidase (MAO) inhibitors exert antidepressant effects by inhibiting the breakdown of norepinephrine by the enzyme monoamine oxidase

TABLE 16.3   Foods Containing Tyramine

Fruits	avocados, bananas, raisins, papaya products (including meat tenderizers), canned figs
Dairy products	cheese (cottage cheese is okay), sour cream, yogurt
Alcohol	beer, wine (especially red wine)
Meats	beef or chicken liver, pâté, meat extracts, pickled or kippered herring, pepperoni, salami, sausage, bologna/hot dogs
Vegetables	pods of broad beans (e.g., fava beans)
Sauces	soy sauce
Yeast	all yeast and yeast extracts
Other foods to avoid	chocolate

which is found in many common foods (see Table 16.3). MAO inhibitors should be used with caution in epilepsy as they may lower the seizure threshold.

The nurse should obtain a careful drug history; common drugs that may interact with an MAO inhibitor include other MAO inhibitors, insulin, caffeine-containing products, other antidepressants, meperidine, and possibly opioids and methyldopa. There must be at least a 14-day interval between the use of MAO inhibitors and these other drugs.

Some clients may not achieve the full therapeutic benefits of an MAO inhibitor for 4 to 8 weeks. Because depression continues during this time, clients may discontinue the drug if they do not feel it is helping them.

Because of the serious side effects possible with MAO inhibitors, client education is vital. The client's ability to comprehend restrictions and be compliant with them may be impaired in a severely depressed state. Client education should include goals, reasons for obtaining baseline data such as vital signs and laboratory studies, and a dietary consult for possible side effects. In addition, include the follow-

ing points when educating clients and their caregivers about MAO inhibitors:

- Avoid foods containing tyramine (provide a list).
- Do not take any prescription or OTC drugs or herbal products without first consulting with the healthcare provider.
- Refrain from caffeine intake.
- Wear a MedicAlert bracelet identifying the MAO inhibitor medication.
- Be aware that it may take several weeks or more to obtain the full therapeutic effect of drug.
- Maintain follow-up appointments with healthcare provider.
- Do not drive or engage in hazardous activities until sedative effect is known; drug may be taken at bedtime if sedation occurs.
- Observe for and report signs of impending stroke or MI.

Pr PROTOTYPE DRUG | Phenelzine (Nardil)

ACTIONS AND USES

Phenelzine produces its effects by irreversible inhibition of monoamine oxidase; therefore, it intensifies the effects of norepinephrine in adrenergic synapses. It is used to manage symptoms of depression not responsive to other types of pharmacotherapy and is occasionally used for panic disorder. Drug effects may persist for 2 to 3 weeks after therapy is discontinued.

ADMINISTRATION ALERTS

- Wash-out periods of 2 to 3 weeks are required before introducing other drugs.
- Abrupt discontinuation of this drug may cause rebound hypertension.
- Phenelzine is pregnancy category C.

PHARMACOKINETICS

Phenelzine is well absorbed from the GI tract. It is widely distributed, crosses the placenta, and enters breast milk. It is mostly metabolized by the liver. Its half-life is unknown.

ADVERSE EFFECTS AND INTERACTIONS

Common side effects are constipation, dry mouth, orthostatic hypotension, insomnia, nausea, and loss of appetite. It may increase heart rate and neural activity leading to delirium, mania, anxiety, and convulsions. Severe hypertension may occur when ingesting foods containing tyramine. Seizures, respiratory depression, circulatory collapse, and coma may occur in cases of severe overdose. Many other drugs affect the action of phenelzine. Concurrent use of TCAs and SSRIs should be avoided since the combination can cause temperature elevation and seizures. Opiates, including meperidine, should be avoided due to increased risk of respiratory failure or hypertensive crisis.

Use with caution with herbal supplements, such as ginseng, which could cause headache, tremors, mania, insomnia, irritability, and visual hallucinations. Concurrent use with ephedra, St. John's wort, or ma huang could lead to hypertensive crisis.

 See the Companion Website for a Nursing Process Focus specific to this drug.

NURSING PROCESS FOCUS Clients Receiving Antidepressant Therapy

Assessment	Potential Nursing Diagnoses/Identified Patterns
Prior to administration: ■ Obtain complete health history including allergies, drug history, and possible drug interactions. ■ Obtain history of cardiac (including recent MI), renal, biliary, liver, and mental disorders including ECG and blood studies: CBC, platelets, glucose, BUN, creatinine, electrolytes, liver function tests and enzymes, and urinalysis. ■ Assess neurological status, including seizure activity and identification of recent mood and behavioural patterns.	■ Ineffective coping ■ Powerlessness ■ Disturbed thought processes related to side effects of drug ■ Adjustment difficulties ■ Need for knowledge related to drug therapy ■ Risk for self-directed violence ■ Urinary retention related to anticholinergic side effects of drug

Planning: Client Goals and Expected Outcomes

The client will:
- Report mood elevation and effectively engage in activities of daily living
- Report an absence of suicidal ideations and improvement in thought processes
- Demonstrate a decrease in anxiety (e.g., ritual behaviours)
- Demonstrate an understanding of the drug's action by accurately describing drug effects and precautions

Implementation

Interventions (Rationales)	Client Teaching/Discharge Planning
■ Monitor vital signs especially pulse and blood pressure. (Imipramine may cause orthostatic hypotension.)	Instruct client to: ■ Report any change in sensorium particularly impending syncope ■ Avoid abrupt changes in position ■ Monitor vital signs (especially blood pressure), ensuring proper use of home equipment ■ Consult the nurse regarding "reportable" blood pressure readings (e.g., lower than 80/50)
■ Observe for serotonin syndrome in SSRI use. If suspected, discontinue drug and initiate supportive care. Respond according to ICU/emergency department protocols.	■ Inform client about the signs of serotonin syndrome, which can occur with overdosage and can be life-threatening (see page 177 for description).
■ Monitor for paradoxical diaphoresis, which must be considered a significant sign, especially serious when coupled with nausea/vomiting or chest pain.	■ Instruct client to seek immediate medical attention for dizziness, headache, tremor, nausea/vomiting, anxiety, disorientation, hyperreflexia, diaphoresis, and fever.
■ Monitor cardiovascular status. Observe for hypertension and signs of impending stroke or MI and heart failure.	■ Instruct client to immediately report severe headache, dizziness, paresthesias, bradycardia, chest pain, tachycardia, nausea/vomiting, or diaphoresis.
■ Monitor neurological status. Observe for somnolence and seizures. (TCAs may cause somnolence related to CNS depression and may reduce the seizure threshold.)	Instruct client to: ■ Report significant changes in neurological status, such as seizures, extreme lethargy, slurred speech, disorientation, or ataxia and to discontinue the drug ■ Take dose at bedtime to avoid daytime sedation
■ Monitor mental and emotional status. Observe for suicidal ideation. (Therapeutic benefits may be delayed. Outpatients should have no more than a 7-day medication supply.) ■ Monitor for underlying or concomitant psychoses such as schizophrenia or bipolar disorders. (Antidepressants may trigger manic states.)	Instruct client: ■ To immediately report dysphoria or suicidal impulses ■ To commit to a "no self-harm" verbal contract ■ That it may take 10 to 14 days before improvement is noticed, and about 1 month to achieve full therapeutic effect
■ Monitor sleep-wake cycle. Observe for insomnia and/or daytime somnolence.	Instruct client to: ■ Take drug very early in the morning if insomnia occurs to promote normal timing of sleep onset ■ Avoid driving or performing hazardous activities until effects of drug are known ■ Take drug at bedtime if daytime drowsiness persists

continued

NURSING PROCESS FOCUS   Clients Receiving Antidepressant Therapy   *(Continued)*

Interventions (Rationales)	Client Teaching/Discharge Planning
▪ Monitor renal status and urinary output. (Antidepressants may cause urinary retention due to muscle relaxation in urinary tract. Imipramine is excreted through the kidneys. Fluoxetine is slowly metabolized and excreted, increasing the risk of organ damage. Urinary retention may exacerbate existing symptoms of prostatic hypertrophy.)	Instruct client to: ▪ Monitor fluid intake and output ▪ Notify the healthcare provider of edema, dysuria (hesitancy, pain, diminished stream), changes in urine quantity or quality (e.g., cloudy, with sediment) ▪ Report fever or flank pain that may be indicative of a urinary tract infection related to urine retention
▪ Use cautiously with older adults and the young. (Diminished kidney and liver function related to aging can result in higher serum drug levels and may require lower doses. Children, due to an immature CNS, respond paradoxically to CNS drugs.)	Instruct client that: ▪ Older adults may be more prone to side effects such as hypertension and dysrhythmias ▪ Children on imipramine for nocturnal enuresis may experience mood alterations
▪ Monitor gastrointestinal status. Observe for abdominal distention. (Muscarinic blockade reduces tone and motility of intestinal smooth muscle and may cause paralytic ileus.)	Instruct client to: ▪ Exercise, drink adequate amounts of fluid, and add dietary fibre to promote stool passage ▪ Consult the nurse regarding a bulk laxative or stool softener if constipation becomes a problem
▪ Monitor liver function. Observe for signs and symptoms of hepatotoxicity. ▪ Monitor blood studies including CBC, differential, platelets, PT, PTT, and liver enzymes.	Instruct client to: ▪ Report nausea, vomiting, diarrhea, rash, jaundice, epigastric or abdominal pain or tenderness, or change in colour of stool ▪ Adhere to laboratory testing regimen for blood tests and urinalysis as directed
▪ Monitor hematological status. Observe for signs of bleeding. (Imipramine may cause blood dyscrasias. Use with warfarin may increase bleeding time.)	▪ Instruct client to report excessive bruising, fatigue, pallor, shortness of breath, frank bleeding, and/or tarry stools. ▪ Demonstrate guaiac testing on stool for occult blood.
▪ Monitor immune/metabolic status. Use with caution in clients with diabetes mellitus or hyperthyroidism. (If given in hyperthyroidism agranulocytosis can occur. Imipramine may either increase or decrease serum glucose. Fluoxetine may cause initial anorexia and weight loss, but with prolonged therapy may result in weight gain of up to 10 kilograms/20 pounds.)	▪ Instruct diabetics to monitor glucose level daily and consult nurse regarding reportable serum glucose levels (e.g., less than 70 and more than 140). ▪ Instruct client that anorexia and weight loss will diminish with continued therapy.
▪ Observe for extrapyramidal and anticholinergic effects. In overdosage, 12 hours of anticholinergic activity is followed by CNS depression. ▪ Do not treat overdosage with quinidine, procainamide, atropine, or barbiturates. (Quinidine and procainamide can increase the possibility of dysrhythmia, atropine can lead to severe anticholinergic effects, and barbiturates can lead to excess sedation.)	Instruct client to: ▪ Immediately report involuntary muscle movement of the face or upper body (e.g., tongue spasms), fever, anuria, lower abdominal pain, anxiety, hallucinations, psychomotor agitation, visual changes, dry mouth, and difficulty swallowing ▪ Relieve dry mouth with (sugar-free) hard candies, chewing gum, and fluids ▪ Avoid alcohol-containing mouthwashes, which can further dry oral mucous membranes
▪ Monitor visual acuity. Use with caution in narrow-angle glaucoma. (Imipramine may cause an increase in intraocular pressure. Anticholinergic effects may produce blurred vision.)	Instruct client to: ▪ Report visual changes, headache, or eye pain ▪ Inform eye care professional of imipramine therapy
▪ Ensure client safety. (Dizziness caused by postural hypotension increases the risk of fall injuries.)	Instruct client to: ▪ Call for assistance before getting out of bed or attempting to ambulate alone ▪ Avoid driving and performing hazardous activities until blood pressure is stabilized and effects of the drug are known

Evaluation of Outcome Criteria

Evaluate effectiveness of drug therapy by confirming that client goals and expected outcomes have been met (see "Planning").

See Tables 16.1 (page 173) and 16.2 (page 174) for a list of drugs to which these nursing actions apply.

16.7 Atypical Antidepressants

Several antidepressants have been classified as **atypical antidepressants** because of their unique or atypical structural or functional properties. Their efficacy in relieving depression is similar to the TCAs and SSRIs.

Bupropion, a norepinephrine and dopamine reuptake inhibitor (NDRI), is a unique agent that inhibits dopamine and norepinephrine reuptake without significant effects on the activity of monoamine oxidase, serotonin, or other neurotransmitters. One of the metabolites of bupropion that is concentrated in the brain may be an even more effective NDRI. Bupropion and its metabolites have no appreciable affinity for histamine, alpha-adrenergic, beta-adrenergic, dopamine, acetylcholine, or serotonin postsynaptic receptors. Therefore, side effects are generally more tolerable. Adverse effects include seizures, agitation, insomnia, tremor, headache, dry mouth, nausea, and vomiting.

Serotonin and norepinephrine reuptake inhibitors (SNRIs), such as venlafaxine, inhibit serotonin and norepinephrine reuptake. Venlafaxine has greater efficacy at higher doses. Depressive symptoms may improve earlier than with other antidepressants, often within 2 weeks of use. Common side effects include anxiety, headache, insomnia, abnormal dreams, dry mouth, drowsiness, dizziness, constipation, nervousness, sweating, chills, paresthesia, sexual dysfunction, loss of appetite, and nausea. Venlafaxine should be taken with meals to minimize nausea. Increased blood pressure occurs in some clients, so blood pressure should be monitored before and periodically during therapy.

Mirtazapine is a unique agent in that it does not inhibit the reuptake of norepinephrine, dopamine, or serotonin. Its most potent action is blocking histamine H_1-receptors. Through direct effects on specific serotonin and adrenergic subreceptors, norepinephrine and serotonin levels increase in the synapse. The antihistamine action of mirtazapine contributes to sedation, a common side effect. Increased appetite, weight gain, constipation, and dry mouth are other common side effects.

Norepinephrine reuptake inhibitors (NRIs), such as reboxetine, increase the action of norepinephrine by inhibiting the reuptake of norepinephrine into presynaptic neurons. These agents may improve symptoms in depressed clients who experience fatigue, apathy, impaired concentration, and slowness in information processing. Adverse effects include increased heart rate and other symptoms associated with excessive sympathetic nervous system stimulation. These agents are currently available only through Health Canada's Special Access Program.

Nurses should monitor clients for unusual responses when newer drugs are being used. Clients should be advised against using alcohol when taking atypical antidepressants to avoid harmful drug interactions. Caution clients not to drive if sedation effects persist.

BIPOLAR DISORDER

Bipolar disorder, once known as **manic depression**, is characterized by a shift between extreme and opposite moods, such as euphoria and depression. Clients may oscillate rapidly between both extremes, or there may be prolonged periods where mood is normal.

16.8 Characteristics of Bipolar Disorder

During the depressive stages of bipolar disorder, clients exhibit the symptoms of major depression described earlier in this chapter. To meet the DSM-IV criteria for bipolar I disorder, clients must have at least one episode of **mania**, an emotional state characterized by high psychomotor activity and irritability, for at least 1 week. Hypomania is characterized by the same symptoms, but they are less severe. Mania and hypomania may result from abnormal functioning of neurotransmitters or receptors in the brain. Hypomania may involve an excess of excitatory neurotransmitters, such as norepinephrine, or a deficiency of inhibitory neurotransmitters, such as GABA. It is important to distinguish mania from the effects of drug use or abuse and also from schizophrenia. Symptoms of mania, as shown in the following list, are generally opposite of depressive symptoms:

- Inflated self-esteem or grandiosity
- Decreased need for sleep (e.g., feels rested after only 3 hours of sleep)
- Increased talkativeness
- Flight of ideas or the subjective feeling that thoughts are racing
- Distractibility (i.e., attention too easily drawn to unimportant or irrelevant stimuli) or agitation
- Seeking attention from others at work or school or seeking sexual attention

NATURAL THERAPIES

St. John's Wort for Depression

St. John's wort (*Hypericum perforatum*) is an herb found throughout Britain, Asia, Europe, and North America that is commonly used as an antidepressant. It gets its name from a legend that red spots once appeared on its leaves on the anniversary of St. John's beheading. The word *wort* is a British term for "plant." Researchers once claimed that it produced its effects the same way MAO inhibitors do, by increasing the levels of serotonin, norepinephrine, and dopamine in the brain. More recent evidence suggests that it may inhibit serotonin reuptake. Some claim that it is just as effective as fluoxetine (Prozac), paroxetine (Paxil), and sertraline (Zoloft) for mild to moderate depression and with milder side effects. It may also be used as an anti-infective agent for conditions such as *Staphylococcus* and *Streptococcus* infections, for nerve pain such as neuralgia and sciatica, and for mental burnout. St. John's wort should not be taken concurrently with antidepressant medications.

An active ingredient in St. John's wort is a photoactive compound that, when exposed to light, produces substances that can damage myelin. Clients have reported feeling stinging pain on the hands after sun exposure while taking this herbal remedy. Advise clients who take this herb to apply sunscreen or to wear protective clothing when outdoors.

- Excessive involvement in pleasurable activities that have a high potential for painful consequences (e.g., unrestrained buying sprees, sexual indiscretions, or foolish business investments)

Bipolar disorder is an episodic, long-term illness with a variable course. In evaluating the individual client in order to make immediate clinical recommendations and decisions, as well as in beginning to formulate a long-term treatment plan, a number of longitudinal issues must be considered. These include the number of prior episodes, the average length of episodes and inter-episodes, the length of interval since the last episode of mania or depression, the level of psychosocial and symptomatic functioning between episodes, and the response to prior treatment.

MOOD STABILIZERS

Drugs for bipolar disorder are called **mood stabilizers** because they have the ability to moderate extreme shifts in emotions between mania and depression. Some antiseizure drugs are also used for mood stabilization in bipolar clients.

16.9 Pharmacotherapy of Bipolar Disorder

The mainstay for the treatment of bipolar disorder is lithium, as monotherapy or in combination with other drugs. Other drugs that stabilize mood have multiple uses. For example, carbamazepine and valproic acid are antiseizure drugs that have adjunct uses in bipolar disease. Table 16.4 shows select drugs used to treat bipolar disorder.

Lithium has a narrow therapeutic index and is monitored via serum levels every 1 to 3 days when beginning therapy, and every 2 to 3 months thereafter. To decrease risk of toxicity, a range of 0.6 to 0.8 mEq/L may be targeted. Close monitoring encourages adherence and helps to avoid toxicity. Lithium acts like sodium in the body, so conditions where sodium is lost (e.g., excessive sweating or dehydration) can cause lithium toxicity. If identified early, withholding the drug may prevent acute toxicity. Lithium overdose may be treated with hemodialysis and supportive care.

It is not unusual for other drugs to be used in combination with lithium for the control of bipolar disorder. During the depressed stage, a TCA or bupropion may be necessary. During the manic phases, a benzodiazepine will moderate manic symptoms. In cases of extreme agitation, delusions, or hallucinations, an antipsychotic agent may be indicated. Continued client adherence is essential to achieve successful pharmacotherapy; some clients do not perceive their condition as abnormal.

NURSING CONSIDERATIONS

Lithium is the only drug in this class. See "Nursing Process Focus: Clients Receiving Lithium" for information on this prototype drug. Lithium is classified as an antimanic agent as well as a mood stabilizer. Refer to chapters on antiseizure drugs (Chapter 15), antipsychotics (Chapter 17), and anxiolytics (Chapter 14) for additional nursing considerations on adjunct medications.

ATTENTION DEFICIT–HYPERACTIVITY DISORDER

Attention deficit–hyperactivity disorder (ADHD) is a condition characterized by poor attention span, behaviour control issues, and/or hyperactivity. Although normally diagnosed in childhood, symptoms of ADHD may extend into adulthood.

16.10 Characteristics of ADHD

ADHD affects as many as 5% of all children. Most children diagnosed with this condition are between the ages of 3 and 7 years, and boys are four to eight times more likely to be diagnosed than girls.

ADHD is characterized by developmentally inappropriate behaviours involving difficulty in paying attention or focusing on tasks. ADHD may be diagnosed when the child's hyperactive behaviours significantly interfere with normal

TABLE 16.4	Drugs for Bipolar Disorder: Mood Stabilizers
Drug	*Route and Adult Dose*
lithium (carbolith)	PO; Initial: 300–600 mg tid; maintenance 300 mg tid (max 2.4 g/day)
Antiseizure Drugs	
carbamazepine (Tegretol)	PO; 200 mg bid, gradually increased to 800–1200 mg/day in three to four divided doses
lamotrigine (Lamictal)	PO; 50 mg/day for 2 weeks, then 50 mg bid for 2 weeks; may increase gradually up to 300–500 mg/day in two divided doses (max 700 mg/day)
valproic acid (Depakene) (see page 165 for the Prototype Drug box)	PO; 250 mg tid (max 60 mg/kg/day)

Pr PROTOTYPE DRUG | Lithium (Carbolith)

ACTIONS AND USES

Although the exact mechanism of action is not clear, lithium is thought to alter the activity of neurons containing dopamine, norepinephrine, and serotonin by influencing the release, synthesis, and reuptake of the neurotransmitters. Therapeutic actions are stabilization of mood during periods of mania and antidepressant effects during periods of depression. Lithium has neither antimanic nor antidepressant effects in clients without bipolar disorder. After taking lithium for 2 to 3 weeks, clients are better able to concentrate and function in self-care.

PHARMACOKINETICS

Lithium is completely absorbed from the GI tract. It is widely distributed, crosses the placenta, and enters breast milk and CSF. It is excreted unchanged by the kidneys. Its half-life is 27 hours. Therapeutic serum lithium levels are from 0.6 to 0.8 mEq/L for prophylaxis of mania or depression, and from 0.8 to 1.5 mEq/L for clients in acute phases of mania.

ADMINISTRATION ALERTS

- Lithium has a narrow therapeutic/toxic ratio; risk of toxicity is high.
- Acute overdosage may be treated by hemodialysis.
- Lithium is pregnancy category D.

ADVERSE EFFECTS AND INTERACTIONS

Lithium may cause dizziness, fatigue, short-term memory loss, increased urination, nausea, vomiting, loss of appetite, abdominal pain, diarrhea, dry mouth, muscular weakness, and slight tremors. Some drugs increase the rate at which the kidneys remove lithium from the bloodstream, including diuretics, sodium bicarbonate, and potassium citrate. Other drugs, such as methyldopa and probenecid, inhibit the rate of lithium excretion. Clients should not have a salt-free diet when taking this drug because it reduces lithium excretion. Diuretics enhance excretion of sodium and increase the risk of lithium toxicity. Concurrent administration of anticholinergic drugs can cause urinary retention that, coupled with the polyuria effect of lithium, may cause a medical emergency. Alcohol can potentiate drug action.

WHERE**NURSING PROCESS FOCUS**   Clients Receiving Lithium (Carbolith)

Assessment	Potential Nursing Diagnoses/Identified Patterns
Prior to administration: - Obtain complete health history including allergies, drug history, and possible drug interactions. - Assess mental and emotional status, including any recent suicidal ideation. - Obtain cardiac history (including ECG and vital signs), history of renal or liver disorders, and blood studies: glucose, BUN, creatinine, electrolytes, and liver enzymes.	- Risk for self-directed violence - Disturbed thought processes - Disturbed sleep pattern - Sleep deprivation (in mania) - Risk for fluid volume imbalance - Self-care deficit: dressing/grooming

Planning: Client Goals and Expected Outcomes

The client will:
- Demonstrate stabilization of mood, including absence of mania and suicidal depression
- Engage in normal activities of daily living and report subjective improvement in mood
- Demonstrate understanding of drug action by accurately describing drug effects and precautions

Implementation

Interventions (Rationales)	Client Education/Discharge Planning
- Monitor mental and emotional status. Observe for mania and/or extreme depression. (Lithium should prevent mood swings.)	- Instruct client to keep a symptom log to document response to medication.
- Monitor electrolyte balance. (Lithium is a salt affected by dietary intake of other salts such as sodium chloride. Insufficient dietary salt intake causes the kidneys to conserve lithium, increasing serum lithium levels.)	Instruct client to: - Monitor dietary salt intake; consume sufficient quantities, especially during illness or physical activity - Avoid activities that cause excessive perspiration
- Monitor fluid balance. (Lithium causes polyuria by blocking effects of antidiuretic hormone.) - Measure intake and output. Weigh client daily. (Short-term changes in weight are a good indicator of fluctuations in fluid volume. Excess fluid volume increases the risk of HF; pitting edema may signal HF.)	Instruct client to: - Increase fluid intake by 1 to 1.5 L per day - Limit or eliminate caffeine consumption (caffeine has a diuretic effect that can cause lithium sparing by the kidneys) - Notify healthcare provider of excessive weight gain or loss, or pitting edema

continued

NURSING PROCESS FOCUS Clients Receiving Lithium (Carbolith) *(Continued)*

Interventions (Rationales)	Client Education/Discharge Planning
■ Monitor renal status. (Lithium may cause degenerative changes in the kidney which increases drug toxicity.) ■ Monitor laboratory tests: CBC, differential, BUN, creatinine, uric acid, and urinalysis. Use with caution in kidney disease.	Instruct client to: ■ Immediately report anuria, especially accompanied by lower abdominal tenderness, distention, headache, and diaphoresis ■ Inform healthcare provider of nausea, vomiting, diarrhea, flank pain or tenderness, and changes in urinary quantity and quality (e.g., sediment)
■ Monitor cardiovascular status. (Lithium toxicity may cause muscular irritability resulting in cardiac dysrhythmias or angina.) ■ Monitor vital signs including apical pulse. ■ Use with caution in clients with a history of CAD or heart disease.	Instruct client to: ■ Immediately report palpitations, chest pain, or other symptoms suggestive of myocardial infarction ■ Monitor vital signs, ensuring proper use of home equipment
■ Monitor gastrointestinal status. (Lithium may cause dyspepsia, diarrhea, or metallic taste.)	■ Instruct client to take drug with food to reduce stomach upset and to report distressing GI symptoms.
■ Monitor metabolic status. (Lithium may cause goiter with prolonged use and false-positive results on thyroid tests.)	■ Instruct client to report symptoms of goiter or hypothyroidism: enlarged mass on neck, fatigue, dry skin or edema.

Evaluation of Outcome Criteria

Evaluate effectiveness of drug therapy by confirming that patient goals and expected outcomes have been met (see "Planning").

play, sleep, or learning activities. Symptoms of ADHD include the following:

- Easy distractibility
- Failure to receive or follow instructions properly
- Inability to focus on one task at a time and jumping from one activity to another
- Difficulty remembering
- Frequent loss or misplacement of personal items
- Excessive talking and interrupting other children in a group
- Inability to sit still when asked to do so repeatedly
- Impulsiveness
- Sleep disturbance

The etiology of ADHD is not clear. Often a specific cause is not identified. A variety of physical and neurological disorders have been implicated. Causes may include contact with high levels of lead in childhood and prenatal exposure to alcohol and drugs. Genetic factors may also play a role, although a single gene has not been isolated and a specific mechanism of genetic transmission is not known. Recent evidence suggests that hyperactivity may be related to a deficit or dysfunction of dopamine, norepinephrine, and serotonin in the reticular activating system of the brain. Although once thought to be the culprits, sugars, chocolate, high-carbohydrate foods and beverages, and certain food additives have been disproved as causative or aggravating factors for ADHD. The nurse is often involved in the screening and the mental health assessment of children with suspected ADHD.

When a child is referred for testing, both the child and family are assessed. Data are collected on the child's physical, psychological, and developmental health situation to create an individualized plan of care.

Once ADHD is diagnosed, the nurse is instrumental in educating the parents and child, based on his or her developmental level, about the disorder and the importance of medication management and adherence. Parents should be educated about the importance of appropriate expectations and behavioural consequences and coping mechanisms that might be used to manage the demands of a child who is hyperactive. Self-esteem must be fostered in the child so that ego strengths can develop.

One-third to one-half of children diagnosed with ADHD also experience symptoms of attention dysfunction in their adult years. Symptoms of ADHD in adults appear similar

PHARMFACTS

Attention Deficit–Hyperactivity Disorder

- ADHD is the major reason why children are referred for mental health treatment.
- About one-half are also diagnosed with oppositional defiant or conduct disorder.
- About one-fourth are also diagnosed with anxiety disorder.
- About one-third are also diagnosed with depression.
- And about one-fifth also have a learning disability.

LIFESPAN CONSIDERATIONS

Zero Tolerance in Schools

Methylphenidate is an effective drug to treat ADHD and is often promoted by teachers and school counsellors as an adjunct to improving academic performance and social adjustment. However, schools may have a "zero drug tolerance" policy that creates a hostile environment for students who must take this drug. Zero tolerance policies generally prohibit the possession of *any* drug and define the school's right to search and seizure and the right to demand that students submit to random drug testing or screening as a condition of participating in sports and extracurricular activities. In some districts, students found in violation of such policies may be expelled or arrested.

Methylphenidate is a Schedule III controlled substance considered to have a high abuse potential. Students who take this drug should be made aware of the academic and social consequences of unauthorized possession of this medication. Most schools have strict guidelines regarding medication administration and require original prescriptions and containers of drugs to be supplied to the school health office. Students should carry an official notice from the healthcare provider regarding methylphenidate therapy that may be produced in the event of random drug testing.

to mood disorders. Symptoms include anxiety, mania, restlessness, and depression, which can cause difficulties in interpersonal relationships. Some clients have difficulty holding jobs and may have increased risk for alcohol and drug abuse. Untreated ADHD has been linked to low self-esteem, diminished social success, and criminal or violent behaviours.

DRUGS FOR ATTENTION DEFICIT–HYPERACTIVITY DISORDER

The traditional drugs used to treat ADHD in children have been CNS stimulants. These drugs stimulate specific areas of the CNS that heighten alertness and increase focus. A non–CNS stimulant has also been approved to treat ADHD. Agents for treating ADHD are shown in Table 16.5.

16.11 Pharmacotherapy of ADHD

CNS stimulants are the main course of treatment for ADHD. Stimulants reverse many of the symptoms, helping clients to focus on tasks. The most widely prescribed drug for ADHD is methylphenidate (Ritalin). Another CNS stimulant that is rarely prescribed due to its abuse potential is dextroamphetamine. These are Schedule III controlled substances and pregnancy category C.

Clients taking CNS stimulants must be carefully monitored. CNS stimulants used to treat ADHD may create paradoxical hyperactivity. Adverse reactions include insomnia, nervousness, anorexia, and weight loss. Occasionally, a client may suffer from dizziness, depression, irritability, nausea, or abdominal pain.

Non–CNS stimulants have been tried for ADHD; however, they exhibit less efficacy. Clonidine is sometimes prescribed when clients are extremely aggressive, active, or have difficulty falling asleep. Atypical antidepressants, such as bupropion, and TCAs, such as desipramine and imipramine, are considered second-choice drugs when CNS stimulants fail to work or are contraindicated.

A recent addition to the treatment of ADHD in children and adults is atomoxetine. Although its exact mechanism is not known, it is classified as a norepinephrine reuptake inhibitor. Clients on atomoxetine showed improved ability to focus on tasks and reduced hyperactivity. Efficacy appears to be equivalent to methylphenidate, although the drug is too new for long-term comparisons. Common side effects include headache, insomnia, upper abdominal pain, decreased appetite, and cough. Unlike methylphenidate, it is not a scheduled drug; thus, parents who are hesitant to place their child on stimulants now have a reasonable alternative.

NURSING CONSIDERATIONS

Methylphenidate is the only drug in its class. See "Nursing Process Focus: Clients Receiving Methylphenidate" and the Prototype Drug box for more information.

MediaLink Adults with ADD

TABLE 16.5 Drugs for Attention Deficit–Hyperactivity Disorder

Drug	Route and Adult Dose
CNS Stimulants	
dextroamphetamine (Dexedrine)	3–5 years old: PO; 2.5 mg qd to bid; may increase by 2.5 mg at weekly intervals > 6 years old: PO; 5 mg qd to bid; increase by 5 mg at weekly intervals (max 40 mg/day)
methylphenidate (Ritalin)	PO; 5–10 mg before breakfast and lunch, with gradual increase of 5–10 mg/week as needed (max 60 mg/day)
Non-stimulants for ADHD	
atomoxetine (Strattera)	PO; Start with 40 mg in AM; may increase after 3 days to target dose of 80 mg/day given either once in the morning or divided morning and late afternoon/early evening; may increase to max of 100 mg/day if needed

Pr PROTOTYPE DRUG | Methylphenidate (Ritalin)

ACTIONS AND USES

Methylphenidate activates the reticular activating system, causing heightened alertness in various regions of the brain, particularly those centres associated with focus and attention. Activation is partially achieved by the release of neurotransmitters such as norepinephrine, dopamine, and serotonin. Impulsiveness, hyperactivity, and disruptive behaviour are usually reduced within a few weeks. These changes promote improved psychosocial interactions and academic performance.

PHARMACOKINETICS

Methylphenidate is slowly and incompletely absorbed from the GI tract. Distribution is unknown. It is mostly metabolized by the liver. Its half-life is 2 to 4 hours.

ADMINISTRATION ALERTS

- Sustained-release tablets must be swallowed whole. Breaking or crushing these tablets causes immediate release of the entire dose.
- Methylphenidate is pregnancy category C.

ADVERSE EFFECTS AND INTERACTIONS

In a non-ADHD client, methylphenidate causes nervousness and insomnia. All clients are at risk for irregular heart beat, high blood pressure, and liver toxicity. Methylphenidate is a Schedule III drug, indicating its potential to cause dependence when used for extended periods. Periodic drug-free "holidays" are recommended to reduce drug dependence and to assess the client's condition.

Methylphenidate interacts with many drugs. For example, it may decrease the effectiveness of antiseizure medications, anticoagulants, and guanethidine. Concurrent therapy with clonidine may increase adverse effects. Antihypertensives or other CNS stimulants could potentiate the vasoconstrictive action of methylphenidate. MAO inhibitors may produce hypertensive crisis.

NURSING PROCESS FOCUS   Clients Receiving Methylphenidate (Ritalin)

Assessment	Potential Nursing Diagnoses/Identified Patterns
Prior to administration: ■ Obtain complete health history including allergies, drug history, and possible drug interactions. ■ Obtain history of neurological, cardiac, renal, biliary, and mental disorders including blood studies: CBC, platelets, liver enzymes. ■ Assess neurological status, including identification of recent behavioural patterns. ■ Assess growth and development.	■ Risk for growth retardation related to methylphenidate ■ Risk for unsuccessful interpersonal relationships ■ Inadequate nutrition ■ Need for knowledge regarding drug therapy ■ Disturbed sleep pattern

Planning: Client Goals and Expected Outcomes

The client will:
- Experience subjective improvement in attention/concentration and reduction in impulsivity and/or psychomotor symptoms ("hyperactivity")
- Demonstrate understanding of the drug's action by accurately describing drug effects and precautions

Implementation

Interventions (Rationales)	Client Education/Discharge Planning
■ Monitor mental status and observe for changes in level of consciousness and adverse effects such as persistent drowsiness, psychomotor agitation or anxiety, dizziness, trembling, or seizures.	■ Instruct client to report any significant increase in motor behaviour, changes in sensorium, or feelings of dysphoria.
■ Use with caution in epilepsy. (Drug may lower the seizure threshold.)	■ Instruct client to discontinue drug immediately if seizures occur and to notify healthcare provider.
■ Monitor vital signs. (Stimulation of the CNS induces the release of catecholamines with a subsequent increase in heart rate and blood pressure.)	Instruct client to: ■ Immediately report rapid heartbeat, palpitations, or dizziness ■ Monitor blood pressure and pulse, ensuring proper use of home equipment
■ Monitor gastrointestinal and nutritional status. (CNS stimulation causes anorexia and elevates BMR, producing weight loss.) Other GI side effects include nausea/vomiting and abdominal pain.	Instruct client to: ■ Report any distressing GI side effects ■ Take drug with meals to reduce GI upset and counteract anorexia; eat frequent small nutrient- and calorie-dense snacks ■ Weigh self weekly and report significant losses over 0.5 kg

continued

NURSING PROCESS FOCUS   Clients Receiving Methylphenidate (Ritalin)   *(Continued)*

Interventions (Rationales)	Client Education/Discharge Planning
■ Monitor laboratory tests such as CBC, differential, and platelet count. (Drug is metabolized in the liver and excreted by the kidneys; impaired organ function can increase serum drug levels. Drug may cause leukopenia and/or anemia.)	Instruct client to: ■ Report shortness of breath, profound fatigue, pallor, bleeding or excessive bruising (these are signs of blood disorder) ■ Report nausea; vomiting; diarrhea; rash; jaundice; abdominal pain, tenderness, or distention; or change in colour of stool (these are signs of liver disease) ■ Adhere to laboratory testing regimen for blood tests and urinalysis as directed
■ Monitor effectiveness of drug therapy.	Instruct client to: ■ Schedule regular drug holidays ■ Not discontinue drug abruptly as rebound hyperactivity or withdrawal symptoms may occur; taper the dose prior to starting a drug holiday ■ Keep a behaviour diary to chronicle symptoms and response to drug ■ Safeguard medication supply due to abuse potential
■ Monitor growth and development. (Growth rate may stall in response to nutritional deficiency caused by anorexia.)	■ Instruct client that reductions in growth rate are associated with drug usage. Drug holidays may decrease this effect.
■ Monitor sleep-wake cycle. (CNS stimulation may disrupt normal sleep patterns.)	Instruct client that: ■ Insomnia may be adverse reaction ■ Sleeplessness can sometimes be counteracted by taking the last dose no later than 4 PM. ■ Drug is not intended to treat fatigue; warn the patient that fatigue may accompany wash-out period

Evaluation of Outcome Criteria

Evaluate effectiveness of drug therapy by confirming that client goals and expected outcomes have been met (see "Planning").

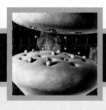

CHAPTER REVIEW

KEY CONCEPTS

The numbered key concepts provide a succinct summary of the important points from the corresponding numbered section within the chapter. If any of these points are not clear, refer to the numbered section within the chapter for review. Expanded versions can be found on the Companion Website.

16.1 Depression has many causes and methods of classification. The identification of depression and its etiology is essential for proper treatment.

16.2 Major depression may be treated with medications, psychotherapeutic techniques, or electroconvulsive therapy.

16.3 The two basic mechanisms of action are blocking the enzymatic breakdown of norepinephrine and slowing the reuptake of serotonin.

16.4 TCAs are older medications used mainly for the treatment of major depression, obsessive-compulsive disorder, and panic attacks.

16.5 SSRIs act by selectively blocking the reuptake of serotonin in nerve terminals. Because of more tolerable side effects, SSRIs are drugs of choice in the pharmacotherapy of depression.

16.6 MAO inhibitors are usually prescribed in cases when other antidepressants have not been successful. They have more serious side effects than other antidepressants.

16.7 Atypical antidepressants are newer drugs that may be used as first-choice drugs or when other drugs are not successful.

16.8 Clients with bipolar disorder display not only signs of depression, but also mania, a state characterized by excessive psychomotor activity and irritability.

16.9 Mood stabilizers such as lithium are used to treat both the manic and depressive stages of bipolar disorder.

16.10 The most efficacious drugs for symptoms of ADHD are the CNS stimulants such as methylphenidate. A newer, non-stimulant drug, atomoxetine, has shown promise in clients with ADHD.

REVIEW QUESTIONS

1 Identify the classes of drugs used to treat major depression. Which class is the most effective? Which exhibits the fewest side effects?

2 A sexually active man insists on discontinuing his SSRI due to his inability to achieve erections for intercourse. What are his options for controlling depression?

3 A client with bipolar disorder becomes physically abusive during manic episodes and denies his behaviour is abnormal. What advice would you give, and what treatment options are available?

4 The frustrated parents of a 9-year-old insist that their son be medicated for ADHD. What assessment would be needed? What therapeutic options are available?

CRITICAL THINKING QUESTIONS

1. A teacher approaches the school nurse regarding her concerns about Sean, a 10-year-old Aboriginal boy in her class who has been diagnosed with ADHD. What behaviours, school performance, and developmental issues could have prompted the inquiry by the teacher? What does the nurse need to know about Sean from the teacher and from his parents? What drug therapy may be prescribed for children with ADHD and why? How might the nurse promote an optimal experience with the medication (considering safety, efficacy, cultural factors, and holistic care)?

2. A 66-year-old Caucasian female client has been diagnosed with clinical depression following the death of her husband. She says that she has not been able to sleep for weeks and that she is "living on coffee and cigarettes." The healthcare provider prescribes fluoxetine (Prozac). How should the nurse respond to the client's query about when she should begin feeling "more like myself"? What information does the client require to promote safety and efficacy with antidepressant therapy? What community resources might she find helpful? What cultural factors should be taken into consideration in providing holistic care?

3. A 26-year-old Vietnamese mother of three children comes to the prenatal clinic suspecting a fourth pregnancy. She tells the nurse that she got "real low" after her third baby and that she was prescribed sertraline (Zoloft). She tells the nurse that she is really afraid of "going crazy" if she has to stop taking the drug because of this pregnancy. What factors should the nurse take into account in assessing and planning care for this client? What community resources may be available?

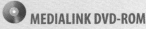 **EXPLORE MediaLink**

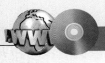 www.pearsoned.ca/adams-king

MEDIALINK DVD-ROM
- **Audio Glossary**
- **CRNE Review**
- **Videos**
  Bipolar Disorder 1
  Bipolar Disorder 2
  Bipolar Disorder 3
- **Animations**
  Mechanism of Action: Fluoxetine (*Prozac*)
  Mechanism of Action: Methylphenidate (*Ritalin*)
  Mechanism of Action: Venlafaxine (*Effexor*)

COMPANION WEBSITE
- **CRNE Review**
- **Case Study:** Client taking an SSRI
- **Dosage Calculations**
- **Nursing Process Focus Charts**

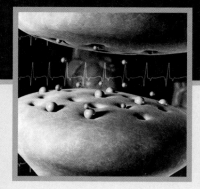

CHAPTER 17

Drugs for Psychoses

DRUGS AT A GLANCE

CONVENTIONAL (TYPICAL) ANTIPSYCHOTICS
Phenothiazines
  chlorpromazine (Apo-Chlorpromazine)
Non-phenothiazines
  haloperidol (Haldol)

ATYPICAL ANTIPSYCHOTICS
  clozapine (Clozaril)

OBJECTIVES

After reading this chapter, the student should be able to do the following:

1. Identify drug classes used for treating psychoses.
2. Explain the therapeutic action of antipsychotic drugs in relation to physiological aspects of neurotransmission.
3. For each of the drug classes listed in Drugs at a Glance, identify a representative drug and explain its mechanism of action, primary actions, and important adverse effects.
4. Discuss the rationale for selecting a specific antipsychotic drug for the treatment of schizophrenia.
5. Explain the importance of client drug adherence in the pharmacotherapy of schizophrenia.
6. Describe the nurse's role in the pharmacological management of schizophrenia.
7. Explain the symptoms associated with extrapyramidal side effects of antipsychotic drugs and the nurse's role in preventing and managing these side effects.
8. Describe and explain, based on pharmacological principles, the rationale for nursing assessment, planning, and interventions for clients with psychoses.
9. Use the nursing process to care for clients receiving drug therapy for psychoses.

MediaLink

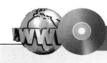 www.pearsoned.ca/adams-king

CRNE review, case studies, and other interactive resources for this chapter can be found on the Companion Website at **www.pearsoned.ca/adams-king**. Click on "Chapter 17" to select the activities for this chapter. For animations, more CRNE review questions, and an audio glossary, access the accompanying DVD-ROM in this textbook.

KEY TERMS

akathisia   page 194

atypical antipsychotics   page 198

conventional (typical) antipsychotics
    page 194

delusions   page 192

dopamine D_2-receptor   page 193

dystonias   page 194

extrapyramidal signs (EPS)   page 194

hallucinations   page 192

illusions   page 192

negative symptoms   page 193

neuroleptics   page 194

neuroleptic malignant syndrome (NMS)
    page 195

paranoia   page 192

pseudo-Parkinsonism   page 194

positive symptoms   page 193

psychosis   page 192

schizo-affective disorder   page 193

schizophrenia   page 192

tardive dyskinesia   page 194

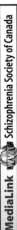

MediaLink Schizophrenia Society of Canada

Severe mental illness can be incapacitating for the client and intensely frustrating for relatives and those dealing with the client on a regular basis. Before the 1950s, clients with acute mental dysfunction were institutionalized, often for their entire lives. The introduction of chlorpromazine in the 1950s, and the development of newer agents, revolutionized the treatment of mental illness.

17.1 The Nature of Psychoses

A **psychosis** is a mental health condition characterized by **delusions** (firm ideas and beliefs not founded in reality), **hallucinations** (seeing, hearing, or feeling something that is not there), **illusions** (distorted perceptions of actual sensory stimuli), disorganized behaviour, and difficulty relating to others. Behaviour may range from total inactivity to extreme agitation and combativeness. Some psychotic clients exhibit **paranoia**, an extreme suspicion and delusion that they are being followed and that others are trying to harm them. Because they are unable to distinguish what is real from what is illusion, they are often viewed as insane.

Psychoses may be classified as acute or chronic. Acute psychotic episodes occur over hours or days, whereas chronic psychoses develop over months or years. Sometimes a cause may be attributed to the psychosis, such as brain damage, overdoses of certain medications, extreme depression, chronic alcoholism, or drug addiction. Genetic factors are known to play a role in some psychoses. Unfortunately, the vast majority of psychoses have no identifiable cause.

People with psychosis are usually unable to function normally in society without long-term drug therapy. Clients must see their healthcare provider periodically and medication usually must be taken for life. Family members and social support groups are important sources of help for clients who cannot function without continuous drug therapy.

SCHIZOPHRENIA

Schizophrenia is a type of psychosis characterized by abnormal thoughts and thought processes, disordered communication, withdrawal from other people and the outside environment, and a high risk for suicide. Several subtypes of schizophrenic disorders are based on clinical presentation.

17.2 Signs and Symptoms of Schizophrenia

Schizophrenia is the most common psychotic disorder, affecting 0.5% to 1% of the population. Symptoms generally begin to appear in early adulthood, with a peak incidence in men 15 to 24 years of age and women 25 to 34 years of age. Symptoms may be mild with no lasting impairment, but the majority experience repeated episodes with worsening symptoms and outcomes. Clients experience

LIFESPAN CONSIDERATIONS

Schizophrenia across the Lifespan

- Schizophrenia can occur in childhood, but it usually begins in early adulthood.
- Incidence is slightly higher in males.
- Symptoms may compromise the ability of adults to fulfill role expectations and maintain employment.
- Rates of suicide are 15% to 25% higher among teens and adults than the national average.
- Drug dosages may require adjustment due to age-related changes in pharmacokinetics.
- Side effects may decrease drug adherence in all age groups.
- Older adults may experience more severe adverse effects.

many different symptoms that may change over time. The following symptoms may appear quickly or take several months or years to develop:

- Hallucinations, delusions, or paranoia
- Strange behaviour, such as communicating in rambling statements or made-up words
- Alternating rapidly between extreme hyperactivity and stupor
- Attitude of indifference or detachment toward life activities
- Acting strangely or irrationally
- Deterioration of personal hygiene and job or academic performance
- Marked withdrawal from social interactions and inter-personal relationships

When observing clients with schizophrenia, nurses should look for both positive and negative symptoms. **Positive symptoms** are those that add on to normal behaviour. These include hallucinations, delusions, and a disorganized thought or speech pattern. **Negative symptoms** are those that subtract from normal behaviour. These symptoms include a lack of interest, motivation, responsiveness, or pleasure in daily activities. Negative symptoms are characteristic of the indifferent personality exhibited by many schizophrenics. Proper diagnosis of positive and negative symptoms is important for selection of the appropriate antipsychotic drug.

The cause of schizophrenia has not been determined, although several theories have been proposed. There appears to be a genetic component to schizophrenia since many clients suffering from schizophrenia have family members who have been afflicted with the same disorder. Another theory suggests the disorder is caused by imbalances in neurotransmitters in specific areas of the brain. This theory suggests the possibility of overactive dopaminergic pathways in the basal nuclei, an area of the brain that controls motor activity. The basal ganglia (nuclei) are responsible for starting and stopping synchronized motor activity, such as leg and arm motions during walking.

Symptoms of schizophrenia seem to be associated with the **dopamine D_2-receptor**. The basal nuclei are particularly rich in D_2-receptors, while the cerebrum contains very few. All antipsychotic drugs act by entering dopaminergic synapses and competing with dopamine for D_2-receptors. By blocking about 65% of the D_2-receptors, antipsychotic drugs reduce the symptoms of schizophrenia. If 80% are blocked, motor abnormalities begin to occur (Seeman & Seeman, 2002). Figure 17.1 illustrates antipsychotic drug action at the dopaminergic receptor.

Schizo-affective disorder is a condition in which the client exhibits symptoms of both schizophrenia and mood disorder. For example, an acute schizo-affective reaction may include distorted perceptions, hallucinations, and delusions followed by extreme depression. Over time, both positive and negative psychotic symptoms will appear. It is challenging to differentiate schizo-affective disorder from

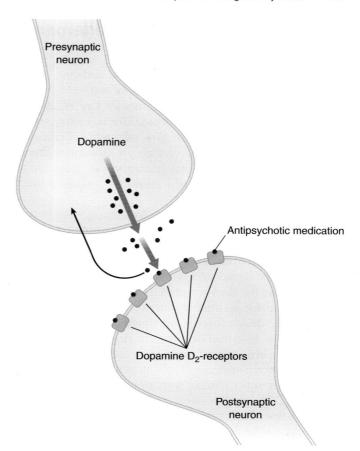

● **Figure 17.1** Mechanism of action of antipsychotics: antipsychotic drug molecules occupy D_2-receptors on the postsynaptic neuron, preventing dopamine from stimulating the receptors

bipolar disorder or major depression with psychotic features, as clients with affective disorders may also experience psychotic episodes.

Many conditions can cause bizarre behaviour, and these should be distinguished from schizophrenia. Chronic use of amphetamines or cocaine can create a paranoid syndrome. Certain complex partial seizures (Chapter 15) can cause unusual symptoms that are sometimes mistaken for psychoses. Brain neoplasms, infections, and hemorrhage can also cause bizarre, psychotic-like symptoms.

SPECIAL CONSIDERATIONS

Cultural Views and Treatment of Mental Illness

Some cultures have very different perspectives on the cause and treatment of mental illness. The foundation of many of these mental health treatments involves herbs and spiritual healing methods. Aboriginal Peoples may be treated by the community traditional "medicine man," who may treat mental symptoms with a sweat lodge and herbs. Some African Canadians may be treated by a traditional voodoo priest or other traditional healer, and herbs are frequently used to treat mental symptoms. Amulets, or charms, that are worn on a string or chain may be used by members of some cultures to protect the wearer from evil spirits that are believed to cause mental illness.

17.3 Pharmacological Management of Psychoses

Management of severe mental illness is difficult. Many clients do not see their behaviour as abnormal and have difficulty understanding the need for medication. When that medication produces undesirable side effects, such as severe twitching or loss of sexual function, adherence diminishes and clients exhibit symptoms of their pre-treatment illness. Agitation, distrust, and extreme frustration are common as clients cannot comprehend why others are unable to think and see the same as them.

From a pharmacological perspective, therapy has both a positive and a negative side. While many symptoms of psychosis can be controlled with current drugs, adverse effects are common and often severe. The antipsychotic agents do not cure mental illness, and symptoms remain in remission only as long as the client chooses to take the drug. In terms of efficacy, there is little difference among the various antipsychotic drugs; there is no single drug of choice for schizophrenia. Selection of a specific drug is based on the needs of the client, the occurrence of side effects, and clinician experience. For example, clients with Parkinson's disease need an antipsychotic with minimal extrapyramidal side effects. Those who operate machinery would need a drug that does not cause sedation. Men who are sexually active may want a drug without negative effects on ejaculation. The experience and skills of the physician and mental health nurse are particularly valuable in achieving successful psychiatric pharmacotherapy.

CONVENTIONAL (TYPICAL) ANTIPSYCHOTIC AGENTS

The two basic categories of drug for psychoses are conventional antipsychotics and atypical antipsychotics. The conventional antipsychotic agents include the phenothiazines and phenothiazine-like drugs. They are most effective at treating the positive signs of schizophrenia, such as hallucinations and delusions, and have been the treatment of choice for psychoses for 50 years. Antipsychotic drugs are sometimes referred to as **neuroleptics.**

PHENOTHIAZINES

17.4 Treating Psychoses with Phenothiazines

The **conventional antipsychotics**, sometimes called first generation or **typical antipsychotics**, include the phenothiazine and phenothiazine-like agents. They are listed in Table 17.1. Within each category, agents are named by their chemical structure.

The first effective drug used to treat schizophrenia was chlorpromazine, a low-potency phenothiazine agent. Several phenothiazines are now available to treat mental illness. All are efficacious at blocking the excitement associated with the positive symptoms of schizophrenia, although they differ in their potency and side effect profiles. False perceptions, such as hallucinations and delusions, often begin to diminish within days. Other symptoms, however, may require as long as 7 to 8 weeks of pharmacotherapy to improve. Because of the high rate of recurrence of psychotic episodes, pharmacotherapy should be considered long term, often for the life of the client. Phenothiazines are thought to act by preventing dopamine and serotonin from occupying their receptor sites in certain regions of the brain. This mechanism is illustrated in Figure 17.1.

Although they revolutionized the treatment of severe mental illness, the phenothiazines exhibit numerous adverse effects that can limit pharmacotherapy. These are listed in Table 17.2. Anticholinergic effects such as dry mouth, postural hypotension, and urinary retention are common. Ejaculation disorders occur in a high percentage of clients taking phenothiazines; delay in achieving orgasm (in both men and women) is a common cause for non-adherence. Menstrual disorders are common. Each phenothiazine has a slightly different side effect spectrum. For example, perphenazine has a lower incidence of anticholinergic effects. Thioridazine frequently causes sedation, whereas this side effect is less common with trifluoperazine.

Unlike many other drugs whose primary action is on the CNS (e.g., amphetamines, barbiturates, anxiolytics, alcohol), antipsychotic drugs do not cause dependence. They also have a wide safety margin between a therapeutic and a lethal dose; deaths due to overdoses of antipsychotic drugs are uncommon.

One particularly serious set of adverse reactions to anti-psychotic drugs is called extrapyramidal signs. **Extrapyramidal signs (EPS)** include acute dystonia, akathisia, pseudo-parkinsonism, and tardive dyskinesia. Acute **dystonias** occur early in the course of pharmacotherapy and involve severe muscle spasms, particularly of the back, neck, tongue, and face. **Akathisia**, the most common, is an inability to rest or relax. The client paces, has trouble sitting or remaining still, and has difficulty sleeping. Symptoms of antipsychotic-induced **pseudo-parkinsonism** include tremor, muscle rigidity, stooped posture, and a shuffling gait. Long-term use of phenothiazines may lead to **tardive dyskinesia**, which is characterized by unusual tongue and face movements such as lip smacking and wormlike motions of the tongue. If extrapyramidal effects are reported early and the drug is withdrawn or the dosage is reduced, the side effects can be reversible. With higher doses given for prolonged periods, the extrapyramidal symptoms may become permanent. The nurse must be vigilant in observing and reporting EPS, as prevention is the best treatment.

With the conventional antipsychotics, it is not always possible to control the disabling symptoms of schizophrenia without producing some degree of extrapyramidal effects. In these clients, drug therapy may be warranted to treat EPS. Concurrent pharmacotherapy with an anticholinergic drug may prevent some of the extrapyramidal signs (see Chapter 18). For acute dystonia, benztropine may be given parenterally. Levodopa is usually avoided since its ability to increase dopamine function antagonizes the action of the phenothiazines. Beta-adrenergic blockers and benzodi-

TABLE 17.1	Conventional Antipsychotic Drugs: Phenothiazines
Drug	**Route and Adult Dose**
℗ chlorpromazine HCl (Apo-Chlorpromazine)	PO; 25–100 mg tid or qid (max 1000 mg/day) IM/IV; 25–50 mg (max 600 mg q4–6h)
fluphenazine HCl (Apo-Fluphenazine)	PO; 0.5–10 mg/day (max 20 mg/day)
perphenazine (Apo-Perphenazine)	PO; 4–16 mg bid to qid (max 64 mg/day)
promazine HCl (Apo-Promazine)	PO/IM; 10–200 mg every 4–6 hours (max 1000 mg/day)
thioridazine HCl (Apo-Thioridazine)	PO; 50–100 mg tid (max 800 mg/day)
trifluoperazine HCl (Apo-Trifluoperazine)	PO; 1–2 mg bid; (max 20 mg/day)

azepines are sometimes given to reduce signs of akathisia. Amantadine, an antiviral, may be given to reduce signs of tardive dyskinesia.

NURSING CONSIDERATIONS

The role of the nurse in phenothiazine therapy involves careful monitoring of the client's condition and providing education as it relates to the prescribed drug regimen. Assessment information that must be gathered on clients beginning antipsychotic pharmacotherapy includes a complete health history such as any long-term physical problems (e.g., seizure disorders, cardiovascular disease), medication use, allergies, and lifestyle information (e.g., use of alcohol, illegal drugs, caffeine, tobacco, herbal preparations). This allows the physician to individualize treatment and minimize the possibility of adverse reactions.

Assessment also includes a complete physical examination, including liver and kidney function tests, vision screening, and mental status to provide a baseline of the client's health status. If the client is a child, the nurse should assess for hyperexcitability, dehydration, and gastroenteritis as well as chicken pox or measles because such conditions increase the chance of EPS. If possible, phenothiazines should not be given to children under 12 years of age. If the client is elderly, the nurse should also determine whether a lower dose may be indicated due to the slower metabolism in older adults.

Contraindications to the use of phenothiazine and phenothiazine-like drugs include CNS depression, bone marrow suppression, coma, alcohol withdrawal syndrome, lactation, age (children under age 6 months), and presence of Reye's syndrome. This class of drug must be used with caution in asthma, emphysema, respiratory infections, pregnancy (only when benefits outweigh risks), and in older adults and children.

The nurse should monitor the client for extrapyramidal symptoms. Symptoms include lip smacking; spasms of the face, tongue, or back muscles; facial grimacing; involuntary upward eye movements; jerking motions; extreme restlessness; stooped posture; shuffling gait; and tremors at rest. Observations of EPS by the nurse should be reported to the physician immediately. These symptoms may be reason to discontinue the drug.

A possible life-threatening side effect of antipsychotic drugs is **neuroleptic malignant syndrome (NMS)**. In this condition, the client suffers a toxic reaction to therapeutic doses of an antipsychotic drug. The client exhibits elevated temperature, unstable blood pressure, profuse sweating, dyspnea, muscle rigidity, and incontinence. The nurse should observe for these symptoms and report them immediately to the healthcare provider.

In addition, the nurse should assess the client for drowsiness and sedation, which are both common side effects of this type of medication due to CNS depression. The nurse should evaluate the client's safety and ability to function.

MediaLink   Animation: Extrapyramidal Signs

TABLE 17.2	Adverse Effects of Conventional Antipsychotic Agents
Effect	**Description**
acute dystonia	severe spasms, particularly the back muscles, tongue, and facial muscles; twitching movements
akathisia	constant pacing with repetitive, compulsive movements
pseudo-Parkinsonism	tremor, muscle rigidity, stooped posture, shuffling gait
tardive dyskinesia	bizarre tongue and face movements such as lip smacking and wormlike motions of the tongue; puffing of cheeks; uncontrolled chewing movements
anticholinergic effects	dry mouth, tachycardia, blurred vision
sedation	usually diminishes with continued therapy
hypotension	particularly severe when quickly moving from a recumbent to an upright position
sexual dysfunction	impotence and diminished libido
neuroleptic malignant syndrome	high fever, confusion, muscle rigidity, and high serum creatine kinase; can be fatal

Client and family education is an especially important aspect of care for clients with mental illness. Client education as it relates to phenothiazines should include goals, reasons for obtaining baseline data, and possible side effects. The nurse should educate the family regarding symptoms indicative of EPS and NMS and instruct them to report such symptoms to the physician immediately. If adherence is a problem, the nurse can supply clients and families with dose calendars and reminder signs. Because these drugs are prescribed for long-term use, the nurse should teach the client the importance of taking the drug as directed and to contact the healthcare provider immediately if side effects occur or if symptoms begin to return. See "Nursing Process Focus: Clients Receiving Conventional Phenothiazines and Non-Phenothiazine Therapy" on page 198 for additional specific points that the nurse should include when teaching clients and caregivers about these drugs.

NON-PHENOTHIAZINES

17.5 Treating Psychoses with Conventional Antipsychotics: Non-Phenothiazines

The conventional non-phenothiazine antipsychotic class consists of drugs whose chemical structures are dissimilar to the phenothiazines. They are listed in Table 17.3. Introduced shortly after the phenothiazines, initial expectations were that non-phenothiazines would produce fewer side effects. Unfortunately, this appears to not be the case. The spectrum of side effects for the non-phenothiazines is identical to that for the phenothiazines, although the degree to which a particular effect occurs depends on the specific drug. In general, the non-phenothiazine agents cause less sedation and fewer anticholinergic side effects than chlorpromazine, but they exhibit an equal or even greater incidence of extrapyramidal signs. Concurrent therapy with other CNS depressants must be carefully monitored due to the potential additive effects.

Drugs in the non-phenothiazine class have the same therapeutic effects and efficacy as the phenothiazines. They are also believed to act by the same mechanism as the phenothiazines, that is, by blocking postsynaptic D_2-receptors. As a class, they offer no significant advantages over the phenothiazines in the treatment of schizophrenia.

NURSING CONSIDERATIONS

The role of the nurse in conventional non-phenothiazine therapy involves careful monitoring of the client's condition and providing education as it relates to the prescribed drug regimen. Assessment of clients taking a conventional non-phenothiazine antipsychotic includes a complete drug history, including current and past medications to establish any previous allergic reactions or adverse effects from these medications. Elderly clients must be assessed more carefully than younger clients due to the possibility of unusual adverse

---

Pr PROTOTYPE DRUG | Chlorpromazine (Apo-Chlorpromazine)

ACTIONS AND USES

Chlorpromazine provides symptomatic relief of positive symptoms of schizophrenia and controls manic symptoms in clients with schizo-affective disorder. Many clients must take chlorpromazine for 7 or 8 weeks before they experience improvement. Extreme agitation may be treated with IM or IV injections, which begin to act within minutes. Chlorpromazine can also control severe nausea and vomiting.

ADMINISTRATION ALERTS

- Sustained-release forms should not be crushed or opened.
- When the drug is administered IM, give deep IM, only in the upper outer quadrant of the buttocks; client should remain supine for 30 to 60 minutes after injection, and then rise slowly.
- The drug must be gradually withdrawn over 2 to 3 weeks, and nausea/vomiting, dizziness, tremors, or dyskinesia may occur.
- IV forms should be used only during surgery or for severe hiccups.
- Chlorpromazine is pregnancy category C (contraindicated during lactation).

PHARMACOKINETICS

Chlorpromazine PO is variably absorbed. Chlorpromazine IM is well absorbed. It is widely distributed, crosses the blood-brain barrier and placenta, and enters breast milk. It is about 90% protein bound. It is highly metabolized by the liver and GI mucosa. Its half-life is 30 hours.

ADVERSE EFFECTS AND INTERACTIONS

Strong blockade of alpha-adrenergic receptors and weak blockade of cholinergic receptors explain some of chlorpromazine's adverse effects. Common side effects are dizziness, drowsiness, and orthostatic hypotension.

EPS occur mostly in older adults, women, and pediatric clients who are dehydrated. NMS may also occur. Clients taking chlorpromazine and exposed to warmer temperatures should be monitored more closely for symptoms of NMS.

Chlorpromazine interacts with several drugs. For example, concurrent use with sedative medications such as phenobarbital can cause excessive sedation and should be avoided. Taking chlorpromazine with tricyclic antidepressants can elevate blood pressure. Concurrent use of chlorpromazine with antiseizure medication can lower the seizure threshold.

Herbal supplements should be used only on the advice of the healthcare provider. Some products, such as kava and St. John's wort, increase the risk and severity of dystonia.

 See the Companion Website for a Nursing Process Focus Chart specific to this drug.

TABLE 17.3	Conventional Antipsychotic Drugs: Non-Phenothiazines
Drug	**Route and Adult Dose**
haloperidol (Haldol)	PO; 0.2–5 mg bid or tid
loxapine succinate (Apo-Loxapine)	PO; Start with 20 mg/day and rapidly increase to 60–100 mg/day in divided doses (max 250 mg/day)
pimozide (Orap)	PO; 1–2 mg/day in divided doses; gradually increase every other day to 7–16 mg/day (max 10 mg/day)
thiothixene HCl (Navane)	PO; 2 mg tid; may increase up to 15 mg/day (max 60 mg/day)

reactions such as confusion, depression, and hallucinations that are drug induced.

A complete baseline assessment, including physical assessment, mental status (orientation, affect, cognition), vital signs, lab studies (CBC, liver and renal function tests), pre-existing medical conditions (especially cardiac, kidney, and liver function), and vision screening should be performed. The nurse should also assess the available support system because many psychiatric clients are unable to self-manage their drug regimen. Contraindications for this class of drug include Parkinson's disease, CNS depression, alcoholism, seizure disorders, and age less than 3 years.

When monitoring and teaching about side effects, the nurse should inform the client and caregivers that sedation is a less severe side effect than with phenothiazines, but there is a greater EPS incidence with non-phenothiazine antipsychotics. A possible life-threatening adverse effect of antipsychotic drugs is NMS. Refer to information under "Nursing Considerations" for phenothiazine drugs for information regarding EPS and NMS.

Because of the anticholinergic side effect the nurse should monitor for dry mouth, u constipation, and hypotension with resultant tach Adherence with this classification of drug is equally as important as with the phenothiazines. The nurse should assess for alcohol and illegal drug use, which cause an increased depressant effect when used with antipsychotic drugs. The nurse should also caution the client that any form of caffeine used with these drugs would likely increase anxiety.

When assessing older clients, the nurse should check for unusual reactions to haloperidol. Older adults need smaller doses and more frequent monitoring with a gradual dose increase. There is a great occurrence of tardive dyskinesia in elderly women. This category of drug is not safe for use in children under 2 years of age.

Client education as it relates to conventional non-phenothiazines should include goals, reasons for obtaining baseline data, and possible side effects. The nurse should instruct the family regarding symptoms indicative of EPS

Pr PROTOTYPE DRUG | Haloperidol (Haldol)

ACTIONS AND USES

Haloperidol is classified chemically as a butyrophenone. Its primary use is for the management of acute and chronic psychotic disorders. It may be used to treat clients with Tourette's syndrome and children with severe behaviour problems such as unprovoked aggressiveness and explosive hyperexcitability. It is approximately 50 times more potent than chlorpromazine, but it has equal efficacy in relieving symptoms of schizophrenia. Haldol LA is a long-acting preparation that lasts for approximately 3 weeks following IM or SC administration. This is particularly beneficial for clients who are uncooperative or unable to take oral medications.

ADMINISTRATION ALERTS

- The drug must not be abruptly discontinued, or severe adverse reactions may occur.
- The client must take medication as ordered for therapeutic results to occur.
- If the client does not comply with oral therapy, injectable extended-release haloperidol should be considered.
- Haloperidol is pregnancy category C.

PHARMACOKINETICS

Haloperidol is well absorbed after oral or IM administration. It is widely distributed, crosses the placenta, and enters breast milk. It is about 90% protein bound. It is mostly metabolized by the liver. Its half-life is 21 to 24 hours.

ADVERSE EFFECTS AND INTERACTIONS

Haloperidol produces less sedation and hypotension than chlorpromazine, but the incidence of EPS is high. Elderly clients are more likely to experience side effects and often are prescribed half the adult dose until the side effects of therapy can be determined. Although the incidence of NMS is rare, it can occur.

Haloperidol interacts with many drugs. For example, the following drugs decrease the effects/absorption of haloperidol: aluminum- and magnesium-containing antacids, levodopa (also increases chance of levodopa toxicity), lithium (increases chance of severe neurological toxicity), phenobarbital, phenytoin (also increases chance of phenytoin toxicity), rifampin, and beta-blockers (may increase blood levels of haloperidol thus leading to possible toxicity). Haloperidol inhibits the action of centrally acting antihypertensives.

Herbal supplements, such as kava, may increase the effect of haloperidol. Herbal supplements should be used only on the advice of the healthcare provider.

 See the Companion Website for a Nursing Process Focus Chart specific to this drug.

and NMS, telling them to report such symptoms to the healthcare provider immediately. See "Nursing Process Focus: Clients Receiving Conventional Phenothiazine and Non-Phenothiazine Therapy" for additional teaching points.

ATYPICAL ANTIPSYCHOTIC AGENTS

Atypical antipsychotics treat both positive and negative symptoms of schizophrenia. They have become drugs of choice for treating psychoses. These agents are listed in Table 17.4.

NURSING PROCESS FOCUS Clients Receiving Conventional Phenothiazine and Non-Phenothiazine Therapy

Assessment	Potential Nursing Diagnoses/Identified Patterns
Prior to administration: ■ Obtain complete health history (medical and psychological) including allergies, drug history, and possible drug interactions. ■ Obtain baseline lab studies (electrolytes, CBC, BUN, creatinine, WBC, liver enzymes, drug screens). ■ Assess for hallucinations, level of consciousness, mental status. ■ Assess client support systems.	■ Ineffective therapeutic regimen management related to non-adherence with medication regimen, presence of side effects, and need for long-term medication use ■ Anxiety related to symptoms of psychosis ■ Risk for injury related to side effects of medication ■ Non-adherence, related to length of time before medication reaches therapeutic levels, desire to use alcohol or illegal drugs ■ Deficient knowledge related to no previous contact with psychosis or its treatment

Planning: Client Goals and Expected Outcomes

The client will:
■ Report a reduction of psychotic symptoms, including delusions, paranoia, irrational behaviour, hallucinations
■ Demonstrate an understanding of the drug's action by accurately describing side effects, precautions, and measures to take to decrease any side effects
■ Immediately report side effects or adverse reactions
■ Adhere to recommended treatment regimen

Implementation

Interventions (Rationales)	Client Education/Discharge Planning
■ Monitor for decrease of psychotic symptoms. (If client continues to exhibit symptoms of psychosis, he or she may not be taking drug as ordered, may be taking an inadequate dose, or may not be affected by the drug; it may need to be discontinued and another antipsychotic begun.)	Instruct client and caregiver to: ■ Notice increases or decreases in symptoms of psychosis, including hallucinations, abnormal sleep patterns, social withdrawal, delusions, and paranoia ■ Contact physician if no decrease of symptoms occurs over a 6-week period
■ Monitor for side effects such as drowsiness, dizziness, lethargy, headaches, blurred vision, skin rash, diaphoresis, nausea/vomiting, anorexia, diarrhea, menstrual irregularities, depression, hypotension, and hypertension.	■ Instruct client and caregiver to report side effects. ■ Inform client and caregiver that impotence, gynecomastia, amenorrhea, and enuresis may occur.
■ Monitor for anticholinergic side effects such as orthostatic hypotension, constipation, anorexia, genitourinary problems, respiratory changes, and visual disturbances.	Instruct client to: ■ Avoid abrupt changes in position ■ Not drive or perform hazardous activities until effects of the drug are known ■ Report vision changes ■ Comply with required laboratory tests ■ Increase dietary fibre, fluids, and exercise to prevent constipation ■ Relieve symptoms of dry mouth with sugarless hard candy or gum and frequent drinks of water ■ Notify physician immediately if urinary retention occurs
■ Monitor for EPS and NMS. (Presence of EPS may be sufficient reason for client to discontinue antipsychotic. NMS is life-threatening and must be reported and treated immediately.)	Instruct client and caregiver to: ■ Recognize tardive dyskinesia, dystonia, akathisia, pseudo-Parkinsonism ■ Immediately seek treatment for elevated temperature, unstable blood pressure, profuse sweating, dyspnea, muscle rigidity, incontinence
■ Monitor for alcohol/illegal drug use. (Client may decide to use alcohol or illegal drugs as a means of coping with symptoms of psychosis so may stop taking the antipsychotic. Used concurrently, these will cause increased CNS depressant effect.)	■ Instruct client to refrain from alcohol and illegal drug use. Refer client to community support groups for persons with addictions, as appropriate, and to mental health support groups for general support.

continued

NURSING PROCESS FOCUS Clients Receiving Conventional Phenothiazine and Non-Phenothiazine Therapy (Continued)

Interventions (Rationales)	Client Education/Discharge Planning
■ Monitor caffeine use. (Use of caffeine-containing substances will negate effects of antipsychotics.)	Instruct client or caregiver of: ■ Common caffeine-containing products ■ Acceptable substitutes, such as decaffeinated coffee and tea, caffeine-free colas
■ Monitor for cardiovascular changes, including hypotension, tachycardia, and ECG changes. (Haloperidol has fewer cardiotoxic effects than other antipsychotics, and may be preferred for client with existing CV problems.)	■ Instruct client and caregiver that dizziness and falls, especially upon sudden position changes, may indicate CV changes. Teach safety measures.
■ Monitor for smoking. (Heavy smoking may decrease metabolism of haloperidol, leading to decreased efficacy.)	■ Instruct client to stop or decrease smoking. Refer to smoking cessation programs, if indicated.
■ Monitor elderly clients closely. (Older adults may need lower doses and a more gradual dosage increase. Elderly women are at greater risk for developing tardive dyskinesia.)	■ Instruct caregiver to observe for unusual reactions such as confusion, depression, and hallucinations and for symptoms of tardive dyskinesia and to report immediately. ■ Instruct elderly client or caregiver on ways to counteract anticholinergic effects of medication, while taking into account any other existing medical problems.
■ Monitor lab results, including RBC and WBC counts, and drug levels.	■ Advise client and caregiver of necessity of having regular lab studies done.
■ Monitor for use of medication. (All antipsychotics must be taken as ordered for therapeutic results to occur.)	■ Instruct client and caregiver that medication must be continued as ordered, even if no therapeutic benefits are felt, because it may take several months to achieve full therapeutic benefits.
■ Monitor for seizures. (Drug may lower seizure threshold.)	■ Instruct client and caregiver that seizures may occur and review appropriate safety precautions.
■ Monitor client's environment. (Drug may cause client to perceive a brownish discoloration of objects or photophobia. Drug may also interfere with the ability to regulate body temperature.)	Instruct client and caregiver to: ■ Wear dark glasses to avoid discomfort from photophobia ■ Avoid temperature extremes ■ Be aware that perception of brownish discoloration of objects may appear, but it is not harmful

Evaluation of Outcome Criteria

Evaluate effectiveness of drug therapy by confirming that client goals and expected outcomes have been met (see "Planning").

See Tables 17.1 and 17.3 on page 195 for lists of drugs to which these nursing actions apply.

TABLE 17.4 Atypical Antipsychotic Drugs

Drug	Route and Adult Dose
clozapine (Clozaril)	PO; start at 25–50 mg/day and titrate to a target dose of 50–450 mg/day in 3 days; may increase further (max 900 mg/day)
olanzapine (Zyprexa)	Adult: PO; start with 5–10 mg/day; may increase by 2.5–5 mg every week (range 10–15 mg/day, max 20 mg/day) Geriatric: PO; start with 5 mg/day
quetiapine fumarate (Seroquel)	PO; start with 25 mg bid; may increase to a target dose of 300–400 mg/day in divided doses
risperidone (Risperdal)	PO; 1–6 mg bid; increase by 2 mg daily to an initial target dose of 6 mg/day

17.6 Treating Psychoses with Atypical Antipsychotics

The approval of clozapine, the first atypical antipsychotic, marked the first major advance in the pharmacotherapy of psychoses since the discovery of chlorpromazine decades earlier. Clozapine and the other drugs in this class are called atypical, or second generation, antipsychotics because they have a broader spectrum of action than the conventional antipsychotics, controlling both the positive and negative symptoms of schizophrenia. Furthermore, at therapeutic doses they exhibit their antipsychotic actions without producing the EPS effects of the conventional agents. Some drugs, such as clozapine, are especially useful for clients in whom other drugs have proven unsuccessful.

The mechanism of action of the atypical agents is largely unknown, but they are thought to act by blocking several different receptor types in the brain. Like the phenothiazines, the atypical agents block dopamine D$_2$-receptors. However, the atypical agents also block serotonin (5-HT) and alpha-adrenergic receptors, which is thought to account for some of their properties. Because they are only loosely bound to D$_2$-receptors, fewer extrapyramidal side effects occur than with the conventional antipsychotics.

Although there are fewer side effects with atypical antipsychotics, adverse effects are still significant and clients must be carefully monitored. Although most antipsychotics cause weight gain, the atypical agents are associated with obesity and its risk factors. Risperidone and some of the other antipsychotic drugs increase prolactin levels, which can lead to menstrual disorders, decreased libido, and osteoporosis in women. In men, high prolactin levels can cause lack of libido and impotence. There is also concern that some atypical agents alter glucose metabolism, which could lead to type 2 diabetes.

NURSING CONSIDERATIONS

The role of the nurse in atypical antipsychotic therapy involves careful monitoring of the client's condition and providing education as it relates to the prescribed drug regimen. Assessments of the client taking atypical antipsychotics include a complete health history, including seizure activity, cardiovascular status, psychological disorders, and neurological and blood diseases. Baseline lab tests, including CBC, WBC with differential, electrolytes, blood urea nitrogen (BUN), creatinine, and liver enzymes, should be obtained. A WBC with differential should be continued every week for the first 6 months, then every 2 weeks for the next 6 months, then every 4 weeks until the drug is discontinued. The nurse should assess for hallucinations, mental status, dementia, and bipolar disorder, initially and throughout therapy. The nurse should obtain the client's drug history to determine possible drug interactions and allergies.

Atypical antipsychotics are contraindicated during pregnancy and lactation as they can cause harm to the developing fetus and the infant. The nurse should instruct female clients to have a negative pregnancy test within 6 weeks of beginning therapy and to use reliable birth control during treatment. Female clients should also be instructed to notify their physician if they plan to become pregnant. In addition, clozapine is contraindicated in coma or severe CNS depression, uncontrolled epilepsy, history of clozapine-induced agranulocytosis, and leukopenia (WBC count less than 5000/mm^3).

Precautions must be taken when atypical antipsychotics are given to clients with cardiovascular disorders and conditions that predispose the client to hypotension. Additional precautions include the concurrent use of other CNS depressants (including alcohol), renal or hepatic disorders, exposure to extreme heat, older and younger age (older adults and children), prostatic hypertrophy, glaucoma, and a history of paralytic ileus.

Client education as it relates to atypical antipsychotic drugs should include goals, reasons for obtaining baseline data, and possible side effects. The nurse should include the following points when educating clients and their families about atypical antipsychotic medications:

- Avoid abrupt changes in position to decrease dizziness and postural hypotension.

Pr PROTOTYPE DRUG | Clozapine (Clozaril)

ACTIONS AND USES

Therapeutic effects of clozapine include remission of a range of psychotic symptoms, including delusions, paranoia, and irrational behaviour. Of severely ill clients, 25% show improvement within 6 weeks of starting clozapine; 60% show improvement within 6 months. Clozapine acts by interfering with the binding of dopamine to its receptors in the limbic system. Clozapine also binds to alpha-adrenergic, serotonergic, and cholinergic sites throughout the brain.

ADMINISTRATION ALERTS

- The client should be given only a 1-week supply of clozapine at a time, to ensure return for weekly lab studies.
- Dose must be increased gradually.
- Clozapine is pregnancy category B.

PHARMACOKINETICS

Clozapine is well absorbed after oral administration. It is widely distributed and crosses the placenta and blood-brain barrier. It is about 95% protein bound. It is mostly metabolized on first pass by the liver. Its half-life is 8 to 12 hours.

ADVERSE EFFECTS AND INTERACTIONS

Because seizures and agranulocytosis are associated with clozapine use, a course of therapy with conventional antipsychotics is recommended before starting clozapine therapy. Common side effects are dizziness, drowsiness, headache, constipation, transient fever, salivation, flu-like symptoms, and tachycardia. As with the conventional agents, elderly clients exhibit a higher incidence of orthostatic hypotension and anticholinergic side effects. Clozapine may also cause bone marrow suppression, which has proven fatal in some cases.

Clozapine interacts with many drugs. For example, it should not be taken with alcohol, other CNS depressants, or with drugs that suppress bone marrow function, such as anticancer drugs.

Concurrent use with antihypertensives may lead to hypotension. Benzodiazepines taken with clozapine may lead to severe hypotension and a risk for respiratory arrest. Concurrent use of digoxin or warfarin may cause increased levels of those drugs, which could lead to increased cardiac problems or hemorrhage, respectively. If phenytoin is taken concurrently with clozapine, seizure threshold will be decreased.

Use with caution with herbal supplements, such as kava, which may increase CNS depression.

 See the Companion Website for a Nursing Process Focus Chart specific to this drug.

- Take drug strictly as prescribed; do not make any dosage changes or stop taking the medication without approval of the healthcare provider. Medication may take a minimum of 6 weeks before any therapeutic effects are noted.
- Have routine lab studies performed as ordered.
- Call the physician if no improvement in behaviour is noted after 6 weeks of therapy.

- Avoid use of alcohol, illegal drugs, caffeine, and tobacco.
- If significant side effects occur, continue taking the medication, but contact the physician immediately.
- Increase intake of fruits, vegetables, and fluids if constipation occurs.

NURSING PROCESS FOCUS Clients Receiving Atypical Antipsychotic Therapy	
Assessment	**Potential Nursing Diagnoses/Identified Patterns**
Prior to administration: ■ Obtain complete health history (medical and psychological) including allergies, drug history, and possible drug interactions. ■ Obtain baseline lab studies, especially RBC and WBC counts. ■ Assess for hallucinations, mental status, level of consciousness. ■ Assess client support systems.	■ Anxiety related to symptoms of psychosis, side effects of medication ■ Risk for injury related to side effects of medication, psychosis ■ Non-adherence related to lack of understanding or knowledge, desire to use alcohol and caffeine-containing products ■ Risk for violence, self-directed or directed at others

Planning: Client Goals and Expected Outcomes

The client will:
- Adhere to recommended treatment regimen
- Report a reduction of psychotic symptoms, including delusions, paranoia, irrational behaviour, hallucinations
- Demonstrate an understanding of the drug's actions by accurately describing side effects, precautions, and measures to take to decrease any side effects

Implementation

Interventions (Rationales)	Client Education/Discharge Planning (Rationales)
■ Monitor RBC and WBC counts. (If WBC levels drop below 3500 mm^3, the client may be developing life-threatening agranulocytosis; drug will need to be stopped immediately.)	■ Advise client and caregiver of importance of having weekly lab studies performed.
■ Monitor for hematological side effects. (Neutropenia, leukopenia, agranulocytosis, and thrombocytopenia may occur secondary to possible bone marrow suppression caused by drug.)	■ Instruct client to report immediately any sore throat, signs of infection, fatigue without apparent cause, bruising.
■ Observe for side effects such as drowsiness, dizziness, depression, anxiety, tachycardia, hypotension, nausea/vomiting, excessive salivation, urinary frequency or urgency, incontinence, weight gain, muscle pain or weakness, rash, fever.	■ Instruct client and caregiver to report side effects.
■ Monitor for anticholinergic side effects, such as mouth dryness, constipation, and urinary retention. (Severe urinary retention may be corrected only by use of an indwelling catheter.)	Instruct client and caregiver to: ■ Increase dietary fibre, fluids, and exercise to prevent constipation ■ Relieve symptoms of dry mouth with sugarless hard candy or chewing gum and frequent drinks of water ■ Notify physician immediately if urinary retention occurs
■ Monitor for decrease of psychotic symptoms. (If client continues to exhibit symptoms of psychosis, he or she may not be taking medication as ordered, may be taking an inadequate dose, or may not be affected by the drug; it may need to be discontinued and another antipsychotic begun.)	Instruct client and caregiver to: ■ Notice increases or decreases in symptoms of psychosis, including hallucinations, abnormal sleep patterns, social withdrawal, delusions, and paranoia ■ Contact physician if no decrease of symptoms occurs over a 6-week period
■ Monitor for alcohol or illegal drug use. (Used concurrently, these will cause increased CNS depression. Client may decide to use alcohol or illegal drugs as a means of coping with symptoms of psychosis so may stop taking the drug.)	■ Instruct client to refrain from alcohol or illegal drug use. Refer client to AA, NA, or other support group as appropriate.
■ Monitor caffeine use. (Use of caffeine-containing substances will inhibit effects of antipsychotics.)	Instruct client and caregiver of: ■ Common caffeine-containing products ■ Acceptable substitutes, including decaffeinated coffee and tea, caffeine-free soda
■ Monitor for smoking. (Heavy smoking may decrease blood levels of drug.)	■ Instruct client to stop or decrease smoking. Refer to smoking cessation programs if indicated.

continued

NURSING PROCESS FOCUS Clients Receiving Atypical Antipsychotic Therapy *(Continued)*	
Interventions (Rationales)	**Client Education/Discharge Planning**
■ Monitor elderly closely. (Older clients may be more sensitive to anticholinergic side effects.) ■ Monitor for EPS and NMS. (Presence of EPS may be sufficient reason for client to discontinue medication. NMS is life-threatening and must be reported and treated immediately.)	■ Instruct elderly clients on ways to counteract anticholinergic effects of medication, while taking into account any other existing medical problems. Instruct client and caregiver to: ■ Recognize tardive dyskinesia, dystonia, akathisia, pseudo-Parkinsonism ■ Seek immediate treatment for elevated temperature, unstable blood pressure, profuse sweating, dyspnea, muscle rigidity, incontinence

Evaluation of Outcome Criteria
Evaluate effectiveness of drug therapy by confirming that client goals and expected outcomes have been met (see "Planning").

See Table 17.4 (page 199) for a list of drugs to which these nursing actions apply.

17.7 Treating Psychoses with Dopamine System Stabilizers

Due to side effects caused by conventional and atypical antipsychotic medications, a new drug class was developed to better meet the needs of clients with psychoses. The drugs in this class are called dopamine system stabilizers (DSSs). Clients with schizophrenia and schizo-affective disorder may exhibit fewer extrapyramidal symptoms when treated with a DSS than with haloperidol. Known side effects include headache, nausea/vomiting, fever, constipation, and anxiety.

PHARMFACTS

Psychoses

- Symptoms of psychosis are often associated with other mental health problems, including substance abuse, depression, and dementia.
- Psychotic disorders are among the most misunderstood mental health disorders in North America.
- An estimated 300 000 Canadians have schizophrenia.
- Clients with psychosis often develop symptoms between the age of 13 and the early 20s.
- As many as 50% of homeless people have schizophrenia.
- The probability of acquiring schizophrenia is 1 in 137 for the general population, 1 in 10 if one parent has the disorder, and 1 in 4 if both parents are schizophrenic.

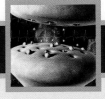

CHAPTER REVIEW

KEY CONCEPTS

The numbered key concepts provide a succinct summary of the important points from the corresponding numbered section within the chapter. If any of these points are not clear, refer to the numbered section within the chapter for review. Expanded versions can be found on the Companion Website.

17.1 Psychoses are severe mental and behavioural disorders characterized by disorganized mental capacity and an inability to recognize reality.

17.2 Schizophrenia is a type of psychosis characterized by abnormal thoughts and thought processes, disordered communication, withdrawal from other people and the outside environment, and a high risk for suicide.

17.3 Pharmacological management of psychoses is difficult because the adverse effects of the drugs may be severe, and clients often do not understand the need for medication.

17.4 The phenothiazines have been effectively used for the treatment of psychoses for over 50 years; however, they

have a high incidence of side effects. Extrapyramidal signs (EPS) and the neuroleptic malignant syndrome (NMS) are two particularly serious conditions.

17.5 The non-phenothiazine conventional antipsychotics have the same therapeutic applications and side effects as the phenothiazines.

17.6 Atypical antipsychotics are often preferred because they address both positive and negative symptoms of schizophrenia and produce less dramatic side effects.

17.7 Dopamine system stabilizers are the newest antipsychotic class. It is hoped that this new class will have equal efficacy to other antipsychotic classes, with fewer serious side effects.

REVIEW QUESTIONS

1 What are extrapyramidal signs (EPS)? What do EPS indicate? What can the nurse do to limit EPS?

2 What is the major difference between a conventional and an atypical antipsychotic?

3 How does each drug class generally affect positive and negative symptoms of schizophrenia?

4 Explain why the pharmacological management of severe mental illness is so difficult. What can the nurse do to improve the success of antipsychotic pharmacotherapy?

CRITICAL THINKING QUESTIONS

1. A 22-year-old male client has been on haloperidol (Haldol LA) for 2 weeks for the treatment of schizophrenia. During a follow-up assessment, the nurse notices that the client keeps rubbing his neck and is complaining of neck spasms. What is the potential cause of the sore neck and what would be the potential treatment? What is the nurse's initial action? What teaching is appropriate for this client?

2. A 68-year-old client has been put on olanzapine (Zyprexa) for treatment of acute psychosis. What is a priority of care for this client? What teaching is important for this client?

3. A 20-year-old, newly diagnosed schizophrenic client has been on chlorpromazine and is doing well. Today the nurse notices that the client appears more anxious and is demonstrating increased paranoia. What is the potential problem? What is the nurse's initial action? What client teaching is important?

4. You firmly believe that the medication prescribed for your client with schizophrenia is in your client's best interest. You explained to the client the benefits of taking the medication. The client clearly understands your explanation. The client states that the side effects are unacceptable and refuses to take the medication. What should you do? What factors should you consider in making your decision?

EXPLORE
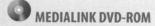 MediaLink

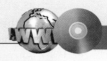 www.pearsoned.ca/adams-king

 MEDIALINK DVD-ROM
- **Audio Glossary**
- **CRNE Review**
- **Videos**
  Extrapyramidal Side Effects: Akathisia
  Extrapyramidal Side Effects: Forward Tremor
  Extrapyramidal Side Effects: Grasping Tremor
  Extrapyramidal Side Effects: Lateral Tremor
  Extrapyramidal Side Effects: Torticollis
  Schizophrenia: Hallucinations
  Schizophrenia: Hearing Voices
  Schizophrenia: When Did It Begin?
  Tardive Dyskinesia: Ambulation
  Tardive Dyskinesia: Choreoathetoid
  Tardive Dyskinesia: Oral

COMPANION WEBSITE
- **CRNE Review**
- **Case Study:** Client taking antipsychotics
- **Dosage Calculations**
- **Nursing Process Focus Charts**

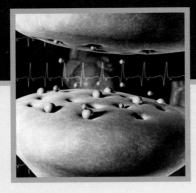

CHAPTER 18

Drugs for Degenerative Diseases of the Nervous System

DRUGS AT A GLANCE

DRUGS FOR PARKINSON'S DISEASE

Dopaminergics

  ℞ *carbidopa-levodopa (Sinemet)*

Anticholinergics

  ℞ *benztropine (Apo-Benztropine)*

DRUGS FOR ALZHEIMER'S DISEASE

Acetylcholinesterase Inhibitors

  ℞ *donepezil (Aricept)*

OBJECTIVES

After reading this chapter, the student should be able to do the following:

1. Identify drug classes used for treating Parkinson's disease.
2. Explain the therapeutic action of anti-Parkinson's drugs, focusing on the roles of dopamine and acetylcholine in the brain.
3. For each of the drug classes listed in Drugs at a Glance, identify a representative drug and explain its mechanism of action, primary actions, and important adverse effects.
4. Explain the therapeutic action of drugs used for treating Alzheimer's disease and the efficacy of existing medications.
5. Discuss the nurse's role in the pharmacological management of clients with Parkinson's disease and Alzheimer's disease.
6. Describe and explain, based on pharmacological principles, the rationale for nursing assessment, planning, and interventions for clients receiving drug therapy for degenerative diseases of the CNS.
7. Use the nursing process to care for clients receiving drug therapy for degenerative diseases of the CNS.

MediaLink

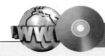 www.pearsoned.ca/adams-king

CRNE review, case studies, and other interactive resources for this chapter can be found on the Companion Website at **www.pearsoned.ca/adams-king**. Click on "Chapter 18" to select the activities for this chapter. For animations, more CRNE review questions, and an audio glossary, access the accompanying DVD-ROM in this textbook.

Degenerative diseases of the CNS are often difficult to deal with pharmacologically. Medications are unable to stop or reverse the progressive nature of these diseases; they can only offer symptomatic relief. Parkinson's disease and Alzheimer's disease, the two most common debilitating and progressive conditions, are the focus of this chapter.

18.1 Degenerative Diseases of the Central Nervous System

Degenerative diseases of the CNS include a diverse set of disorders that differ in their causes and outcomes. Some, such as Huntington's disease, are quite rare, affect younger clients, and are caused by chromosomal defects. Others, such as Alzheimer's disease, affect millions of people, mostly elderly clients, and have a devastating economic and social impact. Table 18.1 lists the major degenerative disorders of the CNS.

The etiology of most neurological degenerative diseases is unknown. Most progress from very subtle signs and symptoms early in the course of the disease to profound neurological and cognitive deficits. In their early stages, these disorders may be quite difficult to diagnose. With the exception of Parkinson's disease, pharmacotherapy provides only minimal benefit. Currently, medication is unable to cure any of the degenerative diseases of the CNS.

PARKINSON'S DISEASE

Parkinson's disease is a degenerative disorder of the CNS caused by death of neurons that produce the brain neurotransmitter dopamine. It is the second most common degenerative disease of the nervous system, affecting nearly 100,000 Canadians. Pharmacotherapy is often successful at reducing some of the distressing symptoms of this disease.

PHARMFACTS

Degenerative Diseases of the Central Nervous System

- There is no cure for degenerative diseases of the nervous system.
- Drugs alleviate the symptoms but do not halt the progression.
- As symptoms advance, more medication is needed. While treatment enables people to function better, it can cause unpleasant side effects.
- Clients often require assistance to ensure they receive their medications.
- Safety is an important consideration as physical and cognitive changes increase risk of falls and other injuries.

TABLE 18.1 Degenerative Diseases of the Central Nervous System

Disease	Description
Alzheimer's disease	progressive loss of brain function characterized by memory loss, confusion, and dementia
amyotrophic lateral sclerosis	progressive weakness and wasting of muscles caused by destruction of motor neurons
Huntington's disease	autosomal dominant genetic disorder resulting in progressive dementia and involuntary, spasmodic movements of limb and facial muscles
multiple sclerosis	demyelination of neurons in the CNS resulting in progressive weakness, visual disturbances, mood alterations, and cognitive deficits
Parkinson's disease	progressive loss of dopamine in the CNS causing tremor, muscle rigidity, and abnormal movement and posture

LIFESPAN CONSIDERATIONS

Age-Related Incidence

- The incidence of Parkinson's disease increases with age. Most clients with Parkinson's disease are over the age of 50; 20% may be diagnosed under the age of 50, and 5% to 10% under the age of 40.
- Nearly 300,000 Canadians over age 65 have Alzheimer's disease.
- One in 20 Canadians over age 65 is affected by Alzheimer's disease:
  - 1 in 100 from age 65 to 74
  - 1 in 14 from age 75 to 84
  - 1 in 4 from age 85 onward

PHARMFACTS

Parkinson's and Alzheimer's Diseases

- Nearly 100,000 Canadians have Parkinson's disease.
- More men than women develop Parkinson's disease.
- More women than men develop Alzheimer's disease.
- Alzheimer's disease accounts for about 65% of all dementia.
- Half of Canadians with dementia live in the community; half live in institutions.
- Degenerative diseases of the CNS affect all ethnic groups.

18.2 Characteristics of Parkinson's Disease

Parkinson's disease affects primarily clients older than 50 years of age; however, even teenagers can develop the disorder. Men are affected slightly more than women. The disease is progressive, with the expression of full symptoms often taking many years. The symptoms of Parkinson's disease, or Parkinsonism, are summarized as follows:

- Tremors: The hands and head develop a palsy-like motion or shakiness when at rest; pill-rolling is a common behaviour in progressive states, in which clients rub the thumb and forefinger together in a circular motion.
- Muscle rigidity: Stiffness may resemble symptoms of arthritis; clients often have difficulty bending over or moving limbs. Some clients develop a rigid poker face. These symptoms may be less noticeable at first but progress to become obvious in later years.
- Bradykinesia: **Bradykinesia** is the most noticeable of all symptoms; clients may have difficulty chewing, swallowing, or speaking. Clients with Parkinson's disease have difficulties initiating movement and controlling fine muscle movements. Walking often becomes difficult. Clients shuffle their feet without taking normal strides.
- Postural instability: Clients may be humped over slightly and easily lose their balance. Stumbling results in frequent falls with associated injuries.

Although Parkinson's disease is a progressive, neurological disorder primarily affecting muscle movement, other health problems often develop in these clients, including anxiety, depression, sleep disturbances, dementia, and disturbances of the autonomic nervous system such as difficulty urinating and performing sexually. Several theories have been proposed to explain the development of **Parkinsonism**. Because some clients with Parkinson's symptoms have a family history of this disorder, a genetic link is highly probable. Numerous environmental toxins also have been suggested as a cause, but results have been inconclusive. Potentially harmful agents include carbon monoxide, cyanide, manganese, chlorine, and pesticides. Viral infections, head trauma, and stroke have also been proposed as causes of Parkinsonism.

Symptoms of Parkinsonism develop due to the degeneration and destruction of dopamine-producing neurons within an area of the brain known as the substantia nigra. Under normal circumstances, neurons in the **substantia nigra** supply dopamine to the **corpus striatum**, a region of the brain that controls unconscious muscle movement.

Balance, posture, muscle tone, and involuntary muscle movement depend on the proper balance of the neurotransmitters dopamine (inhibitory) and acetylcholine (stimulatory) in the corpus striatum. If dopamine is absent, acetylcholine has a more dramatic stimulatory effect in this area. For this reason, drug therapy for Parkinsonism focuses not only on restoring dopamine function, but also on blocking the effect of acetylcholine within the corpus striatum. Thus, when the brain experiences a loss of dopamine within the substantia nigra, or an overactive cholinergic influence in the corpus striatum, Parkinsonism results.

Extrapyramidal signs (EPS) develop for the same neurochemical reasons as Parkinson's disease. Recall from Chapter 17 that antipsychotic drugs act through a blockade of dopamine receptors. Treatment with certain antipsychotic drugs may induce Parkinsonism-like symptoms, or EPS, by interfering with the same neural pathway and functions affected by the lack of dopamine.

EPS may occur suddenly and become a medical emergency. With acute EPS, the client's muscles may spasm or become locked up. Fever and confusion are other signs and symptoms of this reaction. For acute EPS in a healthcare facility, short-term medical treatment can be provided by administering diphenhydramine (Benadryl). If recognized outside the healthcare setting, the client should immediately be taken to the emergency room as untreated acute episodes of EPS can be fatal.

DRUGS FOR PARKINSONISM

Anti-Parkinsonism agents are given to restore the balance of dopamine and acetylcholine in specific regions of the brain. These drugs include dopaminergic agents and anticholinergics (cholinergic blockers).

DOPAMINERGICS

18.3 Treating Parkinsonism with Dopaminergic Drugs

The goal of pharmacotherapy for Parkinson's disease is to increase the ability of the client to perform normal daily activities such as eating, walking, dressing, and bathing. Although pharmacotherapy does not cure this disorder, symptoms may be dramatically reduced in some clients.

Drug therapy attempts to restore the functional balance of dopamine and acetylcholine in the corpus striatum of the brain. Dopaminergic drugs are used to increase dopamine levels in this region. These agents are listed in Table 18.2. The drug of choice for Parkinsonism is levodopa, in combination with carbidopa. Levodopa, a dopaminergic drug, has been used more extensively than any other medication for this disorder. As shown in Figure 18.1, levodopa is a precursor for dopamine synthesis. Supplying it directly leads to increased biosynthesis of dopamine within the nerve terminals. Whereas levodopa can cross the blood-brain barrier, dopamine cannot; thus, dopamine itself is not used for therapy. The effectiveness of levodopa can be "boosted" by combining it with carbidopa. Carbidopa does not cross the blood-brain barrier but acts outside the CNS to decrease the metabolism of levodopa to dopamine. Thus, the combination of levodopa and carbidopa makes more levodopa available to enter the CNS.

Several additional approaches to enhancing dopamine are used in treating Parkinsonism. Entacapone and selegiline inhibit enzymes that normally destroy levodopa and/or dopamine. Bromocriptine, pergolide, pramipexole, and ropinirole directly activate the dopamine receptor and are called dopamine agonists. Amantadine, an antiviral agent, causes the release of dopamine from its nerve terminals. All of these drugs are considered adjuncts to the pharmacotherapy of Parkinson's disease because they are not as effective as levodopa.

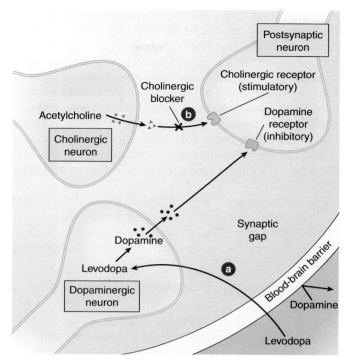

● **Figure 18.1** Mechanism of action of anti-Parkinsonism drugs: (a) levodopa therapy increases dopamine production; (b) anticholinergic (cholinergic blocker) decreases the amount of acetylcholine reaching the receptor

NURSING CONSIDERATIONS

The role of the nurse in dopaminergic therapy involves careful monitoring of the client's condition and providing education as it relates to the prescribed drug regimen. Prior to the initiation of drug therapy, the client's health history should be taken. Those with narrow-angle glaucoma, undiagnosed skin lesions, or history of hypersensitivity should not take dopaminergic agents. Dopaminergics should be used cautiously in clients with severe cardiac, renal, liver, or endocrine diseases, mood disorders, a history of seizures or ulcers, or those who are pregnant or lactating. Initial lab testing should include a complete blood count and liver and renal function studies. These tests should be obtained throughout the treatment regimen. Baseline information should include vital signs, especially blood pressure, mental status, and symptoms of Parkinson's disease. Lastly, all other medications taken by the client should be fully evaluated for compatibility with dopaminergic agonists.

During initial treatment, blood pressure, pulse, and respirations should be closely monitored because these drugs may cause hypotension and tachycardia. Additional

TABLE 18.2   Dopaminergic Drugs Used for Parkinsonism

Drug	Route and Adult Dose
amantadine (Symmetrel)	PO; 100 mg qd or bid
bromocriptine (Parlodel)	PO; 1.25–2.5 mg/day up to 100 mg/day in divided doses
carbidopa-levodopa (Sinemet)	PO; 1 tablet containing 10 mg carbidopa/100 mg levodopa or 25 mg carbidopa/100 mg levodopa tid (max 6 tabs/day)
pergolide (Permax)	PO; Start with 0.05 mg daily for 2 days; increase by 0.1 or 0.15 mg/day every 3 days for 12 days; then increase by 0.25 mg every third day (max 5 mg/day)
pramipexole dihydrochloride (Mirapex)	PO; Start with 0.125 mg tid for 1 week; double this dose for the next week; continue to increase by 0.25 mg/dose tid every week to a target dose of 1.5 mg tid
ropinirole hydrochloride (Requip)	PO; Start with 0.25 mg tid; may increase by 0.25 mg/dose tid every week to a target dose of 1 mg tid
selegiline hydrochloride (Apo-Selegiline)	PO; 5 mg/dose bid; doses greater than 10 mg/day are potentially toxic

lab testing for diabetes and acromegaly should be done if the client is expected to take the drug long term. The nurse should especially monitor clients for excessive daytime sleepiness, eye twitching, involuntary movements, hand tremors, fatigue, anxiety, mood changes, confusion, agitation, nausea, vomiting, anorexia, dry mouth, and constipation. Muscle twitching and mood changes may indicate toxicity and should be reported at once. The nurse may need to assist clients with drug administration and activities of daily living, including ambulation, at least initially. It is normal for the client's urine and perspiration to darken in colour.

Client education as it relates to dopaminergic drugs should include goals, reasons for obtaining baseline data, and possible side effects. The following are additional points to include when instructing the client and caregivers regarding dopaminergics:

- Increase fibre and fluid consumption to prevent constipation.
- Avoid foods high in pyridoxine (vitamin B$_6$) such as beef, liver, ham, pork, egg yolks, sweet potatoes, and oatmeal because they will decrease the effects of these medications.
- Report significant reactions or side effects immediately.
- It may be several months before the full therapeutic effect of pharmacotherapy is achieved.
- Do not abruptly discontinue taking the drug because Parkinsonian crisis may occur.
- Change positions slowly to prevent dizziness and fainting.

ANTICHOLINERGICS

18.4 Treating Parkinsonism with Anticholinergics

A second approach to changing the balance between dopamine and acetylcholine in the brain is to give anticholinergics, or cholinergic blockers. By blocking the effect of acetylcholine, anticholinergics inhibit the hyperactivity of this neurotransmitter in the corpus striatum of the brain. These agents are shown in Table 18.3 on page 210.

Anticholinergics such as atropine were the first agents used to treat Parkinsonism. The numerous peripheral side effects have limited the uses of this drug class. The anticholinergics now used for Parkinsonism are centrally acting and produce fewer side effects. Although they act on the CNS, autonomic effects such as dry mouth, blurred vision, tachycardia, urinary retention, and constipation are still troublesome. The centrally acting anticholinergics are not as effective as levodopa at relieving severe symptoms of Parkinsonism. They are used early in the course of the disease when symptoms are less severe, in clients who cannot tolerate levodopa, and in combination therapy with other anti-Parkinsonism drugs.

NURSING CONSIDERATIONS

The following content provides nursing considerations that apply to anticholinergics when given to treat Parkinsonism. For the complete nursing process applied to anticholinergic therapy, see "Nursing Process Focus: Clients Receiving Anticholinergic Therapy" in Chapter 13 on page 135.

Pr PROTOTYPE | Carbidopa-Levodopa (Sinemet)

ACTIONS AND USES

Levodopa restores the neurotransmitter dopamine in extrapyramidal areas of the brain, thus relieving some Parkinson's symptoms. To increase its effect, levodopa is combined with carbidopa, which prevents its enzymatic breakdown in the periphery. As long as 6 months may be needed to achieve maximum therapeutic effects.

ADMINISTRATION ALERTS

- The client may be unable to self-administer medication and may need assistance.
- Administer exactly as ordered.
- Abrupt withdrawal of the drug can result in Parkinsonism crisis or neuroleptic malignant syndrome (NMS).
- Carbidopa-levodopa is pregnancy category C.

PHARMACOKINETICS

Levodopa is well absorbed after oral administration. It is widely distributed, crosses the blood-brain barrier and placenta, and enters breast milk. Carbidopa does not cross the blood-brain barrier but enters breast milk. Levodopa (half-life 1 hour) and carbidopa (half-life 1 to 2 hours) are mostly metabolized by the liver.

ADVERSE EFFECTS AND INTERACTIONS

Side effects of levodopa include uncontrolled and purposeless movements such as extending the fingers and shrugging the shoulders, involuntary movements, loss of appetite, nausea, and vomiting. Muscle twitching and spasmodic winking are early signs of toxicity. Orthostatic hypotension is common in some clients. The drug should be discontinued gradually since abrupt withdrawal can produce acute Parkinsonism.

Levodopa interacts with many drugs. For example, tricyclic antidepressants decrease effects of levodopa, increase postural hypotension, and may increase sympathetic activity, with resulting hypertension and sinus tachycardia. Levodopa cannot be used if a monoamine oxidase (MAO) inhibitor was taken within 14 to 28 days because concurrent use may precipitate hypertensive crisis. Haloperidol taken concurrently may antagonize therapeutic effects of levodopa. Methyldopa may increase toxicity. Antihypertensives may cause increased hypotensive effects. Antiseizure drugs may decrease therapeutic effects of levodopa. Antacids containing magnesium, calcium, or sodium bicarbonate may increase levodopa absorption, which could lead to toxicity. Pyridoxine reverses the anti-Parkinsonism effects of levodopa.

Use with caution with herbal supplements, such as kava, which may worsen symptoms of Parkinson's disease.

NURSING PROCESS FOCUS   Clients Receiving Carbidopa-Levodopa (Sinemet)

Assessment	Potential Nursing Diagnoses/Identified Patterns
Prior to administration: ■ Obtain complete health history including allergies, drug history, and possible drug interactions. ■ Obtain baseline evaluation of severity of Parkinson's disease to determine medication effectiveness. ■ Obtain baseline vital signs, especially blood pressure and pulse.	■ Risk for falls ■ Need for knowledge related to drug therapy ■ Impaired physical mobility ■ Self-care deficit: feeding, toileting ■ Constipation

Planning: Client Goals and Expected Outcomes

The client will:
■ Report increased ease of movement and decreased symptoms of Parkinson's disease
■ Demonstrate an understanding of the drug's action by accurately describing drug side effects, precautions, and measures to take to decrease any side effects
■ Immediately report side effects and adverse reactions
■ Adhere to the medication regimen

Implementation

Interventions (Rationales)	Client Education/Discharge Planning
■ Monitor vital signs closely when dose is being adjusted. (Hypotension could occur as a result of dose adjustment. Dysrhythmias can occur in clients predisposed to cardiac problems.)	Instruct client and caregiver to: ■ Report signs of hypotension: dizziness, light-headedness, feeling that heart is racing or skipping beats, and dyspnea ■ Have ECGs and vital signs taken periodically
■ Provide for client safety. (Orthostatic hypotension may occur.)	Instruct client: ■ To change position slowly and to resume normal activities slowly ■ How to prevent and protect self from falls
■ Monitor for behaviour changes. (Drug increases risk of depression and suicidal thoughts and may cause other mood disturbances such as aggressiveness and confusion.)	Instruct client and caregiver to: ■ Watch for and report immediately any signs of changes in behaviour or mood ■ Seek counselling or a support group to help deal with these feelings; assist client to find such resources if needed
■ Monitor for symptoms of overdose. (Muscle twitching and blepharospasm are early symptoms.)	■ Instruct client and caregiver to be aware of newly occurring muscle twitching, including muscles of eyelids, and to report it immediately.
■ Monitor for improved functional status followed by a loss of therapeutic effects (on-off phenomenon) due to changes in dopamine levels that may last only minutes, or days. (Usually this occurs in clients on long-term levodopa therapy.)	■ Instruct client and caregiver to report rapid, unpredictable changes in motor symptoms to healthcare provider immediately, and that this can be corrected with changes in levodopa dosage schedule.
■ Evaluate diet. (Absorption of levodopa decreases with high-protein meals and high consumption of pyridoxine-containing foods.)	Instruct client to: ■ Take drug on empty stomach, but food may be eaten 15 minutes after, to decrease GI upset ■ Avoid taking levodopa with high-protein meals ■ Avoid high consumption of foods containing vitamin B_6 (pyridoxine) such as bananas, wheat germ, green vegetables, liver, legumes ■ Watch for vitamin B_6 in multivitamins, fortified cereals, and antinauseants, and avoid such products
■ Monitor glucose levels in clients with diabetes mellitus. (Loss of glycemic control may occur in the diabetic client.)	Instruct diabetic client to: ■ Consistently monitor blood glucose both by self and with periodic lab studies ■ Report symptoms of hypo- or hyperglycemia
■ Monitor for decreased kidney or liver function. (Decrease in these functions may slow metabolism and excretion of drug, possibly leading to overdose or toxicity.)	■ Instruct client to keep all appointments for liver and kidney function tests during therapy.
■ Monitor for side effects in older adults. (Elderly clients may experience more rapid and severe side effects, especially those affecting the cardiovascular system.)	■ Instruct elderly clients to report any symptoms involving cardiovascular system: changes in heart rate, dizziness, faintness, edema, palpitations.

continued

NURSING PROCESS FOCUS   Clients Receiving Carbidopa-Levodopa (Sinemet)   *(Continued)*

Interventions (Rationales)	Client Education/Discharge Planning
▪ Monitor for other drug-related changes. (Drug may cause urine and perspiration to darken in colour, but it is not a sign of overdose or toxicity.)	▪ Inform client that urine may darken and sweat may be dark coloured, but not to be alarmed.

Evaluation of Outcome Criteria

Evaluate effectiveness of drug therapy by confirming that client goals and expected outcomes have been met (see "Planning").

TABLE 18.3   Anticholinergic Drugs Used for Parkinsonism

Drug	Route and Adult Dose
benztropine mesylate (Apo-Benztropine)	PO; 0.5–1 mg/day; gradually increase as needed (max 6 mg/day)
biperiden hydrochloride (Akineton)	PO; 2 mg qd to qid
diphenhydramine hydrochloride (Benadryl) (see page 412 for the Prototype Drug box)	PO; 25–50 mg tid or qid (max 300/day)
procyclidine hydrochloride (PMS-Procyclidine)	PO; 2.5 mg tid pc; may be increased to 5 mg tid if tolerated with an additional 5 mg at hs (max 45–60 mg/day)
trihexyphenidyl hydrochloride (PMS-Trihexyphenidyl)	PO; 1 mg for day 1; double this for day 2; then increase by 2 mg every 3–5 days up to 6–10 mg/day (max 15 mg/day)

The role of the nurse in anticholinergic therapy for Parkinsonism involves careful monitoring of the client's condition and providing education as it relates to the prescribed drug regimen. As with clients taking dopaminergic drugs, the nurse needs to carefully evaluate and monitor clients taking anticholinergic drugs. Before a client begins treatment, a thorough health history should be obtained. Clients under the age of 3 years and those with known hypersensitivity, narrow-angle glaucoma, myasthenia gravis, or obstruction of the urinary or gastrointestinal tract should not take cholinergic blockers. These drugs should be used carefully in older adults (due to slowed metabolism), in clients who have dysrhythmias or benign prostatic hypertrophy (BPH), and in pregnant or lactating women. Before treatment begins, the nurse should obtain a medication history and a complete physical that includes complete blood count, liver and renal function studies, vital signs, mental status, and progression of Parkinson's disease to establish baseline data. These tests should be repeated throughout the treatment to help determine effectiveness of the drug.

Client education as it relates to anticholinergics should include goals, reasons for obtaining baseline data, and possible

---

Pr PROTOTYPE | Benztropine (Apo-Benztropine)

ACTIONS AND USES

Benztropine acts by blocking excess cholinergic stimulation of neurons in the corpus striatum. It is used for relief of Parkinsonism symptoms and for the treatment of EPS brought on by antipsychotic pharmacotherapy. This medication suppresses tremors but does not affect tardive dyskinesia.

ADMINISTRATION ALERTS

▪ The client may be unable to self-administer medication and may need assistance.

▪ Benztropine may be taken in divided doses, two to four times a day, or the entire day's dose may be taken at bedtime.

▪ If muscle weakness occurs, dose should be reduced.

▪ Benztropine is pregnancy category C.

PHARMACOKINETICS

Benztropine is well absorbed after oral or IM administration. Distribution, metabolism, excretion, and half-life are unknown.

ADVERSE EFFECTS AND INTERACTIONS

As expected from its autonomic action, benztropine can cause typical anticholinergic side effects such as sedation, dry mouth, constipation, and tachycardia.

Benztropine interacts with many drugs. For example, benztropine should not be taken with tricyclic antidepressants, MAO inhibitors, phenothiazines, procainamide, or quinidine because of combined sedative effects. OTC cold medicines and alcohol should be avoided. Other drugs that enhance dopamine release or activation of the dopamine receptor may produce additive effects. Haloperidol will cause decreased effectiveness.

Antihistamines, phenothiazines, tricyclics, disopyramide, and quinidine may increase anticholinergic effects, and antidiarrheals may decrease absorption.

 See the Companion Website for a Nursing Process Focus Chart specific to this drug.

side effects. The following are important points to include when teaching clients and caregivers about anticholinergics:

- To help relieve dry mouth, take frequent drinks of cool liquids, suck on sugarless hard candy or ice chips, and chew sugarless gum.
- Take with food or milk to prevent GI upset.
- Be evaluated by an eye specialist periodically as anticholinergics may promote glaucoma development.
- Avoid driving and other hazardous activities because drowsiness may occur. Do not abruptly discontinue taking the drug as withdrawal symptoms such as tremors, insomnia, and restlessness may occur.
- Avoid use of alcohol.
- Notify the healthcare provider if the following side effects or adverse reactions occur: disorientation, depression, hallucinations, confusion, memory impairment, nervousness, psychoses, vision changes, nausea/vomiting, urinary retention, dysuria.
- Wear dark glasses and avoid bright sunlight as necessary.

ALZHEIMER'S DISEASE

Alzheimer's disease is a devastating, progressive, degenerative disease that generally begins after age 60. By age 85, as many as 25% of the population may be affected. Pharmacotherapy has limited success in improving the cognitive function of clients with Alzheimer's disease.

18.5 Characteristics of Alzheimer's Disease

An estimated 290,000 Canadians over age 65 have Alzheimer's disease. **Alzheimer's disease (AD)** is responsible for about 65% of all dementia. **Dementia** is a degenerative disorder characterized by progressive memory loss, confusion, and inability to think or communicate effectively. Consciousness and perception are usually unaffected. Known causes of dementia include multiple cerebral infarcts, severe infections, and toxins. Although the cause of most dementia is unknown, it is usually associated with cerebral atrophy or other structural changes within the brain. The client generally lives 5 to 10 years following diagnosis; AD is the fourth leading cause of death.

Despite extensive, ongoing research, the etiology of Alzheimer's disease remains unknown. The early-onset familial form of this disorder, accounting for about 10% of cases, is associated with gene defects on chromosome 1, 14, or 21. Chronic inflammation and excess free radicals may cause neuron damage. Environmental, immunological, and nutritional factors, as well as viruses, are considered possible sources of brain damage.

Although the cause may be unknown, structural damage in the brain of Alzheimer's clients has been well documented. **Amyloid plaques** and **neurofibrillary tangles** found within the brain at autopsy are present in nearly all clients with AD.

It is suspected that these structural changes are caused by chronic inflammatory or oxidative cellular damage to the surrounding neurons. There is a loss in both the number and function of neurons.

Alzheimer's clients experience a dramatic loss of ability to perform tasks that require acetylcholine as the neurotransmitter. Because acetylcholine is a major neurotransmitter within the **hippocampus**, an area of the brain responsible for learning and memory, and other parts of the cerebral cortex, neuronal function within these brain areas is especially affected. Thus, an inability to remember and to recall information is among the early symptoms of AD. Symptoms of this disease are as follows:

- Impaired memory and judgment
- Confusion or disorientation
- Inability to recognize family or friends
- Aggressive behaviour
- Depression
- Psychoses, including paranoia and delusions
- Anxiety

DRUGS FOR ALZHEIMER'S DISEASE

Drugs are used to slow memory loss and other progressive symptoms of dementia. Some drugs are given to treat associated symptoms such as depression, anxiety, or psychoses. The acetylcholinesterase inhibitors are the most widely used class of drug for treating AD. These agents are shown in Table 18.4. Memantine, the first of a new class of drug called glutamergic inhibitors, was approved in 2003.

ACETYLCHOLINESTERASE INHIBITORS

18.6 Treating Alzheimer's Disease with Acetylcholinesterase Inhibitors

Health Canada has approved only a few drugs for AD. The most effective of these medications act by intensifying the effect of acetylcholine at the cholinergic receptor, as shown in Figure 18.2. Acetylcholine is naturally degraded in the synapse by the enzyme acetylcholinesterase (AchE). When acetylcholinesterase is inhibited, acetylcholine levels become elevated and produce a more profound effect on the receptor. As described in Chapter 13, the acetylcholinesterase inhibitors are indirect-acting cholinergics.

When treating AD, the goal of pharmacotherapy is to improve function in three domains: activities of daily living, behaviour, and cognition. Although the acetylcholinesterase inhibitors improve all three domains, their efficacy is modest, at best. These agents do not cure AD—they only slow its progression. Therapy is begun as soon as the diagnosis of AD is established. These agents are ineffective in treating the severe stages of this disorder, probably because so many neurons have died; increasing the levels of acetylcholine is only effective if there are functioning neurons present. Often, as the disease progresses, the acetylcholinesterase inhibitors are discontinued; their therapeutic benefit is not

Table 18.4	Acetylcholinesterase Inhibitors Used for Alzheimer's Disease
Drug	**Route and Adult Dose**
donepezil hydrochloride (Aricept)	PO; 5–10 mg at hs
galantamine (Reminyl)	PO; Start with 4 mg bid at least 4 weeks; if tolerated, may increase by 4 mg bid q4wk to target dose of 12 mg bid (max 8–16 mg bid)
rivastigmine tartrate (Exelon)	PO; Start with 1.5 mg bid with food; may increase by 1.5 mg bid q2wk if tolerated; target dose 3–6 mg bid (max 12 mg bid)

enough to outweigh their expense or the risk of side effects.

All acetylcholinesterase inhibitors used to treat AD have equal efficacy. Side effects are those expected of drugs that enhance the parasympathetic nervous system (Chapter 13). The GI system is most affected, with nausea, vomiting, and diarrhea being reported. Of the agents available for AD, rivastigmine is associated with weight loss, a potentially serious side effect in some elderly clients. When discontinuing therapy, doses of the acetylcholinesterase inhibitors should be lowered gradually.

Although acetylcholinesterase inhibitors are the mainstay of treatment for AD dementia, several other agents are being investigated for their possible benefit in delaying the progression of AD. Because at least some of the neuronal changes in AD are caused by oxidative cellular damage, antioxidants such as vitamin E are being examined for their effects in AD clients. Other agents currently being examined are anti-inflammatory agents, such as the COX-2 inhibitors, estrogen, and *Ginkgo biloba*.

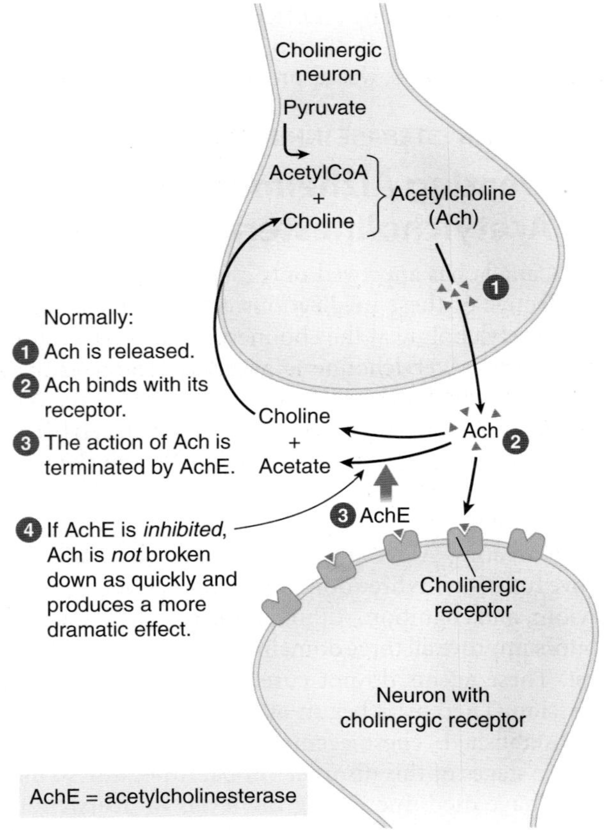

Agitation occurs in the majority of clients with AD. This may be accompanied by delusions, paranoia, hallucinations, or other psychotic symptoms. Atypical antipsychotic agents such as risperidone and olanzapine may be used to control these episodes. Conventional antipsychotics such as haloperidol are occasionally prescribed, though extrapyramidal side effects often limit their use. The pharmacotherapy of psychosis is presented in Chapter 17.

Although not as common as agitation, anxiety and depression may occur in AD clients. Anxiolytics such as buspirone or some of the benzodiazepines are used to control excessive anxiousness (Chapter 14). Mood stabilizers, such as sertraline, citalopram, or fluoxetine, are given when major depression interferes with daily activities (Chapter 16).

NURSING CONSIDERATIONS

The following content provides nursing considerations that apply to acetylcholinesterase inhibitors when given to treat Alzheimer's disease. For the complete nursing process applied to acetylcholinesterase inhibitor therapy, see "Nursing Process Focus: Clients Receiving Cholinergic Therapy" in Chapter 13 on page 131.

The role of the nurse in acetylcholinesterase inhibitor therapy involves carefully monitoring the client's condition and providing education as it relates to the prescribed drug regimen. Prior to the initiation of drug therapy, the client's health history should be taken. Young children and those with hypersensitivity should not take acetylcholinesterase inhibitors. Clients with narrow-angle glaucoma or undiagnosed skin lesions should not take rivastigmine. All acetylcholinesterase inhibitors should be used cautiously in clients with severe cardiac, renal, liver, or respiratory diseases (such as asthma or COPD), a history of seizures, GI bleeding or peptic ulcers, and those who are pregnant or lactating. Lab testing, including a complete blood count and liver and renal function tests, should be done initially and throughout the treatment regimen. Baseline vital signs should be taken. During initial treatment, vital signs should be closely monitored as these medications may cause hypotension. A full assessment of mental status and other signs of Alzheimer's disease should be done to provide a baseline and determine effectiveness of medication. All other medications taken by the client should be fully evaluated for interactions with acetylcholinesterase inhibitors.

The nurse should monitor clients for side effects or reactions such as changes in mental status, mood changes, dizziness, confusion, insomnia, nausea, vomiting, and anorexia. Additionally, those taking tacrine should be mon-

Normally:

1. Ach is released.
2. Ach binds with its receptor.
3. The action of Ach is terminated by AchE.
4. If AchE is *inhibited*, Ach is *not* broken down as quickly and produces a more dramatic effect.

AchE = acetylcholinesterase

● **Figure 18.2** Alzheimer's disease drugs work by intensifying the effect of acetylcholine at the receptor

itored for urinary frequency, hepatotoxicity, and GI bleeding. Client education as it relates to acetylcholinesterase inhibitors should include goals, reasons for obtaining baseline data, and possible side effects.

Nurses may care for clients with AD in acute or long-term care facilities or may provide support and education for caregivers in the home. Families and clients who are able to understand must be made aware that currently available medications may slow the progression of the disease but not effect a cure. In addition, the nurse should include the following points when educating clients and caregivers about acetylcholinesterase inhibitors:

- Take with food or milk to decrease GI upset.
- Take drug strictly as prescribed or serious side effects may result.
- Report any changes in mental status or mood.
- Report the following side effects to the healthcare provider: dizziness, confusion, insomnia, constipation, nausea, urinary frequency, GI bleeding, vomiting, seizures, and anorexia.
- Make appointments with the healthcare provider on a regular basis.
- To help relieve dry mouth, take frequent drinks of cool liquids, suck on sugarless hard candy, or chew sugarless gum.
- Increase fibre and fluid consumption to prevent constipation.
- Recognize symptoms of overdose: severe nausea/vomiting, sweating, salivation, hypotension, bradycardia, convulsions, and increased muscle weakness, including respira-

NATURAL THERAPIES

Ginkgo biloba for Treatment of Dementia

Ginkgo biloba has been used for many years to improve memory. In Europe, an extract of this herb is already approved for the treatment of dementia. In one study, 120 mg of ginkgo taken daily was shown to improve mental functioning and stabilize Alzheimer's disease. In other studies, clinical results were seen between 4 weeks and 6 months of treatment and were found to be relevant. Clients need to speak with their healthcare provider before taking this herb. Although most clients can take ginkgo without problems, those on anticoagulants may have an increased risk for bleeding.

SPECIAL CONSIDERATIONS

Living with Alzheimer's or Parkinson's Disease

Both Alzheimer's and Parkinson's disease are progressive, degenerative, neurological disorders. While Alzheimer's disease leads to impairments in memory, thinking, and reasoning, Parkinson's disease can lead to the inability to hold small items due to tremors and rigidity. It is because of these progressive symptoms that clients need all the help and support that caregivers can provide. While non-pharmacological management such as providing a safe environment can help, medications are available to slow the progression and minimize symptoms. Caregivers will need to provide assistance with activities of daily living, including making sure that these clients receive their medications.

For clients with Alzheimer's, the side effects of some drugs used to control dementia can disrupt sleep. Additionally, people with dementia often suffer sleep apnea. In addition to providing a routine and structured environment, new research suggests that as little as a few hours of bright light, especially in the evening, may help people living with Alzheimer's maintain a normal sleeping pattern. Clients who received light therapy in the evening also experienced an improvement in their sleep cycle.

tory muscles; if noted, contact healthcare provider immediately.

Pr PROTOTYPE DRUG | Donepezil (Aricept)

ACTIONS AND USES

Donepezil is an acetylcholinesterase inhibitor that improves memory in cases of mild to moderate Alzheimer's dementia by enhancing the effects of acetylcholine in neurons in the cerebral cortex that have not yet been damaged. Clients should receive pharmacotherapy for at least 6 months prior to assessing maximum benefits of drug therapy. Improvement in memory may be observed as early as 1 to 4 weeks following initiation of the medication. The therapeutic effects of donepezil are often short-lived, and the degree of improvement is modest, at best. An advantage of donepezil over other drugs in its class is that its long half-life permits it to be given once daily.

ADMINISTRATION ALERTS

- Give medication prior to bedtime.
- Medication is most effective when given on a regular schedule.
- Donepezil is pregnancy category C.

PHARMACOKINETICS

Donepezil is well absorbed after oral administration. Distribution is unknown. It is about 96% protein bound. It is mostly metabolized by the liver, with less than 20% excreted unchanged by the kidneys. Its half-life is 70 hours.

ADVERSE EFFECTS AND INTERACTIONS

Common side effects of donepezil are vomiting, diarrhea, and darkened urine. CNS side effects include insomnia, syncope, depression, headache, and irritability. Musculoskeletal side effects include muscle cramps, arthritis, and bone fractures. Generalized side effects include headache, fatigue, chest pain, increased libido, hot flashes, urinary incontinence, dehydration, and blurred vision. Unlike tacrine, hepatotoxicity has not been observed. Clients with bradycardia, hypotension, asthma, hyperthyroidism, or active peptic ulcer disease should be monitored carefully. Anticholinergics will be less effective. Donepezil interacts with several other drugs. For example, bethanechol causes a synergistic effect. Phenobarbital, phenytoin, dexamethasone, and rifampin may speed elimination of donepezil. Quinidine or ketoconazole may inhibit metabolism of donepezil. Because donepezil acts by increasing cholinergic activity, other drugs with cholinergic effects should not be administered concurrently.

 See the Companion Website for a Nursing Process Focus Chart specific to this drug.

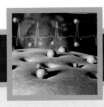

CHAPTER REVIEW

KEY CONCEPTS

The numbered key concepts provide a succinct summary of the important points from the corresponding numbered section within the chapter. If any of these points are not clear, refer to the numbered section within the chapter for review. Expanded versions can be found on the Companion Website.

18.1 Degenerative diseases of the nervous system such as Parkinson's disease and Alzheimer's disease cause a progressive loss of neuron function.

18.2 Parkinson's disease is characterized by symptoms of tremors, muscle rigidity, and postural instability and ambulation caused by the destruction of dopamine-producing neurons within the corpus striatum. The underlying biochemical problem is lack of dopamine activity and a related hyperactivity of acetylcholine.

18.3 The most commonly used medications for Parkinsonism attempt to restore levels of dopamine in the corpus striatum

of the brain. Levodopa, enhanced by combination with carbidopa, is the drug of choice for Parkinson's disease.

18.4 Centrally acting anticholinergic drugs are sometimes used to relieve symptoms of Parkinsonism, although they are less effective than levodopa.

18.5 Alzheimer's disease is a progressive, degenerative disease of older adults. Primary symptoms include disorientation, confusion, and memory loss.

18.6 Acetylcholinesterase inhibitors are used to slow the progression of Alzheimer's disease symptoms. These agents have minimal efficacy, and do not cure the dementia.

REVIEW QUESTIONS

1 What is the major pathology of Parkinson's disease? What brain neurotransmitters are affected and how?

2 What major drug category can produce Parkinsonism symptoms with over-medication? What are Parkinson-like symptoms called?

3 Describe the two basic approaches for restoring neurotransmitter balance in clients with Parkinson's disease.

4 Alzheimer's disease is a dysfunction of which brain neurotransmitters? How do drugs for Alzheimer's disease restore neurotransmitter function and improve Alzheimer's symptoms?

CRITICAL THINKING QUESTIONS

1. A 58-year-old Parkinson's client is started on levodopa-carbidopa (Sinemet). In obtaining her health history, the nurse notes that the client takes Mylanta on a regular basis for mild indigestion, takes multivitamins daily (vitamins A, B_6, D, and E), and has a history of diabetes mellitus type 2. What should the nurse include in teaching for this client?

2. A client is on levodopa-carbidopa (Sinemet) and benztropine. During a regular office follow-up, the client tells

the nurse that she is going to Arizona in July to visit her grandchildren. What teaching is important for this client?

3. A 67-year-old Alzheimer's client has been started on donepezil (Aricept) and has a history of heart failure, type 2 diabetes mellitus, and hypertension. The client's wife asks the nurse if this new medicine is appropriate for her husband to take. How should the nurse respond? What teaching should be done?

EXPLORE
MediaLink

 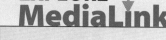 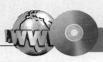

Ewww.pearsoned.ca/adams-king

MEDIALINK DVD-ROM
- Audio Glossary
- CRNE Review
- Videos
  Alzheimer's Disease
  Parkinson's Disease
- Animation
  Multiple Sclerosis

COMPANION WEBSITE
- CRNE Review
- Case Study: Client taking dopaminergic drug for parkinsonism
- Dosage Calculations
- Nursing Process Focus Charts

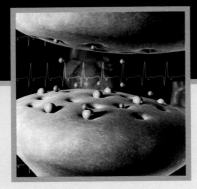

CHAPTER 19

Drugs for the Control of Pain

DRUGS AT A GLANCE

OPIOID (NARCOTIC) ANALGESICS

Opioid agonists
 ℞ morphine (Epimorph, others)

Opioids with mixed agonist-antagonist activity

Opioid antagonists
 ℞ naloxone (Narcan)

NON-OPIOID ANALGESICS

Acetaminophen

Non-steroidal anti-inflammatory drugs (NSAIDs)

Salicylates
 ℞ acetylsalicylic acid (Aspirin, others)

Ibuprofen and ibuprofen-like drugs

Selective COX-2 inhibitors

Centrally acting agents

ANTIMIGRAINE AGENTS

Triptans
 ℞ sumatriptan (Imitrex)

Ergot alkaloids

Miscellaneous antimigraine agents

OBJECTIVES

After reading this chapter, the student should be able to do the following:

1. Identify drug classes used for treating pain.
2. Explain the therapeutic action of analgesics in relation to physiological mechanisms of pain.
3. For each of the drug classes listed in Drugs at a Glance, identify a representative drug and explain its mechanism of action, primary actions, and important adverse effects.
4. Relate the importance of pain assessment to effective pharmacotherapy.
5. Discuss the nurse's role in using pharmacological and non-pharmacological therapies for clients experiencing pain.
6. Compare and contrast the types of opioid receptors and their importance to pharmacology.
7. Explain the role of opioid antagonists in the diagnosis and treatment of acute opioid toxicity.
8. Describe the long-term treatment of opioid dependence.
9. Compare the pharmacotherapeutic approaches of preventing migraines to those of aborting migraines.
10. Describe and explain, based on pharmacological principles, the rationale for nursing assessment, planning, and interventions for clients experiencing pain.
11. Use the nursing process to care for clients receiving analgesics and antimigraine drugs.

MediaLink

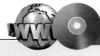 www.pearsoned.ca/adams-king

CRNE review, case studies, and other interactive resources for this chapter can be found on the Companion Website at **www.pearsoned.ca/adams-king**. Click on "Chapter 19" to select the activities for this chapter. For animations, more CRNE review questions, and an audio glossary, access the accompanying DVD-ROM in this textbook.

KEY TERMS

Pain is a physiological and emotional experience characterized by unpleasant feelings, usually associated with trauma or disease. On a simple level, pain may be viewed as a defence mechanism that helps people to avoid potentially damaging situations and encourages them to seek medical help. Although the neural and chemical mechanisms for pain are straightforward, many psychological and emotional processes can modify this sensation. Anxiety, fatigue, and depression can increase the perception of pain. Positive attitudes and support from caregivers may reduce the perception of pain. Clients are more likely to tolerate their pain if they know the source of the sensation and the medical course of treatment designed to manage the pain. For example, if clients know that the pain is temporary, such as during labour or after surgery, they are more likely to be accepting of the pain.

19.1 Assessment and Classification of Pain

The psychological reaction to pain is a subjective experience. The same degree and type of pain may be described as excruciating and unbearable by one client, while not mentioned during physical assessment by another. Several numerical scales and survey instruments are available to help healthcare providers standardize the assessment of pain and measure the progress of subsequent drug therapy. Successful pain management depends on accurate assessment of both the degree of pain experienced by the client and the potential underlying disorders that may be causing the pain. Selection of the correct therapy is dependent on the nature and character of the pain.

Pain can be classified as either acute or chronic. Acute pain is an intense pain occurring over a defined time, usually from injury to recovery. Chronic pain persists longer than 6 months, can interfere with daily activities, and is associated with feelings of helplessness or hopelessness.

Pain can also be classified as to its source. Injury to *tissues* produces **nociceptor pain**. This type of pain may be further subdivided into somatic pain, which produces sharp, localized sensations, or visceral pain, which is described as a generalized dull, throbbing, or aching pain. In contrast, **neuropathic pain** is caused by injury to *nerves* and typically is described as burning, shooting, or numb pain. Whereas nociceptor pain responds quite well to conventional pain relief medications, neuropathic pain has less therapeutic success.

PHARMFACTS

Pain

Pain is a common symptom:

- Over 50% of adults experience muscle pain each year.
- Approximately 4 million Canadians experience chronic arthritic pain.
- Approximately 7.5% of working-age Canadians are limited in their activities due to pain or discomfort; 70% of this group report constant pain.
- Pain-related disability increases gradually with age.
- Up to 40% of people with cancer report moderate to severe pain.

LIFESPAN CONSIDERATIONS

Pain in Infants and Older Adults

■ Infants and older adults are the most likely Canadians to be under-medicated for pain.

■ Infants older than 1 month can clear opioids as well as adults.

■ Premature infants can experience severe pain; they receive normal pain signals but have underdeveloped mechanisms to moderate pain signals.

■ Due to age-related changes in pharmacokinetics, older adults may experience more frequent and serious side effects from analgesics.

CULTURAL CONSIDERATIONS

Cultural Influences on Pain Expression and Perception

How a person responds to pain and the type of pain management chosen may be culturally determined. Establishment of a therapeutic relationship is of the utmost importance in helping a client attain pain relief. Respect the client's attitudes and beliefs about pain as well as the preferred treatment. An assessment of the client's needs, beliefs, and customs by listening, showing respect, and allowing the client to help develop and choose treatment options to attain pain relief is the most culturally sensitive approach.

When assessing pain, the nurse must remember that some clients may openly express their feelings and need for pain relief while others believe that the expression of pain symptoms, such as crying, is a sign of weakness. Pain management also varies according to cultural and religious beliefs. Traditional pain medications may or may not be the preferred method for pain control. For example, some Aboriginal Peoples and some Asian Canadians may prefer to use alternative therapies such as herbs, thermal therapies, acupuncture, massage, and meditation. Prayer plays an important role within some Canadian cultural groups, including some African Canadians.

19.2 Non-Pharmacological Techniques for Pain Management

Although drugs are quite effective at relieving pain in most clients, they can have significant side effects. For example, at high doses, acetylsalicylic acid (ASA) causes gastrointestinal (GI) bleeding, and the opioids cause significant drowsiness and have the potential for dependence. Non-pharmacological techniques may be used in place of drugs or as an adjunct to pharmacotherapy to assist clients in obtaining adequate pain relief. When used concurrently with medication, non-pharmacological techniques may allow for lower doses and possibly fewer drug-related adverse effects. Some techniques used for reducing pain are as follows:

- Acupuncture
- Biofeedback therapy
- Massage
- Heat or cold
- Meditation
- Relaxation therapy
- Art or music therapy
- Imagery
- Chiropractic manipulation
- Hypnosis
- Therapeutic touch
- Transcutaneous electrical nerve stimulation (TENS)
- Energy therapies such as reiki and qigong

Clients with intractable cancer pain sometimes require more invasive techniques, as rapidly growing tumours press on vital tissues and nerves. Furthermore, chemotherapy and surgical treatments for cancer can cause severe pain. Radiation therapy may provide pain relief by shrinking solid tumours that may be pressing on nerves. Surgery may be used to reduce pain by removing part or all of the tumour. Injection of alcohol or another neurotoxic substance into neurons is occasionally performed to cause nerve blocks. Nerve blocks irreversibly stop impulse transmission along the treated nerves and have the potential to provide total pain relief.

19.3 The Neural Mechanisms of Pain

The process of pain transmission begins when pain receptors are stimulated. These receptors, called **nociceptors**, are free nerve endings strategically located throughout the body. The nerve impulse signalling the pain is sent to the spinal cord along two types of sensory neurons, called A-delta and C fibres. **A-delta fibres** are wrapped in myelin, a lipid substance that speeds nerve transmission. **C fibres** are unmyelinated; thus they carry information more slowly. The A-delta fibres signal sharp, well-defined pain, whereas the C fibres conduct dull, poorly localized pain.

Once pain impulses reach the spinal cord, neurotransmitters are responsible for passing the message along to the next neuron. Here, a neurotransmitter called **substance P** is thought to be responsible for continuing the pain message, although other neurotransmitter candidates have been proposed. Spinal substance P is critical because it controls whether pain signals will continue to the brain. The activity of substance P may be affected by other neurotransmitters released from neurons in the CNS. One group of neurotransmitters called **endogenous opioids** includes endorphins, dynorphins, and enkephalins. Figure 19.1 shows one point of contact where endogenous opioids modify sensory information at the level of the spinal cord. If the pain impulse reaches the brain, it may respond to the sensation with many possible actions, ranging from signalling the skeletal muscles to jerk away from a sharp object, to mental depression caused by thoughts of death or disability in those suffering from chronic pain.

The fact that the pain signal begins at nociceptors located within peripheral tissues and proceeds through the CNS provides several targets for the pharmacological intervention of pain transmission. In general, the two main classes of pain medication act at different locations: the non-steroidal anti-inflammatory drugs (NSAIDs) act at the peripheral level, and the opioids act in the CNS.

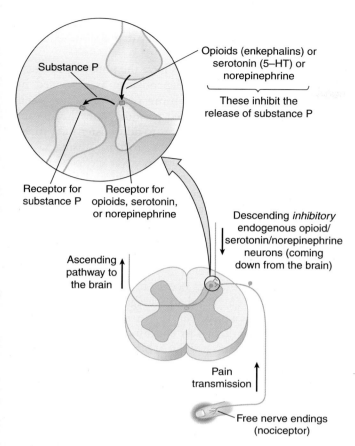

Substance P

Opioids (enkephalins) or serotonin (5–HT) or norepinephrine

These inhibit the release of substance P

Receptor for substance P

Receptor for opioids, serotonin, or norepinephrine

Descending *inhibitory* endogenous opioid/serotonin/norepinephrine neurons (coming down from the brain)

Ascending pathway to the brain

Pain transmission

Free nerve endings (nociceptor)

● **Figure 19.1** Neural pathways for pain

OPIOID (NARCOTIC) ANALGESICS

Analgesics are medications used to relieve pain. The two basic categories of analgesics are the opioids and the non-opioids. An opioid analgesic is a natural or synthetic morphine-like substance capable of reducing severe pain. Opioids are **narcotic** substances, meaning that they produce numbness and stupor-like symptoms.

19.4 Classification of Opioids

Terminology associated with the narcotic analgesic medications is often confusing. Several of these drugs are obtained from opium, a milky extract from the unripe seeds of the poppy plant that contains over 20 different chemicals with pharmacological activity. These natural substances are called **opiates**. Opium consists of 9% to 14% morphine and 0.8% to 2.5% codeine. In a search for safer analgesics, chemists have created several dozen synthetic drugs with activity similar to that of the opiates. **Opioid** is a general term referring to any of these substances, natural or synthetic, and is often used interchangeably with the term *opiate*.

Narcotic is a general term used to describe morphine-like drugs that produce analgesia and CNS depression. Narcotics may be natural, such as morphine, or synthetic, such as meperidine (Demerol). In common usage, a narcotic analgesic is the same as an opioid, and the terms are often used

interchangeably. In the context of drug enforcement, however, the term narcotic is often used to describe a much broader range of illegal drugs of addiction such as hallucinogens, heroin, amphetamines, and marijuana. In medical environments, restrict the use of the term *narcotic* to specifically refer to opioid substances. Because narcotics have addictive and high abuse potential, drug products that contain narcotics are designated Controlled Drugs and Substances Act (CDSA) Schedule I, and their administration is documented on the narcotic control record.

Opioids exert their actions by interacting with at least six types of receptors: mu (types one and two), kappa, sigma, delta, and epsilon. From the perspective of pain management, the **mu** and **kappa receptors** are the most important. Drugs that stimulate a particular receptor are called opioid agonists; those that block a receptor are called opioid antagonists. The types of actions produced by activating mu and kappa receptors are shown in Table 19.1.

Some opioid agonists, such as morphine, activate both mu and kappa receptors. Other opioids, such as pentazocine, exert mixed opioid agonist-antagonist effects by activating the kappa receptor but blocking the mu receptor. Opioid blockers such as naloxone inhibit both the mu and kappa receptors. This is the body's natural way of providing the mechanism for a diverse set of body responses from one substance. Figure 19.2 illustrates opioid actions on the mu and kappa receptors.

19.5 Pharmacotherapy with Opioids

Opioids are drugs of choice for moderate to severe pain that cannot be controlled with other classes of analgesics. Over 20 different opioids are available as medications, which may be classified by similarities in their chemical structure, by their mechanism of action, or by their efficacy, as shown in Table 19.2. The most clinically useful method is by efficacy, which places opiates into categories of strong or moderate narcotic activity. Morphine is the prototype drug for severe pain, and the drug to which all other opiates are compared.

Opiates produce many important effects other than analgesia. They are effective at suppressing the cough reflex

Table 19.1	Responses Produced by Activation of Specific Opioid Receptors	
Response	**Mu Receptor**	**Kappa Receptor**
analgesia	X	X
decreased GI motility	X	X
euphoria	X	
miosis		X
physical dependence	X	
respiratory depression	X	
sedation	X	X

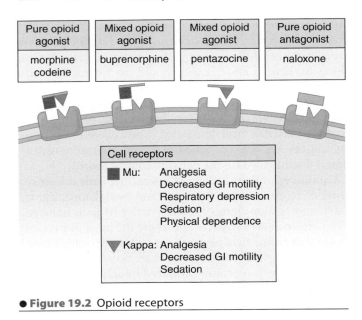

● **Figure 19.2** Opioid receptors

reasons why opiates are sometimes abused. There are many adverse effects, including respiratory depression, sedation, nausea, and vomiting.

All of the narcotic analgesics have the potential to cause physical and psychological dependence, as discussed in Chapter 12. Dependence is more likely to occur when taking high doses for extended periods. Many healthcare providers and nurses are hesitant to administer the proper amount of opioid analgesics for fear of causing client dependence or of producing serious adverse effects such as sedation or respiratory depression. Because of this under-medication, clients may not receive complete pain relief. When used according to accepted medical practice, clients can, and indeed should, receive the pain relief they need without fear of addiction or adverse effects. Clients who are addicted to narcotics will often need higher doses of the drugs for adequate pain relief. Because tolerance to the respiratory depression effects occurs rapidly when narcotics are taken regularly, higher than average doses can safely be given. Pain relief is a priority.

It is common practice to combine opioids and non-narcotic analgesics into a single tablet or capsule. The two classes of analgesics work synergistically to relieve pain, and the dose of narcotic can be kept small to avoid dependence and opioid-related side effects. Combination products containing narcotics are designated CDSA Schedule I. Caffeine

and at slowing the motility of the GI tract for cases of severe diarrhea. As powerful CNS depressants, opioids can cause sedation, which may be either a therapeutic effect or a side effect depending on the client's disease state. Some clients experience euphoria and intense relaxation, which are

TABLE 19.2 Opioids for Pain Management	
Drug	**Route and Adult Dose**
Opioid Agonists with Moderate Efficacy	
codeine	PO; 15–60 mg qid
hydrocodone bitartrate (Hycodan)	PO; 5–10 mg q4–6h prn (max 15 mg/dose)
oxycodone hydrochloride (OxyContin)	PO; 5–10 mg qid prn (supplied 5–80 mg/tablet)
oxycodone terephthalate (Percocet)	PO; 5–10 mg qid prn (supplied 5–80 mg/tablet)
propoxyphene napsylate (Darvon-N)	PO; 100 mg q4h prn (max 600 mg/day)
Opioid Agonists with High Efficacy	
hydromorphone hydrochloride (Dilaudid)	PO; 1–8 mg q4–6h prn
meperidine hydrochloride (Demerol)	PO; 50–150 mg q3–4h prn
methadone hydrochloride (Metadol)	PO; 2.5–10 mg q3–4h prn (supplied 1–25 mg/tablet)
⊙ morphine sulfate (Epimorph, Statex, others)	PO; 10–30 mg q4h prn (also SR, PR, SC/IM/IV)
Opioids with Mixed Agonist-Antagonist Effects	
butorphanol tartrate (Apo-Butorphanol)	Nasal spray; 1–2 mg q3–4h prn
nalbuphine hydrochloride (Nubain)	SC/IM/IV; 10–20 mg q3–6h prn (max 160 mg/day)
pentazocine hydrochloride (Talwin)	PO; 50–100 mg q3–4h (max 600 mg/day) SC/IM/IV; 30 mg q3–4h (max 360 mg/day)
Opioid Antagonists	
⊙ naloxone hydrochloride (Narcan)	IV; 0.4–2 mg; may be repeated every 2–3 min up to 10 mg if necessary
naltrexone hydrochloride (ReVia)	PO; 50 mg followed by another 50 mg in 1 hour if no withdrawal response (max 800 mg/day)

is often added to enhance absorption and distribution of the analgesic. Caffeine may also help relieve headache by constricting cerebral blood vessels. Some common combination analgesics are as follows:

- Percocet (oxycodone HCl, 5 mg; acetaminophen, 325 mg)
- Percodan (oxycodone HCl, 4.5 mg; oxycodone terephthalate, 0.38 mg; acetylsalicylic acid, 325 mg)
- Darvocet-N 50 (propoxyphene napsylate, 50 mg; acetaminophen, 325 mg)
- A.C. & C Tablets (acetylsalicylic acid, 325 mg; caffeine, 15 mg; codeine phosphate, 8 mg)
- Atasol 30 (acetaminophen, 325 mg; caffeine, 30 mg; codeine phosphate, 30 mg)
- Tylenol with Codeine No. 2 (acetaminophen, 300 mg; caffeine, 15 mg; codeine phosphate, 15 mg)

Some opioids are used primarily for conditions other than pain. For example, alfentanil, fentanyl, remifentanil, and sufentanil are used for general anesthesia; these are discussed in Chapter 20. Codeine is most often prescribed as a cough suppressant and is covered in Chapter 29. Opiates used in treating diarrhea are presented in Chapter 37.

NURSING CONSIDERATIONS

The role of the nurse involves careful monitoring of the client's condition and providing education as it relates to the prescribed drug regimen. When providing care for clients taking opioids, perform an initial assessment to determine the presence or history of severe respiratory disorders, increased intracranial pressure (ICP), seizures, and liver or renal disease. Obtain an allergy history before administering these drugs. A complete blood count and liver and renal studies, including aspartate aminotransferase (AST), alanine aminotransferase (ALT), amylase, and bilirubin, should be obtained to rule out the presence of disease. The character, duration, location, and intensity of pain should be determined before the administration of these agents. Obtain a history of current medication usage, especially alcohol and other CNS depressants because these drugs will increase respiratory depression and sedation. Contraindications include hypersensitivity and conditions precluding IV opioid administration, such as acute asthma or upper airway obstruction.

Through activation of primarily mu receptors, opioids may cause profound respiratory depression. Vital signs, especially respirations, should be obtained prior to and throughout the treatment regimen. Opioids should not be administered if respirations are below 12 per minute. Narcotic antagonists such as naloxone should be readily available if respirations fall below 10 per minute. Watch for decreasing level of consciousness and ensure safety by keeping the bed in a low position with side rails raised. Assistance may be needed with ambulation and activities of daily living (ADL).

LIFESPAN CONSIDERATIONS

The Influence of Age on Pain Expression and Perception

Pain control in both children and older adults can be challenging. Knowledge of developmental theories, the aging process, behavioural cues, subtle signs of discomfort, and verbal and nonverbal responses to pain are a must when it comes to effective pain management. Older clients may have a decreased perception of pain or simply ignore pain as a "natural" consequence of aging. Because these clients frequently go under-medicated, a thorough assessment is a necessity. As with adults, it is important that the nurse believe children's self-reports when assessing for pain. Developmentally appropriate pain rating tools are available and should be used on a continuous basis. Comfort measures should also be used.

When administering opioids for pain relief, always closely monitor older adults and children. Smaller doses are usually indicated, and side effects may be heightened. Closely monitor decreased respirations, loss of consciousness (LOC), and dizziness. Body weight should be taken prior to the start of opioid administration and doses calculated accordingly. Bed/crib rails should be kept raised, and the bed should be in the low position at all times to prevent injury from falls. Some opioids, such as meperidine, should be used cautiously in children. Many older adults take multiple drugs (polypharmacy); therefore, it is important to obtain a complete list of all medications taken and check for interactions.

Another severe adverse reaction, increased ICP, occurs as an indirect result of the respiratory depression effect. When respiration is suppressed, the CO_2 content of blood is increased, which dilates the cerebral blood vessels and causes ICP to rise. Similarly, orthostatic hypotension may also occur due to the blunting of the baroreceptor reflex and dilation of the peripheral arterioles and veins.

The nurse should continually monitor urinary output for urinary retention. This may occur due to the effect of increasing tone in the bladder sphincter and through suppression of the bladder stimuli.

Side effects such as constipation, nausea, and vomiting occur due to a combination of actions on the GI tract. By suppressing intestinal contractions, increasing the tone of the anal sphincter, and inhibiting secretion of fluids into the intestine, constipation may occur. Nausea or vomiting may occur due to the direct stimulation of the chemoreceptor trigger zone of the medulla. If this occurs, an antiemetic may be indicated. Opioids may be contraindicated for clients suffering from diarrhea caused by infections, especially following antibiotic therapy (pseudomembranous colitis). Pathogens in the GI tract produce toxins that are shed during diarrhea; constipation causes toxins to build up in the body.

Client education as it relates to opioids should include goals, reasons for obtaining baseline data such as vital signs and laboratory tests and procedures, and possible side effects. See "Nursing Process Focus: Clients Receiving Opioid Therapy" on page 223 for important points to include when teaching clients regarding this class of drug.

Pr **PROTOTYPE DRUG** | Morphine (Epimorph, others)

ACTIONS AND USES

Morphine binds with both mu and kappa receptor sites to produce profound analgesia. It causes euphoria, constriction of the pupils, and stimulation of cardiac muscle. It is used for symptomatic relief of serious acute and chronic pain after non-narcotic analgesics have failed, as a pre-anesthetic medication, to relieve shortness of breath associated with heart failure and pulmonary edema, and for acute chest pain connected with myocardial infarction.

ADMINISTRATION ALERTS

- Oral solution may be given sublingually.
- Oral solution comes in multiple strengths; carefully observe drug orders and labels before administering.
- Morphine causes peripheral vasodilation, which results in orthostatic hypotension and flushing of the face and neck.
- Morphine is pregnancy category D in long-term use or with high doses.

PHARMACOKINETICS

Morphine is variably absorbed following PO administration. It is well absorbed by other routes. It is widely distributed, crosses the placenta, and enters breast milk. It is up to 35% protein bound. It is mostly metabolized by the liver. The half-life of morphine is 2 to 4 hours in adults. Half-life is 10 to 20 hours in premature neonates, 7.6 hours in neonates, 6.2 hours in infants 1 to 3 months, 3 hours in children 6 months to 2.5 years, and 1 to 2 hours in children 3 to 6 years.

ADVERSE EFFECTS AND INTERACTIONS

Morphine may cause dysphoria (restlessness, depression, and anxiety), hallucinations, nausea, constipation, dizziness, and an itching sensation. Overdose may result in severe respiratory depression or cardiac arrest. Tolerance develops to the analgesic, sedative, and euphoric effects of the drug. Cross-tolerance also develops between morphine and other opioids such as heroin, methadone, and meperidine. Physical and psychological dependence develop when high doses are taken for prolonged periods of time. Morphine may intensify or mask the pain of gallbladder disease, due to biliary tract spasms.

Morphine interacts with several drugs. For example, concurrent use of CNS depressants such as alcohol, other opioids, general anesthetics, sedatives, and antidepressants such as MAO inhibitors and TCAs potentiates the action of opiates, increasing the risk of severe respiratory depression and death.

Use with caution with herbal supplements, such as yohimbe, which may potentiate the effect of morphine.

 See the Companion Website for a Nursing Process Focus Chart specific to this drug.

OPIOID ANTAGONISTS

19.6 Pharmacotherapy with Opioid Antagonists

Opioid overdose can occur as a result of overly aggressive pain therapy or as a result of substance abuse. Any opioid may be abused for its psychoactive effects; however, morphine, meperidine, and heroin are preferred due to their potency. Although heroin is currently available as a legal analgesic in many countries, it is deemed too dangerous for therapeutic use by Health Canada and is a major drug of addiction. Once injected or inhaled, heroin rapidly crosses the blood-brain barrier to the brain, where it is metabolized to morphine. Thus, the effects and symptoms of heroin administration are actually caused by the activation of mu and kappa receptors by morphine. The initial effect is an intense euphoria, called a rush, followed by several hours of deep relaxation.

Acute opioid intoxication is a medical emergency, with respiratory depression being the most serious problem. Infusion with the opioid antagonist naloxone may be used to reverse respiratory depression and other acute symptoms. In cases when the client is unconscious and the healthcare provider is unclear what drug has been taken, opioid antagonists may be given to diagnose the overdose. If the opioid antagonist fails to quickly reverse the acute symptoms, the overdose was likely due to a non-opioid substance.

NURSING CONSIDERATIONS

The role of the nurse in opioid antagonist therapy involves careful monitoring of the client's condition and providing education as it relates to the prescribed drug regimen. The primary indication for use of an opioid antagonist is established or suspected opioid-induced respiratory depression. An opioid antagonist may also be used to reverse opioid-induced pruritis. The primary nursing response is to assess the client's respiratory status and administer the opioid antagonist if respirations are below 10 breaths per minute (bpm). Resuscitative equipment should be immediately accessible. Obtaining key medical information is a priority; the presence/history of cardiovascular disease should be included. Opioids increase cardiac workload, so they must be used with caution in clients with cardiovascular disease. Assess the social context of the client's environment for the potential for opioid dependency. Opioid antagonists should be used cautiously in clients who are physically dependent on opioids because drug-induced withdrawal may be more severe than spontaneous opioid withdrawal. Caution is also advised in pregnant or lactating women and in children.

The nurse should assess the client's pain level before administration of these drugs and during therapy. During and immediately after the administration of opioid antagonists, check vital signs every 3 to 5 minutes (especially respiratory function and blood pressure). Obtain an arterial blood gas and ECG when ordered. Monitor for the following side

Pr PROTOTYPE DRUG | Naloxone (Narcan)

ACTIONS AND USES

Naloxone is a pure opioid antagonist, blocking both mu and kappa receptors. It is used for complete or partial reversal of opioid effects in emergency situations when acute opioid overdose is suspected. Given IV, it will immediately cause opioid withdrawal symptoms in clients physically dependent on opioids. It is also used to treat postoperative opioid depression and opioid pruritis. It is occasionally given as adjunctive therapy to reverse hypotension caused by septic shock.

PHARMACOKINETICS

Naloxone is well absorbed following IM or SC administration. Given intravenously, it begins to reverse opioid-initiated CNS and respiratory depression within minutes. It is widely distributed and crosses the blood-brain barrier and placenta. It is metabolized by the liver. Half-life is 60 to 90 minutes in adults and up to 3 hours in neonates.

ADMINISTRATION ALERTS

- Administer for respiratory rate of fewer than 10 breaths per minute. Keep resuscitative equipment accessible.
- Naloxone is pregnancy category B.

ADVERSE EFFECTS AND INTERACTIONS

Naloxone itself has minimal toxicity. However, in reversing the effects of opioids, the client may experience rapid loss of analgesia, increased blood pressure, tremors, hyperventilation, nausea/vomiting, and drowsiness. It should not be used for respiratory depression caused by non-opioid medications.

Drug interactions include a reversal of the analgesic effects of opioid agonists and agonist-antagonists.

 See the Companion Website for a Nursing Process Focus Chart specific to this drug.

effects: drowsiness, tremors, hyperventilation, ventricular tachycardia, and loss of analgesia. If giving these drugs to drug-dependent clients, monitor for signs of opioid withdrawal such as cramping, vomiting, hypertension, and anxiety.

Opioid antagonists such as naltrexone are also used for the treatment of opioid addiction. The nurse must monitor for side effects during treatment, many of which reflect the opioid withdrawal syndromes. Symptoms include increased thirst, chills, fever, joint/muscle pain, CNS stimulation, drowsiness, dizziness, confusion, seizures, headache, nausea,

vomiting, diarrhea, rash, rapid pulse and respirations, pulmonary edema, and wheezing. Vital signs should be taken every 3 to 5 minutes. Respiratory function should be continually assessed, and cardiac status should be monitored for tachycardia and hypertension. As with naloxone, resuscitative equipment should always be available.

Client education regarding opioid antagonists should include goals, reasons for obtaining baseline data such as vital signs and tests and procedures, and possible drug side effects. See "Nursing Process Focus: Clients Receiving Opioid Therapy" for specific teaching points.

NURSING PROCESS FOCUS   Clients Receiving Opioid Therapy

Assessment	Potential Nursing Diagnoses/Identified Patterns
Prior to administration: ■ Obtain complete health history including allergies, drug history, and possible drug interactions. ■ Assess pain (quality, intensity, location, duration). ■ Assess respiratory function. ■ Assess level of consciousness before and after administration. ■ Obtain vital signs.	■ Need for knowledge related to drug therapy ■ Acute pain, related to injury, disease, or surgical procedure ■ Ineffective breathing pattern related to action of medication ■ Constipation ■ Disturbed sleep pattern related to surgical pain

Planning: Client Goals and Expected Outcomes

The client will:
- Report pain relief or a reduction in pain intensity
- Demonstrate an understanding of the drug's action by accurately describing drug side effects and precautions
- Immediately report effects such as untoward or rebound pain, restlessness, anxiety, depression, hallucination, nausea, dizziness, and itching

Implementation

Interventions (Rationales)	Client Education/Discharge Planning
■ Opioids may be administered PO, SC, IM, IV, or PR. ■ Opioids are CDSA Schedule I controlled substances. (Opioids produce both physical and psychological dependence.)	Instruct client: ■ To take necessary steps to safeguard drug supply; avoid sharing medications with others ■ That oral *capsules* may be opened and mixed with cool foods; extended-release *tablets*, however, may not be chewed, crushed, or broken ■ That oral solution given sublingually may be in a higher concentration than solution for swallowing

continued

NURSING PROCESS FOCUS Clients Receiving Opioid Therapy *(Continued)*

Interventions (Rationales)	Cient Education/Discharge Planning
■ Monitor liver function via laboratory tests. (Opioids are metabolized in the liver. Hepatic disease can increase blood levels of opioids to toxic levels.)	Instruct client to: ■ Report nausea; vomiting; diarrhea; rash; jaundice; abdominal pain, tenderness, or distention; or change in colour of stool ■ Adhere to laboratory testing regimen for liver function as ordered by the healthcare provider
■ Monitor vital signs, especially depth and rate of respirations and pulse oximetry. ■ Withhold the drug if the client's respiratory rate is below 12, and notify the healthcare provider. ■ Keep resuscitative equipment and a narcotic-antagonist such as naloxone accessible. (Opioid antagonists may be used to reverse respiratory depression, decreased level of consciousness, and other symptoms of narcotic overdose.)	Instruct client or caregiver to: ■ Monitor vital signs regularly, particularly respirations ■ Withhold medication for any difficulty in breathing or respirations below 12 breaths per minute; report symptoms to the healthcare provider
■ Monitor neurological status; perform neurochecks regularly. ■ Monitor changes in level of consciousness. (Decreased LOC and sluggish pupillary response may occur with high doses.) ■ Observe for seizures. (Drug may increase ICP.)	Instruct client to: ■ Report headache or any significant change in sensorium, such as an aura or other visual affects that may indicate an impending seizure ■ Recognize seizures and methods to ensure personal safety during a seizure ■ Report any seizure activity immediately
■ If ordered prn, administer medication upon client request or when nursing observations indicate client expressions of pain.	Instruct client to: ■ Alert the nurse immediately upon the return or increase of pain ■ Notify the nurse regarding the drug's effectiveness
■ Monitor renal status and urinary output. (These drugs may cause urinary retention, which may exacerbate existing symptoms of prostatic hypertrophy.)	Instruct client or caregiver to: ■ Measure and monitor fluid intake and output ■ Report symptoms of dysuria (hesitancy, pain, diminished stream), changes in urine quality, or scanty urine output ■ Report fever or flank pain, which may be indicative of a urinary tract infection
■ Monitor for other side effects such as restlessness, dizziness, anxiety, depression, hallucinations, nausea, and vomiting. (Hives or itching may indicate an allergic reaction due to the production of histamine.)	Instruct client or caregiver to: ■ Recognize side effects and symptoms of an allergic or anaphylactic reaction ■ Immediately report any shortness of breath, tight feeling in the throat, itching, hives or other rash, feelings of dysphoria, nausea, or vomiting ■ Avoid the use of sleep-inducing OTC antihistamines without first consulting the healthcare provider
■ Monitor for constipation. (Drug slows peristalsis.)	Instruct client to: ■ Maintain an adequate fluid and fibre intake to facilitate stool passage ■ Use a stool softener or laxative as recommended by the healthcare provider
■ Ensure client safety. ■ Monitor ambulation until response to drug is known. (Drug can cause sedation and dizziness.)	Instruct client to: ■ Request assistance when getting out of bed ■ Avoid driving and performing hazardous activities until effects of the drug are known
■ Monitor frequency of requests and stated effectiveness of narcotic administered. (Opioids cause tolerance and dependence.)	Instruct client and caregiver: ■ Regarding cross-tolerance issues ■ To monitor medication supply to observe for hoarding, which may signal an impending suicide attempt ■ When educating clients suffering from terminal illnesses, address the issue of drug dependence from the perspective of reduced life expectancy.

Evaluation of Outcome Criteria

Evaluate effectiveness of drug therapy by confirming that client goals and expected outcomes have been met (see "Planning").

See Table 19.2 (page 220) for a list of drugs to which these nursing actions apply.

19.7 Treatment for Opioid Dependence

Although effective at relieving pain, the opioids have a greater risk for dependence than almost any other class of medication. Tolerance develops relatively quickly to the euphoric effects of opioids, causing users to escalate their doses and take the drug more frequently. The higher and more frequent doses can rapidly cause physical dependence.

When physically dependent clients attempt to discontinue drug use, they experience extremely uncomfortable symptoms that convince many to continue their drug-taking behaviour in order to avoid the suffering. As long as the drug is continued, they feel "normal," and many can continue work and social activities. In cases when the drug is abruptly discontinued, about 7 days of withdrawal symptoms are experienced before the client overcomes the physical dependence.

The intense craving characteristic of psychological dependence may occur for many months, and even years, following discontinuation of opioids. This often results in a return to drug-seeking behaviour unless significant support systems are established.

One common method of treating opioid dependence is to switch the client from IV and inhalation forms of illegal drugs to methadone. Although an opioid, oral methadone does not cause the euphoria of the injectable opioids. Methadone does not cure the dependence, and the client must continue taking the drug to avoid withdrawal symptoms. This therapy, called **methadone maintenance**, may continue for many months or years until the client decides to enter a total withdrawal treatment program. Methadone maintenance allows clients to return to productive work and social relationships without the physical, emotional, and criminal risks of illegal drug use.

A newer treatment approach that is used in some countries is to administer buprenorphine, an opioid agonist-antagonist, by the sublingual route. Buprenorphine is used early in opioid addiction therapy to prevent opioid withdrawal symptoms. A combination agent, Suboxone, contains both buprenorphine and naloxone, and is used later in the maintenance of opioid addiction.

NON-OPIOID ANALGESICS

The non-opioid analgesics include acetaminophen, the non-steroidal anti-inflammatory drugs (NSAIDs), and a few centrally acting agents.

NON-STEROIDAL ANTI-INFLAMMATORY DRUGS (NSAIDS)

The NSAIDs inhibit **cyclooxygenase**, which is an enzyme responsible for the formation of prostaglandins. When cyclooxygenase is inhibited, inflammation and pain are reduced.

19.8 Pharmacotherapy with NSAIDs

NSAIDs are the drugs of choice for mild to moderate pain, especially for pain associated with inflammation. These drugs have many advantages over the opioids. Acetylsalicylic acid (ASA) and ibuprofen are available OTC and are inexpensive. They are available in many different formulations, including those designed for children. They are safe and produce adverse effects only at high doses. The NSAIDs have antipyretic and anti-inflammatory activity, as well as analgesic properties. Some of the NSAIDs, such as the selective COX-2 inhibitors, are used primarily for their anti-inflammatory properties. The role of the NSAIDs in the treatment of inflammation and fever is discussed in Chapter 31. Table 19.3 highlights the common non-opioid analgesics.

The NSAIDs act by inhibiting pain mediators at the nociceptor level. When tissue is damaged, chemical mediators are released locally, including histamine, potassium ion, hydrogen ion, bradykinin, and prostaglandins. Bradykinin is associated with the sensory impulse of pain. Prostaglandins can induce pain through the formation of free radicals.

Prostaglandins are formed with the help of two enzymes called cyclooxygenase type one (COX-1) and cyclooxygenase type two (COX-2). ASA inhibits both COX-1 and COX-2. Because the COX-2 enzyme is more specific for the synthesis of those prostaglandins that cause pain and inflammation, the selective COX-2 inhibitors provide more specific pain relief and produce fewer side effects than ASA. Figure 19.3 on page 227 illustrates the mechanisms involved in pain at the nociceptor level.

Several important non-opioid analgesics are not classified as NSAIDs. Acetaminophen is a non-opioid analgesic that has equal efficacy to ASA and ibuprofen in relieving pain. Acetaminophen is one of the most widely used analgesics, yet its mechanism of action remains unclear. Possible mechanisms of action, including potential interaction with opioid, serotonergic, adrenergic, cholinergic, and COX systems, are currently being investigated. Acetaminophen is featured as an antipyretic Prototype Drug in Chapter 31. Clonidine and tramadol are centrally acting analgesics. Tramadol has weak opioid activity, though it is not thought to relieve pain by this mechanism.

NURSING CONSIDERATIONS

The role of the nurse in NSAID therapy involves careful monitoring of the client's condition and providing education as it relates to prescribed drug regimen. Because NSAIDs are readily available, inexpensive, and taken orally, clients sometimes forget that these medications can have serious side effects. The inhibition of COX-1 by ASA makes it more likely to cause gastric ulcers and bleeding and acute renal failure. Ibuprofen exerts less of an effect on COX-1 inhibition, so it produces less gastric bleeding than ASA.

When caring for clients taking high doses of these drugs, a thorough assessment for pregnancy and the presence/history of hypersensitivity, bleeding disorders, gastric ulcers, and severe renal/hepatic disease should be done. NSAIDs are not recommended for clients with these conditions. Hemoglobin and renal and liver function studies (BUN, creatinine,

TABLE 19.3 Non-Opioid Analgesics	
Drug	*Route and Adult Dose*
acetaminophen (Tylenol) (see page 408 for the Prototype Drug box)	PO; 325–650 mg q4–6h
NSAIDs	
Selective COX-2 Inhibitors	
celecoxib (Celebrex)	PO; 100–200 mg bid or 200 mg qid
Ibuprofen and Ibuprofen-Like: Non-Salicylates	
diclofenac (Voltaren)	PO; 50 mg bid to qid (max 200 mg/day)
diflunisal (Apo-Diflunisal)	PO; 1000 mg followed by 500 mg bid to tid
etodolac (Ultradol)	PO; 200–400 mg tid to qid
flurbiprofen (Ansaid)	PO; 50–100 mg tid to qid (max 300 mg/day)
ibuprofen (Advil, Motrin)	PO; 400 mg tid to qid (max 1200 mg/day)
indomethacin (Indocin)	PO; 25–50 mg bid or tid (max 200 mg/day) or 75 mg sustained release one to two times/day
ketoprofen (Rhodis)	PO; 12.5–50 mg tid to qid (also IM/IV 100 mg/mL)
ketorolac tromethamine (Toradol)	PO; 10 mg qid prn (max 40 mg/day) (also IM 10–30 mg/mL)
meloxicam (Mobicox)	PO; 7.5–15 mg qd (max 15 mg/day)
naproxen (Naprosyn)	PO; 500 mg followed by 200–250 mg tid to qid (max 1000 mg/day)
naproxen sodium (Anaprox)	PO; 250–500 mg bid (max 1000 mg/day)
piroxicam (Apo-Piroxicam)	PO; 10–20 mg qd to bid (max 20 mg/day)
sulindac (Apo-Sulin)	PO; 150–200 mg bid (max 400 mg/day)
Salicylates	
acetylsalicylic acid (Aspirin, others)	PO; 325–500 mg q4h (max 4 g/day)
Centrally Acting Agents	
clonidine (Catapres)	PO; 0.1 mg bid to tid (max 0.8 mg/day)
tramadol (Tramacet)	PO; 37.5 mg tramadol combined with 325 mg acetaminophen q4–6h prn (max 400 mg/day tramadol)

AST, ALT) should be performed before and during pharmacotherapy. An assessment of the location, character, and intensity of pain should be done initially for baseline data and throughout treatment to determine drug effectiveness. ASA has many drug interactions, therefore a complete client drug list should be obtained (see "Nursing Process Focus: Clients Receiving NSAID Therapy" on page 228). Contraindications include hypersensitivity to ASA or other NSAIDs and bleeding disorders such as hemophilia, von Willebrand's disease, telangiectasia, and favism (due to a genetic G6PD enzyme deficiency). When taking high doses of these medications, it is important that clients are monitored for nephrotoxicity (dysuria, hematuria, oliguria), blood dyscrasias, hepatitis, and allergic responses (rash and urticaria). Monitor clients for the following side effects: nausea, abdominal pain, anorexia, dizziness, and drowsiness. To decrease GI upset, the medication may be taken with food and plenty of fluids. Tablets with enteric coating should not be crushed.

Nurses should exercise extreme caution in administering ASA to children and teenagers. ASA has been implicated in the development of Reye's syndrome in conjunction with flu-like illnesses. Febrile, dehydrated children can rapidly develop ASA toxicity. Use ASA with caution in clients who are pregnant or lactating. Pregnancy category C (D in third trimester) denotes potential harm to the fetus.

Client education for non-opioid analgesics should include goals; reasons for obtaining baseline data such as vital signs, diagnostic procedures, and laboratory tests; and possible side effects. See "Nursing Process Focus: Clients Receiving NSAID Therapy" on page 228 for specific points to include when teaching clients regarding this class of drug.

TENSION HEADACHES AND MIGRAINES

Headaches are some of the most common complaints of clients. Living with headaches can interfere with activities of daily life, thus causing great distress. The pain and the inability to focus and concentrate result in work-related absences and the inability to take care of home and family. When the headaches are persistent, or occur as migraines, drug therapy is warranted.

19.9 Classification of Headaches

Of the several varieties of headache, the most common is the **tension headache.** This occurs when muscles of the head and neck become very tight due to stress, causing a steady and lingering pain. Although quite painful, tension

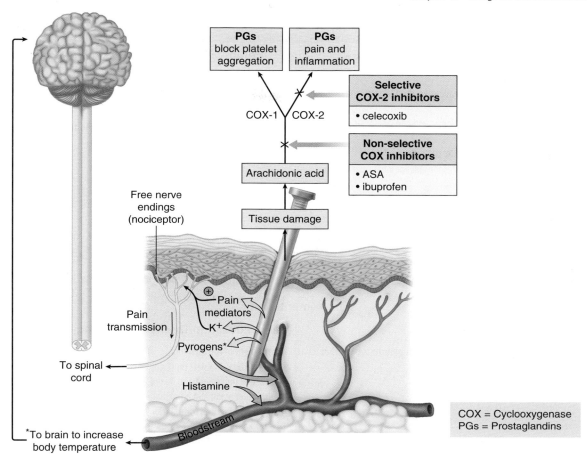

Pr **PROTOTYPE DRUG** | Acetylsalicylic Acid (Aspirin, others)

ACTIONS AND USES

Acetylsalicylic acid (ASA) inhibits prostaglandin synthesis involved in the processes of pain and inflammation and produces mild to moderate relief of fever. It has limited effects on peripheral blood vessels, causing vasodilation and sweating. ASA has significant anticoagulant activity, and this property is responsible for its ability to reduce the risk of mortality following MI and to reduce the incidence of stroke. ASA has also been found to reduce the risk of colorectal cancer, although the mechanism by which it affords this protective effect is unknown.

ADMINISTRATION ALERTS

- Platelet aggregation inhibition caused by ASA is irreversible. ASA should be discontinued 1 week prior to elective surgery.
- ASA is excreted in the urine and affects urine testing for glucose and other metabolites, such as vanillylmandelic acid (VMA).
- ASA is pregnancy category D.

PHARMACOKINETICS

ASA is well absorbed after oral administration. It is widely distributed, crosses the placenta, and enters breast milk. It is mostly metabolized by the liver. The amount excreted unchanged in urine varies according to urine pH (increases as urinary pH increases). Its half-life is 2 to 3 hours for low doses but can be up to 30 hours at high doses if liver metabolism is saturated.

ADVERSE EFFECTS AND INTERACTIONS

At high doses, such as those used to treat severe inflammatory disorders, ASA may cause gastric discomfort and bleeding because of its antiplatelet effects. Enteric-coated tablets and buffered preparations are available for clients who experience GI side effects.

Because ASA increases bleeding time, it should not be given to clients receiving anticoagulant therapy such as warfarin, heparin, and plicamycin. ASA may potentiate the action of oral hypoglycemic agents. The effects of NSAIDs, uricosuric agents (such as probenecid), beta-blockers, spironolactone, and sulfa drugs may be decreased when combined with ASA.

Concurrent use of phenobarbital, antacids, and glucocorticoids may decrease ASA effects. Insulin, methotrexate, phenytoin, sulfonamides, and penicillin may increase effects. When taken with alcohol, pyrazolone derivatives, steroids, or other NSAIDs, there is an increased risk for gastric ulcers.

Use with caution with herbal supplements, such as feverfew, which may increase the risk of bleeding.

 See the Companion Website for a Nursing Process Focus Chart specific to this drug.

NURSING PROCESS FOCUS   Clients Receiving NSAID Therapy

Assessment	Potential Nursing Diagnoses/Identified Patterns
Prior to administration: ■ Obtain complete health history including allergies, drug history, and possible drug interactions. ■ Determine pain history and preferred analgesic and non-analgesic pain management strategies. ■ Determine current pain and analgesic usage patterns. ■ Identify infectious agents or other factors responsible for inflammation or pain.	■ Acute pain related to injury or surgical procedure ■ Chronic pain related to back injury ■ Need for knowledge related to drug therapy ■ Ineffective health maintenance related to chronic pain

Planning: Client Goals and Expected Outcomes

The client will:
■ Report pain relief or a reduction in pain intensity
■ Demonstrate an understanding of the drug's action by accurately describing drug side effects and precautions
■ Report ability to manage activities of daily living
■ Immediately report effects such as unresolved, untoward, or rebound pain; persistent fever; blurred vision; tinnitus; bleeding; changes in colour of stool or urine

Implementation

Interventions (Rationales)	Client Education/Discharge Planning
■ NSAIDs may be administered PO or PR. When using suppositories, monitor integrity of rectum; observe for rectal bleeding.	Inform client of the following: ■ Enteric-coated tablets must not be cut or crushed. Regular tablets may be broken or pulverized and mixed with food. ■ Administer liquid ASA immediately after mixing because it breaks down rapidly. ■ Different drugs and formulations, such as ibuprofen and naproxen, should not be taken concurrently. Consult the healthcare provider regarding appropriate OTC analgesics for specific types of pain. ■ ASA is an anticoagulant. The body needs time to manufacture new platelets to make clots that promote wound healing. Consult the nurse regarding ASA therapy following surgery. ■ Advise laboratory personnel of ASA therapy when providing urine samples.
■ Monitor vital signs, especially temperature. (Increased pulse and blood pressure may indicate discomfort; increased pulse and decreased blood pressure accompanied by pallor and/or dizziness may indicate bleeding.)	Instruct client to: ■ Report rapid heartbeat, palpitations, dizziness, or pallor ■ Monitor blood pressure and temperature ensuring proper use of home equipment
■ Monitor for signs of GI bleeding or hepatic toxicity. (NSAIDs can be a local irritant to the GI tract and are metabolized in the liver.) ■ Monitor gastrointestinal elimination; conduct guaiac stool testing for occult blood. ■ Monitor CBC for signs of anemia related to blood loss.	Instruct client to: ■ Report any bleeding, abdominal pain, anorexia, heartburn, nausea, vomiting, jaundice, or a change in the colour or character of stools ■ Know the proper method of obtaining stool samples and home testing for occult blood ■ Adhere to a regimen of laboratory testing as ordered by the healthcare provider ■ Take NSAIDs with food to reduce stomach upset
■ Assess for character, duration, location, and intensity of pain and the presence of inflammation.	■ Instruct client to notify nurse if pain and/or inflammation remains unresolved. ■ Advise client to take only the prescribed amount to decrease the potential for adverse effects.
■ Monitor for hypersensitivity reaction. ■ Monitor urinary output and edema in feet/ankles. (Medication is excreted through the kidneys. Long-term use may lead to renal dysfunction.) ■ Monitor for sensory changes indicative of drug toxicity: tinnitus, blurred vision. ■ Evaluate blood salicylate levels.	Advise client to: ■ Immediately report shortness of breath, wheezing, throat tightness, itching, or hives. If these occur, stop taking ASA immediately and inform the healthcare provider. ■ Immediately report changes in urination, flank pain, or pitting edema ■ Return to healthcare provider for prescribed follow-up appointments ■ Immediately report any sensory changes in sight or hearing, especially blurred vision or ringing in the ears

Evaluation of Outcome Criteria

Evaluate effectiveness of drug therapy by confirming that client goals and expected outcomes have been met (see "Planning").

See Table 19.3 (page 226) under "NSAIDs" for a list of drugs to which these nursing actions apply.

headaches are self-limiting and generally considered an annoyance rather than a medical emergency. Tension headaches can usually be effectively treated with OTC analgesics such as ASA, acetaminophen, or ibuprofen.

The most painful type of headache is the **migraine**, which is characterized by throbbing or pulsating pain, sometimes preceded by an aura. **Auras** are sensory cues that let the client know that a migraine attack is coming. Examples of sensory cues are jagged lines, flashing lights, and special smells, tastes, or sounds. Most migraines are accompanied by nausea and vomiting. Triggers for migraines include nitrates, monosodium glutamate (MSG) found in many Asian foods, red wine, perfumes, food additives, caffeine, chocolate, and aspartame. By avoiding foods containing these substances, some clients can prevent the onset of a migraine attack.

19.10 Drug Therapy for Migraine Headaches

There are two primary goals for the pharmacological therapy of migraines. The first is to stop migraines in progress, and the second is to prevent migraines from occurring. For the most part, the drugs used to abort migraines are different from those used for prophylaxis. Drug therapy is most effective if it is started before a migraine has reached a severe level. Drugs for migraines are listed in Table 19.4.

The two major drug classes used as antimigraine agents, the triptans and the ergot alkaloids, are both serotonin (5-HT) agonists. Serotonergic receptors are found throughout the CNS and in the cardiovascular and GI systems. At least five receptor subtypes have been identified. In addition to the triptans, other drugs acting at serotonergic receptors include the popular antianxiety agents fluoxetine and buspirone.

Pharmacotherapy of migraine termination generally begins with acetaminophen or NSAIDs. If OTC analgesics are unable to abort the migraine, the drugs of choice are often the triptans. The first of the triptans, sumatriptan, was marketed in the 1990s. Triptans are selective for the 5-HT$_1$ receptor subtype, and they are thought to act by constricting certain intracranial vessels. They are effective in aborting migraines with or without aura. Although oral forms of the triptans are most convenient, clients who experience nausea and vomiting during the migraine may require an alternate dosage form. Intranasal formulations and prefilled syringes of triptans are available for clients who are able to self-administer the medication.

For clients who are unresponsive to triptans, the ergot alkaloids may be used to abort migraines. The first purified alkaloid, ergotamine, was isolated from the ergot fungus in 1920, although the actions of the ergot alkaloids had been known for thousands of years. Ergotamine is an inexpensive drug that is available in oral, sublingual, and suppository forms. Modification of the original molecule has produced a number of other pharmacologically useful drugs, such as dihydroergotamine. Dihydroergotamine is given parenterally and as a nasal spray. Because the ergot alkaloids interact

with adrenergic and dopaminergic receptors, as well as serotonergic receptors, they produce multiple actions and side effects. Many ergot alkaloids are pregnancy category X drugs.

Drugs for migraine prophylaxis include various classes of drug that are discussed in other chapters of this textbook. These include beta-adrenergic blockers, calcium channel blockers, antidepressants, and antiseizure drugs. Because all of these drugs have the potential to produce side effects, prophylaxis is only initiated if the incidence of migraines is high and the client is unresponsive to the drugs used to abort migraines. Of the various drugs, propranolol is one of the most commonly prescribed. Amitriptyline is preferred for clients who may have a mood disorder or suffer from insomnia in addition to their migraines.

PHARMFACTS

Migraines

- About 15% of Canadians suffer from migraines.
- Incidence is slightly higher in the Prairie and Maritime provinces.
- Caucasians are more likely to experience migraines than Asians or Africans.
- Most people experience their first attack in childhood or adolescence.
- Before puberty, more boys have migraines than girls.
- After puberty, females have 4 to 8 times more migraines than males.
- Persons with a family history of headache or migraine have a higher chance of developing these disorders.
- Of all migraines, 95% are controlled by drug therapy and other measures.

NURSING CONSIDERATIONS

The role of the nurse in antimigraine therapy involves careful monitoring of the client's condition and providing education as it relates to the prescribed drug regimen. Before starting clients on antimigraine medications, gather information about the frequency and intensity of the migraine headaches and the presence/history of MI, angina, and hypertension. Also determine pregnancy status and gather information about the presence/history of renal and liver disease and diabetes. Laboratory tests to determine renal and liver disease should be obtained.

The baseline frequency of migraine headaches along with apical pulse, respirations, and blood pressure should be obtained. Because migraines may be stress related, the client's stress level and coping mechanisms should be investigated. Always assess for hypersensitivity and the use of other medications. With triptans, clients should not take MAO inhibitors or SSRIs, which cause an increase in effect.

The nurse should assess the client's neurological status, including LOC, blurred vision, nausea and vomiting, and tingling in the extremities. These signs or symptoms may indicate a migraine is beginning. A quiet, calm environment with decreased noise and subdued lighting should be provided, and care should be organized to limit disruptions

TABLE 19.4   Antimigraine Drugs

Drug	Route and Adult Dose
DRUGS FOR TERMINATING MIGRAINES	
Ergotamine Alkaloids	
dihydroergotamine mesylate (D.H.E. 45, Migranal)	IM; 1 mg; may be repeated at 1-hour intervals to a total of 3 mg (max 6 mg/week)
ergotamine tartrate ergotamine with caffeine (Cafergot, Ercaf, others)	PO; 1–2 mg followed by 1–2 mg every 30 minutes until headache stops (max of 6 mg/day or 10 mg/week)
Triptans	
almotriptan (Axert)	PO; 6.25–12.5 mg, may repeat in 2 hours if necessary (max 2 tabs/day)
eletriptan (Relpax)	PO; 20–40 mg, may repeat in 2 hours if necessary (max 80 mg/day)
naratriptan (Amerge)	PO; 1–2.5 mg; may repeat in 4 hours if necessary (max 5 mg/day)
rizatriptan (Maxalt)	PO; 5–10 mg, may repeat in 2 hours if necessary (max 30 mg/day); 5 mg with concurrent propranolol (max 15 mg/day)
sumatriptan (Imitrex)	PO; 25 mg for 1 dose (max 100 mg)
zolmitriptan (Zomig)	PO; 2.5–5 mg; may repeat in 2 hours if necessary (max 10 mg/day)
DRUGS FOR PREVENTING MIGRAINES	
almotriptan (Axert)	PO; 6–12.5 mg, may repeat in 2 hours if necessary (max 2 tabs/day)
eletriptan (Relpax)	PO; 20–40 mg, may repeat in 2 hours if necessary (max 80 mg/day)
Beta-Adrenergic Blockers	
atenolol (Tenormin) (see page 295 for the Prototype Drug box)	PO; 25–50 mg qd (max 100 mg/day)
metoprolol (Lopresor) (see page 295 for the Prototype Drug box)	PO; 50–100 mg qd–bid (max 450 mg/day)
propranolol hydrochloride (Inderal) (see page 324 for the Prototype Drug box)	PO; 80–240 mg qd in divided doses; may need 160–240 mg/day
timolol (Apo-Timolol)	PO; 10 mg bid; may increase to 60 mg/day in 2 divided doses
Calcium Channel Blockers	
nifedipine (Adalat) (see page 261 for the Prototype Drug box)	PO; 10–20 mg tid (max 180 mg/day)
nimodipine (Nimotop)	PO; 60 mg q4h for 21 days, start therapy within 96 hours of subarachnoid hemorrhage
verapamil hydrochloride (Isoptin) (see page 327 for the Prototype Drug box)	PO; 40–80 mg tid (max 360 mg/day)
Tricyclic Antidepressants	
amitriptyline hydrochloride (Elavil)	PO; 75–100 mg/day
imipramine (Tofranil) (see page 176 for the Prototype Drug box)	PO; 75–100 mg/day (max 300 mg/day)
Miscellaneous Agents	
valproic acid (Depakene, Depakote) (see page 165 for the Prototype Drug box)	PO; 250 mg bid (max 1000 mg/day)
methysergide (Sansert)	PO; 4–8 mg/day in divided doses
riboflavin (vitamin B_2)	As a supplement: PO; 5–10 mg/day For deficiency: PO; 5–30 mg/day in divided doses

and decrease neural stimulation. Cold packs can be applied to help lessen the uncomfortable effects of the migraine. Monitor for possible side effects, including dizziness, drowsiness, vasoconstriction, warming sensations, tingling, light-headedness, weakness, and neck stiffness. Use with caution during pregnancy or lactation. Sumatriptan is excreted in breast milk. Advise the client that the drug could be harmful to the fetus or infant. Because of the vasoconstriction action of the drugs, they are contraindicated in the following conditions: hypertension; myocardial ischemia and coronary artery disease (CAD); history of MI, dysrhythmias, or heart failure; high-risk CAD profile; and diabetes.

The ergot alkaloids promote vasoconstriction, which terminates ongoing migraines. Side effects may include nausea, vomiting, weakness in the legs, myalgia, numbness and tingling in fingers and toes, angina-like pain, and tachycardia. Toxicity may be evidenced by constriction of peripheral arteries: cold, pale, numb extremities and muscle pain. Sumatriptan is metabolized in the liver and excreted by the kidneys; impaired organ function can increase serum drug levels. The client should be advised against, and monitored for, constant usage because these medications can cause physical dependence.

Client education regarding drug therapy for migraines should include goals; reasons for obtaining baseline data such as vital signs, laboratory tests, and procedures (such as computed tomography or magnetic resonance images of the brain, or lumbar puncture for samples of CSF); and possible side effects. Following are teaching points to include when educating clients regarding the ergot alkaloids:

- Take dose immediately after onset of symptoms.
- Control, avoid, or eliminate factors that trigger a headache or migraine, such as fatigue, anxiety, and alcohol.
- Report the signs of ergot toxicity, which may include muscle pain, numbness, and cold extremities.

NATURAL THERAPIES

Feverfew for Migraines

Feverfew (*Tanacetum parthenium*) is an herb that originated in southeastern Europe and is now found all over Europe, Australia, and North America. The common name feverfew is derived from its antipyretic properties. The leaves contain the active ingredients, the most prevalent of which is a lactone known as parthenolide. Standardization of this herb is based on the percent of parthenolide in the product.

Feverfew has an overall spectrum of action resembling that of ASA. The herb has been shown to exert anti-inflammatory and antispasmodic effects, as well as to inhibit platelet aggregation. Feverfew extract has also been shown to contain a novel type of mast cell inhibitor that inhibits anti-IgE-induced histamine release. In clinical trials, feverfew was associated with a reduction in the number and severity of migraine attacks, as well as a reduction in vomiting. The most common adverse effect is mouth ulceration, which occurs in about 10% of feverfew users.

- Do not overuse any of these drugs as physical dependence may result.

See "Nursing Process Focus: Clients Receiving Triptan Therapy" for specific teaching points about this subclass.

Pr PROTOTYPE DRUG | Sumatriptan (Imitrex)

ACTIONS AND USES

Sumatriptan belongs to a relatively new group of antimigraine drugs known as the triptans. The triptans act by causing vasoconstriction of cranial arteries; this vasoconstriction is moderately selective and does not usually affect overall blood pressure. This medication is available in oral, intranasal, and SC forms. SC administration terminates migraine attacks in 10 to 20 minutes; the dose may be repeated 60 minutes after the first injection, to a maximum of two doses per day. If taken orally, sumatriptan should be administered as soon as possible after the migraine is suspected or has begun.

PHARMACOKINETICS

Sumatriptan is well absorbed after SC and intranasal administration. Absorption is variable after oral administration due to first-pass metabolism. Distribution is unknown. It is mostly metabolized by the liver. Its half-life is 2 hours.

ADMINISTRATION ALERTS

- Sumatriptan may produce cardiac ischemia in susceptible persons with no previous cardiac events. Healthcare providers may opt to administer the initial dose of sumatriptan in the healthcare setting.
- The drug's systemic vasoconstrictor activity may cause hypertension and result in dysrhythmias or myocardial infarction. Keep resuscitative equipment accessible.
- Sumatriptan selectively reduces carotid arterial blood flow. Monitor changes in LOC and observe for seizures.
- Sumatriptan is pregnancy category C.

ADVERSE EFFECTS AND INTERACTIONS

Some dizziness, drowsiness, or a warming sensation may be experienced after taking sumatriptan; however, these effects are not normally severe enough to warrant discontinuation of therapy. Because of its vasoconstricting action, the drug should be used cautiously, if at all, in clients with recent myocardial infarction or a history of angina pectoris, hypertension, or diabetes.

Sumatriptan interacts with several drugs. For example, an increased effect may occur when taken with MAO inhibitors or SSRIs. Further vasoconstriction can occur when taken with ergot alkaloids and other triptans.

 See the Companion Website for a Nursing Process Focus Chart specific to this drug.

NURSING PROCESS FOCUS   Clients Receiving Triptan Therapy

Assessment	Potential Nursing Diagnoses/Identified Patterns
Prior to administration: ■ Obtain complete health history including allergies, drug history, and possible drug interactions. ■ Determine pain and analgesic usage patterns. ■ Identify infectious agents or other factors responsible for inflammation or pain. ■ Assess level of consciousness before and after administration.	■ Acute pain related to severe headache ■ Need for knowledge related to drug therapy ■ Ineffective coping related to chronic pain ■ Ineffective health maintenance related to inability to manage ADL

Planning: Client Goals and Expected Outcomes

The client will:
■ Report pain relief or a reduction in pain intensity
■ Demonstrate an understanding of the drug's action by accurately describing drug side effects and precautions
■ Immediately report effects such as shortness of breath, chest tightness or pressure, jaw pain, untoward or worsened rebound headache, seizures or other neurological changes

Implementation

Interventions (Rationales)	Client Education/Discharge Planning
■ Administer the first dose of the medication under supervision.	■ Instruct client that the first dose may need to be given under medical supervision because of potential cardiac side effects. Reassure client that this is merely a precautionary measure.
■ Monitor vital signs, especially blood pressure and pulse. (Triptans have vasoconstrictor action.)	■ Instruct client to monitor vital signs, especially blood pressure and pulse, ensuring proper use of home equipment.
■ Observe for changes in severity, character, or duration of headache. (Sudden severe headaches of "thunderclap" quality can signal subarachnoid hemorrhage. Headaches that differ in quality and are accompanied by such signs as fever, rash, or stiff neck may herald meningitis.)	■ Instruct client that changes in the character of migraines could signal other potentially more serious disorders. ■ Provide the client with written materials on warning signs of stroke; discuss other conditions such as meningitis, which may cause headache.
■ Monitor neurological status; perform neurochecks regularly	Instruct client: ■ That feeling dizzy or light-headed can be the result of the drug's action on the CNS or coronary ischemia ■ To immediately report episodes of severe dizziness or impending syncope ■ To review emergency response and safety measures in the event of a seizure
■ Monitor for possible side effects: dizziness, drowsiness, warming sensation, tingling, lightheadedness, weakness, or neck stiffness due to vasoconstriction. (Such symptoms can result from decreased blood flow to the brain related to reduced carotid arterial blood supply.)	Advise client: ■ To immediately report side effects to the healthcare provider ■ Regarding emergent symptoms suggestive of stroke or MI that may require immediate emergency intervention and transport to a hospital
■ Monitor dietary intake of foods that contain tyramine. (These foods may trigger an acute migraine.)	■ Instruct client to avoid or limit foods containing tyramine such as pickled foods, beer, wine, and aged cheeses. Provide client with a list of tyramine-containing foods.
■ Monitor kidney and liver function via laboratory tests.	Instruct client to: ■ Report nausea; vomiting; diarrhea; rash; jaundice; abdominal pain, tenderness, distention; or change in colour of stool ■ Adhere to laboratory testing regimen for liver function as ordered by healthcare provider

Evaluation of Outcome Criteria

Evaluate effectiveness of drug therapy by confirming that client goals and expected outcomes have been met (see "Planning").

See Table 19.4 (page 230) under "Triptans" for a list of drugs to which these nursing actions apply.

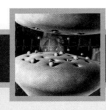

CHAPTER REVIEW

KEY CONCEPTS

The numbered key concepts provide a succinct summary of the important points from the corresponding numbered section within the chapter. If any of these points are not clear, refer to the numbered section within the chapter for review. Expanded versions can be found on the Companion Website.

19.1 The ways to assess and classify pain include acute or chronic and nociceptor or neuropathic.

19.2 Non-pharmacological techniques such as massage, biofeedback therapy, and meditation are often important adjuncts to effective pain management.

19.3 Neural mechanisms include the pain transmission via A-delta or C fibres and the release of substance P.

19.4 Opioids are natural or synthetic substances extracted from the poppy plant that exert their effects through interaction with mu and kappa receptors.

19.5 Opioids are the drugs of choice for severe pain. They also have other important therapeutic effects including dampening of the cough reflex and slowing of the motility of the GI tract.

19.6 Opioid antagonists may be used to reverse the symptoms of opioid toxicity or overdose, such as sedation and respiratory depression.

19.7 Opioid withdrawal can result in severe symptoms, and dependence is often treated with methadone maintenance.

19.8 Non-opioid analgesics, such as ASA, acetaminophen, and the selective COX-2 inhibitors, are effective in treating mild to moderate pain, inflammation, and fever.

19.9 Headaches are classified as tension headaches or migraines. Migraines may be preceded by auras, and symptoms include nausea and vomiting.

19.10 The goals of pharmacotherapy for migraine headaches are to stop migraines in progress and to prevent them from occurring. Triptans, ergot alkaloids, and a number of drugs from other classes are used for migraines.

REVIEW QUESTIONS

1 What questions should the nurse ask during an assessment to identify a client's type of pain? How would the nurse distinguish between acute pain and chronic pain? Which is the most difficult type of pain to treat?

2 What is a nociceptor? Describe how pain is regulated, considering substance P and endogenous opioids.

3 Distinguish between the following terms: *opioid, opiate,* and *narcotic.* Name the classes of opioid receptors and identify those that are connected with analgesia. Under what conditions should opioid drugs be used?

4 Name three common types of disorder controlled by non-opioid analgesics. Which non-opioid analgesic controls fever but not inflammation? Which control both fever and inflammation?

CRITICAL THINKING QUESTIONS

1. A client is on a client-controlled analgesia (PCA) pump to manage postoperative pain related to recent orthopedic surgery. The PCA is set to deliver morphine 6 mg per hour basal rate. The nurse discovers the client to be unresponsive with a respiratory rate of 8 and oxygen saturation of 84%. What is the nurse's initial response? What are the nurse's subsequent actions?

2. A 64-year-old client has had a long-standing history of migraine headaches as well as coronary artery disease, diabetes mellitus type 2, and hypertension. Upon review of the medical history, the nurse notes that this client has recently started on sumatriptan (Imitrex), prescribed by the client's new neurologist. What intervention and/or teaching should be done for this client?

3. A 58-year-old client with a history of a recent myocardial infarction is on beta-blocking medications and anticoagulant therapy. The client also has a history of arthritis and during a recent flare-up began taking ASA since this medication has helped in the past. What teaching or recommendation would the nurse have for this client?

EXPLORE
MediaLink

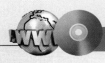

www.pearsoned.ca/adams-king

MEDIALINK DVD-ROM
- Audio Glossary
- CRNE Review
- Animations
  Mechanism of Action: Morphine
  Mechanism of Action: Oxycodone

COMPANION WEBSITE
- CRNE Review
- **Case Study:** Pain Management
- Dosage Calculations
- Nursing Process Focus Charts

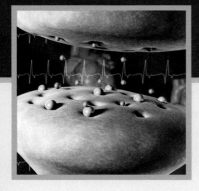

CHAPTER 20

Drugs for Local and General Anesthesia

DRUGS AT A GLANCE

LOCAL ANESTHETICS
Amides
  🔊*lidocaine (Xylocaine)*
Esters
Miscellaneous agents

GENERAL ANESTHETICS
Inhalation agents
Gasses
  🔊*nitrous oxide*
Volatile liquids
  🔊*halothane (Fluothane)*
Intravenous agents
Barbiturate and barbiturate-like agents
  🔊*thiopental (Pentothal)*
Opioids
Benzodiazepines

ADJUNCTS TO ANESTHESIA
Barbiturate and barbiturate-like agents
Opioids
Neuromuscular blocking agents
  🔊*succinylcholine (Quelicin)*
Miscellaneous agents

OBJECTIVES

After reading this chapter, the student should be able to do the following:

1. Identify drug classes used for local and general anesthesia.
2. Compare and contrast the five major clinical techniques for administering local anesthetics.
3. Describe differences in therapeutic action between the two major chemical classes of local anesthetics.
4. Explain why epinephrine and sodium hydroxide are sometimes included in local anesthetic cartridges.
5. Explain the therapeutic action of drugs used for general anesthesia with reference to effects on the CNS.
6. Compare and contrast the two primary ways that general anesthesia may be induced.
7. For each of the drug classes listed in Drugs at a Glance, identify a representative drug and explain its mechanism of action, primary actions, and important adverse effects.
8. Discuss the nurse's role in the pharmacological management of clients receiving anesthetics.
9. Describe and explain, based on pharmacological principles, the rationale for nursing assessment, planning, and interventions for clients receiving anesthetics.
10. Use the nursing process to care for clients receiving anesthetics.

MediaLink

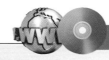 **www.pearsoned.ca/adams-king**

CRNE review, case studies, and other interactive resources for this chapter can be found on the Companion Website at **www.pearsoned.ca/adams-king**. Click on "Chapter 20" to select the activities for this chapter. For animations, more CRNE review questions, and an audio glossary, access the accompanying DVD-ROM in this textbook.

Anesthesia is a state achieved by administering drugs that cause a loss of sensation. Local anesthesia occurs when sensation is lost to a limited part of the body without loss of consciousness. General anesthesia requires different classes of drugs that cause loss of sensation to the entire body, usually resulting in a loss of consciousness. This chapter will examine drugs used for both local and general anesthesia.

LOCAL ANESTHESIA

Local anesthesia is loss of sensation to a relatively small part of the body without loss of consciousness. This technique may be necessary when a relatively brief dental or medical procedure is performed.

20.1 Regional Loss of Sensation Using Local Anesthetics

Although local anesthesia often results in a loss of sensation to a small, limited area, it sometimes affects relatively large portions of the body, such as an entire limb. Because of this, some local anesthetic treatments are more accurately called surface anesthesia or regional anesthesia, depending on how the drugs are administered and their resulting effects.

The five major routes for applying local anesthetics are shown in Figure 20.1. The method employed is dependent on the location and extent of the desired anesthesia. For example, some local anesthetics are applied topically before a needle stick or minor skin surgery. Others are used to block sensations to large areas such as a limb or the lower abdomen. The different methods of local and regional anesthesia are summarized in Table 20.1.

LOCAL ANESTHETICS

Local anesthetics are drugs that produce a rapid loss of sensation to a limited part of the body. They produce their therapeutic effect by blocking the entry of sodium ions into neurons.

20.2 Mechanism of Action of Local Anesthetics

The mechanism of action of local anesthetics is well known. Recall that the concentration of sodium ions is normally higher on the outside of neurons than on the inside. A rapid influx of sodium ions into cells is necessary for neurons to fire and conduct an action impulse.

Local anesthetics act by blocking sodium channels, as illustrated in Figure 20.2. Because the blocking of sodium channels is a non-selective process, both sensory and motor impulses are affected. Thus, both sensation and muscle activity will

TABLE 20.1	Methods of Local Anesthetic Administration	
Route	**Formulation/Method**	**Description**
topical (surface)	creams, sprays, suppositories, drops, and lozenges	applied to mucous membranes including the eyes, lips, gums, nasal membranes, and throat; very safe unless absorbed
infiltration (field block)	direct injection into tissue immediate to the surgical site	drug diffuses into tissue to block a specific group of nerves in a small area close to the surgical site
nerve block	direct injection into tissue that may be distant from the operation site	drug affects nerve bundles serving the surgical area; used to block sensation in a limb or large area of the face
spinal	injection into the CSF	drug affects large, regional area such as the lower abdomen and legs
epidural	injection into epidural space of spinal cord	most commonly used in obstetrics during labour and delivery

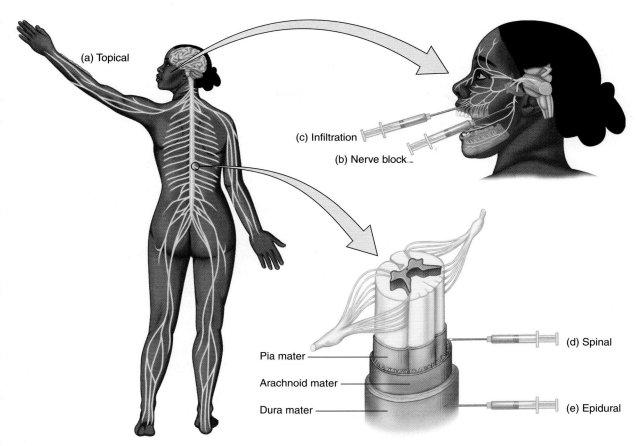

(a) Topical

(c) Infiltration

(b) Nerve block

Pia mater

Arachnoid mater

Dura mater

(d) Spinal

(e) Epidural

● **Figure 20.1** Techniques for applying local anesthesia: (a) topical; (b) nerve block; (c) infiltration; (d) spinal; (e) epidural

PHARMFACTS

Anesthesia and Anesthetics

- Thousands of people receive general anesthetics each year in Canada.
- General anesthetics are sometimes administered by a nurse anesthetist.
- The first medical applications of anesthetics were in 1842 with ether and in 1846 with nitrous oxide.
- Herbal products may interact with anesthetics; St. John's wort may intensify or prolong the effects of some opioids and anesthetics.

Sodium hydroxide is sometimes added to anesthetic solutions to increase the effectiveness of the anesthetic in regions that have extensive local infection or abscesses. Bacteria tend to acidify an infected site, and local anesthetics are less effective in an acidic environment. Adding alkaline substances such as sodium hydroxide or sodium bicarbonate neutralizes the region and creates a more favourable environment for the anesthetic.

temporarily diminish in the area treated with the local anesthetic. Because of their mechanism of action, local anesthetics are sometimes called sodium channel blockers.

During a medical or surgical procedure, it is essential that the duration of action of the anesthetic last long enough to complete the procedure. Small amounts of epinephrine are sometimes added to the anesthetic solution to constrict blood vessels in the immediate area where the local anesthetic is applied. In addition to reducing bleeding in the area, this keeps the anesthetic in the area longer, thus extending the duration of action of the drug. The addition of epinephrine to lidocaine, for example, increases the duration of the local anesthetic effect from 20 minutes to as long as 60 minutes. This is important for dental or surgical procedures that take longer than 20 minutes; otherwise, a second injection of the anesthetic would be necessary.

NATURAL THERAPIES

Clove and Anise as Natural Dental Remedies

One natural remedy for tooth pain is oil of clove. Extracted from the plant *Eugenia*, eugenol is the chemical in clove that is thought to produce its numbing effect. It works especially well for cavities. The herb is applied by soaking a piece of cotton and packing it around the gums close to the painful area. Dentists sometimes recommend it for temporary relief of a toothache. Clove oil has an antiseptic effect that has been reported to kill bacteria, fungi, and helminths.

Another natural remedy is oil of anise, from *Pimpinella anisum,* that is used for jaw pain caused by nerve pressure or gritting of teeth. Anise oil is an antispasmodic agent, which means it relaxes intense muscular pressure around the jaw angle, cheeks, and throat area. It has extra benefits in that it is also a natural expectorant, cough suppressant, and breath freshener. The pharmacological effects of anise are thought to be due to the chemical anethole, which is similar in structure to natural catecholamines.

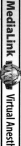

MediaLink   Virtual Anesthesia Textbook

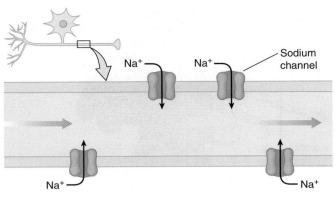

(a) Normal nerve conduction

(b) Local anesthetic blocking sodium channels

● **Figure 20.2** Mechanism of action of local anesthetics: (a) Na⁺ enters neuron for normal nerve conduction; (b) local anesthetic blocks sodium channels and prevents nerve conduction

20.3 Classification of Local Anesthetics

Local anesthetics are classified by their chemical structure; the two major classes are **esters** and **amides**. The terms *ester* and *amide* refer to types of chemical linkages found within the anesthetic molecules, as illustrated in Figure 20.3. Although esters and amides have equal efficacy, important differences exist. A small number of miscellaneous agents are neither esters nor amides. Local anesthetic agents are listed in Table 20.2.

Cocaine was the first local anesthetic widely used for medical procedures. Cocaine is a natural ester found in the leaves of the *Erythroxylon coca* plant native to the Andes Mountains of Peru. As late as the 1880s, cocaine was routinely used for eye surgery, nerve blocks, and spinal anesthesia. Although still available for local anesthesia, cocaine is a CDSA Schedule I drug and is rarely used therapeutically in Canada. The abuse potential of cocaine is discussed in Chapter 12.

Another ester, procaine, was the drug of choice for dental procedures from the mid-1900s to the 1960s, until the development of the amide anesthetics led to a significant decline in its use. One ester, benzocaine (Solarcaine, others) is used as a topical, OTC agent for treating a large number of painful conditions, including sunburn, insect bites, hemorrhoids, sore throat, and minor wounds.

Amides have largely replaced the esters because they produce fewer side effects and generally have a longer duration of action. Lidocaine is the most widely used amide for short surgical procedures requiring local anesthesia.

Adverse effects of local anesthetics are uncommon. Allergy is rare. When it does occur, it is often due to sulfites, which are added as preservatives to prolong the shelf life of the anesthetic, or to methylparaben, which may be added to retard bacterial growth in anesthetic solutions. Early signs of adverse effects of local anesthetics include symptoms of CNS stimulation such as restlessness or anxiety. Later effects, such as drowsiness and unresponsiveness, are due to CNS depression. Cardiovascular effects, including hypotension and dysrhythmias, are possible. Clients with a history of cardiovascular disease are often given forms of local anesthetics that contain no epinephrine in order to reduce the potential effects of this sympathomimetic on the heart and blood pressure. CNS and cardiovascular side effects are not expected unless the local anesthetic is absorbed rapidly or is accidentally injected directly into a blood vessel.

NURSING CONSIDERATIONS

The role of the nurse in local anesthetic administration involves careful monitoring of the client's condition and providing education as it relates to the prescribed drug

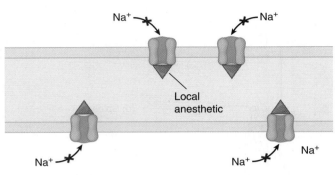

● **Figure 20.3** Chemical structure of ester and amide local anesthetics

TABLE 20.2   Select Local Anesthetics

Chemical Classification	Drug
esters	benzocaine (Solarcaine, others)
	chloroprocaine (Nesacaine)
	cocaine
	procaine (Novocain)
	tetracaine (Pontocaine)
amides	articaine (Septanest)
	bupivacaine (Marcaine)
	dibucaine (Nupercaine, Nupercainal)
	Pr lidocaine (Xylocaine)
	mepivacaine (Carbocaine)
	prilocaine (Citanest)
	ropivacaine (Naropin)
miscellaneous agents	dyclonine (Cepacol)
	pramoxine (Tronothane)

regimen. Although these medications are usually administered by the physician to anesthetize an area for medical procedures, the nurse often assists. The nurse's role may include preparing the area to be anesthetized and monitoring the effectiveness of the medication by assessing pain and comfort levels. Document the presence of broken skin, infection, burns, and wounds at the site of anesthetic administration.

LIFESPAN CONSIDERATIONS

Effects of Anesthesia on Children and Older Adults

Children are usually more sensitive to anesthesia than adults because their body systems are not fully developed. Therefore, medication dosages must be carefully calculated. Some drugs used for anesthesia, such as neuromuscular blockers, are not recommended for use by children under the age of 2 years.

Children who are undergoing surgery have fears and concerns about surgery and anesthesia. A child's age and developmental level play a role in his or her thoughts about receiving anesthesia. Children younger than 1 year are usually not concerned about what will be happening and will easily separate from family members. Fear of needles, the unknown, and being separated from primary caregivers begins to happen during the toddler stage and continues throughout childhood. Children are often perceptive to the anxieties of their parents; therefore, it is imperative that caregivers remain calm. Holding the child during induction of anesthesia might help alleviate fears. Local anesthetic creams can be applied to the skin to decrease the pain of needle sticks.

Older adults are also more affected by anesthesia than younger adults. Because of the changes in drug metabolism that occur with advancing age, these clients are particularly sensitive to the effects of barbiturate and general anesthetics. This increases the chance of side effects; therefore, elderly clients should be monitored closely. Older adults are also especially sensitive to the effects of local anesthetics. Sedative-hypnotic drugs used preoperatively may cause increased confusion or excitement in older adults.

Contraindications for these drugs include hypersensitivity to local anesthetics; sepsis and blood dyscrasias; untreated sinus bradycardia; and severe degrees of atrioventricular,

---

Pr PROTOTYPE DRUG | Lidocaine (Xylocaine)

ACTIONS AND USES

Lidocaine, the most frequently used injectable local anesthetic, acts by blocking neuronal pain impulses. It is injected as a nerve block for spinal and epidural anesthesia. Its actions are achieved by blocking sodium channels located within the membranes of neurons.

Lidocaine may be given IV, IM, or SC to treat dysrhythmias, as discussed in Chapter 25. A topical form is also available.

PHARMACOKINETICS

Lidocaine is well absorbed. It is widely distributed, crosses the blood-brain barrier and placenta, and concentrates in adipose tissue. Lidocaine is mostly metabolized by the liver. Its half-life is biphasic, with an initial phase from 7 to 30 minutes and a final phase from 1.5 to 2 hours.

ADMINISTRATION ALERTS

- Solutions of lidocaine containing preservatives or epinephrine are intended for local anesthesia only and must never be given parenterally for dysrhythmias.
- Topical lidocaine should not be applied to large skin areas or to broken or abraded areas as significant absorption may occur. It should not be allowed to come in contact with the eyes.
- For spinal or epidural block, use only preparations specifically labelled for IV use.
- Lidocaine is pregnancy category B.

ADVERSE EFFECTS AND INTERACTIONS

When used for anesthesia, side effects are uncommon. An early symptom of toxicity is CNS excitement, leading to irritability and confusion. Serious adverse effects include convulsions, respiratory depression, and cardiac arrest. Until the effect of the anesthetic diminishes, clients may injure themselves by biting or chewing areas of the mouth that have no sensation following a dental procedure.

Barbiturates may decrease activity of lidocaine. Increased effects of lidocaine occur if taken concurrently with cimetidine, quinidine, and beta-blockers. If lidocaine is used on a regular basis, its effectiveness may diminish when used with other medication.

 See the Companion Website for a Nursing Process Focus Chart specific to this drug.

MediaLink   Mechanism of Action: Lidocaine

sinoatrial, and intraventricular heart block in the absence of a pacemaker. Local anesthetics should be used with caution over large body areas, in clients with extensive surface trauma, and in severe skin disorders because the medication may be absorbed and result in systemic effects. Unless specifically formulated for optic use, local anesthetics should not be used on the eyes.

Although adverse reactions are rare, clients should be monitored for cardiac palpitations and difficulty breathing or swallowing. Assess vital signs during the procedure and report any changes immediately. The client should be monitored for reactions such as irritation, rash, and signs of CNS excitation such as restlessness or anxiety.

Clients should be instructed to use benzocaine cautiously on inflamed skin or mucous membranes as it may increase irritation. Lidocaine viscous is used to anesthetize the throat for some procedures, such as those that require an endoscope to be passed down the throat. After such procedures, the client should be monitored for return of the gag reflex before drinking or eating. Advise clients to wait at least 1 hour before eating.

GENERAL ANESTHESIA

General anesthesia is a loss of sensation occurring throughout the entire body, accompanied by a loss of consciousness. General anesthetics are applied when it is necessary for clients to remain still and without pain for a longer period of time than could be achieved with local anesthetics.

20.4 Characteristics of General Anesthesia

The goal of general anesthesia is to provide a rapid and complete loss of sensation. Signs of general anesthesia

NURSING PROCESS FOCUS Clients Receiving Local Anesthesia	
Assessment	**Potential Nursing Diagnoses/Identified Patterns**
Prior to administration: ■ Assess for allergies to amide-type local anesthetics. ■ Check for the presence of broken skin, infection, burns, and wounds where medication is to be applied. ■ Assess for character, duration, location, and intensity of pain where medication is to be applied.	■ Risk for aspiration ■ Risk for injury ■ Need for knowledge related to drug use
Planning: Client Goals and Expected Outcomes	
The client will: ■ Experience no pain during surgical procedure ■ Experience no side effects or adverse reactions to anesthesia	
Implementation	
Interventions (Rationales)	**Client Education/Discharge Planning**
■ Monitor for cardiovascular side effects. (These may occur if anesthetic is absorbed.) ■ Monitor skin or mucous membranes for infection or inflammation. (Condition could be worsened by drug.) ■ Monitor for length of effectiveness. (Local anesthetics are effective for 1 to 3 hours.) ■ Obtain information about and monitor use of other medications. ■ Provide for client safety. (There is potential for injury related to lack of sensation in the area being treated.) ■ Monitor for gag reflex. (Xylocaine viscous may interfere with swallowing reflex.)	■ Instruct client to report any unusual heart palpitations. If using medication on a regular basis, instruct client to see a healthcare provider regularly. ■ Instruct client to report irritation or increase in discomfort in areas where medication is used. ■ Instruct client to report any discomfort during procedure. ■ Instruct client to report use of any medication to healthcare provider. ■ Inform client about having no feeling in anesthetized area and taking extra caution to avoid injury, including heat-related injury. Instruct client to: ■ Not eat within 1 hour of administration ■ Not chew gum while any portion of mouth or throat is anesthetized to prevent biting injuries
Evaluation of Outcome Criteria	
Evaluate the effectiveness of drug therapy by confirming that client goals and expected outcomes have been met (see "Planning").	

See Table 20.2 (p. 239) for a list of drugs to which these nursing actions apply.

TABLE 20.3	Stages of General Anesthesia
Stage	**Characteristics**
1	Loss of pain: The client loses general sensation but may be awake. This stage proceeds until the client loses consciousness.
2	Excitement and hyperactivity: The client may be delirious and try to resist treatment. Heart rate and breathing may become irregular and blood pressure can increase. IV agents are administered here to calm the client.
3	Surgical anesthesia: Skeletal muscles become relaxed and delirium stabilizes. Cardiovascular and breathing activities stabilize. Eye movements slow and the client becomes still. Surgery is performed during this stage.
4	Paralysis of the medulla region in the brain (responsible for controlling respiratory and cardiovascular activity): If breathing or the heart stops, death could result. This stage is usually avoided during general anesthesia.

include total analgesia and loss of consciousness, memory, and body movement. Although these signs are similar to those of sleeping, general anesthesia and sleep are not exactly the same. General anesthetics depress all nervous activity in the brain, whereas sleeping depresses only very specific areas. In fact, some brain activity actually increases during sleep, as described in Chapter 14.

General anesthesia is rarely achieved with a single drug. Instead, multiple medications are used to rapidly induce unconsciousness, cause muscle relaxation, and maintain deep anesthesia. This approach, called **balanced anesthesia**, allows the dose of inhalation anesthetic to be lower, thus making the procedure safer for the client.

General anesthesia is a progressive process that occurs in distinct phases. The most efficacious medications can quickly induce all four stages, whereas others are only able to induce stage 1. Stage 3 is where most major surgery occurs; thus, it is called **surgical anesthesia**. When seeking surgical anesthesia, it is desirable to progress through stage 2 as rapidly as possible since this stage produces distressing symptoms. These stages are shown in Table 20.3.

GENERAL ANESTHETICS

General anesthetics are drugs that rapidly produce unconsciousness and total analgesia. These drugs are usually administered by the IV or inhalation routes. To supplement the effects of a general anesthetic, adjunct drugs are given before, during, and after surgery.

20.5 Pharmacotherapy with Inhaled General Anesthetics

There are two primary methods of inducing general anesthesia. Intravenous agents are usually administered first because they act within a few seconds. After the client loses consciousness, inhaled agents are used to maintain the anesthesia. During short surgical procedures or those requiring lower stages of anesthesia, the IV agents may be used alone.

Inhaled general anesthetics, shown in Table 20.4, may be gasses or volatile liquids. These agents produce their effects by preventing the flow of sodium into neurons in the CNS, thus delaying nerve impulses and producing a dramatic reduction in neural activity. The exact mechanism for how

this occurs is not exactly known, although it is likely that GABA receptors in the brain are activated. It is not the same mechanism known for local anesthetics. There is some evidence suggesting that the mechanism may be related to how some antiseizure drugs work; however, this is still not conclusive. There is not a specific receptor that binds to general anesthetics, and they do not seem to affect neurotransmitter release.

Gaseous General Anesthetics The only gas used routinely for anesthesia is nitrous oxide, commonly called laughing gas. Nitrous oxide is used for dental procedures and for brief obstetrical and surgical procedures. It may also be used in conjunction with other general anesthetics, making it possible to decrease their dosages with greater effectiveness.

Nitrous oxide should be used cautiously in myasthenia gravis as it may cause respiratory depression and prolonged hypnotic effects. Clients with cardiovascular disease, especially those with increased intracranial pressure, should be monitored carefully because the hypnotic effects of the drug may be prolonged or potentiated.

NURSING CONSIDERATIONS

Nitrous oxide has a rapid onset and recovery with minimal side effects (e.g., nausea and vomiting). The nurse's responsibilities are to determine the knowledge level of the client and to reassure the client to alleviate anxiety. Postoperatively, monitor the client's LOC, vital signs, and pain level and give medication to prevent nausea and vomiting. See "Nursing Process Focus: Clients Receiving General Anesthesia" p. 244 for more information, including specific teaching points.

TABLE 20.4	Inhaled General Anesthetics
Type	*Drug*
volatile liquid	desflurane (Suprane)
	enflurane (Ethrane)
	🅟 halothane (Fluothane)
	isoflurane (Forane)
	sevoflurane (Sevorane)
gas	🅟 nitrous oxide

Volatile Liquid General Anesthetics The volatile anesthetics are liquid at room temperature but are converted into a vapour and inhaled to produce their anesthetic effects. Commonly administered volatile agents are halothane, enflurane, and isoflurane. The most potent of these is halothane. Some general anesthetics enhance the sensitivity of the heart to drugs such as epinephrine, norepinephrine, dopamine, and serotonin. Most volatile liquids depress cardiovascular and respiratory function. Because it has less effect on the heart and does not damage the liver, isoflurane has become the most widely used inhalation anesthetic. The volatile anesthetics are excreted almost entirely by the lungs, through exhalation.

NURSING CONSIDERATIONS

General anesthesia is primarily used for lengthy surgical procedures, and it involves significant risks. The client should be informed that anesthesia will be administered by highly trained personnel, either an anesthesiologist or a nurse anesthetist, and that the nurse will have a major role in monitoring the client and ensuring client safety. A comprehensive assessment must be done in each phase of surgical experience. General preoperative information should be obtained such as vital signs, lab tests, health history, level of knowledge concerning the procedure, and the presence of anxiety. Preoperatively, the client should be assessed for the use of alcohol or other CNS depressants within the previous 24 hours as these substances will enhance anesthetic effects. Information concerning the use of other medications should also be obtained.

Use of halothane is contraindicated in clients who have had this drug within the previous 14 to 21 days as it can cause halothane hepatitis if used frequently. Halothane is also contraindicated in pregnancy (category D) and in clients with diminished hepatic functioning as it can be hepatotoxic. Caution should be used in clients with cardiac conditions, especially bradycardia and dysrhythmias, as the medication decreases blood pressure and sensitizes the myocardium to catecholamines, which can lead to serious dysrhythmias.

In the immediate postoperative period, monitor the client for side effects of the general anesthesia such as nausea and vomiting, CNS depression, respiratory difficulty, and vital sign changes. Also monitor for complications related to the procedure, such as bleeding or impeding shock.

See "Nursing Process Focus: Clients Receiving General Anesthesia" on page 244 for more details, including specific teaching points.

IV ANESTHETICS

20.6 Pharmacotherapy with IV Anesthetics

Intravenous anesthetics, shown in Table 20.5, are important supplements to general anesthesia. Although occasionally used alone, they are often administered with inhaled general anesthetics. Concurrent administration of IV and inhaled anesthetics allows the dose of the inhaled agent to be reduced, thus lowering the potential for serious side effects. Furthermore, when combined, IV anesthetics provide more analgesia and muscle relaxation than could be provided by the inhaled anesthetic alone. When IV anesthetics are administered without other anesthetics, they are generally reserved for medical procedures that take less than 15 minutes.

Drugs employed as IV anesthetics include barbiturates, opioids, and benzodiazepines. Opioids offer the advantage of superior analgesia. Combining the opioid fentanyl with the antipsychotic agent droperidol produces a state known

---

Pr PROTOTYPE DRUG | Halothane (Fluothane)

ACTIONS AND USES

Halothane produces a potent level of surgical anesthesia that is rapid in onset. Although potent, halothane does not produce as much muscle relaxation or analgesia as other volatile anesthetics. Therefore, halothane is primarily used with other anesthetic agents including muscle relaxants and analgesics. Nitrous oxide is sometimes combined with halothane. Clients recover from anesthesia rapidly after halothane is discontinued.

PHARMACOKINETICS

Halothane is rapidly absorbed. It is widely distributed and crosses the blood-brain barrier. Elimination is primarily by the lungs and kidneys. Half-life is variable.

ADVERSE EFFECTS AND INTERACTIONS

Halothane moderately sensitizes the heart muscle to epinephrine; therefore, dysrhythmias are a concern. This agent lowers blood pressure and respiration rate. It also increases the risk of aspirating stomach contents into the lungs. Because of potential hepatotoxicity, use of halothane has declined.

Malignant hyperthermia is rare but can be a fatal adverse effect triggered by all inhalation anesthetics. It causes muscle rigidity and severe temperature elevation (up to 43°C). This risk is greatest when halothane is used with succinylcholine.

Levodopa taken concurrently increases the level of dopamine in the CNS and should be discontinued 6 to 8 hours before halothane administration.

Skeletal muscle weakness, respiratory depression, or apnea may occur if halothane is administered concurrently with polymyxins, lincomycin, or aminoglycosides.

 See the Companion Website for a Nursing Process Focus Chart specific to this drug.

Pr PROTOTYPE DRUG | Nitrous Oxide

ACTIONS AND USES

The main action of nitrous oxide is analgesia caused by suppression of pain mechanisms in the CNS. It causes cerebral vasodilation and increased cerebral blood flow. This agent has a low potency and does not produce complete loss of consciousness or profound relaxation of skeletal muscle. Because nitrous oxide does not induce surgical anesthesia (stage 3), it is commonly combined with other surgical anesthetic agents. Nitrous oxide is ideal for dental procedures because the client remains conscious and can follow instructions while experiencing full analgesia.

PHARMACOKINETICS

Nitrous oxide is rapidly absorbed. It is widely distributed and crosses the blood-brain barrier and placenta. (It can cause CNS depression in the fetus.) Elimination is primarily by the lungs and kidneys. Half-life is variable.

ADMINISTRATION ALERT

- Establish an IV if one is not already in place in case emergency medications are needed.

ADVERSE EFFECTS

When used in low to moderate doses, nitrous oxide produces few adverse effects. At higher doses, clients exhibit some adverse signs of stage 2 anesthesia such as anxiety, excitement, and combativeness. Lowering the inhaled dose will quickly reverse these adverse effects. As nitrous oxide is exhaled, the client may temporarily have some difficulty breathing at the end of a procedure. Nausea and vomiting following the procedure are more common with nitrous oxide than with other inhalation anesthetics. Nitrous oxide has the potential to be abused (sometimes by medical personnel) because of the relaxed, sedated state that it produces.

See the Companion Website for a Nursing Process Focus Chart specific to this drug.

---

as **neurolept analgesia**. In this state, clients are conscious but insensitive to pain and unconnected with surroundings. The premixed combination of these two agents is marketed as Innovar. A similar conscious, dissociated state is produced with ketamine. For this reason, ketamine has been misused as a **date rape drug** and is now reclassified from a Schedule F to a CDSA Schedule I drug in Canada. Clients who receive these drugs therapeutically or illicitly may express awareness of events that occurred while under the drug's influence, yet at the same time have a sense of uncertainty and unreality about them. Nurses play an important role in assessing and educating clients who may unwittingly be exposed to these drugs.

NURSING CONSIDERATIONS

The role of the nurse in drug therapy with IV anesthetics involves careful monitoring of the client's condition and providing education as it relates to the anesthetic in use. IV sedation is used to decrease anxiety and fear secondary to confinement of the mask used for inhalation anesthesia. A thorough, complete assessment must be completed prior to selecting an anesthetic or combination of anesthetics. Clients may be given medications other than anesthesia during preoperative, perioperative, or postoperative periods, including antianxiety agents, sedatives, analgesics, opioids, and anticholinergics. Obtain a complete medical history from the client. IV anesthetics are contraindicated in clients with drug sensitivity since allergic reactions can result, ranging from hives to respiratory arrest. Because they are administered intravenously, suitability of an IV access site should be assessed.

Clients with cardiovascular disease should be monitored carefully as IV anesthetics can cause depression of the

TABLE 20.5   Intravenous Anesthetics

Chemical Classification	Drug
barbiturate and barbiturate-like agents	propofol (Diprivan)
	thiopental sodium (Pentothal)
benzodiazepines	diazepam (Valium)
	lorazepam (Ativan)
	midazolam hydrochloride (Apo-Midazolam)
opioids	alfentanil hydrochloride (Alfenta)
	fentanyl citrate (Duragesic)
	remifentanil hydrochloride (Ultiva)
	sufentanil citrate (Sufenta)
others	ketamine (Ketalar)

myocardium, leading to dysrhythmias. Clients with respiratory disorders should also be monitored carefully because respiratory depression may result in high levels of anesthetic in the blood. Thiopental should be used with caution in clients with seizure disorders, increased intracranial pressure, neurological disorders, and myxedema.

The use of general anesthetics results in CNS depression. During the postoperative period, monitor the client for vital sign changes, hallucinations, confusion, and excitability. Other side effects or reactions that should be assessed include respiratory difficulties, shivering and trembling, nausea or vomiting, headache, and somnolence. Preoperative teaching is vital to understanding the anesthetic and the entire surgical experience. It also helps allay fears and anxiety of the client and caregivers.

See "Nursing Process Focus: Clients Receiving General Anesthesia" for specific teaching points.

Pr PROTOTYPE DRUG | Thiopental (Pentothal)

ACTIONS AND USES

Thiopental is the oldest IV anesthetic. It is used for brief medical procedures or to rapidly induce unconsciousness prior to administering inhaled anesthetics. It is classified as an ultrashort-acting barbiturate, having an onset time of less than 30 seconds and a duration of only 10 to 30 minutes. Unlike some anesthetic agents, it has very low analgesic properties.

ADMINISTRATION ALERT

- Thiopental is pregnancy category C.

PHARMACOKINETICS

Thiopental is rapidly absorbed. It is widely distributed. It is metabolized in the liver and forms an active metabolite, pentobarbital. Elimination is by the kidneys. Half-life is 3 to 11.5 hours.

ADVERSE EFFECTS AND INTERACTIONS

Like other barbiturates, thiopental can produce severe respiratory depression when used in high doses. It is used with caution in clients with cardiovascular disease because of its ability to depress the myocardium and cause dysrhythmias. Clients may experience emergence delirium postoperatively. This causes hallucinations, confusion, and excitability.

Thiopental interacts with many other drugs. For example, use of CNS depressants potentiate respiratory and CNS depression. Phenothiazines increase the risk of hypotension.

Use with caution with herbal supplements, such as kava and valerian, which may potentiate sedation.

 See the Companion Website for a Nursing Process Focus Chart specific to this drug.

NURSING PROCESS FOCUS   Clients Receiving General Anesthesia

Assessment	Potential Nursing Diagnoses/Identified Patterns
Prior to administration: ■ Obtain complete health history including allergies, drug history, and possible drug interactions. ■ Assess for presence/history of severe respiratory, cardiac, renal, or liver disorders. ■ Obtain baseline vital signs. ■ Assess for any musculoskeletal disorders or injuries that may impair movement and require special positioning during anesthesia. ■ Obtain blood work: complete blood count and chemistry panel. ■ Assess client's knowledge of procedure and level of anxiety.	■ Anxiety related to surgical procedure ■ Impaired gas exchange ■ Need for knowledge related to drug use ■ Nausea, related to drug side effect ■ Disturbed sensory perception ■ Ineffective breathing pattern ■ Decreased cardiac output

Planning: Client Goals and Expected Outcomes

The client will:
- Experience adequate anesthesia during surgical procedure
- Experience no side effects or adverse reaction to anesthesia
- Demonstrate an understanding of perioperative procedures

Implementation

Interventions (Rationales)	Client Education/Discharge Planning
■ Preoperatively, assess knowledge level of pre- and postoperative procedures. Ensure that client has accurate information and questions are answered. (Teaching will reduce client anxiety.)	■ Give pre- and postoperative instructions. ■ Explain what the client will see, hear, and feel prior to surgery. ■ Explain the recovery room process. ■ Explain what the client and family will see and hear postoperatively. ■ Take client on tour of operative facilities, if possible.
■ Preoperatively, assess emotional state. (Clients who are fearful or extremely anxious may be more difficult to induce and maintain under anesthesia.) ■ Monitor preoperative status.	■ Instruct client about using stress-reduction techniques such as deep breathing, imagery, and distraction. Instruct client to: ■ Remain NPO as ordered prior to surgery to prevent risk of aspiration, nausea, and vomiting ■ Stop taking medications 24 hours prior to surgery as ordered by healthcare provider ■ Refrain from alcohol 24 hours prior to surgery

continued

NURSING PROCESS FOCUS	Clients Receiving General Anesthesia *(Continued)*
Interventions (Rationales)	**Client Education/Discharge Planning**
■ Postoperatively, monitor for respiratory difficulty and adequate O_2-CO_2 exchange. (Anesthetics cause respiratory depression.) ■ Monitor recovery from anesthesia. Evaluate LOC, nausea, vomiting, and pain. ■ Monitor vital signs. (Respiratory status may be impaired leading to prolonged apnea, respiratory depression, and cyanosis. Blood pressure may drop to shock levels.)	■ Inform client to report shortness of breath, difficulty breathing, or dizziness. ■ Instruct client about possible side effects and to report any discomfort immediately. ■ Advise client to report heart palpitations, dizziness, difficulty breathing, or faintness.

Evaluation of Outcome Criteria
Evaluate the effectiveness of drug therapy by confirming that client goals and expected outcomes have been met (see "Planning").
See Tables 20.4 (p. 241) and 20.5 (p. 243) for lists of drugs to which these nursing actions apply.

20.7 Non-Anesthetic Drugs as Adjuncts to Surgery

A number of drugs are used either to complement the effects of general anesthetics or to treat anticipated side effects of the anesthesia. These agents, shown in Table 20.6, are called adjuncts to anesthesia. They may be given prior to, during, or after surgery.

The preoperative drugs given to relieve anxiety and provide mild sedation include barbiturates and benzodiazepines. Opioids such as morphine may be given to counteract pain that the client will experience after surgery. Anticholinergics such as atropine may be administered to dry secretions and to suppress the bradycardia caused by some anesthetics.

During surgery, the primary adjuncts are the **neuromuscular blockers**. So that surgical procedures can be carried out safely, it is necessary to administer drugs that cause skeletal muscles to totally relax. Administration of these drugs also allows the amount of anesthetic to be reduced. Neuromuscular blocking agents are classified as depolarizing blockers or non-depolarizing blockers. The only depolarizing blocker is succinylcholine, which works by binding to acetylcholine receptors at neuromuscular junctions to cause total skeletal muscle relaxation. Succinylcholine is used in surgery for ease of tracheal intubation. Mivacurium is the shortest acting of the non-depolarizing blockers, whereas tubocurarine is a longer acting neuromuscular blocking agent. The non-depolarizing blockers cause muscle paralysis by competing with acetylcholine for cholinergic receptors at neuromuscular junctions. Once on the receptor, the non-polarizing blockers prevent muscle contraction. When drugs that decrease sensation and cause skeletal muscles to relax are administered, the client is unable to resist being positioned in a way that would otherwise cause discomfort and perhaps injury. It is important that the nurse assess for and document any musculoskeletal disorders or injuries and limitations to joint movement that may require special positioning during anesthesia.

Postoperative drugs include analgesics for pain and antiemetics such as promethazine or ondansetron for the nausea and vomiting that sometimes occur during recovery

TABLE 20.6	Select Adjuncts to Anesthesia
Chemical Classification	**Drug**
barbiturate and barbiturate-like agents	butabarbital sodium (Butisol)
	pentobarbital (Nembutal)
	secobarbital (Novo-Secobarb)
opioids	alfentanil hydrochloride (Alfenta)
	fentanyl citrate (Duragesic)
	fentanyl/droperidol (Innovar)
	remifentanil hydrochloride (Ultiva)
	sufentanil citrate (Sufenta)
miscellaneous agents	bethanechol chloride (Urecholine): anticholinergic
	droperidol (Inapsine): dopamine blocker
	promethazine (Phenergan): dopamine blocker
	⊕ succinylcholine chloride (Quelicin): neuromuscular blocker
	tubocurarine: neuromuscular blocker

from the anesthetic. Occasionally a cholinergic such as bethanechol is administered to stimulate the smooth muscle of the bladder wall to contract to expel urine and the smooth muscle of the bowel to begin peristalsis following surgery.

NURSING CONSIDERATIONS

The role of the nurse in neuromuscular blocker therapy involves careful monitoring of the client's condition and providing education as it relates to the drug therapy. Neuromuscular blocking agents are used so that the client experiences complete skeletal muscle relaxation during the surgical procedure. Continuous use is not recommended because of potential side effects. Clients should be aware that these drugs are used only in a controlled acute care setting, usually surgery, by a skilled professional.

In preparation for use of succinylcholine, assess for the presence/history of hepatic or renal dysfunction, neuro-

muscular disease, fractures, myasthenia gravis, malignant hyperthermia, glaucoma, and penetrating eye injuries. Use of this drug is contraindicated in these conditions. Use in children under 2 years is contraindicated because it can cause dysrhythmias and malignant hyperthermia.

Mivacurium is used for intubation and is contraindicated for persons with renal or hepatic disease, fluid and electrolyte imbalances, neuromuscular disorders, respiratory disease, and obesity. It should be used cautiously in older adults and children. It should not be used during pregnancy or lactation. An anesthesiologist may administer it during cesarean section.

Prior to use of any neuromuscular blocker, assess physical status to rule out potential expected problems, including vital signs, reflexes, muscle tone and response, pupil size and reactivity, ECG, lung sounds, bowel sounds, affect, and LOC. Monitor for a decrease in blood pressure, tachycardia, prolonged apnea, bronchospasm, respiratory depression, paralysis, and hypersensitivity.

Pr PROTOTYPE DRUG | Succinylcholine (Quelicin)

ACTIONS AND USES

Like the natural neurotransmitter acetylcholine, succinylcholine acts on cholinergic receptor sites at neuromuscular junctions. At first, depolarization occurs and skeletal muscles contract. After repeated contractions, however, the membrane is unable to repolarize as long as the drug stays on the receptor. Effects are first noted as muscle weakness and muscle spasms. Eventually paralysis occurs. Succinylcholine is rapidly broken down by the enzyme pseudocholinesterase; when the IV infusion is stopped, the duration of action is only a few minutes. Use of succinylcholine reduces the amount of general anesthetic needed for procedures.

ADMINISTRATION ALERT

- Succinylcholine is pregnancy category C.

PHARMACOKINETICS

Succinylcholine is widely distributed. It is metabolized mostly by the liver. A small amount is excreted unchanged in the urine. Its half-life is unknown.

ADVERSE EFFECTS AND INTERACTIONS

Succinylcholine can cause complete paralysis of the diaphragm and intercostal muscles; thus, mechanical ventilation is necessary during surgery. Bradycardia and respiratory depression are expected adverse effects. If doses are high, the ganglia are affected, causing tachycardia, hypotension, and urinary retention. Clients with certain genetic mutations may experience rapid onset of extremely high fever with muscle rigidity—a serious condition known as malignant hyperthermia.

Additive skeletal muscle blockade will occur if succinylcholine is given concurrently with clindamycin, aminoglycosides, furosemide, lithium, quinidine, or lidocaine.

Increased effect of succinylcholine may occur if given concurrently with phenothiazines, oxytocin, promazine, tacrine, or thiazide diuretics. Decreased effect of succinylcholine occurs if given with diazepam.

If this drug is given concurrently with halothane or nitrous oxide, an increased risk of bradycardia, dysrhythmias, sinus arrest, apnea, and malignant hyperthermia exists. If succinylcholine is given concurrently with cardiac glycosides, there is increased risk of cardiac dysrhythmias. If narcotics are given concurrently with succinylcholine, there is increased risk of bradycardia and sinus arrest.

 See the Companion Website for a Nursing Process Focus Chart specific to this drug.

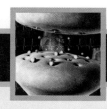

CHAPTER REVIEW

KEY CONCEPTS

The numbered key concepts provide a succinct summary of the important points from the corresponding numbered section within the chapter. If any of these points are not clear, refer to the numbered section within the chapter for review. Expanded versions can be found on the Companion Website.

20.1 Regional loss of sensation is achieved by administering local anesthetics topically or through the infiltration, nerve block, spinal, or epidural methods.

20.2 Local anesthetics act by blocking sodium channels in neurons. Epinephrine is sometimes added to prolong the duration of anesthetic action.

20.3 Local anesthetics are classified as amides or esters. The amides, such as lidocaine, have generally replaced the esters due to their greater safety.

20.4 General anesthesia produces a complete loss of sensation accompanied by loss of consciousness. This is usually achieved through the use of multiple medications.

20.5 Inhaled general anesthetics are used to maintain surgical anesthesia. Some, such as nitrous oxide, have low efficacy, while others, such as halothane, can induce deep anesthesia.

20.6 IV anesthetics are used either alone, for short procedures, or to supplement inhalation anesthetics.

20.7 Numerous non-anesthetic medications, including opioids, antianxiety agents, barbiturates, and neuromuscular blockers, are administered as adjuncts to surgery.

REVIEW QUESTIONS

1 What is local anesthesia? Name the five general methods of local and regional anesthesia.

2 How does a local anesthetic work? How does the anesthetic action of lidocaine given with epinephrine differ from that of lidocaine without epinephrine?

3 What is the role of IV anesthetics in surgical anesthesia? Why are these drugs not used alone for general anesthesia?

4 What role do adjunct medications serve in anesthesia?

CRITICAL THINKING QUESTIONS

1. An elderly client requires local anesthesia during suturing of a 3 cm laceration to the distal fourth metacarpal of the left hand. The healthcare provider requests lidocaine (Xylocaine) 1% with epinephrine. What is the nurse's response?

2. A client who has a history of heart failure is on digoxin (Lanoxin) and has a history of mild renal failure. The healthcare provider requests the nurse to prepare succinyl-

choline IV as an anesthetic for this client who is having an outpatient procedure. What is the nurse's response?

3. The nurse is reviewing the chart of a client who has recently had abdominal surgery. The client is 67 years old and has been on digoxin (Lanoxin), ibuprofen, and Maalox daily. Which of these medications is an indication that this client may require closer monitoring (and why)? What are some nursing priorities?

EXPLORE
MediaLink

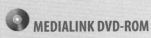

www.pearsoned.ca/adams-king

MEDIALINK DVD-ROM

- Audio Glossary
- CRNE Review
- Animation
  Mechanism of Action: Lidocaine

COMPANION WEBSITE

- CRNE Review
- **Case Study:** Client receiving local anesthetic
- Dosage Calculations
- Nursing Process Focus Charts

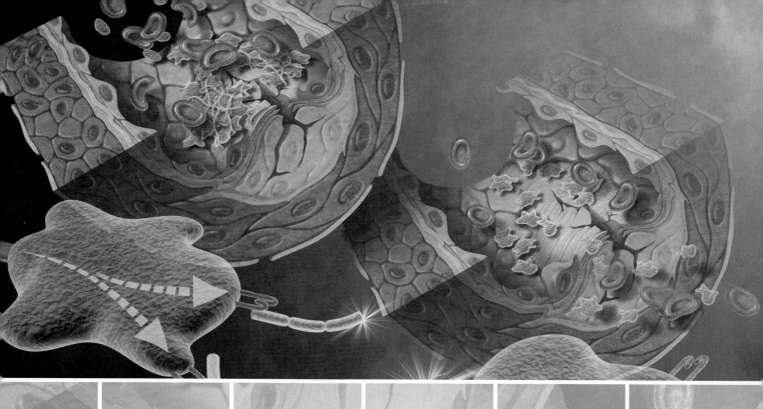

Unit 5

The Cardiovascular and Respiratory Systems

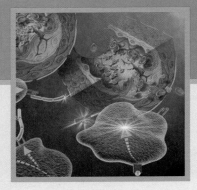

CHAPTER 21

Drugs for Hypertension

DRUGS AT A GLANCE

DIURETICS
> hydrochlorothiazide (HCTZ, Urozide)

CALCIUM CHANNEL BLOCKERS
> nifedipine (Adalat, Apo-Nifed)

DRUGS AFFECTING THE RENIN-ANGIOTENSIN SYSTEM
Angiotensin-converting enzyme (ACE) inhibitors
> enalapril (Vasotec)

Angiotensin II receptor blockers

ADRENERGIC AGENTS
Alpha-blockers
> doxazosin (Cardura)

Beta-blockers
Centrally acting agents

DIRECT VASODILATORS
> hydralazine (Apo-Hydralazine)

OBJECTIVES

After reading this chapter, the student should be able to do the following:

1. Identify drug classes used for treating hypertension.
2. Explain the therapeutic action of each class of antihypertensive drug in relation to the pathophysiology of hypertension.
3. Discuss the role of the nurse regarding the non-pharmacological control of hypertension through client teaching.
4. Describe the nurse's role in the pharmacological management of clients receiving drugs for hypertension.
5. For each of the drug classes listed in Drugs at a Glance, identify a representative drug and explain its mechanism of action, therapeutic effects, and important adverse effects.
6. Describe and explain, based on pharmacological principles, the rationale for nursing assessment, planning, and interventions for clients with hypertension.
7. Use the nursing process to care for clients receiving drug therapy for hypertension.

MediaLink

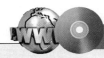

www.pearsoned.ca/adams-king

KEY TERMS

Cardiovascular disease, which includes all conditions affecting the heart and blood vessels, is the most common cause of death in Canada. **Hypertension** (HTN), or high blood pressure, is the most common of the cardiovascular diseases. About one in five Canadians has hypertension, yet more than 40% don't know they have it. Although mild HTN can often be controlled with lifestyle modifications, moderate to severe HTN requires pharmacotherapy. Because nurses encounter numerous clients with this disease, having an understanding of the underlying principles of antihypertensive therapy is critical. Nurses play a vital role in teaching the client safe principles of pharmacotherapy as it relates to hypertension.

21.1 Risk Factors for Hypertension

Hypertension having no identifiable cause is called primary, idiopathic, or essential. This classification accounts for 90% of all cases. Secondary hypertension, accounting for only 10% of all cases, is caused by identifiable factors such as excessive secretion of epinephrine by the adrenal glands or by narrowing of the renal arteries.

Because chronic hypertension may produce no identifiable symptoms for as long as 10 to 20 years, many people are not aware of their condition. Convincing clients to control their diets, buy costly medications, and take drugs on a regular basis when they are feeling healthy is an important, yet challenging task for the nurse. In addition, many clients do not take HTN medications because of their undesirable side effects. Failure to control this condition, however, can result in serious consequences. Prolonged or improperly controlled HTN can damage small blood vessels, leading to accelerated narrowing of the arteries that can result in angina, myocardial infarction, and peripheral vascular disease. One of the most serious consequences of chronic hypertension is that the heart must work harder to pump blood to the various organs and tissues. This excessive cardiac workload can cause the heart to fail and the lungs to fill with fluid, a condition known as heart failure (HF). Drug therapy of HF is covered in Chapter 24.

PHARMFACTS

Hypertension Statistics

- Approximately 5 million, or one in five, Canadians have high blood pressure, but about 40% of them are not aware of their condition.
- Only about 16% of those diagnosed have adequate control of their blood pressure (BP).
- More than one-half of people with hypertension require two or more drugs, and about one-fifth require three or more drugs to achieve control of their BP.
- The World Health Organization predicts a 60% increase in the number of adults with hypertension over the next 20 years.
- An obese person is three to five times more likely to develop hypertension than someone of a healthy weight.
- People with diabetes are two to three times more likely to have hypertension than those who do not have diabetes.
- Hypertension is more prevalent in Aboriginal Peoples and those of African or South Asian descent.
- Hypertension increases with age, with the following approximate incidences:
  - 30% of those over age 50
  - 64% of men over age 65
  - 75% of women over age 75
- Hypertension is the most common complication of pregnancy.

Source: Canadian Hypertension Society, www.hypertension.ca/chs/; Heart and Stroke Foundation, www.heartandstroke.ca.

Damage to the vessels that supply blood and oxygen to the brain can result in transient ischemic attacks and cerebral vascular accidents or strokes. Renal damage and retinal damage are also common sequelae of sustained hypertension.

The death rate from cardiovascular-related diseases has dropped significantly over the past 20 years due, in large part, to the recognition and treatment of hypertension, as well as the acceptance of healthier lifestyle habits. Early treatment is essential as the long-term cardiovascular damage caused by hypertension may be irreversible if the disease is allowed to progress unchecked.

21.2 Factors Responsible for Blood Pressure

Although many factors can influence blood pressure, the three factors truly responsible for creating the pressure are cardiac output, peripheral resistance, and blood volume. These are shown in Figure 21.1.

The volume of blood pumped per minute is called the **cardiac output**. The higher the cardiac output, the higher the blood pressure. Cardiac output is determined by heart rate and **stroke volume**, which is the amount of blood pumped by a ventricle in one contraction. This is important to pharmacology because drugs that change the cardiac output, stroke volume, or heart rate have the potential to influence a client's blood pressure.

As blood flows at high speeds through the vascular system, it exerts force against the walls of the vessels. Although the inner layer of the blood vessel lining, known as the **endothelium**, is extremely smooth, this friction reduces the velocity of the blood. This turbulence-induced friction in the arteries is called **peripheral resistance**. Arteries have smooth muscle in their walls which, when constricted, will cause the inside diameter (lumen) to become smaller, thus creating more resistance and higher pressure. A large number of drugs affect vascular smooth muscle, causing vessels to constrict and raising blood pressure. Other drugs cause the smooth muscle to relax, thereby opening the lumen and lowering blood pressure. Chapter 13 presents the role of the autonomic nervous system in controlling peripheral resistance.

The third factor responsible for blood pressure is the total amount of blood in the vascular system, or blood volume.

While the average person maintains a relatively constant blood volume of approximately 5 L, this can change due to many regulatory factors and certain disease states. More blood in the vascular system will exert additional pressure on the walls of the arteries and raise blood pressure. For example, high sodium diets may cause water to be retained by the body, thus increasing blood volume and raising blood pressure. On the other hand, substances known as **diuretics** can cause fluid loss through urination, thus decreasing blood volume and lowering blood pressure. Loss of blood volume during hemorrhage or shock also lowers blood pressure (see Chapter 27).

21.3 Normal Regulation of Blood Pressure

It is critical that the body maintain a normal range of blood pressure and that it have the ability to safely and rapidly change pressure as it proceeds through daily activities such as sleep and exercise. Low blood pressure can cause dizziness and lack of adequate urine formation, whereas excessively high pressure can cause vessels to rupture. How the body maintains homeostasis of blood pressure during periods of change is shown in Figure 21.2.

Blood pressure is regulated on a minute-to-minute basis by a cluster of neurons in the medulla oblongata called the **vasomotor centre**. Nerves travel from the vasomotor centre to the arteries, where the smooth muscle is instructed to either constrict (raise blood pressure) or relax (lower blood pressure). Potent vasoconstrictors, such as angiotensin II and endothelin, and potent vasodilators, such as nitric oxide and vasodilator prostaglandins, that are released in the vascular endothelium exert local effects on blood pressure.

Receptors in the aorta and the internal carotid artery act as sensors to provide the vasomotor centre with vital information on conditions in the vascular system. **Baroreceptors** have the ability to sense pressure within large vessels, and **chemoreceptors** recognize pH and levels of oxygen and carbon dioxide in the blood. The vasomotor centre reacts to information from baroreceptors and chemoreceptors by raising or lowering blood pressure accordingly.

Emotions can also have a profound effect on blood pressure. Anger and stress can cause blood pressure to rise,

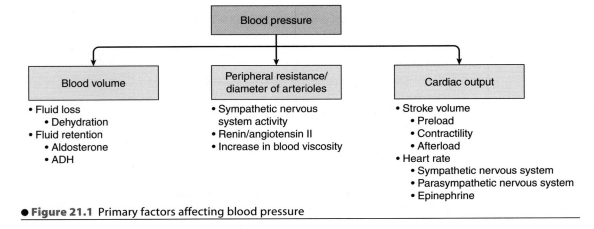

● **Figure 21.1** Primary factors affecting blood pressure

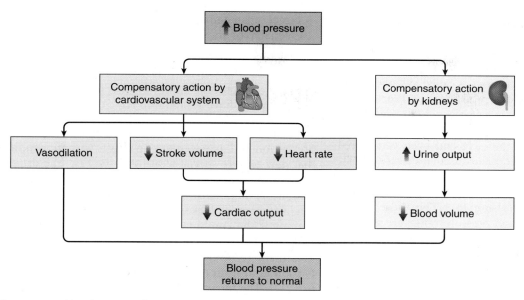

● **Figure 21.2** Blood pressure homeostasis

whereas mental depression and lethargy may cause it to fall. Strong emotions, if present for a prolonged time period, may become important contributors to chronic hypertension.

A number of hormones and other endogenous agents affect blood pressure on a daily basis. When given as medications, some of these agents may have a profound effect on blood pressure. For example, injection of epinephrine or norepinephrine will immediately raise blood pressure. **Antidiuretic hormone (ADH)** is a potent vasoconstrictor that can also increase blood pressure by raising blood volume. The **renin-angiotensin system** is particularly important in the pharmacotherapy of hypertension and is discussed later in this chapter. A summary of the various nervous and hormonal factors influencing blood pressure is shown in Figure 21.3.

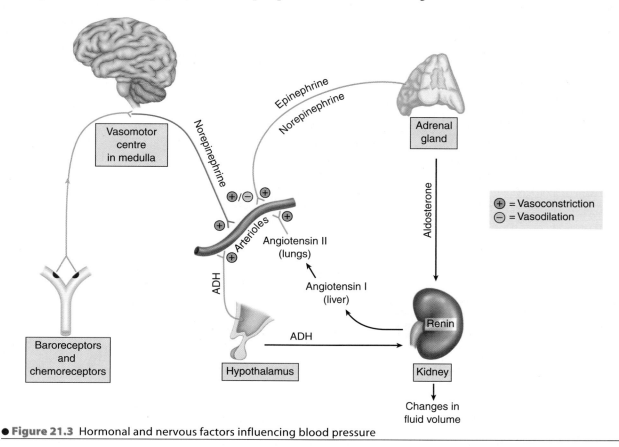

● **Figure 21.3** Hormonal and nervous factors influencing blood pressure

21.4 Indications for Hypertension Therapy

When the ventricles of the heart contract and eject blood, the pressure created in the arteries is called **systolic blood pressure**. When the ventricles relax and the heart is not ejecting blood, pressure in the arteries will fall, and this is called **diastolic blood pressure**. For many years, blood pressure measuring 120/80 mm Hg had been considered optimal. However, the risk of cardiovascular disease (CVD) beginning at 115/75 mm Hg *doubles* with each increment of 20/10 mm Hg. Individuals with prehypertension are at increased risk for progression to HTN; those in the 130–139/80–89 mm Hg blood pressure range are at twice the risk of developing hypertension as those with lower values. Individuals with systolic blood pressure of 120 to 139 mm Hg or diastolic blood pressure of 80 to 89 mm Hg may be considered as *prehypertensive*. These clients should be strongly encouraged by the nurse to adopt health-promoting lifestyle modifications to prevent CVD.

The diagnosis of chronic HTN is rarely made on a single blood pressure measurement. A client having a sustained systolic pressure of 140 to 159 mm Hg or diastolic pressure of 90 to 99 mm Hg, after multiple measurements made over several clinic visits, is said to have stage 1 hypertension. In low-risk patients with stage 1 hypertension, lifestyle modification can be the sole therapy. The *Canadian Hypertension Education Program Recommendations* (2007) state that pharmacotherapy for HTN is indicated in clients with any of the following:

- Other cardiovascular risk factors, if blood pressure remains equal to or above 140/90 mm Hg with lifestyle modification

- Target organ damage (e.g., proteinuria), if blood pressure is equal to or above 140/90 mm Hg
- Known atherosclerotic disease (e.g., previous stroke), even if blood pressure is normal
- Diabetes or chronic kidney disease, if blood pressure is equal to or above 130/80 mm Hg

Lifestyle modification is the cornerstone of hypertension prevention and management. In clients without conditions that may require special treatment, the first-line drugs are thiazide diuretics, angiotensin-converting enzyme (ACE) inhibitors, angiotensin II receptor blockers (ARBs), and calcium channel blockers. An example of dual combination therapy is the combination of a thiazide diuretic with an ACE inhibitor or ARB for an additive hypotensive effect. Treatment recommendations from the Canadian Hypertension Education Program (2007) are summarized in Figure 21.4. The nurse should check the website for annually revised recommendations.

21.5 Non-Pharmacological Therapy of Hypertension

When a client is first diagnosed with hypertension, a comprehensive medical history is necessary to determine if the disease can be controlled by non-pharmacological means. In many cases, modifying certain health-related lifestyle habits, such as increasing physical activity, lowering salt consumption, eating a balanced diet, minimizing the consumption of alcohol, avoiding smoking, and maintaining a healthy body weight, may eliminate the need for pharmacotherapy. Even if pharmacotherapy is required to manage the hypertension, it is important that the client continue

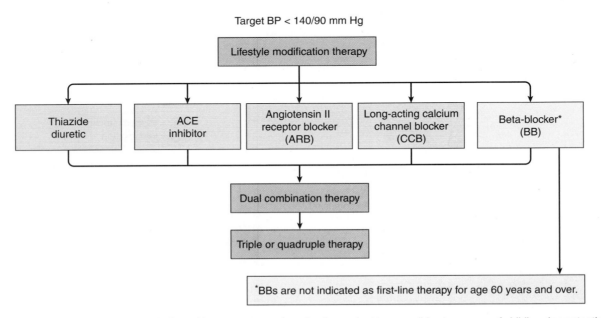

ACE inibitors and ARBs are contraindicated in pregnancy and caution is required in prescribing to women of childbearing potential.

● **Figure 21.4** Guidelines for the management of hypertension

Source: Adapted from the 2007 Canadian Hypertension Education Program Recommendations with the permission of the Canadian Cardiovascular Society.

SPECIAL CONSIDERATIONS

Lifestyle Recommendations for the Mangement of Hypertension

1. Healthy diet in accordance with the DASH diet: high in fresh fruits and vegetables and low-fat dairy products; low in saturated fat and salt

2. Regular physical activity: 30 to 60 minutes of moderate cardiorespiratory activity (such as walking, jogging, cycling, or swimming) four to seven times per week

3. Limited alchohol intake: no more than 2 standard drinks per day (less than 14 per week for men and less than 9 per week for women)

4. Healthy weight: maintain an ideal body weight (BMI 18.5–24.9 kg/m^2; waist circumference < 102 cm for men and < 88 cm for women)

5. Restricted salt intake: less than 100 mmol/day for individuals considered salt-sensitive (such as those over age 45, of African descent, or with impaired renal function or diabetes)

6. Smoke-free environment

7. Stress management

Source: Adapted from the 2006 Canadian Hypertension Education Program Recommendations

positive lifestyle changes so that dosages can be minimized, thus lowering the potential for drug side effects. The nurse is key to educating clients about controlling their HTN. Non-pharmacological methods for controlling hypertension are presented in the box above, "Special Considerations: Lifestyle Recommendations for the Mangement of Hypertension."

21.6 Risk Factors and Selection of Antihypertensive Drugs

The goal of antihypertensive therapy is to reduce blood pressure in order to avoid serious, long-term consequences of HTN. Keeping blood pressure within acceptable limits reduces the risk of hypertension-related diseases such as stroke and heart failure. Several strategies that are used to achieve this goal are summarized in Figure 21.5.

The pharmacological management of hypertension is individualized with regard to the client's risk factors, concurrent medical conditions, and degree of blood pressure elevation. Once the appropriate drug has been chosen, a low dose is prescribed. Depending on the expected response time of the drug, the client will be re-evaluated, and the dosage may be adjusted. A second drug from a different class may be added if the client has not responded to the initial medication.

It is common practice for healthcare providers to prescribe two antihypertensives concurrently to manage resistant HTN. The advantage of using two drugs is that lower doses may be used, resulting in fewer side effects and better client adherence. Unfortunately, adherence decreases when clients need to take more than one drug or need to take them more often. In an effort to minimize non-adherence, drug manufacturers sometimes combine two drugs into a single pill or capsule. These combination drugs are quite common in the treatment of hypertension. It is important for the client to receive education on all the drugs in combination formulas. Select combination drugs are shown in

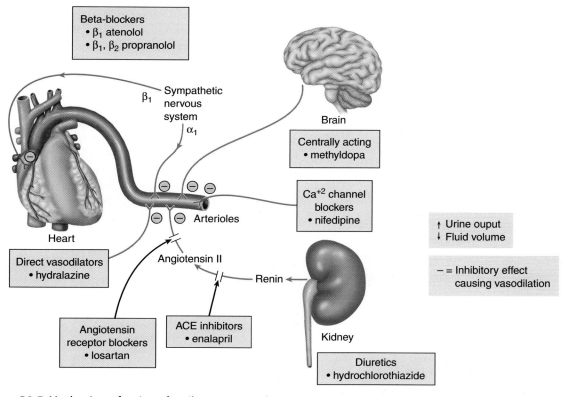

● **Figure 21.5** Mechanism of action of antihypertensive drugs

TABLE 21.1   Combination Drugs Commonly Used to Treat Hypertension

Trade Name	Thiazide Diuretic	Adrenergic Agent	Potassium-Sparing Diuretic	ACE Inhibitor or Angiotensin II Receptor Blocker	Other
Aldactazide	hydrochlorothiazide		spironolactone		
Aini-Hydro	hydrochlorothiazide		amiloride		
Hyzaar	hydrochlorothiazide			losartan	
Lopresor	hydrochlorothiazide	metoprolol			
Lotensin	hydrochlorothiazide			benazepril	
Moduret	hydrochlorothiazide		amiloride		
Riva-Zide	hydrochlorothiazide		triamterene		
Tarka				trandolapril	verapamil
Vaseretic	hydrochlorothiazide			enalapril	
Zestoretic	hydrochlorothiazide			lisinopril	

Table 21.1. Strategies that may be used to promote adherence with antihypertensive therapy are summarized in the box "Special Considerations: Strategies to Promote Adherence with HTN Pharmacotherapy."

The types of drugs used to treat chronic hypertension generally fall into five primary classes, as follows:

1. Diuretics
2. Calcium channel blockers
3. Agents affecting the renin-angiotensin system
4. Adrenergic agents
5. Direct-acting vasodilators

SPECIAL CONSIDERATIONS

Strategies to Promote Adherence with HTN Pharmacotherapy

- Teach clients to take their pills on a regular schedule that is associated with a routine daily activity such as brushing the teeth.
- Help clients get more involved in their treatment, for example, by measuring their own blood pressure.
- Teach clients and their families about the disease/treatment regimens, verbally and in writing (audio recordings are often helpful).
- Assess adherence to pharmacological and non-pharmacological therapy.
- Simplify medication regimens (e.g., by using long-acting, once-daily, or fixed-dose combination tablets).
- Utilize unit-of-use packaging such as blister packs.
- Follow up with telephone contact, particularly during the first 3 months of therapy.
- Collaborate with other healthcare providers to promote adherence with pharmacological and lifestyle modification prescriptions.

Source: Adapted from the 2006 Canadian Hypertension Education Program

DIURETICS

Diuretics act by increasing the volume of urine production. They are widely used in the treatment of hypertension and heart failure. These agents are shown in Table 21.2.

21.7 Treating Hypertension with Diuretics

Diuretics were the first class of drug used to treat hypertension in the 1950s. Despite many advances in pharmacotherapy, diuretics are still considered first-line drugs for this disease because they produce few adverse effects and are very effective at controlling mild to moderate hypertension. Although sometimes used alone, they are frequently prescribed with other antihypertensive drugs to enhance their effectiveness. Diuretics are also used to treat heart failure (Chapter 24) and kidney disorders (Chapter 43).

Although many different diuretics are available for hypertension, all produce a similar result: the reduction of blood volume through the urinary excretion of water and electrolytes. **Electrolytes** are ions such as sodium (Na^+), calcium (Ca^{+2}), chloride (Cl^-), and potassium (K^+). The mechanism by which diuretics reduce blood volume (specifically where and how the kidney is affected) differs among the various classes of diuretic. Details on the mechanisms of action of the diuretic classes are discussed in Chapter 43.

When a drug changes urine composition or output, electrolyte depletion is possible; the specific electrolyte lost is dependent on the mechanism of action of the particular drug. Potassium loss (hypokalemia) is of particular concern for loop and thiazide diuretics. Others such as triamterene have less tendency to cause potassium depletion and, for this reason, are called potassium-sparing diuretics. Taking potassium supplements with potassium-sparing diuretics may result in dangerously high potassium levels in the blood (hyperkalemia), leading to cardiac conduction abnormalities.

TABLE 21.2   Diuretics for Hypertension

Drug	Route and Adult Dose
Potassium-Sparing Type	
amiloride (Midamor)	PO; 5–20 mg in one to two divided doses (max 20 mg/day)
spironolactone (Aldactone) (see page 623 for the Prototype Drug box)	PO; 25–100 mg qd (max 200 mg/day)
triamterene (Apo-Triazide)	PO; 100 mg bid (max 300 mg/day)
Thiazide and Thiazide-Like Agents	
chlorothiazide (Diuril) (see page 622 for the Prototype Drug box)	PO; 250–500 mg qd (max 2 g/day)
chlorthalidone (Apo-Chlorthalidone)	PO; 50–100 mg qd (max 100 mg/day)
hydrochlorothiazide (HCTZ, Urozide)	PO; 12.5–100 mg qd (max 5 mg/day)
indapamide (Lozide)	PO; 2.5–5.0 mg qd
metolazone (Zaroxolyn)	PO; 5–20 mg qd
Loop (High-Ceiling) Type	
bumetanide (Burinex)	PO; 0.5–2.0 mg qd (max 10 mg/day)
furosemide (Lasix) (see page 314 for the Prototype Drug box)	PO; 20–80 mg qd (max 600 mg/day)

NURSING CONSIDERATIONS

The role of the nurse in diuretic therapy for HTN involves careful monitoring of the client's condition and providing education as it relates to the prescribed drug regimen. Diuretics decrease circulating blood volume, causing the potential development of dehydration and hypovolemia. **Orthostatic** (postural) **hypotension** may occur because of the reduced blood volume. The client may experience dizziness and faintness after rising too quickly from a sitting or lying position.

Because diuretics act by altering the physiological balance of fluid and electrolytes in the body, careful monitoring of laboratory values and body weight are essential. The client should be weighed daily and changes reported. The nurse must measure fluid intake and output and assess insensible losses that may occur due to exercise or illness, such as high fever. The ankles and lower legs should be examined for signs of pitting edema, which signifies fluid retention. Auscultate breath and heart sounds when taking vital signs; rales or rhonchi may indicate pulmonary edema, and "crackles" and murmurs may indicate impending heart failure. Electrolyte levels, particularly sodium and potassium, should be monitored carefully during diuretic therapy. Diuretics can reduce the renal excretion of lithium, causing this drug to build up to toxic levels. Most diuretics are contraindicated in clients who are unable to produce urine (anuria).

Because diuretics cause frequent urination, assess the client's ability to safely go to the bathroom, or secure a urinal or bedside commode as needed. Diuretics should be administered early in the day so sleep is not interrupted by frequent urination.

Photosensitivity is also a side effect of many diuretics. Photosensitization occurs when a drug, absorbed into the bloodstream, enters the skin. Sunlight, also absorbed by the skin, chemically changes the drug, and the new compound triggers a reaction in the body.

Potassium-Sparing Diuretics   Potassium-sparing diuretics should not be used in clients with renal insufficiency or hyperkalemia since potassium levels may rise to life-threatening levels. Potassium-sparing diuretics are not normally used for pregnant or lactating women as they range from pregnancy category B (triamterene) to category D (spironolactone). Uric acid levels may increase, and clients with a history of gout or kidney stones may not tolerate these diuretics. Complete blood counts should be obtained periodically throughout therapy as agranulocytosis and other hematological disorders may occur. Because white blood cell levels may be too low to combat infections, clients should report fever, rash, and sore throat. Spironolactone can cause gynecomastia (breast enlargement) and androgenic effects such as testicular atrophy or accelerated hair growth (hirsutism) in females. Clients should avoid excess potassium in their diet and salts that contain potassium (e.g., KCl).

Thiazide and Thiazide-Like Diuretics   Because thiazide and thiazide-like diuretics alter blood chemistry, including fluid and electrolyte balance, laboratory values (K^+, Cl^-, Na^+, Ca^{+2}, Mg^{+2}, CBC, BUN, creatinine, cholesterol, and serum lipids) should be closely monitored. These drugs may cause excess potassium excretion; therefore, clients should increase potassium in their diet. Potassium supplements may be necessary. These diuretics can cause hyperglycemia and decrease the effectiveness of oral antidiabetic drugs. Because uric acid levels may increase, clients should be monitored for signs and symptoms of gout.

Pr PROTOTYPE DRUG | Hydrochlorothiazide (HCTZ, Urozide)

ACTIONS AND USES

Hydrochlorothiazide is the most widely prescribed diuretic for hypertension, belonging to a large class known as the thiazides. Like many diuretics, it produces few adverse effects and is effective at producing a 10 to 20 mm Hg reduction in blood pressure. Clients with severe HTN, however, may require the addition of a second drug from a different class to control their blood pressure.

HCTZ acts on the kidney tubule to decrease the reabsorption of sodium. Normally, over 99% of the sodium entering the kidney is reabsorbed by the body so that very little leaves via the urine. When HCTZ blocks this reabsorption, more sodium is sent into the urine. When sodium moves across the tubule, water flows with it; thus, blood volume decreases and blood pressure falls. The volume of urine produced is directly proportional to the amount of sodium reabsorption blocked by the diuretic.

ADMINISTRATION ALERTS

- Administer the drug early in the day to prevent nocturia.
- Hydrochlorothiazide is pregnancy category B.

PHARMACOKINETICS

HCTZ is rapidly absorbed, widely distributed, and excreted mainly unchanged by the kidneys. It has a half-life of 6 to 15 hours.

ADVERSE EFFECTS AND INTERACTIONS

The most common side effects of HCTZ involve potential electrolyte imbalances; potassium is lost along with the sodium. Because hypokalemia may cause conduction abnormalities in the heart, clients must closely monitor their dietary potassium and are usually asked to increase their potassium intake as a precaution.

HCTZ potentiates the action of other antihypertensives and increases responsiveness to skeletal muscle relaxants. Thiazides may reduce the effectiveness of anticoagulants, sulfonylureas, antigout drugs, and antidiabetic drugs including insulin. Cholestyramine, colestipol, and NSAIDs reduce the effectiveness of HCTZ.

CNS depressants such as alcohol, barbiturates, and opioids may exacerbate the orthostatic hypotension caused by HCTZ. Steroids or amphotericin B increase potassium loss when given with HCTZ, leading to hypokalemia.

HCTZ increases the risk of serum toxicity of the following drugs: digitalis, lithium, allopurinol, diazoxide, anesthetics, and antineoplastics. HCTZ alters vitamin D metabolism and causes calcium conservation; use of calcium supplements may cause hypercalcemia.

Use with caution with herbal supplements, such as ginkgo, which may produce a paradoxical increase in blood pressure.

 See the Companion Website for a Nursing Process Focus Chart specific to this drug.

Because thiazides may increase blood lipids, these agents should be used cautiously in clients with existing hyperlipidemia. Cautious use is advised during pregnancy (category B) and lactation as these diuretics cross the placenta and are secreted into breast milk. Thiazides may exacerbate systemic lupus erythematosus (SLE) and therefore are contraindicated in this condition. Elderly clients are at increased risk of electrolyte imbalances due to physiological changes in the kidneys related to aging. Losses of potassium and magnesium caused by thiazide diuretics increase the risk of digoxin toxicity.

Loop (High-Ceiling) Diuretics The efficacious loop, or high-ceiling, group of diuretics is more likely to cause severe potassium loss, hypovolemia, and hypotension compared to other diuretic classes. The client's blood pressure should be monitored frequently, especially with IV administration.

Loop diuretics are ototoxic—an effect more likely to occur in clients with renal insufficiency or when high doses are administered. Hearing loss usually reverses when the drug is discontinued. Loop diuretics may also increase glucose and uric acid levels; therefore, these laboratory values should be monitored during therapy.

See "Nursing Process Focus: Clients Receiving Diuretic Therapy" for specific teaching points.

CALCIUM CHANNEL BLOCKERS

Calcium channel blockers exert a number of beneficial effects on the heart and blood vessels by blocking calcium ion channels. They are widely used in the treatment of hypertension and other cardiovascular diseases. These agents are shown in Table 21.3 on page 260.

NURSING PROCESS FOCUS Clients Receiving Diuretic Therapy

Assessment	Potential Nursing Diagnoses/Identified Patterns
Prior to administration: ■ Obtain complete health history including allergies, drug history, and possible drug interactions. ■ Obtain vital signs; assess in context of client's baseline values. ■ Obtain baseline weight. ■ Auscultate chest sounds for rales or rhonchi indicative of pulmonary edema. ■ Assess lower limbs for edema; note character/level (e.g., "+ + pitting"). ■ Obtain blood and urine specimens for laboratory analysis.	■ Need for knowledge regarding drug therapy ■ Risk for fluid and electrolyte imbalance ■ Increased urinary elimination related to diuretic use ■ Fatigue

continued

NURSING PROCESS FOCUS   Clients Receiving Diuretic Therapy   *(Continued)*

Planning: Client Goals and Expected Outcomes

The client will:
- Exhibit a reduction in systolic/diastolic blood pressure
- Demonstrate an understanding of the drug's action by accurately describing drug side effects and precautions
- Maintain normal serum electrolyte levels during drug therapy.

Implementation

Interventions (Rationales)	Client Education/Discharge Planning
■ Monitor laboratory values. (Diuretic therapy affects the results of laboratory tests.)	Instruct client to: ■ Inform laboratory personnel of diuretic therapy when providing blood or urine samples ■ Carry a wallet card or wear medical identification jewellery to indicate diuretic therapy
■ Monitor vital signs, especially blood pressure. (Diuretics reduce circulating blood volume, resulting in lowered blood pressure.)	Instruct client to: ■ Monitor vital signs as specified by the nurse, particularly blood pressure, ensuring proper use of home equipment ■ Withhold medication for severe hypotensive readings as specified by the nurse (e.g., "hold for levels below 88/50")
■ Observe for changes in level of consciousness, dizziness, fatigue, postural hypotension. (These are caused by reduction in circulating blood volume.)	Instruct client to: ■ Report dizziness or light-headedness ■ Rise slowly from prolonged periods of sitting or lying down ■ Obtain blood pressure readings in sitting, standing, and supine positions to monitor fluctuations in blood pressure
■ Monitor for fluid overload and signs of heart failure. (Increased blood volume causes increased cardiac workload and pulmonary edema.) ■ Measure intake and output and daily body weight.	Instruct client: ■ To immediately report any severe shortness of breath, frothy sputum, profound fatigue, and edema in extremities ■ To measure and monitor fluid intake and output and to weigh self daily ■ To consume enough *plain* water to remain adequately, but not over, hydrated ■ To avoid excessive heat, which contributes to excessive sweating and fluid loss ■ That increased urine output and decreased weight indicate that the drug is working
■ Monitor nutritional status. (Electrolyte imbalances may be counteracted by dietary measures.)	For clients taking potassium-wasting diuretics, instruct to: ■ Eat foods high in potassium, such as bananas, apricots, kidney beans, sweet potatoes, and peanut butter For clients taking potassium-sparing diuretics, instruct to: ■ Avoid foods high in potassium ■ Consult with nurse before using vitamin/mineral supplements or electrolyte-fortified sports drinks
■ Observe for signs of hyperglycemia. Use drug with caution in diabetics.	■ Instruct client to report signs and symptoms of diabetes mellitus to health-care provider.
■ Monitor liver and kidney function. (Drugs are metabolized by the liver and excreted by the kidneys.)	Instruct client to: ■ Immediately report symptoms of metabolic imbalances: nausea and vomiting, profound weakness, lethargy, muscle cramps, depression/disorientation, hallucinations, heart spasms, palpitations, numbness or tingling in limbs, extreme thirst, changes in urine output ■ Adhere to laboratory testing regimen as ordered by the healthcare provider
■ Observe for hypersensitivity reaction.	■ Instruct client to immediately report difficulty breathing, throat tightness, hives or rash, muscle cramps, or tremors.
■ Observe for signs of infection.	■ Instruct client or caregiver to report any flu-like symptoms: shortness of breath, fever, sore throat, malaise, joint pain, or profound fatigue.

continued

NURSING PROCESS FOCUS Clients Receiving Diuretic Therapy *(Continued)*

Interventions (Rationales)	Client Education/Discharge Planning
■ Monitor hearing and vision. (Loop diuretics such as furosemide are ototoxic. Thiazide diuretics increase serum digitalis levels, which may produce visual changes.)	Instruct client to: ■ Report changes in hearing such as ringing or buzzing in the ears or becoming "hard of hearing" ■ Report dimness of sight, seeing halos, or "yellow vision"
■ Monitor for alcohol and caffeine use. (Alcohol potentiates the hypotensive action of some thiazide diuretics. Caffeine is a mild diuretic that could increase diuresis.)	■ Instruct client to restrict consumption of alcohol and caffeine.
■ Ensure client safety. Monitor ambulation until effects of drug are known. (Postural hypotension can be caused by drug.)	Instruct client to: ■ Obtain help before getting out of bed or attempting to walk alone ■ Avoid sudden changes of position to prevent dizziness caused by postural hypotension ■ Avoid driving and other activities requiring mental alertness or physical coordination until effects of the drug are known
■ Monitor reactivity to light exposure. (Drug causes photosensitivity.)	Instruct client to: ■ Limit exposure to the sun ■ Wear dark glasses and light-coloured, loose-fitting clothes when outdoors

Evaluation of Outcome Criteria

Evaluate the effectiveness of drug therapy by confirming that client goals and expected outcomes have been met (see "Planning").

See Table 21.2 (page 257) for a list of drugs to which these nursing actions apply.

TABLE 21.3 **Calcium Channel Blockers for Hypertension**	
Drug	*Route and Adult Dose*
Selective: for Blood Vessels	
amlodipine (Norvasc, caduet)	PO; 5–10 mg qd (max 10 mg/day)
felodipine (Plendil, Renedil)	PO; 5–10 mg qd (max 20 mg/day)
nifedipine (Adalat, Apo-Nifed)	PO; 10–20 mg tid (max 180 mg/day)
Non-Selective: for Blood Vessels and Heart	
diltiazem (Cardizem, Novo-Diltiazem) (see page 296 for the Prototype Drug box)	PO; 60–120 mg sustained release bid
verapamil (Isoptin, Apo-Verap) (see page 327 for the Prototype Drug box)	PO; 80–160 mg tid (max 360 mg/day)

21.8 Treating Hypertension with Calcium Channel Blockers

Calcium channel blockers (CCBs) comprise a group of drugs used to treat a number of cardiovascular diseases, including angina pectoris, dysrhythmias, and hypertension. After CCBs were first approved for the treatment of angina in the early 1980s, it was quickly noted that a "side effect" was the lowering of blood pressure in hypertensive clients. CCBs have since become a widely prescribed class of drug for hypertension.

Contraction of muscle is regulated by the amount of calcium ion inside the cell. When calcium enters the cell through channels in the plasma membrane, muscular contraction is initiated. CCBs block these channels and inhibit calcium from entering the cell, limiting muscular contrac-

tion. At low doses, CCBs cause the smooth muscle in arterioles to relax, lowering peripheral resistance and decreasing blood pressure. Some CCBs such as nifedipine are selective for calcium channels in arterioles, while others such as verapamil affect channels in both arterioles and the myocardium. CCBs vary in their potency and by the frequency and types of side effects they produce. Uses of CCBs in the treatment of angina and dysrhythmias are discussed in Chapters 23 and 25, respectively.

NURSING CONSIDERATIONS

The role of the nurse in CCB therapy for HTN involves careful monitoring of the client's condition and providing education as it relates to the prescribed drug regimen. CCBs

Pr **PROTOTYPE DRUG** | Nifedipine (Adalat, Apo-Nifed)

ACTIONS AND USES

Nifedipine is a CCB generally prescribed for HTN and variant or vasospastic angina. It is occasionally used to treat Raynaud's phenomenon and hypertrophic cardiomyopathy. Nifedipine acts by selectively blocking calcium channels in myocardial and vascular smooth muscle, including that in the coronary arteries. This results in less oxygen utilization by the heart, an increase in cardiac output, and a fall in blood pressure. Nifedipine is as effective as diuretics and beta-adrenergic blockers at reducing blood pressure.

ADMINISTRATION ALERTS

- Do not administer immediate-release formulations of nifedipine if an impending MI is suspected or within 2 weeks following a confirmed MI.
- Administer nifedipine capsules or tablets whole. If capsules or extended-release tablets are chewed, divided, or crushed, the entire dose will be delivered at once.
- Nifedipine is pregnancy category C.

PHARMACOKINETICS

Nifedipine is well absorbed, but bioavailability is reduced due to first-pass metabolism. It is 92% to 98% protein bound and is mostly metabolized by the liver. It has a half-life of 2 to 5 hours.

ADVERSE EFFECTS AND INTERACTIONS

Side effects of nifedipine are generally minor and related to vasodilation, such as headache, dizziness, and flushing. Fast-acting forms of nifedipine can cause reflex tachycardia. To avoid rebound hypotension, discontinuation of the drug should occur gradually. In rare cases, nifedipine may cause a paradoxical increase in anginal chest pain possibly related to hypotension or heart failure.

Nifedipine may increase serum levels of digitalis, cimetidine, and ranitidine. Nifedipine may potentiate the effects of warfarin, resulting in increased INR. Potentiation may also occur with fentanyl anesthesia, resulting in severe hypotension and increased fluid volume requirements. Grapefruit juice may cause enhanced absorption of nifedipine. Nifedipine may reduce serum levels of quinidine.

Alcohol potentiates the vasodilating action of nifedipine and could lead to syncope caused by a severe drop in blood pressure. Nicotine causes vasoconstriction, counteracting the desired effect of nifedipine.

Use with caution with melatonin, which may increase blood pressure and heart rate.

 See the Companion Website for a Nursing Process Focus Chart specific to this drug.

---

affect the coronary arteries and myocardial conductivity and contractility. ECG, heart rate, and blood pressure should be assessed prior to therapy; vital signs should be monitored regularly thereafter. CCBs reduce myocardial contractility and can increase the risk of, and worsen, heart failure. CCBs are contraindicated in clients with certain types of heart conditions such as sick sinus syndrome or third-degree AV block without the presence of a pacemaker. Due to their potent vasodilating effects, CCBs can cause reflex tachycardia, a condition that occurs when the heart rate increases due to the rapid fall in blood pressure created by the drug. CCBs are pregnancy category C.

Tachycardia and hypotension are most pronounced with IV administration of CCBs. Grapefruit juice increases absorption of these drugs from the GI tract, causing greater than expected effects from the dose. Grapefruit juice taken with a sustained-release CCB could result in rapid toxic overdose, which is a medical emergency.

Teaching strategies regarding calcium channel blockers should include goals; reasons for obtaining baseline data such as vital signs, tests for cardiac and renal disorders (including ECG), and laboratory values; and possible side effects. See "Nursing Process Focus: Clients Receiving Calcium Channel Blocker Therapy" for specific teaching points.

NURSING PROCESS FOCUS Clients Receiving Calcium Channel Blocker Therapy

Assessment	Potential Nursing Diagnoses/Identified Patterns
Prior to administration: ■ Obtain complete health history including data on recent cardiac events, allergies, drug history, and possible drug interactions. ■ Obtain ECG and vital signs; assess in context of client's baseline values. ■ Assess neurological status and level of consciousness. ■ Auscultate chest sounds for rales or rhonchi indicative of pulmonary edema. ■ Assess lower limbs for edema; note character/level.	■ Need for knowledge regarding to drug therapy ■ Decreased cardiac output ■ Altered tissue perfusion

Planning: Client Goals and Expected Outcomes

The client will:
- Exhibit a reduction in systolic/diastolic blood pressure
- Demonstrate an understanding of the drug's action by accurately describing drug side effects and precautions.

continued

NURSING PROCESS FOCUS Clients Receiving Calcium Channel Blocker Therapy *(Continued)*

Implementation

Interventions and (Rationales)	Client Education/Discharge Planning
■ Monitor vital signs.	Instruct client to: ■ Monitor vital signs as specified by the nurse, particularly blood pressure, ensuring proper use of home equipment ■ Withhold medication for severe hypotensive readings as specified by the nurse (e.g., "hold for levels below 88/50") ■ Immediately report palpitations or rapid heartbeat
■ Observe for changes in level of consciousness, dizziness, fatigue, postural hypotension (caused by vasodilation). ■ Observe for paradoxical increase in chest pain or angina symptoms (related to severe hypotension). ■ Obtain blood pressure readings in sitting, standing, and supine positions to monitor fluctuations in blood pressure.	Instruct client to: ■ Report dizziness or light-headedeness ■ Report chest pain or other angina-like symptoms ■ Rise slowly from prolonged periods of sitting or lying
■ Monitor for signs of heart failure. (CCBs can decrease myocardial contractility, increasing the risk of heart failure.)	■ Instruct client to immediately report any severe shortness of breath, frothy sputum, profound fatigue, and swelling. These may be signs of heart failure or fluid accumulation in the lungs.
■ Monitor for fluid accumulation. ■ Measure intake and output and daily body weight. (Edema is a side effect of some CCBs.)	Instruct client to: ■ Avoid excessive heat, which contributes to excessive sweating and fluid loss ■ Measure and monitor fluid intake and output and to weigh self daily ■ Consume enough *plain* water to remain adequately, but not over, hydrated
■ Observe for hypersensitivity reaction.	■ Instruct client to immediately report difficulty breathing, throat tightness, hives or rash, muscle cramps, or tremors.
■ Monitor liver and kidney function. (CCBs are metabolized in the liver and excreted by the kidneys.)	Instruct client to: ■ Report signs of liver toxicity: nausea, vomiting, anorexia, bleeding, severe upper or abdominal pain, heartburn, jaundice, or a change in the colour or character of stools ■ Report signs of renal toxicity: fever, flank pain, changes in urine output, colour or character (e.g., cloudy, with sediment) ■ Adhere to laboratory testing regimens as ordered by the healthcare provider
■ Observe for constipation. Client may need an increase in dietary fibre, or laxatives.	Advise client to: ■ Maintain adequate fluid and fibre intake to facilitate stool passage ■ Use a bulk laxative or stool softener, as recommended by the healthcare provider
■ Ensure client safety. ■ Monitor ambulation until response to drug is known (due to postural hypotension caused by drug).	■ Instruct client to avoid driving and other activities requiring mental alertness or physical coordination until effects of the drug are known

Evaluation of Outcome Criteria

Evaluate the effectiveness of drug therapy by confirming that client goals and expected outcomes have been met (see "Planning").

See Table 21.3 (page 260) for a list of drugs to which these nursing actions apply.

DRUGS AFFECTING THE RENIN-ANGIOTENSIN SYSTEM

Drugs that affect the renin-angiotensin pathway decrease blood pressure and increase urine volume. They are widely used in the treatment of hypertension, heart failure, and myocardial infarction. These agents are shown in Table 21.4.

21.9 Pharmacotherapy with ACE Inhibitors and Angiotensin II Receptor Blockers

The renin-angiotensin system is a key homeostatic mechanism that controls blood pressure and fluid balance. This mechanism is illustrated in Figure 21.6. Renin is an enzyme

TABLE 21.4 ACE Inhibitors and Angiotensin II Receptor Blockers for Hypertension

Drug	Route and Adult Dose
ACE Inhibitors	
benazepril (Lotensin)	PO; 10–40 mg in one to two divided doses (max 40 mg/day)
captopril (Capoten)	PO; 6.25–25 mg tid (max 450 mg/day)
enalapril (Vasotec)	PO; 5–40 mg in one to two divided doses (max 40 mg/day)
fosinopril (Monopril)	PO; 5–40 mg qd (max 80 mg/day)
lisinopril (Prinivil, Zestril) (see page 309 for the Prototype Drug box)	PO; 10 mg qd (max 80 mg/day)
quinapril (Accupril)	PO; 10–20 mg qd (max 80 mg/day)
ramipril (Altace)	PO; 2.5–5 mg qd (max 20 mg/day)
trandolapril (Mavik)	PO; 1–4 mg qd (max 8 mg/day)
Angiotensin II Receptor Blockers	
candesartan (Atacand)	PO; Start at 16 mg qd (range 8–32 mg divided once or twice daily)
eprosartan (Teveten)	PO; 600 mg qd or 400 mg PO qid–bid (max 800 mg/day)
irbesartan (Avapro, Avalide)	PO; 150–300 mg qd (max 300 mg/day)
losartan (Cozaar)	PO; 25–50 mg in one to two divided doses (max 100 mg/day)
telmisartan (Micardis)	PO; 40 mg qd; may increase to 80 mg/day
valsartan (Diovan)	PO; 80 mg qd (max 320 mg/day)

secreted by specialized cells in the kidney when blood pressure falls or when there is a decrease in sodium flowing through the kidney tubules. Once in the blood, renin converts the inactive liver protein angiotensinogen to angiotensin I. When passing through the lungs, angiotensin I is converted to **angiotensin II**, one of the most potent natural vasoconstrictors known. The enzyme responsible for the final step in this system is **angiotensin-converting enzyme (ACE)**. The intense vasoconstriction of arterioles caused by angiotensin II raises blood pressure by increasing peripheral resistance.

Angiotensin II also stimulates the secretion of two hormones that markedly affect blood pressure: aldosterone and ADH. **Aldosterone**, a hormone from the adrenal cortex, increases sodium reabsorption in the kidney. The enhanced sodium reabsorption helps the body retain water, thus increasing blood volume and raising blood pressure. ADH, a hormone from the posterior pituitary, enhances the conservation of water by the kidneys. This raises blood pressure by increasing blood volume. Pharmacotherapy with ADH is discussed in Chapter 39.

First detected in the venom of pit vipers in the 1960s, ACE inhibitors have been approved as drugs for hypertension since the 1980s. Since then, drugs in this class have become key agents in the treatment of hypertension. ACE inhibitors block the effects of angiotensin II, decreasing blood pressure through two mechanisms—lowering peripheral resistance and decreasing blood volume. Some ACE inhibitors have also been approved for the treatment of myocardial infarction and heart failure, as discussed in Chapters 23 and 24, respectively.

Side effects of ACE inhibitors are usually minor and include persistent cough and postural hypotension, particularly

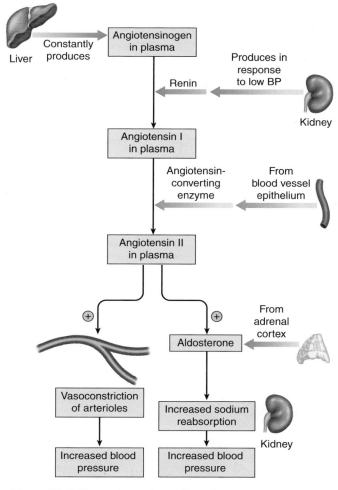

● **Figure 21.6** The renin-angiotensin pathway

following the first few doses of the drug. The most serious adverse effect is the development of angioedema, an acute hypersensitivity reaction featuring non-inflammatory swelling of the skin, mucous membranes, and other organs. Angioedema may be life-threatening; laryngeal swelling can lead to asphyxia and death. The development of angioedema usually occurs within days of taking an ACE inhibitor; however, it can occur as a delayed reaction months or even years into therapy.

A second method of altering the renin-angiotensin pathway is by blocking the action of angiotensin II *after* it is formed. The **angiotensin II receptor blockers (ARBs)** block receptors for angiotensin II in arteriolar smooth muscle and in the adrenal gland, thus causing blood pressure to fall. Their effects of arteriolar dilation and increased sodium excretion by the kidneys are similar to those of the ACE inhibitors. ARBs differ in how they are distributed and eliminated from the body. Some ARBs need to be converted to an active form in the body before they can lower blood pressure. Drugs in this class are often combined with drugs from other classes for the management of HTN.

The most common side effects of ARBs are cough, elevated potassium levels, low blood pressure, dizziness, headache, drowsiness, diarrhea, abnormal taste sensation (metallic or salty taste), and rash. Since ARBs may increase blood levels of potassium, the use of potassium supplements, salt substitutes that contain potassium, or other drugs that increase potassium may result in excessive blood potassium levels. ARBs may also increase the blood concentration of lithium. Compared to ACE inhibitors, cough occurs less often with ARBs. ARBs may cause birth defects if used in pregnancy.

New drugs that use different methods of altering the renin-angiotensin system are in clinical trials and show promise for the pharmacotherapy of HTN. Aldosterone receptor blockers prevent aldosterone from reaching its receptors in the kidneys, resulting in less sodium reabsorption and a fall in blood pressure. Vasopeptidase inhibitors have dual inhibition of both ACE and the enzyme neutral endopeptidase (NEP). Inhibiting NEP leads to a buildup of natriuretic peptides, which causes both vasodilation and diuresis.

NURSING CONSIDERATIONS

The role of the nurse in ACE inhibitor therapy for HTN involves careful monitoring of the client's condition and providing education as it relates to the prescribed drug regimen. ACE inhibitors act on the vasodilator bradykinin, causing a chronic, dry or "tickling," non-productive cough. Because cough is a significant symptom, it should always be investigated. For example, dry cough may result from vasovagal stimulation related to angina or impending MI. Severe paroxysms of dry cough may indicate laryngeal swelling and the onset of life-threatening angioedema. Suspected angioedema requires immediate discontinuance of ACE inhibitor therapy. Due to the risk of angioedema, resuscitative equipment and oxygen apparatus should remain accessible during initiation of ACE inhibitor therapy, especially during IV administration. Intravenous administration may initiate an immediate, profound hypotensive response and possible loss of consciousness.

Contraindications to ACE inhibitors include hypersensitivity and any history of angioedema (idiopathic, familial, or drug induced). They should not be given to clients with heart failure who are presently taking a potassium-sparing diuretic. ACE inhibitors increase the risk of stroke, angina, peripheral artery disease (PAD), and GI bleeding.

Pr PROTOTYPE DRUG | Enalapril (Vasotec)

ACTIONS AND USES

Enalapril is one of the most frequently prescribed ACE inhibitors for hypertension. Unlike captopril (Capoten)—the first ACE inhibitor to be marketed—enalapril has a prolonged half-life, which permits administration once or twice daily. Enalapril acts by reducing angiotensin II and aldosterone levels to produce a significant reduction in blood pressure with few side effects. Enalapril may be used by itself or in combination with other antihypertensives to minimize side effects.

ADMINISTRATION ALERTS

- Enalapril may produce a first-dose phenomenon resulting in profound hypotension, which may lead to syncope.
- Enalapril is pregnancy category D.

PHARMACOKINETICS

Enalapril is converted by the liver to its active metabolite, enalaprilat. All ACE inhibitors cross the placenta. Enalapril and enalaprilat have a half-life of 11 hours and are excreted by the kidneys.

ADVERSE EFFECTS AND INTERACTIONS

ACE inhibitors such as enalapril can cause potassium and creatine levels in the blood to increase. They cause fewer cardiac side effects than beta-adrenergic blockers. Enalapril may cause orthostatic hypotension when moving quickly from a supine to an upright position. A rapid fall in blood pressure may occur following the first dose. Other side effects include headache and dizziness.

ACE inhibitors can cause life-threatening angioedema, neutropenia, and agranulocytosis. Renin-releasing antihypertensives potentiate the action of enalapril and can cause profound hypotension.

Thiazide diuretics increase potassium loss; potassium-sparing diuretics increase serum potassium and may be prescribed with thiazide diuretics to decrease risk of hypokalemia. Enalapril may induce lithium toxicity by reducing renal clearance of lithium. NSAIDs may reduce the effectiveness of ACE inhibition.

 See the Companion Website for a Nursing Process Focus Chart specific to this drug.

ACE inhibitors are also contraindicated in pregnancy (category D), lactation, and in clients with renal insufficiency.

See "Nursing Process Focus: Clients Receiving ACE Inhibitor Therapy" for specific teaching points.

ADRENERGIC AGENTS

The adrenergic receptor has been a site of pharmacological action in the treatment of hypertension since the first such drugs were developed in the 1950s. Blockade of adrenergic receptors results in a number of beneficial effects on the heart and blood vessels, and these autonomic drugs are used

SPECIAL CONSIDERATIONS

Ethnicity and ACE Inhibitor Action

ACE inhibitors can have unique idiosyncratic effects on individuals of particular racial and/or ethnic groups. In particular, African Canadian clients experience reduced efficacy and a higher incidence of angioedema. Inform clients of African descent of the variations in drug effectiveness and increased risk of angioedema.

for a wide variety of cardiovascular disorders. Table 21.5 (p. 267) shows the adrenergic agents used for hypertension.

NURSING PROCESS FOCUS   Clients Receiving ACE Inhibitor Therapy

Assessment	Potential Nursing Diagnoses/Identified Patterns
Prior to administration: ■ Obtain complete health history including data on recent cardiac events and any incidence of angioedema, allergies, drug history, and possible drug interactions. ■ Obtain ECG and vital signs; assess in context of client's baseline values. ■ Assess neurological status and level of consciousness. ■ Obtain blood and urine specimens for laboratory analysis.	■ Need for knowledge regarding drug therapy ■ Risk for injury related to orthostatic hypotension ■ Ineffective tissue perfusion ■ Risk for hyperkalemia

Planning: Client Goals and Expected Outcomes

The client will:
■ Exhibit a reduction in systolic/diastolic blood pressure
■ Maintain normal serum electrolyte levels during drug therapy
■ Demonstrate an understanding of the drug's action by accurately describing drug side effects and precautions

Implementation

Interventions (Rationales)	Client Education/Discharge Planning
■ Monitor for first-dose phenomenon of profound hypotension.	■ Warn the client about the first-dose phenomenon; reassure that this effect diminishes with continued therapy. Instruct client: ■ That changes in consciousness may occur due to rapid reduction in blood pressure; immediately report a feeling of faintness ■ That the drug takes effect in approximately 1 hour and peaks in 3 to 4 hours; rest in the supine position beginning 1 hour after administration and for 3 to 4 hours after the first dose ■ Always arise slowly, avoiding sudden posture changes
■ Observe for hypersensitivity reaction, particularly angioedema. (Angioedema may arise at any time during ACE inhibitor therapy but is generally expected shortly after initiation of therapy.)	Instruct client: ■ To immediately report difficulty breathing, throat tightness, muscle cramps, hives or rash, and tremors. These symptoms can occur with the first dose or much later as a delayed reaction ■ That angioedema can be life-threatening and to call emergency medical services if severe dyspnea or hoarseness is accompanied by swelling of the face or mouth
■ Monitor for the presence of blood dyscrasia. ■ Observe for signs of infection: fever, sore throat, malaise, joint pain, ecchymoses, profound fatigue, shortness of breath, or pallor. (Bruising is a sign of bleeding, which can indicate the presence of a serious blood disorder.)	Instruct client to: ■ Immediately report any flu-like symptoms ■ Observe for bruising; signs of bleeding from the nose, mouth, or GI tract ("coffee grounds" vomit or tarry stools); menstrual flooding; or bright red rectal bleeding
■ Monitor for changes in level of consciousness, dizziness, drowsiness, or lightheadedness. (Signs of decreased blood flow to the brain are due to the drug's vasodilating hypotensive action. Sudden syncopal collapse is possible.)	Instruct client to: ■ Report dizziness or fainting that persists beyond the first dose, as well as unusual sensations (e.g., numbness and tingling) or other changes in the face or limbs ■ Contact the healthcare provider, before the next scheduled dose of the drug, if fainting occurs

continued

NURSING PROCESS FOCUS   Clients Receiving ACE Inhibitor Therapy   *(Continued)*

Interventions (Rationales)	Client Education/Discharge Planning
■ Monitor for persistent dry cough. (This may be triggered by bradykinin's proinflammatory action.) ■ Monitor changes in cough pattern. (This may indicate another disease process.)	Instruct client to: ■ Expect persistent dry cough ■ Report any change in the character or frequency of cough. Any cough accompanied by shortness of breath, fever, or chest pain should be reported *immediately* because it may indicate MI ■ Sleep with head elevated if cough becomes troublesome when in supine position ■ Use non-medicated, sugar-free lozenges or hard candies to relieve cough
■ Monitor for dehydration or fluid overload. (Dehydration causes low circulating blood volume and will exacerbate hypotension. Severe dehydration may trigger syncope and collapse. Pitting edema indicates fluid retention and can be a sign of heart failure; it may also indicate reduced drug efficacy.)	Instruct client to: ■ Observe for signs of dehydration such as oliguria, dry lips and mucous membranes, or poor skin turgor ■ Report any bodily swelling that leaves sunken marks on the skin when pressed ■ Measure and monitor fluid intake and output and to weigh self daily ■ Monitor increased need for fluid caused by vomiting, diarrhea, or excessive sweating ■ Avoid excessive heat, which contributes to sweating and fluid loss ■ Consume adequate amounts of *plain* water
■ Monitor for hyperkalemia (may occur due to reduced aldosterone levels).	Instruct client to: ■ Immediately report signs of hyperkalemia: nausea, irregular heartbeat, profound fatigue or muscle weakness, and slow or faint pulse ■ Avoid consuming electrolyte-fortified snacks or sports drinks that may contain potassium ■ Avoid using salt substitute (KCl) to flavour foods ■ Consult the healthcare provider before taking any nutritional supplements containing potassium
■ Monitor for liver and kidney function. (ACE inhibitors are metabolized by the liver and excreted by the kidneys.)	Instruct client to: ■ Report signs of liver toxicity: nausea; vomiting; anorexia; diarrhea; rash; jaundice; abdominal pain, tenderness, or distention; or change in the colour or character of stools ■ Discontinue drug immediately and contact the healthcare provider if jaundice occurs ■ Adhere to laboratory testing regimen as ordered by the healthcare provider
■ Ensure client safety (due to postural hypotension caused by drug). ■ Monitor ambulation until response to the drug is known.	Instruct client to: ■ Obtain help prior to getting out of bed or attempting to walk alone ■ Avoid driving or other activities that require mental alertness or physical coordination until effects of the drug are known

Evaluation of Outcome Criteria

Evaluate the effectiveness of drug therapy by confirming that client goals and expected outcomes have been met (see "Planning").

See Table 21.4 (page 263) under "ACE Inhibitors" for a list of drugs to which these nursing actions apply.

21.10 Pharmacotherapy with Adrenergic Agents

As discussed in Chapter 13, the autonomic nervous system controls involuntary functions of the body such as heart rate, pupil size, and smooth muscle contraction, including that in the arterial walls. Stimulation of the sympathetic division causes fight-or-flight responses such as faster heart rate, an increase in blood pressure, and bronchodilation. Peripheral blood vessels are innervated only by sympathetic nerves.

Antihypertensive drugs have been developed that affect the sympathetic division through a number of distinct mechanisms, although they all have in common the effect of lowering blood pressure. These mechanisms include the following:

- Blockade of alpha$_1$-receptors in the arterioles
- Selective blockade of beta$_1$-receptors in the heart
- Non-selective blockade of both beta$_1$- and beta$_2$-receptors
- Non-selective blockade of both alpha- and beta-receptors

TABLE 21.5 Adrenergic Agents for Hypertension

Drug	Route and Adult Dose
Beta-Blockers	
atenolol (Tenormin): beta$_1$ (see page 295 for the Prototype Drug box)	PO; 25–50 mg qd (max 100 mg/day)
bisoprolol (Apo-Bisoprolol): beta$_1$	PO; 2.5–5 mg qd (max 20 mg/day)
metoprolol (Lopresor): beta$_1$ (see page 295 for the Prototype Drug box)	PO; 50–100 mg qd–bid (max 450 mg/day)
propranolol (Inderal): beta$_1$ and beta$_2$ (see page 324 for the Prototype Drug box)	PO; 10–30 mg tid or qd (max 320 mg/day) IV; 0.5–3.0 mg q4h prn
timolol (Apo-Timolol): beta$_1$ and beta$_2$ (see page 692 for the Prototype Drug box)	PO; 15–45 mg tid (max 60 mg/day)
Alpha$_1$-Blockers	
Ⓟ doxazosin (Cardura)	PO; 1 mg hs; may increase to 16 mg/day in one to two divided doses (max 16 mg/day)
prazosin (Minipress) (see page 139 for the Prototype Drug box)	PO; 1 mg hs; may increase to 1 mg bid–tid (max 20 mg/day)
terazosin (Apo-Terazosin)	PO; 1 mg hs; may increase 1–5 mg/day (max 20 mg/day)
Alpha$_2$-Adrenergic Agonists	
clonidine (Catapres)	PO; 0.1 mg bid–tid (max 0.8 mg/day)
methyldopa (Aldomet)	PO; 250 mg bid or tid (max 3 g/day)
Alpha$_1$- and Beta-Blockers (Centrally Acting)	
labetalol (Trandate, Normodyne)	PO; 100 mg bid; may increase to 200–400 mg bid (max 1200–2400 mg/day)
Adrenergic Neuron Blockers (Peripherally Acting)	
guanethidine (Ismelin, Apo-Guanethidine)	PO; 10 mg qd; may increase by 10 mg q5–7d up to 300 mg/day (start with 25–50 mg/day in hospitalized patients, increase by 25–50 mg q1–3d)

- Stimulation of alpha$_2$-receptors in the brainstem (centrally acting)
- Blockade of peripheral adrenergic neurons

The earliest drugs for hypertension were non-selective agents, blocking nerve transmission at the ganglion or blocking both alpha- and beta-receptors. Although these non-selective agents revolutionized the treatment of hypertension, they produced significant side effects. They are rarely used today because the selective agents are more efficacious and better tolerated by clients.

The side effects of adrenergic blockers are generally predictable extensions of the fight-or-flight response. The alpha$_1$-adrenergic blockers tend to cause orthostatic hypotension when moving quickly from a supine to an upright position. Dizziness, nausea, bradycardia, and dry mouth are also common. Less common, though sometimes a major cause for non-adherence, is their adverse effect on male sexual function. These agents can cause decreased libido and erectile dysfunction (impotence). Non-selective beta-blockers will slow the heart rate and cause bronchoconstriction. They should be used with caution in clients with asthma or heart failure. Some beta-blockers are associated with clinical depression.

Some adrenergic agents cause blood pressure reduction by acting on alpha$_2$-receptors in the CNS. Methyldopa is converted to a "false" neurotransmitter in the brainstem,

thus causing a shortage of the "real" neurotransmitter and inhibition of the sympathetic nervous system. Clonidine, an alpha$_2$-agonist, affects alpha-adrenergic receptors in the cardiovascular control centres in the brainstem. The centrally acting agents have a tendency to produce sedation and may cause depression. They are not considered first-line drugs in the pharmacotherapy of HTN.

NURSING CONSIDERATIONS

The role of the nurse in adrenergic agent therapy for HTN involves careful monitoring of the client's condition and providing education as it relates to the prescribed drug regimen. Because of their widespread therapeutic applications, discussions of adrenergic antagonists appear in many chapters in this text. Prototype Drugs include atenolol and metoprolol in Chapter 23, carvedilol in Chapter 24, propranolol in Chapter 25, and timolol in Chapter 48.

Alpha$_1$-Antagonists Alpha$_1$-antagonists are indicated for hypertension. These drugs are also used to treat benign prostatic hyperplasia (BPH) and urinary obstruction because they relax smooth muscle in the prostate and bladder neck, thus reducing urethral resistance. The client may experience hypotension with the first few doses of these medications, and orthostatic hypotension may persist throughout treatment. The first-dose phenomenon, especially syncope, can occur. Therefore, it remains important to assess blood pressure prior to and routinely during therapy in order to maintain client safety. Assess for common side effects such as weakness, dizziness, headache, and GI complaints such as nausea and vomiting. Older adults are especially prone to the hypotensive and hypothermic effects related to vasodilation caused by these drugs. Drugs in this group range from pregnancy category B (prazosin) to C (terazosin). See "Nursing Process Focus: Clients Receiving Adrenergic Antagonist Therapy" in Chapter 13 for more information.

Alpha$_2$-Agonists   Alpha$_2$-agonists are centrally acting and have multiple side effects. These drugs are usually reserved to treat hypertension uncontrolled by other drugs. Assess for the presence of common adverse effects such as orthostatic hypotension, sedation, decreased libido, impotence, sodium/water retention, and dry mouth. Alpha$_2$-agonists are pregnancy category C; these drugs are distributed into breast milk.

Beta-Blockers   Adrenergic antagonists may be cardioselective (beta$_1$) or non-specific (beta$_1$ and beta$_2$) receptor blockers. Cardioselective beta-blockers decrease heart rate and affect myocardial conduction and contractility. Reduction in myocardial contractility reduces myocardial oxygen demand. Non-specific beta-blockers produce the same effects but also act on the respiratory system and the blood vessels, producing vasoconstriction and bronchoconstriction. Be alert for signs of respiratory distress, including shortness of breath and wheezing, in clients on non-specific beta-blocking drugs. These side effects tend to occur at high doses and with older drugs. Beta-blockers have several other important therapeutic applications. By decreasing the cardiac workload, beta-blockers can ease the symptoms of angina pectoris (Chapter 23). By slowing conduction through the myocardium, beta-blockers are able to treat certain types of dysrhythmia (Chapter 25). Other therapeutic uses include the treatment of heart failure (Chapter 24), myocardial infarction (Chapter 23), and migraines (Chapter 19).

Because all beta-blockers affect myocardial contractility, monitor heart rate, rhythm, and sounds, as well as the ECG. Beta-blockers can produce bradycardia and heart block. Reduction in heart rate can also contribute to fatigue and activity intolerance. Beta-blockers cause the heart rate to become less responsive to exertion. Clients should be advised to monitor their pulse as well as blood pressure daily. Because beta-blockers inhibit the sympathetic response to low blood glucose, diabetic clients should be warned that symptoms of hypoglycemia (diaphoresis, nervousness, and palpitation) may be less observable while on beta-blocker therapy.

See "Nursing Process Focus: Clients Receiving Beta-Adrenergic Antagonist Therapy" for more information.

DIRECT VASODILATORS

Drugs that directly affect arteriolar smooth muscle are highly effective at lowering blood pressure but produce too many side effects to be drugs of first choice. These agents are shown in Table 21.6.

21.11 Treating Hypertension with Direct Vasodilators

All antihypertensive classes discussed thus far lower blood pressure through indirect means by affecting enzymes (ACE inhibitors), autonomic nerves (alpha- and beta-blockers), or fluid volume (diuretics). It would seem that a more efficient way to reduce blood pressure would be to cause a direct relaxation of arteriolar smooth muscle; unfortunately, the direct vasodilator drugs have the potential to produce serious adverse effects. All direct vasodilators can produce **reflex tachycardia** as a compensatory response to the sudden decrease in blood pressure. Hydralazine can induce a lupus-like syndrome. Pericardial effusions have been reported with minoxidil use. Because safer drugs are available, oral direct vasodilators are rarely prescribed.

Pr PROTOTYPE DRUG | Doxazosin (Cardura)

ACTIONS AND USES

Doxazosin is a selective alpha$_1$-adrenergic blocker available only in oral form. Because it is selective for alpha$_1$-receptors in vascular smooth muscle, it has few adverse effects on other autonomic organs and is preferred over non-selective beta-blockers. Doxazosin dilates arteries and veins and is capable of causing a rapid, profound fall in blood pressure. Clients who have difficulty urinating due to an enlarged prostate (e.g., BPH) sometimes receive this drug to relieve symptoms of dysuria.

PHARMACOKINETICS

Doxazosin is well absorbed and is 98% protein bound. It is extensively metabolized by the liver. It has a half-life of 22 hours.

ADMINISTRATION ALERTS

- Doxazosin may produce a first-dose phenomenon resulting in profound hypotension, which may lead to syncope.
- The first-dose phenomenon can recur when medication is resumed after a period of withdrawal and with dosage increases.
- Doxazosin is pregnancy category B.

ADVERSE EFFECTS AND INTERACTIONS

Upon starting doxazosin therapy, some clients experience orthostatic hypotension, although tolerance normally develops to this side effect after a few doses. Dizziness and headache are also common side effects, although they are rarely severe enough to cause discontinuation of therapy.

Oral cimetidine may cause a mild increase (10%) in the half-life of doxazosin. This increase is not considered to be clinically significant.

 See the Companion Website for a Nursing Process Focus Chart specific to this drug.

NURSING PROCESS FOCUS   Clients Receiving Beta-Adrenergic Antagonist Therapy

Assessment	Potential Nursing Diagnoses/Identified Patterns
Prior to administration: ■ Obtain complete health history including allergies, drug history, and possible drug interactions. ■ Assess vital signs, urinary output, and cardiac output (initially and throughout therapy). ■ Assess for presence of respiratory disease, including asthma and COPD.	■ Need for knowledge regarding drug therapy ■ Decreased cardiac output ■ Risk for injury related to orthostatic hypotension ■ Sexual dysfunction ■ Non-adherence with therapeutic regimen

Planning: Client Goals and Expected Outcomes

The client will:
■ Exhibit a reduction in systolic/diastolic blood pressure
■ Report a decrease in cardiac symptoms such as chest pain and dyspnea on exertion
■ Demonstrate an understanding of the drug's action by accurately describing drug side effects and precautions

Implementation

Interventions (Rationales)	Client Education/Discharge Planning
■ Monitor vital signs and pulse; observe for signs of bradycardia, heart failure, and pulmonary edema. (Beta-blockers affect heart rate.) ■ Monitor for orthostatic hypotension when assisting client up from a supine position.	■ Instruct client to monitor vital signs as specified by the nurse, particularly blood pressure, ensuring proper use of home equipment. Instruct client to: ■ Withhold medication for severe hypotensive readings as specified by the nurse (e.g., "hold for levels below 88/50") ■ Always arise slowly, avoiding sudden posture changes
■ Observe for additional side effects such as fatigue and weakness.	■ Instruct client to report side effects such as slow pulse, difficulty breathing, dizziness, confusion, fatigue, weakness, and impotence.
■ In diabetic clients, monitor for hypoglycemia. (Beta-adrenergic blockers may prevent clients from experiencing common signs of low blood glucose levels.) ■ Observe for side effects such as drowsiness.	■ Instruct the diabetic client to check blood glucose levels and be more alert for and report signs of hypoglycemia. ■ Instruct client to avoid driving and other activities requiring mental alertness or physical coordination until effects of the drug are known.
■ Measure intake and output; measure daily weight.	Instruct client to: ■ Measure and monitor fluid intake and output and to weigh self daily ■ Consume enough *plain* water to remain adequately, but not over, hydrated

Evaluation of Outcome Criteria

Evaluate the effectiveness of drug therapy by confirming that client goals and expected outcomes have been met (see "Planning").

See Table 21.5 (page 267) under "Beta-Blockers" for a list of drugs to which these nursing actions apply.

TABLE 21.6   Direct-Acting Vasodilators for Hypertension

Drug	Route and Adult Dose
diazoxide (Proglycem)	PO; 100 mg bid or tid (max 300 mg/day)
hydralazine (Apo-Hydralazine)	PO; 25–50 mg qid (max 300 mg/day)
minoxidil (Loniten)	PO; 5–40 mg/day in a single or divided doses (max 100 mg/day)
nitroprusside (Nitropress, Nipride)	IV; 1.5–10 µg/kg/min

One direct-acting vasodilator, nitroprusside, is specifically used for those clients who have aggressive, life-threatening hypertension that must be quickly controlled. Nitroprusside, with a half-life of only 2 minutes, has the capability of lowering blood pressure almost instantaneously upon IV administra- tion. It is essential to continuously monitor clients receiving this drug in order to avoid hypotension because of over-treatment. In conditions such as malnutrition or surgery or high rates of infusion, nitroprusside may lead to depletion of sulfur stores and accumulation of cyanide and its toxic metabolites.

NURSING CONSIDERATIONS

Direct vasodilators are primarily utilized in emergency situations when it is necessary to reduce blood pressure quickly. In the critical care or emergency department setting, the client will likely undergo continuous monitoring of vital signs, ECG, and pulse oximetry. The nurse may also be expected to auscultate blood pressures every 5 to 15 minutes during the drug infusion. Closely observe monitoring equipment to assess heart rate/ECG for reflex tachycardia.

Contraindications include hypersensitivity, coronary artery disease, rheumatic mitral valve disease, cerebrovascular disease, renal insufficiency, and systemic lupus erythematosus. Direct vasodilators can cause priapism, a sustained, painful penile erection unrelieved by orgasm. Clients may feel embarrassed by priapism and be reluctant to report this side effect. They should be warned that priapism constitutes a medical emergency; if not treated promptly, permanent impotence may result.

There are specific considerations for the various types of direct vasodilators. For minoxidil therapy, monitor blood pressure and pulse in both arms while the client is lying, sitting, and standing to assess for orthostatic hypotension. The client should be informed that these agents may cause elongation, thickening, and increased pigmentation of body hair. This is normal and will stop when the drug is discontinued.

For IV diazoxide, be aware that repeated IV use can result in sodium and water retention; sodium, BUN, and the presence of edema and heart failure should be monitored. Diuretics may be used to counteract this effect when used during labour and delivery. However, fetal or neonatal hyperbilirubinemia, thrombocytopenia, or altered carbohydrate metabolism may be complications.

NATURAL THERAPIES

Hawthorn for Hypertension

A number of botanicals have been reported to possess antihypertensive activity, including hawthorn, which is sometimes called mayflower. Hawthorn (*Crataegus laevigata*) is a thorny shrub or small tree that is widespread in North America, Europe, and Asia. In some cultures, the shrub is surrounded in magic and religious rites and is thought to ward off evil spirits. The ship *Mayflower* was named after this shrub.

Leaves, flowers, and berries of the plant are dried or extracted in liquid form. Active ingredients are flavonoids and procyanidins. Hawthorn has been purported to lower blood pressure after 4 weeks or longer of therapy, although the effect has been small. The mechanism of action may be inhibition of ACE or reduction of cardiac workload. Clients taking cardiac glycosides should avoid hawthorn because it has the ability to decrease cardiac output. Clients should be advised not to rely on any botanical for the treatment of hypertension without frequent measurements of blood pressure to be certain therapy is effective.

Intravenous nitroprusside is a chemically unstable solution. The only diluent compatible with nitroprusside is 5% dextrose in water (D5W). This drug should never be mixed with any other drugs or diluents. Once dissolved in the vial, nitroprusside solution should be further diluted (in a 250 mL to 1 L bag of D5W) to prevent phlebitis. Reconstituted nitroprusside solution is brown and considered stable for up to 24 hours, but the drug is exceptionally light-sensitive. Once reconstituted, wrap the IV bag and tubing in an opaque substance (e.g., aluminum foil); labelling should appear on the wrap as well as on the bag itself. The drug solution should be checked periodically and the drug discarded if the colour of the solution changes.

See "Nursing Process Focus: Clients Receiving Direct Vasodilator Therapy" for specific teaching points.

Pr PROTOTYPE DRUG | Hydralazine (Apo-Hydralazine)

ACTIONS AND USES

Hydralazine was one of the first oral antihypertensive drugs marketed in North America. It acts through direct vasodilation of vascular smooth muscle. Although it produces an effective reduction in blood pressure, drugs in other antihypertensive classes have largely replaced hydralazine. The drug is available in both oral and parenteral formulations.

ADMINISTRATION ALERTS

- Abrupt withdrawal of the drug may cause rebound hypertension and anxiety.
- Hydralazine is pregnancy category C.

PHARMACOKINETICS

Hydralazine is rapidly absorbed, widely distributed, and mostly metabolized by the GI mucosa and liver. It has a half-life of 2 to 8 hours.

ADVERSE EFFECTS AND INTERACTIONS

Hydralazine may produce serious side effects, including severe reflex tachycardia. Clients taking hydralazine sometimes receive a beta-adrenergic blocker to counteract this effect on the heart. The drug may produce a lupus-like syndrome with extended use. Sodium and fluid retention is a potentially serious adverse effect. Because of these side effects, the use of hydralazine is mostly limited to clients whose HTN cannot be controlled with other, safer medications.

MAO inhibitors may potentiate hypotensive action. Other antihypertensive drugs given concomitantly can cause profound hypotension. NSAIDs may decrease the antihypertensive response.

 See the Companion Website for a Nursing Process Focus Chart specific to this drug.

NURSING PROCESS FOCUS   Clients Receiving Direct Vasodilator Therapy

Assessment	Potential Nursing Diagnoses/Identified Patterns
Prior to administration: ■ Obtain complete health history including allergies, drug history, and possible drug interactions. ■ Obtain ECG and vital signs; assess in context of client's baseline values. ■ Auscultate heart and chest sounds. ■ Assess neurological status and level of consciousness. ■ Obtain blood and urine specimens for laboratory analysis.	■ Need for knowledge regarding drug therapy ■ Risk for fluid and electrolyte imbalance ■ Ineffective tissue perfusion ■ Excess fluid volume ■ Risk for injury related to orthostatic hypotension ■ Risk for impaired skin integrity (e.g., IV vasodilators)

Planning: Client Goals and Expected Outcomes

The client will:
■ Exhibit a reduction in systolic/diastolic blood pressure
■ Demonstrate an understanding of the drug's action by accurately describing drug side effects and precautions

Implementation

Intervention (Rationales)	Client Education/Discharge Planning
■ Observe for signs and symptoms of lupus.	■ Instruct client to report classic "butterfly rash" over the nose and cheeks, muscle aches, and fatigue when taking hydralazine.
■ Monitor client vital signs every 5 to 15 minutes and titrate infusion based on prescribed parameters. (These drugs cause rapid hypotension.)	■ Instruct client to report any burning or stinging pain, swelling, warmth, redness, or tenderness at the IV insertion site, which may signal phlebitis.
■ Use with caution with impaired cardiac/cerebral circulation. (The hypotension produced by vasodilators may further compromise individuals who already suffer from ischemia.)	Instruct client to: ■ Report angina-like symptoms: chest, arm, back and/or neck pain, palpitations ■ Report faintness; dizziness; drowsiness; any sensation of cold, numbness, or tingling; pale or dusky look to the hands and feet ■ Report headache or signs of stroke: facial drooping, visual changes, limb weakness, or paralysis ■ Monitor vitals signs (especially blood pressure) daily or as often as advised by the nurse
■ Monitor for dizziness. (This is a sign of hypotension that occurs because the brain is not getting enough blood flow.)	Instruct client to: ■ Avoid driving and other activities requiring mental alertness or physical coordination until effects of the drug are known ■ Always arise slowly, avoiding sudden posture changes
■ Evaluate need for lifestyle modifications.	■ Instruct client to comply with additional interventions for HTN such as weight reduction, modification of sodium intake, smoking cessation, exercise, and stress management.
■ Discontinue medication gradually. (Abrupt withdrawal of drug may cause rebound hypertension and anxiety.)	■ Instruct client to not suddenly stop taking the drug.

Evaluation of Outcome Criteria

Evaluate the effectiveness of drug therapy by confirming that client goals and expected outcomes have been met (see "Planning").

See Table 21.6 (page 269) for a list of drugs to which these nursing applications apply.

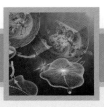

CHAPTER REVIEW

KEY CONCEPTS

The numbered key concepts provide a succinct summary of the important points from the corresponding numbered section within the chapter. If any of these points are not clear, refer to the numbered section within the chapter for review. Expanded versions can be found on the Companion Website.

21.1 High blood pressure is classified as essential (primary) or secondary. Uncontrolled hypertension can lead to chronic and debilitating disorders such as stroke, heart attack, and heart failure.

21.2 The three primary factors controlling blood pressure are cardiac output, peripheral resistance, and blood volume.

21.3 Many factors help to regulate blood pressure, including the vasomotor centre, baroreceptors and chemoreceptors in the aorta and internal carotid arteries, and the renin-angiotensin system.

21.4 Hypertension has been recently redefined as a sustained blood pressure of 140/90 mm Hg after multiple measurements made over several clinic visits. A person with sustained blood pressure of 120–139/80–89 mm Hg is said to be prehypertensive and is at increased risk of developing hypertension.

21.5 Because antihypertensive medications may have uncomfortable side effects, lifestyle changes such as proper diet and exercise should be implemented prior to and during pharmacotherapy to allow lower drug doses.

21.6 Pharmacotherapy of HTN often begins with low doses of a single medication. If ineffective, a second agent from a different class may be added to the regimen.

21.7 Diuretics are often the first-line medications for HTN because they have few side effects and can control minor to moderate hypertension.

21.8 Calcium channel blockers block calcium ions from entering cells and cause smooth muscle in arterioles to relax, thus reducing blood pressure. CCBs have emerged as major drugs in the treatment of hypertension.

21.9 Drugs blocking the renin-angiotensin system prevent the intense vasoconstriction caused by angiotensin II. These drugs also decrease blood volume, which enhances their antihypertensive effect.

21.10 Antihypertensive autonomic agents are available to block $alpha_1$-, $beta_1$-, and/or $beta_2$-receptors, or stimulate $alpha_2$-receptors in the brainstem (centrally acting).

21.11 A few medications lower blood pressure by acting directly to relax arteriolar smooth muscle, but these are not widely used due to their numerous side effects.

REVIEW QUESTIONS

1 Describe strategies that the nurse can use to promote adherence with antihypertensive medications in a client who experiences no symptoms.

2 State the major reasons why a client should continue lifestyle changes, even though the antihypertensive drug appears to be effective.

3 Why is it important for clients to weigh themselves on a regular basis when taking antihypertensive drugs?

CRITICAL THINKING QUESTIONS

1. A 74-year-old client has a history of hypertension, mild renal failure, and angina. The client is on a low-sodium, low-protein diet. The most recent blood pressure (BP) is 106/84 mm Hg. Should the nurse give the client benazepril (Lotensin) as scheduled? Why or why not?

2. A client with diabetes is on atenolol (Tenormin) for hypertension. What teaching should be done for this client?

3. A client is having a hypertensive crisis (230/130 mm Hg), and the BP needs to be lowered. The client has an IV drip of nitroprusside (Nitropress) initiated. How much would the nurse want to lower this client's BP? Name three nursing factors that are crucial when administering this drip.

EXPLORE
MediaLink

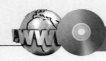

 MEDIALINK DVD-ROM
- **Audio Glossary**
- **CRNE Review**
- **Animations**
  Mechanism of Action: Doxazosin
  Mechanism of Action: Nifedipine

 COMPANION WEBSITE
- **CRNE Review**
- **Case Study:** Client with hypertension
- **Dosage Calculations**
- **Nursing Process Focus Charts**

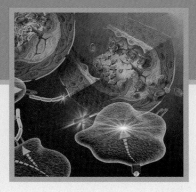

CHAPTER 22

Drugs for Lipid Disorders

DRUGS AT A GLANCE

HMG-COA REDUCTASE INHIBITORS
> *atorvastatin (Lipitor)*

BILE ACID RESINS
> *cholestyramine (Novo-Cholamine, PMS-Cholestyramine)*

NICOTINIC ACID

FIBRIC ACID AGENTS
> *gemfibrozil (Lopid)*

OBJECTIVES

After reading this chapter, the student should be able to do the following:

1. Identify drug classes used for treating lipid disorders.
2. Explain the therapeutic action of each class of drug used for lipid disorders in relation to the pathophysiology of the disorder requiring treatment.
3. Discuss the role of the nurse in teaching clients regarding control of cholesterol and LDL levels through non-pharmacological means.
4. Describe the nurse's role in the pharmacological management of clients receiving drugs for lipid disorders.
5. For each of the drug classes listed in Drugs at a Glance, identify a representative drug and explain its mechanism of action, therapeutic effects, and important adverse effects.
6. Describe and explain, based on pharmacological principles, the rationale for nursing assessment, planning, and interventions for clients with lipid disorders.
7. Use the nursing process to care for clients receiving drug therapy for lipid disorders.

MediaLink

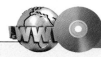 www.pearsoned.ca/adams-king

CRNE review, case studies, and other interactive resources for this chapter can be found on the Companion Website at **www.pearsoned.ca/adams-king**. Click on "Chapter 22" to select the activities for this chapter. For animations, more CRNE review questions, and an audio glossary, access the accompanying DVD-ROM in this textbook.

Research during the 1960s and 1970s brought about a nutritional revolution as new knowledge about lipids and their relationship to obesity and cardiovascular disease allowed people to make more intelligent lifestyle choices. Since then, advances in the diagnosis of lipid disorders have helped to identify those clients at greatest risk for cardiovascular disease and those most likely to benefit from pharmacological intervention. Research in pharmacology has led to safe, effective drugs for lowering lipid levels, thus decreasing the risk of cardiovascular-related diseases. As a result of this knowledge and advancement in pharmacology, the incidence of death due to most cardiovascular diseases has been declining, although cardiovascular disease remains the leading cause of death in North America.

22.1 Types of Lipid

The three types of lipid important to humans are illustrated in Figure 22.1. The most common are the **triglycerides**, which form a large family of different lipids all having three fatty acids attached to a chemical backbone of glycerol. Triglycerides are the major storage form of fat in the body and the only type of lipid that serves as an important energy source. They account for 90% of total lipids in the body.

The **phospholipids** are formed when a phosphorous group replaces one of the fatty acids in a triglyceride. These lipids are essential for building plasma membranes. The best-known phospholipids are **lecithins**, which are found in high concentration in egg yolks and soybeans. Lecithins were once promoted as a natural treatment for high cholesterol levels, but controlled studies have not shown lecithin to be of any benefit for this disorder. Likewise, lecithin has been proposed as a remedy for nervous system diseases such as Alzheimer's disease and bipolar disorder, but there is no definite evidence to support these claims.

The **steroids** are a diverse group of substances having a common chemical structure called the **sterol nucleus**, or ring. **Cholesterol** is the most widely known of the steroids, and its role in promoting atherosclerosis has been clearly demonstrated. Cholesterol is a natural and vital component of plasma membranes. Unlike the triglycerides that provide fuel for the body during times of energy need, cholesterol serves as the building block for a number of essential biochemicals, including vitamin D, bile acids, cortisol, estrogen, and testosterone. While clearly essential for life, the body only needs minute amounts of cholesterol. The liver is able to synthesize adequate amounts of cholesterol from other chemicals; it is not necessary to provide additional cholesterol in the diet. Dietary cholesterol is obtained solely from animal products; humans do not metabolize the sterols produced by plants. Health Canada recommends less than 300 mg of dietary cholesterol per day.

PHARMFACTS

High Blood Cholesterol

- The incidence of high blood cholesterol increases until age 65.
- Over 43% of adult Canadians have elevated total blood cholesterol.
- Moderate alcohol intake does not reduce LDL cholesterol, but it does increase HDL cholesterol.
- Prior to menopause, high blood cholesterol occurs more frequently in men, but after age 50, the condition is more common in women.
- To lower blood cholesterol, both dietary cholesterol and saturated fat must be reduced.
- Familial hypercholesterolemia affects 1 in 500 people. It is a genetic disease that predisposes people to high cholesterol levels.

MediaLink   How Can I Lower My Cholesterol by Changing My Diet?

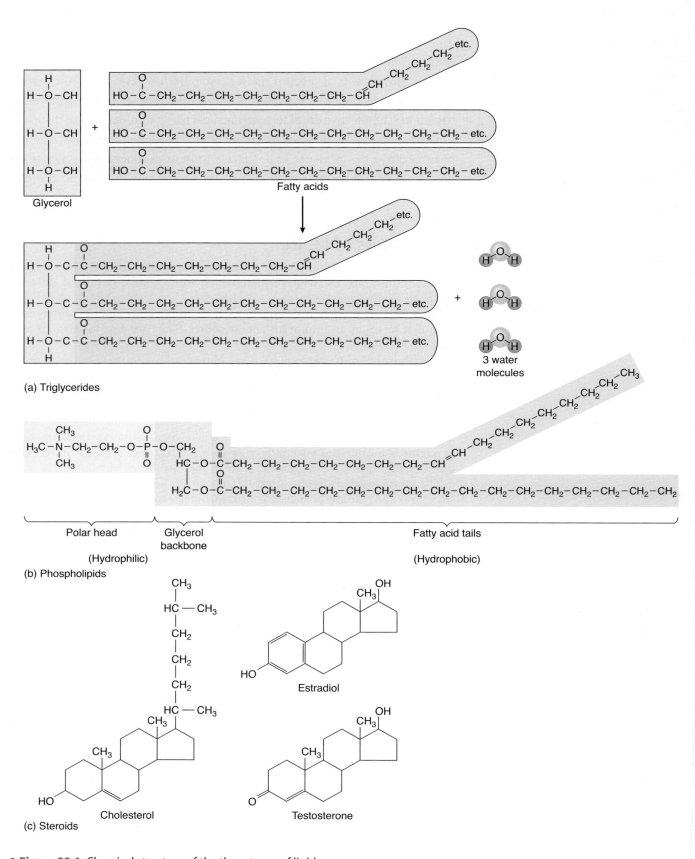

(a) Triglycerides

(b) Phospholipids

(c) Steroids

● **Figure 22.1** Chemical structure of the three types of lipid

22.2 Lipoproteins

Because lipid molecules are not soluble in plasma, they must be specially packaged for transport through the blood. To accomplish this, the body forms complexes called **lipoproteins** that consist of various amounts of cholesterol, triglycerides, and phospholipids, along with a protein carrier. The protein component is called an **apoprotein** (*apo-* means "separated from" or "derived from").

The three most common lipoproteins are classified according to their composition, size, and weight or density, which comes primarily from the amount of apoprotein present in the complex. Each type varies in lipid and apoprotein makeup and serves a different function in transporting lipids from sites of synthesis and absorption to sites of utilization. For example, **high-density lipoprotein (HDL)** contains the most apoprotein, up to 50% by weight. The highest amount of cholesterol is carried by **low-density lipoprotein (LDL)**. Figure 22.2 illustrates the three basic lipoproteins and their compositions.

To understand the pharmacotherapy of lipid disorders, it is important to learn the functions of the major lipoproteins and their roles in transporting cholesterol. LDL transports cholesterol from the liver to the tissues and organs, where it is used to build plasma membranes or to synthesize other steroids. Once in the tissues, it can also be stored for later use. Storage of cholesterol in the lining of blood vessels, however, is not desirable because it contributes to plaque buildup and atherosclerosis. LDL is often called "bad" cholesterol because this lipoprotein contributes significantly to plaque deposits and coronary artery disease. Lowering LDL levels in the blood has been shown to decrease the incidence of coronary artery disease. **Very low–density lipoprotein (VLDL)** is the primary carrier of triglycerides in the blood. Through a series of steps, VLDL is reduced in size to become LDL.

HDL is manufactured in the liver and small intestine and assists in the transport of cholesterol away from the body tissues and back to the liver in a process called **reverse cholesterol transport**. The cholesterol component of the HDL is then broken down to unite with bile that is subsequently excreted in the feces. Excretion via bile is the only route the body uses to remove cholesterol. Because HDL transports cholesterol for destruction and removes it from the body, it is considered "good" cholesterol.

Hyperlipidemia, the general term meaning "high levels of lipids in the blood," is a major risk factor for cardiovascular disease. Elevated blood cholesterol, or **hypercholesterolemia**, is the type of hyperlipidemia that is most familiar to the general public. **Dyslipidemia** refers to abnormal (excess or deficient) levels of lipoproteins. The etiology may be inherited and/or acquired.

22.3 Achieving and Maintaining Desirable Lipid Levels

Achieving and maintaining optimal lipid levels are important for the prevention of cardiovascular disease. It is not adequate

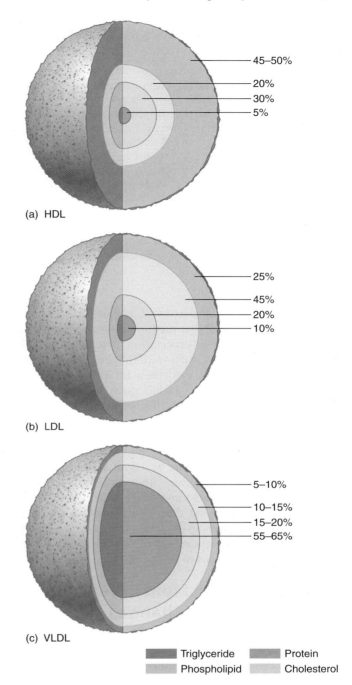

(a) HDL — 45–50% / 20% / 30% / 5%

(b) LDL — 25% / 45% / 20% / 10%

(c) VLDL — 5–10% / 10–15% / 15–20% / 55–65%

Triglyceride   Protein
Phospholipid   Cholesterol

● **Figure 22.2** Composition of the lipoproteins

to simply measure total cholesterol in the blood. Because some cholesterol is being transported for destruction, a more accurate profile is obtained by measuring LDL cholesterol and the ratio of total cholesterol to HDL cholesterol in the blood. The goal in maintaining normal cholesterol levels is to maximize the HDL and minimize the LDL. The target LDL cholesterol level is less than 2.5 mmol/L. The target total cholesterol to HDL cholesterol ratio is less than 4.0. Triglyceride levels may also be assessed. The optimal serum triglyceride concentration is less than 1.7 mmol/L.

Scientists have further divided LDL into subclasses of lipoproteins. For example, one variety called lipoprotein

LIFESPAN CONSIDERATIONS

Pediatric Dyslipidemia

Most people consider dyslipidemia a condition that occurs with advancing age. Dyslipidemias, however, are also a concern for some pediatric clients. Children at risk include those with a family history of premature coronary artery disease or dyslipidemia and those who have hypertension, diabetes, or are obese. Lipid levels fluctuate in children, and they tend to be higher in girls. Nutritional intervention, regular physical activity, and risk factor management are warranted when the LDL cholesterol level reaches 2.85 to 3.34 mmol/L. More aggressive dietary therapy and pharmacotherapy may be warranted in pediatric clients with LDL cholesterol levels above 3.37 mmol/L. The long-term effects of lipid-lowering drugs in children have not been clearly established; therefore, drug therapy is not recommended for children under 10 years of age. Cholestyramine and colestipol are the only approved drugs for hypercholesterolemia in children, although side effects sometimes result in poor adherence. Research into the use of niacin and low-dose statin pharmacotherapy in children is continuing.

(a) has been strongly associated with plaque formation and heart disease. It is likely that further research will discover other varieties, with the expectation that drugs will be designed to be more selective toward the "bad" lipoproteins.

Establishing treatment guidelines for dyslipidemia has been difficult as the condition has no symptoms and the progression to cardiovascular disease may take decades. Based on years of research, the Canadian Working Group on Hypercholesterolemia and other Dyslipidemias recently revised the recommended treatment guidelines for dyslipidemia. The new guidelines are based on accumulated evidence that reducing "borderline" high cholesterol levels can result in fewer heart attacks and fewer deaths. In addition, the guidelines recommend that high cholesterol levels be treated more aggressively in diabetic clients and other high-risk groups. These guidelines will likely lead to more widespread use of medications to treat dyslipidemia.

22.4 Controlling Lipid Levels through Lifestyle Changes

Lifestyle changes should always be included in any treatment plan for reducing blood lipid levels. Many clients with borderline laboratory values can control their dyslipidemia entirely through non-pharmacological means. It is important to note that all the lifestyle factors for reducing blood lipid levels also apply to cardiovascular disease in general. Because many clients taking lipid-lowering drugs also have underlying cardiovascular disease, these lifestyle changes are particularly important. Following are the most important lipid-reduction interventions:

- Monitor blood lipid levels regularly, as recommended by the healthcare provider.
- Maintain weight and waist circumference at an optimum level.
- Implement a medically supervised exercise plan.
- Reduce dietary saturated fat, trans fatty acids, and cholesterol to less than 7% of total calories, while increasing the proportion of monounsaturated and polyunsaturated fats.
- Increase soluble fibre in the diet, as found in oat bran, apples, beans, grapefruit, and broccoli.
- Limit alcohol use to no more than two standard drinks per day.
- Reduce or eliminate tobacco use.

Nutritionists recommend that the intake of dietary fat be less than 30% of the total caloric intake. Cholesterol intake should be reduced as much as possible and should not exceed 300 mg/day. It is interesting to note that restriction of dietary cholesterol alone will not result in a significant reduction in blood cholesterol levels. This is because the liver reacts to a low-cholesterol diet by making more cholesterol and by inhibiting its excretion when saturated fats are present. Thus, the client must reduce saturated fat in the diet, as well as cholesterol, to control the amount made by the liver and to ultimately lower blood cholesterol levels.

The use of plant sterols and stanols is now approved in some countries to reduce blood cholesterol levels. These plant lipids have a similar structure to cholesterol and therefore compete with that substance for absorption in the digestive tract. When the body absorbs the plant sterols, cholesterol is excreted from the body. When less cholesterol is delivered to the liver, LDL uptake increases, thereby decreasing the serum LDL level. Plant sterols and stanols may be obtained from a variety of sources, including wheat, corn, rye, oats, and rice, as well as nuts and olive oil. In countries where they are approved, they may be found in some margarines, salad dressings, cereals, and fruit juices. The daily intake of plant sterols or stanols should not exceed 3 g. Health Canada advises that sterols may pose health risks for certain groups such as pregnant women, children, people predisposed to hemorrhagic strokes, and people on cholesterol-lowering medication. Investigations are in progress to assess the safety of plant sterols and stanols.

HMG-COA REDUCTASE INHIBITORS (STATINS)

The statin class of antihyperlipidemics interferes with a critical enzyme in the synthesis of cholesterol. Cholesterol is manufactured in the liver by a series of more than 25 metabolic steps, beginning with acetyl CoA, a two-carbon unit that is produced from the breakdown of fatty acids. Of the many enzymes involved in this complex pathway, **HMG-CoA reductase** (3-hydroxy-3-methylglutaryl coenzyme A reductase) serves as the primary regulatory site for cholesterol biosynthesis. Under normal conditions, this enzyme is controlled through negative feedback: high levels of LDL cholesterol in the blood will shut down production of HMG-CoA reductase, thus turning off the cholesterol pathway. Figure 22.3 illustrates selected steps in cholesterol biosynthesis and the importance of HMG-CoA reductase.

The statins, which are also known as HMG-CoA reductase inhibitors, are shown in Table 22.1 on page 280. They are first-line drugs in the treatment of lipid disorders.

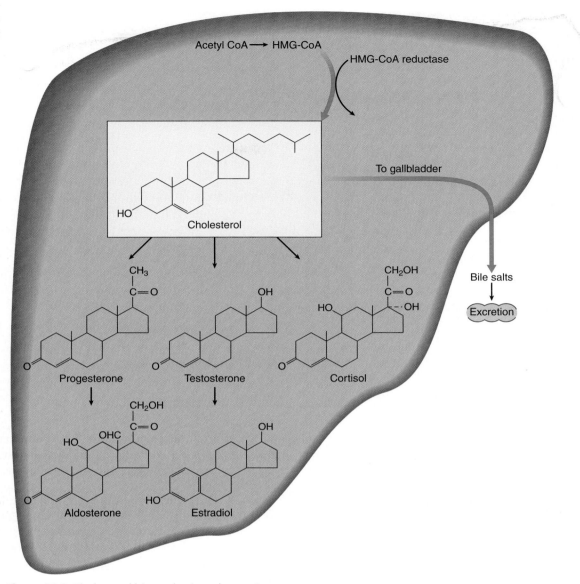

● **Figure 22.3** Cholesterol biosynthesis and excretion

22.5 **Pharmacotherapy with Statins**

In the late 1970s, compounds isolated from various species of fungi were found to inhibit cholesterol production in human cells in the laboratory. This class of drug, known as the statins, has since revolutionized the treatment of lipid disorders. Statins can produce a dramatic 20% to 40% reduction in LDL cholesterol levels. In addition to reducing the LDL cholesterol level in the blood, statins can also lower triglyceride and VLDL levels and raise the level of "good" HDL cholesterol.

The statins act by inhibiting HMG-CoA reductase, which results in less cholesterol biosynthesis. As the liver makes less cholesterol, it responds by making more LDL receptors on the surface of liver cells. The greater number of LDL receptors in liver cells results in increased removal of LDL from the blood. Blood levels of both LDL and cholesterol are reduced. The drop in lipid levels is not permanent,

however, so clients need to remain on these drugs during the remainder of their lives or until their hyperlipidemia can be controlled through dietary or lifestyle changes. Statins have been shown to slow the progression of coronary artery disease and to reduce mortality from cardiovascular disease. The mechanisms of action of the statins and other drugs for dyslipidemia are illustrated in Figure 22.4.

All the statins are given orally and are tolerated well by most clients. Many of them should be administered in the evening since cholesterol biosynthesis in the body is higher at night. Atorvastatin is effective regardless of the time of day it is taken.

Much research is ongoing to determine other therapeutic effects of drugs in the statin class. For example, statins block the vasoconstrictive effect of the A-beta protein, a significant protein involved in Alzheimer's disease. Cholesterol and A-beta protein have similar effects on blood vessels, causing them to constrict. Preliminary research suggests that the

TABLE 22.1	Drugs for Dyslipidemia
Drug	**Route and Adult Dose**
HMG-CoA Reductase Inhibitors	
atorvastatin (Lipitor)	PO; 10–80 mg qd
fluvastatin (Lescol)	PO; 20–80 mg qd (max 80 mg/day)
lovastatin (Advicor, Apo-Lovastatin, Mevacor)	PO; 20–80 mg qd–bid
pravastatin (Pravachol)	PO; 10–40 mg qd
rosuvastatin (Crestor)	PO; 10–40 mg qd
simvastatin (Zocor)	PO; 10–80 mg qd
Bile Acid–Binding Agents	
cholestyramine (Novo-Cholamine, PMS-Cholestyramine)	PO; 4–9 g bid–qid ac and hs
colestipol (Colestid)	PO; 5–15 g bid–qid ac and hs
fenofibrate (Lipidil, Apo-Fenofibrate)	PO; 100–200 mg qd (max 200 mg/day)
Fibric Acid Agents	
fenofibrate (Lipidil, Apo-Fenofibrate)	PO; 100–200 mg qd (max 200 mg/day)
gemfibrozil (Lopid)	PO; 300–600 mg bid (max 1500 mg/day)
Other Agents	
ezetimibe (Ezetrol)	PO; 10 mg/day
niacin (Niacin, Niacin SR)	Hyperlipidemia: PO; 1.5–3.0 g/day in divided doses (max 6 g/day) Niacin deficiency: PO; 50–500 mg/day
orlistate (Xenical)	PO; 120 mg tid with meals

statins may protect against dementia by inhibiting the protein and thus slowing dementia caused by blood vessel constriction.

NURSING CONSIDERATIONS

The role of the nurse in statin therapy involves careful monitoring of the client's condition and providing education as it relates to the prescribed drug regimen. Although statin drugs are effective in reducing blood lipid levels, there can be serious adverse effects in some clients. Statins are pregnancy category X and should not be used in clients who are pregnant or breastfeeding or who may become pregnant. Women taking statin drugs should utilize effective birth control and stop taking the medication if they suspect pregnancy.

Because liver dysfunction may occur with the use of statin drugs, the nurse should monitor liver function tests before and during therapy. Statin drugs should not be used in clients with active liver disease or unexplained elevations in liver function tests. This drug class should be used cautiously in clients who drink large quantities of alcohol, and alcohol use should be restricted or discontinued while on the medication. Because myopathy has been reported by some clients, the nurse should assess the client for muscle pain, tenderness, and weakness. Creatinine phosphokinase (CPK) levels should be obtained if myopathy is suspected and, if elevated, statin therapy should be discontinued. The drug may be discontinued if muscle weakness persists even without CPK elevation.

Nausea, vomiting, heartburn, dyspepsia, abdominal cramping, and diarrhea are common, though less serious, side effects. The statins can be taken with the evening meal to help alleviate GI upset.

Client education as it relates to these drugs should include goals, reasons for obtaining baseline data such as vital signs and tests for cardiac and hepatic disorders, and possible side effects. Following are the important points the nurse should include when teaching clients regarding HMG-CoA reductase inhibitors:

- Keep all scheduled laboratory visits for liver function tests.
- Do not take other prescription drugs, OTC medications, herbal remedies, or vitamins/minerals without notifying the healthcare provider.
- Practise reliable contraception and notify the healthcare provider if pregnancy is planned or suspected.
- Immediately report unexplained muscle pain, tenderness, or weakness, especially if accompanied by malaise or fever.
- Immediately report unexplained numbness, tingling, weakness, or pain in feet or hands.
- Take drug with the evening meal to prevent GI disturbances.

BILE ACID RESINS

Bile acid resins bind bile acids, thus increasing the excretion of cholesterol. They are sometimes used in combination with the statins. These agents are shown in Table 22.1.

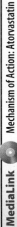

MediaLink | Mechanism of Action: Atorvastatin

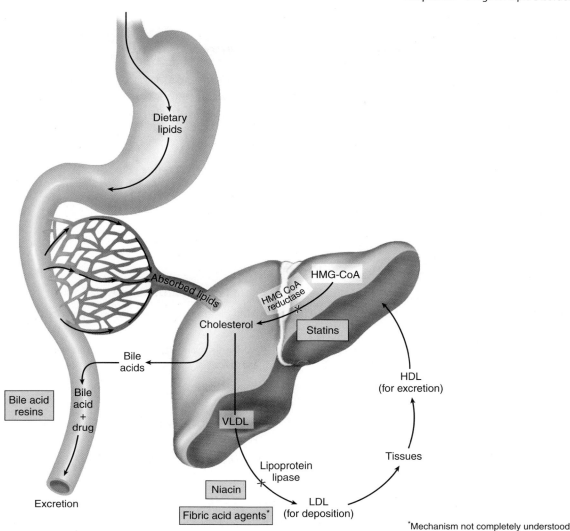

● **Figure 22.4** Mechanisms of action of lipid-lowering drugs

---

Pr PROTOTYPE DRUG | Atorvastatin (Lipitor)

ACTIONS AND USES

The primary indication for atorvastatin is hypercholesterolemia. The statins act by inhibiting HMG-CoA reductase. As the liver makes less cholesterol, it responds by making more LDL receptors on the surface of liver cells. The greater number of LDL receptors in liver cells results in increased removal of LDL from the blood. Blood levels of both LDL and cholesterol are reduced, although at least 2 weeks of therapy are required before these effects are realized.

ADMINISTRATION ALERTS

- Administer with food to decrease GI discomfort.
- Drug may be taken at any time of day.
- Atorvastatin is pregnancy category X.

PHARMACOKINETICS

Atorvastatin is rapidly absorbed. Bioavailability is 14% due to first-pass metabolism. It is excreted mostly in bile and feces. It has a half-life of 14 hours.

ADVERSE EFFECTS AND INTERACTIONS

Side effects of atorvastatin are rarely severe enough to cause discontinuation of therapy and include GI complaints such as intestinal cramping, diarrhea, and constipation. A small percentage of clients experience liver damage; thus, hepatic function is monitored during the first few months of therapy.

Atorvastatin interacts with many other drugs. For example, it may increase digoxin levels by 20%, as well as increase levels of norethindrone and ethinyl estradiol (oral contraceptives). Erythromycin may increase atorvastatin levels by 40%.

Grapefruit juice inhibits the metabolism of statins, allowing them to reach toxic levels. Since HMG-CoA reductase inhibitors also decrease the synthesis of coenzyme Q10 (CoQ10), clients may benefit from CoQ10 supplements.

 See the Companion Website for a Nursing Process Focus Chart specific to this drug.

NURSING PROCESS FOCUS Clients Receiving HMG-CoA Reductase Inhibitor Therapy

Assessment	Potential Nursing Diagnoses/Identified Patterns
Prior to administration: ■ Obtain a complete health history including allergies, drug history, and possible drug interactions. ■ Obtain baseline liver function tests, lipid studies, and a pregnancy test in women of childbearing age.	■ Need for knowledge regarding drug therapy and lifestyle modifications ■ Non-adherence related to dietary and drug regimen ■ Chronic pain related to drug-induced myopathy

Planning: Client Goals and Expected Outcomes

The client will:
■ Immediately report skeletal muscle pain, unexplained muscle soreness, or weakness
■ Demonstrate adherence with appropriate lifestyle changes
■ Demonstrate an understanding of the drug's action by accurately describing drug side effects and precautions

Implementation

Interventions (Rationales)	Client Education/Discharge Planning
■ Monitor blood cholesterol and triglyceride levels at intervals during therapy (to determine effectiveness of therapy).	■ Advise client of the importance of keeping appointments for laboratory testing.
■ Monitor client adherence with dietary regimen. (Maintenance of controlled saturated fat in the diet is essential to effectiveness of medications.)	■ Provide client with information needed to maintain a diet low in saturated fat and cholesterol
■ Monitor client for alcohol abuse. (Excessive alcohol intake may result in liver damage and interfere with drug effectiveness.)	■ Instruct client to avoid or limit alcohol use.
■ Monitor CPK level. (Elevated CPK may be indicative of impending myopathy.) ■ Monitor liver function. (Liver dysfunction may occur with these drugs.)	■ Instruct client to report symptoms of leg or muscle pain to the healthcare provider.
■ Obtain client's smoking history. (Smoking increases risk of cardiovascular disease and may decrease HDL levels.)	■ Encourage smoking cessation if appropriate.

Evaluation of Outcome Criteria

Evaluate the effectiveness of drug therapy by confirming that client goals and expected outcomes have been met (see "Planning").

See Table 22.1 (page 280) for a list of drugs to which these nursing actions apply.

22.6 Bile Acid Resins for Reducing Cholesterol and LDL Levels

Prior to the discovery of the statins, the primary means of lowering blood cholesterol was through use of bile acid–binding drugs called bile acid resins or sequestrants. These drugs bind bile acids, which contain a high concentration of cholesterol. Because of their large size, resins are not absorbed from the small intestine and the bound bile acids and cholesterol are eliminated in the feces. The liver responds to the loss of cholesterol by making more LDL receptors, which removes even more cholesterol from the blood in a mechanism similar to that of the statin drugs.

Although effective at producing a 20% drop in LDL cholesterol, the bile acid sequestrants tend to cause more frequent side effects than statins. Because of this, they are no longer considered first-line drugs for dyslipidemia.

NURSING CONSIDERATIONS

The role of the nurse in bile acid resin therapy involves careful monitoring of the client's condition and providing education as it relates to the prescribed drug regimen. Because bile acid sequestrants act in the GI tract and are not absorbed, they have no systemic side effects. They can, however, cause significant GI effects such as constipation, abdominal pain, bloating, nausea, vomiting, diarrhea, and steatorrhea. The nurse should assess bowel sounds and the presence of GI disturbance. Bile acid resins should be used cautiously in clients with GI disorders such as peptic ulcer disease, hemorrhoids, inflammatory bowel disease, or chronic constipation as they may worsen or aggravate these conditions. These drugs are generally not used during pregnancy or lactation (pregnancy category C).

Bile acid resins decrease the absorption of vitamins and minerals; deficiencies may occur with extended use. Other medications should be taken more than 1 hour before or

4 hours after taking a bile acid sequestrant because of decreased absorption. Cholestyramine powder should be mixed with 60 to 180 mL of water, non-carbonated beverage, highly liquid soup, or pulpy fruit (applesauce, crushed pineapple) to prevent esophageal irritation. The nurse should place the contents of the packet on the surface of the fluid, allow it to stand (without stirring) for 2 minutes, occasionally twirling the glass, and then stir slowly (to prevent foaming) to form a suspension. The client should drink the medication immediately after stirring. The client should not inhale the powder as it may irritate mucous membranes.

Constipation may occur with decreased bowel function. Nausea, vomiting, heartburn, dyspepsia, abdominal cramping, and diarrhea may also occur. Clients with dysphagia or esophageal stricture could develop an obstruction taking this medication.

Client education as it relates to bile acid resins should include goals, reasons for obtaining baseline data such as vital signs and cardiac, hepatic, and renal tests, and possible side effects. Following are important points the nurse should include when teaching clients regarding bile acid resins:

- Take the medication before meals.
- Take other medication 1 hour before or 4 hours after taking bile acid resins to avoid interference with absorption of other drugs.
- A high-bulk diet and adequate fluid intake will help to decrease constipation and bloating.
- Take vitamin supplements to replace folic acid, fat-soluble vitamins, and vitamin K.
- Do not take other prescription drugs, OTC medications, herbal remedies, or vitamins/minerals without notifying the healthcare provider.
- Report the following immediately: yellowing of skin or whites of eyes, severe constipation, flatulence, nausea, heartburn, straining with passing of stools, tarry stools, or abnormal bleeding.

NICOTINIC ACID

Nicotinic acid, or niacin, is a B complex vitamin that is occasionally used to lower lipid levels. It has a number of side effects that limit its use. The dose for nicotinic acid is given in Table 22.1 on page 280.

22.7 Pharmacotherapy with Nicotinic Acid

The ability of nicotinic acid to lower lipid levels is unrelated to its role as a vitamin since much higher doses are needed to produce its antilipidemic effects. For lowering cholesterol, the usual dose is 2 to 3 g/day. When taken as a vitamin, the dose is only 25 mg/day. The primary effect of nicotinic acid is to decrease VLDL levels; since LDL is synthesized from VLDL, the client experiences a reduction in LDL cholesterol levels. It also has the desirable effects of reducing triglycerides and increasing HDL levels. As with other lipid-lowering drugs, maximum therapeutic effect may take a month or longer to achieve.

Although effective at reducing LDL cholesterol by as much as 20%, nicotinic acid produces more side effects than the statins. Flushing and hot flashes occur in almost every client. In addition, a variety of uncomfortable intestinal effects such as nausea, excess gas, and diarrhea are commonly reported. More serious side effects such as hepatotoxicity and gout are possible. Niacin is not usually prescribed for clients with diabetes mellitus because severe hyperglycemia may result. Because of these adverse effects, nicotinic acid is most often used in lower doses in combination with a statin or bile acid sequestrant since the beneficial effects of these drugs are additive.

Pr PROTOTYPE DRUG | Cholestyramine (Novo-Cholamine, PMS-Cholestyramine)

ACTIONS AND USES

Cholestyramine is a powder that is mixed with fluid before being taken once or twice daily. It lowers LDL cholesterol levels by increasing LDL receptors on hepatocytes. The resultant increase in LDL intake from plasma decreases circulating LDL levels.

PHARMACOKINETICS

Cholestyramine is not absorbed or metabolized once it enters the intestine, so it does not produce any systemic effects. It may take 30 days or longer to produce its maximum effect. It is excreted in the feces.

ADMINISTRATION ALERTS

- Mix drug thoroughly with liquid and have the client drink it immediately to avoid potential irritation or obstruction in the GI tract.
- Other drugs should be taken more than 1 hour before or 4 hours after taking cholestyramine.
- Cholestyramine is pregnancy category C.

ADVERSE EFFECTS AND INTERACTIONS

Although cholestyramine rarely produces serious side effects, clients may experience constipation, bloating, gas, and nausea that sometimes limit its use. Because cholestyramine can bind to other drugs and interfere with their absorption, it should not be taken at the same time as other medications. Cholestyramine is sometimes combined with other cholesterol-lowering drugs such as the statins or nicotinic acid to produce additive effects.

 See the Companion Website for a Nursing Process Focus Chart specific to this drug.

Because niacin is available without a prescription, clients should be instructed not to attempt self-medication with this drug. One form of niacin available OTC as a vitamin supplement called nicotinamide has no lipid-lowering effects. Clients should be informed that if nicotinic acid is to be used to lower cholesterol, it should be done under medical supervision.

NURSING CONSIDERATIONS

The role of the nurse in nicotinic acid therapy involves careful monitoring of the client's condition and providing education as it relates to the prescribed drug regimen. Because there is a risk of liver toxicity, niacin therapy must be carefully monitored. This is particularly important with sustained-release versions, which have the highest risk of hepatotoxicity. The nurse should assess liver function prior to and during therapy. Clients with elevated liver enzymes, history of liver disease, or peptic ulcers should not take niacin to lower lipids as this medication can worsen these conditions. In clients predisposed to gout, nicotinic acid may increase uric acid levels and precipitate acute gout.

Clients are most likely to discontinue nicotinic acid therapy due to the intense flushing and pruritus that occur 1 to 2 hours after taking the medication. This response may be caused by prostaglandin release; taking one ASA tablet 30 minutes prior to the nicotinic acid dose will help decrease this effect. The flushing effect decreases with time. Nicotinic acid may affect glycemic control in non-insulin-dependent diabetic clients. Diabetic clients should monitor their blood sugar levels more frequently until the effect of nicotinic acid is known. GI distress is a common side effect that may be decreased by taking the drug with food.

Client education as it relates to nicotinic acid should include goals, reasons for obtaining baseline data such as vital signs and cardiac, hepatic, and renal tests, and possible side effects. Following are important points the nurse should include when teaching clients regarding nicotinic acid:

- Do not take megadoses of niacin due to the risk for serious toxic effects.
- Take niacin with cold water, as hot beverages increase flushing.
- Take with or after meals to prevent GI upset.
- Do not take other prescription drugs, OTC medications, herbal remedies, or vitamins/minerals without notifying the healthcare provider.
- Report the following immediately: flank, joint, or stomach pain; skin colour changes (advise client to stay out of the sun if skin changes occur); and yellowing of the whites of eyes.

FIBRIC ACID AGENTS

Fibric acid agents may be used to lower lipid levels. They are sometimes used in combination with the statins. The fibric acid agents are shown in Table 22.1 on page 280.

22.8 Pharmacotherapy with Fibric Acid Agents

Two fibric acid agents, fenofibrate and gemfibrozil, are sometimes prescribed for clients with excessive triglyceride (VLDL) levels. The mechanism of action of the fibric acid agents is largely unknown.

NURSING CONSIDERATIONS

The role of the nurse in fibric acid therapy involves careful monitoring of the client's condition and providing education as it relates to the prescribed drug regimen. Prior to administering fibric acid, the nurse should assess the client for abdominal pain, nausea, and vomiting, the most common adverse effects. Taking the medication with meals usually decreases GI distress. The nurse should obtain an accurate pharmacological history. The use of fibric acid agents with statin drugs increases the risk of myositis. If a client is taking warfarin, lower dosages will be needed because of competitive protein binding. More frequent monitoring of PT/INR may be necessary until stabilization occurs. Fibric acid is generally not used in lactation or pregnancy (category B).

Client education as it relates to these drugs should include goals, reasons for obtaining baseline data such as vital signs and cardiac and renal tests, and possible side

NATURAL THERAPIES

Coenzyme Q10 and Cardiovascular Disease

Coenzyme Q10 (CoQ10) is a vitamin-like substance found in most animal cells. It is an essential component in the cell's mitochondria for producing energy in the form of adenosine triphosphate (ATP). Because the heart requires high levels of ATP, a sufficient level of CoQ10 is essential to that organ. Supplementation with CoQ10 is especially important to clients taking the HMG-CoA reductase inhibitors because these drugs significantly lower blood levels of CoQ10. CoQ10 and cholesterol share the same metabolic pathways. Inhibition of the enzyme HMG-CoA reductase concurrently decreases CoQ10 levels.

Foods richest in this substance are pork, sardines, beef heart, salmon, broccoli, spinach, and nuts. Older adults appear to have an increased need for CoQ10. Although CoQ10 can be synthesized by the body, many amino acids and other substances are required; therefore, clients with nutritional deficiencies may be in need of supplementation.

In 1978, a Nobel Prize was awarded for research proving the importance of CoQ10 in energy transfer, but it was not until the 1990s that the substance became the top-selling supplement in health food stores. CoQ10 has been purported to aid a wide range of conditions, including heart failure, hypertension, dysrhythmias, angina, diabetes, neurological disorders, cancer, and aging. A considerable body of research has begun to accumulate, particularly regarding the role of CoQ10 in heart disease. Some data have found below-normal levels of CoQ10 in clients with heart failure. Studies suggest that the frequency of pre-ventricular contractions may be reduced in some clients by supplementation with CoQ10. Although most studies have demonstrated positive results, CoQ10 has not been widely accepted in the conventional medical community.

Pr PROTOTYPE DRUG | Gemfibrozil (Lopid)

ACTIONS AND USES

Effects of gemfibrozil include up to a 50% reduction in VLDL with an increase in HDL. The mechanism of action is unknown. It is less effective than the statins at lowering LDL, so it is not a drug of first choice for reducing LDL cholesterol levels. Gemfibrozil is taken orally at 600 to 1200 mg/day.

PHARMACOKINETICS

Gemfibrozil is well absorbed, minimally metabolized by the liver, and eliminated mainly by the kidneys. It has a half-life of 1.5 hours.

ADMINISTRATIVE ALERT

- Administer with meals to decrease GI distress.
- Gemfibrozil is pregnancy category B.

ADVERSE EFFECTS AND INTERACTIONS

Gemfibrozil produces few serious adverse effects, but it may increase the likelihood of gallstones and occasionally affect liver function. The most common side effects are GI related: diarrhea, nausea, and cramping.

Drug interactions with gemfibrozil include oral anticoagulants; concurrent use with gemfibrozil may potentiate anticoagulant effects. Lovastatin increases the risk of myopathy and rhabdomyolysis.

 See the Companion Website for a Nursing Process Focus Chart specific to this drug.

---

effects. Following are the important points the nurse should include when teaching clients about fibric acid agents:

- Keep appointments for medical follow-up and laboratory tests.
- Immediately report the following: unusual bruising or bleeding, right upper quadrant pain, changes in stool colour, or muscle cramping.

MISCELLANEOUS AGENTS

Orlistat (Xenical) is a new class of anti-obesity agent with a unique action. Orlistat is a reversible, long-acting inhibitor of gastrointestinal lipases. These lipases are enzymes that are required for the systemic absorption of dietary triglycerides. By forming a bond with lipases in the stomach and small intestine, orlistat prevents absorption of about 30% of dietary fat, thus producing a weight-loss effect.

22.9 Pharmacotherapy with Orlistat

In addition to contributing to weight loss, orlistat may reduce total cholesterol and LDL cholesterol in the blood.

Orlistat is recommended as an adjunct to a weight-loss program that includes exercise and a healthy diet. The dose is shown in Table 22.1.

Orlistat has negligible systemic absorption. About 97% of unabsorbed drug is excreted by fecal elimination, and less than 2% is excreted in urine. Because it is minimally absorbed, orlistat is a relatively safe anti-obesity drug. Low-dose orlistat is being considered for OTC use. There is concern that OTC availability may lead to abuse by individuals with eating disorders. A multiple vitamin supplement is usually required since orlistat reduces absorption of fat-soluble vitamins.

Side effects of orlistat include oily fecal spotting, oily stools, flatulence, fecal urgency, fecal incontinence, and abdominal pain. Side effects often diminish as the body adjusts. Orlistat is pregnancy category B.

The role of the nurse in orlistat therapy includes client education. Clients should be advised to take orlistat during or immediately following a meal containing fat. A fat-soluble vitamin supplement should be taken at least 2 hours before or after a dose of orlistat. Ways to reduce weight and LDL cholesterol through dietary modification and exercise should be emphasized.

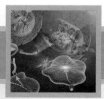

CHAPTER REVIEW

KEY CONCEPTS

The numbered key concepts provide a succinct summary of the important points from the corresponding numbered section within the chapter. If any of these points are not clear, refer to the numbered section within the chapter for review. Expanded versions can be found on the Companion Website.

22.1 Lipids are carried through the blood as lipoproteins; VLDL and LDL are associated with an increased incidence of cardiovascular disease, whereas HDL exerts a protective effect.

22.2 Blood lipid profiles are important diagnostic tools in guiding the therapy of dyslipidemia.

22.3 Before starting pharmacotherapy for hyperlipidemia, clients should seek to control the condition through lifestyle changes such as restriction of dietary saturated fats and cholesterol, increased exercise, and smoking cessation.

22.4 Statins, which inhibit HMG-CoA reductase, a critical enzyme in the biosynthesis of cholesterol, are drugs of first choice for reducing blood lipid levels.

22.5 The bile acid resins bind bile acids (containing cholesterol) and accelerate their excretion. These agents can reduce cholesterol and LDL levels but are not drugs of choice due to their side effects.

22.6 Nicotinic acid, or niacin, can reduce LDL levels, but side effects limit its usefulness.

22.7 Fibric acid agents lower triglyceride levels but have little effect on LDL cholesterol levels. They are not drugs of choice due to their potential side effects.

22.8 Orlistat prevents absorption of triglycerides and may promote weight loss and help lower LDL cholesterol.

REVIEW QUESTIONS

1 Why is the cholesterol in high-density lipoproteins considered to be "good" cholesterol?

2 How does the mechanism of action of the statins differ from that of nicotinic acid?

3 During the assessment of a new client, what kind of information would guide the healthcare provider in determining the need for pharmacotherapy of dyslipidemia?

CRITICAL THINKING QUESTIONS

1. A client has been on atorvastatin (Lipitor) for 3 months with no side effects. The client is now experiencing pain in the muscles of her left leg. She inquires whether this is a cause for concern and whether the pain may be related to her elevated lipid levels or to the atorvastatin therapy. How does the nurse respond?

2. A client is put on cholestyramine (Novo-Cholamine) for elevated lipids. What teaching is important for this client?

3. A male diabetic client presents to the emergency room with complaints of being very red (flushed) and having "hot flashes." The client admits to self-medicating with niacin for elevated lipids. What is the nurse's response?

EXPLORE MediaLink

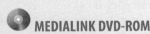

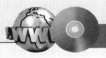   www.pearsoned.ca/adams-king

MEDIALINK DVD-ROM
- Audio Glossary
- CRNE Review
- Animation
  Mechanism of Action: Atorvastatin

 COMPANION WEBSITE
- CRNE Review
- Case Study: Controlling lipid levels
- Dosage Calculations
- Nursing Process Focus Charts

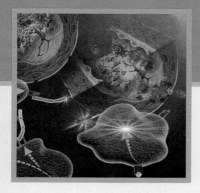

CHAPTER 23

Drugs for Angina Pectoris, Myocardial Infarction, and Cerebrovascular Accident

DRUGS AT A GLANCE

ORGANIC NITRATES
   ◐ nitroglycerin (Nitrostat, others)

BETA-ADRENERGIC BLOCKERS
   ◐ atenolol (Apo-Atenolol, Tenormin)
   ◐ metoprolol (Apo-Metoprolol, Lopresor)

CALCIUM CHANNEL BLOCKERS
   ◐ diltiazem (Cardizem, Novo-Diltazem)

THROMBOLYTICS
   ◐ reteplase (Retavase)

GLYCOPROTEIN IIB/IIIA INHIBITORS

ADJUNCT DRUGS FOR MYOCARDIAL INFARCTION AND CEREBROVASCULAR ACCIDENT

OBJECTIVES

After reading this chapter, the student should be able to do the following:

1. Identify drug classes used for treating angina pectoris, myocardial infarction, and cerebrovascular accident.

2. Explain the therapeutic action of each class of drug used in the treatment of angina, myocardial infarction, and cerebrovascular accident in relation to the pathophysiology of these conditions.

3. Describe the nurse's role in the pharmacological management of clients receiving drugs used in the treatment of angina, myocardial infarction, and cerebrovascular accident.

4. For each of the drug classes listed in Drugs at a Glance, identify a representative drug and explain its mechanism of action, therapeutic effects, and important adverse effects.

5. Describe and explain, based on pharmacological principles, the rationale for nursing assessment, planning, and interventions for clients with angina, myocardial infarction, and cerebrovascular accident.

6. Use the nursing process to care for clients receiving drug therapy for angina, myocardial infarction, and cerebrovascular accident.

MediaLink

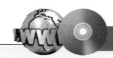

www.pearsoned.ca/adams-king

CRNE review, case studies, and other interactive resources for this chapter can be found on the Companion Website at **www.pearsoned.ca/adams**. Click on "Chapter 23" to select the activities for this chapter. For animations, more CRNE review questions, and an audio glossary, access the accompanying DVD-ROM in this textbook.

KEY TERMS

MediaLink Canadian Cardiovascular Society

MediaLink World Health Organization

The tissues and organs of the body are dependent on the arterial supply of oxygen and other vital nutrients to support life and health. Should the arterial blood supply become compromised, cardiovascular and cerebrovascular functioning may become impaired, resulting in angina pectoris, acute myocardial infarction, or cerebrovascular accident. Such conditions are associated with the development of atherosclerotic plaques or the aggregation of platelets on the intima of blood vessels, with resultant clot formation. Tissues and organs served by the arteries, distal to the site of involvement, become ischemic and suffer varying degrees of damage. This chapter focuses on the pharmacological and nursing interventions related to these conditions.

23.1 Etiology of Coronary Artery Disease and Myocardial Ischemia

Coronary artery disease (CAD) is one of the leading causes of mortality. The primary characteristic defining CAD is narrowing or occlusion of the coronary arteries. The narrowing deprives heart cells of needed oxygen and nutrients, a condition known as **myocardial ischemia**. If it develops over a long period of time, the heart may compensate for its inadequate blood supply and the client may experience no symptoms. Indeed, coronary arteries may be occluded as much as 50% or more and cause no symptoms.

As CAD progresses, however, the heart does not receive enough oxygen to meet the metabolic demands of the myocardium. The oxygen deficiency signals the onset of anaerobic metabolism to generate the energy needed to maintain cardiac function. As a result, lactic acid accumulates. As with any muscle, the buildup of lactic acid produces pain and soreness. When lactic acid activates pericardial pain receptors, the body experiences the sensation of chest pain. Persistent myocardial ischemia may lead to heart attack.

The common etiology of CAD in adults is **atherosclerosis**, which is the presence of plaque within the walls of arteries. **Plaque** is a fatty, fibrous material that accumulates, thus producing varying degrees of intravascular narrowing—a situation that results in partial or total blockage of the blood vessel. In addition, the plaque impairs normal vessel elasticity. In CAD, the atherosclerotic coronary vessel is unable to dilate properly when the myocardium needs additional blood or oxygen. Plaque accumulation occurs gradually, possibly over periods of 40 to 50 years in some individuals, but actually begins to accrue early in life. As the material collects in the intima (inner layer) of a vessel, the cardiac muscle distal to the obstruction receives less oxygen, thus hindering its metabolic functions. The development of atherosclerosis is illustrated in Figure 23.1.

23.2 Blood Supply to the Myocardium

The heart, from the moment it begins to function in utero until death, works to distribute oxygen and nutrients via its non-stop pumping action. Because the heart is a continually working muscle, it needs a steady supply of oxygen and nutrients. Any disturbance in blood flow to the vital organs or the myocardium itself—even for brief episodes—can result in life-threatening consequences.

The myocardium receives its blood via two main arteries that arise within the right and left aortic sinuses at the base of the aorta, called the right and left coronary arteries. These arteries further divide into smaller branches that encircle the heart, bringing the myocardium a continuous supply of oxygen. The numerous smaller vessels serve as natural communication networks among the coronary arteries and are known as **anastomoses**. In the event that one of the vessels becomes restricted or blocked, blood flow to the myocardium may remain relatively uncompromised as a result of these channels functioning to bypass the block.

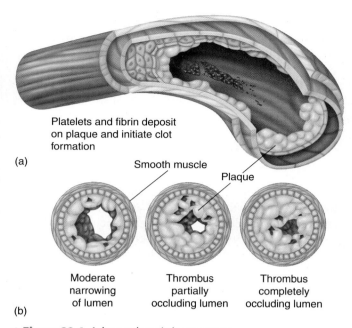

Platelets and fibrin deposit
on plaque and initiate clot
formation

(a)

Smooth muscle

Plaque

| Moderate
narrowing
of lumen | Thrombus
partially
occluding lumen | Thrombus
completely
occluding lumen |

(b)

● **Figure 23.1** Atherosclerosis in an artery

Source: Pearson Education/PH College.

ANGINA PECTORIS

23.3 Pathogenesis of Angina Pectoris

Angina pectoris is acute chest pain caused by insufficient oxygen reaching a portion of the myocardium. About 2% of Canadians have angina pectoris, with over 47,000 new cases each year. It is more prevalent in those over 55 years of age.

The classic presentation of angina pectoris is steady, intense pain, sometimes with a crushing or constricting sensation in the substernal region. Typically, the discomfort radiates to the left shoulder and proceeds down the left arm. It may also extend to the thoracic region of the back or move upward to the jaw. In some clients, the pain is experienced in the midepigastrium or abdominal area. Accompanying the discomfort is severe emotional distress—a feeling of panic with fear of impending death. There is usually pallor, dyspnea with cyanosis, diaphoresis, tachycardia, and elevated blood pressure.

Anginal pain is usually precipitated by physical exertion or emotional excitement—events associated with increased cardiorespiratory oxygen demand. Narrowed coronary arteries containing atherosclerotic deposits block the distribution of oxygen and nutrients to the stressed myocardium. Angina pectoris episodes are usually of short duration. With physical rest and stress reduction, the discomfort subsides within 10 to 15 minutes.

There are three basic types of angina. When anginal occurrences are fairly predictable, as to frequency, intensity, and duration, the condition is described as classic or **stable angina**. The second type of angina, known as atypical or **variant angina** (Prinzmetal's angina), occurs when the decreased myocardial blood flow is caused by spasms of the coronary arteries. It often occurs at the same time each night, during rest or sleep. When episodes of angina arise more frequently, have added intensity, and occur during periods of rest, the condition is termed **unstable angina**. This condition requires more aggressive medical intervention and may be considered a medical emergency as it is associated with an increased risk for myocardial infarction (MI).

Angina pain closely parallels the signs and symptoms of a heart attack. It is extremely important that the nurse know the characteristics that differentiate the two conditions because the pharmacological interventions related to angina differ considerably from those of myocardial infarction. Angina, while painful and distressing, rarely leads to a fatal outcome, and the chest pain is usually immediately relieved by nitroglycerin. Myocardial infarction, however, carries with it a high mortality rate if appropriate treatment is delayed. Pharmacological intervention must be immediately initiated and systematically maintained in the event of myocardial infarction. Females may experience a heart attack as symptoms of fatigue and nausea rather than distressing, crushing chest pain.

Any number of diverse situations—several unrelated to cardiac pathology—may cause chest pain. These include gallstones, peptic ulcer disease, pneumonia, musculoskeletal injuries, and certain cancers. The foremost objective for the healthcare provider when a person presents with chest pain is to quickly determine the cause of the pain so that proper, effective interventions can be delivered. This incorporates a detailed individual and family history, a complete physical examination, and laboratory and other diagnostic tests. All healthcare providers work collaboratively to quickly determine the cause of chest pain.

23.4 Non-Pharmacological Management of Angina

A combination of variables influences the development and progression of angina, including dietary patterns and lifestyle circumstances. The nurse is instrumental in assisting clients to control the rate of recurrence of anginal episodes. Such support includes the formulation of a comprehensive plan of care that incorporates psychosocial support and an individualized teaching plan. The client needs to understand the causes of angina, identify the conditions and situations that trigger it, and develop the motivation to modify behaviours associated with the condition.

In addition to drugs, treatment of angina includes therapies for conditions that worsen coronary artery disease, such as diabetes and hypertension. The practice of healthy lifestyle habits can prevent CAD in many individuals and slow the progression of the disease in those who have plaque buildup. The following factors have been shown to reduce the incidence of CAD:

- Limiting or abstaining from alcohol
- Eliminating foods high in cholesterol or saturated fat
- If blood lipids are high (hyperlipidemia), treating the condition

MediaLink World Heart Federation

- Treating high blood pressure early
- Exercising regularly and maintaining optimum weight
- Not using tobacco

When the coronary arteries are significantly obstructed, the two most common interventions are **percutaneous transluminal coronary angioplasty (PTCA)**, with stent insertion, and **coronary artery bypass graft (CABG)** surgery. PTCA is a procedure whereby the narrowed area of the artery is opened using either a balloon catheter or a laser. The basic concept is to place a catheter, with a small inflatable balloon on the end, within the narrowed section of the artery. Inflation of the balloon causes it to push outward against the narrowed wall of the artery. The stenosis is reduced until it no longer interferes with blood flow. Stenting is done in conjunction with a balloon angioplasty and/or atherectomy, a procedure in which plaque is removed from an artery. Angioplasty with stenting typically leaves less than 10% of the original blockage in the artery.

Coronary bypass surgery is reserved for severe cases of coronary blockage that cannot be dealt with by any other treatment modality. In CABG, a portion of a small blood vessel from the leg or chest is used to create a "bypass

artery." One end of the graft is sewn to the aorta and the other end to the coronary artery beyond the narrowed area. Blood from the aorta then flows through the new grafted vessel to the heart muscle, "bypassing" the blockage in the coronary artery. The result is increased blood flow to the heart muscle, which reduces angina and the risk of heart attack.

23.5 Goals for the Pharmacotherapy of Angina

The pharmacological goals for a client with angina are twofold: to reduce the frequency of angina episodes, and to terminate an incident of acute anginal pain once it is in progress. It is important to remember that interventions are directed toward symptomatic relief and management as there is no drug treatment available to cure the underlying disorder. The primary means by which antianginal drugs accomplish these goals is to reduce the myocardial demand for oxygen. This can be accomplished by at least four different mechanisms:

1. Slowing the heart rate
2. Dilating veins so the heart receives less blood (reduced preload)
3. Causing the heart to contract with less force (reduced contractility)
4. Dilating arterioles to lower blood pressure, thus giving the heart less resistance when ejecting blood from its chambers (reduced afterload)

The pharmacotherapy of angina uses three classes of drug: organic nitrates, beta-adrenergic blockers, and calcium channel blockers. For stable angina, the first line of pharmacotherapy is the rapid-acting organic nitrates that are administered during the anginal episode. If episodes become more frequent or severe, prophylactic treatment is initiated using oral or transdermal organic nitrates, beta-adrenergic blockers, or calcium channel blockers. Persistent angina sometimes requires drugs from two or more classes, such as a beta-blocker combined with a long-acting nitrate or calcium channel blocker. Figure 23.2 illustrates the mechanisms of action of drugs used to prevent and treat angina.

ORGANIC NITRATES

23.6 Treating Angina with Organic Nitrates

Since their medicinal properties were discovered in 1857, organic nitrates have remained the mainstay for the treatment of angina. The primary therapeutic action of the organic nitrates is their ability to relax both arterial and venous smooth muscle. With venous vasodilation, the amount of blood returning to the heart (preload) is reduced, and the chambers contain a smaller volume. With less blood for the ventricles to pump, cardiac output is reduced and the workload of the heart is decreased, thereby lowering

---

SPECIAL CONSIDERATIONS

The Influence of Gender and Ethnicity on Angina

- Angina occurs more frequently in females than in males.
- Among racial-ethnic groups, the incidence of angina is highest among Aboriginal Peoples and people of African decent.
- African females have a risk of angina twice that of their male counterparts.

PHARMFACTS

Angina Pectoris, Myocardial Infarction, and Cerebrovascular Accident

Angina
- The incidence of angina increases steadily with age and peaks in the 80 to 89 age group.
- The onset of angina occurs about 10 years later in women than in men.

Myocardial Infarction
- Rates of ischemic heart disease and myocardial infarction are much higher in Canadian males than females. The rates are similar in Aboriginal and Caucasian males.
- Aboriginal, African, and South Asian Canadian women are at greater risk than Caucasian women of dying from ischemic heart disease and stroke.
- About one-third of the people experiencing MI will die from it.
- About 60% of people who die suddenly of MI had no previous symptoms.
- More than 20% of men and 40% of women will die from MI within 1 year after being diagnosed with ischemic heart disease.

Cerebrovascular Accident
- Stroke is the third leading cause of death, behind heart disease and cancer.
- Of those who suffer a stroke, more than 30% will die within 1 year.
- The incidence increases with age, although 25% of all strokes occur before age 65.

MediaLink **Women and Heart Disease**

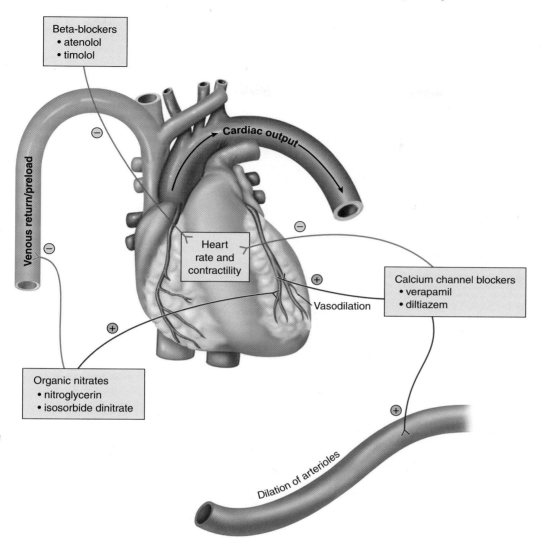

Beta-blockers
• atenolol
• timolol

Cardiac output

Venous return/preload

Heart
rate and
contractility

Calcium channel blockers
• verapamil
• diltiazem

Vasodilation

Organic nitrates
• nitroglycerin
• isosorbide dinitrate

Dilation of arterioles

● **Figure 23.2** Mechanisms of action of drugs used to treat angina

myocardial oxygen demand. The therapeutic outcome is that chest pain is alleviated and episodes of angina become less frequent. The organic nitrates are shown in Table 23.1.

Organic nitrates also have the ability to dilate coronary arteries, which was once thought to be their primary mechanism of action. It seems logical that dilating a partially occluded coronary vessel would allow more oxygen to get to the ischemic tissue. While this effect does indeed occur, it is no longer considered the primary mechanism of nitrate action in treating stable angina. This action, however, is important in treating variant angina, in which the chest pain is caused by coronary artery spasm. The organic nitrates can relax these spasms and terminate the pain.

Organic nitrates are of two types, short acting and long acting. The short-acting nitrates, such as nitroglycerin, are taken sublingually to quickly terminate an acute angina attack in progress. Longer acting nitrates, such as isosorbide dinitrate, are taken orally or delivered through a transdermal patch to decrease the frequency and severity of angina episodes.

TABLE 23.1	Drugs for Angina, Myocardial Infarction, and Cerebrovascular Accident
Drug	**Route and Adult Dose**
Organic Nitrates	
amyl nitrite	Inhalation; 1 ampule (0.18–0.3 mL) Prn
isosorbide dinitrate (Isordil, Novo-Sorbide, Cedocard SR) (see page 311 for the Prototype Drug box)	PO; 2.5–30 mg qid
isosorbide mononitrate (Imdur SR, APO-ISMN)	PO; 20 mg-60 mg qd
nitroglycerin (Nitrostat, Nitro-Dur, Nitrogard SR, others)	SL: 1 tablet (0.3–0.6 mg) or 1 spray (0.4–0.8 mg) q5min Prn
Beta-Adrenergic Blockers	
atenolol (Apo-Atenolol, Tenormin)	PO; 25–50 mg qd (max 100 mg/day)
metoprolol (Apo-Metoprolol, Lopresor)	PO; 100 mg bid (max 400 mg/day)
propranolol (Inderal) (see page 324 for the Prototype Drug box)	PO; 10–20 mg bid–tid (max 320 mg/day)
timolol maleate (Apo-Timolol) (see page 692 for the Prototype Drug box)	PO; 15–45 mg tid (max 60 mg/day)
Calcium Channel Blockers	
amlodipine (Norvasc, Caduet)	PO; 5–10 mg qd (max 10 mg/day)
diltiazem (Cardizem, Novo-Diltazem)	PO; 30 mg qid (max 360 mg/day)
nifedipine (Adalat, Apo-Nifed) (see page 261 for the Prototype Drug box)	PO; 10–20 mg tid (max 180 mg/day)
verapamil (Isoptin, Apo-Verap) (see page 327 for the Prototype Drug box)	PO; 80 mg tid–qid (max 480 mg/day)
Glycoprotein IIb/IIIa Inhibitors	
abciximab (ReoPro)	IV; 0.25 mg/kg initial bolus over 5 min then 10 µg/min for 12 hr
eptifibatide (Integrilin)	IV; 180 µg/kg initial bolus over 1–2 min then 2 µg/kg/min for 24–72 hr
tirofiban HCL (Aggrastat)	IV; 0.4 µg/kg/min for 30 min then 0.1 µg/kg/min for 12–24 hr

Tolerance is a common problem with prolonged use of the long-acting organic nitrates. The magnitude of the tolerance depends on the dosage and the frequency of drug administration. Clients are often instructed to remove the transdermal patch for 6 to 12 hours each day or withhold the nighttime dose of the oral medications to delay the development of tolerance.

Long-acting organic nitrates such as isosorbide dinitrate are also useful in reducing the symptoms of heart failure. Their role in the treatment of this disease is discussed in Chapter 24.

NURSING CONSIDERATIONS

The role of the nurse in nitrate therapy for angina involves careful monitoring of the client's condition and providing education as it relates to the prescribed drug regimen. Because the main action of nitrates is vasodilation, it is vital for the nurse to assess blood pressure prior to administration. IV nitrates have the greatest risk of causing severe hypotension. These drugs are contraindicated in aortic stenosis, pericardial tamponade, and constrictive pericarditis because the heart cannot increase cardiac output to maintain blood pressure as vasodilation occurs. In cases when increased vasodilation would be detrimental to the client (hypotension, shock, head injury with increased intracranial pressure), nitrates are contraindicated since they worsen the conditions. Nitrates should not be taken within 24 hours (before or after) of taking sildenafil (Viagra) because life-threatening hypotension and cardiovascular collapse may occur. Sustained-release forms of these drugs should not be given to clients with glaucoma. Nitrates should be used with caution in clients with severe liver or kidney disease or in early MI.

Assessment should include the client's use of alcohol as this agent can produce an additive vasodilation effect when taken concurrently with nitrates. Taking isosorbide dinitrate or isosorbide mononitrate with alcohol may cause severe hypotension and cardiovascular collapse.

With long-acting nitrates, monitor for orthostatic hypotension and advise clients to change positions gradually. With short-acting forms, ensure that clients are sitting or supine during administration and that blood pressure is taken after each dose. If hypotension occurs, withhold nitrates and remove transdermal forms until blood pressure has returned to normal. Frequent blood pressure measurements are done during therapy to monitor for hypotensive effects. Infusions

Pr PROTOTYPE DRUG | Nitroglycerin (Nitrostat, others)

ACTIONS AND USES

Nitroglycerin, the oldest and most widely used of the organic nitrates, can be delivered by a number of different routes: sublingual, oral (including extended-release forms), translingual, IV, transmucosal, transdermal, and topical. It may be taken while an acute anginal episode is in progress or just prior to physical activity. When given sublingually, it reaches peak plasma levels in approximately 4 minutes, thus terminating angina pain rapidly. Chest pain that does not respond to two or three doses of sublingual nitroglycerin may indicate myocardial infarction.

PHARMACOKINETICS

Nitroglycerin is well absorbed. It is rapidly and almost completely metabolized by the liver and enzymes in the blood. It has a half-life of 1 to 3 minutes.

ADMINISTRATION ALERTS

- For IV administration, use glass IV bottle and special IV tubing because plastic absorbs nitrates significantly, thus reducing client dose.
- Cover IV bottle to reduce degradation of nitrates due to light exposure.
- Use gloves when applying nitroglycerin paste or ointment to prevent self-administration.
- Nitroglycerin is pregnancy category C.

ADVERSE EFFECTS AND INTERACTIONS

The side effects of nitroglycerin are usually cardiovascular in nature and are rarely life-threatening. Because nitroglycerin can dilate cerebral vessels, headache is a common side effect and may be severe. Occasionally, the venodilation created by nitroglycerin causes reflex tachycardia. Some healthcare providers prescribe a beta-adrenergic blocker to diminish this undesirable heart rate increase. The side effects of nitroglycerin often diminish after a few doses.

Concurrent use with sildenafil (Viagra) may cause life-threatening hypotension and cardiovascular collapse. Nitrates should not be taken within 24 hours (before or after) of taking sildenafil.

---

of nitrates are frequently titrated to obtain pain relief for the client or a specific blood pressure level. Hold other forms of nitrates and remove transdermal forms during the infusion.

Client education as it relates to nitrates should include goals, reasons for obtaining baseline data such as vital signs and tests for cardiac and renal disorders, and possible side effects. Following are the important points to include when teaching clients regarding nitrates:

- Refrain from alcohol use; some clients experience flushing, weakness, and fainting.
- If using transdermal patches, rotate the application site and wash skin thoroughly after patch is removed.

- If using a sublingual form, allow the tablet to dissolve under the tongue; do not chew or swallow the tablet.
- If chest pain is not relieved after two doses of nitroglycerin, 5 minutes apart, call emergency medical services (EMS).
- Contact the healthcare provider immediately if blurred vision, dry mouth, or severe headaches occur, which may be signs of overdose.
- Keep medication readily available in its original container, away from excess heat, light, and moisture. Prescription should be replaced every 6 months.

NURSING PROCESS FOCUS   Clients Receiving Nitroglycerin (Nitrostat, others)

Assessment	Potential Nursing Diagnoses/Identified Patterns
Prior to administration: ■ Obtain complete health history including allergies, drug history, and possible drug interactions. ■ Assess vital signs, ECG, frequency and severity of angina, and alcohol use. ■ Obtain history of cardiac disorders and lab tests, including cardiac enzymes, CBC, BUN, creatinine, and liver function tests. ■ Assess if client has taken sildenafil (Viagra) within the last 24 hours.	■ Need for knowledge regarding drug therapy ■ Risk for injury (dizziness or fainting) related to hypotension from drug ■ Ineffective tissue perfusion related to hypotension from drug ■ Acute pain (headache) related to adverse effects of drug

Planning: Client Goals and Expected Outcomes

The client will:
- Experience relief or prevention of chest pain
- Report immediately any chest pain unrelieved by nitroglycerin
- Demonstrate an understanding of the drug's action by accurately describing drug side effects and precautions

continued

NURSING PROCESS FOCUS Clients Receiving Nitroglycerin (Nitrostat, others) (Continued)

Implementation

Interventions (Rationales)	Client Education/Discharge Planning
■ Ask client to describe and rate pain prior to drug administration for description/documentation of anginal episode.	Instruct client to:
	■ Take one tablet every 5 min until pain is relieved during an acute angina attack
■ Obtain 12-lead ECG to differentiate between angina and infarction. (Pharmacotherapy depends on which disorder is presenting.)	■ Call EMS if chest pain is not relieved after two doses
	■ Place SL tablet or spray under tongue; do not inhale spray
■ Monitor blood pressure and pulse. Do not administer drug if client is hypotensive. (Drug will further reduce blood pressure.)	■ Instruct client to sit or lie down before taking medication and to avoid abrupt changes in position.
■ Monitor alcohol use. (Extremely low blood pressure may result, which could cause death.)	■ Emphasize the importance of avoiding alcohol while taking nitroglycerin.
■ Monitor for headache in response to use of nitrates.	Instruct client that:
	■ Headache is a common side effect that usually decreases over time
	■ OTC medicines usually relieve the headache
■ Monitor for use of sildenafil (Viagra) concurrently with nitrates because cardiovascular disease is a major cause of erectile dysfunction in men. (Life-threatening hypotension may result with concurrent use of sildenafil.)	Instruct client to:
	■ Not take sildenafil within 24 hours of taking nitrates
	■ Wait at least 24 hours after taking sildenafil to resume nitrate therapy
■ Monitor need for prophylactic nitrates.	■ Advise client to take medication prior to a stressful event or physical activity to prevent angina.

Evaluation of Outcome Criteria
Evaluate the effectiveness of drug therapy by confirming that client goals and expected outcomes have been met (see "Planning").

BETA-ADRENERGIC BLOCKERS

23.7 Treating Angina with Beta-Blockers

Because of their ability to reduce the workload of the heart by slowing heart rate (negative chronotropic effect) and reducing contractility (negative inotropic effect), beta-blockers are used to decrease the frequency and severity of angina attacks caused by exertion. Unlike the nitrates, tolerance does not develop to the antianginal effects of beta-blockers. They are first-line drugs in the pharmacotherapy of chronic stable angina. Clients should be advised against abruptly stopping beta-blocker therapy as this may result in a sudden increase in cardiac workload and worsen angina. The beta-blockers used for angina are shown in Table 23.1 on page 292. The beta-blockers are widely used in medicine, and additional details may be found in Chapters 13, 21, 24, and 25.

NURSING CONSIDERATIONS

The role of the nurse in beta-blocker therapy for angina involves careful monitoring of the client's condition and providing education as it relates to the prescribed drug regimen. Before administering beta-blockers, assess the client's apical pulse, especially if the client is also taking digoxin,

since both drugs slow atrioventricular (AV) conduction. Because beta-blockers lower blood pressure, vital signs should be monitored. Monitor the client for shortness of breath and respiratory distress. Side effects occur more often with higher doses of beta-blockers.

Because beta-blockers slow heart rate and conduction velocity, they are contraindicated in bradycardia, second- and third-degree heart block, and cardiogenic shock. Beta-blockers should be used with caution in clients with asthma, COPD, or impaired renal function. Diabetic clients should be aware that initial symptoms of hypoglycemia, such as palpitations, diaphoresis, and nervousness, may not be evident with beta-blockade. Blood glucose levels should be monitored frequently in clients with diabetes mellitus because insulin doses may need to be decreased when using beta-blockers.

Beta-blockers should not be abruptly discontinued because with long-term use the heart adapts to the catecholamines blocked by these drugs. When they are withdrawn abruptly, adrenergic receptors are stimulated, causing excitation. This may exacerbate angina and precipitate tachycardia or even an MI in clients with cardiovascular disease. One side effect of beta-blockers is fatigue during exercise because these drugs prevent the heart rate from increasing with activity.

Client education as it relates to beta-blockers should include goals, reasons for obtaining baseline data such as vital signs and tests for cardiac and renal disorders, and possible side effects. Following are important teaching points to include regarding beta-blockers:

- Change positions slowly; report dizziness or light-headedness.
- Do not take OTC medications or herbal products without discussing them with the healthcare provider.
- Do not discontinue medication abruptly.

- If pulse falls below 50 beats/minute (bpm), notify the healthcare provider. This may be 60 beats/minute in some agencies.
- Alternate periods of activity with periods of rest in order to avoid fatigue.
- See also "Nursing Process Focus: Clients Receiving Adrenergic Therapy" in Chapter 13 on page 137 for the complete nursing process applied to caring for clients receiving beta-adrenergic agonists.

Pr PROTOTYPE DRUG | Atenolol (Apo-Atenolol, Tenormin)

ACTIONS AND USES

Atenolol selectively blocks beta$_1$-adrenergic receptors in the heart. Its effectiveness in angina is attributed to its ability to slow heart rate and reduce contractility, both of which lower myocardial oxygen demand. It is also used in the treatment of hypertension and in the prevention of MI. Because of its 6- to 9-hour half-life, it may be taken once a day.

ADMINISTRATION ALERTS

- During IV administration, monitor ECG continuously; blood pressure and pulse should be assessed before, during, and after dose is administered.
- Assess pulse and blood pressure before oral administration. Hold drug if pulse is below 50 beats/minute (60 in some agencies) or if client is hypotensive.
- Initial doses of atenolol may precipitate bronchospasm in susceptible clients.
- Atenolol is pregnancy category C.

PHARMACOKINETICS

Bioavailability of oral atenolol is 50% to 60%. Unabsorbed drug is excreted in the feces and the remainder is excreted by the kidneys. It has a half-life of 6 to 9 hours.

ADVERSE EFFECTS AND INTERACTIONS

Being a cardioselective beta$_1$-blocker, atenolol has few adverse effects on the lung. Like other beta-blockers, therapy generally begins with low doses, which are gradually increased until the therapeutic effect is achieved. The most common side effects of atenolol include fatigue, weakness, and hypotension. Anticholinergics may cause decreased absorption from the GI tract.

Concurrent use with calcium channel blockers may cause excessive cardiac suppression. Concurrent use with digitalis may cause slowed AV conduction, leading to heart block. Clients should avoid concurrent use of this drug with nicotine or caffeine due to their vasoconstricting effects.

In case of beta blocker overdose, glucagon IV may be administered to reduce cardiac depression and increase myocardial contractibility, heart rate, and AV node conduction.

 See the Companion Website for a Nursing Process Focus Chart specific to this drug.

Pr PROTOTYPE DRUG | Metoprolol (Apo-Metoprolol, Lopresor)

ACTIONS AND USES

Metoprolol is a selective beta$_1$-antagonist available in tablet, sustained-release tablet, and IV forms. At high doses, it may also affect beta$_2$-receptors in bronchial smooth muscle. When given IV, it quickly acts to reduce myocardial oxygen demand. Following an acute MI, metoprolol is infused slowly until a target heart rate is reached, usually between 60 and 90 beats/minute. Upon hospital discharge, clients can be switched to oral forms of the drug. Metoprolol is also approved for angina, hypertension, and myocardial infarction.

ADMINISTRATION ALERTS

- During IV administration, monitor ECG, blood pressure, and pulse frequently.
- Assess pulse and blood pressure before oral administration. Hold drug if pulse is below 50 beats/minute (60 in some agencies) or if client is hypotensive.
- Do not crush or chew sustained-release tablets.
- Metoprolol is pregnancy category C.

PHARMACOKINETICS

Metoprolol is well absorbed, widely distributed, and mostly metabolized by the liver. It has a half-life of 3 to 7 hours.

ADVERSE EFFECTS AND INTERACTIONS

Because it is selective for blocking beta$_1$-receptors in the heart, metoprolol has few adverse effects on other autonomic targets and thus is preferred over non-selective beta-blockers, such as propranolol, for clients with lung disorders. Side effects are generally minor and relate to its autonomic activity, such as slowing of the heart rate and hypotension. Because of its multiple effects on the heart, clients with heart failure should be carefully monitored. This agent is contraindicated in cardiogenic shock, sinus bradycardia, and heart block greater than first degree. Concurrent use with digoxin may result in bradycardia. Oral contraceptives may increase metoprolol's effects.

 See the Companion Website for a Nursing Process Focus Chart specific to this drug.

CALCIUM CHANNEL BLOCKERS

23.8 Treating Angina with Calcium Channel Blockers

Blockade of calcium channels has a number of effects on the heart, most of which are similar to those of beta-blockers. Like beta-blockers, the value of calcium channel blockers (CCBs) is presented for several other conditions, including hypertension (Chapter 21) and dysrhythmias (Chapter 25). The first approved use of CCBs was for the treatment of angina. The CCBs used for angina are shown in Table 23.1.

CCBs have several cardiovascular actions that benefit the client with angina. Dihydropyridine CCBs such as amlodipine and nifedipine relax arteriolar smooth muscle, thus lowering blood pressure. This reduction in afterload decreases myocardial oxygen demand. Non-dihydropyridine CCBs such as verapamil and diltiazem also relax arteriolar smooth muscle, but in addition, they slow conduction velocity through the heart, decreasing heart rate and further reducing cardiac workload. An additional effect of the CCBs is their ability to dilate the coronary arteries, bringing more oxygen to the myocardium. Because they are able to relieve the acute vasospasm of variant angina, CCBs are considered drugs of choice for clients with vasospastic angina. For stable angina, they may be used as monotherapy in clients unable to tolerate beta-blockers. In clients with persistent symptoms, dihydropyridine CCBs may be combined with beta-blockers. Non-dihydropyridine CCBs are not generally used with beta-blockers or in heart block because of their effects on conduction.

NURSING CONSIDERATIONS

The role of the nurse in CCB therapy for angina involves careful monitoring of the client's condition and providing education as it relates to the prescribed drug regimen. Because of the effects on blood pressure and heart rate, vital signs should be assessed before administering these medications. Take blood pressure in both arms while the client is lying, sitting, and standing in order to monitor for orthostatic hypotension. Because CCBs, especially when administered IV, can affect myocardial conduction, they are not used in clients with sick sinus syndrome or third-degree AV block without the presence of a pacemaker. The ECG should be assessed prior to initiating therapy for any indication of conduction disturbances.

Some CCBs reduce myocardial contractility and can worsen heart failure (HF). Monitor client for signs and symptoms of worsening HF such as peripheral edema, shortness of breath, and lung congestion. Also monitor the client's weight for a sudden increase, which indicates fluid retention. Bowel function should be assessed as some CCBs cause constipation. Extended-release tablets or capsules should not be crushed or split because this can result in a large dose being released and cause serious hypotension.

Client education as it relates to CCBs should include goals, reasons for obtaining baseline data such as vital signs and tests for cardiac and renal disorders, and possible side effects. Following are important points to include when teaching clients regarding CCBs:

- Take blood pressure and pulse before self-administering the medication. Withhold drug if either pulse or blood pressure is below established parameters and notify the healthcare provider.
- Keep a record of frequency and severity of each angina attack.
- Change positions slowly and be cautious performing hazardous activities until effects of the drug are known.
- Notify the healthcare provider of any symptoms of HF such as shortness of breath, weight gain, and slow heart beat.

Pr PROTOTYPE DRUG | Diltiazem (Cardizem, Novo-Diltazem)

ACTIONS AND USES

Like other calcium channel blockers, diltiazem inhibits the transport of calcium into myocardial cells. It has the ability to relax both coronary and peripheral blood vessels. It is useful in the treatment of atrial dysrhythmias and hypertension as well as angina. When given as extended-release capsules, it can be administered once daily.

ADMINISTRATION ALERTS

- During IV administration, the client must be continuously monitored and cardioversion equipment must be available.
- Extended-release tablets and capsules should not be crushed or split.
- Diltiazem is pregnancy category C.

PHARMACOKINETICS

Diltiazem is well absorbed. It is 70% to 80% protein bound. It is metabolized by the liver. It has a half-life of 3.5 to 9 hours.

ADVERSE EFFECTS AND INTERACTIONS

Side effects of diltiazem are generally not serious and are related to vasodilation: headache, dizziness, and edema of the ankles and feet. Although diltiazem produces few adverse effects on the heart or vessels, it should be used with caution in clients taking other cardiovascular drugs, particularly digoxin or beta-adrenergic blockers. The combined effects of these drugs may cause partial or complete heart block, heart failure, or dysrhythmias.

This drug may increase digoxin and quinidine levels when taken concurrently.

Use with caution with herbal supplements, such as dong quai and ginger, as these products interfere with blood clotting. Calcium chloride can be administered by slow IV push to reverse hypotension or heart block *if* induced by CCBs.

 See the Companion Website for a Nursing Process Focus Chart specific to this drug.

- Do not crush or break extended-release capsules or tablets.
- Avoid grapefruit juice as it can cause CCBs to rise to toxic levels.

See also "Nursing Process Focus: Clients Receiving Calcium Channel Blocker Therapy" in Chapter 21, page 261, for the complete nursing process applied to clients receiving CCBs.

MYOCARDIAL INFARCTION

23.9 Diagnosis of Myocardial Infarction

Heart attack, also known as **myocardial infarction (MI)**, is responsible for a substantial number of deaths each year. Some clients die before reaching a medical facility for treatment, and many others die within 1 to 2 days following the initial MI. Clearly, MI is a serious and frightening disease and one responsible for a large percentage of sudden deaths.

The primary cause of myocardial infarction is advanced coronary artery disease. Plaque buildup can severely narrow one or more branches of the coronary arteries. Pieces of plaque can break off and lodge in a small vessel serving a portion of the myocardium. Deprived of its oxygen supply, this area of myocardium becomes ischemic and the tissue can die unless its blood supply is quickly restored. Figure 23.3 illustrates the pathogenesis and treatment of MI.

Goals for the pharmacological treatment of acute MI are as follows:

- Restore blood supply (perfusion) to the damaged myocardium as quickly as possible through the use of thrombolytics.

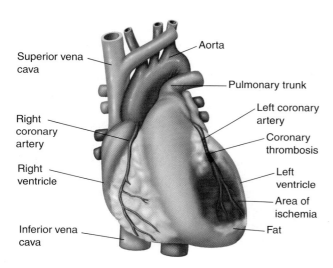

(a) Blockage of left coronary artery with myocardial ischemia

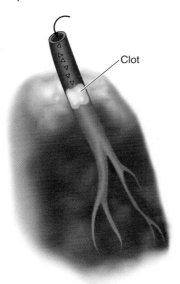

(b) Infusion of thrombolytics

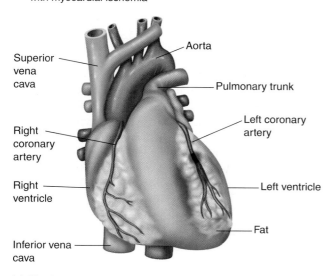

(c) Blood supply restarted to myocardium

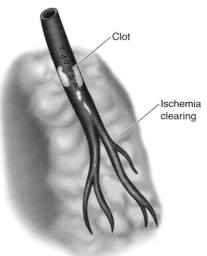

(d) Thrombus dissolving

● **Figure 23.3** Blockage and reperfusion following myocardial infarction: (a) blockage of left coronary artery with resultant myocardial ischemia; (b) infusion of thrombolytics; (c) blood supply returning to the myocardium; (d) thrombus dissolving and ischemia clearing

Source: Figures (a) and (c), Pearson Education/PH College.

TABLE 23.2 Changes in Blood Test Values with Acute MI				
Blood Test	Initial Elevation after MI	Peak Elevation after MI	Duration of Elevation	Normal Range
cholesterol			4 weeks, during stress response	5.2 mmol/L
creatine kinase (CK)	3–8 h	12–24 h	2–4 d	males: 12–80 U/L females: 10–70 U/L
creatinine phosphokinase (CPK)	4–8 h	18–24 h	2–3 d	0–3% of CK
erythrocyte sedimentation rate (ESR)	first week		several weeks	
glucose			duration of stress response	fasting: 3.3–5.8 mmol/L
lactase dehydrogenase (LDH)	8–72 h	3–6 d	8–14 d	95–195 U/L
myoglobin	1–3 h	4–6 h	1–2 d	0–57 µg/mL
troponin I	2–4 h	24–36 h	7–10 d	3.1 µg/L
troponin T	2–4 h	24–36 h	10–14 d	0.01–0.1 µg/L
WBC count	few hours		3–7 d	$4–10 \times 10^9$/L

- Reduce myocardial oxygen demand with organic nitrates and beta-blockers, to prevent further MIs.
- Control or prevent associated dysrhythmias with beta-blockers or other antidysrhythmics.
- Reduce post-MI mortality with ASA and ACE inhibitors.
- Control MI pain and associated anxiety with narcotic analgesics.

Laboratory test results are used to aid in diagnosis and to monitor progress after an MI. Table 23.2 describes important laboratory values.

THROMBOLYTICS

23.10 Treating Myocardial Infarction with Thrombolytics

In the treatment of MI, the goal of thrombolytic therapy is to dissolve clots obstructing the coronary arteries and restore circulation to the myocardium. Quick restoration of cardiac circulation has been found to reduce mortality caused by acute MI. Thrombolytics are most effective when administered from 20 minutes to 12 hours after the onset of MI symptoms. If administered after 24 hours, the drugs are mostly ineffective. After the clot is successfully dissolved, anticoagulant therapy is initiated to prevent the formation of additional clots. Dosages and descriptions of the various thrombolytics are given in Chapter 26.

Thrombolytics have a narrow margin of safety between dissolving "normal" and "abnormal" clots. It must be understood that once infused in the blood, the drugs travel to all vessels and may cause adverse effects anywhere in the body. The primary risk of thrombolytics is excessive bleeding from interference in the normal clotting process. Vital signs must be monitored continuously, and any signs of bleeding generally call for discontinuation of therapy.

Because these drugs are rapidly destroyed in the blood, discontinuation of the drug normally results in the rapid termination of adverse effects.

NURSING CONSIDERATIONS

The role of the nurse in thrombolytic therapy for MI involves careful monitoring of the client's condition and providing education as it relates to the prescribed drug regimen. Assess for conditions that would be contraindicated, including recent trauma or surgery/biopsy, GI bleeding, postpartum (within 10 days), cerebral hemorrhage, bleeding disorders, and thrombocytopenia, because thrombolytics would place the client at risk for increased bleeding. In septic thrombophlebitis, a favourable clot is in place that would be dissolved by thrombolytics, resulting in client injury, so the drugs are contraindicated in this condition. These drugs should be used with caution in any condition where bleeding could be a significant hazard, such as severe renal or liver disease.

IV lines, arterial lines, and Foley catheters should be established prior to beginning thrombolytic therapy to decrease the chance of bleeding from those sites. Monitor vital signs and changes in lab values, including hemoglobin, hematocrit (Hct), platelets, and coagulation studies, that are indicative of bleeding. Because cerebral hemorrhage is a major concern, changes in level of consciousness should be carefully monitored and neurological status assessed. Monitor for dysrhythmias that may occur as cardiac tissue is re-perfused after myocardial infarction. Monitor lab work such as the CBC during and after therapy for indications of blood loss due to internal bleeding. The client has an increased risk of bleeding for 2 to 4 days post-therapy.

Client education as it relates to thrombolytics should include goals, reasons for obtaining baseline data such as vital signs and tests for cardiac and renal disorders, and possible side effects. Following are the important points to include when teaching clients about thrombolytics:

- Keep movement of IV sites to a minimum to prevent bleeding.
- Minimize physical activity during the infusion.
- Report immediately any bleeding from gums, rectum, or vagina during and for at least 4 days following completion of the infusion.

See also "Nursing Process Focus: Clients Receiving Thrombolytic Therapy" in Chapter 26, page 341, for the complete nursing process applied to caring for clients receiving thrombolytics.

ANTIPLATELET AND ANTICOAGULANT DRUGS

23.11 Treating Myocardial Infarction with Antiplatelets and Anticoagulants

Unless contraindicated, 160 to 325 mg of ASA is given as soon as an MI is suspected. ASA use in the weeks following an acute MI dramatically reduces mortality, probably owing to its antiplatelet action. The low doses used in maintenance therapy (75 to 150 mg/day) rarely cause GI bleeding.

Clopidogrel and ticlopidine are antiplatelet agents that block adenosine diphosphate (ADP). They may be used for the prevention of thrombotic stroke and MI. Because these drugs are considerably more expensive than ASA, they are usually considered for clients allergic to ASA or who are at risk for GI bleeding from ASA.

Glycoprotein IIb/IIIa inhibitors are antiplatelet agents with a mechanism of action different from that of ASA. **Glycoprotein IIb/IIIa** is a receptor found on the surface of platelets. Glycoprotein IIb/IIIa inhibitors occupy this receptor and inhibit clot formation. These agents are sometimes used for unstable angina or MI or for clients undergoing PTCA. Abciximab, the most common drug in this class, is infused during PTCA and for 12 hours following the procedure.

Heparin is an anticoagulant that is often initiated following an MI to prevent additional thrombi from forming. Heparin therapy is usually continued for about 3 days after clients are switched to warfarin. An alternative is to administer a low-molecular-weight heparin, such as dalteparin. Refer to Chapter 26 for a comparison of anticoagulants and their dosages.

BETA-ADRENERGIC BLOCKERS

23.12 Treating Myocardial Infarction with Beta-Blockers

The use of the beta-adrenergic blockers in the treatment of cardiovascular disease has been discussed in a number of chapters in this textbook. This section will focus on their use in the treatment of MI. The beta-blockers used for MI are shown in Table 23.1 on page 292.

Beta-blockers have the ability to slow heart rate, decrease contractility, and reduce blood pressure. These three factors reduce myocardial oxygen demand, which is beneficial for clients experiencing a recent MI. In addition, they slow impulse conduction through the heart, which tends to suppress dysrhythmias, which are serious and sometimes fatal complications following an MI. Beta-blockers have been shown to reduce mortality when given within 8 hours of MI onset.

NURSING CONSIDERATIONS

See Nursing Considerations for beta-blockers in Section 23.7.

MediaLink — *Mechanism of Action: Reteplase*

Pr PROTOTYPE DRUG | Reteplase (Retavase)

ACTIONS AND USES

Reteplase acts as a catalyst in the cleavage of plasminogen to plasmin, a substance responsible for degrading the fibrin matrix of a clot. Reteplase is one of the newer thrombolytics. Like other drugs in this class, reteplase should be given as soon as possible after the onset of MI symptoms. It usually acts within 20 minutes, and restoration of circulation to the ischemic site may be faster than with other thrombolytics. After the clot has been dissolved, heparin therapy is often started to prevent additional clots from forming.

PHARMACOKINETICS

Reteplase is rapidly metabolized by the liver and is excreted by the kidneys. It has a half-life of 13 to 16 minutes.

ADMINISTRATION ALERTS

- Drug must be reconstituted just prior to use with diluent provided by the manufacturer; swirl to mix—do not shake.
- Do not give any other drug simultaneously through the same IV line.
- Drug must be administered within 6 hours of onset of MI symptoms and within 3 hours of thrombotic cerebrovascular accident in order to be effective.
- Reteplase is pregnancy category C.

ADVERSE EFFECTS AND INTERACTIONS

Reteplase is contraindicated in clients with active bleeding. The healthcare provider must be vigilant in recognizing and responding to abnormal bleeding during therapy.

Drug interactions with anticoagulants and platelet aggregation inhibitors will produce an additive effect and increase the risk of bleeding.

 See the Companion Website for a Nursing Process Focus Chart specific to this drug.

23.13 Drugs for Symptoms and Complications of Acute Myocardial Infarction

Several additional drugs have proven useful in treating the client presenting with an acute MI. Unless contraindicated, 180 to 325 mg of ASA is given as soon as an MI is suspected. ASA use in the weeks following an acute MI reduces mortality dramatically. Additional actions of ASA may be found in Chapters 19 and 31.

Two ACE inhibitors, captopril and lisinopril, also have been determined to improve survival following acute MI. These drugs are most effective when therapy is started within 1 to 2 days following the onset of symptoms. Oral doses are normally begun after thrombolytic therapy is completed and the client's condition has stabilized. Additional indications for ACE inhibitors may be found in Chapters 21 and 24.

Pain control is essential following acute MI to ensure client comfort and reduce stress. Narcotic analgesics such as morphine sulfate or fentanyl are sometimes given to ease extreme pain associated with acute MI and to sedate the anxious client. The pharmacology of the analgesics is presented in Chapter 19.

CEREBROVASCULAR ACCIDENT

23.14 Pathogenesis of Cerebrovascular Accident

Cerebrovascular accident (CVA), also called **stroke** or **brain attack**, is a major cause of permanent disability. It is the third leading cause of death in North America, following heart disease and cancer. The majority of CVAs are **thrombotic strokes**, which are caused by a thrombus (clot) in a blood vessel serving the brain. Tissues distal to the clot lose their oxygen supply, and neural tissue will die unless circulation is quickly restored. A smaller percentage of CVAs, about 20%, are caused by rupture of a cerebral vessel with associated bleeding into neural tissue, known as a **hemorrhagic stroke**. Symptoms are the same for the two types of stroke. Mortality from CVA is very high: more than 30% of clients die within the first year following the CVA. Most of the risk factors associated with CVA are the same as for other cardiovascular disease, such as hypertension and coronary artery disease.

The signs and symptoms of a CVA depend on a number of factors, the most important of which are the location of the obstruction and how much brain tissue is affected. A stroke affecting one side of the brain will result in neurological deficits on the opposite side of the body. For example, if the stroke occurs in the right side of the brain, the left side of the body will be affected. The five warning signs of stroke are:

1. Paralysis or weakness on one side of the body
2. Vision problems
3. Dizziness
4. Speech/language problems
5. Headache

23.15 Pharmacotherapy of Thrombotic CVA

Drug therapy for thrombotic CVA focuses on two main goals: prevention of CVA through the use of anticoagulants and antihypertensive agents, and restoration of blood supply to the affected neurons as quickly as possible after a CVA through the use of thrombolytics.

Sustained, chronic hypertension is closely associated with CVA. Antihypertensive drugs such as the beta-adrenergic blockers, calcium channel blockers, diuretics, and ACE inhibitors can help control blood pressure and reduce the probability of CVA. Diet and lifestyle factors that reduce blood pressure should be implemented concurrently with antihypertensive pharmacotherapy.

ASA, through its anticoagulant properties, reduces the incidence of stroke. When given in very low doses, ASA discourages the formation of clots by inhibiting platelets. Clients are often placed on a daily regimen of low-dose ASA therapy following a transient ischemic attack (TIA) or following their first CVA. Many healthcare providers recommend low-dose ASA therapy as a prophylactic measure for the prevention of MI and CVA. Ticlopidine is an antiplatelet drug that may be used to provide anticoagulation in clients who cannot tolerate ASA. Other anticoagulants, such as warfarin, may be given to prevent CVA in high-risk individuals, such as those with prosthetic heart valves. More detailed information on anticoagulants can be found in Chapter 26.

The single most important breakthrough in the pharmacotherapy of CVA was the development of the thrombolytic drugs called "clot busters." Prior to the advent of these drugs, the treatment of CVA was largely a passive, wait-and-see strategy. Care was directed at habilitation or rehabilitation after the fact. Stroke is now aggressively treated with thrombolytics as soon as the client arrives at the hospital. Such agents are most effective if administered within 3 hours of the attack. The use of aggressive thrombolytic therapy can completely restore brain function in a significant number of stroke victims. As a result, CVA is now considered a condition that mandates immediate treatment. The condition is often referred to by its newer title, brain attack, which reflects the need for urgent treatment.

SPECIAL CONSIDERATIONS

Cultural, Gender, and Age Considerations in Stroke

- Overall, the incidence and prevalence of stroke are about equal for men and women.
- At all ages, however, more women than men die of stroke.
- Risk of stroke is greater in people who have a family history of stroke.
- Aboriginal Peoples and those of African or South Asian descent have a higher risk of disability and death from stroke than the general population, in part because they have a greater incidence of hypertension, diabetes, and related complications.

NATURAL THERAPIES

Ginseng

Ginseng is one of the oldest known herbal remedies, with at least six species being reported to have medicinal properties. *Panax ginseng* is distributed throughout China, Korea, and Siberia, whereas *Panax quinquefolius* is native to Canada and the United States. The plant's popularity has led to its extinction from certain regions, and much of the available ginseng is now grown commercially.

Standardization of ginseng focuses on a group of chemicals called ginsenosides, although there are many other chemicals in the root, which is the harvested portion of the plant. The *German Commission E Monographs* (a therapeutic guide to herbal medicine) recommend a dose of 20 to 30 mg ginsenosides. This is sometimes reported as a percent, with 5% being the recommended standard amount of ginsenosides.

There are differences in chemical composition among the various species of ginseng: American ginseng is not considered equivalent to Siberian ginseng. Ginseng is reported to be a calcium channel antagonist. By increasing the conversion of L-arginine to nitric oxide, ginseng improves blood flow to the heart in times of low oxygen supply, such as with myocardial ischemia. The Chinese have found that nitric oxide is a potent antioxidant that combats free radical injury to the heart muscle. The nurse should caution clients who take ginseng because herb-drug interactions are possible with warfarin and loop diuretics.

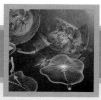

CHAPTER REVIEW

KEY CONCEPTS

The numbered key concepts provide a succinct summary of the important points from the corresponding numbered section within the chapter. If any of these points are not clear, refer to the numbered section within the chapter for review. Expanded versions can be found on the Companion Website.

23.1 Coronary artery disease includes both angina and myocardial infarction. It is caused by narrowing of the arterial lumen due to atherosclerotic plaque.

23.2 The myocardium requires a continuous supply of oxygen from the coronary arteries in order to function properly.

23.3 Angina pectoris is chest pain, usually upon emotional or physical exertion. It is caused by the narrowing of a coronary artery, which results in lack of sufficient oxygen to the heart muscle.

23.4 Angina management may include non-pharmacological therapies such as diet and lifestyle modifications, treatment of underlying disorders, angioplasty, or surgery.

23.5 The pharmacological goals for the treatment of angina are to terminate acute attacks and prevent future episodes. This is usually achieved by reducing cardiac workload.

23.6 The organic nitrates relieve angina by dilating veins and coronary arteries. They are drugs of choice for stable angina.

23.7 Beta-adrenergic blockers relieve angina by decreasing the oxygen demands on the heart. They are sometimes considered first-line drugs for chronic angina.

23.8 Calcium channel blockers relieve angina by dilating the coronary vessels and reducing the workload of the heart. They are drugs of first choice for treating variant angina.

23.9 The early diagnosis of myocardial infarction increases chances of survival. Early pharmacotherapy may include thrombolytics, ASA, beta-blockers, and antidysrhythmics.

23.10 If given within hours after the onset of MI, thrombolytic agents can dissolve clots and restore perfusion to affected regions of the myocardium.

23.11 Glycoprotein IIb/IIIa inhibitors are antiplatelet agents for the treatment of myocardial ischemia.

23.12 When given within 24 hours after the onset of myocardial infarction, beta-adrenergic blockers can improve survival.

23.13 A number of additional drugs are used to treat the symptoms and complications of acute MI. These include analgesics, anticoagulants (including ASA), and ACE inhibitors.

23.14 Cerebrovascular accident, also known as stroke and brain attack, is a major cause of death and disability. CVAs may be caused by a clot or by rupture of a cerebral vessel.

23.15 Aggressive treatment of thrombotic CVA with thrombolytics, to restore perfusion, and anticoagulants, to prevent additional clots from forming, can increase survival.

REVIEW QUESTIONS

1 What are the distinguishing characteristics that differentiate stable, variant, and unstable angina?

2 Why does decreasing the cardiac workload result in the reduction of angina pain?

3 Describe how medication administration with transdermal nitrates can be altered to prevent or delay tolerance in clients with angina pectoris.

4 Why is it important to treat an MI within the first 24 hours after symptoms have begun?

5 What role does ASA play in the pharmacotherapy of myocardial infarction and CVA?

CRITICAL THINKING QUESTIONS

1. A client on the medical unit is complaining of chest pain (4/10), has a history of angina, and is requesting his PRN nitroglycerin spray. The client's BP is 96/60 mm Hg at present. What should the nurse do?

2. A client is recovering from an acute MI and has been put on atenolol (Tenormin). What teaching should the client receive prior to discharge from the hospital?

3. A client with chest pain has been given the calcium channel blocker diltiazem (Cardizem) IV for a heart rate of 118. Blood pressure at this time is 100/60 mm Hg. What precautions should the nurse take?

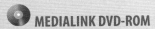

EXPLORE
MediaLink

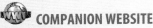

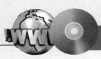

www.pearsoned.ca/adams-king

MEDIALINK DVD-ROM
- **Audio Glossary**
- **CRNE Review**
- **Animations**
  Coronary Artery Disease
  Mechanism of Action: Reteplase

COMPANION WEBSITE
- **CRNE Review**
- **Case Study:** Client receiving nitrates for angina
- **Dosage Calculations**
- **Nursing Process Focus Charts**

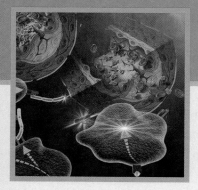

CHAPTER 24

Drugs for Heart Failure

DRUGS AT A GLANCE

ANGIOTENSIN-CONVERTING ENZYME INHIBITORS
- lisinopril (Prinivil, Zestril)

ANGIOTENSIN II RECEPTOR BLOCKERS

BETA-ADRENERGIC BLOCKERS
- carvedilol (Coreg)

VASODILATORS
- isosorbide dinitrate (Isordil, Coronex)

CARDIAC GLYCOSIDES
- digoxin (Lanoxin)

DIURETICS
Loop (high ceiling)
- furosemide (Lasix)

Thiazide and thiazide-like
Potassium-sparing

PHOSPHODIESTERASE INHIBITORS
- milrinone (Apo-Milrinone)

OBJECTIVES

After reading this chapter, the student should be able to do the following:

1. Identify drug classes used for treating heart failure.
2. Explain the therapeutic action of each class of drug used for heart failure in relation to the pathophysiology of heart failure.
3. Describe the nurse's role in the pharmacological management of clients receiving drugs for heart failure.
4. For each of the drug classes listed in Drugs at a Glance, identify a representative drug and explain its mechanism of action, therapeutic effects, and important adverse effects.
5. Describe and explain, based on pharmacological principles, the rationale for nursing assessment, planning, interventions, and teaching for clients with heart failure.
6. Use the nursing process to care for clients receiving drug therapy for heart failure.

MediaLink

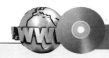

www.pearsoned.ca/adams-king

CRNE review, case studies, and other interactive resources for this chapter can be found on the Companion Website at **www.pearsoned.ca/adams-king.** Click on "Chapter 24" to select the activities for this chapter. For animations, more CRNE review questions, and an audio glossary, access the accompanying DVD-ROM in this textbook.

KEY TERMS

afterload page 305
cardiac output page 305
contractility page 305
Frank-Starling law page 305
heart failure (HF) page 304
peripheral edema page 305
phosphodiesterase page 314
preload page 305

Heart failure is one of the most common and fatal of the cardiovascular diseases, and its incidence is expected to increase as the population ages. Despite the dramatic decline in mortality for most cardiovascular diseases that has occurred over the past two decades, the death rate for heart failure has only recently begun to decrease. Although improved treatment of myocardial infarction and hypertension has led to declines in mortality due to heart failure, approximately one in five clients still dies within 1 year of diagnosis of heart failure, and 50% die within 5 years. Historically, this condition was called *congestive heart failure*; however, because heart failure can be diagnosed without evidence of volume overload or congestion, it is now called heart failure.

PHARMFACTS

Heart Failure

- About 500,000 Canadians have heart failure.
- About one in five dies within a year of diagnosis.
- Heart failure occurs slightly more frequently in men than women.
- African Canadians and Aboriginal Peoples have one and a half to two times the incidence of heart failure as Caucasians.
- Heart failure is twice as frequent in hypertensive clients and five times as frequent in persons who have experienced a heart attack.
- Heart failure increases with age. It affects
    - 2% of those 40 to 59 years old.
    - 5% of those 60 to 69 years old.
    - 10% of those over age 70.

24.1 The Etiology of Heart Failure

Heart failure (HF) is the inability of the ventricles to pump enough blood to meet the body's metabolic demands. HF can be caused by any disorder that decreases the ability of the heart to receive or eject blood. These disorders include:

- Mitral stenosis
- Myocardial infarction
- Chronic hypertension
- Coronary artery disease
- Diabetes mellitus

Because there is no cure for HF, the treatment goals are to prevent, treat, or remove the underlying causes when possible, to improve the client's quality of life. Prevention includes keeping blood pressure and lipid and glucose levels within normal ranges. Effective pharmacotherapy can help to prevent and slow the progression of HF and improve symptoms and quality of life.

24.2 Cardiovascular Changes in Heart Failure

Although a number of diseases can lead to HF, the end result is the same: the heart is unable to pump the volume of blood required to meet the body's metabolic needs. To understand how medications act on the weakened myocardium, it is essential to understand the underlying cardiac physiology.

The right side of the heart receives blood from the venous system and pumps it to the lungs, where the blood receives oxygen and loses its carbon dioxide. The blood returns to the left side of the heart, which pumps it to the rest of the body via the aorta. The amount of blood received by the right side should exactly

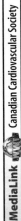

MediaLink The Beating Heart

MediaLink Canadian Cardiovascular Society

equal that sent out by the left side. If this does not happen, HF may occur. The amount of blood pumped by each ventricle per minute is the **cardiac output**. The relationship between cardiac output and blood pressure is explained in Chapter 21.

Although many variables affect cardiac output, the two most important factors are preload and afterload. Just before the chambers of the heart contract (systole), they are filled to their maximum capacity with blood. The degree to which the myocardial fibres are stretched just prior to contraction is called **preload**. The more these fibres are stretched, the more forcefully they will contract, a principle called the **Frank-Starling law**. This is somewhat similar to a rubber band—the more it is stretched, the more forcefully it will snap back. The strength of contraction of the heart is called **contractility**. Drugs that increase preload and contractility help to increase cardiac output. Drugs such as norepinephrine, epinephrine, and thyroid hormone that increase contractility are called positive inotropic agents. Drugs such as beta-adrenergic blockers and quinidine decrease contractility and are called negative inotropic agents.

The second important factor affecting cardiac output is afterload. **Afterload** is the pressure in the aorta that must be overcome for blood to be ejected from the left ventricle. Hypertension increases afterload and workload of the heart. Drugs that treat hypertension are explained in Chapter 21.

In HF, the myocardium becomes weakened, and the heart cannot eject all the blood it receives. This weakening may occur on the left side, the right side, or both sides of the heart. If it occurs on the left side, excess blood accumulates in the left ventricle. The wall of the left ventricle may become thicker (hypertrophies) in an attempt to compensate for the extra blood retained in the chamber. Since the left ventricle has limits to its ability to compensate for the increased preload, blood "backs up" into the lungs, resulting in the classic symptoms of cough and shortness of breath. Left heart failure is sometimes called congestive heart failure (CHF). The pathophysiology of HF is shown in Figure 24.1.

Although left heart failure is more common, the right side of the heart can also weaken, either simultaneously with the left side or independently. In right heart failure, the blood backs up into the peripheral veins, resulting in **peripheral edema** and engorgement of organs such as the liver. The symptoms of HF are listed in Figure 24.2.

PHARMACOTHERAPY OF HEART FAILURE

Drugs can relieve the symptoms of heart failure by a number of different mechanisms, including slowing the heart rate, increasing contractility, and reducing workload. These mechanisms are illustrated in Figure 24.3.

The 2007 Canadian Cardiovascular Society Consensus Conference recommendations for the management of HF are outlined in Figure 24.4. Non-pharmacological recommendations include client education about HF, lifestyle modifications to reduce risk factors and symptoms, and control of salt intake. Pharmacological recommendations include that all HF clients with a left ventricle that ejects less

Source: Adapted from Arnold et al., 2007, with the

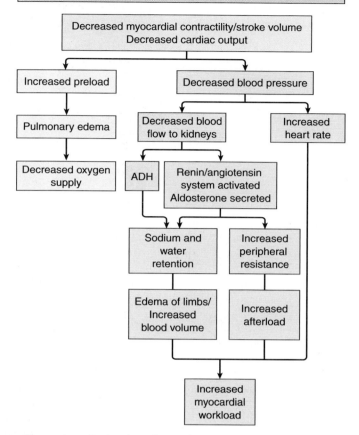

● **Figure 24.1** Pathophysiology of heart failure

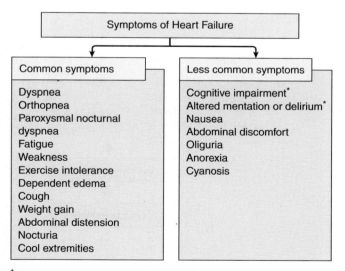

*May be a more common presentation in elderly clients.

● **Figure 24.2** Symptoms of heart failure

Source: Arnold et al., 2006. Reproduced with the permission of the Canadian Cardiovascular Society.

than 40% of received blood should be treated with both an ACE inhibitor and a beta-blocker, unless a specific contraindication exists. Usually, ACE inhibitor therapy is initiated

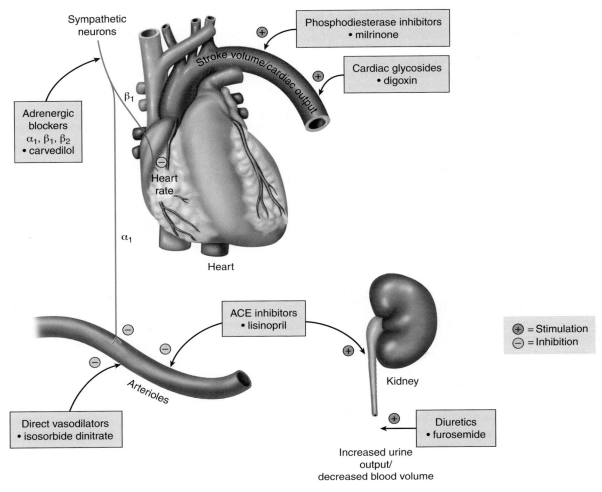

● **Figure 24.3** Mechanisms of action of drugs used for heart failure

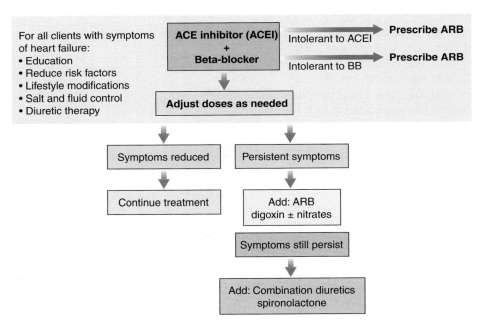

● **Figure 24.4** Treatment of heart failure: recommendations of the Canadian Cardiovascular Society Consensus Conference, Fig. 24.3.

before the beta-blocker is added. Angiotensin-receptor blockers (ARBs) may be used when symptoms persist despite optimal treatment with ACE inhibitors and beta-blockers or when these agents cannot be used. Diuretics should be used for most clients with HF who have peripheral edema or pulmonary congestion. Once acute congestion is cleared, the lowest dose should be used that maintains stable signs and symptoms. Digoxin may be used to relieve symptoms and reduce hospitalizations in clients in sinus rhythm who have persistent moderate to severe symptoms despite optimized therapy with other HF drugs. Also, clients with

HF should be immunized against influenza (annually) and pneumococcal pneumonia (if not done in last 6 years) to reduce the risk of respiratory infections that may seriously aggravate HF.

ACE INHIBITORS AND ANGIOTENSIN RECEPTOR BLOCKERS

Drugs affecting the renin-angiotensin-aldosterone system reduce the afterload on the heart and lower blood pressure. They are often drugs of choice in the treatment of HF. The ACE inhibitors and ARBs used for HF are shown in Table 24.1.

TABLE 24.1   Drugs for Heart Failure

Drug	Route and Adult Dose
ACE Inhibitors	
captopril (Capoten)	PO; 6.25–12.5 mg tid (max 450 mg/day)
enalapril (Vasotec) (see page 264 for the Prototype Drug box)	PO; 2.5 mg qid–bid (max 40 mg/day)
fosinopril (Monopril)	PO; 5–40 mg qd (max 40 mg/day)
lisinopril (Prinivil, Zestril)	PO; 10 mg qd (max 80 mg/day)
quinapril (Accupril)	PO; 10–20 mg qd (max 40 mg/day)
ramipril (Altace)	PO; 2.5–5.0 mg bid (max 10/day)
Angiotensin II Receptor Blockers	
candesartan (Atacand)	PO; start at 16 mg qd (range 8–32 mg divided once or twice daily)
eprosartan (Teveten)	PO; 600 mg qd or 400 mg qid–bid (max 800 mg/day)
irbesartan (Avapro, Avalide)	PO; 150–300 mg qd (max 300 mg/day)
losartan (Cozaar)	PO; 25–50 mg in one to two divided doses (max 100 mg/day)
valsartan (Diovan)	PO; 80 mg qd (max 320 mg/day)
Beta-Adrenergic Blockers	
carvedilol (Coreg)	PO; 3.125 mg bid for 2 wk (max 25 mg bid if < 85 kg or 50 mg bid if > 85 kg)
metoprolol: beta₁ (Lopresor, Lopresor SR)	PO; 12.5–25 mg qd (can be doubled q2wk to max 200 mg/day)
Vasodilators	
hydralazine (Apo-Hydralazine) (see page 270 for the Prototype Drug box)	PO; 10–50 mg qid (max 300 mg/day)
isosorbide dinitrate (Isordil, Coronex)	PO; 2.5–30 mg qid administered ac and hs (max 160 mg/day)
Diuretics	
Loop (High Ceiling)	
bumetanide (Burinex)	PO; 0.5–2.mg qd (max 10 mg/day)
furosemide (Lasix)	PO; 20–80 mg in one or more divided doses (max 600 mg/day)
Thiazide and Thiazide-Like	
hydrochlorothiazide (HCTZ, Urozide) (see page 258 for the Prototype Drug box)	PO; 25–200 mg in one to three divided doses (max 200 mg/day)
Potassium-Sparing	
spironolactone (Aldactone) (see page 623 for the Prototype Drug box)	PO; 5–200 mg in divided doses (max 200 mg/day)
triamterene (Apo-Triazide)	PO; 100 mg bid (max 300 mg/day)
Cardiac Glycosides	
digoxin (Lanoxin)	PO; 0.125–0.5 mg qd
Phosphodiesterase Inhibitors	
milrinone (Apo-Milrinone)	IV; 50 µg/kg over 10 min; then 0.375–0.75 µg/kg/min

24.3 Pharmacotherapy with ACE Inhibitors and ARBs

ACE inhibitors were approved for the treatment of hypertension in the 1980s. Since then, research has shown that they can prevent the occurrence of HF in clients at risk and slow the progression of HF. Because of their relative safety and efficacy, they have replaced digoxin as drugs of choice for the treatment of HF. Unless specifically contraindicated, ACE inhibitors should be given to all clients with HF and many clients at high risk for HF.

The primary action of the ACE inhibitors is to lower blood pressure by their action on the renin-angiotensin-aldosterone system. ACE inhibitors inhibit aldosterone excretion, enhancing the excretion of sodium and water and decreasing blood volume. The resultant reduction in arterial blood pressure reduces the afterload of the heart, thus increasing cardiac output. An additional effect of the ACE inhibitors is dilation of the veins returning blood to the heart. This action, which is probably not directly related to their inhibition of angiotensin, decreases preload and reduces peripheral edema. The combined reductions in preload, afterload, and blood volume substantially decrease the workload of the heart and allow it to work more efficiently for the HF client. Several ACE inhibitors have been shown to reduce mortality following acute myocardial infarction when therapy is started soon after the onset of symptoms (see Chapter 23).

Another mechanism for decreasing the effects of angiotensin is the use of ARBs. The actions of the ARBs are similar to those of the ACE inhibitors, as would be expected since both classes inhibit angiotensin. In clients with HF, ARBs show equivalent efficacy to the ACE inhibitors. Their use in the treatment of HF is usually reserved for clients who are unable to tolerate the side effects of ACE inhibitors or who have persistent HF symptoms despite optimal treatment with ACE inhibitors and beta-blockers. More information on ACE inhibitors and ARBs can be found in Chapter 21.

NURSING CONSIDERATIONS

The role of the nurse in ACE inhibitor or ARB therapy for HF involves careful monitoring of the client's condition and providing education as it relates to the prescribed drug regimen. Prior to beginning therapy, a thorough health history should be taken. These drugs are contraindicated in pregnancy and lactation and in clients with a history of angioedema. A complete blood count should be obtained before starting therapy and repeated every month for the first 3 to 6 months of treatment, then at periodic intervals for 1 year. ACE inhibitors should be withheld if the neutrophil count drops below $1000/mm^3$ because they may cause neutropenia. An increase in serum creatinine of up to 30% is not unexpected when ACE inhibitor or ARB therapy is initiated. Diuretics should be discontinued before the nurse initially administers ACE inhibitors, to prevent severe hypotension. Because ACE inhibitors can cause severe hypotension with initial doses, monitor the client closely for several hours afterward. If severe hypotension does occur, place the client in a supine position and notify the healthcare provider. A lower dose is indicated for elderly clients and those with renal insufficiency. Use with caution in clients with impaired kidney function, hyperkalemia, and those with autoimmune diseases, especially systemic lupus erythematosus (SLE).

Client education as it relates to ACE inhibitors or ARBs used to treat HF should include goals, reasons for obtaining baseline data such as vital signs and tests for cardiac and renal function, and possible side effects. Following are the important points to include when teaching clients regarding ACE inhibitors or ARBs:

- Check with the healthcare provider before taking additional prescription medications or OTC drugs.
- It may take weeks or months for maximum therapeutic response to be reached.
- Follow prescribed dietary modifications, including sodium and potassium restrictions, to prevent side effects of hyponatremia and hyperkalemia.
- Do not take salt or potassium supplements unless ordered by the healthcare provider.
- Avoid driving until the effect of the drug is known.

Refer to "Nursing Process Focus: Clients Receiving ACE Inhibitor Therapy" in Chapter 21 (page 265) for additional information.

SPECIAL CONSIDERATIONS

Points to Consider in Educating Clients with HF

- Regular physical activity is recommended for all clients with stable symptoms and impaired left ventricular systolic function.
- Before starting a physical activity program, all clients should have a graded exercise stress test to assess functional capacity, ischemia, and optimal heart rate.
- Erect and supine blood pressure should be assessed.
- All clients with symptomatic HF should not add salt to their diet, and clients with advanced HF should reduce salt to less than 2 g/day.
- Fluid intake beyond normal needs to prevent thirst is *not* recommended.
- Daily morning weight should be monitored in HF clients with fluid retention or congestion not easily controlled with diuretics and in clients with significant renal dysfunction or hyponatremia.
- Restriction of daily fluid intake to 1.5 to 2 L/day should be considered for clients with fluid retention or congestion not easily controlled with diuretics and in clients with severe renal dysfunction or hyponatremia.
- Clients with HF should be immunized against influenza (annually) and pneumococcal pneumonia (if not done in last 6 years) to reduce the risk of respiratory infections that may seriously aggravate HF.
- Clients should be aware of which symptoms to report immediately to the healthcare provider.

Source: Canadian Cardiovascular Society Consensus Conference recommendations on heart failure (Arnold et al., 2006).

Pr PROTOTYPE DRUG | Lisinopril (Prinivil, Zestril)

ACTIONS AND USES

Due to its value in the treatment of both HF and hypertension, lisinopril has become one of the most commonly prescribed drugs. Like other ACE inhibitors, doses of lisinopril may require 2 to 3 weeks of adjustment to reach maximum efficacy, and several months of therapy may be needed for a client's cardiac function to return to normal. Because of their synergistic hypotensive action, combined therapy with lisinopril and diuretics should be carefully monitored.

PHARMACOKINETICS

Absorption of lisinopril is about 25% but varies. It is excreted unchanged by the kidneys. It has a half-life of 12 hours.

ADMINISTRATION ALERTS

- Measure blood pressure just prior to administering lisinopril to be certain that effects are lasting for 24 hours and to determine if the client's blood pressure is within acceptable range.
- Lisinopril is pregnancy category D.

ADVERSE EFFECTS AND INTERACTIONS

Although lisinopril causes few side effects, hyperkalemia may occur during therapy; thus, electrolyte levels are usually monitored periodically. Other side effects include cough, taste disturbances, headache, dizziness, chest pain, nausea, vomiting, diarrhea, and hypotension.

Lisinopril interacts with indomethacin and other NSAIDs, causing decreased antihypertensive activity. When taken concurrently with potassium-sparing diuretics, hyperkalemia may result. Lisinopril may increase lithium levels and toxicity.

 See the Companion Website for a Nursing Process Focus Chart specific to this drug.

BETA-ADRENERGIC BLOCKERS (ANTAGONISTS)

Only two beta-blockers are approved for the treatment of HF: carvedilol and metoprolol extended-release form. The doses of these agents are shown in Table 24.1 on page 307. They reduce the cardiac workload by decreasing afterload.

24.4 Pharmacotherapy with Beta-Adrenergic Blockers

Beta-adrenergic blockers improve the symptoms of HF by reducing cardiac workload. The negative inotropic effect (decreased heart contractility) of beta-blockers is in contrast to the positive inotropic effect (increased heart contractility) of cardiac glycosides and some other drugs that may be used to treat HF.

Clients with HF have excessive activation of the sympathetic nervous system, which weakens the heart and leads to progression of the disease. Beta-blockers block the cardiac actions of the sympathetic nervous system, thus slowing the heart rate and reducing blood pressure. The decreased afterload that results reduces cardiac workload; after several months of therapy, heart size, shape, and function return to normal in some clients. Extensive clinical research has demonstrated that the proper use of beta-blockers can dramatically reduce HF-associated hospitalizations and deaths.

To benefit clients with HF, however, beta-blockers must be administered in a very specific manner. Initial doses must be one-tenth to one-twentieth of the target dose. Doses are doubled every 2 weeks until the optimum dose is reached. If therapy is begun with too high a dose, or the dose is increased too rapidly, beta-blockers can worsen HF. Beta-blockers are rarely used as monotherapy for HF. The 2007 Canadian Cardiovascular Society Consensus Conference recommends that they be used in combination with ACE inhibitors as first-line therapy for HF.

The basic pharmacology of the beta-blockers is presented in Chapter 13. Other uses of beta-blockers are discussed elsewhere in this text: hypertension in Chapter 21, dysrhythmias in Chapter 25, and angina and myocardial infarction in Chapter 23.

NURSING CONSIDERATIONS

The role of the nurse in beta-blocker therapy involves careful monitoring of the client's condition and providing education as it relates to the prescribed drug regimen. Beta-blockers are contraindicated in clients with decompensated HF, chronic obstructive pulmonary disease (COPD), bradycardia, or heart block. Beta-blockers are also contraindicated in pregnant or lactating clients. These medications should be used with caution in clients with diabetes, peripheral vascular disease, and hepatic impairment. Caution is needed with elderly clients, who may need a reduced dose.

The nurse should monitor for worsening signs and symptoms of HF and for signs of hepatic toxicity. Liver function tests should be assessed periodically. Notify the healthcare provider if signs or symptoms of liver impairment become apparent.

Client education as it relates to beta-blockers should include goals, reasons for obtaining baseline data such as liver function tests, and possible side effects. Following are the important points to include when teaching clients regarding beta-blockers:

- Monitor blood pressure and pulse. Notify the healthcare provider if pulse is less than 50–60 beats/minute.

Pr PROTOTYPE DRUG | Carvedilol (Coreg)

ACTIONS AND USES

Carvedilol is the first beta-blocker approved for the treatment of HF. It has been found to reduce symptoms, slow the progression of the disease, and increase exercise tolerance when combined with other HF drugs such as the ACE inhibitors. Unlike many drugs in this class, carvedilol blocks beta$_1$- and beta$_2$- as well as alpha$_1$-adrenergic receptors. The primary therapeutic effects relevant to HF are a reduction in heart rate and a drop in blood pressure. The lower blood pressure decreases afterload and reduces the workload of the heart.

ADMINISTRATION ALERTS

- To minimize the risk of orthostatic hypotension, give drug with food to slow absorption.
- Carvedilol is pregnancy category C.

PHARMACOKINETICS

The bioavailability of carvedilol is 25% to 35% due to first-pass metabolism. It is 98% protein bound and is excreted mostly in bile and feces. Its half-life is 7 to 10 hours.

ADVERSE EFFECTS AND INTERACTIONS

The ability of carvedilol to decrease the heart rate combined with its ability to reduce contractility has the potential to worsen HF; thus, dosage must be carefully monitored. Because of the potential for adverse cardiac effects, beta-blockers such as carvedilol are not considered first-line drugs alone in the treatment of HF.

Carvedilol interacts with many drugs. For example, levels of carvedilol are significantly increased when taken concurrently with rifampin. MAO inhibitors, clonidine, and reserpine can cause hypotension or bradycardia when given with carvedilol. When given with digoxin, carvedilol may increase digoxin levels. It may also enhance the hypoglycemic effects of insulin and oral hypoglycemic agents.

- Report immediately signs and symptoms of worsening HF, such as shortness of breath, edema of feet and ankles, and chest pain.
- Do not stop taking the drug abruptly without consulting with the healthcare provider.
- Diabetic clients should monitor serum glucose carefully because these drugs may cause changes in blood sugar levels.
- Report significant side effects such as fainting, difficulty breathing, weight gain, and slow, irregular heart rate.

See "Nursing Process Focus: Clients Receiving Beta-Adrenergic Antagonist Therapy" in Chapter 21 (page 269) for additional information.

VASODILATORS

Through their hypotensive effects, vasodilators play a minor role in the pharmacotherapy of HF. They are also used for hypertension and angina pectoris. Doses for the vasodilators are given in Table 24.1 on page 307.

24.5 Pharmacotherapy with Direct Vasodilators

The two drugs in this class, hydralazine and isosorbide dinitrate, act directly to relax blood vessels and lower blood pressure. Hydralazine acts on arterioles, while isosorbide dinitrate acts on veins. Because the two drugs act synergistically, isosorbide dinitrate is usually combined with hydralazine in the treatment of HF. Because of the high incidence of side effects, they are generally reserved for clients who cannot tolerate ACE inhibitors.

NURSING CONSIDERATIONS

The role of the nurse in the care of clients receiving drug therapy with hydralazine for the treatment of hypertension is discussed in Chapter 21 (see "Nursing Considerations" and "Nursing Process Focus: Clients Receiving Direct Vasodilator Therapy" on page 271). The use of isosorbide dinitrate for therapy of angina pectoris is presented in Chapter 23 (see "Nursing Considerations").

CARDIAC GLYCOSIDES

The cardiac glycosides were once used as arrow poisons by African tribes and as medicines by the ancient Egyptians and Romans. The value of the cardiac glycosides in treating heart disorders has been known for over 2000 years. The chemical classification draws its name from three sugars, or glycosides, which are attached to a steroid nucleus. Information on doses of the cardiac glycosides is provided in Table 24.1.

24.6 Pharmacotherapy with Cardiac Glycosides

Extracted from the flowering plants *Digitalis purpurea* (purple foxglove) and *Digitalis lanata* (woolly foxglove), drugs in this class are also called digitalis glycosides. Cardiac glycosides were once the mainstay of HF treatment. Currently, they are reserved for use in clients whose symptoms persist despite first-line therapy with other drugs. The cardiac glycosides cause the heart to beat more forcefully and more slowly, improving cardiac output. The two primary cardiac glycosides—digoxin and digitoxin—are quite similar in effi-

Pr **PROTOTYPE DRUG** | Isosorbide Dinitrate (Isordil, Coronex)

ACTIONS AND USES

Isosorbide dinitrate acts directly and selectively on veins to cause venodilation. This reduces venous return (preload), thus decreasing cardiac workload. The resultant improvement in cardiac output reduces pulmonary congestion and peripheral edema and improves exercise tolerance. Isosorbide dinitrate also dilates the coronary arteries to bring more oxygen to the myocardium. Isosorbide dinitrate belongs to a class of drugs called organic nitrates that are widely used in the treatment of angina.

PHARMACOKINETICS

Isosorbide dinitrate is well absorbed and mostly metabolized by the liver. Its half-life is 50 minutes.

ADMINISTRATION ALERTS

- Do not confuse this drug with isosorbide (Ismotic), which is an oral osmotic diuretic.
- If administered sublingually, advise client not to eat, drink, talk, or smoke while tablet is dissolving.
- Isosorbide dinitrate is pregnancy category C.

ADVERSE EFFECTS AND INTERACTIONS

Common side effects of isosorbide dinitrate include headache and reflex tachycardia. Orthostatic hypotension may cause dizziness and falling, particularly in older adults. Use is contraindicated if the client is also taking sildenafil (Viagra) because serious hypotension may result.

 See the Companion Website for a Nursing Process Focus Chart specific to this drug.

cacy; the primary difference is that the latter has a more prolonged half-life.

The margin of safety between a therapeutic dose and a toxic dose of digitalis is quite narrow, and severe adverse effects may result from unmonitored treatment. Digitalization refers to a procedure in which the dose of cardiac glycoside is gradually increased until tissues become saturated with the drug and the symptoms of HF diminish. If the client is critically ill, digitalization can be accomplished rapidly with IV doses in a controlled clinical environment where side adverse effects are carefully monitored. For outpatients, digitalization with digoxin may occur over a period of 7 days, using oral dosing. In either case, the goal is to determine the proper dose of drug that may be administered without undue adverse effects.

NURSING CONSIDERATIONS

The role of the nurse in cardiac glycoside therapy involves careful monitoring of the client's condition and providing education as it relates to the prescribed drug regimen. Prior to beginning therapy with cardiac glycosides, the client should be evaluated for ventricular dysrhythmias not caused by HF and for any history of hypersensitivity to cardiac glycosides. Renal function should be assessed because the drug is excreted by the kidneys. Administer these drugs with caution in elderly clients; those with acute myocardial infarction, incomplete heart block, and renal insufficiency; and in pregnant or lactating clients.

Side effects that the nurse must monitor for when caring for clients taking these drugs include fatigue, drowsiness, dizziness, visual disturbances, anorexia, nausea, and vomiting. Advise clients to carry or wear identification describing their medical diagnosis and drug regimen. Instruct clients to eat potassium-rich foods as hypokalemia may predispose the client to digoxin toxicity. Antacids and antidiarrheal medications should not be taken within 2 hours of cardiac

glycoside administration because they decrease the absorption of digoxin.

It is common for dysrhythmias to occur when high doses of digoxin are administered. The nurse should be prepared to administer digoxin immune Fab (Digibind) in the case of life-threatening dysrhythmia. This drug binds and subsequently removes digoxin from the body and prevents toxic effects of overdose.

See "Nursing Process Focus: Clients Receiving Cardiac Glycoside Therapy" for specific teaching points.

DIURETICS

Diuretics increase urine flow, thereby reducing blood volume and cardiac workload. They are widely used in the treatment of cardiovascular disease. Select diuretics are shown in Table 24.1 on page 307.

NATURAL THERAPIES

Hawthorn for Heart Failure

Hawthorn (sometimes spelled hawthorne) is a bush found throughout the United States, Canada, Europe, and Asia. This plant is readily available and may be used to treat symptoms of HF. Research supports its use in HF. In a meta-analysis of randomized clinical trials, it was concluded that there is a significant benefit from hawthorn extract as an adjunctive treatment for chronic HF (Pittler et al., 2003). Its cardiovascular effects are believed to be due to its antioxidant flavonoid components, which increase the integrity of the blood vessel walls, improve coronary blood flow, and increase oxygen utilization (Chang et al., 2005).

Reported adverse effects include nausea, vomiting, and dizziness. Because hawthorn is effective at reducing blood pressure, this vital sign must be monitored. Clients who are concurrently taking an antihypertensive medication should especially be aware of this side effect.

Concurrent use with digoxin may be a concern. However, one interaction study showed that at dosages of 0.25 mg of digoxin per day and 450 mg of hawthorn twice daily, hawthorn did not significantly alter the pharmacokinetic parameters of digoxin (Tankanow et al., 2003).

MediaLink

Mechanism of Action: Digoxin

Pr PROTOTYPE DRUG | Digoxin (Lanoxin)

ACTIONS AND USES

The primary benefit of digoxin is its ability to increase the contractility of myocardial contraction—a positive inotropic action. Digoxin accomplishes this by inhibiting Na^+, K^+-ATPase, the critical enzyme responsible for pumping sodium ion out of the myocardial cell in exchange for potassium ion. As sodium accumulates, calcium ions are released from their storage areas in the cell. The release of calcium ion produces a more forceful contraction of the myocardial fibres.

By increasing myocardial contractility, digoxin directly increases cardiac output, thus alleviating symptoms of HF and improving exercise tolerance. The improved cardiac output results in increased urine production and a desirable reduction in blood volume, relieving the distressing symptoms of pulmonary congestion and peripheral edema.

In addition to its positive inotropic effect, digoxin also affects impulse conduction in the heart. Digoxin has the ability to suppress the sinoatrial (SA) node and slow electrical conduction through the atrioventricular (AV) node. Because of these actions, digoxin is sometimes used to treat dysrhythmias, as discussed in Chapter 25.

PHARMACOKINETICS

Digoxin taken orally has 60% to 80% bioavailability and peaks in 2 to 8 hours. It is widely distributed and excreted almost completely unchanged by the kidneys. It has a half-life of 36 to 48 hours.

ADMINISTRATION ALERTS

- Take the client's apical pulse for 1 full minute, noting rate, rhythm, and quality before administering. If pulse is below 60 beats/minute, the drug is usually withheld and the healthcare provider notified.
- Check for recent serum digoxin level results before administering. If level is higher than 1.8, withhold dose and notify healthcare provider.
- Digoxin is pregnancy category C.

ADVERSE EFFECTS AND INTERACTIONS

The most dangerous adverse effect of digoxin is its ability to create dysrhythmias, particularly in clients who have low potassium levels in the blood (hypokalemia). Because diuretics can cause hypokalemia and may also be used to treat HF, concurrent use of digoxin and diuretics must be carefully monitored. Other adverse effects of digoxin therapy include nausea, vomiting, anorexia, fatigue, and visual disturbances such as seeing halos, a yellow/green tinge, or blurring. Periodic serum drug levels should be obtained to determine if the digoxin level is within the therapeutic range, so the dosage may be adjusted based on the laboratory results. Because a small increase in digoxin levels can produce serious adverse effects, the nurse must constantly be on the alert for drug-drug interactions and for changes in renal function.

Digoxin interacts with a number of drugs. Antacids and cholesterol-lowering drugs can decrease absorption of digoxin. If calcium is administered IV together with digoxin, it can increase the risk of dysrhythmias. When the client is also receiving quinidine, verapamil, or flecainide, digoxin levels will be significantly increased, and the digoxin dose should be decreased by 50%.

Use with caution with herbal supplements, such as ginseng, which may increase the risk of digoxin toxicity. Ma huang and ephedra may induce dysrhythmias. Clients on cardiac glycosides should be strongly advised not to take any other prescription or OTC medication or herbal product without notifying the healthcare provider.

 See the Companion Website for a Nursing Process Focus Chart specific to this drug.

NURSING PROCESS FOCUS   Clients Receiving Cardiac Glycoside Therapy

Assessment	Potential Nursing Diagnoses/Identified Patterns
Prior to administration: - Obtain complete health history including allergies, drug history, and possible drug interactions. - Assess vital signs, urinary output, and cardiac output, initially and throughout therapy. - Determine the reason the medication is being administered.	- Need for knowledge regarding drug therapy and lifestyle modifications - Need for knowledge related to dietary and drug regimen - Risk for fluid excess and electrolyte imbalance - Ineffective tissue perfusion related to decreased cardiac output - Risk for injury related to decreased cardiac function - Risk for falls related to drug side effects

Planning: Client Goals and Expected Outcomes

The client will:
- Report decreased symptoms of cardiac decompensation related to fluid overload
- Exhibit evidence of improved organ perfusion, including kidney, heart, and brain
- Demonstrate an understanding of the drug's action by accurately describing drug side effects and precautions
- Immediately report side effects such as nausea, vomiting, diarrhea, heart rate below 50, and vision changes

continued

Implementation

Interventions (Rationales)	Client Education/Discharge Planning
■ Monitor ECG for rate and rhythm changes during initial digitalization therapy. (Drug has a strong positive inotropic effect.)	Instruct client to: ■ Count pulse for 1 full minute and record pulse with every dose ■ Contact healthcare provider if pulse rate is less than 50 or greater than 100 (or as determined by local agency policies; some providers specify reporting pulse less than 60 and withholding the drug)
■ Observe for side effects such as nausea, vomiting, diarrhea, anorexia, shortness of breath, vision changes, and leg muscle cramps.	■ Instruct client to report side effects immediately to prevent toxicity.
■ Weigh client daily.	■ Instruct client to report weight gain of 1 kg or more per day.
■ Administer precise ordered dose at same time each day. (Overdose may cause serious toxicity.)	Instruct client to: ■ Take as directed; do not double dose ■ Not discontinue drug without advice of healthcare provider
■ Monitor serum drug level (to determine therapeutic concentration and toxicity). ■ Report serum drug levels greater than 1.8 ng/mL to healthcare provider.	■ Instruct client to report to laboratory as scheduled by healthcare provider for ongoing drug level determinations.
■ Monitor levels of potassium, magnesium, calcium, BUN, and creatinine. (Hypokalemia predisposes the client to digoxin toxicity.)	■ Instruct client to consume foods high in potassium such as bananas, apricots, kidney beans, sweet potatoes, and peanut butter.
■ Monitor for signs and symptoms of digoxin toxicity.	■ Instruct client to immediately report visual changes, mental depression, palpitations, weakness, loss of appetite, vomiting, and diarrhea.

Evaluation of Outcome Criteria

Evaluate the effectiveness of drug therapy by confirming that client goals and expected outcomes have been met (see "Planning").

See Table 24.1 (page 307) under "Cardiac Glycosides," for a list of drugs to which these nursing actions apply.

24.7 Pharmacotherapy with Diuretics

Diuretics are common drugs for the treatment of clients with HF because they produce few adverse effects and are effective at reducing blood volume, edema, and pulmonary congestion. As diuretics reduce fluid volume and lower blood pressure, the workload of the heart is reduced and cardiac output increases. Diuretics are rarely used alone but are prescribed in combination with ACE inhibitors or other HF drugs.

The mechanism by which diuretics reduce blood volume, specifically where and how the nephron is affected, differs among the various drugs. Differences in mechanisms among the classes of diuretics are discussed in Chapter 43. The role of the thiazide diuretics in the treatment of hypertension is discussed in Chapter 21.

NURSING CONSIDERATIONS

The role of the nurse in diuretic therapy for HF involves careful monitoring of the client's condition and providing education as it relates to the prescribed drug regimen. Prior to initiation of diuretic therapy, the client should be questioned about past history of kidney disease. Diuretics are contraindicated in pregnancy and lactation and in clients with renal dysfunction, fluid and electrolyte depletion, and

hepatic coma. Diuretics should be used cautiously in clients with hepatic cirrhosis or nephritic syndrome and in infants and older adults.

Potassium levels should be monitored closely since nonpotassium-sparing diuretics cause hypokalemia with diuresis. Closely observe older clients for weakness, hypotension, and confusion. Monitor for electrolyte imbalance, elevated BUN, hyperglycemia, and anemia, which can all be side effects of diuretics. Monitor vital signs and carefully monitor intake and output to establish effectiveness of the medication. Rapid and excessive diuresis can result in dehydration, hypovolemia, and circulatory collapse.

Client education as it relates to diuretics should include goals, reasons for obtaining baseline data such as vital signs and tests for renal function, and possible side effects. Following are important points to include when teaching clients about diuretics:

- Monitor total sodium intake daily. The recommended daily intake should be no more than 4000 mg/day.
- Report weight loss of more than 1 kg a week.
- Report fatigue and muscle cramping.
- Change positions slowly because diuretics in combination with other drugs can cause dizziness.

See "Nursing Process Focus: Clients Receiving Diuretic Therapy" in Chapter 21 on page 258 for additional information.

Pr PROTOTYPE DRUG | Furosemide (Lasix)

ACTIONS AND USES

Furosemide is often used in the treatment of acute HF because it has the ability to remove large amounts of edematous fluid from the client in a short period of time. When given IV, diuresis begins within 5 minutes. Clients often experience quick relief from their distressing symptoms. Furosemide acts by preventing the reabsorption of sodium and chloride, primarily in the loop of Henle region of the nephron. Compared to other diuretics, furosemide is particularly beneficial when cardiac output and renal flow are severely diminished.

PHARMACOKINETICS

Furosemide given orally is 60% to 75% bioavailable and 91% to 97% protein bound. It is partly metabolized by the liver and is excreted by the kidneys. It has a half-life of 0.5 to 1 hour.

ADMINISTRATION ALERTS

- Check client's serum potassium levels before administering drug. If potassium levels are falling or are below normal, notify physician before administering.
- Furosemide is pregnancy category C.

ADVERSE EFFECTS AND INTERACTIONS

Side effects of furosemide, like those of most diuretics, involve potential electrolyte imbalances, the most important of which is hypokalemia. Because hypokalemia may cause dysrhythmias in clients taking cardiac glycosides, combination therapy with furosemide and digoxin must be carefully monitored. Because furosemide is so efficacious, fluid loss must be carefully monitored to avoid possible dehydration and hypotension.

When furosemide is given with corticosteroids and amphotericin B, it can potentiate hypokalemia. When given with lithium, elimination of lithium is decreased, causing higher risk of toxicity. When given with sulfonylureas and insulin, furosemide may diminish their hypoglycemic effects.

 See the Companion Website for a Nursing Process Focus Chart specific to this drug.

PHOSPHODIESTERASE INHIBITORS

Phosphodiesterase inhibitors became available in the 1980s. They have a short half-life and are used for the short-term control of acute HF. The dose of milrinone, the prototype, is shown in Table 24.1 on page 307.

24.8 Pharmacotherapy with Phosphodiesterase Inhibitors

Phosphodiesterase inhibitors block the enzyme **phosphodiesterase** in cardiac and smooth muscle. Blocking phosphodiesterase has the effect of increasing the amount of calcium available for myocardial contraction. The inhibition results in two main actions that benefit clients with HF: a positive inotropic response and vasodilation. Cardiac output is increased due to the increase in contractility and the decrease in left ventricular afterload. Due to their toxicity, phosphodiesterase inhibitors are normally reserved for clients who have not responded to ACE inhibitors or cardiac glycosides, and they are generally used only for 2 to 3 days.

NURSING CONSIDERATIONS

The role of the nurse in drug therapy with phosphodiesterase inhibitors involves careful monitoring of the client's condition and providing education as it relates to the prescribed drug regimen. Prior to administration of phosphodiesterase inhibitors, assess potassium levels. If hypokalemia is present, it should be corrected before administering these drugs. Evaluate the client for history of renal impairment and dysrhythmias. Baseline vital signs should be obtained, especially blood pressure, because these drugs can cause hypotension. During IV administration,

the client should be continuously monitored for ventricular dysrhythmias such as ectopic beats, supraventricular dysrhythmias, preventricular contractions (PVCs), ventricular tachycardia, and ventricular fibrillation. If ordered for elderly, pregnant, or pediatric clients, the healthcare provider should be consulted as safety has not been established in these populations or conditions.

Client education as it relates to phosphodiesterase inhibitors should include goals, reasons for obtaining baseline data such as vital signs and tests for cardiac and renal function, and possible side effects. Following are the important points to include when teaching clients about phosphodiesterase inhibitors:

- Report the following immediately: irregular, fast heartbeat; pain or swelling at infusion site; and fever of 38.3°C or higher.
- Report immediately any increase in chest pain that might indicate angina.

SPECIAL CONSIDERATIONS

Psychosocial Issues and Adherence in Clients with HF

Clients with depression and lack of social support who have HF have been shown to be less compliant with their drug therapy regimen. When clients can no longer maintain what they consider an acceptable lifestyle, they may become depressed. Clients are less likely to adhere to lifestyle modifications when depressed. Their choices may place their health and safety at risk. Reduced sexual desire and performance problems are frequently related to side effects of drug therapy and may reduce adherence to drug therapy. Clients may weigh the side effects against the drug's benefits and determine that the risks outweigh the benefits. Assess these issues in all clients with HF. Clients may be referred to cardiac rehabilitation programs, which have been shown to increase adherence.

Pr PROTOTYPE DRUG | Milrinone (Apo-Milrinone)

ACTIONS AND USES

Milrinone is primarily used for the short-term support of advanced HF. It is only given intravenously. Peak effects occur in 2 minutes. Immediate effects of milrinone include an increased force of myocardial contraction and an increase in cardiac output.

PHARMACOKINETICS

Its half-life is 2.3 hours.

ADMINISTRATION ALERTS

- When administering this medication IV, a microdrip set and an infusion pump should be used.
- Milrinone is pregnancy category C.

ADVERSE EFFECTS AND INTERACTIONS

The most serious side effect of milrinone is ventricular dysrhythmia, which may occur in at least 1 of every 10 clients taking the drug. The client's ECG is usually monitored continuously during infusion of the drug. Milrinone interacts with disopyramide, causing excessive hypotension.

In 2001, nesiritide (Natrecor) was approved for treatment of HF. Nesiritide is a small peptide hormone produced through recombinant DNA technology that is structurally identical to endogenous human beta-type natriuretic peptide (hBNP).

When HF occurs, the ventricles begin to secrete hBNP in response to the increased stretch of the ventricular walls. This results in diuresis and renal excretion of sodium and decreased preload. In therapeutic doses, exogenous hBNP also causes vasodilation and afterload. By reducing preload and afterload, hBNP reduces cardiac workload.

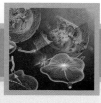

CHAPTER REVIEW

KEY CONCEPTS

The numbered key concepts provide a succinct summary of the important points from the corresponding numbered section within the chapter. If any of these points are not clear, refer to the numbered section within the chapter for review. Expanded versions can be found on the Companion Website.

24.1 The central cause of HF is weakened heart muscle. Diminished contractility reduces cardiac output.

24.2 The three primary characteristics of heart function are force of contraction, heart rate, and speed of impulse conduction.

24.3 ACE inhibitors improve HF by reducing peripheral edema and increasing cardiac output. They are first-line drugs for the treatment of HF.

24.4 Beta-adrenergic blockers play a role in the treatment of HF by slowing the heart rate and decreasing blood pressure. They are used in combination with ACE inhibitors as first-line drugs for HF.

24.5 Vasodilators can help reduce symptoms of HF by reducing preload and decreasing the oxygen demand of the heart.

24.6 Cardiac glycosides increase the force of myocardial contraction and are the traditional drugs of choice for HF. Due to a low safety margin, their use has declined.

24.7 Diuretics relieve symptoms of HF by reducing fluid volume and decreasing blood pressure.

24.8 Phosphodiesterase inhibitors increase the force of contraction and cause vasodilation. They are highly toxic and reserved for acute situations.

24.9 A peptide hormone agent may be used for treatment of heart failure.

REVIEW QUESTIONS

1 How can the Frank-Starling law be used to explain the beneficial effects of the cardiac glycosides in treating heart failure?

2 Why are the ACE inhibitors preferred over both the nitrates and the diuretics in the treatment of heart failure?

3 What is the most dangerous adverse effect of digoxin?

CRITICAL THINKING QUESTIONS

1. A client is newly diagnosed with mild heart failure. The client has been started on digoxin (Lanoxin). What objective evidence would indicate that this drug has been effective?

2. A 69-year-old client has a sudden onset of acute pulmonary edema. The client has no past cardiac history, is allergic to sulfa antibiotics, and routinely takes no medications. The healthcare provider orders furosemide (Lasix) to relieve the pulmonary congestion. What interventions are essential in the care of this client?

3. A client who is diabetic and hypertensive is started on carvedilol (Coreg) for mild heart failure. What teaching is important for this client?

EXPLORE
MediaLink

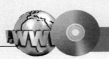

www.pearsoned.ca/adams-king

MEDIALINK DVD-ROM
- **Audio Glossary**
- **CRNE Review**
- **Animations**
  Mechanism of Action: Digoxin
  Mechanism of Action: Furosemide

COMPANION WEBSITE
- **CRNE Review**
- **Case Study:** Client taking cardiac glycosides
- **Dosage Calculations**
- **Nursing Process Focus Charts**

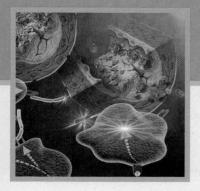

CHAPTER 25

Drugs for Dysrhythmias

DRUGS AT A GLANCE

SODIUM CHANNEL BLOCKERS
  procainamide
    (Apo-Procainamide, Pronestyl)

BETA-ADRENERGIC BLOCKERS
  propranolol (Inderal)

POTASSIUM CHANNEL BLOCKERS
  amiodarone (Cordarone)

CALCIUM CHANNEL BLOCKERS
  verapamil (Isoptin, others)

MISCELLANEOUS DRUGS

OBJECTIVES

After reading this chapter, the student should be able to do the following:

1. Identify drug classes used for treating dysrhythmias.
2. Explain the therapeutic action of each class of antidysrhythmic drug in relation to the pathophysiology of dysrhythmias.
3. Discuss the role of the nurse regarding non-pharmacological therapies for the treatment of dysrhythmias.
4. Describe the nurse's role in the pharmacological management of clients with dysrhythmias.
5. For each of the drug classes listed in Drugs at a Glance, identify a representative drug and explain its mechanism of action, therapeutic effects, and important adverse effects.
6. Describe and explain, based on pharmacological principles, the rationale for nursing assessment, planning, and interventions for clients with dysrhythmias.
7. Use the nursing process to care for clients receiving drug therapy for dysrhythmias.

MediaLink

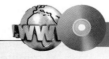

www.pearsonde.ca/adams-king

CRNE review, case studies, and other interactive resources for this chapter can be found on the Companion Website at **www.pearsoned.ca/adams-king**. Click on "Chapter 25" to select the activities for this chapter. For animations, more CRNE review questions, and an audio glossary, access the accompanying DVD-ROM in this textbook.

Dysrhythmias, sometimes called arrhythmias, encompass a number of different disorders that range from harmless to life-threatening. **Dysrhythmias** are abnormalities of electrical conduction that may result in disturbances in heart rate or cardiac rhythm. Diagnosis is often difficult because clients usually must be connected to an electrocardiograph (ECG) and be experiencing symptoms in order to determine the exact type of rhythm disorder. Proper diagnosis and optimum pharmacological treatment can significantly affect the frequency of dysrhythmias and their consequences.

LIFESPAN CONSIDERATIONS

Dysrhythmias

- A large majority of sudden cardiac deaths are thought to be caused by ventricular dysrhythmias.
- Atrial dysrhythmias occur more commonly in men than in women.
- The incidence of atrial dysrhythmias increases with age. They affect
  - Less than 0.5% of those aged 25 to 35.
  - 1.5% of those to age 60.
  - 9% of those over age 75.
- About 15% of strokes occur in clients with atrial dysrhythmias.
- Sudden cardiac death occurs three to four times more frequently in Blacks.
- Atrial fibrillation affects 0.6% of people in Canada.

Source: Statistics Canada; Humphries et al., 2004.

25.1 Frequency of Dysrhythmias in the Population

While some dysrhythmias produce no symptoms and have negligible effects on cardiac function, others are life-threatening and require immediate treatment. Typical symptoms include dizziness, weakness, decreased exercise tolerance, shortness of breath, and fainting. Many clients report palpitations or a sensation that their heart has skipped a beat. Persistent dysrhythmias are associated with increased risk of stroke and heart failure. Severe dysrhythmias may result in sudden death. Since asymptomatic clients may not seek medical attention, it is difficult to estimate the frequency of the disease, although it is likely that dysrhythmias are quite common in the population.

25.2 Classification of Dysrhythmias

Dysrhythmias are classified by a number of different methods. The simplest method is to name dysrhythmias according to the *type* of rhythm abnormality produced and its *location*. Dysrhythmias that originate in the atria are sometimes referred to as **supraventricular**. Those that originate in the ventricles are generally more serious as they more often interfere with the normal function of the heart. **Atrial fibrillation**, a complete disorganization of rhythm, is thought to be the most common type of dysrhythmia. A summary of common dysrhythmias with a brief description of each is given in Table 25.1. Although obtaining a correct diagnosis of the type of dysrhythmia is sometimes difficult, it is essential for effective treatment.

While the actual cause of most dysrhythmias is elusive, dysrhythmias are associated with certain conditions, primarily heart disease and myocardial infarction. The following are diseases and conditions associated with dysrhythmias:

- Hypertension
- Cardiac valve disease such as mitral stenosis
- Coronary artery disease

TABLE 25.1	Types of Dysrhythmia
Dysrhythmia	**Description**
premature atrial contractions or premature ventricular contractions (PVCs)	an extra beat often originating from a source other than the SA node; not normally serious unless it occurs at high frequency
atrial or ventricular tachycardia	rapid heart beat greater than 150 bpm; ventricular is more serious than atrial
atrial or ventricular flutter and/or fibrillation	very rapid, uncoordinated beats; atrial may require treatment but is not usually fatal; ventricular requires immediate treatment
sinus bradycardia	slow heart beat, less than 50 bpm; may require a pacemaker
heart block	area of non-conduction in the myocardium; may be partial or complete; classified as first, second, or third degree

- Medications such as digitalis
- Low potassium levels in the blood
- Myocardial infarction
- Stroke
- Diabetes mellitus
- Congestive heart failure

25.3 Conduction Pathways in the Myocardium

Although there are many types of dysrhythmia, all have in common a defect in the generation or conduction of electrical impulses across the myocardium. These electrical impulses, or **action potentials**, carry the signal for the cardiac muscle cells to contract and must be coordinated precisely for the chambers to beat in a synchronized manner. For the heart to function properly, the atria must contract simultaneously, sending their blood into the ventricles. Following atrial contraction, the right and left ventricles must contract simultaneously. Lack of synchronization of the atria and ventricles or of the right and left sides of the heart may have profound consequences. The total time for the electrical impulse to travel across the heart is about 0.22 seconds. The normal conduction pathway in the heart is illustrated in Figure 25.1.

Normal control of this synchronization begins in a small area of tissue in the wall of the right atrium known as the **sinoatrial (SA) node**. The SA node, or pacemaker, of the heart has a property called **automaticity**, which is the ability to spontaneously generate an action potential without direction from the nervous system. The SA node generates a new action potential approximately 75 times per minute under resting conditions. This is referred to as the normal **sinus rhythm**.

Upon leaving the SA node, the action potential travels quickly across both atria and then to the **atrioventricular (AV) node**. The AV node also has the property of automaticity, although less so than the SA node. Should the SA node malfunction, the AV node has the ability to spontaneously generate action potentials and continue the heart's contraction at a rate of 40 to 60 beats/minute (bpm). Compared to other areas in the heart, impulse conduction through the AV node is slow. This allows the atrial contraction to completely empty blood into the ventricles, thereby optimizing cardiac output.

As the action potential leaves the AV node, it travels rapidly to the **atrioventricular bundle**, or bundle of His. The impulse is then conducted down the right and left **bundle branches** to the **Purkinje fibres**, which carry the action potential to all regions of the ventricles almost simultaneously. Should the SA and AV nodes become nonfunctional, cells in the AV bundle and Purkinje fibres can continue to generate myocardial contractions at a rate of about 30 beats/minute.

Although action potentials normally begin in the SA node and spread across the myocardium in a coordinated manner, other regions of the heart may begin to initiate beats. These areas, known as **ectopic foci** or **ectopic pacemakers**, may begin to send impulses across the myocardium that compete with those from the normal conduction pathway, thereby affecting the normal flow of impulses. Ectopic foci have the potential to cause many of the types of dysrhythmias noted in Table 25.1.

It is important to understand that the underlying purpose of this conduction system is to keep the heart beating in a regular, synchronized manner so that cardiac output can be maintained. Some dysrhythmias occur sporadically, elicit no symptoms, and do not affect cardiac output.

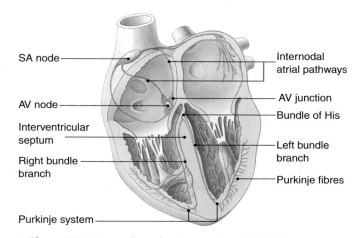

● **Figure 25.1** Normal conduction pathway in the heart
Source: Pearson Education/PH College.

MediaLink ✦ Childhood Dysrhythmias

Others, however, profoundly affect cardiac output, result in client symptoms, and have the potential to produce serious if not fatal consequences. It is these types of dysrhythmias that require pharmacological treatment.

25.4 The Electrocardiograph

The wave of electrical activity across the myocardium can be measured using the electrocardiograph. The graphic recording from this device is an **electrocardiogram (ECG)**, and it is useful in diagnosing many types of heart conditions, including dysrhythmias. An ECG may also be referred to as an EKG.

Three distinct waves are produced on a normal ECG: the P wave, the QRS complex, and the T wave. Changes to the wave patterns or their timing can reveal certain pathologies. For example, an exaggerated R wave suggests enlargement of the ventricles, and a flat T wave indicates ischemia to the myocardium. A normal ECG and its relationship to impulse conduction in the heart are shown in Figure 25.2.

25.5 Sodium, Potassium, and the Myocardial Action Potential

Because most antidysrhythmic drugs act by interfering with myocardial action potentials, a firm grasp of this phenomenon is necessary for understanding drug mechanisms. Action potentials occur in both nervous and cardiac muscle cells due to the changes in specific ions found inside and outside the cell. Under resting conditions, Na^+ and Ca^{+2} are found in higher concentrations *outside* myocardial cells, while K^+ is found in higher concentration *within* these cells. These imbalances are, in part, responsible for the inside of a myocardial cell membrane having a slight negative charge (80 to 90 mV), relative to the outside of the membrane. A cell having this negative membrane potential is said to be **polarized.**

An action potential begins when **sodium ion channels** located in the plasma membrane open and Na^+ rushes into the cell to produce a rapid **depolarization**, or loss of membrane potential. During this period, Ca^{+2} also enters the cell

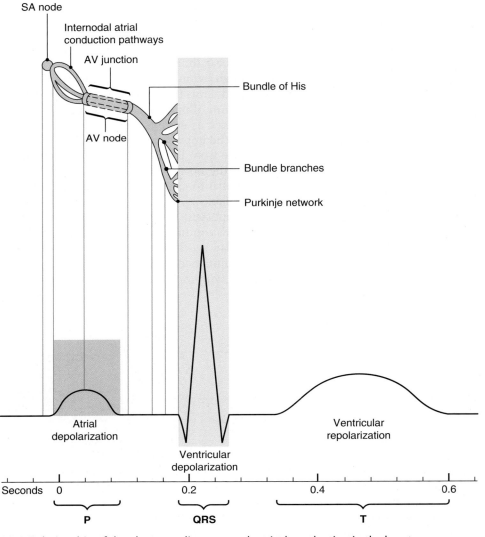

● **Figure 25.2** Relationship of the electrocardiogram to electrical conduction in the heart

Source: Pearson Education/PH College.

through **calcium ion channels**, although the influx is slower than that of sodium. The entry of Ca^{+2} into the cells is a signal for the release of additional calcium that had been held in storage inside the sarcoplasmic reticulum. It is this large increase in intracellular Ca^{+2} that is responsible for the contraction of cardiac muscle.

During depolarization, the inside of the cell membrane temporarily reverses its charge, becoming positive. The cell returns to its polarized state by the removal of K^+ through **potassium ion channels**. In cells located in the SA and AV nodes, it is the influx of Ca^{+2} rather than Na^+ that generates the rapid depolarization of the membrane. Blocking potassium, sodium, or calcium ion channels is a pharmacological strategy used to terminate or prevent dysrhythmias. Figure 25.3 illustrates the flow of ions occurring during the action potential.

During depolarization and most of repolarization, the cell cannot initiate another action potential. This time, known as the **refractory period**, ensures that the action potential finishes and the muscle cell contracts before a second action potential begins. The therapeutic effect of some antidysrhythmic agents is due to their prolongation of the refractory period.

25.6 Non-Pharmacological Therapy of Dysrhythmias

The therapeutic goals of antidysrhythmic pharmacotherapy are to terminate existing dysrhythmias and to prevent abnormal rhythms to reduce the risk of sudden death, stroke, and other complications resulting from the disorder. Because of their potential to cause serious side effects, antidysrhythmic drugs are normally reserved for those clients experiencing overt symptoms or for those whose condition cannot be controlled by other means. There is little or no benefit to the client in treating asymptomatic dysrhythmias with medication. Healthcare providers use several non-pharmacological strategies to eliminate dysrhythmias.

The more serious types of dysrhythmia are corrected through electrical shock of the heart, with treatments such as elective **cardioversion** and **defibrillation**. The electrical shock momentarily stops all electrical impulses in the heart, both normal and abnormal. Under ideal conditions, the temporary cessation of electrical activity will allow the SA node to automatically return conduction to a normal sinus rhythm.

Other types of non-pharmacological treatment include identification and destruction of the myocardial cells

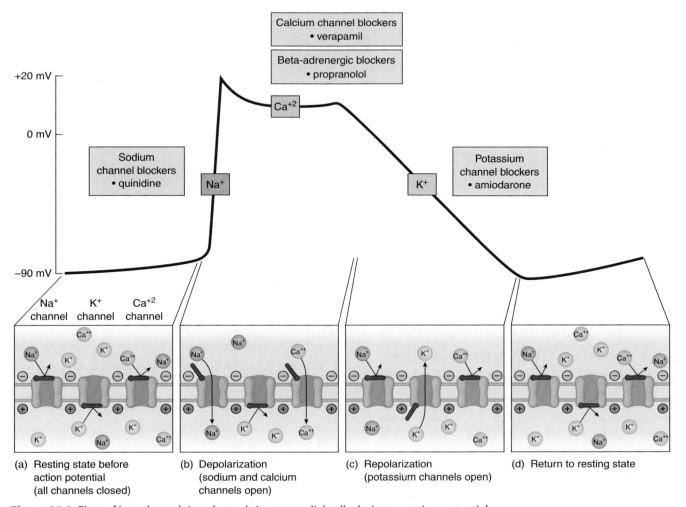

(a) Resting state before action potential (all channels closed)

(b) Depolarization (sodium and calcium channels open)

(c) Repolarization (potassium channels open)

(d) Return to resting state

● **Figure 25.3** Flow of ions through ion channels in myocardial cells during an action potential

responsible for the abnormal conduction through a surgical procedure called catheter ablation. Cardiac pacemakers are sometimes inserted to correct the types of dysrhythmia that cause the heart to beat too slowly. Implantable cardioverter defibrillators (ICDs) are placed in clients to restore normal rhythm by either pacing the heart or giving it an electric shock when dysrhythmias occur. In addition, the ICD is capable of storing information regarding the heart rhythm for the healthcare provider to evaluate.

25.7 Mechanisms and Classification of Antidysrhythmic Drugs

Antidysrhythmic drugs act by altering electrophysiological properties of the heart. They do this in two basic ways: blocking ion flow through ion channels or altering autonomic activity.

Antidysrhythmic drugs are grouped according to the stage in which they affect the action potential. These drugs fall into four primary classes, referred to as I, II, III, and IV, and a fifth group that includes miscellaneous drugs not acting by one of the other four mechanisms. The phases of the action potential at which antidysrhythmic drugs act are shown in Figure 25.3. Categories of antidysrhythmics include the following:

1. Sodium channel blockers (class I)
2. Beta-adrenergic blockers (class II)
3. Potassium channel blockers (class III)
4. Calcium channel blockers (class IV)
5. Miscellaneous antidysrhythmic drugs

Drugs that affect cardiac electrophysiology have a narrow margin between a therapeutic effect and a toxic effect. They not only have the ability to correct dysrhythmias, but also to worsen or even create new dysrhythmias. The nurse must carefully monitor clients taking antidysrhythmic drugs. Often, the client is hospitalized during the initial stages of therapy so that the optimum dose can be accurately determined.

SODIUM CHANNEL BLOCKERS (CLASS I)

The first medical uses of the sodium channel blockers were recorded in the 18th century. This is the largest class of antidysrhythmics, and many are still widely prescribed. The sodium channel blockers are shown in Table 25.2.

25.8 Treating Dysrhythmias with Sodium Channel Blockers

Sodium channel blockers, the class I drugs, are divided into three subgroups, IA, IB, and IC, based on subtle differences in their mechanism of action. Since progression of the action potential is dependent on the opening of sodium ion channels, a blockade of these channels will prevent depolarization. The spread of the action potential across the myocardium will slow, and areas of ectopic pacemaker activity will be suppressed.

NURSING CONSIDERATIONS

The role of the nurse in sodium channel blocker therapy is included in "Nursing Process Focus: Clients Receiving Antidysrhythmic Therapies" on page 327. Additional nursing considerations will vary depending on the drug used.

Because class I antidysrhythmics have profound effects on the heart, a complete health history and physical examination should be obtained before initiating therapy, including baseline ECG, vital signs, hepatic and urinary function tests, and electrolyte values. Assess for heart failure, hypotension, myasthenia gravis, and renal or hepatic impairment as these are contraindicated in class I antidysrhythmic therapy. A thorough drug history should be obtained because these agents interact with a large number of other drugs, including cardiac glycosides, cimetidine, anticonvulsants, nifedipine, and warfarin.

During pharmacotherapy, monitor the client for changes in the ECG such as an increase in PR and QT intervals and widening of the QRS complex. Blood pressure should be monitored frequently as some agents can cause hypotension. Some drugs in this class can cause arterial embolism. This adverse effect is related to the formation of small blood clots in the atrium that occur while the client is being treated for atrial fibrillation. For this reason, current research and 2007 Canadian Consensus Conference guidelines for heart failure and associated atrial fibrillation support the use of anticoagulant (e.g., warfarin) therapy to prevent stroke in clients with atrial fibrillation. Nurses should monitor the client for changes in level of consciousness and respiratory status and report these to the physician immediately.

Monitor drug plasma levels during therapy. Also, the client should be monitored for diarrhea, which occurs in approximately one-third of clients on quinidine. This adverse effect is due to the fact that quinidine is chemically related to quinine in structure and action. Because diarrhea may be intense, implement appropriate interventions related to the diarrhea to maintain fluid and electrolyte balance.

Client education as it relates to sodium channel blockers should include goals, reasons for obtaining baseline data such as vital signs and tests for cardiac and renal function, and possible side effects. Include the following points when teaching clients regarding sodium channel blockers:

- Do not skip doses of the medication, even if feeling well. Do not take two doses at a time if the first dose is missed.
- Avoid the use of alcohol, caffeine, and tobacco.
- Comply with monitoring of lab tests as ordered.
- Report the following symptoms immediately: shortness of breath, signs of bleeding, excessive bruising, fever, nausea, persistent headache, changes to vision or hearing, diarrhea, or dizziness.

BETA-ADRENERGIC BLOCKERS (CLASS II)

Beta-adrenergic blockers are widely used for cardiovascular disorders. Their ability to slow the heart rate and conduction velocity can suppress several types of dysrhythmia. The beta-blockers are shown in Table 25.2.

TABLE 25.2   Antidysrhythmic Drugs

Drug	Route and Adult Dose
Class 1A: Sodium Channel Blockers	
disopyramide phosphate (Rythmodan)	PO; 100–200 mg qid (max 800 mg/day)
procainamide (Apo-Procainamide, Pronestyl)	PO; 1 g loading dose followed by 250–500 mg every 3 hours
quinidine gluconate (Apo-Quin-G)	PO; 200–600 mg tid or qid (max 3–4 g/day)
quinidine polygalacturonate (Cardioquin)	PO; 275–825 mg q3–4h for four or more doses until dysrhythmia terminates, then 137.5–275 mg bid or tid
quinidine sulfate (Biquin Durules)	PO; 200–600 mg tid or qid (max 3–4 g/day)
Class 1B: Sodium Channel Blockers	
lidocaine (Xylocaine) (see page 239 for the Prototype Drug box)	IV; 1–4 mg/min infusion; no more than 200–300 mg should be infused in a 1-hour period
mexiletine (Novo-Mexiletine)	PO; 200–300 mg tid (max 1200 mg/day)
phenytoin (Dilantin) (see page 164 for the Prototype Drug box)	IV; 50–100 mg every 10–15 min until dysrhythmia is terminated (max 1 g/day)
Class 1C: Sodium Channel Blockers	
flecainide (Tambocor)	PO; 50–100 mg bid; increase by 500 mg bid every 4 days (max 400 mg/day)
propafenone (Rythmol)	PO; 150–300 mg tid (max 900 mg/day)
Class II: Beta-Blockers	
acebutolol (Monitan, Sectral)	PO; 200–600 mg bid (max 1200 mg/day)
esmolol (Brevibloc)	IV; 50 µg/kg/min maintenance dose (max 200 µg/kg/min)
propranolol (Inderal)	PO; 10–30 mg tid or qid (max 320 mg/day); IV; 0.5–3.1 mg q4h or prn
Class III: Potassium Channel Blockers	
amiodarone (Cordarone)	PO; 400–600 mg/day in one to two divided doses (max 1600 mg/day as loading dose)
sotalol (Rylosol)	PO; 80 mg bid (max 320 mg/day)
Class IV: Calcium Channel Blockers	
diltiazem (Cardizem, others) (see page 296 for the Prototype Drug box)	IV; 5–10 mg/hr continuous infusion (max 15 mg/hr) for a maximum of 24h
verapamil (Isoptin, others)	PO; 240–480 mg/d in divided doses IV direct; 5–10 mg; may repeat in 15–30 min if needed
Miscellaneous Antidysrhythmics	
adenosine (Adenocard, Adenoscan)	IV; 6–12 mg given as a bolus injection
digoxin (Lanoxin) (see page 312 for the Prototype Drug box)	PO; 0.125–0.5 mg qid
ibutilide (Corvert)	IV; 1 mg infused over 10 min

25.9 Treating Dysrhythmias with Beta-Adrenergic Blockers

Beta-blockers are used to treat a large number of cardiovascular diseases, including hypertension, MI, heart failure, and dysrhythmias. Because of potentially serious side effects, however, only a few beta-blockers are approved to treat dysrhythmias. Beta-blockers slow the heart rate (negative chronotropic effect) and decrease conduction velocity through the AV node. Myocardial automaticity is reduced, and many types of dysrhythmias are stabilized. The main value of beta-blockers as antidysrhythmic agents is to treat atrial dysrhythmias associated with heart failure. Abrupt discontinuation of beta-blockers can lead to dysrhythmias

and hypertension. The basic pharmacology of beta-adrenergic blockers is explained in Chapter 13.

NURSING CONSIDERATIONS

The role of the nurse caring for clients receiving beta-adrenergic antagonists for dysrhythmias is included in "Nursing Process Focus: Clients Receiving Antidysrhythmic Therapies" in this chapter. For additional nursing considerations, refer to "Nursing Process Focus: Clients Receiving Beta-Adrenergic Antagonist Therapy" in Chapter 21.

All drugs in this class are contraindicated in clients with heart block, severe bradycardia, AV block, and asthma. The action of beta-blockers is to decrease the contractions of the

Pr PROTOTYPE DRUG | Procainamide (Apo-Procainamide, Pronestyl)

ACTIONS AND USES

Procainamide blocks sodium ion channels in myocardial cells, thus reducing automaticity and slowing conduction of the action potential across the myocardium. This slight delay in conduction velocity prolongs the refractory period and can suppress dysrhythmias. Procainamide is referred to as a broad-spectrum drug because it has the ability to correct many different types of atrial and ventricular dysrhythmia. Procainamide is available in capsule, extended-release tablet, IV, and IM formulations. The therapeutic serum drug level is 4 to 8 µg/mL.

PHARMACOKINETICS

Procainamide is well absorbed and is 75% to 90% protein bound. It is mostly metabolized by the liver and excreted by the kidneys. It has a half-life of 3 hours.

ADMINISTRATION ALERTS

- The supine position should be used during IV administration because severe hypotension may occur.
- Do not break or crush extended-release tablets
- Procainamide is pregnancy category C.

ADVERSE EFFECTS AND INTERACTIONS

Nausea, anorexia, diarrhea, hypotension, abdominal pain, and headache are common adverse effects. Like all antidysrhythmic drugs, procainamide has the ability to produce new dysrhythmias or worsen existing ones. A lupus-like syndrome may occur in 30% to 50% of clients taking the drug over a year. High doses may produce CNS effects such as confusion or psychosis. Hypotension due to overdosage may be treated with vasopressors. Procainamide is contraindicated in clients with complete AV block, severe HF, blood dyscrasias, and myasthenia gravis.

---

myocardium and to lessen the speed of conduction through the AV node. This action predisposes clients with certain existing heart problems to experience a significant decrease in heart rate that may not be well tolerated. The most common adverse reaction to these drugs is hypotension.

Monitor elderly clients for cognitive dysfunction and depression, as well as hallucinations and psychosis, which are more likely with higher doses. These reactions appear to be related to the lipid solubility of this medication and its ability to cross the blood-brain barrier. Monitor for hypoglycemia. There is an increased incidence of hypoglycemia in clients with type 1 diabetes mellitus because beta-blockers may inhibit glycogenolysis.

Client education as it relates to beta-adrenergic blockers should include goals, reasons for obtaining baseline data such as vital signs and tests for cardiac and renal function, and possible side effects. Provide the following information when teaching clients about beta-adrenergic blockers:

- Take pulse prior to drug administration. Report pulse rate less than 50 to the healthcare provider.
- Slowly rise from a sitting or lying position to avoid dizziness.
- Report the following symptoms immediately: shortness of breath, feeling of skipping a heartbeat, painful or difficult urination, frequent nighttime urination,

Pr PROTOTYPE DRUG | Propranolol (Inderal)

ACTIONS AND USES

Propranolol is a non-selective beta-adrenergic blocker, affecting beta$_1$-receptors in the heart and beta$_2$-receptors in pulmonary and vascular smooth muscle. Propranolol reduces heart rate, slows conduction velocity, and lowers blood pressure. Propranolol is most effective against tachycardia caused by excessive sympathetic stimulation. It is approved to treat a wide variety of diseases, including hypertension, angina, and migraine headaches, and to prevent myocardial infarction.

ADMINISTRATION ALERTS

- Abrupt discontinuation may cause myocardial infarction, severe hypertension, and ventricular dysrhythmias because of a potential rebound effect.
- If pulse is less than 50 beats/minute (or as per agency policy), withhold the dose and notify the physician.
- Propranolol is pregnancy category C.

PHARMACOKINETICS

Propranolol undergoes extensive first-pass metabolism and is 93% protein bound. It is almost completely metabolized by the liver. Its onset of action is 30 minutes, and the half-life is 3 to 6 hours.

ADVERSE EFFECTS AND INTERACTIONS

Common side effects of propranolol include fatigue, hypotension, and bradycardia. Because of its ability to slow the heart rate, clients with other cardiac disorders such as heart failure must be carefully monitored. Side effects such as diminished libido and impotence may result in non-adherence in male clients.

Propranolol interacts with many other drugs, including phenothiazines, which have additive hypotensive effects. Propranolol should not be given within 2 weeks of an MAO inhibitor. Beta-adrenergic agonists such as albuterol antagonize the actions of propranolol.

Intravenous glucagon reverses the cardiac depression caused by beta blocker overdose by increasing myocardial contractibility, heart rate, and improving AV node conduction.

 See the Companion Website for a Nursing Process Focus Chart specific to this drug.

Asian Clients' Sensitivity to Propranolol

Studies have shown that due to genetic polymorphisms, Asians metabolize and excrete propranolol more quickly than Caucasians and are also much more sensitive to propranolol. The drug has a significantly greater effect on heart rate in Asian people, and some may require doses up to 50% lower than Caucasians. The nurse should assess this population for possible overdosage and monitor for possible adverse reactions due to high drug levels.

weight gain of 1 kg or more, dizziness, insomnia, drowsiness, or confusion.

POTASSIUM CHANNEL BLOCKERS (CLASS III)

Although a small drug class, the potassium channel blockers have important applications to the treatment of dysrhythmias. These drugs prolong the refractory period, which stabilizes certain types of dysrhythmia. The potassium channel blockers are shown in Table 25.2.

25.10 Treating Dysrhythmias with Potassium Channel Blockers

The drugs in class III exert their actions by blocking potassium ion channels in myocardial cells. After the action potential has passed and the myocardial cell is in a depolarized state, repolarization depends on removal of potassium from the cell. The class III medications delay repolarization of the myocardial cells and lengthen the refractory period, which tends to stabilize dysrhythmias. In addition to blocking potassium channels, sotalol is also a beta-adrenergic

blocker. Drugs in this class generally are not first-line therapy due to potentially serious side effects.

NURSING CONSIDERATIONS

The role of the nurse caring for clients receiving potassium channel blockers for dysrhythmias is included in "Nursing Process Focus: Clients Receiving Antidysrhythmic Therapies" on page 327. Additional nursing considerations will vary depending on the specific drug. Be aware of the specific mechanism of action, side effects, administration requirements, and client teaching for each drug prescribed. These drugs are not recommended for use during pregnancy (category C) or lactation.

Client education as it relates to potassium channel blockers should include goals, reasons for obtaining baseline data such as vital signs and tests for liver and renal function, and possible side effects. Provide the following information when teaching clients about potassium channel blockers:

- Have regular eye exams, due to possible vision changes.
- Avoid prolonged sun exposure and use sunscreen.
- Take medication with meals or a small snack.
- Report the following symptoms immediately: shortness of breath, feeling that the heart has skipped a beat, cough, vision changes, yellow eyes and skin (jaundice), right upper abdominal pain, and dizziness.

CALCIUM CHANNEL BLOCKERS (CLASS IV)

Like the beta-blockers, the calcium channel blockers are widely prescribed for various cardiovascular disorders. By

---

Pr PROTOTYPE DRUG | Amiodarone (Cordarone)

ACTIONS AND USES

Amiodarone is structurally similar to thyroid hormone. It is approved for the treatment of resistant ventricular tachycardia that may prove life-threatening, and it has become a drug of choice for the treatment of atrial dysrhythmias in clients with heart failure. In addition to blocking potassium ion channels, some of this drug's actions on the heart relate to its blockade of sodium ion channels.

PHARMACOKINETICS

Amiodarone is 96% protein bound, accumulates in body tissues, and is metabolized by the liver. Its onset of action may take several weeks when taken orally. The therapeutic serum level of amiodarone is 0.5 to 2.5 μg/mL. Its effects can last 4 to 8 weeks after the drug is discontinued since it has a long half-life that may exceed 100 days.

ADMINISTRATION ALERTS

- Hypokalemia and hypomagnesemia should be corrected prior to initiating therapy.
- Amiodarone is pregnancy category D.

ADVERSE EFFECTS AND INTERACTIONS

The most serious adverse effect of amiodarone occurs in the lung; the drug causes a pneumonia-like syndrome. The drug also causes blurred vision, rashes, photosensitivity, nausea, vomiting, anorexia, fatigue, dizziness, and hypotension. Amiodarone is stored in certain tissues; thus, adverse effects may be slow to resolve. As with other antidysrhythmics, clients must be closely monitored to avoid serious toxicity.

Amiodarone interacts with many other drugs and herbals. For example, it increases digoxin levels in the blood and enhances the actions of anticoagulants. Use with beta-adrenergic blockers may potentiate sinus bradycardia, sinus arrest, or AV block. Amiodarone may increase phenytoin levels two- to threefold. Use with echinacea may cause an increase in hepatotoxicity. Aloe may cause an increased effect of amiodarone. Grapefruit juice may decrease metabolism and worsen hypotension.

 See the Companion Website for a Nursing Process Focus Chart specific to this drug.

slowing conduction velocity, they are able to stabilize certain dysrhythmias. The antidysrhythmic calcium channel blockers are shown in Table 25.2.

25.11 Treating Dysrhythmias with Calcium Channel Blockers

Although about 10 calcium channel blockers (CCBs) are available to treat cardiovascular disease, only a limited number have been approved for dysrhythmias. A few CCBs such as diltiazem and verapamil block calcium ion channels in the heart; the remainder are specific to calcium channels in vascular smooth muscle. The basic pharmacology of this drug class is presented in Chapter 21.

Blockade of calcium ion channels has a number of effects on the heart, most of which are similar to those of beta-adrenergic blockers. Effects include reduced automaticity in the SA node and slowed impulse conduction through the AV node. This prolongs the refractory period and stabilizes many types of dysrhythmia. CCBs are only effective against supraventricular dysrhythmias.

NURSING CONSIDERATIONS

The role of the nurse caring for clients receiving CCBs for dysrhythmias is included in "Nursing Process Focus: Clients Receiving Antidysrhythmic Therapies" in this chapter. For additional nursing considerations, refer to "Nursing Process Focus: Clients Receiving Calcium Channel Blocker Therapy" in Chapter 21 on page 261.

CCB therapy should never be initiated in clients with sick sinus syndrome, heart block, severe hypotension, cardiogenic shock, or severe heart failure. The desired action of this drug class is to decrease oxygen demand, reduce cardiac workload, and increase oxygen to the myocardium. These therapeutic actions may cause clients with existing heart abnormalities to experience adverse effects on the heart. These drugs may produce lethal ventricular dysrhythmias. Calcium chloride may be administered by slow IV push to reverse hypotension or heart block *if* induced by CCBs.

Because CCBs cause vasodilation of peripheral arterioles and decrease total peripheral vascular resistance, some clients, especially older adults, may not be able to tolerate the rapid decrease in blood pressure and are at increased risk of falls. Older clients should be informed about the importance of changing positions slowly and using hand rails and other safety devices as required. Because constipation is a common side effect of these drugs, the nurse also should instruct the client to eat foods high in fibre. These drugs are not recommended for use during pregnancy (category C) or lactation.

Client education as it relates to CCBs used to treat dysrhythmias should include goals, reasons for obtaining baseline data such as vital signs, and possible side effects. Provide the following information when teaching clients about CCBs:

- Report any feelings that the heart has skipped a beat.
- Take blood pressure frequently and report changes: either low blood pressure or elevated blood pressure.
- Take pulse frequently and notify healthcare provider if it falls below 60 beats/minute.
- Observe for swelling (edema).
- Report any shortness of breath.

25.12 Treating Dysrhythmias with Digoxin and Miscellaneous Drugs

Several other drugs are occasionally used to treat specific dysrhythmias but do not act by the mechanisms previously described. These miscellaneous agents are shown in Table 25.2. Although digoxin is primarily used to treat heart failure, it is also prescribed for certain types of atrial dysrhythmia because of its ability to decrease automaticity of the SA node and slow conduction through the AV node. Because excessive levels of digoxin can produce serious dysrhythmias, and interactions with other medications are common, clients must be carefully monitored during therapy. Additional information on the mechanism of action and the adverse effects of digoxin may be found in Chapter 24.

Adenosine and ibutilide are two additional drugs used for specific dysrhythmias. Adenosine is a naturally occurring nucleoside. When given as a 1- to 2-second bolus IV injection, adenosine terminates serious atrial tachycardia by slowing conduction through the AV node and decreasing automaticity of the SA node. Although dyspnea is common, side effects are generally self-limiting because of its 10-second half-life.

Ibutilide is also used as a short-acting IV intervention, infused over 10 minutes to terminate atrial flutter and fibrillation by prolonging the duration of the cardiac action potential. The infusion is stopped as soon as the dysrhythmia is terminated.

NATURAL THERAPIES

Magnesium for Dysrhythmias

Magnesium has been shown to be effective in the treatment of certain cardiac dysrhythmias in those clients who are magnesium deficient. Magnesium deficiency is associated with a number of dysrhythmias, including atrial fibrillation, premature atrial and ventricular beats, ventricular tachycardia, and ventricular fibrillation. The mechanism of magnesium's antidysrhythmic action is not fully understood, but it may be related to its role in maintaining intracellular potassium. It may also be related to its role as a natural calcium channel blocker. Magnesium may be administered intravenously or in liquid or capsule form. Foods that are rich in magnesium include unpolished grains, nuts, and green vegetables.

Pr PROTOTYPE DRUG | Verapamil (Isoptin, others)

ACTIONS AND USES

Verapamil, a CCB, acts by inhibiting the flow of Ca^{+2} into both myocardial cells and vascular smooth muscle cells. In the heart, this action slows conduction velocity and stabilizes dysrhythmias. In the vessels, calcium ion channel inhibition lowers blood pressure, which reduces cardiac workload. Verapamil also dilates the coronary arteries, an action that is important when the drug is used to treat angina (see Chapter 23).

PHARMACOKINETICS

Verapamil is readily absorbed, but its bioavailability is less than 25% due to rapid metabolism by the liver. It is 90% protein bound. When taken PO, its onset of action is 1 to 2 hours. Its therapeutic serum level is 0.08 to 0.3 μg/mL. Its half-life is 4.5 to 12 hours.

ADMINISTRATION ALERTS

- Capsule contents should not be dissolved or chewed.
- For IV administration, inspect drug preparation to make sure solution is clear and colourless.
- Verapamil is pregnancy category C.

ADVERSE EFFECTS AND INTERACTIONS

Side effects are generally minor and may include headache, constipation, and hypotension. Because verapamil can cause bradycardia, clients with heart failure should be carefully monitored. Clients should notify their healthcare provider if their heart rate falls below 50 beats/minute or if systolic blood pressure falls below 90 mm Hg. Like many other antidysrhythmics, verapamil has the ability to elevate blood levels of digoxin. Since both digoxin and verapamil have the effect of slowing conduction through the AV node, their concurrent use must be carefully monitored.

Grapefruit juice may decrease metabolism of CCBs and increase their serum concentration, thus worsening hypotension. Use with caution with herbal supplements, such as hawthorn, which may have additive hypotensive effects.

 See the Companion Website for a Nursing Process Focus Chart specific to this drug.

NURSING PROCESS FOCUS   Clients Receiving Antidysrhythmic Therapies

Assessment	Potential Nursing Diagnoses/Identified Patterns
Prior to administration: ■ Obtain complete health history including allergies, drug history, and possible drug interactions. ■ Assess to determine if cardiac alteration is producing a symptomatic effect on cardiac output, including vital signs, level of consciousness, urinary output, skin temperature, and peripheral pulses. ■ Obtain baseline ECG to compare throughout therapy.	■ Need for k nowledge regarding drug therapy and adverse effects ■ Safety from injury related to decreased cardiac output and cardiac conduction abnormalities

Planning: Client Goals and Expected Outcomes

The client will:
- Exhibit improved cardiac output as evidenced by stabilization of heart rate, heart rhythm, sensorium, urinary output, and vital signs
- State expected outcomes of drug therapy
- Demonstrate an understanding of the drug's action by accurately describing drug side effects and precautions

Implementation

Interventions (Rationales)	Client Education/Discharge Planning
■ Monitor cardiac rate and rhythm continuously if administering drug IV. (IV route is used when rapid therapeutic effects are needed. Constant monitoring is needed to detect any potential serious dysrhythmias.)	■ Explain the need for continuous ECG monitoring when administering the medication intravenously.
■ Monitor IV site. Administer all parenteral medication via infusion pump.	■ Instruct client to report any burning or stinging pain, swelling, warmth, redness, or tenderness at the IV insertion site.
■ Investigate possible causes of the dysrhythmia such as electrolyte imbalances, hypoxia, pain, anxiety, caffeine ingestion, and tobacco use.	Instruct client to: ■ Maintain a diet low in sodium and fat, with sufficient potassium ■ Report illness such as flu, vomiting, diarrhea, and dehydration to healthcare provider to avoid adverse effects ■ Restrict use of caffeine and tobacco products

continued

NURSING PROCESS FOCUS Clients Receiving Antidysrhythmic Therapies *(Continued)*

Interventions (Rationales)	Client Education/Discharge Planning
▪ Observe for side effects specific to the antidysrhythmic used.	Instruct client to: ▪ Report adverse effects specific to prescribed antidysrhythmic ▪ Report palpitations, chest pain, dyspnea, unusual fatigue, weakness, and visual disturbances
▪ Monitor for proper use of medication.	Instruct client to: ▪ Never discontinue the drug abruptly ▪ Take the drug exactly as prescribed, even if feeling well ▪ Take pulse prior to taking the drug. (Instruct client regarding the normal range and rhythm of pulse; instruct to consult the healthcare provider regarding "reportable" pulse.)

Evaluation of Outcome Criteria

Evaluate the effectiveness of drug therapy by confirming that client goals and expected outcomes have been met (see "Planning").

See Table 25.2 for a list of drugs (Class I–IV) to which these nursing actions apply.

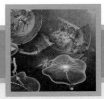

CHAPTER REVIEW

KEY CONCEPTS

The numbered key concepts provide a succinct summary of the important points from the corresponding numbered section within the chapter. If any of these points are not clear, refer to the numbered section within the chapter for review. Expanded versions can be found on the Companion Website.

25.1 The frequency of dysrhythmias in the population is difficult to predict because many clients experience no symptoms. Persistent or severe dysrhythmias may be lethal.

25.2 Dysrhythmias are classified by location (atrial or ventricular) or type of rhythm abnormality produced (flutter, fibrillation, block).

25.3 The electrical conduction pathway from the SA node, to the AV node, to the bundle branches and Purkinje fibres keeps the heart beating in a synchronized manner. Some myocardial cells in these regions have the property of automaticity.

25.4 The electrophysiological events in the heart can be measured with an electrocardiograph.

25.5 Changes in sodium and potassium levels generate the action potential in myocardial cells. Depolarization occurs when sodium (and calcium) rushes in; repolarization occurs when potassium is removed.

25.6 Non-pharmacological therapy of dysrhythmias, including cardioversion, ablation, and implantable cardioverter defibrillators, are often the treatments of choice.

25.7 Antidysrhythmic drugs are classified by their mechanism of action into classes I through IV.

25.8 Sodium channel blockers are the largest group of antidysrhythmics and act by slowing the rate of impulse conduction across the heart.

25.9 Beta-adrenergic blockers act by reducing automaticity as well as slowing conduction velocity across the myocardium.

25.10 Potassium channel blockers act by prolonging the refractory period of the heart.

25.11 Calcium channel blockers act by reducing automaticity and by slowing myocardial conduction velocity. Their actions and effects are similar to the beta-blockers.

25.12 Digoxin, adenosine, and ibutilide are used for specific dysrhythmias but do not act by blocking ion channels.

REVIEW QUESTIONS

1 Trace the flow of electrical conduction through the heart. What would happen if the impulse never reached the AV node?

2 Why does slowing the speed of the electrical impulse across the myocardium sometimes correct a dysrhythmia?

3 Why are selective alpha-adrenergic blockers such as doxazosin (Cardura) of no value in treating dysrhythmias?

4 Remembering the effects of digoxin on the heart from Chapter 24, explain why most antidysrhythmic drugs have the potential to cause serious side effects in clients taking cardiac glycosides.

CRITICAL THINKING QUESTIONS

1. A client with a history of COPD and tachycardia has recently been placed on propranolol (Inderal) to control the tachydysrhythmia. What is a priority for the nurse in monitoring this client?

2. A client is started on amiodarone (Cordarone) for cardiac dysrhythmia. This client is also on digoxin (Lanoxin), warfarin (Coumadin), and insulin. What is a priority teaching for this client?

3. A client is on verapamil (Isoptin) and digoxin (Lanoxin). What are the priority assessments for this client? What teaching should be provided?

EXPLORE MediaLink

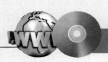

www.pearsoned.ca/adams-king

MEDIALINK DVD-ROM
- **Audio Glossary**
- **CRNE Review**
- **Animations**
  Dysrhythmia
  Mechanism of Action: Propranolol
  Mechanism of Action: Amiodarone

COMPANION WEBSITE
- **CRNE Review**
- **Case Study:** Client taking a sodium channel blocker
- **Dosage Calculations**
- **Nursing Process Focus Charts**

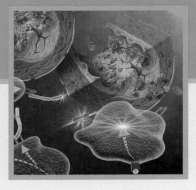

CHAPTER 26

Drugs for Coagulation Disorders

DRUGS AT A GLANCE

ANTICOAGULANTS
Parenteral anticoagulants
  heparin (Hepalean)
Oral anticoagulants
  warfarin (Coumadin, Warfilone)

ANTIPLATELET AGENTS
ADP receptor blockers
  clopidogrel (Plavix)
Glycoprotein IIb/IIIa receptor blockers

THROMBOLYTICS
  alteplase (Activase)

ANTIFIBRINOLYTICS
  aminocaproic acid (Amicar)

OBJECTIVES

After reading this chapter, the student should be able to do the following:

1. Identify drug classes used for treating coagulation disorders.
2. Explain the therapeutic action of each class of drug used in relation to the pathophysiology of coagulation (thromboembolic) disorders.
3. Explain how laboratory testing of coagulation parameters is used to monitor anticoagulant pharmacotherapy.
4. Describe the nurse's role in the pharmacological management of clients with coagulation disorders.
5. For each of the drug classes listed in Drugs at a Glance, identify a representative drug and explain its mechanism of action, therapeutic effects, and important adverse effects.
6. Describe and explain, based on pharmacological principles, the rationale for nursing assessment, planning, and interventions for clients with coagulation disorders.
7. Use the nursing process to care for clients receiving drug therapy for coagulation disorders.

MediaLink

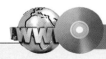

www.pearsoned.ca/adams-king

CRNE review, case studies, and other interactive resources for this chapter can be found on the Companion Website at **www.pearsoned.ca/adams-king**. Click on "Chapter 26" to select the activities for this chapter. For animations, more CRNE review questions, and an audio glossary, access the accompanying DVD-ROM in this textbook.

The process of **hemostasis**, or the stopping of blood flow, is an essential mechanism protecting the body from both external and internal injury. Without efficient hemostasis, bleeding from wounds or internal injuries would lead to shock and perhaps death. Too much clotting, however, can be just as dangerous. The physiological processes of hemostasis must maintain a delicate balance between fluidity and coagulation.

A number of diseases and conditions can affect hemostasis, including myocardial infarction, cerebrovascular accident, venous thrombus, valvular heart disease, and indwelling catheters. Because these disorders are so prevalent, nurses will have frequent occasions to administer and monitor coagulation-modifying drugs.

PHARMFACTS

Clotting Disorders

- Liver disease is a common cause of coagulation disorders as this organ supplies many of the clotting factors.
- Deep vein thrombosis (DVT) and pulmonary emboli are common among clients with reduced mobility.
- Von Willebrand's disease (vWD) is the most common hereditary bleeding disorder. It is caused by a deficiency of von Willebrand factor (vWF), which plays a role in platelet aggregation and acts as a carrier for factor VIII.
- Hemophilia A is a hereditary bleeding disorder caused by a lack of clotting factor VIII; it accounts for 80% of all hemophilia cases.
- Hemophilia B is a hereditary bleeding disorder caused by a lack of clotting factor IX.
- Both hemophilia A and B are very rare disorders. Hemophilia A and B together affect fewer than 1 in 60,000 Canadians (about 3000 people).

Source: Canadian Hemophilia Society.

26.1 The Process of Hemostasis

The process of hemostasis is complex, involving a number of substances called **clotting factors**. Hemostasis occurs in a series of sequential steps, sometimes referred to as a cascade. Drugs can be used to modify several of these steps.

When a blood vessel is injured, a series of events initiate the clotting process. The vessel spasms, causing constriction, which limits blood flow to the injured area. Platelets have an affinity for the damaged vessel. They become sticky, adhering to each other and to the injured area. Aggregation is facilitated by adenosine diphosphate (ADP), the enzyme thrombin, and thromboxane A_2, while adhesion is made possible by platelet receptor sites and von Willebrand's factor. As the bound platelets break down, they release substances that attract more platelets to the area. Blood flow is further slowed, thus allowing the process of **coagulation**, which is the formation of an insoluble clot. The basic steps of hemostasis are shown in Figure 26.1.

When collagen is exposed at the site of vascular injury and platelets adhere to the damaged cells, a series of complex reactions called the **coagulation cascade** is initiated. Coagulation occurs when fibrin threads form to create a meshwork that fortifies the blood constituents so that they develop the clot. During the cascade, various plasma proteins that are circulating in an inactive state are converted to their active forms. Two separate pathways, along with numerous biochemical processes, lead to coagulation. The intrinsic pathway is activated in response to injury. The extrinsic pathway is activated when blood leaks out of a vessel and

MediaLink Canadian Hemophilia Society

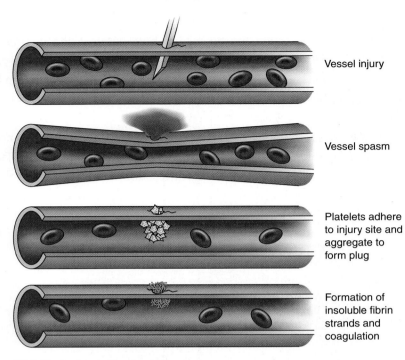

Vessel injury

Vessel spasm

Platelets adhere to injury site and aggregate to form plug

Formation of insoluble fibrin strands and coagulation

● **Figure 26.1** Basic steps of hemostasis

enters tissue spaces. There are common steps between the two pathways and the outcome is the same—the formation of the fibrin clot. The steps in each coagulation cascade are shown in Figure 26.2.

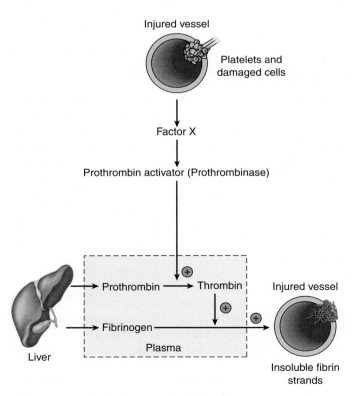

Injured vessel

Platelets and damaged cells

Factor X

Prothrombin activator (Prothrombinase)

Liver

Prothrombin → Thrombin

Injured vessel

Fibrinogen

Plasma

Insoluble fibrin strands

● **Figure 26.2** Major steps in the coagulation cascade: common pathway

Near the end of the common pathway, a chemical called **prothrombin activator**, or prothrombinase, is formed. Prothrombin activator converts the clotting factor **prothrombin** to an enzyme called **thrombin**. Thrombin then converts **fibrinogen**, a plasma protein, to long strands of **fibrin**. The fibrin strands provide a framework for the structure of the clot. Thus, two of the factors essential to clotting, thrombin and fibrin, are only formed after injury to the vessel. The fibrin strands form an insoluble web over the injured area to stop blood loss. Normal blood clotting occurs in approximately 6 minutes.

It is important to note that several clotting factors, including thromboplastin and fibrinogen, are proteins made by the liver that are constantly circulating through the blood in an inactive form. Vitamin K, which is made by bacteria residing in the large intestine, is required for the liver to make four of the clotting factors. Because of the crucial importance of the liver in creating these clotting factors, clients with serious liver disorders often have abnormal coagulation.

26.2 Removal of Blood Clots

Hemostasis has been achieved once a blood clot is formed, protecting the body from excessive hemorrhage. The clot, however, stops most or all of the blood flow to the affected area; circulation must eventually be restored so that the tissue can resume normal activities. The process of clot removal is called **fibrinolysis**. It is initiated within 24 to 48 hours of clot formation and continues until the clot is dissolved.

Fibrinolysis also involves several cascading steps. When the fibrin clot is formed, nearby blood vessel cells secrete

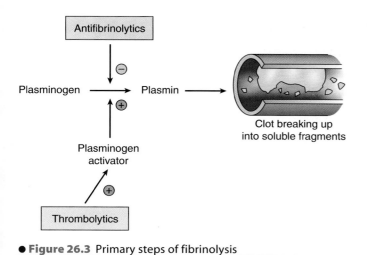

● **Figure 26.3** Primary steps of fibrinolysis

the enzyme **tissue plasminogen activator (t-PA)**, which converts the inactive protein **plasminogen** in the fibrin clot to its active enzymatic form called **plasmin**. Plasmin then digests the fibrin strands to remove the clot. The body normally regulates fibrinolysis such that unwanted fibrin clots are removed but fibrin present in wounds is left to maintain hemostasis. The steps of fibrinolysis are shown in Figure 26.3.

26.3 Diseases of Hemostasis

To diagnose bleeding disorders, a thorough health history and physical examination is necessary. Laboratory tests measuring coagulation must be obtained. These usually include a whole blood clotting time, **prothrombin time (PT)**, thrombin time, **activated partial thromboplastin time (aPTT)**, liver function tests, and in some instances a bleeding time. Platelet count is also of interest in assessing bleeding disorders. Additional tests may be indicated based on the results of these laboratory analyses.

Thromboembolic disorders occur when undesirable clots are formed. Once a stationary clot, called a **thrombus**, forms in a vessel, it often grows larger as more fibrin is added. Arterial thrombi are particularly problematic as they deprive an area of blood flow. Cessation of blood flow results in an infarction and tissue death will result. This is the case in myocardial infarctions and many cerebrovascular accidents (CVAs).

Pieces of a thrombus may break off and travel in the bloodstream to affect other vessels. A travelling clot is called an **embolus**. Thrombi in the venous system usually form in the veins of the legs in susceptible clients, a condition called **deep vein thrombosis (DVT)**. Thrombi can also form in the atria during atrial fibrillation. A thrombus in the right atrium can dislodge and travel to the lung, causing a pulmonary embolism. A thrombus in the left atrium can dislodge and cause a CVA or an arterial infarction elsewhere in the body. Arterial thrombi and emboli can also result from procedures involving arterial punctures, such as angiography. Thromboembolic disorders are the most common indications for pharmacotherapy with anticoagulants.

PHARMFACTS

Secondary Causes of Thrombocytopenia

Diseases
AIDS
Alcoholism
Anemia (aplastic, folic acid, vitamin B_{12})
Disseminated intravascular coagulation (DIC)
Infectious mononucleosis
Leukemia
Viral infections

Drugs

ASA	heparin
cimetidine	naproxen
digitalis	ibuprofen
indomethacin	quinidine
furosemide	sulfonamides
morphine sulfate	thiazide diuretics

Therapeutic Regimens
Chemotherapy
Radiation therapy

Bleeding disorders are characterized by abnormal clot formation. The most common bleeding disorder is a deficiency of platelets known as **thrombocytopenia**, which results from any condition that suppresses bone marrow function. Certain drugs such as immunosuppressants and most anticancer agents can cause this condition.

Hemophilias are bleeding disorders caused by genetic deficiencies in certain clotting factors. They are typified by prolonged coagulation times that result in persistent bleeding that can be acute. The classic form, hemophilia A, is caused by a lack of clotting factor VIII and accounts for approximately 80% of all cases. Hemophilia B, or Christmas disease, is caused by a deficiency of factor IX and makes up about 20% of cases. Hemophilia is treated with the administration of the absent clotting factor and, in acute situations, transfusions of fresh frozen plasma. Of the other inherited bleeding disorders, **von Willebrand's disease (vWD)** is the most common. This disorder results in a decrease in the quantity or quality of von Willebrand factor (vWF), which has a role in platelet aggregation. This type of bleeding disorder is treated with factor VIII concentrate as well as desmopressin, which promotes the release of stored vWF. For the most severely affected clients, plasma products containing vWF may be required.

26.4 Mechanisms of Coagulation Modification

Drugs can modify hemostasis by four basic mechanisms, as summarized in Table 26.1. The most commonly prescribed coagulation modifiers are the **anticoagulants**, which are used to prevent the formation of clots. To accomplish clot prevention, drugs can either inhibit specific clotting factors in the coagulation cascade or diminish the clotting action of platelets. Regardless of the mechanism, all anticoagulant

TABLE 26.1	Mechanisms of Coagulation Modification	
Type of Modification	**Mechanism**	**Drug Classification**
prevention of clot formation	inhibition of specific clotting factors	anticoagulant
prevention of clot formation	inhibition of platelet actions	anticoagulant/antiplatelet
removal of an existing clot	dissolving of the clot	thrombolytic
promotion of clot formation	inhibition of the destruction of fibrin	antifibrinolytic

drugs will increase the normal time the body takes to form clots.

Once an abnormal clot has formed in a blood vessel, it may be critical to quickly remove it to restore normal function. This is particularly important for vessels serving the heart, lungs, and brain. A specific class of drug, the **thrombolytics**, has been developed to dissolve such life-threatening clots.

Occasionally, it is necessary to actually promote the formation of clots. These drugs, called **antifibrinolytics**, inhibit the normal removal of fibrin, thus keeping the clot in place for a longer period of time. Antifibrinolytics are primarily used to speed clot formation in order to limit bleeding from a surgical site.

Since hemostasis involves a delicate balance of factors favouring clotting versus those inhibiting clotting, pharmacotherapy with coagulation modifiers is individualized to each client. Clients receiving coagulation-modifying drugs require regular physical and laboratory assessments.

ANTICOAGULANTS

Anticoagulants are drugs used to prolong bleeding time in order to prevent blood clots from forming. They are widely used in the treatment of thromboembolic disease.

26.5 Pharmacotherapy with Parenteral and Oral Anticoagulants

Anticoagulants lengthen clotting time and prevent thrombi from forming or growing larger by inhibiting certain clotting factors. Thromboembolic disease can be life-threatening; thus, therapy is often begun by administering anticoagulants intravenously or subcutaneously to achieve a rapid onset of action. The most commonly prescribed parenteral anticoagulant is heparin. As the disease stabilizes, the client is switched to an oral anticoagulant, with careful monitoring of appropriate laboratory coagulation studies. Warfarin is the most commonly prescribed oral anticoagulant.

Anticoagulants act by a number of different mechanisms, as illustrated in Figure 26.4. These drugs are often referred to as blood thinners, which is actually not the case, because they do not change the viscosity of the blood. Instead, anticoagulants exert a negative charge on the surface of the platelets, so the clumping action or aggregation of these cells is inhibited. Heparin acts by enhancing the inhibitory actions of **antithrombin III**. Warfarin acts by inhibiting the hepatic synthesis of coagulation factors II, VII, IX, and X. Table 26.2 lists the primary anticoagulants.

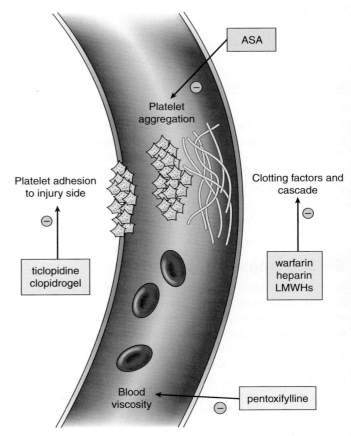

● **Figure 26.4** Mechanisms of action of anticoagulants

In recent years, the heparin molecule has been shortened and modified to create a new class of drug called **low molecular weight heparins (LMWHs)**. The mechanism of action of these agents is similar to that of heparin, except their inhibition is more specific to active factor X (see Figure 26.2). LMWHs possess the same degree of anticoagulant activity as heparin but have several advantages. LMWHs are less likely to cause thrombocytopenia. The duration of action of LMWHs is two to four times longer, and they produce a more stable response than heparin; therefore, fewer follow-up lab tests are needed, and the client or family members can be trained to give the necessary SC injections at home. LMWHs have become the drugs of choice for a number of clotting disorders, including the prevention of DVT following surgery.

Other parenteral anticoagulants include the direct thrombin inhibitors argatroban, bivalirudin, and lepirudin.

TABLE 26.2   Anticoagulants

Drug	Route and Adult Dose
🔁 heparin (Hepalean)	IV; infusion: 5000–40,000 units/day SC; 15,000–20,000 units bid
pentoxifylline (Apo-Pentoxifylline, Trental)*	PO; 400 mg tid
🔁 warfarin (Coumadin, warfilone)	PO; 2–15 mg/day
Low Molecular Weight Heparins (LMWHs)	
dalteparin (Fragmin)	SC; 2500–5000 units/day for 5–10 days
danaparoid (Orgaran)	SC; 750 units bid for 7–10 days
enoxaparin (Lovenox)	SC; 40 mg bid for 7–10 days
tinzaparin (Innohep)	SC; 175 units/kg qd for at least 6 days
Direct Thrombin Inhibitors	
argatroban (Acova, Novastan)	IV; 2 μg/kg/min (max 10 μg/kg/min)
bivalirudin (Angiomax)	IV; 1 mg/kg initial bolus followed by 2.5 mg/kg/h for 4 h (continue at 0.2 mg/kg/h up to 20 h)
lepirudin (Refludan)	IV; 0.4 mg/kg initial bolus (max 44 mg) followed by 0.15 mg/kg/h (max 16.5 mg/h) for 2–10 days

*Sometimes classified as a hemorrheological drug.

Thrombin inhibitors bind to both clot-bound and circulating thrombin, preventing the formation of fibrin clots. The therapeutic aPTT value for these drugs is usually one and a half to three times the control value. Bivalirudin is administered in combination with ASA to prevent thrombi in clients undergoing angioplasty. Argatroban and lepirudin are indicated for prevention or treatment of thrombocytopenia induced by heparin therapy. There is no specific antidote for these agents. Blood transfusion may be required if excessive bleeding occurs.

An experimental oral anticoagulant, ximelagatran (Exanta), was in the final stages of clinical trials in 2008. It is the first new oral anticoagulant in the last 50 years and the first in a new class of anticoagulant, called the direct thrombin inhibitors. The primary advantage of this drug is that it is given at a fixed dose with no titrating or coagulation monitoring. Compared to available anticoagulants, it has low potential for food and drug interactions.

NURSING CONSIDERATIONS

The role of the nurse in anticoagulant therapy involves careful monitoring of the client's condition and providing education as it relates to the prescribed drug regimen. The most serious side effect of anticoagulants is bleeding. Assess the client for signs of bleeding, including bruising, nosebleeds, excessive menstrual flow, "coffee grounds" emesis, tarry stools, tea-coloured urine, bright red bleeding from the rectum, dizziness, fatigue, or pale, pasty-looking skin. The risk of bleeding is dose dependent—the higher the dose, the higher the risk.

Hypotension accompanied by declining CBC values (RBCs, platelets, hemoglobin, and hematocrit) may signal internal bleeding. Lumbar pain and unilateral abdominal wall bulges or swelling could indicate retroperitoneal hemorrhage. Guaiac tests can be performed on stool to identify occult blood. Use of heparin during breastfeeding can trigger bleeding from the nipples and should be avoided. Use of warfarin during pregnancy is contraindicated as it can cause hemorrhage or other abnormalities in the fetus.

Monitoring of laboratory values during anticoagulant therapy is essential to client safety. For heparin, aPTT is measured, with normal values ranging from 25 to 40 seconds. For therapeutic anticoagulation, the aPTT should be one to two times the client's baseline. During continuous intravenous heparin therapy, the aPTT is measured daily and 6 to 8 hours after any changes in dosage.

Prothrombin time (PT) is a laboratory test used to monitor the effectiveness of warfarin. The normal PT range is 12 to 15 seconds. During therapeutic anticoagulation, PT should increase to one to two times the client's baseline. Because laboratory testing methods for PT vary, PT is also reported as an international normalized ratio (INR) value; INR values of 2.0 to 3.5 are considered therapeutic. PT is measured daily until the therapeutic dose is determined, and then the frequency of testing is decreased to weekly or monthly as therapy progresses.

When transitioning from IV heparin to PO warfarin, the two drugs must be administered simultaneously for 2 to 3 days. Heparin has a brief half-life (90 minutes) and warfarin has a long one (1 to 3 days). The aPTT returns to normal within 2 to 3 hours following discontinuation of heparin, so concomitant pharmacotherapy is necessary to ensure continuous therapeutic anticoagulation. During this transition, there is increased risk of bleeding due to the potentiated action of the combined drugs.

LMWHs are given subcutaneously, with dosage calculations based on the client's weight rather than laboratory values. Follow the manufacturer's recommendations for sites of injection. There is an increased risk of bleeding if injected into muscle. For example, enoxaparin is given in

Mechanism of Action: Warfarin   MediaLink

the subcutaneous tissue of the anterolateral or posterolateral abdominal wall (the "love handles"). To administer safely, gently grasp a skinfold between the thumb and forefinger, insert a 1 cm (3/8 inch) needle fully at a 90-degree angle, and hold the skinfold throughout the injection. For exceptionally lean clients, a longer needle is used and is carefully inserted at a 45-degree angle to avoid inadvertent IM injection of the medication. To prevent tissue injury and bruising, an injection site should never be massaged.

Client education should include goals, reasons for obtaining baseline data such as vital signs and blood tests, and possible side effects. Following are important points to include when teaching clients about heparin and warfarin:

- Immediately report burning, stinging, tightness, tenderness, warmth, or other pain at heparin injection or IV insertion sites; these signs may signal drug infiltration into sensitive tissues.

- Notify the nurse of excessive bruising or evidence of swelling at a heparin injection site.

- Take warfarin at the same time each day.

- Moderate daily intake of vitamin K–rich foods when taking warfarin.

- Avoid strenuous and hazardous activities that could result in bleeding injury.

General teaching strategies for anticoagulants can be found in "Nursing Process Focus: Clients Receiving Anticoagulant Therapy" in this chapter.

Health Canada: Warfarin Interactions   MediaLink

ANTIPLATELET AGENTS

Antiplatelet drugs cause an anticoagulant effect by interfering with various aspects of platelet function—primarily platelet aggregation. Unlike the anticoagulants, which are used primarily to prevent thrombosis in veins, antiplatelet agents are used to prevent clot formation in arteries. The antiplatelet agents are shown in Table 26.3.

26.6 Inhibition of Platelet Function

Platelets are a central component of the hemostasis process, and too few platelets or diminished platelet function can profoundly increase bleeding time. The antiplatelet drugs are classified as such due to their inhibition of platelet function:

- ASA
- Adenosine diphosphate (ADP) receptor blockers
- Glycoprotein IIb/IIIa receptor blockers
- Drugs for intermittent claudication

ASA deserves special mention as an antiplatelet agent. Because it is available over the counter, clients may not consider ASA a potent medication; however, its anticoagulant activity is well documented. ASA acts by binding irreversibly to the enzyme cyclooxygenase in platelets. This binding inhibits the formation of thromboxane A_2, a powerful inducer of platelet aggregation. The anticoagulant effect of a single dose of ASA may persist for as long as a week.

The Miracles of ASA   MediaLink

Pr PROTOTYPE DRUG | Heparin (Hepalean)

ACTIONS AND USES

Heparin is a natural substance found in the liver and the lining of blood vessels. Its normal function is to prolong coagulation time, thereby preventing excessive clotting within blood vessels. As a result, it prevents the enlargement of existing clots and the formation of new ones. The binding of heparin to antithrombin III inactivates several clotting factors and inhibits thrombin activity.

ADMINISTRATION ALERTS

- Heparin is poorly absorbed by the GI mucosa because of rapid metabolism by the hepatic enzyme heparinase. Therefore, it must be given either SC or through IV bolus injection or continuous infusion.

- When administering heparin SC, never draw back the syringe plunger once the needle has entered the skin, and never massage the site after injection. Doing either can contribute to bleeding or tissue damage.

- IM administration is contraindicated due to bleeding risk.

- Heparin is pregnancy category C.

PHARMACOKINETICS

The onset of action for IV heparin is immediate, whereas SC heparin may take up to 1 hour for maximum therapeutic effect. It does not cross the placenta or enter breast milk. It is metabolized by the liver and reticulo-endothelial system (lymph nodes, spleen). Half-life is 1.5 hours.

ADVERSE EFFECTS AND INTERACTIONS

Abnormal bleeding is not uncommon with heparin therapy. Should aPTT become prolonged or toxicity be observed, discontinuation of the drug will result in loss of anticoagulant activity within hours. If serious hemorrhage occurs, a specific antagonist, protamine sulfate, may be administered to neutralize the anticoagulant activity of heparin. Protamine sulfate has an onset of action of 5 minutes and is also an antagonist to the LMWHs.

Oral anticoagulants, including warfarin, potentiate the action of heparin. Drugs that inhibit platelet aggregation, such as ASA, indomethacin, and ibuprofen, may induce bleeding. Nicotine, digitalis, tetracyclines, and antihistamines may inhibit anticoagulation.

Use with caution with herbal supplements, such as arnica, which contains a coumarin component and may increase the anticoagulant effect.

 See the Companion Website for a Nursing Process Focus Chart specific to this drug.

Pr PROTOTYPE DRUG | Warfarin (Coumadin, Warfilone)

ACTIONS AND USES

Unlike heparin, the anticoagulant activity of warfarin can take several days to reach its maximum effect. This explains why heparin and warfarin therapy are overlapped. Warfarin inhibits the action of vitamin K. Without adequate vitamin K, the synthesis of clotting factors II, VII, IX, and X is diminished. Because these clotting factors are normally circulating in the blood, it takes several days for their plasma levels to fall and for the anticoagulant effect of warfarin to appear. Another reason for the slow onset is that 99% of the warfarin is bound to plasma proteins and is thus unavailable to produce its effect.

PHARMACOKINETICS

The onset of action is 36 to 72 hours. Warfarin crosses the placenta but does not enter breast milk. Protein binding is 99%. It is metabolized by the liver. Half-life is 42 hours.

ADMINISTRATION ALERTS

- Should life-threatening bleeding occur during therapy, the anticoagulant effects of warfarin can be reduced in 6 hours through the IM or SC administration of its antagonist, vitamin K_1.
- Warfarin is pregnancy category D.

ADVERSE EFFECTS AND INTERACTIONS

The most serious adverse effect of warfarin is abnormal bleeding. Upon discontinuation of therapy, the anticoagulant activity of warfarin may persist for up to 10 days.

Extensive protein binding is responsible for numerous drug-drug interactions, some of which include NSAIDs, diuretics, SSRIs and other antidepressants, steroids, antibiotics, vaccines, and vitamins (e.g., vitamin K). Concurrent use with NSAIDs may increase bleeding risk.

Use with caution with herbal supplements, such as arnica, feverfew, garlic, and ginger, which may increase the risk of bleeding.

 See the Companion Website for a Nursing Process Focus Chart specific to this drug.

NURSING PROCESS FOCUS   Clients Receiving Anticoagulant Therapy

Assessment	Potential Nursing Diagnoses/Identified Patterns
Prior to administration: ■ Obtain complete health history including recent surgeries or trauma, allergies, drug history, and possible drug interactions. ■ Obtain vital signs; assess in context of client's baseline values.	■ Adequate knowledge regarding drug therapy and adverse effects ■ Safety from injury (bleeding, bruising) related to adverse effects of anticoagulant therapy ■ Safety from physical injury such as falls ■ Effective tissue perfusion ■ Tissue integrity ■ Safety from Infection

Planning: Client Goals and Expected Outcomes

The client will:
- Experience a decrease in blood coagulability as evidenced by laboratory values and signs of effective blood circulation
- Experience a safe environment with no evidence of physical injury
- Demonstrate an understanding of the drug's action by accurately describing drug side effects and precautions

Implementation

Interventions (Rationales)	Client Education/Discharge Planning
■ Monitor for adverse clotting reactions. (Heparin can cause thrombus formation with thrombocytopenia, or "white clot syndrome." Warfarin may cause cholesterol microemboli, which result in gangrene, localized vasculitis, or "purple toes syndrome.") ■ Observe for signs of skin necrosis such as blue or purple mottling of the feet that blanches with pressure or fades when the legs are elevated. (Clients on anticoagulant therapy remain at risk of developing emboli, resulting in CVA or PE.) ■ Use with caution in clients with GI, renal and/or liver disease, alcoholism, diabetes, hypertension, hyperlipidemia, and in the elderly and premenopausal women. (Clients with CAD risk factors are at increased risk of developing cholesterol microemboli.)	Instruct client to: ■ Immediately report sudden dyspnea, chest pain, temperature or colour change in the hands, arms, legs, and feet (Gangrene may occur between day 3 and 8 of warfarin therapy. Purple toes syndrome usually occurs within weeks 3 to 10 or later.) ■ Feel pedal pulses daily to check circulation ■ Protect feet from injury by wearing loose-fitting socks; avoid going barefoot ■ Instruct elderly clients, menstruating women, and those with peptic ulcer disease, alcoholism, or kidney or liver disease that they have an increased risk of bleeding. ■ Diabetics and clients with high blood pressure or cholesterol are at risk of developing microscopic clots despite anticoagulant therapy.

continued

NURSING PROCESS FOCUS Clients Receiving Lithium (Eskalith) *(Continued)*	
Interventions (Rationales)	**Client Education/Discharge Planning**
▪ Monitor for signs of bleeding: flu-like symptoms, excessive bruising, pallor, epistaxis, hemoptysis, hematemesis, menorrhagia, hematuria, melena, frank rectal bleeding, or excessive bleeding from wounds or in the mouth. (Bleeding is a sign of anticoagulant overdose.)	Advise client to: ▪ Immediately report flu-like symptoms (dizziness, chills, weakness, pale skin); blood coming from a cough, the nose, mouth, or rectum; menstrual "flooding"; "coffee grounds" vomit; tarry stools; excessive bruising; bleeding from wounds that cannot be stopped within 10 minutes; all physical injuries ▪ Avoid all contact sports and amusement park rides that cause intense or violent bumping or jostling ▪ Use a soft toothbrush and an electric shaver ▪ Keep a "pad count" during menstrual periods to estimate blood loss
▪ Monitor vital signs. (Increase in heart rate accompanied by low blood pressure or subnormal temperature may signal bleeding.)	▪ Instruct client to immediately report palpitations, fatigue, or feeling faint, which may signal low blood pressure related to bleeding.
▪ Monitor laboratory values (aPTT, PTT) for therapeutic values. (Because heparin is metabolized by the liver and may cause significant elevations of SGOT [S-AST] and SGPT [S-ALT], also assess these enzyme values.) ▪ Monitor CBC, especially in premenopausal women.	Instruct client to: ▪ Always inform laboratory personnel of heparin therapy when providing samples ▪ Carry a wallet card or wear medical ID jewellery indicating heparin therapy
Evaluation of Outcome Criteria	
Evaluate the effectiveness of drug therapy by confirming that client goals and expected outcomes have been met (see "Planning").	
See Table 26.2 for a list of drugs to which these nursing actions apply.	

TABLE 26.3   Antiplatelet Agents

Drug	Route and Adult Dose
ASA (Aspirin, others) (see page 227 for the Prototype Drug box)	PO; 80 mg qd to 650 mg bid
dipyridamole (Persantine)	PO; 75–100 mg qd
ADP Receptor Blockers	
ⓟ clopidogrel (Plavix)	PO; 75 mg qd
ticlopidine (Apo-Ticlopidine)	PO; 250 mg bid
Glycoprotein IIb/IIIa Receptor Blockers	
abciximab (ReoPro)	IV; 0.25 mg/kg initial bolus over 5 min then 10 μg/kg/min for 12 hr
eptifibatide (Integrilin)	IV; 180 μg/kg initial bolus over 1–2 min then 2 μg/kg/min for 24–72 hr
tirofiban (Aggrastat)	IV; 0.4 μg/kg/min for 30 min then 0.1 μg/kg/min for 12–24 hr

Concurrent use of ASA with other coagulation modifiers should be avoided unless medically approved. The primary uses of ASA are described in relation to several conditions in this textbook: pain relief in Chapter 19, prevention of strokes and myocardial infarction in Chapter 23, and reduction of inflammation in Chapter 31.

The ADP receptor blockers comprise a small group of drugs that irreversibly alter receptors for ADP on the plasma membrane of platelets. ADP is unable to bind to the altered receptors and thus the platelets are unable to receive the chemical signals required for them to aggregate. Both ticlopidine and clopidogrel are given orally to prevent thrombi formation in clients who have experienced a recent thromboembolic event such as a stroke or MI. Ticlopidine can cause life-threatening neutropenia and agranulocytosis.

Clopidogrel is much safer, having side effects comparable to those of ASA.

Glycoprotein IIb/IIIa inhibitors are relatively new additions to the treatment of thromboembolic disease. **Glycoprotein IIb/IIIa** is an enzyme necessary for platelet aggregation. Inhibition of this enzyme has the effect of preventing thrombus formation in clients experiencing a recent MI, stroke, or percutaneous transluminal coronary angioplasty (PTCA). Although these drugs are the most efficacious antiplatelet agents, they are very expensive. Another major disadvantage is that they can be given only by the IV route.

Intermittent claudication (IC) is a condition caused by insufficient blood flow to skeletal muscles in the lower limbs. Ischemia of skeletal muscles causes severe pain on walking, particularly in the calf muscles. Although some of the therapies for myocardial ischemia are beneficial in treating IC, two drugs are used *only* for this disorder. Pentoxifylline has antiplatelet action and acts on RBCs to reduce their viscosity and increase their flexibility, thus allowing them to enter vessels that are partially occluded and reduce hypoxia and pain in the muscle. Cilostazol inhibits platelet aggregation and promotes vasodilation, which brings additional blood to ischemic muscles. Both drugs are given orally and show only modest improvement in IC symptoms. Exercise and therapeutic lifestyle changes are necessary for maximum benefit.

NURSING CONSIDERATIONS

The role of the nurse in antiplatelet therapy involves careful monitoring of the client's condition and providing education as it relates to the prescribed drug regimen. Drugs affecting platelet aggregation increase the risk of bleeding when the client sustains trauma or undergoes medical procedures or surgery. These drugs are sometimes given in addition to anticoagulants, which further increases bleeding risk. Injection or venipuncture wounds will require prolonged direct pressure to control bleeding. Observe for ecchymoses and monitor bleeding time following venipunctures. Bleeding lasting more than 10 minutes may require special medical or nursing interventions, such as suturing or "sand-bagging" a large venipuncture site.

ASA may cause gastritis or GI bleeding due to inhibition of prostaglandins in the GI tract (prostaglandins increase bicarbonate and mucous layer production). ASA and ticlopidine may cause nausea and GI upset. Nursing interventions for ASA therapy can be found in "Nursing Process Focus: Clients Receiving NSAID Therapy" in Chapter 19.

Client education as it relates to antiplatelet agents should include goals; reasons for obtaining baseline data such as vital signs, diagnostic procedures, and laboratory tests; and possible side effects. Following are important points to include when teaching clients regarding antiplatelet agents:

- Avoid strenuous and hazardous activities that could result in bleeding injury.
- Do not take OTC products containing ASA, due to increased risk of bleeding, unless otherwise directed by healthcare provider.
- If taking antiplatelet agents concurrently with anticoagulants, be aware that the risk of bleeding is greater.
- Report spontaneous nosebleeds, bleeding gums, excessive bruising, and other signs of bleeding to the healthcare provider.

THROMBOLYTICS

Thrombolytics promote fibrinolysis, or clot destruction, by converting plasminogen to plasmin. The enzyme plasmin digests fibrin and breaks down fibrinogen, prothrombin, and other plasma proteins and clotting factors. Unlike the anticoagulants, thrombolytics actually bring about dissolution (lysis) of the insoluble fibrin within intravascular

NATURAL THERAPIES

Garlic for Cardiovascular Health

Garlic (*Allium sativum*) is one of the best-studied herbs. Purported indications for garlic include arteriosclerosis, common cold, cough/bronchitis, high cholesterol, hypertension, and tendency to infection. It has been proven to be of value in only a few of these disorders.

Several different substances, known as alliaceous oils, have been isolated from garlic and shown to have pharmacological activity. Dosage forms include eating prepared garlic oil or the fresh bulbs from the plant.

Garlic has been shown to decrease the aggregation or "stickiness" of platelets, thus producing an anticoagulant effect. Platelet aggregation on roughened walls of arteries damaged by atherosclerosis commonly initiates the formation of blood clots that lead to heart attacks and strokes. Claims that garlic can reduce heart disease and the incidence of stroke may be related to this action. Clients taking anticoagulant medications should limit their intake of garlic to avoid bleeding complications.

Pr PROTOTYPE DRUG | Clopidogrel (Plavix)

ACTIONS AND USES

Clopidogrel prolongs bleeding time by inhibiting platelet aggregation. It is used to prevent thrombi formation in clients at risk of stroke or MI and to prevent postoperative DVT. Because the drug is expensive but has anticoagulant activity similar to ASA, it is usually prescribed for clients unable to tolerate ASA. It is given orally.

PHARMACOKINETICS

The onset of action is less than 24 hours. The active metabolite of clopidogrel rather than the parent compound is responsible for the antiplatelet action. The active metabolite is 94% protein bound and, once metabolized, it is excreted in urine and feces. Half-life of the active metabolite is 8 hours.

ADMINISTRATION ALERTS

- Do not crush or split tablets.
- Discontinue drug 1 week before surgery.
- Clopidogrel is pregnancy category B.

ADVERSE EFFECTS AND INTERACTIONS

Side effects are similar to ASA and include headache, dizziness, rash, pruritus, and cough. Upon discontinuation of therapy, the anticoagulant activity may persist for up to 5 days. Overdose with risk of hemorrhage may be treated with platelet infusions.

Numerous drug-drug and drug-herbal interactions may occur. Increased risk of bleeding may occur with concurrent use of NSAIDs, other anticoagulants, and natural products such as arnica, chamomile, clove, feverfew, ginger, ginkgo, garlic, ginseng, and others.

TABLE 26.4	Thrombolytics
Drug	**Route and Adult Dose**
alteplase (Activase)	IV; begin with 60 mg and then infuse 20 mg/h over next 2 h
anistreplase (Eminase)	IV; 30 units over 2–5 min
reteplase (Retavase) (see page 299 for the Prototype Drug box)	IV; 10 units over 2 min; repeat dose in 30 min
streptokinase (Streptase)	IV; 250,000–1.5 million units over a short time
urokinase (Abbokinase)	IV; 4400–6000 units administered over several minutes to 12 h

emboli and thrombi. Their therapeutic effect is proportional to the time frame in which they are administered—they are more effective when given as soon as possible after clot formation occurs, preferably within 4 hours.

26.7 Pharmacotherapy with Thrombolytics

It is often mistakenly believed that the purpose of anticoagulants such as heparin or warfarin is to dissolve pre-existing clots, but this is not the case. A totally different class of drugs is needed for this purpose. The thrombolytics, shown in Table 26.4, are administered quite differently than the anticoagulants and produce their effects by different mechanisms. Thrombolytics are prescribed for disorders in which an intravascular clot has already formed, such as acute myocardial infarction, pulmonary embolism, acute ischemic cerebrovascular accident, and deep vein thrombosis (DVT).

Thrombolytics are non-specific; that is, they will dissolve whatever clots they encounter. Because clotting is a natural and desirable process to prevent excessive bleeding, thrombolytics have a narrow margin of safety between dissolving "abnormal" and "normal" clots. Vital signs must be monitored continuously and any signs of bleeding may call for discontinuation of therapy. Because these drugs are rapidly destroyed in the bloodstream, discontinuation normally results in immediate termination of thrombolytic activity. After the clot is successfully dissolved with the thrombolytic, anticoagulant therapy is generally initiated to prevent the reformation of clots.

Since the discovery of streptokinase, the first thrombolytic, there have been a number of ensuing generations of thrombolytics. The newer drugs such as tenecteplase, or TNK t-PA, are more fibrin specific and are reported to have fewer side effects than streptokinase. Tissue plasminogen activator (t-PA), marketed as alteplase, has replaced urokinase as the drug of choice in clearing thrombosed central intravenous lines. Urokinase was removed from the market due to the possibility of viral contamination, because it is obtained from pooled human donors.

Pr PROTOTYPE DRUG | Alteplase (Activase)

ACTIONS AND USES

Produced through recombinant DNA technology, alteplase is identical to the enzyme human tissue plasminogen activator (t-PA). Like other thrombolytics, the primary action of alteplase is to convert plasminogen to plasmin, which then dissolves fibrin clots. To achieve maximum effect, therapy should begin immediately after the onset of symptoms. Alteplase does not exhibit the allergic reactions seen with streptokinase. An unlabelled use is for restoration of patency of IV catheters.

PHARMACOKINETICS

The onset of action for IV alteplase is 5 to 10 minutes. It is rapidly metabolized by the liver. Half-life is 0.5 hours.

ADMINISTRATION ALERTS

- Drug must be given within 6 hours of the onset of symptoms of MI and within 3 hours of thrombotic CVA for maximum effectiveness.
- Avoid IM injections, IV punctures, and arterial punctures during infusion to decrease the risk of bleeding.
- Alteplase is pregnancy category C.

ADVERSE EFFECTS AND INTERACTIONS

Thrombolytics such as alteplase are contraindicated in clients with active bleeding or with a history of recent trauma. Trauma may include, but is not limited to, physical injury, surgery, biopsies, or childbirth (within the 10-day postpartum period). The nurse must carefully monitor the client for signs of bleeding every 15 minutes for the first hour of therapy and every 30 minutes thereafter. Signs of bleeding such as spontaneous ecchymoses, hematomas, or epistaxis should be reported to the healthcare provider immediately.

Use with caution with herbal supplements, such as ginkgo, which may cause an increased thrombolytic effect.

 See the Companion Website for a Nursing Process Focus Chart specific to this drug.

NURSING CONSIDERATIONS

The role of the nurse in thrombolytic therapy involves careful monitoring of the client's condition and providing education as it relates to the prescribed drug regimen. Thrombolytics are generally administered in the critical care or emergency department setting. Identify conditions that exclude the client from receiving thrombolytics, such as recent trauma, surgery, biopsy, arterial emboli, cerebral embolism, hemorrhage, thrombocytopenia, septic thrombophlebitis, or childbirth (within 10 days). Baseline coagulation tests (aPTT, bleeding time, PT, and/or INR) should be obtained prior to therapy. Baseline Hct, hemoglobin, and platelet counts should be obtained so they may be compared to later values to assess for bleeding. Cerebral hemorrhage is a major concern; thus, assess for changes in level of consciousness and check neurological status. When given for myocardial infarction, observe for dysrhythmias that may occur as cardiac tissue perfusion is re-established. IM injections are contraindicated during thrombolytic therapy due to the risk of bleeding.

See "Nursing Process Focus: Clients Receiving Thrombolytic Therapy" for specific teaching points.

These drugs are often given in acute situations when time for client teaching may be limited and the client may be unable to focus on information due to the stress of the situation. This information can be discussed further when the client is ready.

ANTIFIBRINOLYTICS

Antifibrinolytics have an action opposite to that of anticoagulants: to shorten bleeding time. They are used to prevent excessive bleeding following surgery.

NURSING PROCESS FOCUS   Clients Receiving Thrombolytic Therapy

Assessment	Potential Nursing Diagnoses/Identified Patterns
Prior to administration: ■ Obtain complete health history including recent surgeries or trauma, allergies, drug history, and possible drug interactions. ■ Obtain vital signs; assess in context of client's baseline values. ■ Assess lab values: aPTT, PT, Hgb, Hct, platelet count.	■ Adequate knowledge regarding drug therapy and adverse effects ■ Safety from injury (bleeding) related to adverse effects of thrombolytic therapy ■ Effective tissue perfusion with decrease in size of thrombus

Planning: Client Goals and Expected Outcomes

The client will:
■ Experience dissolving of pre-existing blood clot(s) as evidenced by laboratory values ordered by the healthcare provider
■ Demonstrate an understanding of the drug's action by accurately describing drug side effects and precautions

Implementation

Interventions (Rationales)	Client Education/Discharge Planning
■ If necessary, start IV lines, arterial line, and Foley catheter prior to beginning therapy. (This decreases the risk of bleeding from those sites.) ■ Monitor vital signs every 15 minutes during first hour of infusion, then every 30 minutes during remainder of infusion. ■ Client should be moved as little as possible during the infusion. (This is done to prevent internal injury.) ■ If given for thrombotic CVA, monitor neurological status frequently. ■ Monitor cardiac response while medication is infusing. (Dysrhythmias may occur with reperfusion of myocardium.) ■ Monitor blood tests (Hct, Hgb, platelet counts) during and after therapy for indications of blood loss due to internal bleeding. (Client has increased risk of bleeding for 2 to 4 days post-infusion.)	■ Instruct client about procedures and why they are necessary prior to beginning thrombolytic therapy. Advise client: ■ Of the need for frequent taking of vital signs ■ That activity will be limited during infusion, and a pressure dressing may be needed to prevent any active bleeding ■ Advise client about assessments and why they are necessary. ■ Advise client that cardiac rhythm will be monitored during therapy. ■ Instruct client of increased risk for bleeding and need for activity restriction and frequent monitoring during this time.

Evaluation of Outcome Criteria

Evaluate the effectiveness of drug therapy by confirming that client goals and expected outcomes have been met (see "Planning").

See Table 26.4 for a list of drugs to which these nursing actions apply.

26.8 Pharmacotherapy with Antifibrinolytics

The final class of coagulation modifiers, the antifibrinolytics, is a small group of drugs used to prevent and treat excessive bleeding from surgical sites. All of the antifibrinolytics have very specific indications for use and none are commonly prescribed. Although their mechanisms differ, all drugs in this class prevent fibrin from dissolving, thus enhancing the stability of the clot. Because of their ability to slow blood flow, they are sometimes classified as hemostatic agents.

Desmopressin differs from the others in being a hormone similar to vasopressin, a hormone naturally present in the body that promotes the renal conservation of water. Unlike the other antifibrinolytics, it has uses beyond hemostasis that include the control of excessive or nocturnal urination (enuresis). The antifibrinolytics are listed in Table 26.5.

NURSING CONSIDERATIONS

The role of the nurse in antifibrinolytic therapy involves careful monitoring of the client's condition and providing education as it relates to the prescribed drug regimen. Assess for clotting. Changes in peripheral pulses, paresthesias, positive Homans' sign, and prominence of superficial veins indicate clotting occurring in peripheral arterial or venous vasculature. Chest pain and shortness of breath may indicate pulmonary thrombus or embolus. Use is contraindicated in clients with disseminated intravascular clotting and severe renal impairment.

Antifibrinolytics are administered intravenously. Monitor injection sites frequently for thrombophlebitis and extravasation. Antifibrinolytics may affect the muscles, causing wasting and weakness. Identify and report the presence of myopathy and myoglobinuria, manifesting as reddish-brown urine.

Client education as it relates to antifibrinolytic agents should include goals; reasons for obtaining baseline data such as vital signs, diagnostic procedures, and laboratory tests; and possible side effects. Following are important points to include when teaching clients regarding antifibrinolytic agents:

- Report renewed bleeding episodes.
- Avoid the use of ASA and OTC medications containing ASA.
- Report the following immediately: excessive bleeding following a medical or dental procedure, altered colour vision, decreased amounts of urine, and pain, numbness, or tingling in the extremities.

TABLE 26.5 Antifibrinolytics	
Drug	**Route and Adult Dose**
aminocaproic acid (Amicar)	IV; 4–5 g for 1 hour, then 1–1.25 g/h until bleeding is controlled
aprotinin (Trasylol)	IV; 15,000 units as a test dose, then give 500,000 units during surgery
tranexamic acid (Cyklokapron)	PO; 25 mg/kg qid

Pr PROTOTYPE DRUG | Aminocaproic Acid (Amicar)

ACTIONS AND USES

Aminocaproic acid acts by inactivating plasminogen, the precursor of the enzyme plasmin that digests the fibrin clot. Aminocaproic acid is prescribed in situations where there is excessive bleeding due to clots being dissolved prematurely. During acute hemorrhages, it can be given IV to reduce bleeding in 1 to 2 hours. It is most commonly prescribed following surgery to reduce postoperative bleeding. The therapeutic serum level is 100 to 400 µg/mL.

PHARMACOKINETICS

The onset and duration of action and half-life for oral aminocaproic acid are unknown. It is widely distributed and excreted mostly unchanged by the kidneys.

ADMINISTRATION ALERTS

- This drug may cause hypotension and bradycardia when given IV. Assess vital signs frequently and place client on cardiac monitor to assess for dysrhythmias.
- Aminocaproic acid is pregnancy category C.

ADVERSE EFFECTS AND INTERACTIONS

Since aminocaproic acid tends to stabilize clots, it should be used cautiously in clients with a history of thromboembolic disease. Side effects are generally mild.

Drug interactions include hypercoagulation with concurrent use of estrogens and oral contraceptives.

 See the Companion Website for a Nursing Process Focus Chart specific to this drug.

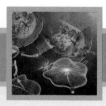

CHAPTER REVIEW

KEY CONCEPTS

The numbered key concepts provide a succinct summary of the important points from the corresponding numbered section within the chapter. If any of these points are not clear, refer to the numbered section within the chapter for review. Expanded versions can be found on the Companion Website.

26.1 Hemostasis is a complex process involving multiple steps and a large number of enzymes and factors. The final product is a fibrin clot that stops blood loss.

26.2 Fibrinolysis, or removal of a blood clot, is an enzymatic process initiated by the release of t-PA. Plasmin digests the fibrin strands, thus restoring circulation to the injured area.

26.3 Diseases of hemostasis include thromboembolic disorders caused by thrombi and emboli and bleeding disorders such as hemophilia and von Willebrand's disease.

26.4 The normal coagulation process can be modified by a number of different mechanisms, including inhibiting clotting factors, dissolving fibrin, and influencing platelet function.

26.5 Anticoagulants prevent clot formation. The primary drugs in this category are heparin (parenteral) and warfarin (oral).

26.6 Several drugs prolong bleeding time by interfering with the aggregation of platelets. Antiplatelet agents include ASA, ADP blockers, and glycoprotein IIb/IIIa receptor blockers.

26.7 Thrombolytics are used to dissolve existing intravascular clots in clients with MI and CVA.

26.8 Antifibrinolytics are used to promote the formation of clots in clients with excessive bleeding from surgical sites.

REVIEW QUESTIONS

1 Which clotting factors are always circulating in the blood? Which are only formed after coagulation has been initiated?

2 Both warfarin and heparin are effective anticoagulants. Why would a healthcare provider choose heparin over warfarin?

3 Explain why the commonly used term for anticoagulants, *blood thinners,* is not correct.

4 A client has begun to hemorrhage while being infused with alteplase (t-PA). What action should be taken?

CRITICAL THINKING QUESTIONS

1. The nurse is working on a medical unit where a client suddenly develops left-sided weakness and garbled speech. The nurse calls the physician. Since the client appears to be having a CVA, heparin 5000 units IV to infuse continuously at 1000 units per hour is ordered. What nursing actions are required in carrying out this order? What additional care is required for the client and the client's family?

2. A client has had an acute myocardial infarction and is to receive alteplase (Activase) to lyse the clot. What nursing action should be taken prior to the client receiving the medication? What are some priorities for care once the drug is commenced?

3. A client is receiving enoxaparin SC after being diagnosed with thrombophlebitis. What precautions should be taken when giving this medication?

EXPLORE
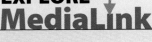
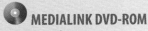

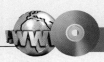

www.pearsoned.ca/adams-king

MEDIALINK DVD-ROM
- Audio Glossary
- CRNE Review
- Animations
  Mechanism of Action: Heparin
  Mechanism of Action: Warfarin

COMPANION WEBSITE
- CRNE Review
- Case Study: Client taking anticoagulants
- Dosage Calculations

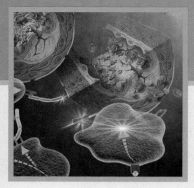

CHAPTER 27

Drugs for Shock

DRUGS AT A GLANCE

FLUID REPLACEMENT AGENTS
Blood and blood products
Crystalloid solutions
Colloid solutions
> *normal human serum albumin (Albuminar, others)*

VASOCONSTRICTORS
> *norepinephrine (Levophed, Norepinephrine Bitartrate)*

CARDIOTONIC AGENTS
> *dopamine (Dopastat, others)*

OBJECTIVES

After reading this chapter, the student should be able to do the following:

1. Relate the symptoms of the different types of shock to their physiological causes.
2. Explain the initial treatment for a client who is in shock.
3. Identify drug classes used for treating shock.
4. Explain the therapeutic action of each class of drug used for shock in relation to the pathophysiology of shock.
5. Compare and contrast the use of colloids and crystalloids in fluid replacement therapy.
6. Describe the nurse's role in the pharmacological management of clients receiving drugs for shock.
7. For each of the drug classes listed in Drugs at a Glance, identify a representative drug and explain its mechanism of action, therapeutic effects, and important adverse effects.
8. Describe and explain, based on pharmacological principles, the rationale for nursing assessment, planning, and interventions for clients being treated for shock.
9. Use the nursing process to care for clients receiving drug therapy for shock.

MediaLink

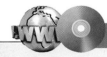

www.pearsoned.ca/adams-king

CRNE review, case studies, and other interactive resources for this chapter can be found on the Companion Website at **www.pearsoned.ca/adams-king**. Click on "Chapter 27" to select the activities for this chapter. For animations, more CRNE review questions, and an audio glossary, access the accompanying DVD-ROM in this textbook.

Shock is a condition in which vital tissues are not receiving enough blood to function properly. Without adequate oxygen and other nutrients, cells cannot carry out normal metabolic processes. Shock is considered a medical emergency; failure to reverse the causes and symptoms of shock may lead to irreversible organ damage and death. This chapter examines how drugs are used to aid in the treatment of different types of shock.

PHARMFACTS

Shock

- Cardiogenic shock, because it responds poorly to treatment, is the most lethal form of shock and has an 80% to 100% mortality rate.
- Hypovolemic shock carries a 10% to 31% mortality rate.
- With anaphylactic or distributive shock, death can ensue within minutes if treatment is not available.
- Septic or "warm" shock, usually caused by gram-negative bacteria, has a mortality rate of 40% to 70% but can be as high as 90%, depending on the causative organism.

27.1 Characteristics of Shock

Shock is a collection of signs and symptoms, many of which are non-specific, that occur when vital tissues are not receiving enough blood to function. Although symptoms vary somewhat among the different kinds of shock, some similarities exist. The client appears pale and may claim to feel sick or weak without reporting specific complaints. Behavioural changes are often some of the earliest symptoms and may include restlessness, anxiety, confusion, depression, and apathy. Lack of sufficient blood flow to the brain may result in fainting. Thirst is a common complaint. The skin may feel cold or clammy. Without immediate treatment, multiple body systems will be affected and respiratory failure or renal failure may result. Figure 27.1 shows common symptoms of a client in shock.

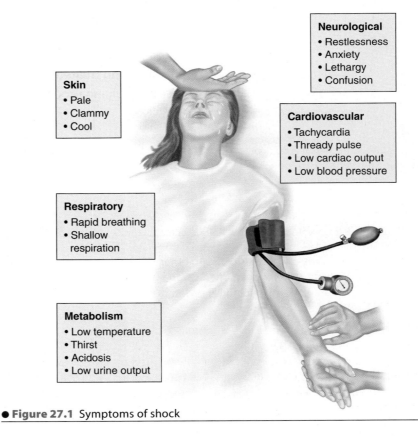

Neurological
- Restlessness
- Anxiety
- Lethargy
- Confusion

Skin
- Pale
- Clammy
- Cool

Cardiovascular
- Tachycardia
- Thready pulse
- Low cardiac output
- Low blood pressure

Respiratory
- Rapid breathing
- Shallow respiration

Metabolism
- Low temperature
- Thirst
- Acidosis
- Low urine output

● **Figure 27.1** Symptoms of shock

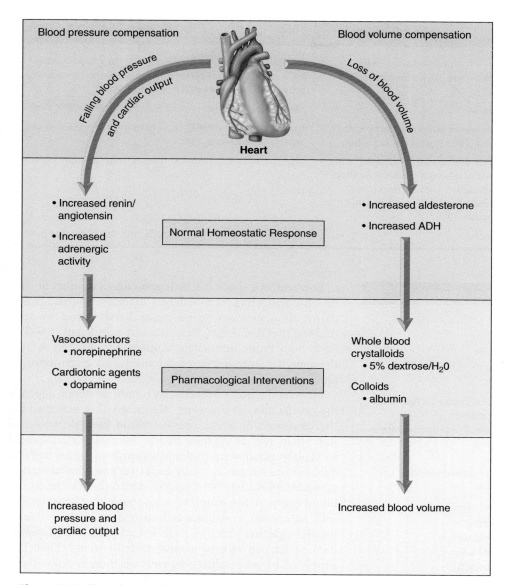

● **Figure 27.2** Physiological changes during circulatory shock and pharmacological intervention

The central problem in most types of shock is the inability of the cardiovascular system to send sufficient blood to the vital organs, with the heart and brain being affected early in the progression of the condition. Assessing the client's cardiovascular status will often give important indications for a diagnosis of shock. Blood pressure is usually low and cardiac output diminished. Heart rate may be rapid with a weak pulse. Breathing is usually rapid and shallow. Figure 27.2 illustrates the physiological changes that occur during circulatory shock.

27.2 Causes of Shock

Shock is often classified by naming the underlying pathological process or organ system causing the condition. Table 27.1 lists the different types of shock and their primary causes.

Diagnosis of shock is rarely based on non-specific symptoms. A careful medical history, however, may give the nurse valuable clues as to what type of shock may be present.

For example, obvious trauma or bleeding would suggest **hypovolemic shock**, related to volume depletion. If trauma to the brain or spinal cord is evident, **neurogenic shock**, a type of distributive shock caused by a sudden loss of nerve impulse communication, may be suspected. A history of heart disease would suggest **cardiogenic shock**, which is caused by a loss of adequate cardiac output due to pump failure. A recent infection may indicate **septic shock**, a type of distributive shock caused by the presence of bacteria and toxins in the blood. A history of allergy with a sudden onset of symptoms following food or drug intake may suggest **anaphylactic shock**, the most severe type I allergic response.

FLUID REPLACEMENT AGENTS

Certain agents are used to replace blood or other fluids lost during hypovolemic shock. Fluid replacement therapy includes blood, blood products, colloids, and crystalloids, as shown in Table 27.2.

TABLE 27.1	Common Types of Shock	
Type of Shock	**Definition**	**Underlying Pathology**
cardiogenic	failure of the heart to pump sufficient blood to tissues	left heart failure, myocardial ischemia, myocardial infarction, dysrhythmias, pulmonary embolism, myocardial or pericardial infection
hypovolemic	loss of blood volume	hemorrhage, burns, profuse sweating, excessive urination, vomiting, diarrhea
neurogenic	vasodilation due to overstimulation of the parasympathetic or understimulation of the sympathetic nervous systems	trauma to spinal cord or medulla, severe emotional stress or pain, drugs that depress the central nervous system
septic	multiple organ dysfunction as a result of pathogenic organisms in the blood resulting in vasodilation and changes in permeability of capillaries; often a precursor to acute respiratory distress syndrome (ARDS) and disseminated intravascular coagulation (DIC)	widespread inflammatory response to bacterial, fungal, or parasitic infection
anaphylactic	acute allergic reaction	severe reaction to allergen such as penicillin, nuts, shellfish, or animal proteins

TABLE 27.2	Fluid Replacement Agents
Agent	**Examples**
blood products	• whole blood • plasma protein fraction • fresh frozen plasma • packed red blood cells
colloids	• plasma protein fraction (Plasmanate, Plasma-Plex, Plasmatein, PPF, Protenate) • dextran 40 (Gentran 40, Hyskon, Rheomacrodex) or dextran 70 (Macrodex) • hetastarch (Hespan) • normal human serum albumin (Albuminar, Buminate, Plasbumin)
crystalloids	• normal saline (0.9% sodium chloride) • lactated Ringer's solution • Plasmalyte (hypertonic solution) • hypertonic saline (3% sodium chloride) • 5% dextrose in water (D5W)

27.3 Treatment Priorities for Shock

Shock is treated as a medical emergency, and the first goal is to maintain basic life support. Rapid identification of the underlying cause, followed by aggressive treatment, is essential since the client's condition may deteriorate rapidly without specific, emergency measures. The initial nursing interventions consist of keeping the client quiet and warm and offering psychological support and reassurance. Maintaining the ABCs of life support—airway, breathing, and circulation—to sustain normal blood pressure is critical. The client is immediately connected to a cardiac monitor and a pulse oximeter is applied. Blood pressure readings are taken on the opposite arm of the pulse oximeter since peripheral vasoconstriction with the inflation of the cuff will alter oximetry readings. Unless contraindicated, oxygen is administered at 15 L/min via a non-rebreather mask. Neurological status and level of consciousness are monitored.

Hypovolemic shock can be triggered by a number of conditions, including hemorrhage, extensive burns, severe dehydration, persistent vomiting or diarrhea, and intensive diuretic therapy. If the client has lost significant blood or other body fluids, immediate maintenance of blood volume through the administration of fluid and electrolytes or blood products is essential.

Blood and blood products may be administered, depending on the clinical situation. Whole blood is indicated for the treatment of acute, massive blood loss (depletion of more than 30% of the total volume) when there is the need to replace plasma volume and supply red blood cells to increase the oxygen-carrying capacity. The administration of whole blood has been largely replaced with the use of blood components. A unit of whole blood can be separated into its specific constituents (red and white blood cells, platelets, plasma proteins, fresh frozen plasma, and globulins), which can be used to treat more than one client. The supply of blood products depends on human donors and requires careful crossmatching to ensure compatibility between the donor and the recipient. Whole blood, while carefully screened, has the potential to transmit serious infections such as hepatitis and HIV.

CRYSTALLOIDS AND COLLOIDS

27.4 Treating Shock with Crystalloids and Colloids

Because it is safer to administer only the needed components, rather than whole blood, other products are used to provide volume expansion and to sustain blood pressure. These are of two basic types: colloids and crystalloids. Colloid and crystalloid infusions are often used when up to one-third of an adult's blood volume has been lost.

Colloids are proteins or other large molecules that stay suspended in the blood for a long period because they are too large to cross membranes. While circulating, they draw water molecules from the cells and tissues into the blood vessels through their ability to increase **oncotic pressure**.

Blood product colloids include normal human serum albumin, plasma protein fraction, and serum globulins. The non-blood product colloids are dextran (40, 70, and high molecular weight) and hetastarch. These agents are indicated to provide life-sustaining support following massive hemorrhage, for plasma exchange, and to treat shock, burns, acute liver failure, and neonatal hemolytic disease.

Crystalloids are IV solutions that contain electrolytes in concentrations resembling those of plasma. Unlike colloids, crystalloid solutions can readily leave the blood and enter cells. They are used to replace fluids that have been lost and to promote urine output. Common crystalloids include normal saline, hypertonic saline, lactated Ringer's solution, and 5% dextrose in water (D5W).

NURSING CONSIDERATIONS

The role of the nurse in crystalloid and colloid therapy for shock involves careful monitoring of the client's condition and providing education as it relates to the prescribed drug regimen. Because of the ability of all colloids to pull fluid into the vascular space, circulatory overload is a serious adverse outcome. Monitoring for blood pressure changes is essential; pressure may increase with a healthy heart, or decrease if the heart fails with fluid overload. Lung sounds must also be monitored; crackles will be heard with pulmonary congestion. Pulse oximetry can be utilized to monitor for changes in oxygenation that may become evident before lung sounds change. Monitoring intake, output, and body weight will assist in assessing fluid retention or loss.

These products are used with caution in lactation and pregnancy (category C).

Anaphylactic reactions may occur with the use of plasma protein fraction, dextran 75, dextran 70, and hetastarch. Signs and symptoms of an allergic response may include periorbital edema, urticaria, wheezing, and difficulty breathing. The use of dextran, a high molecular weight polysaccharide, is further limited because it can interfere with coagulation and platelet adhesion. Hetastarch, a synthetic starch resembling human glycogen, can increase the PT, PTT, and bleeding time when given in large doses, thus limiting its use in conditions where normal clotting is essential. Clients with renal failure who are exhibiting anuria or oliguria are at great risk for fluid overload because of the fluid shift that will occur and their inability to rid the body of excess fluid through urination.

Client education as it relates to fluid replacement therapy should include goals, reasons for obtaining baseline data such as vital signs and tests for cardiac and renal function, and possible side effects. Instruct the client to immediately report difficulty breathing, wheezing, and itching as they may indicate an allergic response. See "Nursing Process Focus: Clients Receiving Fluid Replacement Therapy" in this chapter for more teaching points.

VASOCONSTRICTORS

In some types of shock, the most serious medical challenge facing the client is hypotension, which may become so profound as to cause collapse of the circulatory system. Vasoconstrictors are drugs for maintaining blood pressure when fluid replacement agents have proven ineffective. These agents are shown in Table 27.3.

Pr PROTOTYPE DRUG | Normal Human Serum Albumin (Albuminar, others)

ACTIONS AND USES

Normal serum **albumin** is a protein extracted from whole blood, plasma, or placental human plasma that contains 96% albumin and 4% globulins and other proteins. Albumin naturally comprises about 60% of all blood proteins. Its normal functions are to maintain plasma osmotic pressure and to shuttle certain substances through the blood, including a substantial number of drug molecules. After extraction from blood or plasma, it is sterilized to remove possible contamination by the hepatitis viruses or HIV.

Administered IV, albumin increases the osmotic pressure of the blood and moves fluid from the tissues to the general circulation. It is used to restore plasma volume in hypovolemic shock or to restore blood proteins in clients with hypoproteinemia. It has an immediate onset of action and is available in concentrations of 5% and 25%.

PHARMACOKINETICS

Albumin is confined to the intravascular space, unless vascular permeability is increased. Its half-life is 2 to 3 weeks.

ADMINISTRATION ALERTS

- Higher concentrations must be infused more slowly because the risk of a large, rapid fluid shift is greater.
- Use a large gauge (16–20) IV cannula for administration of drug.
- Albumin is pregnancy category C.

ADVERSE EFFECTS AND INTERACTIONS

Because albumin is a natural blood product, allergic reactions are possible. However, coagulation factors, antibodies, and most other blood proteins have been removed; therefore, the incidence of allergic reactions from albumin is not high. Signs of allergy include fever, chills, rash, dyspnea, and possibly hypotension. Protein overload may occur if excessive albumin is infused.

No clinically significant drug interactions have been established.

 See the Companion Website for a Nursing Process Focus Chart specific to this drug.

NURSING PROCESS FOCUS   Clients Receiving Fluid Replacement Therapy

Assessment	Potential Nursing Diagnoses/Identified Patterns
Prior to administration: ■ Obtain complete health history including allergies, drug history, and possible drug interactions. ■ Assess lung sounds. ■ Obtain vital signs. ■ Assess level of consciousness. ■ Assess renal function (BUN and creatinine).	■ Adequate knowledge regarding drug therapy and adverse effects ■ Safety from physical injury related to adverse effects of drug therapy ■ Effective tissue perfusion ■ Fluid and electrolyte balance ■ Comfort

Planning: Client Goals and Expected Outcomes

The client will:
■ Immediately report difficulty breathing
■ Report itching, flushing
■ Maintain urinary output at least 50 ml/h
■ Have vital signs within normal range for client
■ Experience a safe environment with no evidence of physical injury
■ Demonstrate an understanding of drug therapy by accurately describing intended effects, side effects, and precautions

Implementation

Interventions (Rationales)	Client Education/Discharge Planning
■ Monitor respiratory status. (Effects of drugs and rapid infusion may result in fluid overload.) ■ Monitor intake and output for changes in renal function. ■ Monitor electrolytes. (Crystalloid drugs may cause hypernatremia and resulting fluid retention.) ■ Observe client for signs of allergic reactions. (Administration of blood and blood products could cause allergic reactions.) ■ Observe urine for changes in colour. (Adverse reaction to blood could cause hematuria.)	Instruct client to: ■ Report any signs of respiratory distress ■ Report changes in sensorium such as light-headedness, drowsiness, or dizziness ■ Instruct client concerning rationale for Foley catheter insertion. ■ Instruct client to report any evidence of edema. Instruct client: ■ To report itching, rash, chills, and difficulty breathing ■ That frequent blood draws are necessary to monitor possible complications of drug administration ■ Instruct client to notify the healthcare provider if changes in urine colour occur.

Evaluation of Outcome Criteria

Evaluate the effectiveness of drug therapy by confirming that client goals and expected outcomes have been met (see "Planning").

See Table 27.2 for a list of the drugs to which these nursing actions apply.

TABLE 27.3	Vasoconstrictors for Shock
Drug	**Route and Adult Dose**
Non-Specific Alpha- and Beta-Adrenergic Agonists	
Ⓟ norepinephrine (Levophed, Norepinephrine Bitartrate)	IV; 2–12 μg/min until pressure stabilizes, then 2–4 μg/min for maintenance
Specific Alpha-Adrenergic Agonists	
methoxamine (Vasoxyl) phenylephrine (Neo-Synephrine, others)	IV; 3–5 mg over 5–10 min IV; 0.1–0.18 mg/min until pressure stabilizes, then 0.04–0.06 mg/min for maintenance

27.5 Treating Shock with Vasoconstrictors

In the early stages of shock, the body compensates for the fall in blood pressure by increasing the activity of the sympathetic nervous system. This sympathetic activity results in vasoconstriction, thus raising blood pressure and increasing the rate and force of myocardial contraction. The purpose of these compensatory measures is to maintain blood flow to vital organs such as the heart and brain and to decrease flow to other organs, including the kidneys and liver.

The body's ability to compensate is limited, however, and profound hypotension may develop as shock progresses. In severe cases, fluid replacement agents alone are not effective at raising blood pressure and other medications are indicated. Historically, sympathomimetic vasoconstrictors have been used to stabilize blood pressure in shock clients. When given intravenously, these drugs will immediately raise blood pressure. Because of side effects and potential organ damage due to the rapid and extreme vasoconstriction, these drugs are used as a last resort. These emergency drugs are considered critical care agents. Sympathomimetics used for shock include norepinephrine, isoproterenol, methoxamine, and phenylephrine. The basic pharmacology of the beta-adrenergic agonists, or sympathomimetics, is presented in Chapter 13.

NURSING CONSIDERATIONS

The role of the nurse in vasoconstrictor therapy for shock involves careful monitoring of the client's condition and providing education as it relates to the prescribed drug regimen. Prior to administration, assess for history of narrow-angle glaucoma and cardiovascular disease, and obtain an ECG reading. Vasoconstrictors are contraindicated in clients with severe cardiovascular disease and narrow-angle glaucoma as they may worsen these conditions. Assess blood pressure, pulse, and urine output.

In addition to many of the adverse effects described in the Prototype Drug box for norepinephrine, other drugs in this class could cause additional side effects. Phenylephrine will cause necrosis of tissue if extravasation occurs. Ensure IV patency prior to beginning the infusion and observe the IV site during the entire infusion. Monitor blood pressure and titrate the drip if blood pressure is elevated. Urine output should be monitored because extreme vasoconstriction may lead to decreased renal perfusion.

Monitor the client for chest pain and ECG changes. Dosages are usually reduced if the heart rate exceeds 110 beats/minute. Monitor mental status, skin temperature of extremities, and colour of ear lobes, nail beds, and lips.

Client education as it relates to vasoconstrictor therapy should include goals, reasons for obtaining baseline data such as vital signs and tests for cardiac function, and possible side effects. Explain to the client the use of medication and the rationale for frequent monitoring. Instruct the client to immediately report any pain or burning at the IV site. See "Nursing Process Focus: Clients Receiving Adrenergic Therapy" in Chapter 13, page 317, for the complete nursing process applied to caring for clients receiving beta-adrenergic agonists (sympathomimetics).

CARDIOTONIC AGENTS

Cardiotonic drugs increase the force of contraction of the heart. In the treatment of shock, they are used to increase

---

Pr PROTOTYPE DRUG | Norepinephrine (Levophed, Norepinephrine Bitartrate)

ACTIONS AND USES

Norepinephrine (NE) is an adrenergic that acts directly on alpha-adrenergic receptors in vascular smooth muscle to immediately raise blood pressure. It also stimulates $beta_1$-receptors in the heart, thus producing a positive inotropic response that increases cardiac output. The primary indications for NE are acute shock and cardiac arrest. NE is the vasopressor of choice for septic shock because research has demonstrated that it significantly decreases mortality.

PHARMACOKINETICS

NE is administered by IV infusion, with an onset of action within 2 minutes. It is widely distributed. It is metabolized by the liver and kidneys. Its half-life is 1 minute. Because its duration of action is only 1 to 2 minutes after the infusion is terminated, discontinuing the drug in the case of overdose may be sufficient.

ADMINISTRATION ALERTS

- Infusion is started only after patency of the IV is ensured. Monitor the infusion rate continuously.
- Phentolamine should be available in case of extravasation.
- Do not abruptly discontinue infusion.
- Norepinephrine is pregnancy category D.

ADVERSE EFFECTS AND INTERACTIONS

NE is a powerful vasoconstrictor, so continuous monitoring of blood pressure is required to detect hypertension. NE should not be administered if hypertension is present. When first administered, reflex bradycardia is sometimes experienced. It also has the ability to produce various types of dysrhythmia. Monitor heart rate and rhythm. Blurred vision and photophobia are signs of overdose.

NE interacts with many drugs, including alpha- and beta-blockers, which may antagonize the drug's vasopressor effects. Conversely, ergot alkaloids and tricyclic antidepressants may potentiate vasopressor effects. Halothane, digoxin, and cyclopropane may increase the risk of dysrhythmias.

 See the Companion Website for a Nursing Process Focus Chart specific to this drug.

TABLE 27.4   Cardiotonic Drugs for Shock

Drug	Route and Adult Dose
digoxin (Lanoxin, Apo-, PMS–Digoxin) (see page 312 for the Prototype Drug box)	IV; digitalizing dose 2.5–5 μg q6h for 24 h; maintenance dose 0.125–0.5 mg qd
dobutamine (Dobutamine, Dobutrex)	IV; infused at a rate of 2.5–40 μg/kg/min for a max of 72 h
dopamine hydrochloride (Dopastat, Inotropin, Revimine)	IV; 1–50 μg/kg/min initial dose; may be increased to 30 μg/kg/min

the cardiac output. The cardiotonic agents are shown in Table 27.4.

27.6 Treating Shock with Cardiotonic Agents

As shock progresses, the heart may begin to fail; cardiac output decreases, lowering the amount of blood reaching vital tissues and deepening the degree of shock. Cardiotonic drugs, also known as **inotropic agents**, have the potential to reverse the cardiac symptoms of shock by increasing the strength of myocardial contraction. Digoxin increases myocardial contractility and cardiac output, thus quickly bringing critical tissues their essential oxygen. Chapter 24 should be reviewed because digoxin and other medications prescribed for heart failure are sometimes used for the treatment of shock.

Dobutamine is a beta$_1$-adrenergic agonist that has value in the short-term treatment of certain types of shock due to its ability to cause the heart to beat more forcefully. Dobutamine is especially beneficial in cases when the primary cause of shock is related to heart failure, not hypovolemia. The resulting increase in cardiac output assists in maintaining blood flow to vital organs. Dobutamine has a half-life of only 2 minutes, and it is only given as an IV infusion.

Dopamine is both an alpha- and beta-receptor agonist. Dopamine is utilized at different dosage levels and will have different effects based on what receptors are most affected. It is primarily used in shock conditions to increase blood pressure by causing peripheral vasoconstriction (alpha$_1$ stimulation) and increasing the force of myocardial contraction (beta$_1$ stimulation). Dopamine has the potential to cause dysrhythmias.

NURSING CONSIDERATIONS

The role of the nurse in cardiotonic therapy for shock involves careful monitoring of the client's condition and providing education as it relates to the prescribed drug regimen. Prior to administration, assess for history of cardiovascular disease, and obtain an ECG. Blood pressure, pulse, urine output, and body weight should also be assessed.

Cardiotonic agents are contraindicated in clients with ventricular tachycardia, because they will worsen dysrhythmia, and in hypertrophic idiopathic subaortic stenosis, because increasing contractility will precipitate heart fail-

ure. Safe use during pregnancy and lactation has not been established (category C). They should be used cautiously in clients who are hypertensive since they increase blood pressure. With atrial fibrillation, a rapid ventricular response may increase heart rate excessively. Hypovolemia should be corrected with whole blood or plasma prior to the start of dopamine infusion.

Cardiotonic medications may be used separately or concurrently with other antishock agents. They are only given as a continuous infusion, and dosage is based on micrograms per kilogram per minute. Careful calculations must be done to arrive at the appropriate number of millilitres per hour in order to set the IV pump to deliver the correct dosage. IV pump technology is such that some will automate calculations, and most have the ability to deliver dosages to a tenth of a millilitre. The IV rate can be found by multiplying the ordered dose times the client's weight in kilograms times 60 (to get micrograms per hour), then dividing this amount by the concentration of the infusion (micrograms per millilitre). The result will be the millilitres per hour the client should receive. Weigh the client each morning. The client's dose is recalculated each day, based on that weight.

Clients should be connected to a cardiac monitor prior to and during the infusion of cardiotonic drugs. Monitor the client's blood pressure frequently. If a pressure monitoring catheter is in place, pulmonary wedge pressure and cardiac output should be assessed to keep these parameters within normal ranges. Initiate the IV in a large vein; a central line is preferable. Extravasation of dopamine can cause severe, localized vasoconstriction resulting in sloughing of tissue and tissue necrosis if not reversed with phentolamine injections at the site of the infiltration. If extravasation occurs, discontinue the IV, restart it in another site, and administer the antidote. If infiltration occurs, dobutamine can be irritating to the vein and surrounding tissues, although it causes less severe vasoconstriction than dopamine.

Monitor renal function closely, including urine output, BUN, and creatinine levels. With improved cardiac output, renal function should improve and urine output increase. Low doses of dopamine increase renal perfusion and should enhance urine output. Foley catheters are frequently employed to ensure accurate measurement of urine output.

Client education as it relates to cardiotonic therapy should include goals, reasons for obtaining baseline data such as vital signs and tests for cardiac and renal function, and possible side effects. Advise the client that continuous cardiac monitoring will occur while receiving the medica-

Pr PROTOTYPE DRUG | Dopamine (Dopastat, others)

ACTIONS AND USES

Dopamine is the immediate metabolic precursor to norepinephrine. While classified as a sympathomimetic, dopamine's mechanism of action is dependent on the dose. At low doses, the drug selectively stimulates dopaminergic receptors, especially in the kidneys, leading to vasodilation and an increased blood flow through the kidneys. This makes dopamine of particular value in treating hypovolemic and cardiogenic shock. At higher doses, dopamine stimulates $beta_1$-adrenergic receptors, causing the heart to beat more forcefully and increasing cardiac output. Another beneficial effect of dopamine when given in higher doses is its ability to stimulate alpha-adrenergic receptors, thus causing vasoconstriction and raising blood pressure.

PHARMACOKINETICS

Dopamine is administered IV only. It is widely distributed but does not cross the blood-brain barrier. It is metabolized rapidly by the liver and kidneys. Its half-life is 2 minutes. Thus, discontinuing the drug in the case of overdose may suffice.

ADMINISTRATION ALERTS

- Drug is given as a continuous infusion only.
- Ensure patency of IV site prior to beginning infusion.
- Phentolamine is the antidote for extravasation of the drug and should be readily available.
- Dopamine is pregnancy category C.

ADVERSE EFFECTS AND INTERACTIONS

Because of its profound effects on the cardiovascular system, the nurse must continuously monitor clients receiving dopamine for signs of dysrhythmias and hypotension. Side effects are normally self-limiting because of the short half-life of the drug. Dopamine is a vesicant drug that can cause severe, irreversible damage if it escapes from the vein into surrounding tissues.

Dopamine interacts with many other drugs. Concurrent administration with MAO inhibitors and ergot alkaloids increases alpha-adrenergic effects. Phenytoin may decrease dopamine action. Beta-blockers may antagonize cardiac effects. Alpha-blockers antagonize peripheral vasoconstriction. Halothane increases the risk of hypertension and ventricular dysrhythmias.

 See the Companion Website for a Nursing Process Focus Chart specific to this drug.

tion. Following are additional points to include when teaching clients regarding cardiotonic agents:

- Report chest pain, difficulty breathing, palpitations, or headache.
- Immediately report burning or pain at IV site.

- Immediately report chest pain or numbness or tingling in the extremities.

See "Nursing Process Focus: Clients Receiving Adrenergic Therapy" in Chapter 13, page 137, for the complete nursing process applied to caring for clients receiving beta-adrenergic agonists.

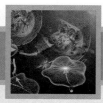

CHAPTER REVIEW

KEY CONCEPTS

The numbered key concepts provide a succinct summary of the important points from the corresponding numbered section within the chapter. If any of these points are not clear, refer to the numbered section within the chapter for review. Expanded versions can be found on the Companion Website.

27.1 Shock is a clinical syndrome characterized by the inability of the cardiovascular system to pump enough blood to meet the metabolic needs of the tissues.

27.2 Shock is often classified by the underlying pathological process or by the organ system that is primarily affected. Types of shock include cardiogenic, hypovolemic, neurogenic, septic, and anaphylactic.

27.3 The initial treatment of shock involves administration of basic life support and replacement of lost fluid. Whole blood may be indicated in cases of massive hemorrhage.

27.4 During hypovolemic shock, crystalloids replace lost fluids and electrolytes; colloids expand plasma volume and maintain blood pressure.

27.5 Vasoconstrictors are critical care drugs sometimes needed during severe shock to maintain blood pressure.

27.6 Cardiotonic drugs are useful in reversing the decreased cardiac output resulting from shock.

REVIEW QUESTIONS

1 How would an emergency room nurse who is treating a victim of a motorcycle accident determine the cause of the client's shock?

2 How can cardiotonic drugs reduce the symptoms of shock without causing vasoconstriction?

3 Should the intravenous infusion of dopamine (Inotropin) infiltrate, what nursing intervention is immediately necessary, and why?

CRITICAL THINKING QUESTIONS

1. A client with blood pressure of 84/40 mm Hg is on a norepinephrine (Levophed) drip for cardiogenic shock. Why is this client on this medication? When and how should the norepinephrine drip be discontinued?

2. The healthcare provider orders 3 L of 0.9% normal saline (NS) for a 22-year-old client with vomiting and diarrhea, a heart rate of 122, and blood pressure of 102/54 mm Hg.

Is this an appropriate IV solution for this client? Why or why not?

3. A client with a severe head injury has been put on an IV drip of 5% dextrose in water running at 150 mL/h. The nurse receives this transfer client and is reviewing the healthcare provider's orders. Is the IV solution appropriate for this client? Why or why not?

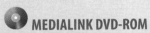

EXPLORE
MediaLink

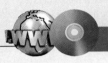

MEDIALINK DVD-ROM
- Audio Glossary
- CRNE Review
- Animations
  Mechanism of Action: Dopamine
  Mechanism of Action: Epinephrine

 COMPANION WEBSITE
- CRNE Review
- **Case Study:** Client with shock
- Dosage Calculations

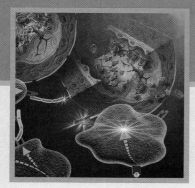

CHAPTER 28

Drugs for Hematopoietic Disorders

DRUGS AT A GLANCE

HEMATOPOIETIC GROWTH FACTORS
Erythropoietin
- *epoetin alfa (Epogen, Eprex)*

Colony-stimulating factors
- *filgrastim (Neupogen)*

Platelet enhancers

ANTIANEMIC AGENTS
- *cyanocobalamin (Anacobin): vitamin B_{12}*

Iron salts
- *ferrous sulfate (Novoferrosulfa, others)*

OBJECTIVES

After reading this chapter, the student should be able to do the following:

1. Identify drug classes used for treating hematopoietic disorders.
2. Explain the therapeutic action of each class of drug used for anemias and hematopoietic disorders in relation to the pathophysiology of the disorder.
3. Explain why hematopoietic agents are often administered to clients following chemotherapy or organ transplant.
4. Explain the role of intrinsic factor in the absorption of vitamin B_{12}.
5. Describe the metabolism, storage, and transfer of iron in the body.
6. Describe the nurse's role in the pharmacological management of clients receiving drugs for hematopoietic disorders.
7. For each of the drug classes listed in Drugs at a Glance, identify a representative drug and explain its mechanism of action, therapeutic effects, and important adverse effects.
8. Describe and explain, based on pharmacological principles, the rationale for nursing assessment, planning, and interventions for clients with hematopoietic disorders.
9. Use the nursing process to care for clients receiving drug therapy for hematopoietic disorders.

MediaLink

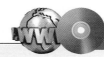

www.pearsoned.ca/adams-king

CRNE review, case studies, and other interactive resources for this chapter can be found on the Companion Website at **www.pearsoned.ca/adams-king**. Click on "Chapter 28" to select the activities for this chapter. For animations, more CRNE review questions, and an audio glossary, access the accompanying DVD-ROM in this textbook.

The blood serves all other cells in the body and is the only fluid tissue. Because of its diverse functions, diseases affecting blood constituents have widespread effects on the body. Correspondingly, drugs for treating blood disorders will affect cells in many different tissues.

PHARMFACTS

Hematopoietic Disorders

- A deficiency of vitamin B_{12}, folate, or vitamin B_6 may increase the blood level of homocysteine, an amino acid normally found in the blood. An elevated blood level of homocysteine is a risk factor for heart disease and stroke.
- Vitamin B_{12} is only present in animal products. Vegetarians who do not eat meats, fish, eggs, milk or milk products, or B_{12}-fortified foods consume no vitamin B_{12} and thus are at high risk of developing a deficiency. Vegetarians may find adequate amounts in fortified cereals, nutritional supplements, and yeast.
- A pregnant woman's body produces 45% more blood because it contains nutrients and oxygen for the growing fetus. The greatest increase in blood production occurs around week 20 of pregnancy when the need for iron is greatest. Many pregnant women feel tired and short of breath around this time.
- Administration of folic acid during pregnancy has been found to reduce birth defects in the nervous system of the baby.
- Heavy menstrual periods may result in significant iron loss.

28.1 Hematopoiesis

Blood is a highly dynamic tissue; over 200 billion new blood cells are formed every day. The process of blood cell formation is called **hematopoiesis** or hemopoiesis. Hematopoiesis occurs primarily in red bone marrow and requires B vitamins, vitamin C, copper, iron, and other nutrients.

Hematopoiesis is responsive to the demands of the body. For example, the production of white blood cells can increase to 10 times the normal number in response to infection. The number of red blood cells can also increase as much as 5 times in response to anemia or hypoxia. Homeostatic control of hematopoiesis is influenced by a number of hormones and growth factors, which allow for points of pharmacological intervention. The process of hematopoiesis is illustrated in Figure 28.1.

The process of hematopoiesis begins with a hematopoietic **stem cell**, which is capable of maturing into any type of blood cell. The specific path taken by the stem cell, whether it becomes an erythrocyte, leukocyte, or platelet, depends on the internal needs of the body. Regulation of hematopoiesis occurs through messages from certain hormones, such as erythropoietin; chemicals secreted by leukocytes, known as colony-stimulating factors; and other circulating substances. Through recombinant DNA technology, some of these growth agents are now available in sufficient quantity to be used as medications.

HEMATOPOIETIC GROWTH FACTORS

Natural hormones that promote some aspect of blood formation are called hematopoietic growth factors. Several growth factors, shown in Table 28.1, are used pharmacologically to stimulate erythrocyte, leukocyte, or platelet production.

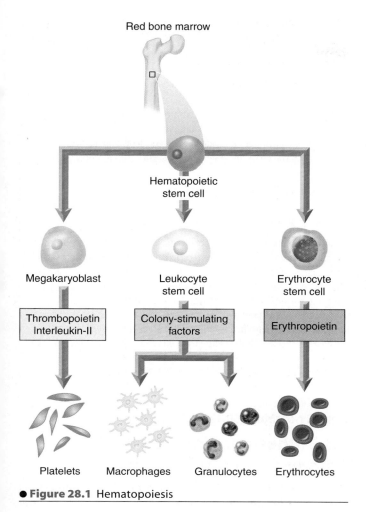

Red bone marrow

Hematopoietic
stem cell

Megakaryoblast

Leukocyte
stem cell

Erythrocyte
stem cell

Thrombopoietin
Interleukin-II

Colony-stimulating
factors

Erythropoietin

Platelets   Macrophages   Granulocytes   Erythrocytes

● **Figure 28.1** Hematopoiesis

HUMAN ERYTHROPOIETIN AND RELATED DRUGS

28.2 Pharmacotherapy with Erythropoietin

The process of red blood cell formation, or erythropoiesis, is primarily regulated by the hormone **erythropoietin**. Secreted by the kidney, erythropoietin travels to the bone marrow where it interacts with receptors on hematopoietic stem cells to increase erythrocyte production. The primary signal for the increased secretion of erythropoietin is a reduction in oxygen reaching the kidney. Serum levels of erythropoietin may increase as much as 1000-fold in response to severe hypoxia. Hemorrhage, chronic obstructive pulmonary disease, anemia, or high altitude may cause this hypoxia. Human erythropoietin is marketed as epoetin alfa.

Darbepoetin alfa is closely related to erythropoietin (epoetin alfa). It has the same pharmacological action, efficacy, and safety profile as these other agents; however, it has an extended duration of action that allows it to be administered once weekly. Darbepoetin alfa is only approved for the treatment of anemia associated with chronic renal failure.

NURSING CONSIDERATIONS

The role of the nurse in hematopoietic growth factor therapy involves careful monitoring of the client's condition and providing education as it relates to the prescribed drug regimen. Since its development, epoetin alfa has significantly improved the quality of life of clients with cancer, AIDS, and chronic renal failure. Although this drug does not cure the primary disease condition, it helps reduce the anemia that dramatically affects the client's ability to perform daily activities. Assess for food or drug allergies because epoetin alfa is contraindicated in individuals who are hypersensitive to many protein-based products. Also assess for a history of uncontrolled hypertension as the drug can raise blood pressure to dangerous levels. Baseline laboratory tests, especially a CBC, and vital signs should be obtained. Hematocrit and hemoglobin levels provide a reference for evaluating the drug's effectiveness. Epoetin alfa should be used with caution in pregnant and lactating clients (pregnancy category C). Premature infants are especially sensitive to benzyl alcohol, which may be used as a preservative in multidose vials; they must be given the preservative-free formulation to prevent "fetal gasping" syndrome.

Table 28.1 Hematopoietic Growth Factors	
Drug	*Route and Adult Dose*
epoetin alfa (Epogen, Eprex): erythropoietin	SC/IV; 3–500 U/kg/dose three times/wk, usually starting with 50–100 U/kg/dose until target Hct range of 30%–33% (max 36%) is reached; Hct should not increase by more than 4 points in any 2-wk period; may increase dose if Hct has not increased 5–6 points after 8 wk of therapy; reduce dose after target range is reached or the Hct increases by greater than 4 points in any 2-wk period; dose usually increased or decreased by 25 U/kg increments
darbepoetin alfa (Aranesp)	SC/IV; 0.45 μg/kg once per week
Colony-Stimulating Factors	
filgrastim (Neupogen): G-CSF	IV; 5 μg/kg/d by 30-min infusion, may increase by 5 μg/kg/d (max 30 μg/kg/d) SC; 5 μg/kg/d as single dose, may increase by 5 μg/kg/d (max 20 μg/kg/d)
sargramostim (Leukine): GM-CSF	IV; 250 μg/m²/d infused over 2 h for 21 d, begin 2–4 h after bone marrow transfusion and not less than 24 h after last dose of chemotherapy or 12 h after last radiation therapy
Platelet Enhancers	
oprelvekin (Neumega)	SC; 50 μg/kg once daily starting 6–24 h after completing chemotherapy

Pr PROTOTYPE DRUG | Epoetin Alfa (Epogen, Eprex)

ACTIONS AND USES

Epoetin alfa is made through recombinant DNA technology and is functionally identical to human erythropoietin. Because of its ability to stimulate erythropoiesis, epoetin alfa is effective in treating specific disorders caused by a deficiency in red blood cell formation. Clients with chronic renal failure often cannot secrete enough endogenous erythropoietin and thus will benefit from epoetin administration. Epoetin is sometimes given to clients undergoing cancer chemotherapy, to counteract the anemia caused by antineoplastic agents. It is occasionally prescribed for clients prior to blood transfusions or surgery and to treat anemia in HIV-infected clients.

PHARMACOKINETICS

Epoetin alfa is administered SC or IV. It is usually administered three times per week until a therapeutic response is achieved. Dose is adjusted according to hematocrit (target is 30% to 36%). Distribution, metabolism, and excretion are unknown. Half-life is 4 to 13 hours.

ADMINISTRATION ALERTS

- The SC route is generally preferred over IV since lower doses are needed and absorption is slower.
- Premature infants are especially sensitive to benzyl alcohol, which may be used as a preservative in multidose vials; therefore, they must be given the preservative-free formulation to prevent "fetal gasping" syndrome.
- Do not shake vial because this may deactivate the drug. Visibly inspect solution for particulate matter.
- Epoetin alfa is pregnancy category C.

ADVERSE EFFECTS AND INTERACTIONS

The most common adverse effect of epoetin alfa is hypertension, which may occur in as many as 30% of clients receiving the drug. Blood pressure should be monitored during therapy, and an antihypertensive drug may be indicated. The risk of thromboembolic events is increased. Clients who are on dialysis may require increased doses of heparin. TIAs, heart attacks, and strokes have occurred in chronic renal failure clients on dialysis who are also being treated with epoetin alfa. The effectiveness of epoetin alfa will be greatly reduced in clients with iron deficiency or other vitamin depleted states since erythropoiesis cannot be enhanced without these vital nutrients. There are no clinically significant drug interactions with epoetin alfa.

Because this drug increases the risk of thromboembolic disease, the client should be monitored for early signs of stroke or heart attack. Clients on dialysis are at higher risk for transient ischemic attack (TIA), stroke, and MI and may need increased doses of heparin while receiving epoetin alfa. Monitor for side effects such as nausea and vomiting, constipation, injection site reaction, and headache.

See "Nursing Process Focus: Clients Receiving Epoetin Alfa (Epogen, Eprex)" for specific teaching points.

COLONY-STIMULATING FACTORS

28.3 Pharmacotherapy with Colony-Stimulating Factors

Control of white blood cell production, or leukopoiesis, is more complicated than erythropoiesis due to the many different types of leukocytes in the blood. The two basic categories of growth factors are interleukins and **colony-stimulating factors (CSFs)**. Because the primary action of

NURSING PROCESS FOCUS   Clients Receiving Epoetin Alfa (Epogen, Eprex)

Assessment	Potential Nursing Diagnoses/Identified Patterns
Prior to administration: - Obtain complete health history including allergies, drug history, and possible drug reactions. - Assess reason for drug administration such as presence/history of anemia secondary to chronic renal failure, malignancy, chemotherapy, autologous blood donation, and treatment with zidovudine in HIV-infected clients . - Assess vital signs, especially blood pressure. - Assess complete blood count, specifically hematocrit and hemoglobin levels, to establish baseline values. - Assess activity tolerance and dietary patterns.	- Adequate knowledge regarding drug therapy and adverse effects - Safety from physical injury such as falls related to anemia symptoms (weakness, dizziness, syncope) - Effective tissue perfusion - Reduced physical activity related to RBC deficiency

Planning: Client Goals and Expected Outcomes

The client will:
- Exhibit an increase in hematocrit level and improvement in anemia-related symptoms
- Immediately report effects such as severe headache, chest pain, confusion, numbness, or loss of movement in an extremity
- Demonstrate an understanding of drug therapy by accurately describing drug's intended effects, side effects, and precautions

continued

NURSING PROCESS FOCUS Clients Receiving Epoetin Alfa (Epogen, Eprex) *(Continued)*

Implementation

Interventions (Rationales)	Client Education/Discharge Planning
■ Monitor vital signs, especially blood pressure. (The rate of hypertension is directly related to the rate of rise of the hematocrit. Clients who have existing hypertension are at higher risk for stroke and seizures. Hypertension is also much more likely in clients with chronic renal failure.)	Instruct client: ■ On the importance of periodic blood pressure monitoring and in the proper use of home blood pressure monitoring equipment ■ On "reportable" blood pressure ranges ("Call healthcare provider when blood pressure is greater than. . . ")
■ Monitor for side effects, especially symptoms of neurological or cardiovascular events.	■ Instruct client to report side effects such as nausea, vomiting, constipation, redness/pain at injection site, confusion, numbness, chest pain, and difficulty breathing.
■ Monitor client's ability to self-administer medication.	Instruct client: ■ In the technique for SC injection if client is to self-administer the medication ■ In proper disposal of needles and syringes
■ Monitor laboratory values such as hematocrit and hemoglobin to evaluate effectiveness of treatment. (Increases in hematocrit and hemoglobin values indicate increased RBC production.)	Instruct client: ■ Of the need for initial and continuing laboratory blood monitoring ■ To keep all laboratory appointments ■ Of latest hematocrit value so that physical activities may be adjusted accordingly
■ Monitor client for signs of seizure activity. (Seizures can result from a rapid rise in hematocrit—especially during first 90 days of treatment.)	■ Instruct client to not drive or perform hazardous activities until the effects of the drug are known.
■ Monitor client for signs of thrombus such as swelling, warmth, and pain in an extremity. (As hematocrit rises, there is an increased chance of thrombus formation, particularly for clients with chronic renal failure.)	Instruct client: ■ To report any increase in size, pain, and/or warmth in an extremity ■ On signs and symptoms of blood clots ■ Not to rub or massage calves and to report leg discomfort
■ Monitor dietary intake. Ensure adequate intake of all essential nutrients. (Response to this medication is minimal if blood levels of iron, folic acid, and vitamin B_{12} are deficient.)	Instruct client to: ■ Maintain adequate dietary intake of essential vitamins and nutrients ■ Continue to follow necessary dietary restrictions if receiving renal dialysis

Evaluation of Outcome Criteria

Evaluate the effectiveness of drug therapy by confirming that client goals and expected outcomes have been met (see "Planning").

---

the interleukins is to modulate the immune system rather than enhance leukopoiesis, they are presented in Chapter 30. One interleukin stimulates the production of platelets and is discussed in Section 28.4.

The leukopoietic growth factors are active at very low concentrations. It is believed that each stem cell stimulated by these growth factors is capable of producing as many as 1000 mature leukocytes. The growth factors not only increase the production of leukocytes, but also activate existing white blood cells. Examples of enhanced functions include increased migration of leukocytes to antigens, increased antibody toxicity, and increased phagocytosis.

CSFs are named according to the types of blood cells they stimulate. For example, granulocyte colony-stimulating factor (G-CSF) increases the production of neutrophils, the most common type of granulocyte. Granulocyte-macrophage colony-stimulating factor (GM-CSF) stimulates both neutrophil and macrophage production. Made through recom-

binant DNA technology, the two CSFs available as medications are filgrastim and sargramostim. Filgrastim is primarily used for chronic neutropenia or neutropenia secondary to chemotherapy. Sargramostim is used specifically to treat non-Hodgkin's lymphoma, acute lymphoblastic leukemia, and clients with Hodgkin's disease who are having autologous bone marrow transplantation.

NURSING CONSIDERATIONS

The role of the nurse in CSF therapy involves careful monitoring of the client's condition and providing education as it relates to the prescribed drug regimen. Prior to administration of filgrastim, assess for hypersensitivity to certain foreign proteins, specifically those in *Escherichia coli*. Due to its structural components, the drug is contraindicated in clients with this type of hypersensitivity. Obtain a health history, especially checking for myeloid cancers such as leukemia because filgrastim may stimulate proliferation of these malignant cells. This drug should not be administered simultaneously with chemotherapy. A baseline CBC with differential and platelet count should be obtained for baseline data to evaluate drug effectiveness. Usage of filgrastim may cause dysrhythmias and tachycardia; therefore, a thorough initial and ongoing cardiac assessment should be performed throughout the treatment regimen.

Assess for both hypertension and skeletal pain, which are adverse effects of filgrastim therapy. The ECG readings should be monitored for abnormal ST segment depression, which is also a side effect of the drug. See "Nursing Process Focus: Clients Receiving Filgrastim (Neupagen)" for further details on this drug.

A CBC should be obtained prior to administration of sargramostim because this drug is contraindicated when excessive leukemic myeloid blasts are present in blood or bone marrow. Obtain a health history, specifically for any known hypersensitivity to GM-CSF or yeast products. Sargramostim should be used cautiously in clients with cardiac disease such as dysrhythmias or heart failure because this agent may cause supraventricular dysrhythmias. This is usually a temporary side effect that disappears when the drug is discontinued. It should also be used with caution in clients with kidney and liver impairment.

It is often difficult to assess the adverse effects of CSF medications because the symptoms may also be attributed to the chemotherapy or the disease itself. A serious side effect of sargramostim is respiratory distress that occurs during the IV infusion, which develops because granulocytes become trapped in the pulmonary circulation. If this occurs, it is recommended that the nurse decrease the infusion rate. Occasionally, clients will develop a syndrome that occurs the first time the drug is administered. The client develops difficulty breathing, tachycardia, low blood pressure, and

light-headedness. This also appears to be related to the trapping of granulocytes in the pulmonary circulation. If these symptoms occur during the first infusion, restart the infusion at half the rate after all symptoms have resolved.

Client education as it relates to CSFs should include goals, reasons for obtaining baseline data such as vital signs, and possible side effects. Include the following general points when teaching clients regarding CSFs:

- Wash hands frequently and avoid people with infections such as colds and flu.
- Immediately report symptoms such as chest pain or palpitations, respiratory difficulty, nausea, vomiting, fever, chills, and malaise.
- Keep all physician and laboratory appointments.

See "Nursing Process Focus: Clients Receiving Filgrastim (Neupogen)" for specific teaching points.

PLATELET ENHANCERS

28.4 Pharmacotherapy with Platelet Enhancers

The production of platelets, or thrombocytopoiesis, begins when megakaryocytes in the bone marrow start shedding membrane-bound packets. These packets enter the bloodstream and become platelets. A single megakaryocyte can produce thousands of platelets.

Megakaryocyte activity is controlled by the hormone **thrombopoietin**, which is produced by the kidneys. Thrombopoietin may be used to increase platelets. Because it is a new drug, clients taking thrombopoietin require careful monitoring for adverse effects.

Oprelvekin is a drug produced through recombinant DNA technology that stimulates the production of megakaryocytes and thrombopoietin. Although it differs slightly from

---

Pr PROTOTYPE DRUG | Filgrastim (Neupogen)

ACTIONS AND USES

Filgrastim is human G-CSF produced through recombinant DNA technology. Its two primary actions are to increase neutrophil production in the bone marrow and to enhance the phagocytic and cytotoxic functions of existing neutrophils. This is particularly important for clients with neutropenia, which is a reduction in circulating neutrophils that often results in severe bacterial and fungal infections. Administration of filgrastim will shorten the length of neutropenia in cancer clients whose bone marrow has been suppressed by antineoplastic agents or in clients following organ transplants. It may also be used in clients with AIDS-related immunosuppression.

PHARMACOKINETICS

Filgrastim is administered daily as a single SC injection or continuously as a slow SC or IV infusion. Dose is adjusted according to absolute neutrophil count (target is sustained count of 1000/mm³). Distribution, metabolism, and excretion are unknown. Half-life is 3.5 hours.

ADMINISTRATION ALERTS

- Do not administer within 24 hours before or after chemotherapy with cytotoxic agents as this will greatly decrease the effectiveness of filgrastim.
- Filgrastim is pregnancy category C.

ADVERSE EFFECTS AND INTERACTIONS

Bone pain is a common side effect of high-dose filgrastim therapy. A small percentage of clients may develop an allergic reaction. Frequent laboratory tests are conducted to ensure that excessive numbers of neutrophils, or leukocytosis, does not occur. Because the antineoplastic drugs and colony-stimulating factors produce opposite effects, filgrastim is not administered until at least 24 hours after a chemotherapy session.

NURSING PROCESS FOCUS   CLIENTS RECEIVING FILGRASTIM (NEUPOGEN)

Assessment	Potential Nursing Diagnoses/Identified Patterns
Prior to administration: ■ Obtain complete health history including allergies, drug history, and possible drug reactions. ■ Assess reason for drug administration such as presence/history of severe bacterial or fungal infections, chemotherapy-induced neutropenia, or AIDS-related immunosuppression. ■ Assess vital signs. ■ Assess complete blood count, specifically WBC with differential, to establish baseline values.	■ Adequate knowledge regarding drug therapy and adverse effects. ■ Safety from injury related to side effects of drug therapy ■ Risk for infection related to impaired immune defence (low WBC)

Planning: Client Goals and Expected Outcomes

The client will:
■ Exhibit an increase in leukocyte levels and experience a decrease in the incidence of infection
■ Demonstrate an understanding of drug therapy by accurately describing drug's intended effects, side effects, and precautions
■ Immediately report significant adverse effects from the medication such as nausea, vomiting, fever, chills, malaise, and skeletal pain, and allergic-type responses such as rash, urticaria, wheezing, and dyspnea

Implementation

Interventions (Rationales)	Client Education/Discharge Planning
■ Monitor vital signs. (Myocardial infarction and dysrhythmias have occurred in a small number of clients because the drug has been known to cause abnormal ST segment depression.)	■ Instruct client to report any chest pain or palpitations.
■ Monitor for signs and symptoms of infection. ■ Limit the client's exposure to pathogenic microorganisms. (Clients are more susceptible to infection until WBC response is achieved.)	Instruct the client to: ■ Wash hands frequently ■ Avoid crowds and people with colds, flu, and infections ■ Cook all foods completely and thoroughly ■ Clean surfaces touched by raw foods ■ Avoid fresh fruits, vegetables, and plants until WBC level is within normal limits ■ Limit exposure to children and animals ■ Increase fluid intake and empty bladder frequently ■ Cough and deep breathe several times per day
■ Monitor complete blood count with differential until WBC count is at an acceptable level.	■ Inform clients of WBC status during the course of the treatment so they may take necessary precautions to avoid infection.
■ Monitor hepatic status during pharmacotherapy. (Filgrastim may cause an elevation in liver enzymes.)	Instruct client: ■ Of the need for initial and continuing laboratory blood monitoring ■ To keep all laboratory appointments
■ Assess for bone pain. (Drug works by stimulating bone marrow cells.)	■ Instruct client to report any pain not relieved by OTC analgesics
■ Monitor for significant side effects and allergic-type reactions. (Client may be hypersensitive to *E. coli*.)	Instruct client to immediately report: ■ Side effects such as nausea, vomiting, fever, chills, and malaise ■ Symptoms of allergic reaction such as rash, urticaria, wheezing, and dyspnea
■ Monitor client's ability to self-administer medication.	Instruct client about: ■ Self-injection technique ■ Proper disposal of needles and syringes

Evaluation of Outcome Criteria

Evaluate the effectiveness of drug therapy by confirming that client goals and expected outcomes have been met (see "Planning").

endogenous interleukin-11, the two are considered functionally equivalent. Oprelvekin is used to stimulate the production of platelets in clients who are at risk for thrombocytopenia caused by cancer chemotherapy. The onset of action is 5 to 9 days, and platelet counts will remain elevated for about 7 days after the last dose. Oprelvekin is only given by the SC route.

NURSING CONSIDERATIONS

The role of the nurse in platelet enhancer therapy involves careful monitoring of the client's condition and providing education as it relates to the prescribed drug regimen. Oprelvekin should not be given to clients with hypersensitivity to this drug. It is used with caution in clients with cardiac disease, especially HF, dysrhythmias, and left ventricular dysfunction, since fluid retention is a common side effect.

As with the colony-stimulating factors, oprelvekin should not be used within 24 hours of chemotherapy because the cytotoxic effects of the antineoplastic agents decrease the effectiveness of the drug. Adverse effects are related to fluid retention and may be severe, including pleural effusion and papilledema. Clients should be advised to report edema to the nurse and to avoid activities that could cause bleeding until the platelet count has returned to normal.

Oprelvekin should be withheld for 12 hours before or after radiation therapy because the breakdown of cells after radiation will decrease the effectiveness of the medication. Monitor clients with a history of edema as this drug aggravates fluid retention and may cause pleural effusion or congestive heart failure.

See "Nursing Process Focus: Clients Receiving Filgrastim (Neupogen)" for additional teaching points.

ANEMIAS

Anemia is a condition in which red blood cells have a diminished capacity to carry oxygen. Although there are many different causes of anemia, they fall into one of the following categories:

- Blood loss due to hemorrhage
- Excessive erythrocyte destruction
- Diminished erythrocyte synthesis due to a deficiency in a substance needed for erythropoiesis

28.5 Classification of Anemias

Classification of anemia is generally based on a description of erythrocyte size and colour. Size is described as normal (normocytic), small (microcytic), or large (macrocytic). Colour is based on the amount of hemoglobin present and is described as normal red (normochromic) or light red (hypochromic). This classification is shown in Table 28.2.

Each type of anemia has specific characteristics, but all have common signs and symptoms. The client often exhibits pallor, which is a paleness of the skin and mucous membranes due to hemoglobin deficiency. Decreased exercise tolerance, fatigue, and lethargy occur because of insufficient oxygen reaching the muscles. Dizziness and fainting are common because the brain is not receiving enough oxygen to properly function. The cardiovascular system attempts to compensate for the oxygen depletion by increasing respiration rate and heart rate. Long-standing or severe disease can result in heart failure.

ANTIANEMIC AGENTS

Several vitamins and minerals are given to enhance the oxygen-carrying capacity of blood in clients with certain anemias. The two most common agents are cyanocobalamin, a purified form of vitamin B_{12}, and ferrous sulfate, an iron supplement. These agents are shown in Table 28.3.

VITAMIN B_{12} AND FOLIC ACID

28.6 Pharmacotherapy with Vitamin B_{12} and Folic Acid

Vitamin B_{12} and folic acid are dietary nutrients essential for rapidly dividing cells. Because erythropoiesis is occurring at a continuously high rate throughout the lifespan, deficiencies in these nutrients often manifest as anemias.

Vitamin B_{12} is an essential component of two coenzymes that are required for normal cell growth and replication. Vitamin B_{12} is not synthesized by either plants or animals; only bacteria serve this function. Because only miniscule amounts of vitamin B_{12} are required (3 μg/day), deficiency

TABLE 28.2 Classification of Anemia		
Morphology	**Description**	**Examples**
normocytic-normochromic	loss of normal erythroblasts or mature erythrocytes	aplastic anemia hemorrhagic anemia sickle cell anemia hemolytic anemia
macrocytic-normochromic	large, abnormally shaped erythrocytes with normal hemoglobin	pernicious anemia folate deficiency anemia
microcytic-hypochromic	small, abnormally shaped erythrocytes with diminished hemoglobin	iron deficiency anemia thalassemia

TABLE 28.3	Antianemic Agents
Drug	**Route and Adult Dose**
cyanocobalamin (Anacobin): vitamin B_{12}	IM/deep SC; 30 μg/d for 5–10 d, then 100–200 μg/mo
folic acid (Apo-Folic, Folvite)	PO/IM/SC/IV; 0.4–1.0 mg/d
Iron Salts	
ferrous fumarate (Palafer, others)	PO; 200 mg tid or qid
ferrous gluconate (Fertinic, others)	PO; 325–600 mg qid, may be gradually increased to 650 mg qid as needed and tolerated
ferrous sulfate (Novoferrosulfa, others)	PO; 750–1500 mg/d in one to three divided doses

of this vitamin is usually not due to insufficient dietary intake. Instead, the most common cause of vitamin B_{12} deficiency is lack of **intrinsic factor**, a protein secreted by stomach cells. Intrinsic factor is required for vitamin B_{12} to be absorbed from the intestine. Figure 28.2 illustrates the metabolism of vitamin B_{12}. Inflammatory diseases of the stomach or surgical removal of the stomach may result in deficiency of intrinsic factor. Inflammatory diseases of the small intestine that affect food and nutrient absorption may also cause vitamin B_{12} deficiency.

The most profound consequence of B_{12} deficiency is a condition called **pernicious**, or **megaloblastic, anemia** that affects both the hematological and nervous systems. The stem cells produce abnormally large erythrocytes that do not fully mature. Red blood cells are most affected, though lack of maturation of all blood cell types may occur in severe disease. Nervous system symptoms may include memory loss, confusion, unsteadiness, tingling or numbness in the limbs, delusions, mood disturbances, and even hallucinations in severe deficiencies. Permanent nervous system damage may result if the disease remains untreated.

Folic acid, or **folate**, is another vitamin essential for normal DNA and RNA synthesis. Like B_{12} deficiency, insufficient folic acid can manifest itself as anemia. In fact, the metabolism of vitamin B_{12} and folic acid are intricately linked: a B_{12} deficiency will create a lack of activated folic acid.

Unlike vitamin B_{12}, folic acid does not require intrinsic factor for intestinal absorption, and the most common cause of folate deficiency is insufficient dietary intake. This is most commonly observed in chronic alcoholism, although other absorption diseases of the small intestine can result in folate anemia. Hematopoietic signs of folate deficiency are the same as those for B_{12} deficiency; however, no neurological signs are present. Folate deficiency during pregnancy has been linked to neural birth defects such as spina bifida; thus, advise pregnant clients and those planning to become pregnant to take adequate amounts of this vitamin. Treatment is often accomplished by increasing the dietary intake of folic acid through fresh green vegetables and wheat products. In cases when adequate dietary intake cannot be achieved, therapy with folate sodium or folic acid is warranted. Folic acid is discussed further in Chapter 38.

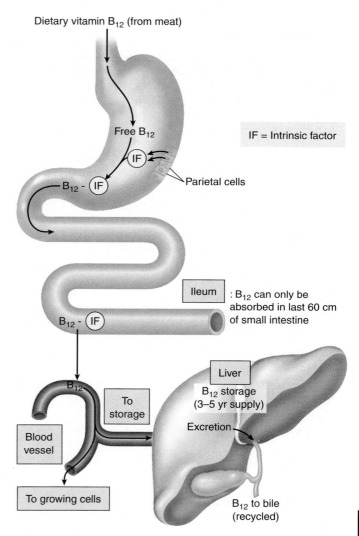

● **Figure 28.2** Metabolism of vitamin B_{12}

NURSING CONSIDERATIONS

The role of the nurse in antianemic therapy involves careful monitoring of the client's condition and providing education as it relates to the prescribed drug regimen. Although most vitamin B_{12} deficiencies are caused by a lack of intrinsic factor, investigate the possibility of inadequate dietary intake of the vitamin, particularly in vegans. Prior to

MediaLink

Raw Liver for Breakfast?

Pr PROTOTYPE DRUG | Cyanocobalamin (Anacobin): Vitamin B$_{12}$

ACTIONS AND USES

Cyanocobalamin is a purified form of vitamin B$_{12}$ that is administered in deficiency states. Treatment of vitamin B$_{12}$ deficiency is most often by weekly, biweekly, or monthly IM or SC injections. Although oral B$_{12}$ supplements are available, they are only effective in clients having sufficient intrinsic factor and normal absorption in the small intestine. Parenteral administration rapidly reverses most signs and symptoms of B$_{12}$ deficiency. If the disease has been prolonged, symptoms may take longer to resolve, and some neurological damage may be permanent. In most cases, treatment must often be maintained for the remainder of the client's life.

PHARMACOKINETICS

Cyanocobalamin is well absorbed after SC, IV, or intranasal administration. Calcium and intrinsic factor are necessary for PO absorption. It is stored in the liver and crosses the placenta and enters breast milk. Excess drug is excreted unchanged in the urine. Half-life is 6 days.

ADMINISTRATION ALERTS

- If PO preparations are mixed with fruit juices, administer quickly because ascorbic acid affects the stability of vitamin B$_{12}$.
- Cyanocobalamin is pregnancy category C when used parenterally.

ADVERSE EFFECTS AND INTERACTIONS

Side effects from cyanocobalamin are uncommon. Hypokalemia is possible, so serum potassium levels are monitored periodically. A small percentage of clients receiving B$_{12}$ exhibit rashes, itching, or other signs of allergy. Anaphylaxis is possible, though rare.

Drug interactions with cyanocobalamin include a decrease in absorption when given concurrently with alcohol, aminosalicylic acid, neomycin, and colchicine. Chloramphenicol may interfere with therapeutic response to cyanocobalamin.

 See the Companion Website for a Nursing Process Focus Chart specific to this drug.

administration, assess for other causes of anemia, including GI dysfunction, GI surgery, tapeworm infestation, and gluten enteropathy.

Prior to and at regular intervals during treatment, a complete blood count is needed to evaluate the effectiveness of vitamin B$_{12}$ therapy. This drug is not an effective treatment for iron deficiency anemias. Cyanocobalamin is contraindicated in clients with severe pulmonary disease and is used cautiously in clients with heart disease.

Potassium levels should be monitored during pharmacotherapy because hypokalemia is a possible side effect of this drug. Assess clients for additional side effects such as itching, rash, or flushing. Clients taking this drug may develop pulmonary edema and heart failure, so cardiovascular status must be monitored.

See "Nursing Process Focus: Clients Receiving Cyanocobalamin (Anacobin): Vitamin B$_{12}$" for specific teaching points.

NURSING PROCESS FOCUS Clients Receiving Cyanocobalamin (Anacobin): Vitamin B$_{12}$

Assessment	Potential Nursing Diagnoses/Identified Patterns
Prior to administration: ■ Obtain complete health history including allergies, drug history, and possible drug reactions. ■ Assess vital signs. ■ Assess for other causes of anemia.	■ Adequate knowledge regarding drug therapy and adverse effects ■ Safety from physical injury such as falls related to anemia symptoms (weakness, dizziness, syncope) ■ Effective tissue perfusion related to effective drug therapy

Planning: Client Goals and Expected Outcomes

The client will:
- Report a decrease in symptoms of vitamin B$_{12}$ deficiency
- Immediately report significant side effects such as dyspnea, palpitations, fatigue, muscle weakness, and dysrhythmias
- Demonstrate an understanding of drug therapy by accurately describing drug's intended effects, side effects, and precautions

Implementation

Interventions (Rationales)	Client Education/Discharge Planning
■ Monitor vital signs. (Altered potassium levels and overexertion may produce cardiovascular complications, especially irregular rhythm.)	■ Instruct client to monitor pulse rate and report irregularities and changes in rhythm.
■ Monitor potassium levels during first 48 hours of therapy. (Conversion to normal red blood cell production increases the need for potassium.)	■ Instruct client on the need for initial and continuing laboratory blood monitoring, and to keep all laboratory appointments.
■ Monitor respiratory pattern. (Pulmonary edema may occur early in therapy related to a possible sensitivity to the drug. Reactions may take up to 8 days to occur.)	■ Instruct client to immediately report any respiratory difficulty.

continued

NURSING PROCESS FOCUS   Clients Receiving Cyanocobalamin (Anacobin): Vitamin B$_{12}$ *(Continued)*

Interventions (Rationales)	Client Education/Discharge Planning
■ Monitor serum vitamin B$_{12}$, RBC, and hemoglobin levels to determine effectiveness of drug. (Initial doses of B$_{12}$ stimulate rapid RBC regeneration, and level should return to near normal within 2 weeks.)	■ Advise client that treatment for pernicious anemia (usually IM injection) must be continued throughout life to prevent neurological damage.
■ Assist client to plan activities and allow for periods of rest to conserve energy.	■ Instruct client to rest when they begin to feel tired and to avoid strenuous activities.
■ Encourage client to maintain adequate dietary intake of essential nutrients and vitamins.	Instruct client: ■ That dietary control, by itself, is not possible in treating pernicious anemia ■ To consume adequate dietary intake of essential nutrients and vitamins
■ Monitor for side effects such as palpitations, fatigue, muscle weakness, and dysrhythmias.	■ Teach client to immediately report side effects to their healthcare provider.

Evaluation of Outcome Criteria

Evaluate the effectiveness of drug therapy by confirming that client goals and expected outcomes have been met (see "Planning").

IRON

Iron is a mineral essential to the function of several biological molecules, the most significant of which is hemoglobin. Of all iron in the body, 60% to 80% is associated with the hemoglobin in erythrocytes. Iron is also essential for a number of mitochondrial enzymes involved in metabolism and energy production in the cell. Because free iron is toxic, the body binds the mineral to the protein complexes **ferritin**, **hemosiderin**, and **transferrin**. Ferritin and hemosiderin maintain iron stores *inside* cells, whereas transferrin *transports* iron to sites in the body where it is needed.

28.7 Pharmacotherapy with Iron

The most common cause of nutritional anemia is iron deficiency. A primary cause of iron deficiency anemia is blood loss, such as may occur from peptic ulcer disease. Certain individuals have an increased demand for iron, including those who are pregnant, experiencing heavy menstruation, or undergoing intensive athletic training. These conditions may require more than the recommended daily intake (RDI) of iron (see Chapter 38). The most significant effect of iron deficiency is a reduction in erythropoiesis, resulting in symptoms of anemia.

After erythrocytes die, nearly all of the iron in their hemoglobin is incorporated into transferrin and recycled for later use. Because of this efficient recycling, only about 1 mg of iron is excreted from the body per day, making daily dietary iron requirements in most individuals quite small. However, the amount of iron lost by some women during menstruation may be significant enough to produce anemic symptoms. Ferrous sulfate, ferrous gluconate, and ferrous fumarate are the most commonly used oral iron preparations.

NURSING CONSIDERATIONS

The role of the nurse in iron therapy involves careful monitoring of the client's condition and providing education as it relates to the prescribed drug regimen. All iron preparations have essentially the same nursing considerations. Before initiating therapy with these medicines, obtain vital signs and a CBC, including hemoglobin and hematocrit levels, to establish baseline values. Obtain a health history, assessing for peptic ulcer, regional enteritis, ulcerative colitis, and cirrhosis of the liver because these drugs are contraindicated in such disorders.

Iron dextran can be given as an IM injection or as an IV infusion and is often used for clients who cannot tolerate oral iron preparations. Prior to administering an infusion, the client must receive a test dose to determine possible allergic reaction, which may cause respiratory arrest and circulatory collapse. Vital signs must be monitored during this initial infusion.

Possible GI reactions such as nausea, vomiting, constipation, and diarrhea are common with the oral iron preparations. Inform the client that these effects will diminish over time and that iron will turn stools a harmless dark green or

LIFESPAN CONSIDERATIONS

Iron Deficiency in Children

Iron deficiency and iron deficiency anemia have been identified as significant problems among children 1 to 2 years of age. Inadequate iron intake and storage is the main reason for this condition. Extremely low levels of iron can cause permanent mental and psychomotor impairment; therefore, prevention is of utmost importance. Primary prevention of iron deficiency can be accomplished by daily supplementation of 10 mg of elemental iron with iron-fortified vitamins, iron drops, or an iron-fortified nutritional drink. Accidental overdose due to ingestion of products containing iron is one of the leading causes of fatal poisoning in children. It is extremely important that iron be kept out of the reach of children. If overdosing occurs, caregivers should call the healthcare provider or poison control centre.

Pr PROTOTYPE DRUG | Ferrous Sulfate (Novoferrosulfa, others)

ACTIONS AND USES

Ferrous sulfate is an iron supplement containing about 30% elemental iron. It is available in a wide variety of dosage forms to prevent or rapidly reverse symptoms of iron deficiency anemia. Other forms of iron include ferrous fumarate, which contains 33% elemental iron, and ferrous gluconate, which contains 12% elemental iron. The doses of these various preparations are based on their iron content.

Laboratory evaluation of hemoglobin or hematocrit values is conducted regularly as excess iron is toxic. Although a positive therapeutic response may be achieved in 48 hours, therapy may continue for several months.

PHARMACOKINETICS

Up to 60% of ferrous sulfate taken PO is absorbed. It crosses the placenta and enters breast milk. It is about 90% protein bound. Ferrous sulfate may be retained in the body for many months because it is mostly recycled, with only small amounts being excreted.

ADMINISTRATION ALERTS

- When administering IV, be careful to prevent infiltration as iron is highly irritating to tissues.
- Use the Z-track method (deep muscle) when giving IM injection.
- Do not crush tablet or empty contents of capsule when administering.
- Do not give tablets or capsules within 1 hour of bedtime.
- Ferrous sulfate is pregnancy category A.

ADVERSE EFFECTS AND INTERACTIONS

The most common side effect of ferrous sulfate is GI upset. Taking the drug with food will diminish GI upset but can decrease the absorption of iron by as much as 70%. In addition, antacids should not be taken with ferrous sulfate because they also reduce absorption of the mineral. Ideally, iron preparations should be administered 1 hour before or 2 hours after a meal. Clients should be advised that iron preparations may darken stools, but this is a harmless side effect. Constipation is also a common side effect. Excessive doses of iron are very toxic, so advise clients to take their medication exactly as directed.

Drug interactions with ferrous sulfate include reduced absorption when given concurrently with antacids. Iron decreases the absorption of tetracyclines, thyroid hormone, levodopa, and methyldopa. It is advisable to take iron supplements *at least* 1 hour before or after other medications.

black colour. Taking oral iron with food reduces GI distress but also greatly reduces absorption. Common adverse reactions of iron dextran are headache and muscle and joint pain; these are more severe when the drug is given IV and are lessened when given IM. Iron dextran appears to increase bone density in the joints, which is the probable cause of the muscle and joint pain.

See "Nursing Process Focus: Clients Receiving Ferrous Sulfate (Novoferrosulfa, others)" for specific teaching points.

NURSING PROCESS FOCUS   Clients Receiving Ferrous Sulfate (Novoferrosulfa, others)

Assessment	Potential Nursing Diagnoses/Identified Patterns
Prior to administration: ■ Obtain complete health history including allergies, drug history, and possible drug reactions. ■ Assess reason for drug administration such as presence/history of anemia or prophylaxis during infancy, childhood, or pregnancy. ■ Assess complete blood count, specifically hematocrit and hemoglobin levels, to establish baseline values. ■ Assess vital signs.	■ Adequate knowledge regarding drug therapy and adverse effects ■ Safety from physical injury such as falls related to anemia symptoms (weakness, dizziness, syncope) ■ Adequate tissue oxygenation (may be impaired related to low RBC count) ■ Balanced intake of iron and other nutrients

Planning: Client Goals and Expected Outcomes

The client will:
- Exhibit an increase in hematocrit level and improvement in anemia-related symptoms
- Demonstrate an understanding of drug therapy by accurately describing drug's intended effects, side effects, and precautions
- Immediately report significant side effects such as gastrointestinal distress

Implementation

Intervention (Rationales)	Client Education/Discharge Planning
■ Monitor vital signs, especially pulse. (Increased pulse is an indicator of decreased oxygen content in the blood.)	■ Instruct client to monitor pulse rate and report irregularities and changes in rhythm.

continued

NURSING PROCESS FOCUS   Clients Receiving Ferrous Sulfate (Novoferrosulfa, others)   *(Continued)*

Interventions (Rationales)	Client Education/Discharge Planning
■ Monitor complete blood count to evaluate effectiveness of treatment. (Increases in hematocrit and hemoglobin values indicate increased RBC production.)	Instruct client: ■ On the need for initial and continuing laboratory blood monitoring ■ To keep all laboratory appointments
■ Monitor changes in stool. (Drug may cause constipation, changes in stool colour, and false positives when stool is tested for occult blood.)	Instruct client: ■ That stool colour may change and this is not a cause for alarm ■ On measures to relieve constipation, such as including fruits and fruit juices in diet and increasing fluid intake and exercise
■ Plan activities and allow for periods of rest to help client conserve energy. (Diminished iron levels result in decreased formation of hemoglobin, leading to weakness.)	Instruct client to: ■ Rest when feeling tired and not to overexert ■ Plan activities to avoid fatigue
■ Administer medication on an empty stomach (if tolerated) at least 1 hour before bedtime. (This maximizes absorption; taking drug closer to bedtime may increase the chance of GI distress.)	Instruct client: ■ Not to crush or chew sustained-release preparations ■ That medication may cause GI upset ■ To take medication with food if GI upset becomes a problem ■ To take at least 1 hour before bedtime
■ Administer liquid iron preparations through a straw or place on the back of the tongue (to avoid staining the teeth).	Instruct client to: ■ Dilute liquid medication before using and to use a straw to take medication ■ Rinse the mouth after swallowing to decrease the chance of staining the teeth
■ Monitor dietary intake to ensure adequate intake of foods high in iron.	■ Instruct client to increase intake of iron-rich foods such as liver, egg yolks, brewer's yeast, wheat germ, and muscle meats.
■ Monitor for potential of child access to medication. (Iron poisoning can be fatal to young children.)	■ Advise parents to store iron-containing vitamins out of reach of children and in childproof containers.

Evaluation of Outcome Criteria

Evaluate the effectiveness of drug therapy by confirming that client goals and expected outcomes have been met (see "Planning").

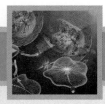

CHAPTER REVIEW

KEY CONCEPTS

The numbered key concepts provide a succinct summary of the important points from the corresponding numbered section within the chapter. If any of these points are not clear, refer to the numbered section within the chapter for review. Expanded versions can be found on the Companion Website.

28.1 Hematopoiesis is the process of erythrocyte production that begins with primitive stem cells in the bone marrow. Homeostatic control of erythropoiesis is through hematopoietic growth factors.

28.2 Erythropoietin is a hormone that stimulates the production of red blood cells and is used, as epoetin alfa, to treat specific anemias.

28.3 Colony-stimulating factors (CSFs) are growth factors that stimulate the production of leukocytes and are used following chemotherapy or organ transplants.

28.4 Platelet enhancers stimulate the activity of megakaryocytes and thrombopoietin and increase the production of platelets.

28.5 Anemias are disorders in which blood has a reduced capacity to carry oxygen, due to hemorrhage, excessive erythrocyte destruction, or insufficient erythrocyte synthesis.

28.6 Deficiencies in either vitamin B_{12} or folic acid can lead to pernicious anemia. Treatment with cyanocobalamin or folate can reverse these anemias in many clients.

28.7 Iron deficiency is the most common cause of nutritional anemia and can be successfully treated with iron supplements.

REVIEW QUESTIONS

1 Colony-stimulating factors are used for various disorders affecting leukocytes. Identify the action and usage for each drug in this class.

2 Although deficiencies of vitamin B$_{12}$ and folic acid produce megaloblastic anemias, distinct differences exist.

Compare and contrast the pharmacotherapy of the two anemias.

3 Explain why iron supplements are not an effective pharmacological treatment for anemias caused by a deficiency of intrinsic factor.

CRITICAL THINKING QUESTIONS

1. A client newly diagnosed with renal failure asks the nurse why he must be on injections of epoetin alfa. How should the nurse respond?

2. A client is receiving filgrastim. The healthcare provider orders vital signs to be taken every shift. Is this an appropriate order? Why or why not?

3. A client is being prescribed ferrous sulfate. What teaching should the nurse provide to this client?

EXPLORE MediaLink

 www.pearsoned.ca/adams-king

MEDIALINK DVD-ROM
- Audio Glossary
- CRNE Review
- Animation
  Mechanism of Action: Epoetin Alfa

COMPANION WEBSITE
- CRNE Review
- Case Study: Erythropoetin and erythrocyte production
- Dosage Calculations

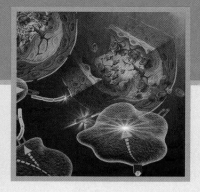

CHAPTER 29

Drugs for Pulmonary Disorders

DRUGS AT A GLANCE

BRONCHODILATORS

Beta-adrenergic agonists
    salmeterol (Serevent Diskhaler Disk)

Methylxanthines

Anticholinergics
    ipratropium bromide (Atrovent, Novo-Ipramide)

ANTI-INFLAMMATORY AGENTS

Glucocorticoids
    beclomethasone (Beclovent, Apo-Beclomethasone)

Mast cell stabilizers

Leukotriene modifiers

COMMON COLD AGENTS

Antitussives
    dextromethorphan (PMS-Dextromethorphan, others)

Expectorants

Mucolytics

OBJECTIVES

After reading this chapter, the student should be able to do the following:

1. List drug classes used for treating pulmonary disorders and discuss differences among their mechanisms of action.
2. Compare the advantages and disadvantages of using the inhalation route of drug administration for pulmonary drugs.
3. Describe the types of devices used to deliver aerosol therapies via the inhalation route.
4. Explain how drugs that modify the autonomic nervous system can be used to modify airflow in the bronchial tree.
5. Describe how drugs can be used to relieve the common symptoms of asthma, chronic bronchitis, and emphysema based on their underlying pathophysiology.
6. Describe the nurse's role in the pharmacological and non-pharmacological treatment of pulmonary disorders.
7. For each of the drug classes listed in Drugs at a Glance, identify a representative drug and explain its mechanism of action, therapeutic effects, and important adverse effects.
8. Describe and explain, based on pharmacological principles, the rationale for nursing assessment, planning, and interventions for clients with pulmonary disorders.
9. Use the nursing process to care for clients receiving drug therapy for pulmonary disorders.

MediaLink

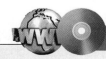

www.pearsoned.ca/adams-king

CRNE review, case studies, and other interactive resources for this chapter can be found on the Companion Website at **www.pearsoned.ca/adams-king**. Click on "Chapter 29" to select the activities for this chapter. For animations, more CRNE review questions, and an audio glossary, access the accompanying DVD-ROM in this textbook.

KEY TERMS

MediaLink   Canadian Lung Association

The respiratory system is one of the most important organ systems—a mere 5 to 6 minutes without breathing may result in death. When functioning properly, the respiratory system provides the body with the oxygen critical for all cells to carry on normal activities. Measurement of the rate and depth of respiration and listening to chest sounds with a stethoscope provide the nurse with valuable clues as to what may be happening internally. The respiratory system also provides a means by which the body can rid itself of excess acids and bases, a topic that is covered in Chapter 44. This chapter examines drugs used in the pharmacotherapy of asthma, the common cold, and chronic obstructive pulmonary disease.

29.1 Physiology of the Respiratory System

The primary function of the respiratory system is to bring oxygen into the body and to remove carbon dioxide. The process by which gasses are exchanged is called **respiration**. The basic structures of the respiratory system are shown in Figure 29.1.

Ventilation is the process of moving air into and out of the lungs. As the diaphragm contracts and lowers in position, it creates a negative pressure that draws air into the lungs, and inspiration occurs. During expiration, the diaphragm relaxes and air leaves the lung passively, with no energy expenditure required. Ventilation is a purely mechanical process that occurs approximately 12 to 18 times per minute in adults, a rate determined by neurons in the brainstem. This rate may

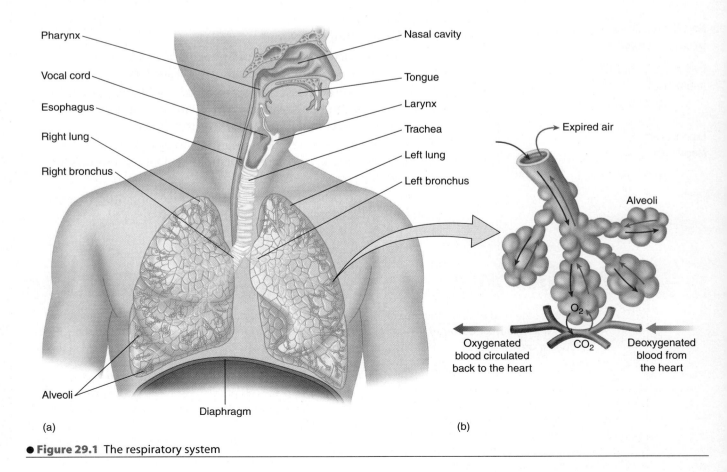

● **Figure 29.1** The respiratory system

be modified by a number of factors, including emotions, fever, stress, the pH of the blood, and certain medication.

Air entering the respiratory system travels through the nose, pharynx, and trachea into the bronchi, which divide into progressively smaller passages called bronchioles. The bronchial tree ends in dilated sacs called alveoli, which have no smooth muscle but are abundantly rich in capillaries. The extremely thin membrane of the alveoli separates the airway from the pulmonary capillaries, allowing gasses to readily move between the internal environment of the blood and the inspired air. As oxygen crosses this membrane, it is exchanged for carbon dioxide, a cellular waste product that travels from the blood to the air. The lung is richly supplied with blood. Blood flow through the lung is called **perfusion**. The process of gas exchange is shown in Figure 29.1.

29.2 Bronchiolar Smooth Muscle

Bronchioles are muscular, elastic structures whose internal diameter, or lumen, varies with the specific needs of the body. Changes in the diameter of the bronchiolar lumen are made possible by smooth muscle controlled by the autonomic nervous system. During the fight-or-flight response, beta$_2$-adrenergic receptors of the sympathetic nervous system are stimulated, the bronchiolar smooth muscle relaxes, and bronchodilation occurs. This allows more air to enter the alveoli, thus increasing the oxygen supply to the body during periods of stress or exercise. Sympathetic nervous system activation also increases the rate and depth of breathing. Drugs that stimulate beta$_2$-adrenergic receptors to cause bronchodilation are some of the most common drugs for treating pulmonary disorders.

When nerves from the parasympathetic nervous system are activated, bronchiolar smooth muscle contracts and the airway diameter narrows, resulting in bronchoconstriction. Bronchoconstriction increases airway resistance, causing breathing to be more laboured and the client to become short of breath. Parasympathetic stimulation also has the effect of slowing the rate and depth of respiration.

29.3 Administration of Pulmonary Drugs via Inhalation

The respiratory system offers a rapid and efficient mechanism for delivering drugs. The enormous surface area of the bronchioles and alveoli and the rich blood supply to these areas results in an almost instantaneous onset of action for inhaled substances.

Pulmonary drugs are delivered to the respiratory system by aerosol therapy. An **aerosol** is a suspension of minute liquid droplets or fine solid particles suspended in a gas. Aerosol therapy can give immediate relief for **bronchospasm**, a condition during which the bronchiolar smooth muscle contracts, leaving the client gasping for breath. Drugs may also be given to loosen viscous mucus in the bronchial tree. The major advantage of aerosol therapy is that it delivers the drugs to their immediate site of action, thus reducing systemic side effects. To produce the same therapeutic action,

an oral drug would have to be given at higher doses, and it would be distributed to all body tissues.

It should be clearly understood that agents delivered by inhalation can produce systemic effects due to absorption. For example, anesthetics such as nitrous oxide and halothane are delivered via the inhalation route and are rapidly distributed to cause CNS depression (see Chapter 20). Solvents such as paint thinners and glues are sometimes intentionally inhaled and can cause serious adverse effects on the nervous system, even death. The nurse must always monitor for systemic effects from inhalation drugs.

Several devices are used to deliver drugs via the inhalation route. **Nebulizers** are small machines that vaporize a liquid medication into a fine mist that can be inhaled using a facemask or handheld device. If the drug is a solid, it may be administered using a **dry powder inhaler (DPI)**. A DPI is a small device that is activated by the process of inhalation to deliver a fine powder directly to the bronchial tree. Turbohalers and rotahalers are types of DPIs. **Metered dose inhalers (MDIs)** are a third type of device commonly used to deliver respiratory drugs. MDIs use a propellant to deliver a measured dose of drug to the lungs during each breath. The client times the inhalation to the puffs of drug emitted from the MDI.

There are disadvantages to administering aerosol therapy. The precise dose received by the client is difficult to measure because it depends on the client's breathing pattern and the correct use of the aerosol device. Even under optimal conditions, only 10% to 50% of the drug actually reaches the bronchial tree. A spacer can improve drug distribution to the lungs: see http://asthma.ca/adults/treatment/spacers.php. The nurse must carefully instruct clients on the correct use of these devices. To reduce the oral absorption of inhaled medicines, clients should rinse their mouth thoroughly following drug use. Two devices used to deliver respiratory drugs are shown in Figure 29.2.

PHARMFACTS

Asthma

- Over 2.2 million Canadians have asthma.
- The prevalence of asthma is continuing to increase in both sexes and in all age and ethnic groups.
- An estimated 10% of children and 5% of adults have active asthma (take medication for asthma or have experienced symptoms in the past 12 months).
- In adults, asthma is slightly more common in females than in males. In children, however, the disease affects twice as many boys as girls.
- Asthma imposes a heavy burden on Canada's healthcare expenditures, reduces productivity, and seriously affects the quality of life for individuals with asthma and their families.
- Despite advances in treatment, there has been only a slight decline in the asthma mortality rate. Failure to further decrease the mortality rate may be a result of non-adherence with medications, inadequate environmental control, and lack of understanding of the consequences of an asthma attack.

Source: Statistics Canada, National Population Health Survey, 1996/97; Canadian Asthma Consensus Conference Guidelines for the Management of Asthma, 2003.

MediaLink — Animation: Small Volume Nebulizer

MediaLink — Animation: Dry Powder Inhaler

MediaLink — Animation: Metered Dose Inhaler

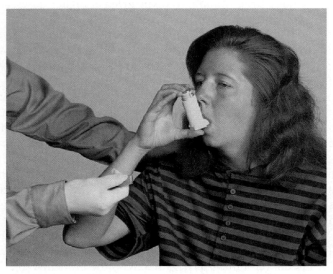

(a) Metered dose inhaler

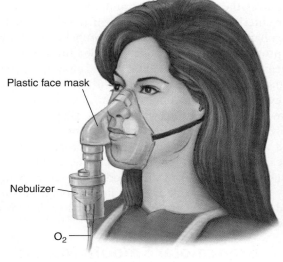

Plastic face mask

Nebulizer

O_2

(b) Nebulizer with attached face mask

● **Figure 29.2** Devices used to deliver respiratory drugs
Source: Pearson Education/PH College.

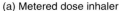

ASTHMA

Asthma is a chronic disease with both inflammatory and bronchospasm components. Drugs may be given to decrease the frequency of asthma attacks or to terminate attacks in progress.

29.4 Pathophysiology of Asthma

Asthma is one of the most common chronic conditions in Canada, affecting more than 2.2 million Canadians. The disease is characterized by acute bronchospasm, causing intense breathlessness, coughing, and gasping for air. Along with bronchoconstriction, the acute inflammatory response is initiated, stimulating mucus secretion and edema in the airways. These conditions are illustrated in Figure 29.3. Status asthmaticus is a severe, prolonged form of asthma unresponsive to drug treatment that may lead to respiratory failure. Typical causes of asthma attacks are listed in Table 29.1.

Although the exact etiology of asthma is unknown, it is believed to be the result of chronic airway inflammation. Controlling environmental factors that contribute to inflammation and asthma, such as dust mites and animal fur, may help slow disease progression and prevent asthma attacks. Because asthma has both a bronchoconstriction component and an inflammation component, pharmacotherapy of the disease focuses on one or both of these mechanisms. The goals of drug therapy are twofold: to terminate bronchospasm during an acute asthma attack and to reduce the frequency of acute asthma attacks and prevent further airway damage. Different medications are usually needed to achieve each of these goals. A summary of the various classes of drug used to treat respiratory diseases is illustrated in Figure 29.4.

According to the Canadian Asthma Consensus Guidelines that were endorsed in 2003, the five fundamental aspects of asthma care are:

1. Achieve acceptable control of the disease.
2. Treatment of asthma should focus on managing inflammation; inhaled glucocorticoids are the first-line anti-inflammatory therapy.
3. Control the environment.
4. A written action plan for guided self-management should be provided for all clients.
5. If acceptable control is not obtained, other drugs can be used in addition to moderate doses of corticosteroid.

BETA-ADRENERGIC AGONISTS

Selective beta$_2$-agonists are effective at relieving acute bronchospasm. They are some of the most frequently prescribed agents for the pharmacotherapy of asthma and other pulmonary diseases. These drugs are listed in Table 29.2.

29.5 Treating Asthma with Beta-Adrenergic Agonists

Beta-adrenergic agonists (sympathomimetics) are drugs of choice in the treatment of acute bronchoconstriction. Sympathomimetics selective for beta$_2$-receptors in the lung have largely replaced the older, non-selective agents such as epinephrine because they produce fewer cardiac side effects. Sympathomimetics act by relaxing bronchial smooth muscle; the resulting bronchodilation lowers airway resistance and makes breathing easier for the client.

A practical method for classifying beta-adrenergic agonists for asthma is by their duration of action. The ultrashort-acting drugs, including isoproterenol and isoetharine, pro-

TABLE 29.1   Common Causes of Asthma

Cause	Sources
air pollutants	tobacco smoke ozone nitrous and sulfur oxides fumes from cleaning fluids or solvents burning leaves
allergens	pollen from trees, grasses, and weeds animal dander household dust and dust mites mould
chemicals and food	drugs, including ASA, ibuprofen, and beta-blockers sulfite preservatives food and condiments, including nuts, monosodium glutamate (MSG), shellfish, and dairy products
respiratory infections	bacterial, fungal, and viral
stress	emotional stress/anxiety exercise in dry, cold climates

duce bronchodilation immediately, but their effects only last 2 to 3 hours. Short-acting agents, such as metaproterenol, terbutaline, and pirbuterol, also act quickly but last 5 to 6 hours. Intermediate-acting sympathomimetics, such as salbutamol last about 8 hours. The longest acting agent, salmeterol, has effects lasting as long as 12 hours. The ultra-short-, short-, and intermediate-acting drugs act quickly enough to terminate acute asthmatic episodes. The onset of action for salmeterol is too long for it to be indicated for acute asthma attack termination. Formoterol is the newest

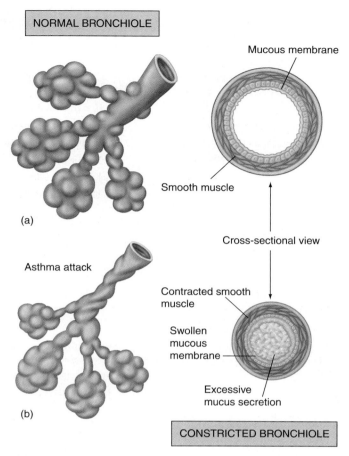

NORMAL BRONCHIOLE

(a)

Mucous membrane

Smooth muscle

Cross-sectional view

Asthma attack

Contracted smooth muscle

Swollen mucous membrane

Excessive mucus secretion

(b)

CONSTRICTED BRONCHIOLE

● **Figure 29.3** Changes in bronchioles during an asthma attack: (a) normal bronchiole; (b) constricted bronchiole

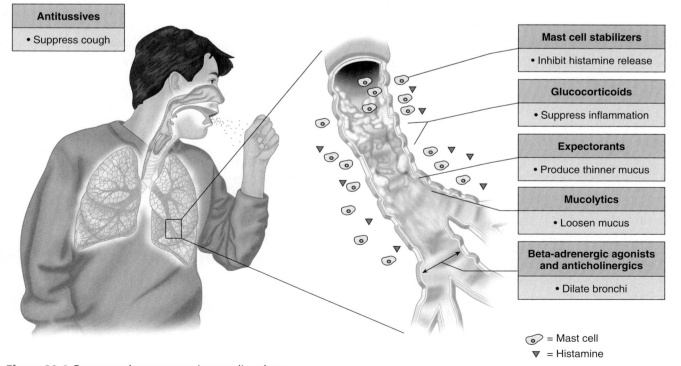

Antitussives

• Suppress cough

Mast cell stabilizers

• Inhibit histamine release

Glucocorticoids

• Suppress inflammation

Expectorants

• Produce thinner mucus

Mucolytics

• Loosen mucus

Beta-adrenergic agonists and anticholinergics

• Dilate bronchi

= Mast cell

▼ = Histamine

● **Figure 29.4** Drugs used to treat respiratory disorders

TABLE 29.2 Bronchodilators Used for Asthma

Drug	Route and Adult Dose
Beta-Adrenergic Agonists	
epinephrine (Adrenalin, Bronkaid, Primatene) (see page 417 for the Prototype Drug box)	SC; 0.1–0.5 mL of 1:1000 q20 min–4h
formoterol fumarate (Foradil)	DPI; 12 μg inhalation capsule q12h
isoproterenol (Isuprel, Medihaler-Iso)	MDI; 1–2 inhalations q4–6h (max 6 inhalations/day)
metaproterenol sulfate (Alupent, Metaprel)	MDI; two to three inhalations q3–4h (max 12 inhalations/day)
salbutamol (Ventolin, DOM-, PMS-Salbutamol, others)	PO; 2–4 mg tid–qid
	Inhalation; 1–2 puffs tid–qid
salmeterol (Serevent)	MDI; two inhalations bid
Methylxanthines	
aminophylline (Aminophylline)	PO; 0.25–0.75 mg/kg/hr divided qid
theophylline (Apo-Theo, Theo-Dur, others)	PO; 0.4–0.6 mg/kg/hr divided tid–qid
Anticholinergics	
ipratropium bromide (Atrovent, Novo-Ipramide)	MDI; Two inhalations qid (max 12 inhalations/day)

beta$_2$-adrenergic agonist, combining a very rapid onset of action (1 to 3 minutes) with a 12-hour duration.

Inhaled beta-adrenergic agonists produce little systemic toxicity because only small amounts of the drugs are absorbed. When given orally, a longer duration of action is achieved, but systemic side effects such as tachycardia are more frequently experienced; these drugs are sometimes contraindicated for clients with dysrhythmias. Tolerance may develop to the therapeutic effects of the beta-adrenergic agonists; therefore, the client must be instructed to seek medical attention should the drugs become less effective with continued use.

NURSING CONSIDERATIONS

The role of the nurse in asthma therapy with beta-adrenergic agonists involves careful monitoring of the client's condition and providing education as it relates to the prescribed drug regimen. Experiencing breathing difficulties can be distressing and greatly impact a client's quality of life. Controlling asthma is vital to a person's ability to perform normal activities of daily living. When beta-adrenergic agonists are used as bronchodilators, they help to reduce respiratory distress.

Assess the client's adherence to medication and the presence of side effects. Assess for the presence/history of bradycardia, dysrhythmias, myocardial infarction, hypothyroidism, decreased renal function, diabetes mellitus, glaucoma, benign prostatic hyperplasia, and tuberculosis. Beta-adrenergic agonists should not be used if the client has a history of dysrhythmia or myocardial infarction. Drugs in this class may cause many undesirable side effects. For clients using isoproterenol, rebound bronchospasm may occur when effects of the drug wear off.

Instruct the client on the use of the inhaler, and observe its use. Instruct the client to hold his or her breath for 10 seconds after inhaling the medication and wait 2 full minutes before the second inhalation.

Client education as it relates to beta-adrenergic agonists should include goals, reasons for obtaining baseline data such as vital signs and tests for cardiac and renal function, and possible side effects. The following are important points to include when teaching clients regarding beta-adrenergic agonists:

- Limit the use of products that contain caffeine.
- Immediately report difficulty breathing, heart palpitations, tremor, vomiting, nervousness, and vision changes.

See "Nursing Process Focus: Clients Receiving Adrenergic Therapy" in Chapter 13, page 137, for the complete nursing process applied to caring for clients receiving beta-adrenergic agonists.

METHYLXANTHINES AND ANTICHOLINERGICS

Although beta-agonists are drugs of choice for treating acute bronchospasm, drugs in the methylxanthine and anticholinergic classes are alternatives for the treatment of asthma. The methylxanthines are older, established drugs. Only one anticholinergic is in widespread use. These agents are shown in Table 29.2.

29.6 Treating Asthma with Methylxanthines and Anticholinergics

The **methylxanthines**, such as theophylline and aminophylline, comprise a group of bronchodilators chemically related to caffeine. Theophylline has a narrow margin of safety and interacts with a large number of other drugs. Side effects such as nausea, vomiting, and CNS stimulation are relatively common, and dysrhythmias may be observed at high doses. Because of their chemical similarities, clients should avoid caffeine-containing foods and beverages when taking methylxanthines. These agents are given by the PO or IV route. Having been largely replaced by safer and more effective drugs, the current use of theophylline is primarily for the long-term, oral prophylaxis of persistent asthma.

Blocking the parasympathetic nervous system produces similar effects to stimulation of the sympathetic nervous system. It is predictable, then, that anticholinergic drugs would cause bronchodilation and have potential use in the pharmacotherapy of asthma and other pulmonary diseases. Ipratropium is the most common anticholinergic prescribed for asthma and COPD pharmacotherapy. It has a slower onset of action than most beta-agonists and produces less intense bronchodilation. Anticholinergic side effects that are associated with drugs in this class are much milder when the drugs are administered by inhalation rather than systemically.

NURSING CONSIDERATIONS

The role of the nurse in asthma therapy with methylxanthines and anticholinergics involves careful monitoring of the client's condition and providing education as it relates to the prescribed drug regimen. Assess respiration rate before and after the first dose from an MDI because the first dose may precipitate bronchospasm. Monitor vital signs and intake and output throughout therapy as these drugs cause diuresis. Elderly clients using methylxanthines should be carefully monitored for toxicity as these clients may exhibit increased sensitivity due to decreased hepatic metabolism.

Methylxanthines may cause dysrhythmias, nausea, vomiting, and irritation of the upper respiratory tract, which may result in cough, drying of mucous membranes, and a bitter taste. To help with dry mouth and bitterness, clients can rinse their mouths frequently or use sugarless, hard candy.

Anticholinergic bronchodilators should be used cautiously in elderly men with benign prostatic hypertrophy and in all clients with glaucoma. The complete nursing process applied to clients receiving anticholinergics is presented in "Nursing Process Focus: Clients Receiving Anticholinergic Therapy" in Chapter 13, page 135.

Client education as it relates to methylxanthines should include goals, reasons for obtaining baseline data such as vital signs and tests for cardiac and renal function, and possible side effects. Instruct the client to immediately report the following: inability to urinate or have a bowel movement, severe headache, heart palpitations, difficulty breathing, changes in vision, and eye pain.

For additional nursing considerations, please refer to "Nursing Process Focus: Clients Receiving Bronchodilators" on page 377.

SPECIAL CONSIDERATIONS

Asthma Management in Schools

Approximately 10% of children have asthma. Researchers suggest that asthma is one of the most common causes of school absenteeism. In a typical class of 30 children or youth, two students suffer from asthma attacks each year while at school. Children cannot learn while experiencing wheezing, coughing, and shortness of breath.

Assisting schools to develop asthma management programs has become the focus of several federal agencies and dozens of professional and client advocacy groups. Many schools are adopting asthma management plans as part of a coordinated school health program. Schools with these programs have established "asthma-friendly" policies, such as allowing students to carry and administer quick-relief asthma medications. Additionally, the schools routinely maintain a copy of the student's asthma action plan from the caregiver or healthcare provider.

The role of the school nurse is to review the plan, determine the student's specific needs, and be sure that the student has immediate access to quick-relief asthma medication. The optimal plan for each student is determined case by case, with input from the student, parents, healthcare provider, and school nurse. Typically, older students are permitted to carry the inhaler and to self-administer as needed. The nurse often keeps a backup supply of the student's medication. For younger children, a supervised health assistant may be delegated to administer the medication.

Pr PROTOTYPE DRUG | Ipratropium Bromide (Atrovent, Novo-Ipramide)

ACTIONS AND USES

Ipratropium is an anticholinergic (muscarinic antagonist) that causes bronchodilation by blocking cholinergic receptors in bronchial smooth muscle. It is administered via inhalation and can relieve acute bronchospasm within minutes after administration. Effects may peak in 1 to 2 hours and continue for up to 6 hours. Ipratropium is less effective than the beta$_2$-agonists but is sometimes combined with beta-agonists or glucocorticoids for their additive effects. It is also prescribed for chronic bronchitis and for the symptomatic relief of nasal congestion.

PHARMACOKINETICS

There is minimal systemic absorption of ipratropium following inhalation. It has a half-life of 2 hours.

ADMINISTRATION ALERTS

- Proper use of the MDI is important to effective delivery of drug. Observe and instruct client in proper use.
- Avoid contact with eyes.
- Ipratropium is pregnancy category B.

ADVERSE EFFECTS AND INTERACTIONS

Because it is not readily absorbed from the lungs, ipratropium produces few systemic side effects. Irritation of the upper respiratory tract may result in cough, drying of the nasal mucosa, or hoarseness. It produces a bitter taste, which may be relieved by rinsing the mouth after use.

See the Companion Website for a Nursing Process Focus Chart specific to this drug.

GLUCOCORTICOIDS

Inhaled glucocorticoids are used for the long-term prevention of asthma attacks. Oral glucocorticoids may be used for the short-term management of acute asthma. The glucocorticoids are shown in Table 29.3.

29.7 Pharmacotherapy of Asthma with Glucocorticoids

Glucocorticoids are first-line therapy for the pharmacotherapy of asthma. When inhaled on a daily schedule, these hormones suppress airway inflammation without major side effects and help prevent acute asthma attacks. Clients should be informed that inhaled glucocorticoids must be taken daily to produce their therapeutic effect and

that these drugs are not effective at terminating episodes in progress. For some clients with mild, persistent asthma who do not wish to take inhaled steroid therapy daily, an as-needed treatment strategy may be acceptable provided it is accompanied by education and an action plan with clear instructions about how and when to increase medication use. Nevertheless, daily inhaled steroid treatment remains the preferred evidence-based therapy for asthma.

For severe, persistent asthma that is unresponsive to other treatments, oral glucocorticoids may be prescribed. If taken for longer than 10 days, oral glucocorticoids can produce significant adverse effects, including adrenal gland atrophy, peptic ulcers, and hyperglycemia. Other uses and adverse effects of glucocorticoids are presented in Chapters 31 and 39.

TABLE 29.3	Anti-Inflammatory Drugs Used for Asthma
Drug	**Route and Adult Dose**
Glucocorticoids	
beclomethasone (Beclovent, Apo-Beclomethasone, others)	MDI; one to two inhalations tid or qid (max 20 inhalations/day)
budesonide (GEN-Budesonide AQ)	DPI; one to two inhalations (100 μg/inhalation) qid (max 800 μg/day)
fluticasone (Flovent) (see page 415 for the Prototype Drug box)	MDI (44 μg); two inhalations bid (max 10 inhalations/day)
methylprednisolone (Medrol, Methylprednisolone Sodium Succinate Inj, Methylprednisolone Acetate Inj, others)	PO; 4–48 mg qd IM/IV; 10–40 mg, repeated if needed
prednisone (Apo-, Novo-Prednisone) (see page 407 for the Prototype Drug box)	PO; 5–60 mg qd
triamcinolone (Nasacort, Nasacort AQ)	MDI; two inhalations tid or qid (max 16 inhalations/day)
Mast Cell Stabilizers	
cromolyn (Apo-, Nu-Cromolyn, Cromolyn Nasal Mist)	MDI; one inhalation qid
Leukotriene Modifiers	
montelukast (Singulair)	PO; 10 mg qd in evening
zafirlukast (Accolate)	PO; 20 mg bid 1 h before or 2 h after meals

NURSING PROCESS FOCUS   Clients Receiving Bronchodilators

Assessment	Potential Nursing Diagnoses/Identified Patterns
Prior to administration: ■ Obtain complete health history including allergies, drug history, and possible drug reactions. ■ Assess for symptoms related to respiratory insufficiency such as dyspnea, orthopnea, cyanosis, nasal flaring, wheezing, and weakness. ■ Obtain vital signs. ■ Auscultate bilateral breath sounds for air movement and adventitious sounds (rales, rhonchi, wheezes). ■ Assess pulmonary function with pulse oximeter, peak expiratory flow meter, and/or arterial blood gasses to establish baseline.	■ Need for knowledge regarding drug therapy, adverse effects, and importance of adherence to treatment ■ Need for knowledge about management of asthma attacks ■ Need for knowledge of environmental modifications to reduce inflammation and disease progression ■ Anxiety related to difficulty breathing ■ Activity intolerance related to ineffective drug therapy ■ Disturbed sleep pattern related to side effects of drugs

Planning: Client Goals and Expected Outcomes

The client will:
■ Exhibit adequate oxygenation as evidenced by improved lung sounds and pulmonary function values
■ Report a reduction in subjective symptoms of respiratory deficiency
■ Demonstrate an understanding of the drug by accurately describing the drug's purpose, action, side effects, and precautions
■ Report at least 6 hours of uninterrupted sleep

Implementation

Interventions (Rationales)	Client Education/Discharge Planning
■ Monitor vital signs including pulse, blood pressure, and respiratory rate.	Instruct client to: ■ Use medication as directed even if asymptomatic ■ Report difficulty with breathing
■ Monitor pulmonary function with pulse oximeter, peak expiratory flow meter, and/or arterial blood gasses. (Monitoring is necessary to assess drug effectiveness.)	■ Instruct client to report symptoms of deteriorating respiratory status such as increased dyspnea, breathlessness with speech, and/or orthopnea.
■ Monitor the client's ability to use inhaler. (Proper use ensures correct dosage.)	Instruct client: ■ In proper use of metered dose inhaler ■ To strictly use the medication as prescribed; do not "double up" on doses ■ To rinse mouth thoroughly following use
■ Observe for side effects specific to the medication used.	■ Instruct client regarding side effects and to report specific drug side effects.
■ Maintain an environment free of respiratory contaminants such as dust, dry air, flowers, and smoke. (These substances may exacerbate bronchial constriction.)	Instruct client to: ■ Avoid respiratory irritants ■ Maintain "clean air environment" ■ Stop smoking and avoid second-hand smoke, if applicable
■ Maintain adequate dietary intake of essential nutrients and vitamins. (Dyspnea interferes with proper nutrition.) ■ Ensure client maintains adequate hydration of 3 to 4 L/day (to liquefy pulmonary secretions).	Instruct client to: ■ Maintain nutrition with foods high in essential nutrients ■ Consume small, frequent meals to prevent fatigue ■ Consume 3 to 4 L of fluid/day if not contraindicated ■ Avoid caffeine (increases CNS irritability)
■ Provide emotional and psychosocial support during periods of shortness of breath.	■ Instruct client in relaxation techniques and controlled breathing techniques.
■ Monitor client adherence. (Maintaining therapeutic drug levels is essential to effective therapy.)	■ Inform the client of the importance of ongoing medication compliance and follow-up.

Evaluation of Outcome Criteria

Evaluate the effectiveness of drug therapy by confirming that client goals and expected outcomes have been met (see "Planning").

See Table 29.2 (page 374) for a list of drugs to which these nursing actions apply.

NURSING CONSIDERATIONS

The role of the nurse in asthma pharmacotherapy with glucocorticoids involves careful monitoring of the client's condition and providing education as it relates to the prescribed treatment. Assess the client for the presence/history of asthma, seasonal rhinitis, hypertension, heart disease, and blood clots. Monitor the client's vital signs and body weight, and assess for signs and symptoms of infection. The steroid inhalers should be used cautiously in clients with hypertension, GI disease, congestive heart failure, or thromboembolic disease.

Since the primary purpose of inhaled glucocorticoids is to *prevent* respiratory distress, the client should be advised that this medication should not be used during an acute asthma attack. Excessive use of a short-acting bronchodilator (more than 3 times per week) for acute asthma attacks, waking with symptoms, or regular dyspnea are signs of uncontrolled asthma requiring adjustment of the glucocorticoid dosage. Additionally, the client should be alert for signs and symptoms of simple infections as glucocorticoids inhibit the inflammatory response and can mask the signs of infection. The client should be advised to rinse the mouth after using steroid inhalers because the drugs may promote fungal infections of the mouth and throat. Glucocorticoids also increase blood glucose levels and should be closely monitored in individuals with diabetes mellitus.

Client education as it relates to glucocorticoids should include goals, reasons for obtaining baseline data such as vital signs and tests for cardiac and renal function, and possible side effects. Following are the important points to include when teaching clients regarding glucocorticoids:

- Monitor temperature and blood pressure daily and report elevation to the healthcare provider.

- If diabetic, monitor blood glucose level closely and report unexplained or consistent elevations.

- Report occurrence of tarry stools, edema, dizziness, or difficulty breathing.

- Do not use these medications to terminate acute asthma attacks. Discuss with healthcare provider the appropriate medication to stop attacks.

See "Nursing Process Focus: Clients Receiving Systemic Glucocorticoid Therapy" in Chapter 39, page 565, for the complete nursing process applied to caring for clients receiving glucocorticoids.

MAST CELL STABILIZERS

Two mast cell stabilizers serve limited though important roles in the prophylaxis of asthma. The mast cell stabilizers act by inhibiting the release of histamine from mast cells. These drugs are shown in Table 29.3.

29.8 Treating Asthma with Mast Cell Stabilizers

Cromolyn and nedocromil are classified as mast cell stabilizers because their action serves to inhibit mast cells from releasing histamine and other chemical mediators of inflammation. By reducing inflammation, they are able to prevent asthma attacks. As with the glucocorticoids, clients must be informed that these agents should be taken on a daily basis and that they are not effective at terminating acute attacks. Maximum therapeutic benefit may take several weeks. Both cromolyn and nedocromil are pregnancy category B.

Cromolyn was the first mast stabilizer discovered. When administered via an MDI or a nebulizer, this drug is a safe alternative to glucocorticoids. An intranasal form of cro-

---

Pr PROTOTYPE DRUG | Beclomethasone (Beclovent, Apo-Beclomethasone)

ACTIONS AND USES

Beclomethasone is a glucocorticoid available through aerosol inhalation (MDI) for asthma or as a nasal spray for allergic rhinitis. For asthma, two inhalations, two to three times per day, usually provide adequate prophylaxis. Beclomethasone acts by reducing inflammation, thus decreasing the frequency of asthma attacks. It is not a bronchodilator and should not be used to terminate asthma attacks in progress.

PHARMACOKINETICS

There is minimal systemic absorption of beclomethasone when inhaled. It has a half-life of 1.5 hours.

ADMINISTRATION ALERTS

- Do not use if the client is experiencing an acute asthma attack.
- Oral inhalation products and nasal spray products are not to be used interchangeably.
- Beclomethasone is pregnancy category C.

ADVERSE EFFECTS AND INTERACTIONS

Inhaled beclomethasone produces few systemic side effects. Because small amounts may be swallowed with each dose, the client should be observed for signs of glucocorticoid toxicity when taking the drug for prolonged periods. Local effects may include hoarseness of the voice. Like all glucocorticoids, the anti-inflammatory properties of beclomethasone can mask signs of infection, and the drug is contraindicated if active infection is present. A large percentage of clients taking beclomethasone on a long-term basis will develop candidiasis, a fungal infection in the throat, due to the constant deposits of drug in the oral cavity.

 See the Companion Website for a Nursing Process Focus Chart specific to this drug.

molyn is used in the treatment of seasonal allergies. Side effects include stinging or burning of the nasal mucosa, irritation of the throat, and nasal congestion. Although not common, bronchospasm and anaphylaxis have been reported. Because of its short half-life (80 minutes), it must be inhaled four to six times per day.

Nedocromil is a newer mast cell stabilizer that has actions and uses similar to cromolyn. Administered with an MDI, the drug produces side effects similar to cromolyn although its longer half-life of 2.3 hours allows less frequent dosing. Clients often experience a bitter, unpleasant taste.

LEUKOTRIENE MODIFIERS

The leukotriene modifiers are newer drugs, approved in the 1990s, that are used to reduce inflammation and ease bronchoconstriction. They modify the action of leukotrienes, which are mediators of the inflammatory response in asthmatic clients. These drugs are shown in Table 29.3.

29.9 Treating Asthma with Leukotriene Modifiers

Leukotrienes are mediators of the immune response that promote airway edema, inflammation, and bronchoconstriction. Zileuton acts by blocking lipoxygenase, the enzyme that converts arachidonic acid into leukotrienes. The remaining two agents in this class, zafirlukast and montelukast, act by blocking leukotriene receptors.

The leukotriene modifiers are approved for the prophylaxis of chronic asthma. They are not bronchodilators and are ineffective in terminating acute asthma attacks. They are all given orally. Because zileuton is taken four times a day, it offers less client convenience than montelukast or zafirlukast, which are taken every 12 hours. Zileuton has a more rapid onset of action (2 hours) than the other two leukotriene modifiers, which take as long as 1 week to obtain therapeutic benefit.

Few serious adverse effects are associated with the leukotriene modifiers. Headache, cough, nasal congestion, or GI upset may occur. Clients over age 55 must be monitored carefully for signs of infection because these clients have been found to experience an increased frequency of infections when taking leukotriene modifiers. These agents may be contraindicated in clients with significant hepatic dysfunction or chronic alcoholism because they are extensively metabolized by the liver.

COMMON COLD

The common cold is a viral infection of the upper respiratory tract that produces a characteristic array of annoying symptoms. It is fortunate that the disorder is self-limiting because there is no cure or effective prevention for colds. Therapies used to relieve symptoms may include the same classes of drugs used for allergic rhinitis (Chapter 31), such as antihistamines, decongestants, and additional drugs such as those that suppress cough and loosen bronchial secretions.

ANTITUSSIVES

Antitussives are drugs used to dampen the cough reflex. They are of value in treating coughs due to allergies or the common cold.

29.10 Pharmacotherapy with Antitussives

Cough is a natural reflex mechanism that serves to forcibly remove excess secretions and foreign material from the respiratory system. In diseases such as emphysema and bronchitis, or when liquids have been aspirated into the bronchi, it is not desirable to suppress the normal cough reflex. Dry, hacking, non-productive cough, however, can be quite irritating to the membranes of the throat and can deprive a client of much needed rest. It is this type of situation in which therapy with antitussives may be warranted. Antitussives are classified as opioids or non-opioids and are shown in Table 29.4.

Opioids, the most efficacious antitussives, act by raising the cough threshold in the CNS. Codeine and hydrocodone are the most frequently used opioid antitussives. Doses needed to suppress the cough reflex are very low, so there is

TABLE 29.4 Agents for the Common Cold and Removal of Excessive Bronchial Mucus

Drug	Route and Adult Dose
Antitussives: Opioids	
codeine	PO; 10–20 mg q4–6h PRN (max 120 mg/24 h)
hydrocodone bitartrate (Hycodan, others)	PO; 5–10 mg q4–6h PRN (max 15 mg/dose)
Antitussives: Non-Opioids	
dextromethorphan (PMS-Dextromethorphan, others)	PO; 10–20 mg q4h or 30 mg q6–8h (max 120 mg/d)
Expectorants	
guaifenesin (Robitussin, others)	PO; 200–400 mg q4h (max 2.4 g/d)
Mucolytics	
acetylcysteine (Mucomyst, Acetylcysteine, Parvolex)	MDI; 1–10 mL of 20% solution q4–6h or 2–20 mL of 10% solution q4–6h

minimal potential for dependence. Most opioid cough mixtures are classified as Schedule III, IV, or V drugs and are reserved for more serious cough conditions. Though not common, overdose from opioid cough remedies may result in significant respiratory depression. Care must be taken when using these medications in clients with asthma or allergies since bronchoconstriction may occur. Opioids may be combined with other agents such as antihistamines, decongestants, and non-opioid antitussives in the therapy of severe cold or flu symptoms. Some of these combinations are shown in Table 29.5.

The most frequently used non-opioid antitussive is dextromethorphan. At low doses, this drug is available in OTC cold and flu medications. Higher doses are available by prescription to treat more severe cough. Dextromethorphan is chemically similar to the opioids and also acts in the CNS to raise the cough threshold. Though not as efficacious as codeine, there is no risk of dependence with dextromethorphan.

Benzonatate is a non-opioid antitussive that acts by a different mechanism. Chemically related to the local anesthetic tetracaine, benzonatate suppresses the cough reflex by anesthetizing stretch receptors in the lungs. If chewed, the drug can cause the side effect of numbing the mouth and pharynx. Side effects are uncommon but may include sedation, nausea, headache, and dizziness.

NURSING CONSIDERATIONS

The role of the nurse in antitussive therapy involves careful monitoring of the client's condition and providing education as it relates to the prescribed drug regimen. The nursing care related to clients receiving antitussive drugs is dependent on the agent used. For all antitussive drugs, assess the client for the presence/history of persistent non-productive cough, respiratory distress, shortness of breath, and/or productive cough.

When codeine or other opioids are prescribed, the client should be monitored for drowsiness. Since cough is a protective mechanism used to clear the lungs of microbes, antitussive drugs should be used in moderation and only to treat cough when it interferes with activities of daily living, rest, or sleep. Extreme caution should be used when administering antitussive drugs to individuals with chronic lung conditions as normal respiratory function is already impaired. Because cough may be a symptom of other serious pulmonary conditions, antitussive drugs should only be used for 3 days, unless otherwise approved by the healthcare provider.

Client education as it relates to antitussives includes goals, reasons for obtaining baseline data such as vital signs and tests for cardiac and renal function, and possible side effects. Following are the specific points to include when teaching clients regarding antitussives:

- Avoid driving and performing hazardous activities while taking opioid antitussives.
- Avoid use of alcohol, which can cause increased CNS depression.
- Immediately report the following: coughing up green- or yellow-tinged secretions, difficulty breathing, excessive drowsiness, constipation, nausea/vomiting.
- Store opioid antitussives away from children.

EXPECTORANTS AND MUCOLYTICS

Certain drugs are available to control excess mucus production. Expectorants increase bronchial secretions, and mucolytics help loosen thick bronchial secretions. These agents are shown in Table 29.4.

TABLE 29.5 Opioid Combination Drugs for Severe Cold Symptoms

Trade Name	Opioid	Non-Opioid Ingredients
Ambenyl Cough Syrup	codeine	bromodiphenhydramine
Calcidrine Syrup	codeine	calcium iodide
Codamine Syrup	hydrocodone	phenylpropanolamine
Codiclear DH Syrup	hydrocodone	guaifenesin
Codimal DH	hydrocodone	phenylephrine, pyrilamine
Hycodan	hydrocodone	homatropine
Hycomine Compound	hydrocodone	phenylephrine, chlorpheniramine, acetaminophen
Hycotuss Expectorant	hydrocodone	guaifenesin
Novahistine DH	codeine	pseudoephedrine, chlorpheniramine
Phenergan with Codeine	codeine	promethazine
Robitussin A-C	codeine	guaifenesin
Tega-Tussin Syrup	hydrocodone	phenylephrine, chlorpheniramine
Triaminic Expectorant DH	hydrocodone	phenylpropanolamine, pyrilamine, pheniramine, guaifenesin
Tussionex	hydrocodone	chlorpheniramine

Pr PROTOTYPE DRUG | Dextromethorphan (PMS-Dextromethorphan, others)

ACTIONS AND USES

Dextromethorphan is a drug included in most cold and flu preparations. It is available in a large variety of formulations, including tablets, liquid-filled capsules, lozenges, and liquids. Like codeine, it acts in the medulla, though it lacks the analgesic and euphoric effects of the opioids and does not produce dependence. Clients whose cough is not relieved by dextromethorphan after several days of therapy should see their healthcare provider.

PHARMACOKINETICS

Dextromethorphan is rapidly absorbed from the GI tract with an onset of action usually within 15 to 30 minutes. It crosses the blood-brain barrier and placenta and enters breast milk. Dextromethorphan and its active metabolite, dextrorphan, are excreted in urine. Its half-life is unknown.

ADMINISTRATION ALERTS

- Avoid pulmonary irritants, such as smoking and other fumes, as these agents may decrease drug effectiveness.
- Dextromethorphan is pregnancy category C.

ADVERSE EFFECTS AND INTERACTIONS

Side effects due to dextromethorphan are rare. Dizziness, drowsiness, and GI upset occur in some clients.

Drug interactions with dextromethorphan include a high risk of excitation, hypotension, and hyperpyrexia when used concurrently with MAO inhibitors. Concurrent use with alcohol may result in increased CNS depression.

 See the Companion Website for a Nursing Process Focus Chart specific to this drug.

29.11 Pharmacotherapy with Expectorants and Mucolytics

Expectorants are drugs that increase bronchial secretions. They act by reducing the thickness, or viscosity, of bronchial secretions, thus increasing mucus flow so that the mucus can more easily be removed by coughing. The most effective OTC expectorant is guaifenesin. Like dextromethorphan, guaifenesin produces few adverse effects and is a common ingredient in many OTC cold and flu preparations. Higher doses of guaifenesin are available by prescription.

Mucolytics are drugs used to break down the chemical structure of mucus molecules. Mucolytics cause thick, viscous bronchial secretions to become thinner and more able to be removed by coughing. Acetylcysteine, one of the few mucolytics available, is delivered by the inhalation route and is not available OTC. It is used in clients who have cystic fibrosis, chronic bronchitis, or other diseases that produce large amounts of thick bronchial secretions. Another mucolytic, dornase alfa, is used to break down DNA molecules in thick bronchial mucus, causing it to become less viscous.

CHRONIC OBSTRUCTIVE PULMONARY DISEASE

Chronic obstructive pulmonary disease (COPD) is a generic term used to describe several pulmonary conditions characterized by cough, mucus production, and impaired gas exchange. Drugs may be used to bring symptomatic relief, but they do not cure the disorders.

29.12 Pharmacotherapy of COPD

COPD is a major cause of death and disability. The three specific COPD conditions are asthma, chronic bronchitis, and emphysema. Chronic bronchitis and emphysema are strongly associated with smoking tobacco products and,

secondarily, with breathing air pollutants. In **chronic bronchitis**, excess mucus is produced in the bronchial tree due to the inflammation and irritation from tobacco smoke or pollutants. The airway becomes partially obstructed with mucus, thus resulting in the classic signs of dyspnea and coughing. An early sign of bronchitis is often a productive cough that occurs upon awakening. Wheezing and decreased exercise tolerance are additional clinical signs. Because microbes enjoy the mucus-rich environment, pulmonary infections are common. Gas exchange may be impaired.

COPD is progressive, with the terminal stage being **emphysema**. After years of chronic inflammation, the bronchioles lose their elasticity and the alveoli dilate to maximum size. The bronchioles collapse during exhalation, which restricts airflow and traps air in the lungs. The client suffers extreme dyspnea from even the slightest physical activity.

Clients with COPD may receive a number of pulmonary drugs for symptomatic relief. The goals of pharmacotherapy are to treat infections, control cough, and relieve bronchospasm. Most clients receive bronchodilators such as ipratropium, beta$_2$-agonists, or inhaled glucocorticoids. Mucolytics and expectorants are sometimes used to reduce the viscosity of the bronchial mucus and to aid in its

SPECIAL CONSIDERATIONS

Respiratory Distress Syndrome

Respiratory distress syndrome (RDS) is a condition, primarily occurring in premature babies, in which the lungs do not produce surfactant. Surfactant forms a thin layer on the inner surface of the alveoli to raise the surface tension. This prevents the alveolus from collapsing during expiration. If birth occurs before the pneumocytes in the lung are mature enough to secrete surfactant, the alveoli collapse and RDS results.

Surfactant medications can be delivered to the newborn either as prophylactic therapy or as rescue therapy after symptoms develop. The two surfactant agents used for RDS are colfosceril and beractant. These drugs are administered intratracheally every 4 to 6 hours, until the client's condition improves.

removal. Oxygen therapy assists breathing in emphysema clients. Antibiotics may be prescribed for clients who experience multiple bouts of pulmonary infection.

Clients should be taught to avoid taking any drugs that have beta-antagonist activity or otherwise cause bronchoconstriction. Respiratory depressants such as opioids and barbiturates should be avoided. It is important to note that none of the pharmacotherapies offer a cure for COPD; they only treat the symptoms of a progressively worsening disease. The most important teaching point for the nurse is to strongly encourage smoking cessation in these clients.

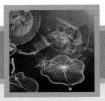

CHAPTER REVIEW

KEY CONCEPTS

The numbered key concepts provide a succinct summary of the important points from the corresponding numbered section within the chapter. If any of these points are not clear, refer to the numbered section within the chapter for review. Expanded versions can be found on the Companion Website.

29.1 The physiology of the respiratory system involves two main processes. Ventilation moves air into and out of the lungs and perfusion allows for gas exchange across capillaries.

29.2 Bronchioles are lined with smooth muscle that controls the amount of air entering the lungs. Dilation and constriction of the airways are controlled by the autonomic nervous system.

29.3 Inhalation is a common route of administration for pulmonary drugs because it delivers drugs directly to the site of action. Nebulizers, MDIs, and DPIs are devices used for aerosol therapies.

29.4 Asthma is a chronic disease that has both inflammation and bronchospasm components. Treatment should focus on the reduction of inflammation. Environmental control can help reduce inflammation and prevent asthma attacks.

29.5 Beta-adrenergic agonists are the most effective drugs for relieving acute bronchospasm. These agents act by activating beta$_2$-receptors in bronchial smooth muscle to cause bronchodilation.

29.6 Methylxanthines and anticholinergics are bronchodilators occasionally used as alternatives to the beta-agonists in asthma therapy.

29.7 Inhaled glucocorticoids are first-line therapy for asthma. They reduce inflammation and provide long-term prophylaxis of attacks. Oral glucocorticoids are also available.

29.8 Cromolyn, a mast cell stabilizer, is a safe drug used for the prophylaxis of asthma, but it is ineffective at relieving acute bronchospasm.

29.9 The leukotriene modifiers, whose primary use is in asthma prophylaxis, act by reducing the inflammatory component of asthma.

29.10 Antitussives are effective at relieving cough due to the common cold. Opioids are used for severe cough. Non-opioids such as dextromethorphan are used for mild or moderate cough.

29.11 Expectorants promote mucus secretion, making the mucus thinner and easier to remove by cough. Mucolytics are agents used to break down thick bronchial secretions.

29.12 Chronic obstructive pulmonary disease (COPD) is a progressive disorder treated with multiple pulmonary drugs. Bronchodilators, expectorants, mucolytics, antibiotics, and oxygen may offer symptomatic relief.

REVIEW QUESTIONS

1 What is the difference between ventilation and perfusion?

2 Name the three types of device used to deliver drugs by the inhalation route. What are the differences between them?

3 Distinguish between the classes of drug that prevent asthma attacks and those that can terminate an attack in progress. Name at least one drug in each class.

4 What is the difference in the mechanism of action between an antitussive and an expectorant?

CRITICAL THINKING QUESTIONS

1. A 72-year-old male client has recently been started on an ipratropium (Atrovent) inhaler. What teaching is important for the nurse to provide?

2. A 65-year-old client has bronchitis and has been coughing for several days. Which is the antitussive of choice for this client, dextromethorphan or codeine? Why?

3. A 45-year-old chronic asthmatic is on glucocorticoids. What assessment and care are required for this client?

EXPLORE MediaLink

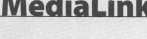

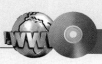

www.pearsoned.ca/adams-king

MEDIALINK DVD-ROM

- **Audio Glossary**
- **CRNE Review**
- **Videos & Animations**
  Mechanism of Action: Salmeterol
  Nursing in Action: Administering Medications by Inhaler
  Acute Respiratory Distress Syndrome (ARDS)
  Asthma
  Metered Dose Inhaler
  Nebulizer

COMPANION WEBSITE

- **CRNE Review**
- **Case Study:** Client with asthma
- **Dosage Calculations**

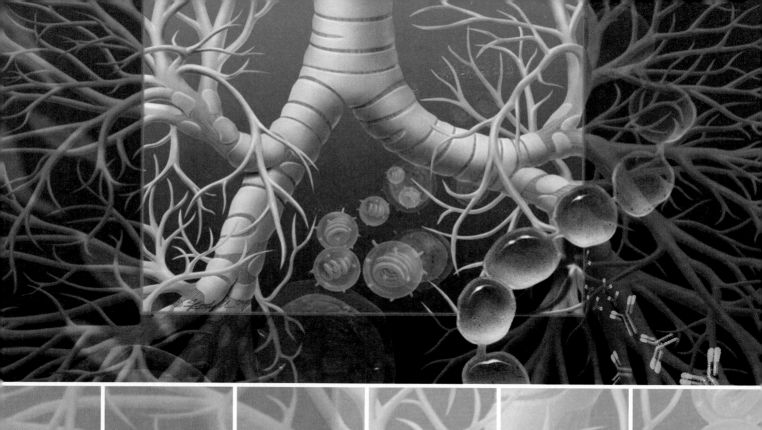

Unit 6

The Immune System

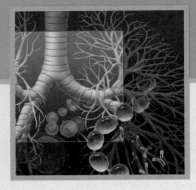

CHAPTER 30

Drugs for Immune System Modulation

DRUGS AT A GLANCE

IMMUNIZATION AGENTS

Vaccines
> *hepatitis B vaccine (Recombivax)*

Immune globulin preparations

IMMUNOSTIMULANTS

Interferons
> *interferon alfa-2 (Intron A)*

Interleukins

Other agents

IMMUNOSUPPRESSANTS

Antibodies

Antimetabolites and cytotoxic agents

Calcineurin inhibitors
> *cyclosporine (Neoral, Sandimmune)*

Glucocorticoids

OBJECTIVES

After reading this chapter, the student should be able to do the following:

1. Identify drug classes used for modifying immune function.
2. Explain the therapeutic action of each class of drugs used for modifying immune function in relation to the pathophysiology of immune disorders.
3. Describe the classes of drugs used as immunosuppressants and explain why they are necessary following organ transplants.
4. Compare and contrast active immunity and passive immunity.
5. For each of the drug classes listed in Drugs at a Glance, identify a representative drug and explain its mechanism of action, therapeutic effects, and important adverse effects.
6. For each of the major vaccines, state the recommended dosage schedule.
7. Describe and explain, based on pharmacological principles, the rationale for nursing assessment, planning, and interventions for clients with immune disorders.
8. Use the nursing process to care for clients receiving drug therapy for immune disorders.

MediaLink

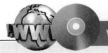

www.pearsoned.ca/adams-king

CRNE review, case studies, and other interactive resources for this chapter can be found on the Companion Website at **www.pearsoned.ca/adams-king**. Click on "Chapter 30" to select the activities for this chapter. For animations, more CRNE review questions, and an audio glossary, access the accompanying DVD-ROM in this textbook.

KEY TERMS

The body comes under continuous attack from a host of foreign agents that include viruses, bacteria, fungi, and single-celled animals. Our extensive body defences are capable of mounting a rapid and effective response against many of these pathogens. In some cases, pharmacotherapy can be used to stimulate body defences so that microbes can be more readily attacked and disease prevented. On other occasions, it is desirable to dampen the immune response, for example, to allow a transplanted organ to survive. This chapter examines the pharmacotherapy of agents affecting the body's immune response to disease.

PHARMFACTS

Vaccines

- Vaccines have eradicated smallpox from the world and the poliovirus from the Western Hemisphere.
- Vaccines lowered the number of diphtheria cases in Canada to 1 or less per year since 1997.
- Vaccines lowered the average annual number of measles cases in Canada by 96% since beginning catch-up and routine two-dose immunization in 1996/97.
- Pertussis is the most prevalent vaccine-preventable disease in Canada, with over 3000 cases per year. It is most severe in children under 1 year of age. Incidence in adolescents and adults is increasing due to waning immunity.
- Vaccines produce few serious adverse effects, while the diseases they help to prevent often have serious or fatal consequences. To make vaccines safer than the disease, the bacterium or virus is killed or weakened.
- About 85% of persons vaccinated develop immunity. Immunity from some vaccines diminishes over time and requires boosters. Blood tests can determine protective levels of several vaccines.
- In 2004, only 61% of 2-year-olds and 41% of 7-year-olds were up-to-date with vaccinations. Under-immunized children and adults are at risk.
- Research is in progress to find ways to combine more antigens in a single vaccine to reduce both the number of injections and office visits for vaccinations.
- A vaccine for human papillomavirus (HPV) is now available in Canada. About 10% to 30% of adults are infected with HPV. The highest incidence is in women aged 20 to 24 years. HPV is believed to be the primary cause of cervical cancer.

Source: Public Health Agency of Canada. (2006). Canadian national report on immunization, 2006. Canada Communicable Disease Report, 32S3, 1–44.

30.1 Non-Specific Body Defences and the Immune Response

The lymphatic system consists of lymphoid cells, tissues, and organs such as the spleen, thymus, tonsils, and lymph nodes. The overall purpose of the lymphatic system is to protect the body from pathogens.

The first line of protection from pathogens is **non-specific defences**, which serve as barriers to microbes and environmental hazards. The non-specific defences are unable to distinguish one type of threat from another; the response or protection is the same regardless of the pathogen. Non-specific defences include physical barriers such as the epithelial lining of the skin and the respiratory and gastrointestinal mucous membranes. These are potential entry points for pathogens. Other non-specific defences are phagocytes, natural killer (NK) cells, the complement system, fever, and interferons. From a pharmacological perspective, one of the most important non-specific defences is inflammation. Because of its significance, inflammation is discussed separately, in Chapter 31.

The body has the capability to mount a second line of defence that is specific to certain pathogens. For example, a specific defence may act against only a single species of bacteria and be ineffective against all others. This defence is known as the **immune response**. Foreign agents that elicit an immune response are called **antigens**. Foreign proteins, such as those present on the surfaces of pollen grains, bacteria, nonhuman cells, and viruses, are the strongest antigens. The primary cell of the immune response that interacts with antigens is the lymphocyte.

The immune response is extremely complex. Basic steps involve recognition of the antigen, communication and coordination with other defence cells, and destruction or suppression of the antigen. A large number of chemical messengers and interactions are involved in the immune response, many of which have yet to be discovered. The two basic divisions of the immune response are antibody-mediated (humoral) immunity and cell-mediated immunity. These are shown in Figure 30.1.

30.2 Humoral Immunity and Antibodies

Humoral immunity is initiated when an antigen encounters a type of lymphocyte known as a **B cell**. The activated B cell divides rapidly to form clones. Most of these cells are called **plasma cells**, whose primary function is to secrete **antibodies** that are specific to the antigen that initiated the challenge. Circulating through the body, antibodies, also known as immunoglobulins, physically interact with the foreign antigen to neutralize it or mark it for destruction by other cells of the immune response. Peak production of antibodies occurs about 10 days after an antigen challenge. The important functions of antibodies are illustrated in Figure 30.2

Some B cells, called *memory B cells,* remember the initial antigen interaction. Should the body be exposed to the same antigen in the future, the immune system will be able to manufacture even higher levels of antibodies in a shorter period, approximately 2 to 3 days. For some antigens, memory can be retained for an entire lifetime. Vaccines are sometimes administered to produce these memory cells in advance of exposure to the antigen so that when the body is exposed to the actual organism, it can mount a fast, effective response.

VACCINES

Vaccines are biological agents used to stimulate the immune system. The goal of vaccine administration is to prevent serious infections by life-threatening pathogens.

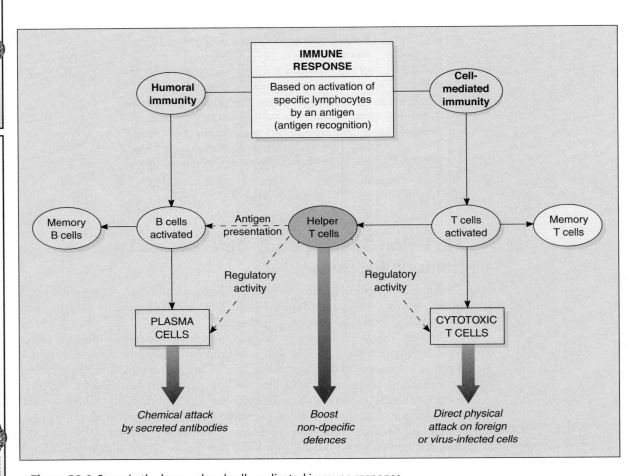

● **Figure 30.1** Steps in the humoral and cell-medicated immune response

Source: Pearson Education/PH College.

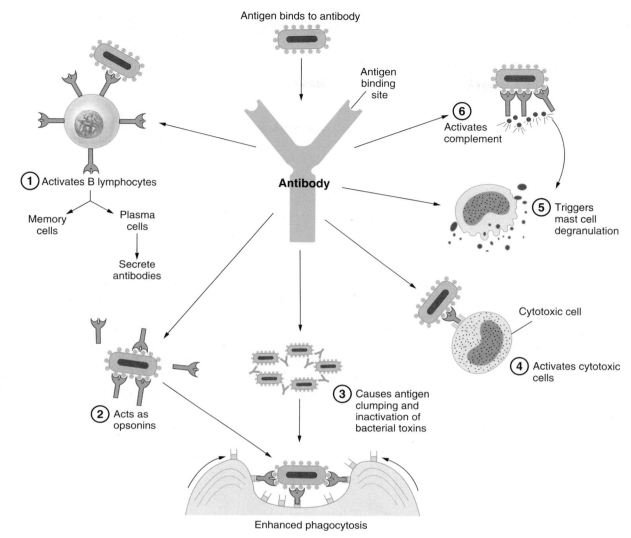

● **Figure 30.2** Functions of antibodies

30.3 Administration of Vaccines

Lymphocytes attack antigens by binding to them through certain receptor proteins on their surface. Sometimes they recognize a toxin or secretion produced by the organism. Scientists have used this knowledge to create vaccines, which are biological products that prevent disease. Vaccines consist of suspensions of one of the following:

• Microbes that have been killed

• Microbes that are alive but weakened (attenuated) so they are unable to produce disease

• Bacterial toxins, called **toxoids**, that have been modified to destroy their hazardous properties

Vaccination, or **immunization**, is performed to expose the client to the modified, harmless pathogen or its toxoid so that an immune response occurs in the following weeks or months. As a result of the vaccination, memory B cells are formed. When later exposed to the actual infectious organism, these cells will react quickly by producing large quantities of antibodies. The protective level of most vac-

cines can be assessed by measuring the amount of antibody in the blood that is produced after the vaccine has been administered, a quantity called **titre**. If the titre falls below the protective level, a follow-up vaccination, called a *booster,* is indicated. While some immunizations are only needed once, most require boosters to provide continuous protection.

The type of immunity achieved through the administration of a vaccine is called **active immunity**. In active immunity, the client's immune system is stimulated to produce antibodies and generate memory cells by exposure to an antigen or a vaccine.

Passive immunity occurs by direct transference of antibodies from one individual to another. Maternal antibodies cross the placenta and provide temporary protection for the fetus and newborn. Agents used to provide passive immunity include infusion of immune globulin following exposure to hepatitis, antivenoms used for snakebites, and sera used to treat botulism, tetanus, and rabies. Because these drugs do not stimulate the client's immune system, memory cells are not produced and the protective effects

TABLE 30.1   Immune Globulin Preparations

Drug	Route and Adult Dose
cytomegalovirus immune globulin (CytoGam)	IV; 150 mg/kg within 72 h of transplantation, then 100 mg/kg for 2, 4, 6, and 8 wk post-transplant, then 50 mg/kg for 12 and 16 wk post-transplant
hepatitis B immune globulin (HyperHep B)	IM; 0.06 mL/kg as soon as possible after exposure, preferably within 24 h, but no later then 7 d, repeat 28–30 d after exposure
immune globulin intramuscular (Gamastan)	IM; 0.02–0.06 mL/kg as soon as possible after exposure if H-BIG is unavailable
immune globulin intravenous (Gammagard, Iveegam)	IV; 100–200 mg/kg/mo IM; 1.2 mL/kg followed by 0.6 mL/kg q2–4wk
rabies immune globulin (Imogam, Hyperab)	IM (gluteal); 20 IU/kg
Rh_o(D) immune globulin (WinRho)	IM/IV; one vial or 300 μg at approximately 28 wk; followed by one vial of minidose or 120 μg within 72 h of delivery if infant is Rh-positive
tetanus immune globulin (HyperTet)	IM; 250 units

last only 2 to 3 weeks. Thus, these drugs are used following exposure or when risk of exposure is high and there is not enough time for the client to develop active immunity. Table 30.1 lists select immune globulin preparations. Figure 30.3 illustrates the development of immunity through vaccines or the administration of antibodies.

Most vaccines are administered with the goal of preventing illness, including measles, polio, whooping cough, tetanus, and hepatitis B. Recently, a vaccine for human papillomavirus (HPV) has become available in Canada. HPV is believed to be the primary cause of cervical cancer. The highest incidence is in women aged 20 to 24 years. In the case of HIV infection, experimental HIV vaccines are given after infection has occurred for the purpose of enhancing the immune system, rather than preventing the disease. Unlike other vaccines, experimental vaccines for

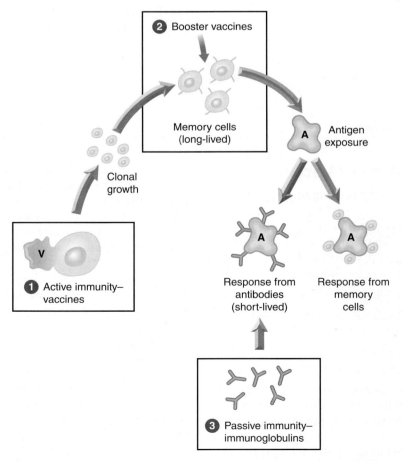

● Figure 30.3 Active and passive immunity: (1) administration of vaccine provides long-lasting active immunity; (2) booster vaccines maintain enough memory cells to provide a quick response; (3) administration of immune globulins provides short-lived passive immunity

TABLE 30.2 **National Advisory Committee on Immunization (NACI) Recommendations for Routine Childhood Vaccination in Canada**

Vaccine	2 Months	4 Months	6 Months	1 Year	18 Months	4–6 Years	14–16 Years
DTaP-IVP	•	•	•		•	•	
Hib	•	•	•		•		
MMR				•	• or	•	
Var				•			
HB	(three doses infancy)			or	2–3 doses pre-teen		
Pneu-C-7	•	•	•	•			
Men-C	•	•	• or	•	• ← 2–3 doses pre-teen →		
Tdap							
Inf	(6–23 months			•	1–2 doses)		
HPV							(3 doses, females, before becoming sexually active)

DTaP-IVP: Diphtheria, tetanus, acellular pertussis, polio vaccine;
Hib: Haemophilus influenza type b vaccine; usually combined with the Dtap-IPV;
MMR: Measles, mumps, rubella vaccine (Administer second dose one month after the first or at age 4–6 years)
Var: Varicella (Chickenpox) vaccine
HB: Hepatitis B Vaccine (Infancy or thereafter. Administer second dose at least 1 month after the first dose, and the third at least 2 months after second dose)
Pneu-C-7: Pneumococcal conjugate vaccine (all children under 2 years of age)

Men-C: Meningococcal C conjugate vaccine (recommended for children under 5 years of age, adolescents and young adults; at least 1 dose after age 5 month.)
Tdap: Tetanus, Diphtheria, acellular pertussis (boosters for tetanus and Diphtheria every 10 years through out lifetime once ≥ 7 years of age)
Inf: Influenza vaccine recommended annually for all children 6–23 months of age and children 2 years and older with chronic health conditions.

Source: Public Health Agency of Canada. (2006). Canadian immunization guide. (7th ed.). Ottawa, ON: Public Works and Government Services.

HIV have thus far been unable to prevent AIDS. Pharmacotherapy of HIV is discussed in Chapter 34.

All vaccines used for routine immunization are effective in preventing disease and have a low risk of serious adverse effects. The diseases, however, can have serious or even fatal consequences. Common side effects of vaccines include redness and discomfort at the site of injection and fever. Although severe reactions are uncommon, anaphylaxis is possible. Vaccinations are contraindicated for clients who have a weak immune system or who are currently experiencing symptoms such as diarrhea, vomiting, or fever.

Effective vaccines have been produced for a number of debilitating diseases, and their widespread use has prevented serious illness in millions of clients, particularly children. One disease, smallpox, has been completely eliminated from the planet through immunization, and others such as polio have diminished to extremely low levels. Immunization is not mandatory in Canada. Immunization is a shared responsibility between federal and provincial/territorial governments. Although some provinces have legislation that requires proof of immunization for school entrance, exceptions are permitted for reasons of conscience, religion, allergies, and medical conditions. Table 30.2 gives some common childhood vaccines and their schedules as recommended by the National Advisory Committee on Immunization (NACI). Nurses should be familiar with recommendations in their jurisdiction as they may differ from those of the NACI.

Although vaccinations have proved a resounding success in children, many adults die of diseases that could be prevented by vaccination. Most mortality from vaccine-preventable disease in adults is from influenza and pneumococcal disease. Hepatitis B is the most important vaccine-preventable infectious occupational disease for healthcare workers. The risk of being infected is a consequence of the prevalence of virus carriers in the population receiving care, the frequency of exposure to blood and other body fluids, and the contagiousness of hepatitis B virus. All Canadian adults require maintenance of immunity to tetanus and diphtheria, preferably with combined (Td) toxoid and a single dose of acellular pertussis vaccine. A vaccine for HPV is newly available in Canada for pre-exposure use in young females to reduce risk of cervical cancer caused by HPV. HPV vaccine is administered in three doses over 6 months at 0, 2, and 6 months. In 2006, the NACI published an adult immunization schedule that contained both age-based and risk-based recommendations. The more common of these are presented in Table 30.3 (see the NACI website for a complete listing).

CULTURAL CONSIDERATIONS

Immunization

Childhood immunizations have proven to be one of the most effective means of preventing and controlling the spread of infectious and communicable diseases, although hundreds of preschool children are not being immunized. In general, immunization levels are lower among Aboriginal Peoples, immigrants, older adults, populations with low socioeconomic status, and some religious groups. According to International Circumpolar Surveillance (ICS), the incidence of invasive pneumococcal disease from 1999 to 2004 was higher among Aboriginals, at 38 per 100,000, than non-Aboriginals, at 9.6 per 100,000 (ICS, unpublished data, 2006). Limited access to preventive services, limited knowledge about vaccination, and attitudes and cultural beliefs about immunization, illness, and healthcare may contribute to these statistics.

Source: Public Health Agency of Canada, INK "http://www.phac-aspc.gc.ca/".

TABLE 30.3 Adult Immunization Schedule: Routine and Specific Risk Situations

Vaccine or Toxoid	Indication	Schedule
tetanus and diphtheria given as Td; and pertussis given as Tdap	Routine for all adults	Td booster every 10 years (doses 1 and 2 given 4–8 weeks apart and dose 3 given 6–12 months later; one of the doses should be given as Tdap for pertussis protection if not previously given)
measles, mumps, and rubella given as MMR	Routine for adults who have no record or an unclear history of prior immunization	1 dose for adults born in or after 1970 without a history of measles or without evidence of immunity to rubella or mumps; second dose for select groups
varicella	Routine for adults who have no record or an unclear history of prior immunization	Doses 1 and 2 at least 4 weeks apart for susceptible adults (no history of natural disease or seronegativity)
influenza	Adults ≥ 65 years; adults < 65 years at high risk of influenza-related complications and their household contacts; healthcare workers	Every autumn using current recommended vaccine formulation
pneumococcal polysaccharide	Adults ≥ 65 years; adults < 65 who have conditions putting them at increased risk of pneumococcal disease	1 dose
hepatitis A	Occupational risk; lifestyle; travel to areas with inadequate sanitation; post-exposure immunoprophylaxis; adults with chronic liver disease	2 doses 6–12 months apart
hepatitis B	Occupational risk; lifestyle; post-exposure immunoprophylaxis; adults with chronic liver disease	3 doses at 0, 1, and 6 months
HPV	Pre-exposure use in young females to reduce risk of cervical cancer caused by HPV	3 doses at 0, 2, and 6 months
bacille Calmette-Guérin (BCG)	Rarely used; consider for high-risk exposure	1 dose
poliomyelitis	Travel to endemic areas; other risk group	Primary series doses 1 and 2 given 4–8 weeks apart and dose 3 given 6–12 months later; 1 booster dose if > 10 years since primary series
meningococcal conjugate	Young adults	1 dose
rabies, pre-exposure use	Occupational; high-risk travellers	3 doses at days 0, 7, and 21

Source: Public Health Agency of Canada. (2006). Canadian immunization guide. (7th ed.). Ottawa, ON: Public Works and Government Services.

Pr PROTOTYPE DRUG | Hepatitis B Vaccine (Recombivax)

ACTIONS AND USES

Hepatitis B vaccine (Recombivax) is used to provide active immunity in individuals who are at risk for exposure to hepatitis B virus (HBV). It is indicated for infants born to HBV-positive mothers and those at high risk for exposure to HBV-infected blood, including nurses, physicians, dentists, dental hygienists, morticians, and paramedics. Because HBV infection is extremely difficult to treat, it is prudent for all healthcare workers to receive the HBV vaccine before beginning their clinical education, unless contraindicated. HBV vaccine does not provide protection against exposure to other (non-B) hepatitis viruses. HBV vaccine is produced by splicing the gene for HBV surface antigen into yeast and harvesting the protein product. It is prepared from recombinant yeast cultures rather than from human blood. Vaccination requires three IM injections; the second dose is given 1 month after the first, and the third dose 6 months after the first.

PHARMACOKINETICS

The pharmacokinetics of HBV vaccine are unknown. The onset of action is 2 weeks, with a peak in 6 months.

ADMINISTRATION ALERTS

- In adults, use the deltoid muscle for the injection site, unless contraindicated.
- Epinephrine (1:1000) should be immediately available to treat a possible anaphylactic reaction.
- Titres should be done a few months after series is completed to confirm immunity.
- HBV vaccine is pregnancy category C.

ADVERSE EFFECTS AND INTERACTIONS

HBV vaccine is well tolerated, and few serious adverse reactions have been reported. Pain and inflammation at the injection site are the most common side effects. Some clients experience transient fever or fatigue. Hypersensitivity reactions such as urticaria or anaphylaxis are possible.

This vaccine is contraindicated in clients with hypersensitivity to yeast or HBV vaccine. The drug should be administered with caution in clients with fever or active infections or in those with compromised cardiopulmonary status.

30.4 Cell-Mediated Immunity and Cytokines

A second branch of the immune response involves lymphocytes called **T cells**. Two major types of T cells are called **helper T cells** and **cytotoxic T cells**. These cells are sometimes named after a protein receptor on their plasma membrane: the helper T cells have a CD4 receptor, and the cytotoxic T cells have a CD8 receptor. The helper T cells are particularly important because they are responsible for activating most other immune cells, including B cells. Cytotoxic T cells travel throughout the body and can directly kill certain bacteria, parasites, virus-infected cells, and cancer cells.

Activated or sensitized T cells rapidly form clones after they encounter their specific antigen. Unlike B cells, however, T cells do not produce antibodies. Instead, activated T cells produce huge amounts of **cytokines**, hormone-like proteins that regulate the intensity and duration of the immune response and mediate cell-to-cell communication. Some cytokines kill foreign organisms directly, while others induce inflammation or enhance the killing power of macrophages. Specific cytokines released by activated T cells include interleukins, gamma interferon, and perforin. Some cytokines are used therapeutically to stimulate the immune system, as discussed in Section 30.5.

As with B cells, some sensitized T cells become memory cells. Should the body encounter the same antigen in the future, the memory T cells will assist in mounting a more rapid immune response.

IMMUNOSTIMULANTS

Despite attempts over many decades to develop effective drugs that stimulate the immune system to fight disease, only a few such drugs have been approved. These agents include interferons and interleukins produced by recombinant DNA technology. Immunostimulants are shown in Table 30.4.

BIOLOGICAL RESPONSE MODIFIERS

30.5 Pharmacotherapy with Biological Response Modifiers

When challenged by specific antigens, certain macrophages, B and T lymphocytes, mast cells, endothelial cells, and stromal cells of the spleen, thymus, and bone marrow secrete cytokines that help defend against the invading organism. These natural cytokines have been identified and, through recombinant DNA technology, large enough quantities can be made available to treat certain disorders. A handful of immunostimulants, sometimes called **biological response modifiers**, have been approved to boost certain functions of the immune system.

Interferons are cytokines secreted by lymphocytes and macrophages that have been infected with a virus. After secretion, interferons attach to uninfected cells and signal them to secrete antiviral proteins. Part of the non-specific defence system, interferons slow the spread of viral infections and enhance the activity of existing leukocytes. The actions of interferons include modulation of immune functions, such as increasing phagocytosis and enhancing the cytotoxic activity of T cells. The two major classes of interferon having clinical utility are alpha and beta. The alpha class has the widest therapeutic application (when used as medications, the spelling is changed to alfa). Indications for interferon alpha therapy include hairy cell leukemia, AIDS-related Kaposi's sarcoma, chronic myelogenous leukemia (alfa-2a), and chronic hepatitis B or C (alfa-2b). Interferon beta is primarily reserved for the treatment of severe multiple sclerosis.

Interleukins are another class of cytokines synthesized by lymphocytes, monocytes, macrophages, and certain other cells that enhance the capabilities of the immune system. At least 20 different interleukins have been identified, though only a few are available as medications. The interleukins have widespread effects on immune function, including stimulation of T-cell function, stimulation of B-cell and plasma cell production, and promotion of inflammation. Interleukin-2, derived from T helper lymphocytes, causes proliferation of T lymphocytes and activated B lymphocytes. It is available as aldesleukin, which is approved for the treatment of metastatic renal carcinoma. Interleukin-11, derived from bone marrow cells, is a growth factor with multiple hematopoietic effects. It is marketed as oprelvekin for its ability to stimulate platelet production in immunosuppressed clients (see Chapter 28).

In addition to interferons and interleukins, a few additional biological response modifiers are available to enhance the immune system. Levamisole is used to stimulate B cells,

TABLE 30.4 Immunostimulants	
Drug	**Route and Adult Dose**
aldesleukin (Proleukin): interleukin-2	IV; 600,000 IU/kg (0.037 mg/kg) q8h by a 15-min IV infusion for a total of 14 doses
bacille Calmette-Guérin (BCG) vaccine	Interdermal; 0.1 mL
interferon alfa-2 (Intron A)	IM/SC; 2 million U/m² three times/wk
interferon beta-1a (Avonex, Rebif)	IM; 30 μg qwk
interferon beta-1b (Betaseron)	SC; 0.25 mg (8 million IU) qod
oprelvekin (Neumega): interleukin-11	SC; 50 μg/kg once daily starting 6–24 h after completing chemotherapy and continuing until platelet count is ≥ 50,000 cells/μL or up to 21 d
peginterferon alfa-2a (Pegasys)	SC; 180 μg once weekly for 48 weeks

T cells, and macrophages in clients with colon cancer. Bacille Calmette-Guérin (BCG) vaccine is an attenuated strain of *Mycobacterium bovis* used for the pharmacotherapy of certain types of bladder cancer.

NURSING CONSIDERATIONS

The role of the nurse in immunostimulant therapy involves careful monitoring of the client's condition and providing education as it relates to the prescribed drug regimen. Immunostimulants are powerful drugs that not only affect target cells, but may also seriously impact other body systems. Prior to starting a client on these drugs, a thorough assessment including a complete health history and present signs and symptoms should be performed because these drugs have serious side effects. The nurse should assess for the presence and/or history of the following diseases or disorders: chronic hepatitis, hairy cell leukemia, malignant melanoma, condylomata acuminata, AIDS-related Kaposi's sarcoma, and renal disorders including cancer. Assessment of infections and cancer verifies the need for these drugs. Immunostimulants are contraindicated for clients with renal or liver disease and in pregnancy. Also before beginning therapy, lab tests, including a complete blood count, electrolytes, renal function, and liver enzymes, should be obtained to provide baseline data. Vital signs and body weight should be measured at the initial assessment and throughout the treatment regimen to monitor progress. As with any drug, the nurse should check for allergies and drug interactions.

Interferon alfa-2b should be used with caution in clients with hepatitis other than hepatitis C, leukopenia, and pulmonary disease. Interferon alfa-2a should be used with caution in cardiac disease, herpes zoster, and recent exposure to chicken pox.

The client should be kept well hydrated during pharmacotherapy. Use of immunostimulants can lead to the development of encephalopathy; therefore, the nurse should assess for changes in mental status. The nurse should be especially vigilant for signs and symptoms of depression and suicidal ideation. Additional nursing interventions may be needed depending on the medication given. When interferon alfa-2b is administered, it may promote development of leukemia because of bone marrow suppression. Periodic blood tests should be obtained to exclude the possibility of leukemia development.

Assessment of a client's pregnancy status prior to beginning interferon beta-1b therapy and throughout therapy should be done as this drug may cause spontaneous abortion. The nurse should instruct the client to use reliable birth control while taking this drug. During the use of interleukin-2, the client should be instructed not to use corticosteroids because these hormones reduce the drug's antitumor effectiveness. Liver, endocrine, or neurological adverse effects that occur during therapy may be permanent.

Unlike most immunostimulants, levamisole restores depressed immune function rather than stimulating the body's immune system above normal levels. While taking this drug, clients should be advised not to consume alcohol because it may induce a disulfiram (Antabuse) reaction. The client should be monitored for depression. Concurrent use of phenytoin (Dilantin) also may produce a possible drug reaction; thus, the nurse will need to monitor phenytoin levels closely.

Because immunostimulants act on fast-growing cells, such as those in the lining of the stomach, nausea and

---

Pr PROTOTYPE DRUG | Interferon Alfa-2 (Intron A)

ACTIONS AND USES

Interferon alfa-2 is a biological response modifier that is available as interferon alfa-2b (Intron A). Interferon 2b is a natural protein that is produced by human lymphocytes 4 to 6 hours after viral stimulation. Indications include hairy cell leukemia, hepatitis C, and malignant melanoma. An unlabelled use is for AIDS-related Kaposi's sarcoma. Interferon 2b affects cancer cells by two mechanisms. First, it enhances or stimulates the immune system to remove antigens. Second, the drug suppresses the growth of cancer cells. As expected from its origin, interferon alfa-2 also has antiviral activity.

PHARMACOKINETICS

Interferon alfa-2 is administered SC or IM. It is metabolized in the liver and kidney and excreted in urine. The half-life is 5 hours.

ADMINISTRATION ALERTS

- The drug should be administered under the careful guidance of a qualified healthcare provider.
- SC administration is recommended for clients at risk for bleeding. (platelet count less than 50×10^9/L)
- Interferon alfa-2 is pregnancy category C.

ADVERSE EFFECTS AND INTERACTIONS

Like many immunostimulants, the most common side effect is a flu-like syndrome of fever, chills, dizziness, and fatigue that usually diminishes as therapy progresses. Nausea, vomiting, diarrhea, and anorexia are relatively common. With prolonged therapy, more serious toxicity such as immunosuppression, hepatotoxicity, and neurotoxicity may be observed.

Interferon alfa-2 interacts with many drugs; for example, it may increase theophylline levels. There is additive myelosuppression with antineoplastics. Zidovudine may increase hematological toxicity.

 See the Companion Website for a Nursing Process Focus Chart specific to this drug.

stomatitis are common side effects. The nurse should provide small, frequent feedings and use non-alcohol-based mouthwash to treat mouth ulcers. Clients taking immunostimulants should immediately report any of the following side effects: hematuria, petechiae, tarry stools, bruising, fever, sore throat, jaundice, dark-coloured urine, clay-coloured stools, feelings of sadness, and nervousness.

See "Nursing Process Focus: Clients Receiving Immunostimulant Therapy" for specific teaching points.

IMMUNOSUPPRESSANTS

Drugs used to inhibit the immune response are called immunosuppressants. They are used for clients who are receiving transplanted tissues or organs. These agents are shown in Table 30.5.

NATURAL THERAPIES

Echinacea for Boosting the Immune System

Echinacea purpurea, or purple coneflower, is a popular medicinal botanical. Native to central Canada and the Midwestern United States, the flowers, leaves, and stems of this plant are harvested and dried. Preparations include dried powder, tincture, fluid extracts, and teas. No single ingredient seems to be responsible for the herb's activity; a large number of active chemicals have been identified from the extracts.

Echinacea was used by Aboriginal Peoples to treat various wounds and injuries. Echinacea is purported to boost the immune system by increasing phagocytosis and inhibiting the bacterial enzyme hyaluronidase. Some substances in echinacea might have antiviral activity, although this has yet to be confirmed by research; thus, the herb is sometimes taken to treat the common cold and influenza. In general, it is used as a supportive treatment for any disease involving inflammation and to enhance the immune system. Side effects are rare; however, it may interfere with drugs that have immunosuppressant effects.

NURSING PROCESS FOCUS   Clients Receiving Immunostimulant Therapy

Assessment	Potential Nursing Diagnose/Identified Patterns
■ Obtain health history including medical conditions, allergies, drug history, and possible drug interactions. ■ Obtain laboratory work: complete blood count, electrolytes, and liver enzymes. ■ Obtain weight and vital signs, especially blood pressure. ■ Assess mental alertness.	■ Safety from physical injury related to side effects of drug ■ Comfort and nutrition (gastrointestinal upset may occour related to side effects of drug) ■ Risk for infection related to bone marrow suppression secondary to drug ■ Need for knowledge regarding drug therapy and adverse effects

Planning: Client Goals and Expected Outcomes

The client will:
- Experience increased immune system function
- Demonstrate an understanding of the drug's action by accurately describing drug side effects and precautions
- Immediately report effects such as fever, chills, sore throat, unusual bleeding, chest pain, palpitations, dizziness, and change in mental status
- Demonstrate the ability to self-administer IM or SC injection

Implementation

Interventions (Rationales)	Client Education/Discharge Planning
■ Monitor for leukopenia, neutropenia, thrombocytopenia, anemia, increased liver enzymes (due to possible bone marrow suppression and liver damage).	Instruct client to: ■ Comply with all ordered laboratory tests ■ Immediately report any unusual bleeding or jaundice ■ Avoid crowds and people with infections ■ Avoid activities that can cause bleeding or impairment of skin integrity
■ Ensure drug is properly administered.	■ Instruct client in proper technique for self-administration of IM or SC injection.
■ Monitor vital signs. (Loss of vascular tone leading to extravasation of plasma proteins and fluids into extravascular spaces may cause hypotension and dysrhythmias.)	Instruct client to: ■ Monitor blood pressure and pulse every day and report any reading outside normal limits ■ Report any palpitations immediately
■ Monitor for common side effects such as muscle aches, fever, weight loss, anorexia, nausea and vomiting, and arthralgia (due to high doses of medications).	Instruct client to: ■ Take medication at bedtime to reduce side effects ■ Use frequent mouth care and small frequent feedings to reduce gastrointestinal disturbances ■ Take acetaminophen for flu-like symptoms
■ Monitor blood glucose levels. (Blood glucose may increase in clients with pancreatitis.)	■ Instruct client to have blood glucose checked at regular intervals.

continued

NURSING PROCESS FOCUS Clients Receiving Immunostimulant Therapy *(Continued)*

Interventions (Rationales)	Client Education/Discharge Planning
■ Monitor for changes in mental status. Drugs may cause depression, confusion, fatigue, visual disturbances, and numbness. (Alpha interferons cause or aggravate neuropsychiatric disorders.)	■ Client should report any mental changes, particularly depression or thoughts of suicide.

Evaluation of Outcome Criteria
Evaluate the effectiveness of drug therapy by confirming that client goals and expected outcomes have been met (see "Planning").

See Table 30.3 (page 392) for a list of drugs to which these nursing actions apply.

TABLE 30.5 Immunosuppressants

Drug	Route and Adult Dose
Antibodies	
alemtuzumab (Maampath)	IV; 3–30 mg/day
basiliximab (Simulect)	IV; 20 mg times two doses (first dose 2 h before surgery, second dose 4 d after transplant)
daclizumab (Zenapax)	IV; 1 mg/kg, start first dose no more than 24 h prior to transplant, then repeat q14d for four more doses
infliximab (Remicade)	IV; 3 mg/kg infused over at least 2 h, followed by 2 mg/kg on weeks 2 and 6, then 2 mg/kg q8wk
lymphocyte immune globulin (Atgam)	IV; 10–30 mg/kg/d
muromonab-CD3 (Orthoclone OKT3)	IV; 5 mg/d administered in < 1 min for 10–14 days
Antimetabolites and Cytotoxic Agents	
azathioprine (Imuran)	PO; 3–5 mg/kg/d initially, may be able to reduce to 1–3 mg/kg/d IV; 3–5 mg/kg/d initially, may be able to reduce to 1–3 mg/kg/d
cyclophosphamide (Cytoxan) (see page 485 for the Prototype Drug box)	PO; initial: 1–5 mg/kg/d; maintenance: 1–5 mg/kg q7–10d IV; initial: 40–50 mg/kg in divided doses over 2–5 d up to 100 mg/kg; maintenance: 10–15 mg/kg q7–10d or 3–5 mg twice weekly
methotrexate (Apo-Methotrexate) (see page 487 for the Prototype Drug box)	PO; 15–30 mg/d for 5 d, repeat q12wk for three courses IM/IV; 15–30 mg/d for 5 d, repeat q12wk for three to five courses
mycophenolate mofetil (CellCept)	PO/IV; start within 24 h of transplant, 1 g bid in combination with corticosteroids and cyclosporine
sirolimus (Rapamune)	PO; 6 mg loading dose immediately after transplant, then 2 mg/d
thalidomide (Thalomid)	PO; 100–300 mg qd (max 400 mg/d) times at least 2 wk
Calcineurin Inhibitors	
cyclosporine (Neoral, Sandimmune)	PO; 250 mg q12h for 2 wk, may increase to 500 mg q12h (max 1 g/d)
tacrolimus (Prograf)	PO; 0.15–0.3 mg/kg/d in two divided doses q12h, start no sooner than 6 h after transplant; give first oral dose 8–12 h after discontinuing IV therapy IV; 0.05–0.1 mg/kg/d as continuous infusion, start no sooner than 6 h after transplant and continue until patient can take oral therapy
Glucocorticoids	
(see Chapter 39 for individual doses)	

30.6 Immunosuppressants to Prevent Transplant Rejection

The immune response is normally viewed as a life saver, protecting individuals from a host of pathogens in the environment. For those receiving organ or tissue transplants, however, the immune response is the enemy. Transplanted organs always contain some antigens that trigger the immune response. This response, called **transplant rejection**, is often acute; antibodies sometimes destroy the transplanted tissue within a few days. The cell-mediated system responds more slowly to the transplant, attacking it about 2 weeks following surgery. Even if the organ survives these attacks, rejection of the transplant may occur months or even years after surgery.

Immunosuppressants are drugs given to dampen the immune response. Transplantation would be impossible without the use of effective immunosuppressant drugs. In addition, these agents may be prescribed for severe cases of rheumatoid arthritis or other inflammatory diseases.

Although the mechanisms of action of the immunosuppressant drugs differ, most are toxic to bone marrow and produce significant adverse effects. Due to the suppressed immune system, infections are common and the client must be protected from situations in which exposure to pathogens is likely. Certain tumours such as lymphomas occur more frequently in transplant recipients than in the general population because their immune systems are suppressed by immunosuppressive drugs.

Drugs used to dampen the immune response include glucocorticoids, antimetabolites, antibodies, and calcineurin inhibitors. The glucocorticoids are potent inhibitors of inflammation that are discussed in detail in Chapters 31 and 39. Antimetabolites such as sirolimus and azathioprine inhibit aspects of lymphocyte replication. Monoclonal and polyclonal antibodies such as basiliximab and muromonab-CD3 interact with specific antigens on the surface of lymphocytes to destroy them. By binding to the intracellular messenger **calcineurin**, cyclosporine and tacrolimus disrupt T-cell function. Because the primary indication for some of these immunosuppressants is to treat specific cancers, the student should also refer to Chapter 35.

NURSING CONSIDERATIONS

The role of the nurse in immunosuppressant therapy involves careful monitoring of the client's condition and providing education as it relates to the prescribed drug regimen. When providing care for clients taking immunosuppressants, an assessment should be done to determine the presence or history of organ transplant or grafting and to verify the need for these drugs. A client with leukemia, metastatic cancer, active infection, or renal or liver disease could be made worse by taking immunosuppressants, so they are contraindicated. They are also contraindicated in pregnancy. These drugs should be used with caution in clients who have pancreatic or bowel dysfunction, hyperkalemia, hypertension, and infection. The nurse should obtain vital signs and lab testing, including a complete blood count, electrolytes, and liver profile, to provide baseline data and reveal any abnormalities.

Many immunosuppressants act on T lymphocytes, suppressing the normal cell-mediated immune reaction. Due to their effect on the immune system, a superimposed infection may occur, causing an increase in the white blood cell count. Monitor vital signs, especially temperature, and laboratory results for indications of infection. The degree of bone marrow suppression (thrombocytopenia and leukopenia) must be carefully monitored as these adverse effects may be life-threatening.

It is important that clients immediately report the following signs and symptoms: alopecia, increased pigmentation, arthralgia, respiratory distress, edema, nausea, vomiting, paresthesia, fever, blood in the urine, black stools, and feelings of sadness. Clients taking azathioprine should be informed and monitored for the development of secondary malignancies.

See "Nursing Process Focus: Clients Receiving Immunosuppressant Therapy" for specific teaching points.

MediaLink · Xenotransplants

Pr **PROTOTYPE DRUG** | Cyclosporine (Neoral, Sandimmune)

ACTIONS AND USES

Cyclosporine is a complex chemical obtained from a soil fungus. Its primary mechanism of action is to inhibit helper T cells. Unlike some of the more cytotoxic immunosuppressants, it is less toxic to bone marrow cells. When prescribed for transplant recipients, it is primarily used in combination with high doses of a glucocorticoid such as prednisone. Cyclosporine is given by the oral route for prevention of transplant rejection, rheumatoid arthritis, and severe psoriasis. An IV form is available for transplant rejection and for severe cases of ulcerative colitis or Crohn's disease. An ophthalmic solution is used to increase tear production for patients with conjunctivitis.

ADMINISTRATION ALERTS

- Neoral (microemulsion) and Sandimmune are not bioequivalent and cannot be used interchangeably without healthcare provider supervision.
- Cyclosporine is pregnancy category C.

PHARMACOKINETICS

The drug is administered PO or IV. Cyclosporine PO undergoes significant first-pass metabolism with about 10% to 60% absorption. Cyclosporine is 90% to 98% protein bound. It is widely distributed and crosses the placenta and enters breast milk. It is extensively metabolized in the liver with small amounts excreted in bile and urine. Half-life is approximately 19 hours.

ADVERSE EFFECTS AND INTERACTIONS

The primary adverse effect of cyclosporine occurs in the kidney, with up to 75% of clients experiencing reduction in urine flow. Other common side effects are tremor, hypertension, and elevated hepatic enzymes. Although infections are common during cyclosporine therapy, they are fewer than with some of the other immunosuppressants. Periodic blood counts are necessary to be certain that WBCs do not fall below 4000/mm^3 or platelets below 75,000/mm^3.

Drugs that decrease cyclosporine levels include phenytoin, phenobarbital, carbamazepine, and rifampin. Drugs that increase cyclosporine levels include antifungal drugs and macrolide antibiotics. Grapefruit juice can raise cyclosporine levels by 50% to 200%.

Use with caution with herbal supplements; for example, the immune-stimulating effects of astragalus and echinacea may interfere with immunosuppressants.

See the Companion Website for a Nursing Process Focus Chart specific to this drug.

NURSING PROCESS FOCUS Clients Receiving Immunosuppressant Therapy

Assessment	Potential Nursing Diagnoses/Identified Patterns
■ Obtain health history including allergies, drug history, and possible drug interactions. ■ Assess for presence of metastatic cancer, active infection, renal or liver disease, and pregnancy. ■ Assess skin integrity; specifically look for lesions and skin colour. ■ Obtain laboratory work: complete blood count, electrolytes, and liver enzymes. ■ Obtain vital signs, especially temperature and blood pressure.	■ Risk for infection related to depressed immune response secondary to drug ■ Risk for injury related to thrombocytopenia secondary to drug

Planning: Client Goals and Expected Outcomes

The client will:
■ Experience no symptoms of organ or allograft rejection
■ Immediately report elevated temperature, unusual bleeding, sore throat, mouth ulcers, and fatigue to healthcare provider
■ Demonstrate an understanding of the drug's action by accurately describing drug side effects and precautions

Implementation

Interventions (Rationales)	Client Education/Discharge Planning
■ Assess renal function. (Drugs cause nephrotoxicity in many clients due to physiological changes in the kidneys such as microcalcifications and interstitial fibrosis.)	Advise client to: ■ Keep accurate record of urine output ■ Report significant reduction in urine flow
■ Monitor liver function. (There is an increased risk for liver toxicity.)	■ Instruct client as to the importance of regular laboratory testing.
■ Watch for signs and symptoms of infection, including elevated temperature. (There is an increased risk of infection due to immune suppression.)	Instruct client to: ■ Use thorough, frequent handwashing ■ Avoid crowds and people with infections
■ Monitor vital signs, especially temperature and blood pressure. (Drugs may cause hypertension, especially in clients with kidney transplants.)	Teach client to: ■ Monitor blood pressure and temperature, ensuring proper use of home equipment ■ Keep all appointments with healthcare provider
■ Monitor for the following possible side effects: hirsutism, leukopenia, gingival hyperplasia, gynecomastia, sinusitis, and hyperkalemia.	Advise client to: ■ See a dentist on a regular basis ■ Comply with regular laboratory assessments (complete blood count, electrolytes, and hormone levels)
■ Monitor client for avoidance of drinking grapefruit juice. (This will increase cyclosporine levels 50% to 200%.)	Instruct client to ■ Completely avoid drinking grapefruit juice ■ Take medication with food to decrease GI upset
■ Assess nutritional status. (Drugs may cause weight gain.)	■ Instruct client regarding a healthy diet that avoids excessive fats and sugars.

Evaluation of Outcome Criteria

Evaluate the effectiveness of drug therapy by confirming that client goals and expected outcomes have been met (see "Planning").

See Table 30.5 (page 396) for a list of drugs to which these nursing actions apply.

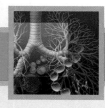

CHAPTER REVIEW

KEY CONCEPTS

The numbered key concepts provide a succinct summary of the important points from the corresponding numbered section within the chapter. If any of these points are not clear, refer to the numbered section within the chapter for review. Expanded versions can be found on the Companion Website.

30.1 Protection from pathogens is provided through non-specific defences that protect the body from general hazards and specific body defences that are activated by antigens.

30.2 Humoral immunity involves the production of antibodies by plasma cells, which neutralize the foreign agent or destroy it.

30.3 Vaccines are biological agents used to prevent illness by boosting antibody production. Vaccines are classified as live, attenuated, or toxoid.

30.4 Cell-mediated immunity involves the activation of specific T cells and the secretion of cytokines such as interferons and interleukins that rid the body of the foreign agent.

30.5 Immunostimulants are biological response modifiers that boost the immune system and are used to treat infections, immunodeficiencies, and cancer.

30.6 Immunosuppressants are used to inhibit the immune system and prevent rejection following organ transplantation.

REVIEW QUESTIONS

1 Why are oral glucocorticoids usually used concurrently with immunosuppressant drugs following a transplant operation?

2 Compare and contrast the type and duration of immunity achieved by administering a vaccine versus gamma globulin.

CRITICAL THINKING QUESTIONS

1. A client is taking sirolimus (Rapamune) following a liver transplant. On the most recent CBC, the nurse noted a marked 50% decrease in platelets and leukocytes. As the client is being examined, what signs and symptoms should the nurse look for, and what are some possible interventions?

2. A client has been exposed to hepatitis A and has been referred for an injection of gamma globulin. The client is hesitant to get a "shot" and says that his immune system is fine. How would the nurse respond?

3. A client had a renal transplant 6 months ago and is taking cyclosporine (Neoral) daily. Name three precautions that the nurse should know when caring for this client.

EXPLORE MediaLink

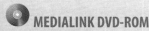

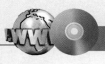 www.pearsoned.ca/adams-king

MEDIALINK DVD-ROM
- Audio Glossary
- CRNE Review
- Animation:
  Mechanism of Action: Interferon alfa-2a

COMPANION WEBSITE
- CRNE Review
- Case Study: Client taking immunostimulants
- Dosage Calculations

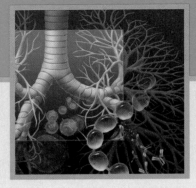

CHAPTER 31

Drugs for Inflammation, Fever, and Allergies

DRUGS AT A GLANCE

ANTI-INFLAMMATORY DRUGS

Non-steroidal anti-inflammatory drugs (NSAIDs)

    📀*ibuprofen (Actiprofen, others)*

Systemic glucocorticoids

    📀*prednisone (Apo-Prednisone)*

ANTIPYRETICS

    📀*acetaminophen (Tylenol)*

ALLERGY DRUGS

H_1-receptor antagonists (antihistamines)

    📀*diphenhydramine (Allerdryl, Benadryl)*

    📀*fexofenadine (Allegra)*

Intranasal glucocorticoids

    📀*fluticasone (Flonase)*

Adrenergics

ANAPHYLAXIS DRUGS

    📀*epinephrine (Adrenalin)*

OBJECTIVES

After reading this chapter, the student should be able to do the following:

1. Explain the therapeutic action of drugs used for treating inflammation in relation to the acute inflammatory response and signs and symptoms of inflammation.
2. Differentiate between histamine H_1- and H_2-receptors.
3. Discuss the role of the nurse regarding the non-pharmacological management of clients receiving drugs for inflammation, fever, and allergies.
4. Describe the nurse's role in the pharmacological management of clients receiving drugs for inflammation, fever, and allergies.
5. For each of the drug classes listed in Drugs at a Glance, identify a representative drug and explain its mechanism of action, therapeutic effects, and important adverse effects.
6. Describe and explain, based on pharmacological principles, the rationale for nursing assessment, planning, and interventions for clients with inflammation, fever, and allergies.
7. Use the nursing process to care for clients receiving drug therapy for inflammation, fever, and allergies.

MediaLink

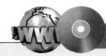

www.pearsoned.ca/adams-king

CRNE review, case studies, and other interactive resources for this chapter can be found on the Companion Website at **www.pearsoned.ca/adams-king.** Click on "Chapter 31" to select the activities for this chapter. For animations, more CRNE review questions, and an audio glossary, access the accompanying DVD-ROM in this textbook.

The pain and redness of inflammation following minor abrasions and cuts is something everyone has experienced. Although there is some discomfort from such scrapes, inflammation is a normal and expected part of our body's defence against injury. For some diseases, however, inflammation can become abnormal and rage out of control, producing severe pain, fever, and other distressing symptoms. It is these sorts of conditions in which pharmacotherapy may be required.

Similarly, the allergy symptoms of nasal congestion, scratchy throat, and postnasal drip are familiar to millions of clients. Allergy symptoms may range from annoying to life-threatening and are common indications for drug therapy.

PHARMFACTS

Inflammatory and Allergic Disorders

- Arthritis, the leading cause of deformity and long-term disability in Canada, affects over 4 million Canadians.
- About 19% of Aboriginal Canadians report having arthritis.
- Inflammatory bowel disease affects about 170,000 Canadians each year; most people are diagnosed between the ages of 15 and 25 or 45 and 55 years.
- Of food allergies, 85% are related to milk, eggs, and nuts.
- About 1% of people are allergic to nuts.
- More than 1% of the population uses NSAIDs on a daily basis.
- Worldwide, more than 30 million people consume NSAIDs daily, and of these, 40% are more than 60 years of age.

INFLAMMATION

Inflammation is a non-specific defence system of the body. Through the process of inflammation, a large number of potentially damaging chemicals and foreign agents may be neutralized.

31.1 The Function of Inflammation

The human body has developed many complex means to defend against injury and invading organisms. Inflammation is one of these defence mechanisms. **Inflammation** is a complex process that may occur in response to a large number of different stimuli, including physical injury, exposure to toxic chemicals, extreme heat, invading microorganisms, or death of cells. It is considered a non-specific defence mechanism because the physiological processes of inflammation proceed in the same manner regardless of the cause. The specific immune defences of the body are presented in Chapter 30.

The central purpose of inflammation is to contain the injury or destroy the foreign agent. By neutralizing the foreign agent and removing cellular debris and dead cells, repair of the injured area can proceed at a faster pace. Signs of inflammation include swelling, pain, warmth, and redness of the affected area.

Inflammation may be classified as acute or chronic. During acute inflammation, such as that caused by minor physical injury, 8 to 10 days are normally needed for the symptoms to resolve and for repair to begin. If the body cannot contain or neutralize the damaging agent, inflammation may continue for prolonged periods and become chronic. In chronic autoimmune disorders such as lupus and rheumatoid arthritis, inflammation may persist for years, with symptoms becoming progressively worse over time. Other disorders such as seasonal allergy arise at predictable times during each year, and inflammation may produce only minor, annoying symptoms.

The pharmacotherapy of inflammation includes drugs that decrease the natural inflammatory response. Most anti-inflammatory drugs are non-specific; this means that whether the inflammation is caused from injury or allergy, the drug will exhibit the same anti-inflammatory actions. A few anti-inflammatory drugs are specific to certain diseases, such as those used to treat gout (see Chapter 46). Following are diseases that have an inflammatory component and that may benefit from anti-inflammatory drugs:

- Allergic rhinitis
- Anaphylaxis
- Ankylosing spondylitis
- Contact dermatitis
- Crohn's disease
- Glomerulonephritis
- Hashimoto's thyroiditis
- Peptic ulcers
- Rheumatoid arthritis
- Systemic lupus erythematosus
- Ulcerative colitis

31.2 The Role of Histamine in Inflammation

Whether the injury is due to pathogens, chemicals, or physical trauma, the damaged tissue releases a number of chemical mediators that act as "alarms" to notify the surrounding area of the injury. Chemical mediators of inflammation include **histamine, leukotrienes, bradykinin, complement,** and **prostaglandins.** Table 31.1 lists the sources and actions of these mediators.

Histamine is a key chemical mediator of inflammation. It is primarily stored within **mast cells** located in tissue spaces under epithelial membranes such as those of the skin, bronchial tree, digestive tract, and blood vessels. Mast cells detect foreign agents or injury and respond by releasing histamine, which initiates the inflammatory response within seconds. In addition to its role in inflammation, histamine also directly stimulates pain receptors and produces symptoms of seasonal allergies.

When released at an injury site, histamine dilates nearby blood vessels, causing capillaries to become more permeable. Plasma and components such as complement proteins and phagocytes can then enter the area to neutralize foreign agents. The affected area may become congested with blood, a condition called **hyperemia,** which can lead to significant swelling and pain. Figure 31.1 illustrates the fundamental steps in acute inflammation.

Rapid release of the chemical mediators of inflammation on a larger scale throughout the body is responsible for the distressing symptoms of **anaphylaxis,** a life-threatening allergic response that may result in shock and death. A number of chemicals, insect stings, foods, and some therapeutic drugs can elicit this widespread release of histamine from mast cells if the person has an allergy to these substances. The pharmacotherapy of anaphylaxis is presented in Chapter 27.

31.3 Histamine Receptors

There are at least two different receptors by which histamine can elicit a response. **H$_1$-receptors** are present in the smooth muscle of the vascular system, the bronchial tree, and the digestive tract. Stimulation of these receptors results in itching, pain, edema, vasodilation, and bronchoconstriction. In contrast, **H$_2$-receptors** are primarily present in the stomach, and their stimulation results in the secretion of large amounts of hydrochloric acid.

LIFESPAN CONSIDERATIONS

NSAID Use

- NSAIDs should be used cautiously in elderly clients because of the potential for drug accumulation and increased bleeding.
- Use may be cautioned in pregnancy and lactation, depending on the specific drug.
- Use ibuprofen with caution in infants younger than 6 months, and use naproxen with caution in children younger than 2 years.
- ASA is contraindicated in children who have or are at risk of varicella or influenza infections because of the possibility of developing Reye's syndrome. **Reye's syndrome** is a rare, though potentially fatal, disorder characterized by an acute increase in intracranial pressure and massive accumulations of lipids in the liver.
- Clients should not breastfeed while taking COX-2 inhibitors as they can be transmitted to the infant through breast milk.

TABLE 31.1	Chemical Mediators of Inflammation
Mediator	**Description**
bradykinin	present in an inactive form in plasma and also stored and released by mast cells; vasodilator that causes pain; effects are similar to those of histamine
complement	series of at least 20 proteins that combine in a cascade fashion to neutralize or destroy an antigen
histamine	stored and released by mast cells; causes dilation of blood vessels, smooth muscle constriction, tissue swelling, and itching
leukotrienes	stored and released by mast cells; effects are similar to those of histamine
prostaglandins	present in most tissues and stored and released by mast cells; increase capillary permeability, attract white blood cells to site of inflammation, and cause pain

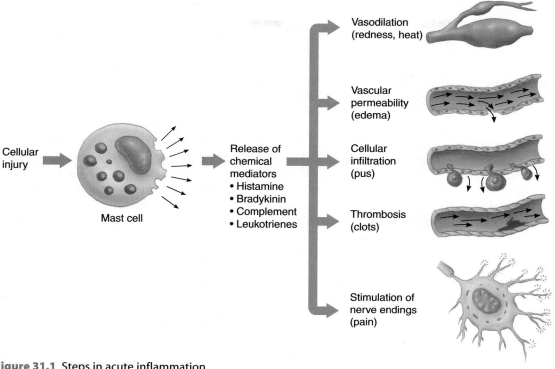

● **Figure 31.1** Steps in acute inflammation

Source: Pearson Education/PH College.

Drugs that act as specific antagonists for H_1- and H_2-receptors are in widespread therapeutic use. H_1-receptor antagonists, used to treat allergies and inflammation, are discussed later in this chapter. H_2-receptor antagonists are used to treat peptic ulcers and are discussed in Chapter 36.

NON-STEROIDAL ANTI-INFLAMMATORY DRUGS

Non-steroidal anti-inflammatory drugs (NSAIDs) such as aspirin and ibuprofen have analgesic, antipyretic, and anti-inflammatory effects. They are drugs of choice in the treatment of mild to moderate inflammation. These agents are shown in Table 31.2.

TABLE 31.2	Select Non-Steroidal Anti-Inflammatory Drugs
Drug	**Route and Adult Dose**
acetylsalicylic acid (Aspirin and others) (see page 227 for the Prototype Drug box)	PO; 350–650 mg q4h (max 4 g/day) for pain/fever
	PO; 3.6–5.4 g/day in 4–6 divided doses for arthritis
	PO; 81–325 mg/day for prevention of acute myocardial infarction or thrombosis
Selective COX-2 Inhibitors	
celecoxib (Celebrex)	PO; 100–200 mg bid (max 400 mg/day)
Ibuprofen and Similar Agents	
diclofenac (Voltaren, PMS-Diclofenac)	PO; 50 mg bid–qid (max 200 mg/day)
diflunisal (Apo-Diflunisal, Novo-Difulnisal)	PO; 250–500 mg bid (max 1500 mg/day)
etodolac (Apo-Etodelac, Gen-Etodolac)	PO; 200–400 mg tid–qid (max 1200 mg/day)
flurbiprofen (Ansaid, Apo-, Nu-Flurbiprofen)	PO; 50–100 mg tid–qid (max 300 mg/day)
ibuprofen (Actiprofen, Advil, others)	PO; 400–800 mg tid–qid (max 3200 mg/day)
ketoprofen (Apo-Keto, Anafen, PMS-Ketoprofen)	PO; 75 mg tid or 50 mg qid (max 300 mg/day)
nabumetone (Apo-, Gen-, Novo-Nabumetone)	PO; 1000 mg qd (max 2000 mg/day)
naproxen (Naprosyn, Apo-Naproxen)	PO; 250–500 mg bid (max 1000 mg/day)
naproxen sodium (Aleve, Anaprox, Apo-Narpro-NA)	PO; 275 mg bid (max 1100 mg/day)
oxaprozin (Daypro, Apo-Oxaprozin)	PO; 600–1200 mg qd (max 1800 mg/day)
piroxicam (Apo-, Dom-, Novo-Piroxicam)	PO; 10–20 mg qd–bid (max 20 mg/day)

31.4 Treating Inflammation with NSAIDs

Because of their high safety margin and availability as OTC drugs, the NSAIDs are first-line drugs for the treatment of mild to moderate inflammation. The NSAID class includes some of the most commonly used drugs in medicine, including ASA, ibuprofen, and the newer COX-2 inhibitors. All NSAIDs have approximately the same efficacy, although the side effect profiles vary among the different drugs. The NSAIDs also exhibit analgesic and antipyretic actions. Although acetaminophen shares the analgesic and antipyretic properties of these other drugs, it has no anti-inflammatory action and is not considered an NSAID.

NSAIDs act by inhibiting the synthesis of prostaglandins. Prostaglandins are lipids that promote inflammation and are found in all tissues. The NSAIDs block inflammation by inhibiting **cyclooxygenase** (COX), the key enzyme in the biosynthesis of prostaglandins. There are two forms of COX, cyclooxygenase-1 (**COX-1**) and cyclooxygenase-2 (**COX-2**). COX-1 is present is all tissues and serves protective functions such as reducing gastric acid secretion, promoting renal blood flow, and regulating smooth muscle tone in blood vessels and the bronchial tree. COX-2, on the other hand, is present only after tissue injury and serves to promote inflammation. Thus, two nearly identical enzymes serve very different functions. The two forms of cyclooxygenase are compared in Table 31.3.

First generation NSAIDs such as ASA and ibuprofen block both COX-1 and COX-2. Although inflammation is reduced, the inhibition of COX-1 results in undesirable side effects such as bleeding, gastric upset, and reduced kidney function.

ASA binds to both COX-1 and COX-2 enzymes, changing their structure and preventing them from forming inflammatory prostaglandins. This inhibition of cyclooxygenase is particularly prolonged in platelets, where a single dose of ASA may cause total inhibition for the entire 8- to 11-day lifespan of the platelet. Because it is readily available, inexpensive, and effective, ASA is often a drug of first choice for treating mild inflammation. The fundamental pharmacology and a Prototype Drug box for ASA (page 227) are presented in Chapter 19.

Unfortunately, large doses of ASA are necessary to suppress severe inflammation, which results in a greater incidence of side effects than when the drug is used for pain or fever. The most common adverse effects observed during high-dose ASA therapy relate to the digestive system. By increasing gastric acid secretion and irritating the stomach lining, ASA may produce epigastric pain, heartburn, and even bleeding due to ulceration. Some ASA formulations are buffered or enteric coated to minimize GI side effects. Because ASA also has a potent anticoagulant effect, the potential for bleeding must be carefully monitored. High doses may produce **salicylism**, a syndrome that includes symptoms such as tinnitus, dizziness, headache, and sweating.

Ibuprofen and a large number of ibuprofen-like drugs are first generation NSAIDs developed as alternatives to ASA. Like ASA, they exhibit their effects through inhibition of both COX-1 and COX-2, although the inhibition by these drugs is reversible. Because they share the same mechanism of action, all drugs in this class have similar efficacy for treating pain, fever, and inflammation. However, the duration of action varies, and clients may respond better to one than another. The most common side effects of ibuprofen-like NSAIDs are nausea and vomiting. These agents have the potential to cause gastric ulceration and bleeding; however, the incidence is less than that of ASA. There is some cross-hypersensitivity between ASA and other first generation NSAIDs. A study of 133,000 California teachers found that taking ibuprofen regularly for five years slightly increased the risk of breast cancer; the study found no increase in the risk of breast cancer among regular users of ASA and acetaminophen (Marshall et al., 2005).

The newest and most controversial class of NSAIDs selectively inhibit COX-2. Inhibition of COX-2 produces the analgesic, anti-inflammatory, and antipyretic actions typical of older NSAIDs without adverse effects on the digestive system and blood coagulation. Thus, these drugs became drugs of choice for the treatment of moderate to severe inflammation. However, in 2004, rofecoxib was withdrawn from the market because data showed that the risk of stroke and heart attack doubled in clients who used the drug for extended periods. Celecoxib is the only drug in this class currently available in Canada. Celecoxib is also used to reduce the number of colorectal polyps in adults with familial adenomatous polyposis (FAP), who have an almost 100% risk of colon cancer.

NURSING CONSIDERATIONS

The role of the nurse in NSAID pharmacotherapy involves careful monitoring of the client's condition and providing education as it relates to the prescribed drug regimen. Assess for sensitivity to NSAIDs, bleeding disorders, peptic

TABLE 31.3	Forms of Cyclooxygenase	
	Cyclooxygenase-1	**Cyclooxygenase-2**
Location	present in all tissues	present at sites of tissue injury
Functions	protects gastric mucosa, supports kidney function, promotes platelet aggregation	mediates inflammation, sensitizes pain receptors, mediates fever in the brain
Inhibition by medications	undesirable: increases risk of gastric bleeding and kidney failure	desirable: results in suppression of inflammation

ulcer disease, anticoagulants (including herbals with anti-coagulant effects), alcoholism, congestive heart failure, fluid retention, hypertension, and renal disease because NSAIDs may be contraindicated in such conditions. NSAIDs promote fluid retention, which may exacerbate hypertension and heart failure. Drugs in this class should not be administered to clients with liver dysfunction because NSAIDs are primarily metabolized in the liver. When the liver is not functioning effectively, metabolites may reach toxic levels and lead to hepatic failure.

Prior to initiation of NSAID therapy, obtain baseline kidney and liver function tests and a CBC. Monitor bleeding time with long-term administration. During therapy, assess for changes in pain (intensity, frequency, and type) and reduction in temperature and inflammation to determine effectiveness. Assess for gastrointestinal bleeding, hepatitis, nephrotoxicity, hemolytic anemia, and salicylate toxicity. Other common side effects may include tinnitus, abdominal cramping, and heartburn.

Client education as it relates to non-steroidal anti-inflammatory drugs should include goals, reasons for obtaining baseline data such as vital signs and laboratory tests, and possible side effects. The following are important points to include when teaching clients regarding NSAIDs:

- Do not give drugs containing ASA to children; Reye's syndrome is a life-threatening disorder.
- Take NSAIDs with food or milk to decrease gastric upset.
- Read labels of OTC drugs carefully as many (e.g., medications for common cold) contain multiple ingredients, including NSAIDs.
- Avoid alcohol.
- Consult a healthcare provider before taking herbal products while taking NSAIDs.

NATURAL THERAPIES

Fish Oils for Inflammation

Fish oils are lipids found primarily in coldwater fish. These oils are rich sources of long-chain polyunsaturated fatty acids of the omega-3 type. The two most studied fatty acids found in fish oils are EPA (eicosapentaenoic acid) and DHA (docosahexaenoic acid). These fatty acids are known for their triglyceride-lowering activity, and they may also have anti-inflammatory actions.

Several mechanisms are believed to account for the anti-inflammatory activity of EPA and DHA. The two competitively inhibit the conversion of arachidonic acid to the proinflammatory prostaglandins, thus reducing their synthesis.

Interactions may occur between fish oil supplements and ASA and other NSAIDs. Although rare, such interactions might be manifested by increased susceptibility to bruising, nosebleeds, hemoptysis, hematuria, and blood in the stool.

- Optimal effects from NSAID therapy may not occur for 1 to 3 weeks.
- Report immediately signs of bleeding such as dark coloured urine or stool, increased bruising, or gingival bleeding; unexplained fatigue; headache or dizziness; changes in hearing (especially ringing in the ears); swelling; itching; or skin rash.

See "Nursing Process Focus: Clients Receiving NSAID Therapy" in Chapter 19 (page 228) for additional teaching points.

SYSTEMIC GLUCOCORTICOIDS

Glucocorticoids have wide therapeutic application. One of their most useful properties is a potent anti-inflammatory action that can suppress severe cases of inflammation. Because of potentially serious adverse effects, however, systemic glucocorticoids are reserved for the short-term treatment of severe disease. These agents are shown in Table 31.4.

Pr PROTOTYPE DRUG | Ibuprofen (Actiprofen, others)

ACTIONS AND USES

Ibuprofen is an older drug used to relieve mild to moderate pain, fever, and inflammation. Its action is due to inhibition of prostaglandin synthesis. Common indications include musculoskeletal disorders such as rheumatoid arthritis and osteoarthritis, mild to moderate pain, reduction of fever, and primary dysmenorrhea. It is available as tablets and as an oral suspension for children.

ADMINISTRATION ALERTS

- Give drug on an empty stomach as tolerated. If nausea, vomiting, or abdominal pain occur, give with food.
- Ibuprofen is pregnancy category B.

PHARMACOKINETICS

Ibuprofen is about 80% absorbed from the GI tract, with minimal distribution into breast milk. It is highly (99%) protein bound. It is mostly metabolized by the liver, and about 1% is excreted unchanged in urine. Half-life is 2 to 4 hours in adults and 1 to 2 hours in children.

ADVERSE EFFECTS AND INTERACTIONS

Side effects of ibuprofen are generally mild and include nausea, heartburn, epigastric pain, and dizziness. Ibuprofen can decrease platelet function. GI ulceration with occult or gross bleeding may occur, especially in clients who take high doses for prolonged periods or regularly consume alcohol. Clients with active peptic ulcers should not take ibuprofen.

Ibuprofen interacts with many other drugs and herbal products. It should be avoided when taking anticoagulants since it competes for plasma binding sites and may significantly increase risk of bleeding. ASA use can decrease the anti-inflammatory action of ibuprofen. Ibuprofen may increase plasma levels of lithium, causing lithium toxicity. The actions of certain diuretics may be diminished when taken concurrently with ibuprofen.

Use with caution with herbal supplements, such as feverfew, garlic, ginger, and ginkgo biloba, which may increase the risk of bleeding.

Ibuprofen is contraindicated in clients with significant renal or hepatic impairment and in those who have nasal polyps, angioedema, or bronchospasm due to ASA or other NSAIDs.

There is no specific treatment for overdose. Administration of an alkaline drug may increase the urinary excretion of ibuprofen.

Table 31.4 **Select Glucocorticoids for Severe Inflammation**	
Drug	*Route and Adult Dose*
betamethasone (Celestone, Betacort)	PO; 0.6–7.2 mg/day
cortisone (Cortisone Acetate, Cortisone Aceticum)	PO; 20–300 mg/day in divided doses
dexamethasone (Apo-Dexamethasone, Decadron)	PO; 0.25–4 mg bid–qid
hydrocortisone (Cortef, A-hydrocort Inj) (see page 564 for the Prototype Drug box)	Topical: 0.5% cream applied qd–qid; PO; 10–320 mg tid–qid PO; 4–48 mg/day in divided doses
methylprednisolone (Depo-Medrol, Medrol,Methylprednisolone)	PO; 5–60 mg qd–qid
prednisolone (PMS-Prednisoline, Prednisolone)	PO; 5–60 mg qd–qid
prednisone (Apo-Prednisone)	PO; 4–48 mg qd–qid
triamcinolone (Kenalog, Triamcinolone Acetonide)	

31.5 Treating Acute or Severe Inflammation with Systemic Glucocorticoids

Glucocorticoids are natural hormones released by the adrenal cortex that have powerful effects on nearly every cell in the body. When used to treat inflammatory disorders, the drug doses are many times higher than those naturally present in the blood. The uses of glucocorticoids include the treatment of neoplasia (Chapter 35), asthma (Chapter 29), arthritis (Chapter 46), and corticosteroid deficiency (Chapter 39).

Glucocorticoids have the ability to suppress histamine release and inhibit the synthesis of prostaglandins by COX-2. In addition, they can inhibit the immune system by suppressing certain functions of phagocytes and lymphocytes. These multiple actions markedly reduce inflammation, making glucocorticoids the most effective medications available for the treatment of severe inflammatory disorders.

Unfortunately, the glucocorticoid drugs have a number of serious adverse effects that limit their therapeutic utility. These include suppression of the normal functions of the adrenal gland (adrenal insufficiency), hyperglycemia, mood changes, cataracts, peptic ulcers, electrolyte imbalances, and osteoporosis. Because of their effectiveness at reducing the signs and symptoms of inflammation, glucocorticoids can mask infections that may be present in the client. This combination of masking signs of infection and suppressing the immune response creates a potential for existing infections to grow rapidly and remain undetected. An active infection is usually a contraindication for glucocorticoid therapy.

Because the appearance of these adverse effects is a function of the dose and duration of therapy, treatment is often limited to the short-term control of acute disease. When longer therapy is indicated, doses are kept as low as possible and alternate-day therapy is sometimes implemented: the medication is taken every other day to encourage the client's adrenal gland to function on the days when no drug is given. During long-term therapy, the nurse must be alert for signs of overtreatment, a condition referred to as **Cushing's syndrome**. Because the body becomes accustomed to high doses of glucocorticoids, clients must discontinue glucocorticoids gradually; abrupt withdrawal can result in acute lack of adrenal function.

NURSING CONSIDERATIONS

The role of the nurse in systemic glucocorticoid therapy involves careful monitoring of the client's condition and providing education as it relates to the prescribed drug regimen. Before beginning therapy, the nurse should screen the client for existing infection. If infection is discovered prior to or during therapy, antibiotics may be required. Glucocorticoids should be used with great caution in clients with HIV or tuberculosis infections.

Prior to therapy, the nurse must also assess the client's metabolic status and fluid and electrolyte balance. Body weight and baseline laboratory data should be obtained, including CBC, serum glucose, sodium and potassium levels. Clients with blood disorders should be observed for possible exacerbation because glucocorticoids promote red blood cell proliferation. These drugs also suppress osteoblast formation, so they should be administered with caution to clients with osteoporosis or other bone disorders. Clients with diabetes mellitus must be monitored carefully because glucocorticoids increase serum glucose. Clients with heart failure, hypertension, or renal disease must be monitored closely due to drug-induced sodium and fluid retention. Glucocorticoids can cross the placenta and affect the developing fetus, so they should be used in pregnancy only when benefits outweigh risks (pregnancy category C). Women receiving high-dose glucocorticoid therapy should be warned against breastfeeding.

The client should be monitored for development of Cushing's syndrome (adrenocortical excess). Signs include bruising and a characteristic pattern of fat deposits in the cheeks (moon face), shoulders (buffalo hump), and abdomen. Clients with existing mental or emotional disorders should be monitored closely: glucocorticoids may trigger mania in bipolar clients. Glucocorticoids may also exacerbate the symptoms of myasthenia gravis, contributing to the risk of respiratory failure.

Glucocorticoids promote the development of gastric ulcers by altering the protective mucous lining of the stomach. Local irritation may be reduced by administering oral doses with food or an antacid. However, the risk of GI bleeding remains, especially with long-term therapy, since changes in the stomach result from *systemic* drug action. Therefore, these drugs should always be administered with caution to clients with a history of peptic ulcer disease. Glucocorticoids also promote capillary fragility; IM injections should be administered deep into the muscle mass to avoid atrophy or abscesses.

Client education as it relates to glucocorticoids should include goals, reasons for obtaining baseline data such as blood tests and body weight, and possible side effects. Following are important points to include when teaching clients regarding glucocorticoids:

- Take the medication at the same time each day.
- Never abruptly discontinue taking the medication.
- Take with food to avoid gastric irritation.
- Guard against infection: avoid persons with infections and wash hands frequently.
- Weigh yourself daily and check ankles/legs for signs of swelling.
- Immediately report the following: difficulty breathing; heartburn; chest, abdominal, or joint/bone pain; nose bleed; bloody cough, vomit, urine or stools; fever; chills; red streaks from wounds or any other sign of infection; increased thirst or urination; fruity breath odour (or significantly elevated daily serum glucose); falls or other accidents (deep lacerations may require antibiotic therapy); and mood swings.

See "Nursing Process Focus: Clients Receiving Systemic Glucocorticoid Therapy" in Chapter 39 (page 565) for additional teaching points.

FEVER

Like inflammation, fever is a natural mechanism in the body's defense system to remove foreign organisms. Many species of bacteria are killed by high fever. The goal of antipyretic therapy is to lower body temperature while treating the underlying cause of the fever, usually an infection. The NSAIDs and acetaminophen are generally safe, effective drugs for reducing fever.

Prolonged, high fever can become quite dangerous, especially in young children in whom fever can stimulate febrile seizures. In adults, excessively high fever can break down body tissues, reduce mental acuity, and lead to delirium or coma, particularly among elderly clients. In rare instances, an elevated fever may be fatal. Often, the healthcare provider must determine whether the fever needs to be dealt with aggressively or allowed to run its course. Drugs used to treat fever are called **antipyretics.**

Pr PROTOTYPE DRUG | Prednisone (Apo-Prednisone)

ACTIONS AND USES

Prednisone is a synthetic glucocorticoid. Its actions are the result of being metabolized to an active form, which is also available as a drug called prednisolone. When used for inflammation, duration of therapy is commonly limited 4 to 10 days. Alternate-day dosing is used for longer term therapy to allow the client's adrenal gland to function. Prednisone is occasionally used to terminate acute bronchospasm in clients with asthma and for clients with certain cancers such as Hodgkin's disease, acute leukemia, and lymphomas.

ADMINISTRATION ALERTS

- IM injections should be administered deep into the muscle mass to avoid atrophy or abscesses.
- Do not use if a systemic infection is present.
- Drug should not be discontinued abruptly.
- Prednisone is pregnancy category C.

PHARMACOKINETICS

Prednisone is well absorbed after oral administration. It is widely distributed, crosses the placenta, and enters breast milk. Prednisone is converted to prednisolone in the liver and then is metabolized by the liver. Its half-life in plasma is about 3.5 hours. Adrenal suppression lasts 30 to 36 hours.

ADVERSE EFFECTS AND INTERACTIONS

When used for short-term therapy, prednisone has few serious adverse effects. Long-term therapy may result in Cushing's syndrome, a condition that includes hyperglycemia, fat redistribution to the shoulders and face, muscle weakness, bruising, and bones that easily fracture. Because glucocorticoids can raise blood glucose levels, diabetic clients may require an adjustment in the doses of insulin or hypoglycedmic agents. Gastric ulcers may occur with long-term therapy and an antiulcer medication may be prescribed prophylactically.

Prednisone interacts with many drugs. For example, barbiturates, phenytoin, and rifampin increase steroid metabolism. Concurrent use with amphotericin B or diuretics increases potassium loss. Prednisone may inhibit antibody response to toxoids and vaccines.

Use with caution with herbal supplements, such as aloe and senna, which may increase potassium loss. Licorice may potentiate the effect of glucocorticoids.

 See the Companion Website for a Nursing Process Focus Chart specific to this drug.

31.6 Treating Fever with Antipyretics

In most clients, fever is more of a discomfort than a life-threatening problem and can be controlled effectively by inexpensive OTC drugs. ASA, ibuprofen, and acetaminophen are all effective antipyretics. Examples of common brand-name drugs taken for fever are Advil, Aleve, Bayer Aspirin, Cope, Excedrin, Motrin, and Tylenol. Many of these drugs are marketed for different age groups, including special, flavoured brands for infants and children. For fast delivery and effectiveness, drugs may come in various forms, including gels, caplets, enteric-coated tablets, and suspensions. ASA and acetaminophen are also available as suppositories. The antipyretics come in various dosages and concentrations, including extra strength.

Until the 1980s, ASA was the most common therapy for fever in children; however, ASA has been implicated in the development of Reye's syndrome. ASA and other salicylates are now contraindicated in children and teenagers with fever. Because of the potential for Reye's syndrome, some healthcare providers also advise against administering *any* NSAID to children or teens. Therefore, acetaminophen has become the antipyretic of choice to treat most fevers.

NURSING CONSIDERATIONS

The role of the nurse in antipyretic therapy involves careful monitoring of the client's condition and providing education as it relates to the prescribed drug regimen. Prior to administering an antipyretic, obtain the client's vital signs, especially temperature. Assess the client's developmental status, the origin of the fever, and associated symptoms to determine the appropriate formulation or route for the antipyretic. For example, clients who are vomiting should receive an antipyretic by suppository, and very young children are generally given flavoured elixirs.

Baseline laboratory data are necessary to assess the client's kidney and liver status; antipyretics may cause toxicity in clients with diminished organ function. Acetaminophen is contraindicated in clients with significant liver disease, including viral hepatitis and cirrhosis, and alcoholism, because it is metabolized by the liver and can greatly increase the risk of hepatotoxicity. Acetaminophen also inhibits warfarin metabolism and may produce toxic accumulation of this drug and cause serious bleeding. NSAIDs may be contraindicated with warfarin as well because they also promote bleeding.

Advise the client or caregiver that liquid forms of acetaminophen and ibuprofen come in different strengths; all children's liquid formulations are not the same. Children

---

Pr PROTOTYPE DRUG | Acetaminophen (Tylenol)

ACTIONS AND USES

Acetaminophen reduces fever by direct action at the level of the hypothalamus and causes dilation of peripheral blood vessels, enabling sweating and dissipation of heat. Acetaminophen and ASA have equal efficacy in relieving pain and reducing fever.

Acetaminophen has no anti-inflammatory action; therefore, it is not effective in treating arthritis or pain caused by tissue swelling following injury. The primary therapeutic usefulness of acetaminophen is for the treatment of fever in children and for relief of mild to moderate pain when aspirin is contraindicated.

PHARMACOKINETICS

Acetaminophen is well absorbed after oral administration. Rectal absorption varies. It is widely distributed in the body, crosses the placenta, and enters breast milk. It is almost completely metabolized in the liver. The metabolites are excreted in urine. The metabolites may also be toxic in overdose. Half-life is 1 to 3 hours.

ADMINISTRATION ALERT

- Liquid forms are available in varying concentrations. For administration in children, the appropriate strength product must be used to avoid toxicity.
- Acetaminophen is pregnancy category B.

ADVERSE EFFECTS AND INTERACTIONS

Acetaminophen is quite safe and adverse effects are uncommon at therapeutic doses. Unlike ASA, acetaminophen has no direct anti-inflammatory effect and does not affect blood coagulation or cause gastric irritation. It is not recommended in clients who are malnourished. In such cases, acute toxicity may result, leading to renal failure, which can be fatal. Other signs of acute toxicity include nausea, vomiting, chills, and abdominal discomfort.

Acetaminophen inhibits warfarin metabolism, causing warfarin to accumulate to toxic levels. High-dose or long-term acetaminophen usage may result in elevated warfarin levels and bleeding. Ingestion of this drug with alcohol is not recommended due to the possibility of liver failure from hepatic necrosis.

The client should avoid taking herbs that have the potential for liver toxicity, including comfrey, coltsfoot, and chaparral.

Acetylcysteine is the antidote for acetaminophen overdose.

 See the Companion Website for a Nursing Process Focus Chart specific to this drug.

NURSING PROCESS FOCUS Clients Receiving Antipyretic Therapy

Assessment	Potential Nursing Diagnoses/Identified Patterns
Prior to administration: ■ Obtain complete health history (mental and physical), including data on origin of fever, recent surgeries, and trauma. ■ Obtain vital signs; assess in context of client's baseline values. ■ Obtain client's complete medication history, including nicotine and alcohol consumption, to determine possible drug allergies and/or interactions.	■ Discomfort ■ Hyperthermia ■ Risk for dehydration ■ Need for knowledge regarding drug therapy and adverse effects ■ Safety from injury related to side effects of drug therapy

Planning: Client Goals and Expected Outcomes

The client will:
■ Experience a reduction in body temperature
■ Demonstrate an understanding of the drug's action by accurately describing drug side effects and precautions

Implementation

Interventions (Rationales)	Client Education/Discharge Planning
■ Assess for intolerance to ASA for possible cross-hypersensitivity to other NSAIDs or acetaminophen. ■ Monitor hepatic and renal function. (Antipyretics are metabolized in the liver and excreted by the kidneys.) ■ Use with caution in clients with a history of excessive alcohol consumption. (Alcohol increases the risk of liver damage associated with acetaminophen or NSAID administration.) ■ Use with caution in diabetics. Observe for signs of hypoglycemia that may occur with acetaminophen usage.	■ Inform client to immediately report any difficulty breathing, itching, or skin rash. Instruct client: ■ To report signs of liver toxicity: nausea, vomiting, anorexia, bleeding, severe upper or lower abdominal pain, heartburn, jaundice, or a change in the colour or character of stools ■ To adhere to laboratory testing regimen for serum blood tests as directed ■ Advise client to abstain from alcohol while taking this medication. ■ Advise clients with diabetes mellitus that acetaminophen may cause low blood sugar and require adjustment of doses of insulin or oral hypoglycemic agents. Instruct client to immediately report: ■ Excessive thirst ■ Large increase or decrease in urine output.

Evaluation of Outcome Criteria

Evaluate the effectiveness of drug therapy by confirming that client goals and expected outcomes have been met (see "Planning").

See Table 31.2 (page 403) for a list of the drugs to which these nursing actions apply. Acetaminophen is also covered in this Nursing Process Focus chart.

---

under 1 year should be given "infant drops" rather than "children's liquid." Acetaminophen is one of the substances most frequently implicated in poisonings of Canadian children less than 6 years of age. Clients should be advised to consult the nurse regarding safe dosages. Inform the client that acetaminophen overdosage can cause hepatic failure.

See "Nursing Process Focus: Clients Receiving Antipyretic Therapy" for additional teaching points.

ALLERGY

Allergies are caused by a hyperresponse of body defences. Because histamine is released during an allergic response, many signs and symptoms of allergy are similar to those of inflammation. Allergies also involve mediators of the immune response.

31.7 Pharmacotherapy of Allergic Rhinitis

Allergic rhinitis, or hay fever, is a common disorder afflicting millions of people annually. Symptoms resemble those of the common cold: tearing eyes, sneezing, nasal congestion, postnasal drip, and itching of the throat. The cause of all allergies is exposure to an antigen. An antigen may be defined as anything that is recognized as foreign by the body. Certain foods, industrial chemicals, drugs, pollen, animal proteins, and even latex gloves can be antigens. A more detailed discussion of the immune system and the pharmacotherapy of immune disorders are included in Chapter 30.

The exact cause of a client's allergic rhinitis is often difficult to pinpoint; however, common causes include pollen from weeds, grasses, and trees; moulds; dust mites; certain foods; and animal dander. Chemical fumes, tobacco

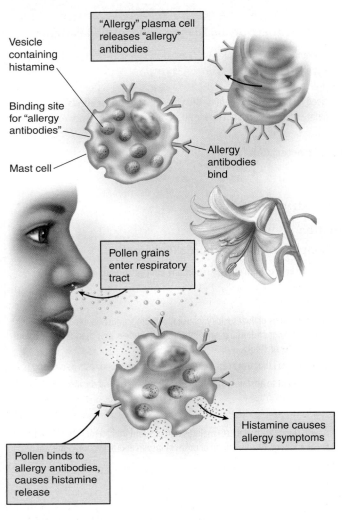

Vesicle containing histamine

"Allergy" plasma cell releases "allergy" antibodies

Binding site for "allergy antibodies"

Mast cell

Allergy antibodies bind

Pollen grains enter respiratory tract

Histamine causes allergy symptoms

Pollen binds to allergy antibodies, causes histamine release

● **Figure 31.2** Allergic rhinitis

smoke, or air pollutants such as ozone are non-allergenic factors that may worsen symptoms. While some clients experience symptoms at specific times of the year, when pollen and mould are at high levels in the environment, other clients are afflicted continuously throughout the year.

The fundamental symptomatic problem of allergic rhinitis is inflammation of the mucous membranes in the nose, throat, and airways. Chemical mediators such as histamine are released that initiate the distressing symptoms. The mechanism of allergic rhinitis is illustrated in Figure 31.2.

Drugs used to treat allergic rhinitis may be grouped into two basic categories: preventers and relievers. Preventers are used for prophylaxis and include antihistamines, glucocorticoids, and mast cell stabilizers. Relievers are used to provide immediate, though temporary, relief of acute allergy symptoms once they have occurred. Relievers include the oral and intranasal adrenergics that are used as nasal decongestants.

H_1-RECEPTOR ANTAGONISTS (ANTIHISTAMINES)

Antihistamines block the actions of histamine at the H_1-receptor. H_1-receptor antagonists are commonly called antihistamines. Because the term *antihistamine* is non-specific and does not indicate which of the two histamine receptors are affected, H_1-receptor antagonist is a more accurate name. These drugs are widely used OTC for relief of allergy symptoms, motion sickness, and insomnia. These agents are shown in Table 31.5.

31.8 Treating Allergic Rhinitis with H_1-Receptor Antagonists

Although a large number of H_1-receptor antagonists are available for use, their efficacies, therapeutic uses, and

TABLE 31.5 H_1-Receptor Antagonists	
Drug	*Route and Adult Dose*
First Generation Agents	
azatadine (Optimine)	PO; 1–2 mg bid
brompheniramine (Dimetapp)	PO; 4–8 mg tid–qid (max 40 mg/day)
chlorpheniramine (Benylin, Chlor-Trimeton)	PO; 2–4 mg tid–qid (max 24 mg/day)
clemastine (Tavist)	PO; 1.34 mg bid (max 8.04 mg/day)
cyproheptadine (EURO-, PMS-Cyproheptadine)	PO; 4 mg tid or qid (max 0.5 mg/kg/day)
dexbrompheniramine (Drixoral)	PO; 6 mg bid
◐ diphenhydramine (Allerdryl, Benadryl)	PO; 25–50 mg tid–qid (max 300 mg/day)
promethazine (Phenergan)	PO; 12.5 mg qd (max 150 mg/day)
triprolidine (Actifed)	PO; 2.5 mg bid or tid
Second Generation Agents	
cetirizine (Zyrtec)	PO; 5–10 mg qd
desloratadine (Aerius)	PO; 5 mg qd
◐ fexofenadine (Allegra)	PO; 60 mg qd–bid (max 120 mg/day)
loratadine (Claritin)	PO; 10 mg qd

side effects are quite similar. These drugs are classified by their generation and their ability to cause sedation, which can be a limiting side effect in some clients. The older, first generation drugs have the potential to cause significant drowsiness, whereas the second generation agents lack this effect in most clients. Care must be taken to avoid alcohol and other CNS depressants when taking antihistamines because their sedating effects may be additive.

The most common therapeutic use of H_1-receptor antagonists is for the treatment of allergies. These medications provide symptomatic relief from the sneezing, runny nose, and itching of the eyes, nose, and throat characteristic of allergic rhinitis. H_1-receptor antagonists are used in OTC cold and sinus medicines, often in combination with other drugs such as decongestants and antitussives. Common OTC antihistamine combinations used to treat allergies are shown in Table 31.6.

Antihistamines are most effective when taken prophylactically to prevent allergic symptoms. Their effectiveness may diminish with long-term use. It should be noted that during severe allergic reactions such as anaphylaxis, histamine is just one of several chemical mediators released; thus, H_1-receptor antagonists alone are not efficacious in treating these acute disorders.

Although most antihistamines are given orally, azelastine was the first to be available by the intranasal route. Azelastine is considered as safe and effective as the oral antihistamines. Although a first generation agent, azelastine causes less drowsiness than others in its class because it is applied locally, and little systemic absorption occurs.

H_1-receptor antagonists are effective in treating a number of other disorders. Motion sickness responds well to these drugs. They are also some of the few drugs available to treat vertigo, a form of dizziness that causes significant nausea. Some of the older antihistamines are marketed as OTC sleep aids, taking advantage of their ability to cause drowsiness.

NURSING CONSIDERATIONS

First Generation H_1-Receptor Antagonists The role of the nurse in drug therapy with first generation H1-receptor antagonists involves careful monitoring of the client's condition and providing education as it relates to the prescribed drug regimen. Before administering a first generation antihistamine, obtain baseline vital signs, including ECG in clients with a history of heart disease. First generation H1-receptor antagonists are contraindicated in clients with a history of dysrhythmias and heart failure. These drugs can cause vasodilation due to H1 stimulation.

First generation H_1-receptor antagonists may cause CNS depression, so they may be contraindicated in clients with a history of depression or sleep disorders, such as narcolepsy and sleep apnea. Because the anticholinergic effects of H_1-receptor antagonists can place clients with narrow-angle glaucoma at risk for injury, they are contraindicated in these clients. Drugs in this class sometimes cause idiosyncratic CNS stimulation; therefore, they may be contraindicated in clients with seizure disorders. Idiosyncratic CNS stimulation, causing hyperactivity, is more common in children.

Elderly clients should be monitored for profound sedation and altered consciousness, which may contribute to falls or other injuries. Prior to initiation of therapy, assess for history of allergy and identify the presence of symptoms such as urticaria, angioedema, nausea, vomiting, motion sickness, and excess mucus production. The agents should be used with caution during pregnancy (pregnancy category C). H_1-antagonists are secreted in breast milk and should not be used by clients who are breastfeeding.

Client education as it relates to first generation H_1-receptor antagonists should include goals; reasons for obtaining baseline data such as vital signs, ECG, and laboratory blood work; and possible side effects.

See "Nursing Process Focus: Clients Receiving Antihistamine Therapy" (page 413) for specific teaching points.

TABLE 31.6	Select OTC Antihistamine Combinations Available for Allergic Rhinitis		
Brand Name	**Antihistamine**	**Decongestant**	**Analgesic**
Actifed Cold and Allergy tablets	triprolidine	pseudoephedrine	–
Actifed Cold and Sinus caplets	chlorpheniramine	pseudoephedrine	acetaminophen
Benadryl Allergy/Cold tablets	diphenhydramine	pseudoephedrine	acetaminophen
Chlor-Trimeton Allergy/ Decongestant tablets	chlorpheniramine	pseudoephedrine	–
Dimetapp Cold and Allergy chewable tablets	brompheniramine	phenylpropanolamine	–
Drixoral Allergy Sinus Extended Relief tablets	dexbrompheniramine	pseudoephedrine	acetaminophen
Sinutab Sinus Allergy tablets	chlorpheniramine	pseudoephedrine	acetaminophen
Sudafed Cold and Allergy tablets	chlorpheniramine	pseudoephedrine	–
Tavist Allergy 12-hour tablets	clemastine	–	–
Triaminic Cold/Allergy softchews	chlorpheniramine	pseudoephedrine	–
Tylenol Allergy Sinus Nighttime caplets	diphenhydramine	pseudoephedrine	acetaminophen

Second Generation H$_1$-Receptor Antagonists The role of the nurse in drug therapy with second generation H$_1$-receptor antagonists involves careful monitoring of the client's condition and providing education as it relates to the prescribed drug regimen. Prior to initiating therapy, assess for the presence/history of allergic rhinitis, conjunctivitis, urticaria, and atopic dermatitis. Baseline vital signs, including ECG in clients with a history of cardiac disease, should be obtained.

Second generation H$_1$-receptor antagonists are generally contraindicated in clients with dysrhythmias because the drugs prolong the QT interval. Due to their anticholinergic effects on the respiratory system, these agents are contraindicated in clients with asthma and in clients who use nicotine. These drugs are metabolized by the liver and excreted by the kidneys; therefore, they are contraindicated in clients with severe liver or renal impairment. Loratadine is most effective when given on an empty stomach.

These drugs should be used with caution in clients with urinary retention due to their anticholinergic effects on the bladder. Anticholinergic activity also affects clients with open-angle glaucoma and hypertension; these clients must be monitored closely. Drugs in this classification are contraindicated in pregnant women in their third trimester due to the possibility of fetal malformation. These drugs should be used with caution in young children because the long-term effects of these drugs on growth and development have not been established.

Client education as it relates to second generation H$_1$-receptor antagonists should include goals; reasons for obtaining baseline data such as vital signs, ECG, and laboratory blood work; and possible side effects.

See "Nursing Process Focus: Clients Receiving Antihistamine Therapy" for specific teaching points.

INTRANASAL GLUCOCORTICOIDS

Glucocorticoids may be applied directly to the nasal mucosa to prevent symptoms of allergic rhinitis. They have begun to replace antihistamines as drugs of choice for the treatment of chronic allergic rhinitis. These drugs are shown in Table 31.7.

31.9 Treating Allergic Rhinitis with Intranasal Glucocorticoids

Section 31.5 presents the importance of the glucocorticoids in treating severe inflammation. As systemic drugs, their use is limited by serious side effects. Intranasal glucocorticoids, however, produce none of the potentially serious adverse effects that are observed when these hormones are given orally or parenterally. Because of their effectiveness and safety, the intranasal glucocorticoids have joined antihistamines as first-line drugs in the treatment of allergic rhinitis.

Intranasal glucocorticoids are administered with a metered-spray device that delivers a consistent dose of drug per spray. When administered properly, their action is limited to the nasal passages. The most frequently reported side effects are an intense burning sensation in the nose immediately after spraying and drying of the nasal mucosa.

Pr PROTOTYPE DRUG | Diphenhydramine (Allerdryl, Benadryl)

ACTIONS AND USES

Diphenhydramine is a first generation H$_1$-receptor antagonist that is a component of some OTC drugs. Its primary use is to treat minor symptoms of allergy and the common cold such as sneezing, runny nose, and tearing of the eyes. OTC preparations may combine diphenhydramine with an analgesic, decongestant, or expectorant. Diphenhydramine is also used as a topical agent to treat rashes, and an IM form is available for severe allergic reactions. Other indications for diphenhydramine include Parkinson's disease, motion sickness, and insomnia.

PHARMACOKINETICS

Diphenhydramine is well absorbed after oral administration. Due to first-pass metabolism, about 50% of an oral dose reaches systemic circulation. It is widely distributed, crosses the placenta, and enters breast milk. It is almost completely metabolized in the liver. Half-life is 2.5 to 7 hours.

ADMINISTRATION ALERTS

- There is an increased risk of anaphylactic shock when this drug is administered parenterally.
- When administering IV, inject at a rate of 25 mg/min to reduce the risk of shock.
- When administering IM, inject deep into the muscle to minimize tissue irritation.
- Antihistamines may cause false positive readings for allergy skin tests.
- Diphenhydramine is pregnancy category C.

ADVERSE EFFECTS AND INTERACTIONS

Older H$_1$-receptor antagonists such as diphenhydramine cause significant drowsiness, although this usually diminishes with long-term use. Occasionally, a client will exhibit CNS stimulation and excitability rather than drowsiness. Anticholinergic effects such as dry mouth, tachycardia, and mild hypotension are seen in some clients. Diphenhydramine may cause photosensitivity.

Diphenhydramine interacts with multiple drugs, particularly CNS depressants (such as alcohol), which enhance sedation. Other OTC cold preparations may increase anticholinergic side effects.

 See the Companion Website for a Nursing Process Focus Chart specific to this drug.

Pr PROTOTYPE DRUG | Fexofenadine (Allegra)

ACTIONS AND USES

Fexofenadine is a second generation H_1-receptor antagonist with efficacy equivalent to that of diphenhydramine. Its primary action is to block the effects of histamine at H_1-receptors. When taken prophylactically, it reduces the severity of nasal congestion, sneezing, and tearing of the eyes. Its long half-life of over 14 hours offers the advantage of being administered once or twice daily. Fexofenadine is only available in oral form. Allegra-D combines fexofenadine with pseudoephedrine, a decongestant.

PHARMACOKINETICS

Fexofenadine is well absorbed after oral administration. Distribution is unknown. It is excreted in urine (80%) and feces. Half-life is 14 hours.

ADMINISTRATION ALERT

- Fexofenadine is pregnancy category C.

ADVERSE EFFECTS AND INTERACTIONS

The major advantage of fexofenadine over first generation antihistamines is that it causes less drowsiness. Although considered non-sedating, the drug can still cause drowsiness in some clients. Other side effects are usually minor and include headache and upset stomach.

No clinically significant drug interactions have been established. However, concurrent use with other antihistamines or CNS depressants may cause synergistic sedative effects.

 See the Companion Website for a Nursing Process Focus Chart specific to this drug.

TABLE 31.7 Intranasal Glucocorticoids

Drug	Route and Adult Dose
beclomethasone (*Beclovent, Apo-Beclomethasone*) (see page 378 for the Prototype Drug box)	Intranasal; one spray bid–qid
budesonide (Rhinocort)	Intranasal; two sprays bid
flunisolide (Nasalide, Nasarel)	Intranasal; two sprays bid; may increase to tid if needed
Pr fluticasone propionate (Flonase)	Intranasal; one spray qd–bid (max qid)
mometasone furoate (Nasonex)	Intranasal; two sprays qd
triamcinolone acetonide (Nasacort AQ)	Intranasal; 2–4 sprays qid

NURSING PROCESS FOCUS Clients Receiving Antihistamine Therapy

Assessment	Potential Nursing Diagnoses/Identified Patterns
Prior to administration: - Obtain complete health history including data on anaphylaxis, asthma, and cardiac disease, plus allergies, drug history, and possible drug interactions. - Obtain ECG and vital signs; assess in context of client's baseline values. - Assess respiratory status: breathing pattern. - Assess neurological status and level of consciousness.	- Presence of somholence, agitation, or disturbed sleep - Altered breathing pattern - Ineffective airway clearance - Thirst - Need for knowledge regarding drug therapy and adverse effects - Safety from injury related to side effects of drug therapy

Planning: Client Goals and Expected Outcomes

The client will:
- Report relief from allergic symptoms such as congestion, itching, or postnasal drip
- Demonstrate an understanding of the drug's action by accurately describing drug side effects and precautions

Implementation

Interventions (Rationales)	Client Education/Discharge Planning
- Auscultate breath sounds before administering. Use with extreme caution in clients with asthma or COPD. Keep resuscitative equipment accessible. (Anticholinergic effects of antihistamines may trigger bronchospasm.) - Monitor vital signs (including ECG) before administering. Use with extreme caution in clients with a history of cardiovascular disease. (Anticholinergic effects can increase heart rate and lower blood pressure. Fatal dysrhythmias and cardiovascular collapse have been reported in some clients receiving antihistamines.)	- Instruct client to immediately report wheezing or difficulty breathing. - Advise asthmatics to consult the nurse regarding the use of injectable epinephrine in emergency situations. Instruct client to: - Immediately report dizziness, palpitations, headache, or chest, arm, or back pain accompanied by nausea/vomiting and/or sweating - Monitor vital signs daily, ensuring proper use of home equipment

continued

NURSING PROCESS FOCUS Clients Receiving Antihistamine Therapy *(Continued)*

Interventions (Rationales)	Client Education/Discharge Planning
▪ Monitor thyroid function. Use with caution in clients with a history of hyperthyroidism. (Antihistamines exacerbate CNS-stimulating effects of hyperthyroidism and may trigger thyroid storm.)	▪ Instruct client to immediately report nervousness or restlessness, insomnia, fever, profuse sweating, thirst, and mood changes.
▪ Monitor for vision changes. Use with caution in clients with narrow-angle glaucoma. (Antihistamines can increase intraocular pressure and cause photosensitivity.)	Instruct client to: ▪ Immediately report head or eye pain and visual changes ▪ Wear dark glasses, use sunscreen, and avoid excessive sun exposure
▪ Monitor neurological status, especially LOC. Use with caution in clients with a history of seizure disorder. (Antihistamines lower the seizure threshold. Older adults are at increased risk of serious sedation and other anticholinergic effects.)	Instruct client to: ▪ Immediately report seizure activity, including any changes in character and pattern of seizures ▪ Avoid driving or performing hazardous activities until effects of the drug are known
▪ Observe for signs of renal toxicity. Measure intake and output. Use with caution in clients with a history of kidney or urinary tract disease. (Antihistamines promote urinary retention.)	▪ Instruct client to immediately report flank pain, difficulty urinating, reduced urine output, and changes in the appearance of urine (cloudy, with sediment, odour, etc.).
▪ Use with caution in clients with diabetes mellitus. Monitor serum glucose levels with increased frequency (e.g., from daily to tid, ac). (Antihistamines decrease serum glucose levels.)	Instruct client to: ▪ Immediately report symptoms of hypoglycemia ▪ Consult the healthcare provider regarding timing of glucose monitoring and reportable results (e.g., "less than 70 mg/dL")
▪ Monitor for GI side effects. Use with caution in clients with a history of GI disorders, especially peptic ulcers or liver disease. (Antihistamines block H_1- receptors, altering the mucosal lining of the stomach. These drugs are metabolized in the liver, increasing the risk of hepatotoxicity.)	Instruct client to: ▪ Immediately report nausea, vomiting, anorexia, bleeding, chest or abdominal pain, heartburn, jaundice, or a change in the colour or character of stools ▪ Avoid substances that irritate the stomach such as spicy foods, alcoholic beverages, and nicotine; take drug with food to avoid stomach upset
▪ Monitor for side effects such as dry mouth; observe for signs of anticholinergic crisis.	Instruct client to: ▪ Immediately report fever or flushing accompanied by difficulty swallowing ("cotton mouth"), blurred vision, and confusion ▪ Avoid mixing OTC antihistamines; always consult the healthcare provider before taking any OTC drugs or herbal supplements ▪ Suck on hard candy to relieve dry mouth, and to maintain adequate fluid intake

Evaluation of Outcome Criteria

Evaluate the effectiveness of drug therapy by confirming that client goals and expected outcomes have been met (see "Planning").

See Table 31.6 for a list of drugs to which these nursing actions apply.

NURSING CONSIDERATIONS

The role of the nurse in drug therapy with intranasal glucocorticoids involves careful monitoring of the client's condition and providing education as it relates to the prescribed drug regimen. Prior to administering glucocorticoid nasal spray, assess the nares for excoriation or bleeding. Broken mucous membranes allow direct access to the bloodstream, increasing the likelihood of systemic effects. The mouth and throat should be examined for signs of infection because glucocorticoids may slow the healing process and mask infections. Intranasal glucocorticoids are contraindicated in clients who demonstrate hypersensitivity to any of the ingredients, including preservatives, in the nasal spray.

Monitor the client for alterations in the nasal and oral mucosa and for signs of upper respiratory (especially oropharyngeal) infection. Signs and symptoms of GI distress should be monitored because swallowing large quantities of the drug may contribute to dyspepsia and systemic drug absorption. Monitor for signs of Cushing's syndrome.

Client education as it relates to intranasal glucocorticoids should include goals, reasons for obtaining baseline data such as vital signs and laboratory blood work, and possible side effects. Instruct the client in the correct use and care of the nasal spray device. Because these medications may take 2 to 4 weeks to be effective, the nurse must advise the client not to discontinue use prematurely. Clients may expect these drugs to act as quickly and effectively as decongestants. All clients, especially children, must be urged not to swallow

Pr PROTOTYPE DRUG | Fluticasone (Flonase)

ACTIONS AND USES

Fluticasone is typical of the intranasal glucocorticoids used to treat seasonal allergic rhinitis. Therapy usually begins with two sprays in each nostril, twice daily, and decreases to one dose per day. Fluticasone acts to decrease local inflammation in the nasal passages, thus decreasing nasal stuffiness.

PHARMACOKINETICS

Less than 2% of fluticasone is absorbed. Small amounts of all glucocorticoids administered intranasally are swallowed. Small amounts cross the placenta and enter breast milk. Fluticasone is rapidly metabolized in the liver. Half-life is 3 hours.

ADMINISTRATION ALERTS

- Directions for use provided by the manufacturer should be carefully followed by the client.
- Fluticasone is pregnancy category C.

ADVERSE EFFECTS AND INTERACTIONS

Side effects of fluticasone are rare. Small amounts of the intranasal glucocorticoids are sometimes swallowed, thus increasing the potential for systemic side effects. Nasal irritation and bleeding occur in a small number of clients. Concomitant use of a local nasal decongestant spray may increase the risk of irritation or bleeding.

Use with caution with herbal supplements, such as licorice, which may potentiate the effects of glucocorticoids.

 See the Companion Website for a Nursing Process Focus Chart specific to this drug.

TABLE 31.8 Sympathomimetics for Allergic Rhinitis	
Drug	**Route and Adult Dose**
ephedrine (Pretz-D, Primatene)	Intranasal (0.1%); one to two drops bid
oxymetazoline (Afrin, Visine LR)	Intranasal (0.05%); two to three sprays bid for up to 3–5 days
phenylephrine (Afrin, Dristan, Neo-Synephrine)	Intranasal (0.1%); two to three drops or sprays q3–4h, as needed
pseudoephedrine (Actifed, Sudafed)	PO; 60 mg 4–6h (max 120 mg/day)
xylometazoline (Otrivin)	Intranasal (0.1%); one to two sprays bid (max three doses/day)

excess amounts of the drug, which is likely to drain down the back of the throat following application. Swallowing large amounts of drug residue increases the risks of systemic side effects. Nasal decongestant sprays are sometimes prescribed with intranasal glucocorticoids for clients with chronic rhinitis. Decongestant sprays should be administered first to clear the nasal passages, allowing for adequate application of the glucocorticoid mist.

Following are other important points to include when teaching clients regarding intranasal glucocorticoids:

- Take the medication exactly as prescribed; additional dosing will not speed relief.
- Shake inhalers thoroughly before spraying.
- Gently clear the nose before spraying. Avoid clearing the nose immediately after spraying.
- Report nosebleeds and nasal burning or irritation that lasts more than a few doses.
- Following administration, spit out the postnasal medication residue.
- Use a humidifier, preservative-free nasal saline spray, or petroleum jelly to ease nasal dryness.

ADRENERGICS

Adrenergics stimulate the sympathetic nervous system. They may be administered orally or intranasally to dry the nasal

mucosa. The agents used for nasal congestion are shown in Table 31.8.

31.10 Treating Nasal Congestion with Adrenergics

As discussed in Chapter 13, adrenergics, or adrenergic agonists, are agents that stimulate the sympathetic branch of the autonomic nervous system. Adrenergics with alpha-adrenergic activity are effective at relieving the nasal congestion associated with allergic rhinitis when given by either the oral or intranasal route. The intranasal preparations such as oxymetazoline are available OTC as sprays or drops and produce an effective response within minutes. Because of their local action, intranasal adrenergics produce few systemic effects. The most serious, limiting side effect of the intranasal preparations is **rebound congestion**. Prolonged use causes hypersecretion of mucus and worsening of nasal congestion once the drug effects wear off. This sometimes leads to a cycle of increased drug use as the condition worsens. Because of this rebound congestion, intranasal adrenergics should be used for no longer than 3 to 5 days.

When administered orally, adrenergics do not produce rebound congestion. Their onset of action by this route, however, is much slower than the intranasal route, and they are less effective at relieving severe congestion. The possibility of systemic side effects is also greater with the oral drugs. Potential side effects include hypertension and CNS stimulation that may lead to insomnia and anxiety. Pseudoephedrine is the most common adrenergic (sympathomimetic) found in oral OTC cold and allergy medicines.

Because the adrenergics only relieve nasal congestion, they are often combined with antihistamines to control the sneezing and tearing of allergic rhinitis. It is interesting to note that some OTC drugs having the same basic name may contain different adrenergics. For example, Neo-Synephrine preparations with a 12-hour duration contain the drug oxymetazoline; Neo-Synephrine preparations that last 4 to 6 hours contain phenylephrine.

NURSING CONSIDERATIONS

The role of the nurse in drug therapy with adrenergics for nasal congestion involves careful monitoring of the client's condition and providing education as it relates to the prescribed drug regimen. Assess for the presence/history of nasal congestion and assess the nares for signs of excoriation or bleeding. Before and during pharmacotherapy, assess vital signs, especially pulse and blood pressure. Oral adrenergics are contraindicated in clients with hypertension due to vasoconstriction caused by stimulation of alpha-adrenergic receptors on systemic blood vessels.

Alpha-adrenergic agonists should be used with caution in clients with prostatic enlargement since these drugs increase smooth muscle activity in the prostate gland and may diminish urinary outflow (see Chapter 42). Clients with thyroid disorders and diabetes mellitus are at risk because adrenergics can increase serum glucose and body metabolism.

These agents should be used with caution in clients with psychiatric disorders, due to an increased risk of agitation. The CNS depression effect of these drugs can seriously exacerbate symptoms of clinical depression.

Client education as it relates to adrenergics for nasal congestion should include goals, reasons for obtaining baseline data such as vital signs and tests for cardiac or metabolic disorders, and possible side effects. The following are important points to include when teaching clients regarding adrenergics:

- Limit use of intranasal preparations to 3 to 5 days to prevent rebound congestion.
- Avoid using other OTC cold or allergy preparations (especially those containing antihistamines) while taking adrenergics because these agents may cause excessive drowsiness.
- Follow the nurse's directions for the use and care of nasal spray dispensers and for proper inhalation technique.
- Report the following immediately: palpitations or chest pain, dizziness or fainting, fever, visual changes, excessively dry mouth, confusion, numbness or tingling in the face or limbs, severe headache, insomnia, restlessness or nervousness, nosebleeds, or persistent intranasal pain or irritation.

See "Nursing Process Focus: Clients Receiving Adrenergic Therapy" in Chapter 13 (page 137) for more information.

ANAPHYLAXIS

Anaphylaxis is a potentially fatal condition in which body defences produce a hyperresponse to an antigen. Upon first exposure, the antigen produces no symptoms; however, the body responds by becoming highly sensitized to a subsequent exposure. During anaphylaxis, the body responds quickly, sometimes within minutes after exposure to the antigen, by releasing massive amounts of histamine and other mediators of the inflammatory response. Shortly after exposure to the antigen, the client may experience itching, hives, and a tightness in the throat or chest. Swelling occurs around the larynx, causing a non-productive cough and the voice to become hoarse. As anaphylaxis progresses, the client experiences a rapid fall in blood pressure and difficulty breathing due to bronchoconstriction. The hypotension causes a rebound speeding up of the heart called reflex tachycardia. Without medical intervention, anaphylaxis leads to a profound shock, which is often fatal. Figure 31.3 illustrates the symptoms of anaphylaxis.

31.11 Pharmacotherapy of Anaphylaxis

Pharmacotherapy of anaphylaxis is symptomatic and involves supporting the cardiovascular system and preventing further hyperresponse by body defences. Various medications are used to treat the symptoms of anaphylaxis depending on the severity of the symptoms. Oxygen is usually administered immediately. Adrenergics such as epinephrine can rapidly reverse hypotension. Antihistamines such as diphenhydramine may be administered IM or IV to prevent stimulation of H_1-receptors. A bronchodilator such as albuterol is sometimes administered by inhalation to relieve the acute shortness of breath caused by histamine. Systemic

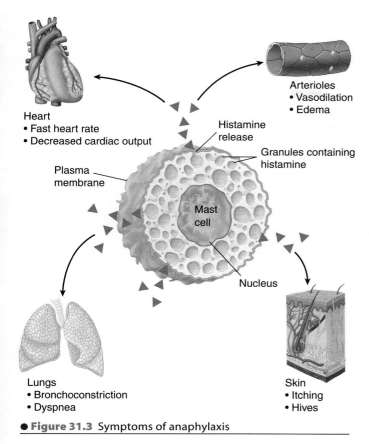

Heart
• Fast heart rate
• Decreased cardiac output

Histamine release

Granules containing histamine

Arterioles
• Vasodilation
• Edema

Plasma membrane

Mast cell

Nucleus

Lungs
• Bronchoconstriction
• Dyspnea

Skin
• Itching
• Hives

● **Figure 31.3** Symptoms of anaphylaxis

glucocorticoids such as hydrocortisone may be administered to dampen the inflammatory response. The pharmacotherapy of shock is presented in Chapter 27.

NURSING CONSIDERATIONS

The role of the nurse in drug therapy with epinephrine involves careful monitoring of the client's condition and providing education as it relates to the drug. Epinephrine is generally administered as an emergency response to severe allergic reactions. Although epinephrine is contraindicated for clients with known hypersensitivity to this drug, in life-threatening situations there are no absolute contraindications to its use.

Epinephrine must be administered with caution to clients with cardiac disease or a history of cerebral atherosclerosis because epinephrine can cause a steep rise in blood pressure, as a result of peripheral vascular constriction combined with cardiac stimulation, that can lead to intracranial bleeding, dysrhythmias, or pulmonary edema. Epinephrine must also be administered with caution to clients with hyperthyroidism; epinephrine exacerbates tachycardia.

Epinephrine is frequently administered in the emergency department setting; resuscitative equipment must be readily accessible. Parenteral epinephrine is irritating to tissues; thus, IV sites must be closely monitored for signs of extravasation. Vital signs, including ECG, are monitored continuously during epinephrine infusions. Auscultate the chest before and after epinephrine injection to monitor improvement in bronchoconstriction (wheezing). Clients with a history of closed-angle glaucoma should be monitored for visual changes as a result of changes in intraocular pressure.

Clients with a history of recurrent anaphylaxis may be prescribed epinephrine to be self-administered intramuscularly via an automatic injectable device (EpiPen). The nurse should instruct these clients regarding safe "pen" storage and disposal and the proper injection technique. Clients should be encouraged to use the medication-free "trainer" pen to practise the technique. Advise the client to expect some medication to remain in the pen following injection and to report all episodes requiring pen usage to the healthcare provider.

Client education as it relates to epinephrine should include goals, reasons for obtaining baseline data such as vital signs and ECG, and possible side effects. Following are

---

Pr **PROTOTYPE DRUG** | Epinephrine (Adrenalin)

ACTIONS AND USES

Subcutaneous or intravenous epinephrine is a drug of choice for anaphylaxis because it can reverse many of the distressing symptoms within minutes. Epinephrine is a non-selective adrenergic agonist, stimulating both alpha- and beta-adrenergic receptors. Almost immediately after injection, blood pressure rises due to stimulation of alpha$_1$-receptors. Activation of beta$_2$-receptors in the bronchi opens the airways and relieves the client's shortness of breath. Cardiac output increases due to stimulation of beta$_1$-receptors in the heart.

PHARMACOKINETICS

Epinephrine is well absorbed after SC injection. It crosses the placenta and enters breast milk but does not cross the blood-brain barrier. Action is rapidly terminated by reuptake into neurons and metabolism.

ADMINISTRATION ALERTS

- Parenteral epinephrine is an irritant that may cause tissue damage if extravasation occurs.
- Epinephrine is pregnancy category C.

ADVERSE EFFECTS AND INTERACTIONS

When administered parenterally, epinephrine may cause serious adverse effects. Hypertension and dysrhythmias may occur rapidly; therefore, the client should be monitored continuously following injection.

Epinephrine interacts with many drugs. For example, it may increase hypotension with phenothiazines and oxytocin. There may be additive toxicities with other adrenergics. MAO inhibitors, tricyclic antidepressants, and alpha- and beta-adrenergic agents inhibit the actions of epinephrine.

 See the Companion Website for a Nursing Process Focus Chart specific to this drug.

the important points to include when teaching clients regarding epinephrine:

- Seek emergency medical attention immediately if a single auto-injection of epinephrine fails to bring relief.
- Report burning, irritation, tenderness, swelling, or hardness at IV or IM injection sites.
- Immediately report changes in level of consciousness, particularly feeling faint.
- Report any of the following: palpitations, chest pain, nausea, vomiting, sweating, weakness, dizziness, confusion, blurred vision, headache, anxiety, or sense of impending doom.

See "Nursing Process Focus: Clients Receiving Adrenergic Therapy" in Chapter 13 (page 137) for more information.

CHAPTER REVIEW

KEY CONCEPTS

The numbered key concepts provide a succinct summary of the important points from the corresponding numbered section within the chapter. If any of these points are not clear, refer to that numbered section within the chapter for review. Expanded versions can be found on the Companion Website.

31.1 Inflammation is a natural, non-specific response that limits the spread of invading microorganisms or injury. Acute inflammation occurs over several days, whereas chronic inflammation may continue for months or years.

31.2 Histamine is a key chemical mediator in inflammation. Release of histamine produces vasodilation, allowing capillaries to become leaky, thus causing tissue swelling.

31.3 Histamine can produce its effects by interacting with two different receptors. The classic antihistamines used for allergies block histamine H_1-receptors in vascular smooth muscle, in the bronchi, and on sensory nerves. The H_2-receptor antagonists are used to treat peptic ulcers.

31.4 Non-steroidal anti-inflammatory drugs (NSAIDs) are the primary drugs for the treatment of simple inflammation. Newer selective COX-2 inhibitors cause less GI distress.

31.5 Systemic glucocorticoids are effective in treating acute or severe inflammation. Overtreatment with these drugs can cause a serious condition called Cushing's syndrome; thus, therapy for inflammation is generally short term.

31.6 Acetaminophen and NSAIDs are the primary agents used to treat fever.

31.7 Allergic rhinitis is a disorder characterized by sneezing, watery eyes, and nasal congestion.

31.8 Antihistamines, or H_1-receptor antagonists, can provide relief from the symptoms of allergic rhinitis. Newer drugs in this class are non-sedating and offer the advantage of once-a-day dosage.

31.9 Intranasal glucocorticoids have become drugs of choice in treating allergic rhinitis due to their high efficacy and wide margin of safety.

31.10 Oral and intranasal adrenergics are used to alleviate the nasal congestion due to allergic rhinitis and the common cold. Intranasal drugs are more efficacious but can only be used for 3 to 5 days due to rebound congestion.

31.11 Anaphylaxis is a serious and often fatal allergic response that is treated with a large number of different drugs, including adrenergics, antihistamines, and glucocorticoids.

REVIEW QUESTIONS

1 Why are antihistamines most effective if given *before* inflammation occurs?

2 The adrenergics are the most effective drugs for relieving nasal congestion, but healthcare providers often prefer to prescribe antihistamines or intranasal glucocorticoids. Why?

3 Why are oral glucocorticoids primarily used concurrently with the immunosuppressant drugs following an organ transplant?

CRITICAL THINKING QUESTIONS

1. A 64-year-old Aboriginal client has a history of diabetes and is on prednisone for rheumatoid arthritis. The client has recently been admitted to the hospital for stabilization of hyperglycemia. What are the nurse's primary concerns when caring for this client?

2. A 44-year-old client is requesting medication for a painful tendonitis of the elbow. This client has mild hypertension, a history of alcohol abuse, and nutritional deficits. This client has a PRN order for acetaminophen (Tylenol), ibuprofen (Motrin), and celecoxib (Celebrex). Which one would the nurse give and why?

3. A 74-year-old male client informs the nurse that he is taking diphenhydramine (Benadryl) to reduce the seasonal allergy symptoms. This client has a history of enlarged prostate and mild glaucoma (controlled by medication). What is the nurse's response?

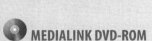

EXPLORE
MediaLink

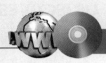

www.pearsoned.ca/adams-king

MEDIALINK DVD-ROM
- **Audio Glossary**
- **CRNE Review**

COMPANION WEBSITE
- **CRNE Review**
- **Case Study:** Client taking anti-inflammatory drugs
- **Dosage Calculations**

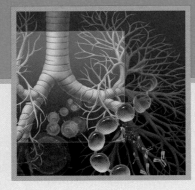

CHAPTER 32

Drugs for Bacterial Infections

DRUGS AT A GLANCE

PENICILLINS
- penicillin G potassium

CEPHALOSPORINS
- cefotaxime (Claforan)

TETRACYCLINES
- tetracycline (Apo-Tetra, others)

MACROLIDES
- erythromycin (Apo-Erythro, others)

AMINOGLYCOSIDES
- gentamicin (Garamycin)

FLUOROQUINOLONES
- ciprofloxacin (Cipro)

SULFONAMIDES
- trimethoprim-sulfamethoxazole (Bactrim, others)

MISCELLANEOUS ANTIBACTERIALS
- vancomycin (PMS-Vancomycin, Vancocin)

ANTITUBERCULAR AGENTS
- isoniazid (Dom-Isoniazid, PMS-Isoniazid)

OBJECTIVES

After reading this chapter, the student should be able to do the following:

1. Identify drug classes used for treating bacterial infections.
2. Explain the therapeutic action of each class of anti-infective drug in relation to the pathophysiology of infection.
3. Explain the differences between *bacteriostatic* and *bactericidal* drugs and when each might be prescribed.
4. Using a specific example, explain how resistance can develop to an anti-infective drug.
5. Explain the importance of culture and sensitivity testing to anti-infective therapy.
6. Identify the mechanism of development and symptoms of superinfections caused by anti-infective therapy.
7. Explain how the pharmacotherapy of tuberculosis differs from that of other infections.
8. Discuss the role of the nurse regarding the non-pharmacological management of bacterial infections, including prevention, promotion of healing, and client teaching.
9. Describe the nurse's role in the pharmacological management of clients receiving drugs for bacterial infections.
10. For each of the drug classes listed in Drugs at a Glance, identify a representative drug and explain its mechanism of action, therapeutic effects, and important adverse effects.
11. Describe and explain, based on pharmacological principles, the rationale for nursing assessment, planning, and interventions for clients with bacterial infections.
12. Use the nursing process to care for clients receiving drug therapy for bacterial infections.

MediaLink

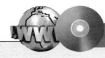

www.pearsoned.ca/adams-king

CRNE review, case studies, and other interactive resources for this chapter can be found on the Companion Website at **www.pearsoned.ca/adams-king.** Click on "Chapter 36" to select the activities for this chapter. For animations, more CRNE review questions, and an audio glossary, access the accompanying DVD-ROM in this textbook.

The human body has adapted quite well to living in a world teeming with microorganisms. Found in air, water, food, and soil, microbes are an essential component of life on the planet. In some cases, such as with microorganisms in the colon, microbes play a beneficial role in human health. In an unnatural environment or when present in unusually high numbers, however, microorganisms can cause a wide variety of ailments ranging from mildly annoying to fatal. The first anti-infective drugs were developed in the mid-1900s. In the last 50 years, researchers have attempted to keep pace with microbes that rapidly become resistant to therapeutic agents. This chapter examines two groups of anti-infectives: the antibacterial agents and the specialized drugs used to treat tuberculosis.

32.1 Pathogenicity and Virulence

An organism that can cause disease is called a **pathogen**. Human pathogens include viruses, bacteria, fungi, unicellular organisms, and multicellular animals. To infect humans, pathogens must bypass a number of elaborate body defences, such as those described in Chapters 30 and 31. Pathogens may enter through broken skin or by ingestion, inhalation, or contact with a mucous membrane such as the nasal, urinary, or vaginal mucosa.

The ability of an organism to cause infection is called pathogenicity. **Pathogenicity** depends on an organism's ability to evade or overcome body defences. Another common word used to describe a pathogen is **virulence**. A highly virulent microbe is one that can produce disease when present in minute numbers.

After gaining entry, pathogens generally cause disease by one of two basic mechanisms. Some pathogens grow rapidly and cause disease by their sheer numbers, which can overcome immune defences and disrupt normal cellular function. A second mechanism is the production of toxins that affect human cells. Even very small amounts of some bacterial toxins may disrupt normal cellular activity and, in extreme cases, result in death.

PHARMFACTS

Antimicrobial Use in Canada from 2000 to 2004

- After cardiovascular and psychotherapeutic drugs, antibiotics were the third most commonly prescribed class of agents.

- The antibacterial classes most frequently dispensed by retail pharmacies in Canada were extended-spectrum penicillins (25%), macrolides (20%), tetracyclines (14%), fluoroquinolones (12%), and second generation cephalosporins (5%).

- Despite a decrease in the total number of antimicrobial prescriptions from 2000 to 2004, costs increased due to use of more costly antimicrobial drugs. Antimicrobials of Very High Human Health Importance (Category I) represented a consistently increasing proportion.

- About 51% of antimicrobials were used for respiratory diseases. The primary antimicrobial classes were extended-spectrum macrolides (32%), amoxicillin (25%), cephalosporins (14%), and oral quinolones (11%).

- It has been estimated that 30% to 40% of endemic institutional antibiotic resistance is caused by the unwashed hands of hospital personnel.

Source: Canadian Integrated Program for Antimicrobial Resistance Surveillance (CIPARS), www.phac-aspc.gc.ca/cipars-picrc/index_e.html; Conly, J. (2002). Antimicrobial resistance in Canada. Canadian Medical Association Journal, 167, 885–891.

Bacterial Infections

- Infectious diseases are the third most common cause of death in North America and first in the world.

- There are 11 to 13 million cases of food-borne illness in Canada every year. Common causes of food-borne illness include *Campylobacter jejuni* (most frequent cause), *Salmonella, Shigella*, and *Escherichia coli*. Symptoms usually start soon after eating contaminated food, but they can occur more than a month later. Most cases can be prevented by using safe food handling practices, cooking meats to a safe internal temperature, and drinking treated water and pasteurized milk.

- Canada has one of the lowest incidence rates of tuberculosis (TB) in the world (about 5.5 per 100,000 Canadians per year). Most cases of active TB occur among certain high-risk groups, including Aboriginal Peoples, foreign-born residents from countries with a high prevalence of TB, disadvantaged inner-city populations, and those with HIV infection.

- Pneumococcal infections are the most common invasive bacterial infections in children and may lead to meningitis.

- *Staphylococcus aureus* is commonly found on the skin and in the nose of healthy people. In the general population, the noses of approximately 25% to 30% of people are colonized (carry the bacteria but do not have an infection). Of these colonized people, 20% to 30% will develop an infection.

- Methicillin-resistant *Staphylococcus aureus* (MRSA) is a strain of *Staphylococcus* that has become resistant to many of the antibiotics usually used to treat it. Although MRSA has mainly been associated with healthcare facilities in the past, in the last few years, MRSA infections are becoming much more common in the community setting.

- Nearly all strains of *S. aureus* in North America are resistant to penicillin.

- Enterococci are bacteria normally found in the lower GI tract. Vancomycin-resistant enterococci (VRE) are strains that have developed resistance to several antibiotics, including vancomycin.

- Urinary tract infection (UTI) is the most common infection acquired in hospitals and nearly all are associated with the insertion of a urinary catheter.

Source: Canadian Food Inspection Agency, 2007; Public Health Agency of Canada.

32.2 Describing and Classifying Bacteria

Because of the enormous number of different bacterial species, several descriptive systems have been developed to simplify their study. It is important for nurses to learn these classification schemes because drugs that are effective against one organism in a class are likely to be effective against other pathogens in the same class. Common bacterial pathogens and the types of diseases they cause are shown in Table 32.1.

One of the simplest methods of classifying bacteria is to examine them microscopically after a crystal violet Gram stain is applied. Some bacteria contain a thick cell wall and retain a purple colour after staining. These are called **gram-positive** bacteria. Examples of gram-positive bacteria include staphylococci, streptococci, and enterococci. Bacteria that have thinner cell walls will lose the violet stain and are called **gram-negative**. Examples of gram-negative bacteria

include bacteroides, *Escherichia coli, Klebsiella, Pseudomonas,* and *Salmonella*. The distinction between gram-positive and gram-negative bacteria is a profound one that reflects important biochemical and physiological differences between the two groups. Some antibacterial agents are effective only against gram-positive bacteria, whereas others are used to treat gram-negative bacteria.

A second descriptive method is based on cellular shape. Bacteria assume several basic shapes that can be readily determined microscopically. Rod shapes are called **bacilli**, spherical shapes are called **cocci**, and spirals are called **spirilla**.

A third factor used to classify bacteria is their ability to use oxygen. Those that thrive in an oxygen environment are **aerobic**; those that grow best without oxygen are **anaerobic**. Some organisms have the ability to change their metabolism and survive in either aerobic or anaerobic conditions, depending on their external environment. Antibacterial drugs differ based on their ability to treat aerobic versus anaerobic bacteria.

32.3 Classification of Anti-Infective Drugs

Any medication that is effective against pathogens is an **anti-infective**. Although **antibiotic** is more frequently used, this term technically refers only to natural substances produced by microorganisms that can kill other microorganisms. In current practice, the terms *antibacterial, anti-infective, antimicrobial,* and *antibiotic* are often used interchangeably, as they are in this textbook.

With over 300 anti-infectives available, it is useful to group these drugs into classes that have similar chemical structures or therapeutic properties. Chemical classes are widely used. Names such as aminoglycoside, fluoroquinolone, and sulfonamide refer to the fundamental chemical structure of a group of anti-infectives. Anti-infectives belonging to the same chemical class share similar antimicrobial properties and side effects.

Another method of classifying anti-infectives is by mechanism of action. Examples include cell wall inhibitors, protein synthesis inhibitors, folic acid inhibitors, and reverse transcriptase inhibitors. These classifications are used in this textbook where appropriate.

32.4 Actions of Anti-Infective Drugs

The primary goal of antimicrobial therapy is to assist in ridding the body of the pathogen. Medications that accomplish this goal by *killing* bacteria are **bactericidal**. Some drugs do not kill the bacteria, but instead slow their growth so that the body's natural defences can dispose of the microorganisms. These *growth-slowing* drugs are **bacteriostatic**.

Bacterial cells are quite different from human cells. Bacteria have cell walls and contain certain enzymes and cellular structures that human cells lack. Antibiotics exert selective toxicity on bacterial cells by targeting these unique

TABLE 32.1   Common Bacterial Pathogens and Diseases

Name of Organism	Disease(s)	Description
Borrelia burgdorferi	Lyme disease	from tick bites
Chlamydia trachomatis	venereal disease, endometriosis	most common cause of sexually transmitted infections
Escherichia coli	traveller's diarrhea, urinary tract infection (UTI), bacteremia, endometriosis	part of host flora in GI tract
Haemophilus	pneumonia, meningitis in children, bacteremia, otitis media, sinusitis	some *Haemophilus* species are host flora in the upper respiratory tract
Klebsiella	pneumonia, UTI	usually infects immunosuppressed patients
Mycobacterium leprae	leprosy	most cases occur in immigrants from Africa or Asia
Mycobacterium tuberculosis	tuberculosis	incidence very high in HIV-infected patients
Mycoplasma pneumoniae	pneumonia	most common cause of pneumonia in clients age 5–35
Neisseria gonorrhoeae	gonorrhea and other sexually transmitted infections, endometriosis, neonatal eye infection	some *Neisseria* species are normal host flora
Neisseria meningitidis	meningitis in children	some *Neisseria* species are normal host flora
Pneumococci	pneumonia, otitis media, meningitis, bacteremia, endocarditis	part of normal flora in upper respiratory tract
Proteus mirabilis	UTI, skin infections	part of host flora in GI tract
Pseudomonas aeroginosa	UTI, skin infections, septicemia	usually infects immunosuppressed patients
Rickettsia rickettsii	Rocky Mountain spotted fever	from tick bites
Salmonella enteritidis	food poisoning	from infected animal products, raw eggs, undercooked meat or chicken
Salmonella typhi	typhoid fever	from inadequately treated food or water supplies
Staphylococcus aureus	pneumonia, food poisoning, impetigo, abscesses, bacteremia, endocarditis, toxic shock syndrome	some *Staphylococcus* species are normal host flora
Streptococcus	pharyngitis, pneumonia, skin infections, septicemia, endocarditis	some *Streptococcus* species are normal host flora
Vibrio cholerae	cholera	from inadequately treated food or water supplies

TABLE 32.2 Mechanism of Action of Antibacterial Drugs

Mechanism of Action	Drug Classification	Examples	Indications
inhibit cell wall synthesis	monobactams	aztreonam	*Pseudomonas*
	beta-lactams	penicillins, cephalosporins, others	
	penicillins	amoxicillin, penicillin G, piperacillin	streptococcal, meningococcal, and pneumococcal infections
	cephalosporins	cefazolin, cefotetan, cefotaxime	respiratory and urinary tract infections
	vancomycin		MRSA
inhibit protein synthesis	aminoglycosides	gentamicin, neomycin, streptomycin	gram-negative coliform infections
	macrolides	clarithromycin, erythromycin	gram-positive cocci, *Legionella, Chlamydia*
	streptogrammins	quinupristin-dalfopristin	*S. aureus,* resistant bacteria
	tetracyclines	oxytetracycline, minocycline	chlamydial and mycoplasmal infections
	chloramphenicol		*Salmonella, Haemophilus influenzae* infections
inhibit DNA or RNA synthesis	fluoroquinolones	ciprofloxacin	urinary tract and respiratory infections
	rifamycins	rifampin	*S. aureus,* meningitis
inhibit metabolic pathways	sulfonamides	sulfamethoxazole, trimethoprim-sulfamethoxazole	urinary tract infections
inhibit nucleic acid synthesis	nitroimidazoles	metronidazole	anaerobic infections, *Helicobacter pylori*

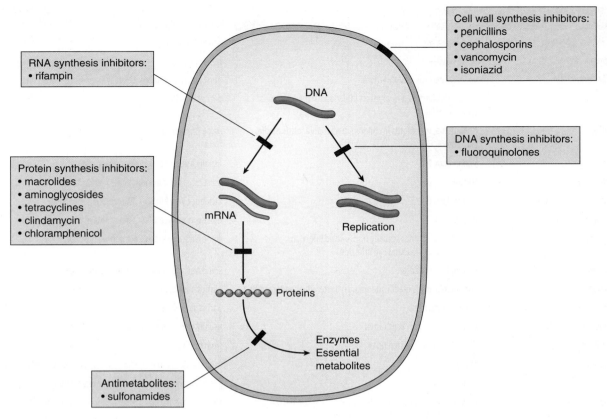

RNA synthesis inhibitors:
• rifampin

Cell wall synthesis inhibitors:
• penicillins
• cephalosporins
• vancomycin
• isoniazid

DNA

Protein synthesis inhibitors:
• macrolides
• aminoglycosides
• tetracyclines
• clindamycin
• chloramphenicol

DNA synthesis inhibitors:
• fluoroquinolones

mRNA

Replication

Proteins

Enzymes
Essential
metabolites

Antimetabolites:
• sulfonamides

● **Figure 32.1** Mechanisms of action of antimicrobial drugs

differences. In this way, bacteria can be killed or their growth severely hampered without major effects on human cells. There are limits to this selective toxicity depending on the specific antibiotic and the dose employed, and side effects can be expected from all the anti-infectives. The basic mechanisms of action of antimicrobial drugs are listed in Table 32.2 and are illustrated in Figure 32.1.

32.5 Antimicrobial Resistance

Microorganisms have the ability to replicate extremely rapidly. During this cell division, bacteria make frequent errors duplicating their genetic code. These **mutations** occur spontaneously and randomly. Although most mutations are harmful to the organism, mutations occasionally result in a bacterial cell that has reproductive advantages over its neighbours. The mutated bacterium may be able to survive in harsher conditions or perhaps grow faster than other cells. Mutations that are of particular importance to medicine are those that confer drug resistance.

Antibiotics help to promote the appearance of drug-resistant bacterial strains by killing populations of bacteria that are sensitive to the drug. Consequently, the only bacteria remaining are those that possess mutations that make them insensitive to the effects of the antibiotic. These antimicrobial-resistant bacteria are then free to grow, without competition from neighbours that were killed by the antibiotic, and the client develops an infection that is resist-

ant to conventional drug therapy. This phenomenon, **acquired resistance**, is illustrated in Figure 32.2. Bacteria may pass the resistance gene to other bacteria through conjugation—the transfer of small pieces of circular DNA called **plasmids.**

It is important to understand that the antibiotic did not create the mutation that caused the bacteria to become resistant. The mutation occurred randomly. The role of the antibiotic is to kill the surrounding cells that were susceptible to the drug, leaving the mutated ones plenty of room to divide and infect the host. It is the bacteria that have become resistant, not the client. Additionally, a client with an infection that is resistant to certain antibacterial agents can transmit the resistant bacteria to others.

The widespread and sometimes unwarranted use of antibiotics has led to a large number of resistant bacterial strains, referred to as **antimicrobial** (or **antibacterial) resistance**. At least 60% of *Staphylococcus aureus* infections are now resistant to penicillin, and resistant strains of *Enterococcus faecalis, Enterococcus faecium,* and *Pseudomonas aeruginosa* are becoming major clinical problems. The longer an antibiotic is used in the population and the more often it is prescribed, the larger the percentage of resistant strains. Infections acquired in a hospital or other healthcare setting, called **nosocomial infections**, are often resistant to common antibiotics.

The Canadian Integrated Program for Antimicrobial Resistance Surveillance (CIPARS) monitors trends in antimicrobial use and antimicrobial resistance in select bacterial organisms from human, animal, and food sources across Canada. Appropriate measures to contain the emergence and spread of resistant bacteria between animals, food, and people in Canada are identified. This information is used to develop evidence-based policies to control antimicrobial use in hospital, community, and agricultural settings and thus to prolong the effectiveness of antimicrobial drugs.

Healthcare providers can play an important role in delaying the emergence of resistance by restricting the use of antibiotics to those conditions deemed medically necessary. In most cases, antibiotics are given when there is clear evidence of bacterial infection. Some clients, however, receive antibiotics to *prevent* an infection, a practice called prophylactic use or chemoprophylaxis. Examples of clients who might receive prophylactic antibiotics include those who have a suppressed immune system, those who have experienced deep puncture wounds such as from dog bites, or those who have prosthetic heart valves, prior to receiving medical or dental surgery.

It is not uncommon for clients to stop taking an antibiotic once they begin to feel better. Discontinuing an antibiotic before all organisms have been killed promotes the emergence of resistant strains. Instruct the client that many organisms still remain, even after the symptoms disappear. The importance of taking the entire drug regimen must be stressed.

32.6 Selection of an Effective Antibiotic

Some antibacterials are effective against a wide variety of different microorganisms. These are called **broad-spectrum antibiotics. Narrow-spectrum antibiotics** are effective against only one or a restricted group of microorganisms.

The selection of an antibiotic therapy effective against a specific organism is an important task of the healthcare provider. Selecting an incorrect drug will delay proper treatment, thus giving the microorganism more time to infect. Prescribing ineffective antibiotics also promotes the development of resistance and may cause unnecessary side effects in the client.

Ideally, laboratory tests should be conducted to identify the organism prior to beginning anti-infective therapy. Lab tests may include examination of body specimens such as urine, sputum, blood, or pus for microorganisms. Organisms isolated from the specimens may be grown in the laboratory and identified. After identification, the laboratory may test several different antibiotics to determine which is most effective against the infecting microorganism. This process of growing the organism and identifying the most effective antibiotic is called **culture and sensitivity testing.**

Proper laboratory testing and identification of bacteria may take several days or, in the case of viruses, several weeks. Some organisms simply cannot be cultured at all. If the infection is severe, the healthcare provider will likely begin

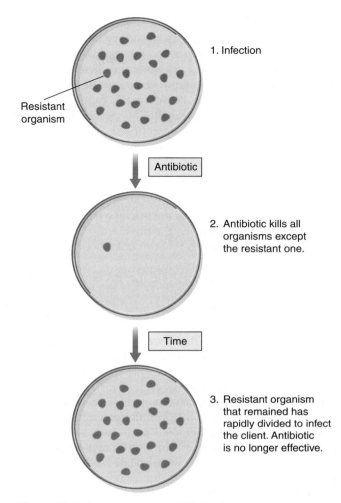

1. Infection

Resistant organism

Antibiotic

2. Antibiotic kills all organisms except the resistant one.

Time

3. Resistant organism that remained has rapidly divided to infect the client. Antibiotic is no longer effective.

● **Figure 32.2** Acquired antimicrobial resistance

therapy immediately with a broad-spectrum antibiotic. After the results of the culture and sensitivity tests are obtained, therapy may be changed to include the antibiotic found to be most effective against the microbe.

In most cases, antibacterial therapy is conducted using a single drug. Combining two antibiotics may actually decrease each drug's efficacy, a phenomenon known as **antagonism.** Use of multiple antibiotics also has the potential to promote resistance. Multidrug therapy may be warranted, however, if several different organisms cause the client's infection or if the infection is so severe that therapy must be started before laboratory tests have been completed. Multidrug therapy is clearly warranted in the treatment of tuberculosis and in clients infected with HIV.

One common side effect of anti-infective therapy is the appearance of secondary infections, known as **superinfections,** which occur when microorganisms normally present in the body are destroyed. These normal microorganisms, or **host flora,** inhabit the skin and the upper respiratory, genitourinary, and intestinal tracts. Some of these organisms serve a useful purpose by producing antibacterial substances and by competing with pathogenic organisms for space and nutrients. Removal of host flora by an antibiotic gives the remaining microorganisms an opportunity to grow, allowing for overgrowth of pathogenic microbes or non-affected host flora. Superinfection should be suspected when a new infection appears while the client is receiving anti-infective therapy. Signs and symptoms of a superinfection may include diarrhea, bladder pain, painful urination, or abnormal vaginal discharge. Broad-spectrum antibiotics are more likely to cause superinfections because they kill so many different species of microorganism.

32.7 Host Factors

The most important factor in selecting an appropriate antibiotic is to be certain that the microbe is sensitive to the effects of the drug. However, the nurse must also take into account certain host factors that can influence the success of antibacterial therapy.

The primary goal of antibiotic therapy is to kill enough bacteria or to slow the growth of the infection such that natural body defences can overcome the invading agent. Unless an infection is highly localized, the antibiotic alone may not be enough: The client's immune system and phagocytic cells will be needed to completely rid the body of the infectious agent. Clients with suppressed immune systems may require aggressive antibiotic therapy with bactericidal agents. These clients include those with AIDS and those being treated with immunosuppressive or anti-neoplastic drugs. Since therapy is more successful when the number of microbes is small, antibiotics may be given on a prophylactic basis to clients whose white blood cell count is extremely low.

Local conditions at the infection site should be considered when selecting an antibiotic because factors that hinder the drug from reaching microbes will limit therapeutic success. Infections of the CNS are particularly difficult to treat because many drugs cannot cross the blood-brain barrier. Injury or inflammation can cause tissues to become acidic or anaerobic and have poor circulation. Excessive pus formation or hematomas can block drugs from reaching their targets. Although most bacteria are extracellular in nature, pathogens such as *Mycobacterium tuberculosis, Salmonella, Toxoplasma,* and *Listeria* may reside intracellularly and thus be resistant to antibacterial action. Consideration of these factors may necessitate a change in the route of drug administration or the selection of a more effective antibiotic specific for the local conditions.

Allergic reactions to antibiotics, while not common, may be fatal. The nurse's assessment must include a thorough drug history; a previous acute allergic incident is highly predictive of future reactions. If severe allergy to a medication is established, it is best to avoid all drugs in the same chemical class. Because the client may have been exposed to an antibiotic unknowingly, through food products or moulds, allergic reactions can occur without previous incident. Penicillins are the class of antibacterials having the highest incidence of allergic reactions; between 0.7% and 4% of all clients who receive the drugs exhibit hypersensitivity.

Other host factors to be considered are age, pregnancy status, and genetics. The very young and very old are often unable to readily metabolize or excrete antibiotics; thus, doses are generally lowered. Some antibiotics cross the placenta. For example, tetracyclines taken by the mother can cause teeth discoloration in the newborn, and aminoglycosides can affect the infant's hearing. The benefits of antibiotic use in pregnant or lactating women must be carefully weighed against the potential risks to the fetus and neonate. Lastly, some clients have a genetic absence of certain enzymes used to metabolize antibiotics. For example, clients with a deficiency of the enzyme glucose-6-phosphate dehydrogenase (G6PD) should not receive sulfonamides, chloramphenicol, or nalidixic acid because their erythrocytes may rupture.

ANTIBACTERIAL AGENTS

Antibacterial agents form a large number of chemical classes. Although drugs within a class have similarities in their mechanisms and spectrum of activity, each is slightly different and learning the differences and therapeutic applications among antibacterial agents can be challenging. Basic nursing assessments and interventions apply to all antibiotic therapies; however, the plan of care should be individualized based on the client's condition, the infection, and the antibacterial agent prescribed.

PENICILLINS

Although not the first anti-infective discovered, penicillin was the first mass-produced antibiotic. Isolated from the fungus *Penicillium* in 1941, the drug quickly became a miracle product by preventing thousands of deaths from infections. Penicillins are indicated for the treatment of pneumonia; meningitis; skin, bone, and joint infections; stomach infections; blood and heart valve infections; gas gangrene; tetanus; anthrax; and sickle cell anemia in infants. The penicillins are shown in Table 32.3.

CULTURAL CONSIDERATIONS

Cultural Beliefs and Antibacterials

People hold beliefs that affect readiness to adopt prescription drugs and therapies. For example, some Aboriginal Canadians may choose to access a sweat lodge to restore health. Many Aboriginals believe that sweating helps to open clogged pores, stimulate the natural flow of sweat, and rid the body of wastes.

Many ethnic groups, including some Chinese, Africans, and Hispanics, believe that illness is caused by an imbalance in hot and cold. In a healthy individual, hot and cold are in balance; when an imbalance occurs, disease results. Illnesses are classified as either hot or cold. For example, sore throat and diarrhea are considered hot diseases; colds, upper respiratory infections, arthritis, and rheumatism are considered cold diseases. Treatment in such cultures is to restore the body's balance through the addition or subtraction of herbs, foods, or medications that are classified as either hot or cold. To treat a hot disease, medications or herbs considered cold are used. For example, penicillin is considered a hot medicine, but amoxicillin is less hot. Using acetaminophen with amoxicillin makes it cooler.

TABLE 32.3 Penicillins

Drug	Route and Adult Dose
Narrow Spectrum/Pencillinase Sensitive	
penicillin G benzathine (Megacillin)	IM; 1.2 million units as a single dose
penicillin G procaine (Ayercillin, Wycillin)	IM; 600,000–1.2 million units qd
penicillin V (Apo-Pen, Pen-Vee)	PO; 125–500 mg qid
Narrow Spectrum/Penicillinase Resistant	
cloxacillin (Orbenin)	PO; 250–500 mg q6h
dicloxacillin (Dynapen)	PO; 125–500 mg qid
Broad Spectrum (Aminopenicillins)	
amoxicillin (Apo-Amoxi, Novomoxin)	PO; 250–500 mg tid
amoxicillin-clavulanate (Clavulin)	PO; 250 or 500 mg tablet (each with 125 mg clavulanic acid) q8–12h
ampicillin (Ampicin, Nu-Ampi)	PO; 250–500 mg bid
Extended Spectrum	
carbenicillin (Pyopen)	PO; 382–764 mg qid
piperacillin sodium (Piperacillin)	IM; 2–4 g tid–qid (max 24 g/day)
piperacillin tazobactam (Tazocin)	IV; 3.375 g qid over 30 min
ticarcillin (Ticar)	IM; 1–2 g qid (max 40 g/day)

32.8 Pharmacotherapy with Penicillins

Penicillins kill bacteria by disrupting their cell walls. Many bacterial cell walls contain a substance called **penicillin-binding protein** that serves as a receptor for penicillin. Penicillin weakens the cell wall and allows water to enter, thus killing the organism. Human cells do not contain cell walls; thus, the actions of the penicillins are specific to bacterial cells.

The portion of the chemical structure of penicillin that is responsible for its antibacterial activity is the **beta-lactam ring**. Some bacteria secrete an enzyme, called **beta-lactamase**, or **penicillinase**, which splits the beta-lactam ring. This structural change causes these bacteria to become resistant to the effects of most penicillins. Since their discovery, large numbers of resistant bacterial strains have appeared that now limit the therapeutic usefulness of the penicillins. The action of penicillinase is illustrated in Figure 32.3.

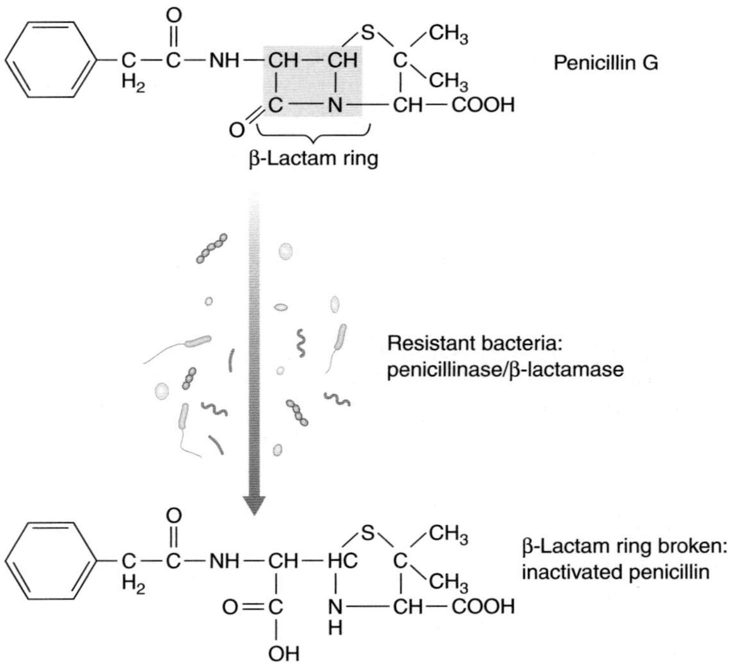

Chemical modifications to the original penicillin molecule produced drugs offering several advantages. Oxacillin and cloxacillin are effective against penicillinase-producing bacteria and are called penicillinase-resistant penicillins. The aminopenicillins such as ampicillin and amoxicillin are effective against a wider range of microorganisms and are called broad-spectrum penicillins. The extended-spectrum penicillins, such as carbenicillin and piperacillin, are effective against even more microbes, including *Pseudomonas, Enterobacter, Klebsiella*, and *Bacteroides fragilis*.

In general, the adverse effects of penicillins are minor; they are one of the safest classes of antibiotic. This has contributed to their widespread use for over 50 years. Allergy to penicillin is the most common adverse effect. Common symptoms of penicillin allergy include rash and fever. Incidence of anaphylaxis ranges from 0.04% to 2%. Allergy to one penicillin increases the risk of allergy to other drugs in the same class.

● Figure 32.3   Action of penicillinase

NURSING CONSIDERATIONS

The role of the nurse in drug therapy with penicillins involves careful monitoring of the client's condition and providing education as it relates to the prescribed drug regimen. Since allergies occur more frequently with penicillins than with any other antibiotic class, it is essential to assess previous drug reactions to penicillin prior to administration. If the client has a history of severe penicillin allergic reaction, cephalosporins should be avoided due to risk of cross-sensitization. Specimens for culture and sensitivity should be obtained prior to the start of antibiotic therapy.

Vital signs, electrolytes, and renal function tests should be obtained prior to and during therapy. Because some penicillin preparations contain high levels of sodium and potassium salts, monitor the client for hyperkalemia and hypernatremia prior to and during therapy. Cardiac status should be monitored, including ECG changes, due to the possibility of worsening an existing heart failure related to the increased sodium intake. Additionally, the client should be monitored for indications of response to therapy, including reduced fever, normal white blood cell count, absence of symptoms such as cough, and improved appetite.

After parenteral administration of penicillins, the client should be observed for 30 minutes for possible allergic reactions, especially with the first dose. Sensitivity may be immediate, accelerated, or delayed.

Clients with impaired renal function may require smaller doses because the majority of penicillin is excreted through the kidneys. Penicillins should be used with caution during lactation because the drug enters breast milk. Monitor for bleeding in those clients on anticoagulant therapy who are receiving high doses of parenteral carbenicillin, piperacillin, or ticarcillin because these drugs may interfere with platelet aggregation.

A small number of clients may develop a serious superinfection called antibiotic-associated pseudomembranous colitis (AAPMC). In this condition, the organism *Clostridium difficile* secretes a toxin that causes severe inflammation of the bowel wall, followed by necrosis. This results in a potentially life-threatening infection. Clients with this condition have two to five semisolid or liquid stools per day. Antidiarrheal drugs should not be administered because these agents cause the toxin to be retained in the bowel. When AAPMC occurs, antibiotic therapy should be discontinued, and fluid/electrolyte replacement is essential.

As with other antibiotics, penicillins may cause other, less severe superinfections with symptoms such as abdominal cramping and diarrhea. Replacement of natural colon flora with probiotic supplements or cultured dairy products such as yogurt or buttermilk may help to alleviate symptoms. Superinfections in elderly, debilitated, or immunosuppressed clients may be serious and require immediate interventions.

Client education as it relates to penicillins should include goals, reasons for obtaining baseline data, and possible side effects. Following are important points to include when teaching clients regarding penicillins:

- Wear a MedicAlert bracelet if allergic to penicillins.
- Take penicillin V, amoxicillin, and amoxicillin-clavulanate with meals to decrease GI distress. Take all other penicillins with a full glass of water, 1 hour before or 2 hours after meals to increase absorption.
- Oral penicillin G should be taken with water because acidic fruit juice can inactivate the drug's antibacterial activity.
- Do not discontinue the drug regimen before the complete prescription has been taken.
- Avoid use of penicillins while breastfeeding.

Pr PROTOTYPE DRUG | Penicillin G Potassium

ACTIONS AND USES

Similar to penicillin V, penicillin G is a drug of choice against streptococci, pneumococci, and staphylococci organisms that do not produce penicillinase. It is also a medication of choice for gonorrhea and syphilis caused by susceptible strains. Penicillin V is more acid stable; over 70% is absorbed after an oral dose compared to the 15% to 30% from penicillin G. Because of its low oral absorption, penicillin G is often given by the IV or IM routes. Penicillinase-producing organisms inactivate both penicillin G and penicillin V.

PHARMACOKINETICS

Penicillin G is administered IM or IV. About 60% is protein bound. It is widely distributed, crosses the placenta, and enters breast milk. It is excreted mostly unchanged in urine. Half-life is 0.5 hours.

ADMINISTRATION ALERTS

- After parenteral administration, observe for possible allergic reactions for 30 minutes, especially following the first dose.
- Do not mix penicillin and aminoglycosides in the same intravenous solution. Give IV medications 1 hour apart to prevent interactions.
- Penicillin G is pregnancy category B.

ADVERSE EFFECTS AND INTERACTIONS

Penicillin G has few side effects. Anaphylaxis is the most serious adverse effect. Diarrhea, nausea, and vomiting are the most common adverse effects and can cause serious complications in certain populations such as children and older adults. Pain at the injection site may occur, and superinfections are possible. Since penicillin G is excreted extensively by the kidneys, renal disease can result in excessive accumulation of the drug.

Penicillin G may decrease the efficacy of oral contraceptives. Colestipol taken with this medication will decrease the absorption of penicillin. Potassium-sparing diuretics may cause hyperkalemia when administered with penicillin G potassium.

 See the Companion Website for a Nursing Process Focus Chart specific to this drug.

TABLE 32.4	Cephalosporins
Drug	**Route and Adult Dose**
First Generation	
cefadroxil (Duricef)	PO; 500 mg–1 g qd–bid (max 2 g/day)
cefazolin (Ancef, Kefzol)	IV/IM; 250 mg–2 g tid (max 12 g/day)
cephalexin (Apo-, Nu-Cephalex, Keflex)	PO; 250–500 mg qid
cephradine (Velosef)	PO; 250–500 mg q6h or 500 mg–1 g q12h (max 4 g/day)
Second Generation	
cefaclor (Ceclor)	PO; 250–500 mg tid
cefotetan (Cefotan)	IV/IM; 1–2 g q12h
cefoxitin (Cefoxitin, Mefoxin)	IV/IM; 1–2 g q6–8h, (max 12 g/day)
cefprozil (Apo-Cefprozil)	PO; 250–500 mg qd–bid
cefuroxime (Ceftin, Kefurox, Zinacef)	PO; 250–500 mg bid
Third Generation	
cefdinir (Omnicef)	PO; 300 mg bid
cefixime (Suprax)	PO; 400 mg qd or 200 mg bid
cefotaxime (Claforan)	IV/IM; 1–2 g bid–tid (max 12 g/day)
ceftazidime (Ceftazdime)	IV/IM; 1–2 mg q8–12h, up to 2 g q6h
ceftriaxone (Ceftriaxone)	IV/IM; 1–2 g q12–24h (max 4 g/d)
Fourth Generation	
cefepime (Maxipime)	IV/IM; 0.5–1.0 g q12h for 7–10 d

- Consult with the nurse about taking probiotic supplements and/or cultured dairy products during antibiotic therapy.
- Report significant side effects immediately, including severe abdominal or stomach cramps, abdominal tenderness, convulsions, decreased urine output, and severe watery or bloody diarrhea.

See "Nursing Process Focus: Clients Receiving Antibacterial Therapy" (p. 439) for the Nursing Process applied to all antibacterials.

CEPHALOSPORINS

Isolated shortly after the penicillins, the four generations of cephalosporins comprise the largest antibiotic class. Like the penicillins, the cephalosporins contain a beta-lactam ring that is mostly responsible for their antimicrobial activity. The cephalosporins are bactericidal and act by attaching to penicillin-binding protein to inhibit cell wall synthesis. The cephalosporins are shown in Table 32.4.

32.9 Pharmacotherapy with Cephalosporins

Over 20 cephalosporins are available and classified by their "generation." First generation cephalosporins contain a beta-lactam ring; bacteria producing beta-lactamase will usually be resistant to these agents. The second generation cephalosporins are more potent, more resistant to beta-lactamase, and exhibit a broader spectrum than the first generation drugs. The third generation cephalosporins generally have a longer duration of action, an even broader spectrum, and are resistant to beta-lactamase. Third generation cephalosporins are sometimes the drugs of choice against infections by *Pseudomonas, Klebsiella, Neisseria, Salmonella, Proteus,* and *Haemophilus influenzae.* Newer, fourth generation drugs are more effective against organisms that have developed resistance to earlier cephalosporins. Third and fourth generation agents are capable of entering the cerebrospinal fluid to treat CNS infections. There are not always clear distinctions among the generations.

The primary therapeutic use of the cephalosporins is for gram-negative infections and for clients who cannot tolerate the less expensive penicillins. Side effects are similar to those of the penicillins, with allergic reactions being the most common adverse effect. The nurse must be alert to the fact that 5% to 10% of the clients who are allergic to penicillin will also be allergic to the cephalosporins. Despite this incidence of cross-sensitivity, the cephalosporins offer a reasonable alternative for clients who are unable to take penicillin. It is common for clients with a mild allergy to penicillin to be given a cephalosporin. Earlier generation cephalosporins exhibited kidney toxicity, but this is diminished with the newer drugs.

NURSING CONSIDERATIONS

The role of the nurse in cephalosporin therapy involves careful monitoring of the client's condition and providing education as it relates to the prescribed drug regimen. The cephalosporins are generally the treatment of choice for clients with gram-negative infections. Assess the

MediaLink

Mechanism of Action: Penicillin

client for the presence/history of bleeding disorders because cephalosporins may reduce prothrombin levels through interference with vitamin K metabolism. Liver function should be assessed because liver function is important in vitamin K production. Renal function should be assessed because most cephalosporins are excreted by the kidney. Culture and sensitivity testing should be performed before and during therapy.

Due to elimination of cephalosporins through the kidneys, it is necessary to monitor intake and output, blood urea nitrogen (BUN), and serum creatinine. If the client is concurrently taking NSAIDs, monitor blood coagulation studies because cephalosporins increase the effect of platelet inhibition.

Cephalosporins should be used with caution in pregnant or lactating clients as they can be transferred to the fetus and infant. Doses should be adjusted appropriately in clients with impaired renal or hepatic function. Certain cephalosporins will cause a disulfiram (Antabuse)–like reaction when alcoholic beverages are consumed. Typical reactions include severe vomiting, weakness, blurred vision, and profound hypotension.

Cephalosporins may predispose clients to pseudomembranous colitis, especially if gastrointestinal pathology pre-exists. Less severe superinfections may also occur. Eating cultured dairy products such as yogurt or kefir may suppress superinfections.

Client education as it relates to cephalosporins should include goals, reasons for obtaining baseline data, and possible side effects. Following are important points to include when teaching clients regarding cephalosporins:

- Avoid alcohol use while taking cephalosporins.
- Eat cultured dairy products to help discourage superinfections.

- Report significant side effects, including diarrhea, onset of flu-like symptoms, blistering or peeling of skin, seizures, decreased urine output, hearing loss, skin rash, breathing difficulty, and unusual tiredness or weakness.

See "Nursing Process Focus: Clients Receiving Antibacterial Therapy" for the Nursing Process applied to all antibacterials.

TETRACYCLINES

The first tetracyclines were extracted from *Streptomyces* soil microorganisms in 1948. Tetracyclines exert a bacteriostatic effect by selectively inhibiting bacterial protein synthesis. The six tetracyclines are effective against a large number of different gram-negative and gram-positive organisms and have one of the broadest spectrums of any class of antibiotic. The tetracyclines are shown in Table 32.5.

32.10 Pharmacotherapy with Tetracyclines

The widespread use of tetracyclines in the 1950s and 1960s resulted in a large number of resistant bacterial strains that now limit their therapeutic utility. They are drugs of choice for only a few diseases: Rocky Mountain spotted fever, typhus, cholera, Lyme disease, ulcers caused by *Helicobacter pylori*, and chlamydial infections. They are occasionally used for the treatment of acne vulgaris. Because of their ability to bind metal ions such as calcium and iron, tetracyclines should not be taken with milk or iron supplements because the drug's absorption may be decreased by as much as 50%. They may also cause yellow-brown teeth discoloration in young children. Some clients experience photosensitivity during therapy, making their skin particularly susceptible to sunburn. Because of their broad spectrum, the risk for superinfection is relatively high.

Pr PROTOTYPE DRUG | Cefotaxime (Claforan)

ACTIONS AND USES

Cefotaxime is a third generation cephalosporin with a broad spectrum of activity against gram-negative organisms. It is effective against many bacteria that have developed resistance to earlier generation cephalosporins and to other classes of anti-infectives. Cefotaxime exhibits bactericidal activity by inhibiting cell wall synthesis. It is prescribed for serious infections of the lower respiratory tract, CNS, genitourinary system, bones, and joints. It may also be used for blood infections such as bacteremia or septicemia. Like many other cephalosporins, cefotaxime is not absorbed from the GI tract and must be given by the IM or IV route.

PHARMACOKINETICS

Cefotaxime is well absorbed after IM administration. It is widely distributed, crosses the placenta, enters breast milk, and enters CSF. It is partly metabolized by the liver. About 50% is excreted unchanged in urine. Half-life is about 1 hour.

ADMINISTRATION ALERTS

- IM injections should be administered deep into a large muscle mass to prevent injury to surrounding tissues.
- Cefotaxime is pregnancy category B.

ADVERSE EFFECTS AND INTERACTIONS

For most clients, cefotaxime and the other cephalosporins are safe medications. Hypersensitivity is the most common adverse effect, although symptoms may include only a minor rash and itching. Anaphylaxis is possible, so the nurse should be alert for this reaction. GI-related side effects such as diarrhea, vomiting, and nausea may occur. Some clients experience considerable pain at the injection site.

Cefotaxime interacts with probenecid, causing decreased renal elimination of the drug. Alcohol interacts with cefotaxime to produce a disulfiram-like reaction. Cefotaxime interacts with NSAIDs to cause an increase in platelet inhibition.

 See the Companion Website for a Nursing Process Focus Chart specific to this drug.

TABLE 32.5   Tetracyclines

Drug	Route and Adult Dose
demeclocycline (Declomycin)	PO; 150 mg q6h or 300 mg q12h (max 2.4 g/day)
doxycycline (Apo-Doxycycline, Vibramycin)	PO/IV; 100 mg bid on day 1, then 100 mg qd (max 200 mg/day)
minocycline (Apo-, PMS-Minocycline, Minocin)	PO; 200 mg as one dose followed by 100 mg bid
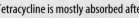 tetracycline (Apo-, Novo-, Nu-Tetra)	PO; 250–500 mg bid–qid (max 2 g/day)

NURSING CONSIDERATIONS

The role of the nurse in tetracycline therapy involves careful monitoring of the client's condition and providing education as it relates to the prescribed drug regimen. Assess the client for presence/history of acne vulgaris, actinomycosis, anthrax, malaria, syphilis, urinary tract infection, rickettsial infection, and Lyme disease. This class of antibiotic can treat all of these disorders. Prior to administration, assess for a history of hypersensitivity to tetracyclines. If possible, culture and sensitivity results should be obtained before therapy is initiated. Lab tests including CBC and kidney and liver function studies should be done. Monitor the client's body temperature, white blood cell count, and culture/sensitivity results to determine the effectiveness of the treatment as well as to observe for superinfections.

Tetracyclines are contraindicated in pregnancy and lactation due to the drug's effect on linear skeletal growth of the fetus and child. They are also contraindicated in children less than 8 years of age due to the drug's ability to cause permanent mottling and discoloration of the teeth. Tetracycline decreases the effectiveness of oral contraceptives, so female clients should use an alternate method of birth control while taking the medication. Tetracyclines should be used with caution in clients with impaired kidney or liver function.

Oral and perineal hygiene care is extremely important to decrease the risk of superinfections due to *Candida*. Tetracyclines cause photosensitivity, which may lead to tingling and burning of the skin, similar to sunburn. Photosensitivity reaction may appear within a few minutes to hours after sun exposure and may persist for several days after pharmacotherapy is completed.

Client education as it relates to tetracyclines should include goals, reasons for obtaining baseline data such as tests for culture and sensitivity, and possible side effects. Following are important points to include when teaching clients regarding tetracyclines:

- Do not save medication because toxic effects may occur if it is taken past the expiration date.
- Do not take these medications with milk products, iron supplements, magnesium-containing laxatives, or antacids.

Pr PROTOTYPE DRUG | Tetracycline (Apo-Tetra, others)

ACTIONS AND USES

Tetracycline is effective against a broad range of gram-positive and gram-negative organisms, including chlamydiae, rickettsiae, and mycoplasma. Tetracycline is given orally, though it has a short half-life that may require administration four times per day. Topical and oral preparations are available for treating acne. An IM preparation is available; injections may cause local irritation and be extremely painful.

PHARMACOKINETICS

Tetracycline is mostly absorbed after PO administration. It is widely distributed, crosses the placenta, enters breast milk, and enters CSF. It is excreted unchanged in urine. Half-life is 6 to 12 hours.

ADMINISTRATION ALERTS

- Administer oral drug with full glass of water to decrease esophageal and GI irritation.
- Administer antacids and tetracycline 1 to 3 hours apart.
- Administer antilipidemic agents at least 2 hours before or after tetracycline.
- Tetracycline is pregnancy category D.

ADVERSE EFFECTS AND INTERACTIONS

Being a broad-spectrum antibiotic, tetracycline has a tendency to affect vaginal, oral, and intestinal flora and cause superinfections. Tetracycline irritates the GI mucosa and may cause nausea, vomiting, epigastric burning, and diarrhea. Diarrhea may be severe enough to cause discontinuation of therapy. Other common side effects include discoloration of the teeth and photosensitivity.

Oral tetracycline interacts with milk products, iron supplements, magnesium-containing laxatives, and antacids. These products reduce the absorption and serum levels of tetracyclines. Tetracycline binds with certain lipid-lowering drugs (colestipol and cholestyramine), thereby decreasing the antibiotic's absorption. This drug decreases the effectiveness of oral contraceptives.

 See the Companion Website for a Nursing Process Focus Chart specific to this drug.

- Wait 1 to 3 hours after taking tetracyclines before taking antacids.
- Take tetracyclines at least 2 hours before or after taking lipid-lowering drugs such as colestipol and cholestyramine.
- Report significant side effects immediately, including increased photosensitivity of skin to sunlight, abdominal pain, loss of appetite, nausea and vomiting, visual changes, and yellowing of skin.

See "Nursing Process Focus: Clients Receiving Antibacterial Therapy" (p. 439) for the Nursing Process applied to all antibacterials.

MACROLIDES

Erythromycin, the first macrolide antibiotic, was isolated from *Streptomyces* in a soil sample in 1952. The macrolide antibiotics inhibit bacterial protein synthesis and may be either bactericidal or bacteriostatic depending on the dose and the target organism.

32.11 Pharmacotherapy with Macrolides

Macrolides are considered safe alternatives to penicillin, although they are drugs of first choice for relatively few diseases. Common uses of macrolides include the treatment of whooping cough, Legionnaire's disease, and infections by *Streptococcus, H. influenzae, Mycoplasma pneumoniae,* and *Chlamydia.* The macrolides are shown in Table 32.6.

The newer macrolides were synthesized from erythromycin. Although their spectrums are similar, the newer agents have a longer half-life and cause less gastric irritation than erythromycin. For example, azithromycin has such an extended half-life that it is administered for only 4 days, rather than the 10 days required for most antibiotics. The shorter duration of therapy is thought to increase client adherence.

NURSING CONSIDERATIONS

The role of the nurse in macrolide therapy involves careful monitoring of the client's condition and providing education as it relates to the prescribed drug regimen. Assess for the presence of respiratory infection, GI tract infection, skin and soft tissue infections, otitis media, gonorrhea, nongonococcal urethritis, and *H. pylori* treatment. Macrolides are indicated for the pharmacological treatment of these disorders. The client should be examined for history of cardiac disorders as macrolides may exacerbate existing heart disease. Due to toxic effects on the liver, hepatic enzymes should be monitored with certain macrolides such as erythromycin estolate.

The client should be assessed for a history of hypersensitivity to macrolides. Rashes or other signs of hypersensitivity should be reported immediately. Culture and sensitivity testing should be performed before initiation of macrolide therapy.

Macrolides are contraindicated in clients with hepatic disease since the liver metabolizes these drugs. These agents should be used with caution in pregnant or breastfeeding women to avoid harm to the fetus or newborn.

Multiple drug-drug interactions occur with macrolides. Certain anesthetic agents (alfentanil) and anticonvulsant drugs (carbamazepine) may interact with macrolides to cause serum drug levels to rise and result in toxicity. Macrolides should be used cautiously with clients receiving cyclosporine, and drug levels must be monitored due to the risk for nephrotoxicity. Clients receiving warfarin need to be monitored closely because macrolides may decrease warfarin metabolism and excretion. Coagulation studies, such as INR, need to be monitored more frequently as dosage adjustments may be required. Clarithromycin and zidovudine must be administered at least 4 hours apart to avoid interaction, which results in a delayed time for peak concentration of zidovudine.

Client education as it relates to macrolides should include goals, reasons for obtaining baseline data such as culture and sensitivity tests, and possible side effects. Following are important points to include when teaching clients regarding macrolides:

- Do not discontinue the medication before the complete prescription has been taken.
- Do not take with or immediately before or after fruit juices.
- Notify the healthcare provider before taking other prescription or OTC medications or herbal products because macrolides interact with many substances.
- Report significant side effects immediately, including severe skin rash, itching, or hives; difficulty breathing or swallowing; yellowing of skin or eyes; dark urine; and pale stools.

See "Nursing Process Focus: Clients Receiving Antibacterial Therapy" for the Nursing Process applied to all antibacterials.

AMINOGLYCOSIDES

The first aminoglycoside, streptomycin, was named after *Streptomyces griseus,* the soil organism from which it was

TABLE 32.6 Macrolides	
Drug	**Route and Adult Dose**
azithromycin (Apo-, Gen-Azithromycin)	PO; 500 mg for one dose, then 250 mg q.d IV; 500 mg qd for one or two doses, then 250 mg qd
clarithromycin (Biaxin)	PO; 250–500 mg bid
erythromycin (Apo-Erythro, Erybid, Erythromid)	PO; 250–500 mg bid or 333 mg tid. IV; 250–500 mg (up to 1 g) q6h

Pr PROTOTYPE DRUG | Erythromycin (Apo-Erythro, others)

ACTIONS AND USES

Erythromycin is inactivated by stomach acid and is thus administered as coated tablets or capsules that are intended to dissolve in the small intestine. Its main application is for clients who are unable to tolerate penicillins or who may have a penicillin-resistant infection. It has a spectrum similar to that of the penicillins and is effective against most gram-positive bacteria. It is often a preferred drug for infections caused by *Bordetella pertussis* (whooping cough) and *Corynebacterium diphtheriae*.

PHARMACOKINETICS

Absorption of erythromycin is variable. It is widely distributed, crosses the placenta, and enters breast milk. It is partly metabolized by the liver and is mostly excreted in bile with a small amount excreted unchanged in urine. Half-life is 1 to 2 hours.

ADMINISTRATION ALERTS

- Administer oral drug on an empty stomach with a full glass of water.
- For suspensions, shake the bottle thoroughly to ensure the drug is well mixed.
- Do not give with or immediately before or after fruit juices.
- Erythromycin is pregnancy category B.

ADVERSE EFFECTS AND INTERACTIONS

The most common side effects of erythromycin are nausea, abdominal cramping, and vomiting, although these are rarely serious enough to cause discontinuation of therapy. Concurrent administration with food may be necessary to reduce these side effects. The most severe adverse effect is hepatotoxicity caused by the estolate form of the drug.

Anesthetic agents and anticonvulsant drugs may interact with erythromycin to cause serum drug levels to rise and result in toxicity. This drug interacts with cyclosporine, increasing the risk for nephrotoxicity. It may increase the effects of warfarin. Erythromycin may interact with medications containing xanthine to cause an increase in theophylline levels.

See the Companion Website for a Nursing Process Focus Chart specific to this drug.

TABLE 32.7	Aminoglycosides
Drug	**Route and Adult Dose**
gentamicin (Garamycin)	IM, IV; 1.5–2.0 mg/kg as a loading dose, then 1–2 mg/kg bid–tid
neomycin (Cicatrin)	IM; 1.3–2.6 mg/kg qid
streptomycin	IM; 15 mg/kg up to 1 g as a single dose
tobramycin (Apo-Tobramycin)	IM, IV; 1–2 mg/kg tid (max 5 mg/kg/day)

isolated in 1942. Once widely used, streptomycin is now usually restricted to the treatment of tuberculosis due to the development of a large number of resistant strains. Although more toxic than other antibiotic classes, aminoglycosides have important therapeutic applications for the treatment of aerobic gram-negative bacteria, mycobacteria, and some protozoans. The aminoglycosides are shown in Table 32.7.

32.12 Pharmacotherapy with Aminoglycosides

Aminoglycosides are bactericidal and act by inhibiting bacterial protein synthesis and by causing the synthesis of abnormal proteins. They are normally reserved for serious systemic infections caused by aerobic gram-negative organisms, including *E. coli*, *Serratia*, *Proteus*, *Klebsiella*, and *Pseudomonas*. When used for systemic bacterial infections, aminoglycosides are given parenterally as they are poorly absorbed from the GI tract. They are occasionally given orally to sterilize the bowel prior to intestinal surgery. Neomycin is available for topical infections of the skin, eyes, and ears. The differences in spelling of some drugs, from

-mycin to -micin, reflects the different organisms from which the drugs were originally isolated.

NURSING CONSIDERATIONS

The role of the nurse in aminoglycoside therapy involves careful monitoring of the client's condition and providing education as it relates to the prescribed drug regimen. Assess the client for a history of previous allergic reaction to aminoglycosides. These anti-infectives are most noted for their toxic effects on the kidneys and vestibular apparatus; therefore, the client should be monitored for ototoxicity and nephrotoxicity during the course of therapy. Baseline audiometry, renal function, and vestibular function need to be assessed prior to the initial administration of aminoglycosides and throughout therapy. Hearing loss may occur after therapy has been completed. Baseline urinalysis is necessary prior to initiation and throughout therapy as renal impairment may increase the risk of toxicity. With streptomycin therapy, caloric tests are assessed for baseline data and to monitor for vestibular toxicity.

Neuromuscular function may also be impaired in clients receiving aminoglycosides. Clients with neuromuscular diseases, such as myasthenia gravis and Parkinson's disease, may experience greater muscle weakness due to neuromuscular blockade caused by aminoglycosides. These antibiotics also should be used with caution in clients receiving anesthetics due to an interaction causing possible neuromuscular blockade.

These drugs should be used with caution in neonates, infants, and older adults. Infants may experience neuromuscular blockade from aminoglycosides due to their immature neurological system. Elderly clients are at a higher risk of nephrotoxicity and ototoxicity because of reduced renal function and may require lower doses. Clients should be instructed to increase fluid intake, unless otherwise contraindicated, to promote excretion of the medications. Superinfection is a side effect of aminoglycoside therapy, and the client should be monitored for diarrhea, vaginal discharge, stomatitis, and glossitis.

Client education as it relates to aminoglycosides should include goals, reasons for obtaining baseline data such as vestibular function tests, and possible side effects. Following are important points to include when teaching clients regarding aminoglycosides:

- Increase fluid intake.
- Report significant side effects immediately, including tinnitus, high-frequency hearing loss, persistent headache, nausea, and vertigo.

See "Nursing Process Focus: Clients Receiving Antibacterial therapy" for the Nursing Process applied to all antibacterials.

FLUOROQUINOLONES

In the past decade, the fluoroquinolones have become an increasingly important class of antibiotic. The first drug in this class, nalidixic acid, was approved in 1962. Classified as a quinolone, the use of nalidixic acid was restricted to urinary tract infections (UTIs) due to its narrow spectrum of activity and a high incidence of bacterial resistance. The development of fluorinated quinolones with a wider spectrum of activity began in the late 1980s and continues today. Four generations of fluoroquinolones are now available, classified by their microbiological activity. All fluoroquinolones have activity against gram-negative pathogens; the later generation agents are significantly more effective against gram-positive agents. The fluoroquinolones are shown in Table 32.8.

32.13 Pharmacotherapy with Fluoroquinolones

The fluoroquinolones are bactericidal and affect DNA synthesis by inhibiting two bacterial enzymes: DNA gyrase and topoisomerase IV. Agents in this class are infrequently first-line drugs, although they are extensively used as alternatives to other antibiotics. Clinical applications include infections of the respiratory, gastrointestinal, and gynecological tracts and some skin and soft tissue infections. The most widely used drug in this class, ciprofloxacin, is an agent of choice for post-exposure prophylaxis of *Bacillus anthracis*. Two newer agents, moxifloxacin and trovafloxacin, are highly effective against anaerobes. Recent studies suggest that some fluoroquinolones may be effective against *M. tuberculosis*.

A major advantage of the fluoroquinolones is that they are well absorbed orally and may be administered either

---

Pr PROTOTYPE DRUG | Gentamicin (Garamycin)

ACTIONS AND USES

Gentamicin is a broad-spectrum, bactericidal antibiotic usually prescribed for serious urinary, respiratory, neurological, or GI infections when less toxic antibiotics are contraindicated. It is often used in combination with other antibiotics or when drugs from other classes have proven ineffective. It is used parenterally, or as drops, for eye infections.

ADMINISTRATION ALERTS

- For IM administration, give deep into a large muscle.
- Use only IM and IV drug solutions that are clear and colourless or slightly yellow. Discard discoloured solutions or those that contain particulate matter.
- Gentamicin is pregnancy category C.

PHARMACOKINETICS

Gentamicin is well absorbed after IM administration. It is widely distributed, crosses the placenta, and enters breast milk. It is mostly excreted in urine. Half-life is 2 to 4 hours.

ADVERSE EFFECTS AND INTERACTIONS

As with other aminoglycosides, adverse effects from gentamicin may be severe. Ototoxicity can produce a loss of hearing or balance, which may become permanent with continued use. Frequent hearing tests should be conducted so that gentamicin may be discontinued if early signs of ototoxicity are detected.

Gentamicin is excreted unchanged, primarily by the kidneys. The nurse must be alert for signs of reduced kidney function, including proteinuria and elevated BUN and creatinine levels. Nephrotoxicity is of particular concern for clients with pre-existing kidney disease and may limit therapy. Resistance to gentamicin is increasing and some cross-resistance among aminoglycosides has been reported.

The risk of ototoxicity increases if the client is currently taking amphotericin B, furosemide, ASA, Bumex, Edecrin, cisplatin, or Humatin.

Concurrent use with amphotericin B, capreomycin, cisplatin, polymyxin B, and vancomycin increases the risk of nephrotoxicity.

 See the Companion Website for a Nursing Process Focus Chart specific to this drug.

TABLE 32.8   Fluoroquinolones

Drug	Route and Adult Dose
First Generation	
cinoxacin (Cinobac)	PO; 250–500 mg bid–qid. PO; chronic therapy: 500 mg qid
Second Generation	
ciprofloxacin (Cipro)	PO; 250–750 mg bid. IV; 400 mg q12h
norfloxacin (Apo-, Novo-Norfloxacin)	PO; 400 mg bid
ofloxacin (Novo-Ofloxacin)	PO/IV; 200–400 mg bid
Third Generation	
levofloxacin (Novo-Levofloxacin)	PO; 250–500 mg/day qd
Fourth Generation	
gemifloxacin (Factive)	PO; 320 mg qd
moxifloxacin (Avelox)	PO/IV; 400 mg qd

once or twice a day. They have a favourable safety profile with nausea, vomiting, and diarrhea being the most common side effects. Although they may be taken with food, they should not be taken concurrently with multivitamins or mineral supplements since calcium, magnesium, iron, and zinc ions can reduce absorption of the antibiotic by as much as 90%.

The most serious adverse effects are dysrhythmias (gatifloxacin and moxifloxacin) and liver failure (trovafloxacin). Central nervous system effects such as dizziness, headache, and sleep disturbances affect 1% to 8% of clients. Because animal studies have suggested that fluoroquinolones affect cartilage development, use in children must be monitored carefully. Use in pregnant or lactating clients should be avoided.

NURSING CONSIDERATIONS

The role of the nurse in fluoroquinolone therapy involves careful monitoring of the client's condition and providing education as it relates to the prescribed drug regimen. Assess for allergic reactions to fluoroquinolones before beginning therapy. Because these agents may decrease leukocytes, the white blood cell count should be carefully monitored. When possible, culture and sensitivity testing should be performed before beginning therapy.

These drugs are contraindicated in clients with a history of hypersensitivity to fluoroquinolones. They should be used with caution in clients with epilepsy, cerebral arteriosclerosis, or alcoholism due to a potential drug interaction that increases the risk of CNS toxicity. Clients with liver and renal dysfunction should be monitored carefully due to the drug being metabolized by the liver and excreted by the kidneys.

Enoxacin and norfloxacin should be taken on an empty stomach. Antacids and ferrous sulfate may decrease the absorption of fluoroquinolones, reducing antibiotic effectiveness. The fluoroquinolones should be administered at least 2 hours before these drugs. Coagulation studies (INR) need to be monitored frequently if these antibiotics are administered concurrently with warfarin due to interactions leading to increased anticoagulation effects.

Monitor urinary output and report quantities of less than 1000 mL in 24 hours to the healthcare provider. The client should be encouraged to drink eight or more glasses of water per day to decrease the risk of crystalluria, which irritates the kidneys. Advise the client to discontinue the drug and notify the healthcare provider if signs of hypersensitivity occur.

The nurse should inform the client that these drugs may cause dizziness and light-headedness and to avoid driving or performing hazardous tasks during drug therapy. These agents should be used with caution during pregnancy and breastfeeding due to untoward effects caused by the passage of antimicrobials to the fetus and newborn. Safety for use by children under 18 years has not been established.

Clients receiving norfloxacin should be informed that photophobia is possible. Some fluoroquinolones, such as ciprofloxacin, may affect tendons, especially in children. The client should refrain from physical exercise if calf, ankle, or Achilles tendon pain occurs.

Client education as it relates to fluoroquinolones should include goals, reasons for obtaining baseline data such as lab work and culture and sensitivity tests, and possible side effects. Following are important points to include when teaching clients regarding fluoroquinolones:

- Wear sunglasses; avoid exposure to bright lights and direct sunlight when taking norfloxacin (Noroxin).
- Report the first signs of tendon pain or inflammation.
- Report the following side effects immediately: dizziness, restlessness, stomach distress, diarrhea, psychosis, confusion, and irregular or fast heart rate.

See "Nursing Process Focus: Clients Receiving Antibacterial Therapy" for the Nursing Process applied to all antibacterials.

Pr **PROTOTYPE DRUG** | Ciprofloxacin (Cipro)

ACTIONS AND USES

Ciprofloxacin, a second generation fluoroquinolone, was approved in 1987 and is the most widely used drug in this class. By inhibiting bacterial DNA gyrase, ciprofloxacin affects bacterial replication and DNA repair. It is more effective against gram-negative than gram-positive organisms. It is prescribed for respiratory infections, bone and joint infections, GI infections, ophthalmic infections, sinusitis, and prostatitis. The drug is rapidly absorbed after oral administration and is distributed to most body tissues. Oral and intravenous forms are available.

PHARMACOKINETICS

Ciprofloxacin is well absorbed after PO administration. It may be given IV. It is widely distributed, crosses the placenta, and enters breast milk. It is partly metabolized by the liver. About 50% is excreted unchanged in urine. Half-life is 4 hours.

ADMINISTRATION ALERTS

- Administer at least 4 hours before antacids and ferrous sulfate.
- Ciprofloxacin is pregnancy category C.

ADVERSE EFFECTS AND INTERACTIONS

GI side effects may occur in as many as 20% of clients. Ciprofloxacin may be administered with food to diminish adverse GI effects. The client should not, however, take this drug with antacids or mineral supplements since drug absorption will be diminished. Some clients report headache and dizziness. Caffeine should be restricted to avoid excessive nervousness, anxiety, and tachycardia.

Concurrent administration with warfarin may increase anticoagulant effects. This drug may increase theophylline levels 15% to 30%. Antacids, ferrous sulfate, and sucralfate decrease the absorption of ciprofloxacin.

 See the Companion Website for a Nursing Process Focus Chart specific to this drug.

SULFONAMIDES

The discovery of the sulfonamides in the 1930s heralded a new era in the treatment of infectious disease. With their wide spectrum of activity against both gram-positive and gram-negative bacteria, the sulfonamides significantly reduced mortality from susceptible microbes and earned its discoverer a Nobel Prize in medicine in 1938. Sulfonamides suppress bacterial growth by inhibiting the essential compound folic acid that is responsible for cellular biosynthesis. Sulfonamides are active against a broad spectrum of microorganisms. The sulfonamides are shown in Table 32.9.

32.14 Pharmacotherapy with Sulfonamides

Several factors have led to a significant decline in the use of sulfonamides. Their widespread use over several decades resulted in a substantial number of resistant strains. The development of the penicillins, cephalosporins, and macrolides gave healthcare providers a larger choice of agents, some of which exhibited an improved safety profile over the sulfonamides. Approval of the combination antibiotic trimethoprim-sulfamethoxazole marked a resurgence in the use of sulfonamides in treating urinary tract infections (UTIs). Agents in this drug class are also given for *Pneumocystis carinii* pneumonia and *Shigella* infections of the small bowel.

Sulfonamides are classified by their absorption and excretion characteristics. Some, such as sulfisoxazole and sulfamethoxazole, are rapidly absorbed when given orally and excreted rapidly by the kidney. Others such as sulfasalazine are poorly absorbed and remain in the alimentary canal to treat intestinal infections. A third group, including sulfadiazine, is used for topical infections. Sulfadoxine has an exceptionally long half-life and is occasionally prescribed for malarial prophylaxis.

In general, the sulfonamides are safe drugs; however, some adverse effects may be serious. Adverse effects include the formation of crystals in the urine, hypersensitivity reactions, nausea, and vomiting. Although not common, sulfonamides can produce potentially fatal blood abnormalities, such as aplastic anemia, acute hemolytic anemia, and agranulocytosis.

NURSING CONSIDERATIONS

The role of the nurse in sulfonamide therapy involves careful monitoring of the client's condition and providing education as it relates to the prescribed drug regimen. Assess for anemia and other hematological disorders because sulfonamides

TABLE 32.9	Sulfonamides
Drug	*Route and Adult Dose*
sulfacetamide (PMS-Sulfacetamide)	Ophthalmic; one to three drops of 10%, 15%, or 30% solution into lower conjunctival sac q2–3h, may increase interval as patient responds or use 1.5–2.5 cm of 10% ointment q6h and at hs
sulfamethoxazole (Apo-Sulfamethoxazole)	PO; 2 g initially followed by 1 g bid–tid
sulfisoxazole (Apo-Sulfisoxazole)	PO; 2–4 g initially followed by 1–2 g qid
Pr trimethoprim-sulfamethoxazole (Bactrim, Novo-Trimel, Septra)	PO; 160 mg TMP/800 mg SMZ bid

Pr PROTOTYPE DRUG | Trimethoprim-Sulfamethoxazole (Bactrim, others)

ACTIONS AND USES

The fixed combination of the sulfonamide sulfamethoxazole (SMZ) with the anti-infective trimethoprim (TMP) is most commonly used in the pharmacotherapy of urinary tract infections. It is also approved for the treatment of *P. carinii* pneumonia, *Shigella* infections of the small bowel, and for acute episodes of chronic bronchitis.

Both SMZ and TMP are inhibitors of the bacterial metabolism of folic acid, or folate. Their action is synergistic: a greater bacterial kill is achieved by the fixed combination than would be achieved with either drug used separately. Because humans obtain the precursors of folate in their diets, these medications are selective for bacterial folate metabolism. Another advantage of the combination is that development of resistance is lower than that observed when either agent is used alone.

PHARMACOKINETICS

This combination is well absorbed after PO administration. It is partly metabolized by the liver. Less than 40% is excreted unchanged in urine. Half-life is 6 to 12 hours.

ADMINISTRATION ALERTS

- Administer oral drugs with a full glass of water.
- Trimethoprim-sulfamethoxazole is pregnancy category C.

ADVERSE EFFECTS AND INTERACTIONS

The most common side effect of TMP-SMZ involves skin rashes, which are characteristic of sulfonamides. Nausea and vomiting are not uncommon. This medication should be used cautiously in clients with pre-existing kidney disease since crystalluria, oliguria, and renal failure have been reported. Periodic laboratory evaluation of the blood is usually performed to identify early signs of agranulocytosis or thrombocytopenia.

TMP and SMZ may enhance the effects of oral anticoagulants. These drugs may also increase methotrexate toxicity.

 See the Companion Website for a Nursing Process Focus Chart specific to this drug.

may cause hemolytic anemia and blood dyscrasias due to a genetically determined deficiency in some clients' red blood cells. Assess renal function as sulfonamides may increase the risk for crystalluria. Culture and sensitivity results should be obtained before initiating sulfonamide therapy. CBC and urinalysis should be obtained during therapy.

Sulfonamides are contraindicated during pregnancy and lactation and for infants less than 2 months of age due to the drug's ability to promote jaundice. Agents in this class must be used with caution in clients with renal impairment. Sulfonamides have a low solubility that may cause crystals to form in urine and obstruct the kidneys or ureters. Encourage increasing fluids to 3000 mL per day to achieve a urinary output of 1500 mL per 24 hours to decrease the possibility of crystalluria.

Cross-sensitivity exists with diuretics, such as acetazolamide and the thiazides, and with sulfonylurea antidiabetic agents. All of these agents should be avoided in clients with a history of hypersensitivity to sulfonamides because this can induce a skin abnormality called Stevens-Johnson syndrome. Instruct the client to stop taking the drug and contact a healthcare provider if rash occurs.

Client education as it relates to sulfonamides should include goals, reasons for obtaining baseline data such as

lab work and culture and sensitivity tests, and possible side effects. Following are the important points to include when teaching clients regarding sulfonamides:

- Avoid exposure to direct sunlight; use sunscreen and protective clothing to decrease effects of photosensitivity.
- Take oral medications with a full glass of water.
- Increase fluid intake to 1500 to 3000 mL per day unless otherwise contraindicated.
- Report significant side effects immediately, including abdominal or stomach cramps or pain, blood in urine, confusion, difficulty breathing, and fever.

See "Nursing Process Focus: Clients Receiving Antibacterial Therapy" for the Nursing Process applied to all antibacterials.

32.15 Miscellaneous Antibacterials

Some anti-infectives cannot be grouped into classes, or the class is too small to warrant separate discussion. That is not to diminish their importance in medicine as some of the miscellaneous anti-infectives are critical drugs in certain situations. The miscellaneous antibiotics are shown in Table 32.10.

MediaLink   Emerging Infectious Diseases

TABLE 32.10 Select Miscellaneous Antibacterials

Drug	Route and Adult Dose
chloramphenicol (Chlorofair, others)	PO; 12.5 mg/kg qid
clindamycin (Dalacin C)	PO; 150–450 mg qid
fosfomycin (Monurol)	PO; 3 g sachet dissolved in 3–4 oz of water as a single dose
methenamine (Mandelamine)	PO; 1 g qid
nitrofurantoin (Apo-Nitrofurantoin)	PO; 50–100 mg qid
quinupristin-dalfopristin (Synercid)	IV; 7.5 mg/kg infused over 60 min q8h
vancomycin (PMS-Vancomycin, Vancocin)	IV; 500 mg qid; 1 g bid; PO, 125–500 mg q6h

Clindamycin is effective against both gram-positive and gram-negative bacteria. Susceptible bacteria include *Fusobacterium* and *Clostridium perfringens*. It is sometimes the drug of choice for oral infections caused by bacteroides. It is considered to be appropriate treatment when less toxic alternatives are not effective options. It is contraindicated in clients with a history of hypersensitivity to clindamycin or lincomycin, regional enteritis, or ulcerative colitis. Clindamycin is limited in use because it is associated with pseudomembranous colitis (AAPMC), the most severe adverse effect of this drug. The client should report significant side effects to the healthcare provider immediately, including diarrhea, rashes, difficulty breathing, itching, and difficulty swallowing.

Quinupristin-dalfopristin is a combination drug that is the first in a new class of antibiotics called streptogramins. Streptogramins are reserved to treat infections caused by antibiotic-resistant gram-positive organisms. Quinupristin-dalfopristin is primarily indicated for treatment of vancomycin-resistant *Enterococcus faecium* infections and is contraindicated in clients with hypersensitivity to this drug. It is used cautiously in clients with renal or hepatic dysfunction. Hepatotoxicity is the most serious adverse effect of this drug. The client should report significant side effects to the healthcare provider immediately, including irritation, pain, or burning at the intravenous infusion site, joint and muscle pain, rash, diarrhea, and vomiting.

Linezolid is significant in being the first drug in a new class of antibiotics called the oxazolidinones. This drug is as effective as vancomycin against methicillin-resistant *S. aureus* (MRSA) infections. Linezolid is administered intravenously or orally. Most clients can be converted from the intravenous to oral route in about 5 days. Linezolid is contraindicated in clients with hypersensitivity to the drug and in pregnancy, and it should be used with caution in clients who have hypertension. Cautious use is also necessary in clients taking MAO inhibitors or serotonin reuptake inhibitors because the drugs can interact, causing a hypertensive crisis. Linezolid can cause thrombocytopenia. The client should report significant side effects to the healthcare provider immediately, including bleeding, diarrhea, headache, nausea, vomiting, rash, dizziness, and fever.

Vancomycin is usually reserved for severe infections from gram-positive organisms such as *S. aureus* and *Streptococcus pneumoniae*. It is often used after bacteria have become resistant to other, safer antibiotics. Vancomycin is the most effective drug for treating MRSA infections. Vancomycin is contraindicated in clients with known hypersensitivity to the drug, and in clients with hearing loss. Due to ototoxicity, hearing must be evaluated frequently throughout the course of therapy. It should not be given to pregnant or lactating clients. Vancomycin can also cause nephrotoxicity leading to uremia.

Vancomycin is administered orally and IV, but not IM. A reaction that can occur with rapid IV administration is known as **red-man syndrome** and includes hypotension with flushing and a red rash on the face and upper body. The client should report significant side effects to the healthcare provider immediately, including superinfections, generalized tingling after IV administration, chills, fever, skin rash, hives, hearing loss, and nausea.

See "Nursing Process Focus: Clients Receiving Antibacterial Therapy" for the Nursing Process applied to all antibacterials.

In September 2003, the first in a new class of antibiotics, the cyclic lipopeptides, was approved. Daptomycin is approved for the treatment of serious skin and skin structure infections such as major abscesses, post-surgical skin wound infections, and infected ulcers caused by *S. aureus*, *Streptococcus pyogenes*, *Streptococcus agalactiae*, and *E. faecalis*. The most common side effects are GI distress, injection site reactions, fever, headache, dizziness, insomnia, and rash.

Pr PROTOTYPE DRUG | Vancomycin (PMS-Vancomycin, Vancocin)

ACTIONS AND USES

Vancomycin is an antibiotic usually reserved for severe infections from gram-positive organisms such as *S. aureus* and *Streptococcus pneumoniae*. It is often used after bacteria have become resistant to other, safer antibiotics. It is bactericidal, inhibiting bacterial cell wall synthesis. Because vancomycin was not used frequently during the first 30 years following its discovery, the incidence of vancomycin-resistant organisms is less than with other antibiotics. Vancomycin is the most effective drug for treating methicillin-resistant *S. aureus* infections, which have become a major problem in North America. Vancomycin resistant strains of *S. aureus*, however, have begun to appear in recent years. Vancomycin is normally given intravenously as it is not absorbed from the GI tract.

ADMINISTRATION ALERTS

- Administer IV slowly at a rate of 10 mg/min over not less than 60 minutes to avoid causing sudden hypotension.
- Vancomycin is pregnancy category C.

ADVERSE EFFECTS AND INTERACTIONS

Frequent, minor side effects include flushing, hypotension, and rash on the upper body, sometimes called the red-man syndrome. More serious adverse effects are possible with higher doses, including nephrotoxicity and ototoxicity. Clients may experience acute allergic reactions, including anaphylaxis.

Vancomycin adds to toxicity of aminoglycosides, amphotericin B, cisplatin, cyclosporine, polymyxin B, and other ototoxic and nephrotoxic medications. It interacts with cholestyramine and colestipol, causing a decrease in absorption of oral vancomycin. It may increase the risk of lactic acidosis when administered with metformin.

 See the Companion Website for a Nursing Process Focus Chart specific to this drug.

NATURAL THERAPIES

The Antibacterial Properties of Goldenseal

Goldenseal (*Hydrastis canadensis*) was once a common plant found in woods in the eastern and midwestern United States. American Indians used the root for a variety of medicinal applications, including wound healing, diuresis, and washes for inflamed eyes. In recent years, the plant has been harvested to near extinction. Goldenseal was reported to mask the appearance of drugs in the urine of clients wanting to hide drug abuse. This claim has since been proven false.

The roots and leaves of goldenseal are dried and available as capsules, tablets, salves, and tinctures. One of the primary active ingredients in goldenseal is hydrastine, which is reported to have antibacterial and antifungal properties. When used topically or locally, it is purported to be of value in treating bacterial and fungal skin infections and oral conditions such as gingivitis and thrush. As an eyewash, it can soothe inflamed eyes. Considered safe for most people, it is contraindicated in pregnancy and hypertension.

TUBERCULOSIS

Tuberculosis is a highly contagious infection caused by *Mycobacterium tuberculosis*. It is treated with multiple anti-infectives for a prolonged period. The antitubercular agents are shown in Table 32.11.

32.16 Pharmacotherapy of Tuberculosis

Tuberculosis (TB) is an infection caused by the organism *M. tuberculosis*. Although the microorganisms typically invade the lung, they may also enter other body systems, particularly bone. Mycobacteria activate cells of the immune response, which attempt to isolate the microorganisms by creating a wall around them. The slow-growing

NURSING PROCESS FOCUS   Clients Receiving Antibacterial Therapy

Assessment	Potential Nursing Diagnoses/Identified Patterns
Prior to administration: ■ Obtain complete health history including allergies, drug history, and possible drug interactions. ■ Obtain specimens for culture and sensitivity before initiating therapy. ■ Perform infection-focused physical examination including vital signs, white blood cell count, and sedimentation rate.	■ Nutritional and fluid intake adequacy ■ Need for knowledge regarding the disease process and transmission ■ Need for knowledge regarding drug therapy, management of side effects, and reporting of adverse effects ■ Need for knowledge regarding the importance of adherence to treatment for healing ■ Potential for injury related to side effects of drug therapy ■ Risk for superinfection

Planning: Client Goals and Expected Outcomes

The client will:
■ Report reduction in symptoms related to the diagnosed infection and have negative results for laboratory and diagnostic tests for the presenting infection
■ Demonstrate an understanding of the drug by accurately describing the drug's purpose, action, side effects, and precautions
■ Immediately report significant side effects such as shortness of breath, swelling, fever, stomatitis, loose stools, vaginal discharge, or cough
■ Complete full course of antibiotic therapy and comply with follow-up care

Implementation

Interventions (Rationales)	Client Education/Discharge Planning
■ Monitor vital signs and symptoms of infection to determine antibacterial effectiveness. (Another drug or different dosage may be required.)	■ Instruct client to notify healthcare provider if symptoms persist or worsen.
■ Monitor for hypersensitivity reaction. (Immediate hypersensitivity reaction may occur within 2 to 30 minutes; accelerated occurs in 1 to 72 hours; and delayed after 72 hours.)	■ Instruct client to discontinue the medication and inform healthcare provider if symptoms of hypersensitivity reaction develop, such as wheezing; shortness of breath; swelling of face, tongue, or hands; and itching or rash.
■ Monitor for severe diarrhea. (The condition may occur due to superinfection or the possible adverse effect of antibiotic associated pseudomembranous colitis, or AAPMC.)	Instruct client to: ■ Consult healthcare provider before taking antidiarrheal drugs, which could cause retention of harmful bacteria ■ Consume cultured dairy products with live active cultures, such as kefir, yogurt, or buttermilk, to help restore and maintain normal intestinal flora
■ Administer drug around the clock (to maintain effective blood levels).	Instruct client to: ■ Take medication on schedule ■ Complete the entire prescription, even if feeling better, to prevent development of resistant bacteria
■ Monitor for superinfection, especially in elderly, debilitated, or immunosuppressed clients. (Increased risk for superinfections is due to elimination of normal flora.)	■ Instruct client to report signs and symptoms of superinfection such as fever; black hairy tongue; stomatitis; loose, foul-smelling stools; vaginal discharge; or cough.

continued

NURSING PROCESS FOCUS Clients Receiving Antibacterial Therapy *(Continued)*

Interventions (Rationales)	Client Education/Discharge Planning
■ Monitor intake of OTC products such as antacids, calcium supplements, iron products, and laxatives containing magnesium. (These products interfere with absorption of many antibiotics.)	■ Advise client to consult with healthcare provider before using OTC medications or herbal products.
■ Monitor for photosensitivity. (Tetracyclines, fluoroquinolones, and sulfonamides can increase client's sensitivity to ultraviolet light and increase risk of sunburn.)	Encourage client to: ■ Avoid direct exposure to sunlight during and after therapy ■ Wear protective clothing, sunglasses, and sunscreen when in the sun
■ Determine the interactions of the prescribed antibiotics with various foods and beverages.	■ Instruct client regarding foods and beverages that should be avoided with specific antibiotic therapies: ■ Avoid acidic fruit juices with penicillins ■ Avoid alcohol intake with cephalosporins ■ Avoid dairy/calcium products with tetracyclines
■ Monitor IV site for signs and symptoms of tissue irritation, severe pain, and extravasation.	■ Instruct client to report pain or other symptoms of discomfort immediately during intravenous infusion.
■ Monitor for side effects specific to various antibiotic therapies. (See "Nursing Considerations" for each antibiotic classification in this chapter.)	■ Instruct client to report side effects specific to antibiotic therapy prescribed.
■ Monitor renal function such as intake and output ratios and urine colour and consistency. Monitor lab work including serum creatinine and BUN. (Some antibiotics such as the aminoglycosides are nephrotoxic.)	■ Explain purpose of required laboratory tests and scheduled follow-up with healthcare provider. ■ Instruct client to increase fluid intake to 2000 to 3000 mL/day.
■ Monitor for symptoms of ototoxicity. (Some antibiotics, such as the aminoglycosides and vancomycin, may cause vestibular or auditory nerve damage.)	Instruct client to notify healthcare provider of: ■ Changes in hearing, ringing in ears, or full feeling in the ears ■ Nausea and vomiting with motion, ataxia, nystagmus, or dizziness
■ Monitor client for compliance with antibiotic therapy.	Instruct client in the importance of: ■ Completing the prescription as ordered ■ Follow-up care after antibiotic therapy is completed

Evaluation of Outcome Criteria

Evaluate the effectiveness of drug therapy by confirming that client goals and expected outcomes have been met (see "Planning").

See Tables 32.3 through 32.10 (pages 427–437) for lists of drugs to which these nursing actions apply.

TABLE 32.11 Antituberculosis Drugs

Drug	Route and Adult Dose
First-Line Agents	
ethambutol (Etibi)	PO; 15–25 mg/kg qd
isoniazid (Dom-, PMS-Isoniazid)	PO; 15 mg/kg qd
	PO/IM; 5 mg/kg/day or 15 mg/kg/2–3 times weekly
pyrazinamide (PMS-Pyrazinamide)	PO; 5–15 mg/kg tid–qid (max 2 g/day)
rifampin (Rifadin, Rofact)	PO/IV; 600 mg qd
rifater: combination of pyrazinamide with isoniazid and rifampin	PO; six tablets qd (for clients weighing 55 kg or more)
streptomycin	IM; 15 mg/kg up to 1.0 g/day as a single dose
Second-Line Agents	
amikacin (Amikin)	IV/IM; 5–7.5 mg/kg as a loading dose, then 7.5 mg/kg bid
ciprofloxacin (Cipro)	PO; 250–750 mg bid. IV; 400 mg q12h
kanamycin (Kantrex)	IM; 5–7.5 mg/kg bid–tid
ofloxacin (Novo-Ofloxacin)	PO; 200–400 mg bid

mycobacteria usually become dormant, existing inside cavities called **tubercles**. They may remain dormant during an entire lifetime, or they may become reactivated if the client's immune system becomes suppressed. When active, tuberculosis can be quite infectious, readily spread by contaminated sputum. With the immune suppression characteristic of AIDS, the incidence of TB has greatly increased; as many as 20% of all AIDS clients develop active tuberculosis infections. Infection by a different species of mycobacterium, *M. leprae*, is responsible for a disease known as leprosy.

Drug therapy of tuberculosis differs from that of most other infections. Mycobacteria have a cell wall that is resistant to penetration by anti-infective drugs. For medications to reach the isolated microorganisms in the tubercles, therapy must continue for 6 to 12 months. Although the client may not be infectious this entire time and may have no symptoms, it is critical that therapy continue for the entire period. Some clients develop multidrug-resistant infections and require therapy for as long as 24 months.

A second difference in the pharmacotherapy of tuberculosis is that at least two, and sometimes four or more, antibiotics are administered concurrently. During the 6- to 24-month treatment period, different combinations of drugs may be used. Multiple-drug therapy is necessary because the mycobacteria grow slowly and resistance is common. Using multiple drugs in different combinations during the long treatment period lowers the potential for resistance and increases the success of the therapy. There are two broad categories of antitubercular agents. One class consists of first-line drugs, which are safer and generally the most effective. A second group of drugs, more toxic and less effective than the first-line agents, are used when resistance develops.

A third difference is that antituberculosis drugs are extensively used for *preventing* the disease in addition to treating it. Chemoprophylaxis is used for close contacts or family members of recently infected tuberculosis clients. Therapy usually begins immediately after a client receives a positive tuberculin test. Clients with immunosuppression, such as those with AIDS or those receiving immunosuppressant drugs, may receive preventive treatment with antituberculosis drugs. A short-term therapy of 2 months, consisting of a combination treatment with isoniazid and pyrazinamide, is approved for tuberculosis prophylaxis in HIV-positive clients.

NURSING CONSIDERATIONS

The role of the nurse in antituberculosis therapy involves careful monitoring of the client's condition and providing education as it relates to the prescribed drug regimen. Before beginning therapy, assess the client for the presence or history of a positive tuberculin skin test, a positive sputum culture, or a close contact with a person recently infected with TB. These conditions are all indications for the use of antituberculosis drugs. Also assess the client for a history of alcohol abuse, AIDS, liver disease, or kidney disease because many antituberculosis drugs are contraindicated in those conditions. They are also contraindicated in clients receiving immunosuppressant drugs. A complete physical exam including vital signs should be performed.

Caution must be observed during pregnancy and lactation and in clients with renal dysfunction or a history of convulsive disorders. The drugs are used with caution in clients with chronic liver disease or alcoholism because of the risk for hepatic injury due to the production of toxic levels of drug metabolites. These drugs may cause asymptomatic hyperuricemia because they can inhibit the renal excretion of uric acid, which may lead to gouty arthritis. Ethambutol is contraindicated in clients with optic neuritis. Some antituberculosis drugs interact with oral contracep-

---

Pr PROTOTYPE DRUG | Isoniazid (Dom-Isoniazid, PMS-Isoniazid)

ACTIONS AND USES

Isoniazid has been a drug of choice for the treatment of *M. tuberculosis* for many years. It is bactericidal for actively growing organisms but bacteriostatic for dormant mycobacteria. It is selective for *M. tuberculosis*. Isoniazid is used alone for chemoprophylaxis or in combination with other antituberculosis drugs for treating active disease.

PHARMACOKINETICS

Isoniazid is well absorbed after PO or IM administration. It is widely distributed, crosses the blood-brain barrier and placenta, and enters breast milk. It is partly metabolized by the liver. About 50% is excreted unchanged in urine. Half-life is 1 to 4 hours.

ADMINISTRATION ALERTS

- Give on an empty stomach, 1 hour after or 2 hours before meals.
- Give with meals if GI irritation occurs.
- For IM administration, administer deep into muscle and rotate sites.
- Isoniazid is pregnancy category C.

ADVERSE EFFECTS AND INTERACTIONS

The most common side effects of isoniazid are numbness of the hands and feet, rash, and fever. Although rare, liver toxicity is a serious adverse effect; thus, be alert for signs of jaundice, fatigue, elevated hepatic enzymes, and loss of appetite. Liver enzyme tests are usually performed monthly during therapy to identify early hepatotoxicity.

Aluminum-containing antacids decrease the absorption of isoniazid. When disulfiram is taken with INH, lack of coordination or psychotic reactions may result. Drinking alcohol with INH increases the risk of hepatotoxicity.

 See the Companion Website for a Nursing Process Focus Chart specific to this drug.

tives and decrease their effectiveness; thus, female clients should use an alternative form of birth control while using these medications.

See "Nursing Process Focus: Clients Receiving Antituberculosis Agents" for specific teaching points.

NURSING PROCESS FOCUS   Clients Receiving Antituberculosis Agents

Assessment	Potential Nursing Diagnoses/Identified Patterns

Prior to administration:
■ Obtain complete health history including allergies, drug history, and possible drug interactions.
■ Perform complete physical examination including vital signs.
■ Assess for presence/history of the following:
  ■ Positive tuberculin skin test
  ■ Positive sputum culture or smear
  ■ Close contact with person recently infected with tuberculosis
  ■ HIV infection or AIDS
  ■ Immunosuppressant drug therapy
  ■ Alcohol abuse
  ■ Liver or kidney disease
■ Assess cognitive ability to comply with long-term therapy.
	■ Nutritional and fluid intake adequacy
	■ Need for knowledge regarding drug therapy and adverse effects
	■ Need for knowledge regarding the importance of adherence to treatment for healing and to protect the community
	■ Potential for injury related to side effects of drug therapy
	■ Risk for superinfection

Planning: Client Goals and Expected Outcomes

The client will:
■ Report reduction in tuberculosis symptoms and have negative results for laboratory and diagnostic tests for TB infection
■ Demonstrate an understanding of the drug by accurately describing the drug's purpose, action, side effects, and precautions
■ Immediately report effects such as visual changes, difficulty voiding, changes in hearing, and symptoms of liver or kidney impairment
■ Complete full course of antitubercular therapy and comply with follow-up care

Implementation

Interventions (Rationales)	Client Education/Discharge Planning
■ Monitor for hepatic side effects. (Antituberculosis agents, such as isoniazid and rifampin, cause hepatic impairment.)	■ Instruct client to report yellow eyes and skin, loss of appetite, dark urine, and unusual tiredness.
■ Monitor for neurological side effects such as numbness and tingling of the extremities. (Antituberculosis agents, such as isoniazid, cause peripheral neuropathy and depletion of vitamin B_6.)	Instruct client to: ■ Report numbness and tingling of extremities ■ Take supplemental vitamin B_6 as ordered to reduce risk of side effects
■ Collect sputum specimens as directed by healthcare provider. (This will determine the effectiveness of the antituberculosis agent.)	■ Instruct the client in technique needed to collect a quality sputum specimen.
■ Monitor for dietary compliance when client is taking isoniazid. (Foods high in tyramine can interact with the drug and cause palpitations, flushing, and hypertension.)	■ Advise clients taking isoniazid to avoid foods containing tyramine, such as aged cheese, smoked and pickled fish, beer and red wine, bananas, and chocolate.
■ Monitor for side effects specific to various antituberculosis drugs.	Instruct client to report side effects specific to antituberculosis therapy prescribed: ■ Blurred vision or changes in colour or vision field (ethambutol) ■ Difficulty in voiding (pyrazinamide) ■ Fever, yellowing of skin, weakness, dark urine (isoniazid, rifampin) ■ Gastrointestinal system disturbances (rifampin) ■ Changes in hearing (streptomycin) ■ Numbness and tingling of extremities (isoniazid) ■ Red discoloration of body fluids (rifampin) ■ Dark concentrated urine, weight gain, edema (streptomycin)
■ Establish infection control measures based on extent of disease condition and established protocol.	■ Instruct client in infectious control measures, such as frequent handwashing, covering the mouth when coughing or sneezing, and proper disposal of soiled tissues.

continued

NURSING PROCESS FOCUS Clients Receiving Antituberculosis Agents *(Continued)*	
Interventions (Rationales)	**Client Education/Discharge Planning**
■ Establish therapeutic environment to ensure adequate rest, nutrition, hydration, and relaxation. (Symptoms of tuberculosis are manifested when the immune system is suppressed.) ■ Monitor client's ability and motivation to comply with therapeutic regimen. (Treatment must continue for the full length of therapy to eliminate all *M. tuberculosis* organisms.)	■ Teach client to incorporate health-enhancing activities, such as adequate rest and sleep, intake of essential vitamins and nutrients, and intake of six to eight glasses of water/day. Explain the importance of complying with the entire therapeutic plan, including: ■ Take all medications as directed by healthcare provider ■ Do not discontinue medication until instructed ■ Wear a medical alert bracelet ■ Keep all appointments for follow-up care
Evaluation of Outcome Criteria	
Evaluate the effectiveness of drug therapy by confirming that client goals and expected outcomes have been met (see "Planning").	

See Table 32.11 (page 440) for a list of drugs to which these nursing actions apply.

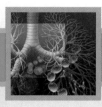

CHAPTER REVIEW

KEY CONCEPTS

The numbered key concepts provide a succinct summary of the important points from the corresponding numbered section within the chapter. If any of these points are not clear, refer to the numbered section within the chapter for review. Expanded versions can be found on the Companion Website.

32.1 Pathogens are organisms that cause disease due to their ability to divide rapidly or secrete toxins.

32.2 Bacteria are described by their shape (bacilli, cocci, or spirilla), their ability to utilize oxygen (aerobic or anaerobic), and by their staining characteristics (gram positive or gram negative).

32.3 Anti-infective drugs are classified by their chemical structures (e.g., aminoglycoside, fluoroquinolone) or by their mechanism of action (e.g., cell wall inhibitor, folic acid inhibitor).

32.4 Anti-infective drugs act by affecting the target organism's metabolism or life cycle and may be bactericidal or bacteriostatic.

32.5 Acquired antimicrobial resistance causes loss of antibiotic effectiveness and is worsened by the overprescribing of these agents.

32.6 Careful selection of the correct antibiotic, through the use of culture and sensitivity testing, is essential for effective pharmacotherapy and to limit adverse effects.

32.7 Host factors such as immune system status, local conditions at the infection site, allergic reactions, age, and genetics influence the choice of antibiotic.

32.8 Penicillins kill bacteria by disrupting the cell wall. Allergies occur most frequently with the penicillins.

32.9 The cephalosporins are similar in structure and function to the penicillins and are one of the most widely prescribed anti-infective classes. Cross-sensitivity may exist with the penicillins in some clients.

32.10 Tetracyclines have some of the broadest spectrums, but they are drugs of choice for relatively few diseases.

32.11 The macrolides are safe alternatives to penicillin for many diseases.

32.12 The aminoglycosides are narrow-spectrum drugs that have the potential to cause serious adverse effects such as ototoxicity, nephrotoxicity, and neuromuscular blockade.

32.13 The use of fluoroquinolones has expanded far beyond their initial role in treating urinary tract infections.

32.14 Once widely prescribed, resistance has limited the usefulness of sulfonamides to urinary tract infections and a few other specific infections.

32.15 A number of miscellaneous antibacterials have specific indications, distinct antibacterial mechanisms, and related nursing care.

32.16 Multiple-drug therapy is needed in the treatment of tuberculosis since the complex microbes are slow growing and commonly develop drug resistance.

REVIEW QUESTIONS

1 Why does antimicrobial resistance become more of a problem when antibiotics are prescribed too often?

2 If penicillins are inexpensive, why might a healthcare provider prescribe a more expensive cephalosporin or macrolide antibiotic?

3 How does drug therapy of tuberculosis differ from conventional anti-infective chemotherapy? What are the rationales for these differences?

CRITICAL THINKING QUESTIONS

1. An 18-year-old female comes to a clinic for prenatal care. She is 8 weeks pregnant. She is healthy and takes no other medication other than low-dose tetracycline for acne. What is a priority of care for this client?

2. A 32-year-old Aboriginal client has a diagnosis of otitis externa, and the healthcare provider has ordered erythromycin PO. This client has a history of hepatitis B, allergies to sulfa and penicillin, and mild hypertension. Should the nurse give the erythromycin? How might the nurse provide culturally competent care for this client?

3. A 66-year-old hospitalized client has MRSA in a cellulitis of the lower extremity and is on gentamicin IV. What is a priority for the nurse to monitor in this client?

EXPLORE
MediaLink

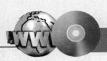 www.pearsoned.ca/adams-king

 MEDIALINK DVD-ROM
- **Audio Glossary**
- **CRNE Review**
- **Videos:** Tuberculosis
- **Animation**
  Mechanism of Action: Ciprofloxacin
  Mechanism of Action: Penicillin

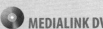 **COMPANION WEBSITE**
- **CRNE Review**
- **Case Study:** Client with tuberculosis
- **Dosage Calculations**

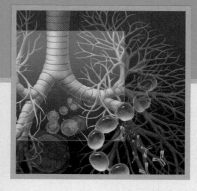

CHAPTER 33

Drugs for Fungal, Protozoan, and Helminthic Infections

DRUGS AT A GLANCE

ANTIFUNGAL DRUGS

Agents for systemic infections
- amphotericin B (Abelcet, others)
- fluconazole (Apo-Fluconazole, Diflucan)

Agents for topical infections
- nystatin (Nadostine, PMS-Nystatin)

ANTIPROTOZOAN DRUGS

Antimalarial agents

Non-malarial antiprotozoan agents
- metronidazole
  (Apo-Metronidazole, Flagyl)

Antiparasitic agents

ANTHELMINTIC DRUGS
- mebendazole (Vermox)

OBJECTIVES

After reading this chapter, the student should be able to do the following:

1. Compare and contrast the pharmacotherapy of superficial and systemic fungal infections.
2. Explain the therapeutic action of each class of drug used for fungal, protozoan, and helminthic infections in relation to the pathophysiology of the infection.
3. Discuss the role of the nurse regarding the non-pharmacological management of fungal infection, including identification of clients who are at greatest risk for acquiring serious fungal infections and client teaching.
4. Explain how an understanding of the *Plasmodium* life cycle is important to the effective pharmacotherapy of malaria.
5. Describe the nurse's role in the pharmacological management of clients receiving drugs for fungal, protozoan, malarial, and helminthic infections.
6. For each of the drug classes listed in Drugs at a Glance, identify a representative drug and explain its mechanism of action, therapeutic effects, and important adverse effects.
7. Describe and explain, based on pharmacological principles, the rationale for nursing assessment, planning, and interventions for clients with fungal infection.
8. Use the nursing process to care for clients receiving drug therapy for fungal infection.

MediaLink

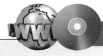

www.pearsoned.ca/adams-king

CRNE review, case studies, and other interactive resources for this chapter can be found on the Companion Website at **www.pearsoned.ca/adams-king.** Click on "Chapter 33" to select the activities for this chapter. For animations, more CRNE review questions, and an audio glossary, access the accompanying DVD-ROM in this textbook.

ungi, protozoans, and multicellular parasites are more complex than bacteria. Because of structural and functional differences, most antibacterial drugs are ineffective against fungi. Although there are fewer drugs to treat fungal, protozoan, and helminthic diseases, the available drugs are usually effective.

PHARMFACTS

Fungal, Protozoan, and Helminthic Diseases

- About 90% of fungal infections in humans are caused by a few dozen species.
- Of all fungal infections, 86% are caused by *Candida albicans*. The second most common (1.3%) is *Aspergillus*.
- Approximately 300 to 500 million cases of malaria occur worldwide each year, with an estimated 2.7 million deaths due to the disease.
- Monotherapy is no longer recommended by the World Health Organization (WHO) for the treatment of malaria due to the increasing problem of drug resistance.
- Fungi cause about 9% of nosocomial infections.
- Chagas disease, caused by *Trypanosoma cruzi*, is the most significant cause of heart disease in some South American countries. It infects 16 million people annually.
- *Ascaris lumbricoides* is the most common intestinal helminthic infection, affecting 1 billion people worldwide.

33.1 Characteristics of Fungi

Fungi are single-celled or multicellular organisms whose primary role on the planet is to serve as decomposers of dead plants and animals, returning the elements to the soil for recycling. Although 100,000 to 200,000 species exist in soil, air, and water, only about 300 are associated with disease in humans. A few species of fungi normally grow on skin and mucosal surfaces as part of the normal host flora.

Unlike bacteria, which grow rapidly to overwhelm hosts' defences, fungi grow slowly, and infections may progress for many months before symptoms develop. Fungi cause disease by replication; they do not secrete toxins like many bacterial species. With a few exceptions, fungal infections are not readily communicable to those in casual contact with the client.

The human body is remarkably resistant to infection by these organisms, and clients with a healthy immune system experience few serious fungal diseases. Clients who have a suppressed immune system, however, such as those infected with HIV, may experience frequent fungal infections, some of which may require aggressive pharmacotherapy.

The species of pathogenic fungi that attack a host with a healthy immune system are somewhat distinct from those that infect clients who are immunocompromised. Clients with intact immune defences are afflicted with *community-acquired* infections such as sporotrichosis, blastomycosis, histoplasmosis, and coccidioidomycosis. *Opportunistic* fungal infections acquired in a nosocomial setting are more likely to be candidiasis, aspergillosis, cryptococcosis, and mucormycosis. Table 33.1 lists the most common fungi that cause disease in humans.

33.2 Classification of Mycoses

Fungal diseases are called **mycoses**. A simple and useful method of classifying fungal infections is to consider them as either superficial or systemic.

Superficial mycoses affect the scalp, skin, nails, and mucous membranes such as the oral cavity and vagina. Mycoses of this type are often treated with topical drugs as the incidence of side effects is much lower using this route of administration. Superficial fungal infections are sometimes called **dermatophytic.**

TABLE 33.1   Fungal Pathogens

Name of Fungus	Description of Disease
Systemic	
Aspergillus fumigatus, others	aspergillosis: opportunistic; most commonly affects lung but can spread to other organs
Blastomyces dermatitidis	blastomycosis: begins in the lungs and spreads to other organs
Candida albicans, others	candidiasis: most common opportunistic fungal infection; may affect nearly any organ
Coccidioides immitis	coccidioidomycosis: begins in the lungs and spreads to other organs
Cryptococcus neoformans	cryptococcosis: opportunistic; begins in the lungs but is the most common cause of meningitis in AIDS patients
Histoplasma capsulatum	histoplasmosis: begins in the lungs and spreads to other organs
Mucorales (various species)	mucormycosis: opportunistic; affects blood vessels; causes sinus infections, stomach ulcers, and others
Pneumocystis carinii	pneumocystis pneumonia: opportunistic; primarily causes pneumonia of the lung but can spread to other organs
Topical	
Candida albicans, others	candidiasis: affects skin, nails, oral cavity (thrush), vagina
Epidermophyton floccosum	athlete's foot (tinea pedis), jock itch (tinea cruris), and other skin disorders
Microsporum audouini, others	ringworm of scalp (tinea capitis)
Sporothrix schenckii	sporotrichosis: primarily affects skin and superficial lymph nodes
Trichophyton (various species)	affects scalp, skin, and nails

Systemic mycoses are those affecting internal organs, typically the lungs, brain, and digestive organs. Although less common than superficial mycoses, systemic fungal infections affect multiple body systems and are sometimes fatal to clients with suppressed immune systems. Mycoses of this type often require aggressive oral or parenteral medications that produce more adverse effects than the topical agents.

Historically, the antifungal drugs used for superficial infections were clearly distinct from those prescribed for systemic infections. In recent years, this distinction has become blurred. Many of the newer antifungal agents may be used for either superficial or systemic infections. Furthermore, some superficial infections may be treated either systemically or topically.

33.3 Mechanism of Action of Antifungal Drugs

Biologically, fungi are classified as eukaryotes; their cellular structure and metabolic pathways are more similar to those of humans than to bacteria. Antibiotics that are efficacious against bacteria are ineffective in treating mycoses. Thus, an entirely different set of agents is needed.

One important difference between fungal cells and human cells is the steroid in their plasma membranes. Whereas cholesterol is essential for animal cell membranes, **ergosterol** is present in fungi. This difference allows antifungal agents such as amphotericin B to be selective for fungal plasma membranes. The largest class of antifungals, the **azoles**, inhibits ergosterol synthesis, causing the fungal plasma membrane to become porous, or leaky.

Some antifungals act by mechanisms that take advantage of enzymatic differences between fungi and humans. For example, in fungi, flucytosine is converted to the toxic antimetabolite 5-fluorouracil, which inhibits both DNA and RNA synthesis. Humans do not have the enzyme necessary for this conversion. Fluorouracil itself is a common antineoplastic drug (see Chapter 35).

DRUGS FOR SYSTEMIC ANTIFUNGAL INFECTIONS

Systemic or invasive fungal disease may require intensive pharmacotherapy for extended periods. Amphotericin B and fluconazole are drugs of choice. Systemic antifungal drugs are shown in Table 33.2.

TABLE 33.2   Drugs for Systemic Mycoses

Drug	Route and Adult Dose
amphotericin B (Abelcet, AmBisome, Fungizone, Amphotec)	IV; 0.25 mg/kg qd; may increase to 1 mg/kg qd or 1.5 mg/kg qod (max 1.5 mg/kg/day)
caspofungin acetate (Cancidas)	IV; loading dose 70 mg infused over 1 hr on day 1, followed by 50 mg infused over 1 hr qid for 30 days
fluconazole (Apo-Fluconazole, Diflucan)	PO; 200–400 mg on day 1, then 100–200 mg qd for 2–4 weeks
flucytosine (Ancotil)	PO; 50–150 mg/kg in divided doses
itraconazole (Sporanox)	PO; 200 mg qd; may increase to 200 mg bid (max 400 mg/day)
ketoconazole (Apo-Ketoconazole, Nizoral)	PO; 200–400 mg qd
terbinafine hydrochloride (Apo-Terbinafine, Lamisil)	PO; 250 mg qd for 6–13 weeks
voriconazole (VFEND)	IV; 6 mg/kg q12h day 1, then 4 mg/kg q12h; may reduce to 3 mg/kg q12h if not tolerated

33.4 Pharmacotherapy of Systemic Fungal Diseases

Opportunistic fungal disease in AIDS clients spurred the development of several new drugs for systemic fungal infections over the past 20 years. Others who may experience systemic mycoses include clients receiving prolonged therapy with corticosteroids, clients with extensive burns or indwelling vascular catheters, clients receiving antineoplastic agents, and clients who received an organ transplant. Pharmacotherapy is often extended, lasting several months. Systemic antifungal drugs have little or no antibacterial activity.

Amphotericin B has been the drug of choice for systemic fungal infections for many years; however, the newer azole drugs such as ketoconazole have replaced amphotericin B for the treatment of less severe systemic infections. Although rarely used as monotherapy, flucytosine is sometimes used in combination with amphotericin B in the pharmacotherapy of severe *Candida* infections. Flucytosine can cause immunosuppression and liver toxicity, and resistance has become a major problem.

NURSING CONSIDERATIONS

The role of the nurse in systemic antifungal therapy involves careful monitoring of the client's condition and providing education as it relates to the prescribed drug regimen. Prior to the initiation of therapy, the client's health history should be taken. This class of drug is contraindicated in clients with hypersensitivity and should be used cautiously in clients with renal impairment or severe bone marrow suppression. Obtain baseline culture and sensitivity tests prior to the beginning of therapy. Baseline and periodic lab tests including BUN, creatinine, CBC, electrolytes, and liver function tests should be obtained. Vital signs, especially pulse and blood pressure, should be obtained for baseline data as clients with heart disease may develop fluid overload.

Amphotericin B causes some degree of kidney damage in 80% of the clients who take it; therefore, weight as well as intake and output should be monitored. Oliguria, changes in intake and output ratios, hematuria, and abnormal renal function tests should be reported to the physician immediately. Because amphotericin B can cause ototoxicity, assess for hearing loss, vertigo, unsteady gait, and tinnitus.

Electrolyte imbalance is a significant side effect due to excretion of the drug in the urine. Hypokalemia is common, so monitor for symptoms of low potassium levels, including dysrhythmias. Also evaluate all other medications taken by the client for compatibility with systemic antifungal medications. Concurrent therapy with medications that reduce liver or renal function is not recommended.

Client education as it relates to systemic antifungal medications should include goals, reasons for obtaining baseline data, and possible side effects. Instruct the client and caregivers to do the following:

- Complete the full course of treatment.
- Avoid drinking alcohol due to its effects on the liver.
- Use effective contraception measures to prevent pregnancy.
- Monitor urinary output and drink plenty of fluids.
- Use caution while performing hazardous activities.

Pr PROTOTYPE DRUG | Amphotericin B (Abelcet, others)

ACTIONS AND USES

Amphotericin B has a wide spectrum of activity that includes most of the fungi pathogenic to humans; thus, it is a drug of choice for most severe systemic mycoses. It may also be indicated as prophylactic antifungal therapy for clients with severe immunosuppression. It acts by binding to ergosterol in fungal cell membranes, causing them to become permeable (leaky). Treatment may continue for several months. Resistance to amphotericin B is not common.

To reduce toxicity, amphotericin B has been formulated with three lipid preparations: liposomal amphotericin B, amphotericin B lipid complex, and amphotericin B cholesteryl sulfate complex. The principal advantage of the lipid formulations is reduced nephrotoxicity and less infusion-related fever and chills. They are generally used only after therapy with other agents has failed, due to their expense.

PHARMACOKINETICS

Because amphotericin B is not absorbed from the GI tract, it is normally given by IV infusion. Topical preparations are available for superficial mycoses. Drug is distributed to most tissues and fluids except for CSF. Half-life with regular dosing is about 2 weeks.

ADMINISTRATION ALERTS

- Infuse slowly. Cardiovascular collapse may result when medication is infused too rapidly.
- Administer premedication to help decrease the chance of infusion reactions.
- Withhold drug if BUN exceeds 40 mg/dL or serum creatinine rises above 3 mg/dL.
- Amphotericin B is pregnancy category B.

ADVERSE EFFECTS AND INTERACTIONS

Amphotericin B can cause a number of serious side effects. Many clients develop fever and chills, vomiting, and headache at the beginning of therapy, which subside as treatment continues. Phlebitis is common during IV therapy. Some degree of nephrotoxicity is observed in most clients, and kidney function tests are normally performed throughout the treatment period.

Amphotericin B interacts with many drugs. For example, concurrent therapy with aminoglycosides, vancomycin, carboplatin, and furosemide, which reduce renal function, is not recommended. Use with corticosteroids, skeletal muscle relaxants, and thiazole may potentiate hypokalemia. If hypokalemia is present, use with digitalis increases the risk of digitalis toxicity.

See also "Nursing Process Focus: Clients Receiving Amphotericin B" opposite for specific points to include when teaching clients regarding this drug.

NURSING PROCESS FOCUS Clients Receiving Amphotericin B (Abelcet, others)	
Assessment	**Potential Nursing Diagnoses/Identified Patterns**
Prior to administration: ■ Obtain complete health history including allergies, drug history, and possible drug interactions. ■ Obtain culture and sensitivity of suspected area of infection to determine need for therapy. ■ Obtain baseline vital signs, especially pulse and blood pressure. ■ Obtain renal function including blood tests (CBC, chemistry panel, BUN, and creatinine).	■ Risk for infection related to drug-induced leukopenia ■ Impaired skin integrity ■ Need for knowledge regarding drug therapy and adverse effects ■ Safety from injury related to side effects of drug therapy

Planning: Client Goals and Expected Outcomes
The client will: ■ Report fewer symptoms of fungal infection ■ Demonstrate an understanding of the drug's action by accurately describing drug side effects and precautions ■ Immediately report effects such as fever, chills, fluid retention, dizziness, or decrease in urine output

Implementation	
Interventions (Rationales)	**Client Education/Discharge Planning**
■ Monitor vital signs, especially pulse and blood pressure, frequently during and after infusion. (Cardiovascular collapse may result when drug is infused too rapidly, which is caused by the drug binding to human cytoplasmic sterols.)	■ Advise client to report dizziness, shortness of breath, heart palpitations, or faintness immediately.
■ Monitor kidney function, including intake and output, urinalysis, and periodic blood work. (Amphotericin B is nephrotoxic. This medication is excreted in the urine and causes significant electrolyte loss from the kidneys.)	Instruct client to: ■ Keep all laboratory appointments for blood work (CBC, electrolytes every 2 weeks; BUN, creatinine weekly) ■ Keep an accurate record of intake and output ■ Drink at least 2.5 L of fluids daily ■ Report a decrease in urinary output, change in the appearance of urine, or weight gain or loss
■ Monitor for GI distress.	Instruct client to: ■ Take an antiemetic prior to drug therapy, if needed ■ Report GI distress such as anorexia, nausea, vomiting, extreme weight loss, and headache
■ Monitor for fluid overload and electrolyte imbalance. (Clients with cardiac disease are at high risk.) ■ Monitor for signs/symptoms of toxicity and hypersensitivity.	■ Advise clients with any form of cardiac disease to report any palpitations, chest pain, swelling of extremities, and shortness of breath. Instruct client to report the following: ■ IV: malaise, generalized pain, confusion, depression, hypotension tachycardia, respiratory failure, evidence of otoxicity such as hearing loss, tinnitus, vertigo, and unsteady gait ■ Topical: irritation, pruritus, dry skin, redness, burning, and itching
■ Monitor IV site frequently for any signs of extravasation. (Medication is irritating to the vein. Use a central line if possible.)	■ Advise client to report any pain at the IV site.

Evaluation of Outcome Criteria
Evaluate the effectiveness of drug therapy by confirming that client goals and expected outcomes have been met (see "Planning").

AZOLES

The azole drug class actually consists of two different chemical classes, the imidazoles and the triazoles. Azole antifungal drugs interfere with the biosynthesis of ergosterol, which is essential for fungal cell membranes. By depleting fungal cells of ergosterol, their growth is impaired. Several new azoles are in the final stages of clinical trials and should become available over the next few years.

33.5 Pharmacotherapy with the Azole Antifungals

Most azoles are given by the topical route, although fluconazole, itraconazole, and ketoconazole may be given orally or parenterally for systemic or superficial infections. Ketoconazole is only available orally, and it is the most hepatotoxic of the azoles. Itraconazole has begun to replace ketoconazole in the therapy of systemic mycoses because it has less hepatotoxicity and may be given either orally or intravenously. It also has a broader spectrum of activity than the other systemic azoles. Clotrimazole is a drug of choice for fungal infections of the skin, vagina, and mouth.

The systemic azole drugs have a spectrum of activity similar to that of amphotericin B, are considerably less toxic, and have the major advantage that they can be administered orally. Topical formulations are available for superficial mycoses, although they may also be given by the oral route for these infections. Common side effects of the oral and parenteral azoles include nausea, vomiting, diarrhea, and rash.

NURSING CONSIDERATIONS

The role of the nurse in azole therapy involves careful monitoring of the client's condition and providing education as it relates to the prescribed drug regimen. Prior to the initiation of pharmacotherapy, the client's health history should be taken. These drugs are contraindicated in clients with hypersensitivity to azole antifungals and should be used with caution in clients with renal impairment. Lab tests, including BUN, creatinine, and liver function tests, should be obtained before therapy begins and throughout the course of treatment. Ketoconazole should not be given to clients with chronic alcoholism because this drug can be toxic to the liver.

Because the azoles can cause GI side effects, assess for nausea, vomiting, abdominal pain, and diarrhea. Monitor for signs and symptoms of hepatotoxicity, such as pruritus, jaundice, dark urine, and skin rash. Azoles may affect glycemic control in diabetic clients, so blood sugar should be monitored carefully in these clients. Evaluate all other medications taken by the client for compatibility with antifungal drugs. Concurrent therapy with drugs that reduce liver or renal function is not recommended. Monitor for alcohol use as it increases the risk of side effects such as nausea and vomiting and increases blood pressure.

Client education as it relates to azole drugs should include goals, reasons for obtaining baseline data, and possible side effects. Instruct the client and caregivers to do the following:

- Complete the full course of treatment.
- Report the use of any other prescription or OTC medications.
- Avoid drinking alcohol due to its effects on the liver.
- Use effective contraception measures to prevent pregnancy.
- Monitor urinary output and drink plenty of fluids.
- Use caution while performing hazardous activities.
- Advise diabetic clients to increase blood glucose monitoring and report hypoglycemia.

DRUGS FOR SUPERFICIAL FUNGAL INFECTIONS

Superficial fungal infections are generally not severe. If possible, superficial infections are treated with topical agents because they are safer than their systemic counterparts. Agents used to treat superficial mycoses are shown in Table 33.3.

Pr PROTOTYPE DRUG | Fluconazole (Apo-Fluconazole, Diflucan)

ACTIONS AND USES

Like other azoles, fluconazole acts by inhibiting the synthesis of ergosterol. Fluconazole, however, offers several advantages over other systemic antifungals. It is rapidly and completely absorbed when given orally. Unlike itraconazole and ketoconazole, it is able to penetrate most body membranes to reach infections in the CNS, bone, eye, urinary tract, and respiratory tract.

A major disadvantage of fluconazole is its relatively narrow spectrum of activity. Although it is effective against *Candida albicans,* it may not be effective against other *Candida* species, which account for a significant percentage of opportunistic fungal infections.

PHARMACOKINETICS

Fluconazole is well absorbed after oral administration. It is widely distributed into CSF, crosses the placenta, and enters breast milk. About 80% is excreted unchanged in urine and the rest is metabolized in the liver. Half-life is 30 hours in adults and 24 hours in children.

ADMINISTRATION ALERTS

- Do not mix IV fluconazole with other drugs.
- Fluconazole is pregnancy category C.

ADVERSE EFFECTS AND INTERACTIONS

Fluconazole causes few serious side effects. Nausea, vomiting, and diarrhea are reported at high doses. Because most of the drug is excreted by the kidneys, it should be used cautiously in clients with pre-existing kidney disease. Unlike ketoconazole, hepatotoxicity with fluconazole is rare.

Fluconazole interacts with several drugs. Use with warfarin may cause increased risk for bleeding. Hypoglycemic reaction may be seen with oral sulfonylureas. Fluconazole levels may be decreased with concurrent rifampin or cimetidine use. The effects of fentanyl, alfentanil, and methadone may be prolonged with concurrent administration of fluconazole.

 See the Companion Website for a Nursing Process Focus Chart specific to this drug.

TABLE 33.3   Drugs for Superficial Mycoses

Drug	Route and Adult Dose)
butoconazole (Gynazole)	Topical; one applicator intravaginally hs for 3 d
ciclopirox olamine (Loprox)	Topical; apply bid for 4 wk
clotrimazole (Canesten, Lotriderm)	Topical; apply bid for 4 wk; for vaginal mycoses, insert one applicator intravaginally hs for 7 d
econazole (Ecostatin)	Topical; apply bid for 4 wk
fluconazole (Apo-Fluconazole, Diflucan)	PO/IV; 200–400 mg on day 1, then 100–200 mg qd for 2–4 wk
griseofulvin (Fulvicin)	PO; 500 mg microsize or 330–375 mg ultra microsize qd
itraconazole (Sporanox)	PO; 200 mg qd; may increase to 200 mg bid (max 400 mg/day)
ketoconazole (Nizoral)	Topical; apply qd–bid to affected area
miconazole (Micatin, Monistat)	Topical; apply bid for 2–4 wk
naftifine (Naftin)	Topical; apply cream qd or gel bid for 4 wk
nystatin (Nadostine, PMS-Nystatin)	PO; 500,000–1,000,000 units tid Intravaginal; one to two tablets daily for 2 wk
terbinafine (Apo-Terbinafine, Lamisil)	Topical; apply qd or bid for 7 wk
terconazole (Terazol)	Topical; insert one applicator intravaginally at hs for 3–7 wk
tolnaftate (Tinactin)	Topical; apply bid for 4–6 wk
undecylenic acid (Desenex, Fungicure)	Topical; apply qd–bid

NATURAL THERAPIES

Remedies for Fungal Infections

Several natural products are reported to have antifungal properties:

- Grape seed extract – taken from the seeds of the grape *Vitis vinifera*; capsules are used orally for 3 to 6 months
- Garlic – in capsule or liquid extract form
- Probiotics – bacteria that compete with the fungi for resources; refrigerated supplements that contain *Lactobacillus acidophilus* and *Bifidobacterium bifidum* are the most potent
- Astragalus root – in capsule and tincture form
- Tea tree oil and thyme oil – used externally for fungal infections of the skin; these oils are powerful and should be diluted with another oil such as olive oil

33.6 Superficial Fungal Infections

Superficial fungal infections of the hair, scalp, nails, and mucous membranes of the mouth and vagina are rarely medical emergencies. Infections of the nails and skin, for example, may be ongoing for months or even years before a client seeks treatment. Unlike systemic fungal infections, superficial infections may occur in any client, not just those who have suppressed immune systems. About 75% of all female clients experience vulvovaginal candidiasis at least once in their lifetime.

Superficial antifungal drugs are much safer than their systemic counterparts because penetration into the deeper layers of the skin is generally poor and only small amounts are absorbed. Many are available as OTC creams, gels, and ointments. If the infection has grown into the deeper skin layers, oral antifungal drugs may be indicated. Extensive superficial mycoses are often treated with oral antifungal drugs along with the topical agents to be certain that the infection is eliminated.

Selection of a particular antifungal agent is based on the location of the infection and characteristics of the lesion. Griseofulvin is an inexpensive, older agent that is indicated for the oral therapy of mycoses of the hair, skin, and nails that have not responded to conventional topical preparations. Itraconazole and terbinafine are oral preparations that have the advantage of accumulating in nail beds, allowing them to remain active many months after therapy is discontinued.

Although nystatin belongs to the same chemical class as amphotericin B, the **polyenes**, nystatin is available in a wider variety of formulations, including cream, ointment, powder, tablet, and lozenge. Too toxic for parenteral administration, it is primarily used topically for *Candida* infections of the vagina, skin, and mouth. When given topically, nystatin produces few adverse effects other than minor skin irritation. It may also be used orally to treat candidiasis of the intestine because it travels through the GI tract without being absorbed. When given orally, it may cause diarrhea, nausea, and vomiting.

NURSING CONSIDERATIONS

The role of the nurse in superficial antifungal therapy involves careful monitoring of the client's condition and providing education as it relates to the prescribed drug regimen. Prior to the initiation of therapy with antifungals, the client's health history should be obtained. Assess for signs of contact dermatitis; if this is present, the drug should be withheld and the physician notified.

Pr PROTOTYPE DRUG | Nystatin (Nadostine, PMS-Nystatin)

ACTIONS AND USES

Nystatin binds to sterols in the fungal cell membrane, allowing leakage of intracellular contents as the membrane becomes weakened. Although it belongs to the same chemical class as amphotericin B, the polyenes, nystatin is available in a wider variety of formulations, including cream, ointment, powder, tablet, and lozenge. It is too toxic for parenteral administration and is primarily used topically for *Candida* infections of the vagina, skin, and mouth. It may also be used orally to treat candidiasis of the intestine because it travels through the GI tract without being absorbed.

PHARMACOKINETICS

Nystatin is poorly absorbed after oral administration. Distribution is unknown. It has a rapid onset and duration of about 2 hours when administered locally.

ADMINISTRATION ALERTS

- Apply with a swab to affected area in infants and children as swishing is difficult or impossible.
- Nystatin is pregnancy category C.

ADVERSE EFFECTS AND INTERACTIONS

When given topically, nystatin produces few adverse effects other than minor skin irritation. There is a high incidence of contact dermatitis, which is related to the preservatives found in many of the formulations.

When given orally, it may cause diarrhea, nausea, and vomiting.

 See the Companion Website for a Nursing Process Focus Chart specific to this drug.

Superficial antifungals, such as nystatin, should not be used vaginally during pregnancy to treat infections caused by *Gardnerella vaginalis* or *Trichomonas* species. They should be used with caution in clients who are lactating.

There are few side effects to antifungals used for superficial mycoses. The medications may be "swished and swallowed" when used to treat oral candidiasis. Monitor for side effects such as nausea, vomiting, and diarrhea when the client is taking high doses. If GI side effects are especially disturbing, the client should be advised to spit out the medication rather than swallowing it. Some orders will be to "swish only" and then to spit out the medication. Monitor for signs of improvement in the mouth and on the tongue to evaluate the effectiveness of the medication.

Client education as it relates to superficial antifungal drugs should include goals, reasons for obtaining baseline data, and possible side effects. Instruct the client and caregivers to do the following:

- Complete the full course of treatment; some infections require pharmacotherapy for several months.

- If self-treating with OTC preparations, follow the directions carefully and notify the healthcare provider if symptoms do not resolve in 7 to 10 days.
- Abstain from sexual intercourse during treatment for vaginal infections.
- Teach clients with vaginal candidiasis the correct method for using vaginal suppositories, creams, and ointments.

See also "Nursing Process Focus: Clients Receiving Pharmacotherapy for Superficial Fungal Infections" for specific points to include when teaching clients regarding this class of drugs.

PROTOZOAN INFECTIONS

Protozoans are single-celled animals. Although only a few of the more than 20,000 species cause disease in humans, they have a significant health impact in Africa, South America, and Asia. Travellers to these continents may acquire these infections overseas and bring them back to the United States and Canada. These parasites often thrive in

---

NURSING PROCESS FOCUS   Clients Receiving Pharmacotherapy for Superficial Fungal Infections

Assessment	Potential Nursing Diagnoses/Identified Patterns
Prior to administration: - Obtain complete health history including allergies, drug history, and possible drug interactions. - Obtain culture and sensitivity of suspected area of infection to determine need for therapy. - Obtain baseline liver function tests.	- Risk for impaired skin integrity (rash) - Need for knowledge regarding drug therapy and adverse effects - Safety from injury related to side effects of drug therapy

Planning: Client Goals and Expected Outcomes
The client will: - Report healing of fungal infection - Demonstrate an understanding of the drug's action by accurately describing drug side effects and precautions - Immediately report adverse effects such as hepatoxicity, GI distress, rash, or decreased urine output

continued

NURSING PROCESS FOCUS   Clients Receiving Pharmacotherapy for Superficial Fungal Infections

Implementation

Interventions (Rationales)	Client Education/Discharge Planning
■ Monitor for possible side effects or hypersensitivity.	Instruct client to report: ■ Burning, stinging, dryness, itching, erythema, urticaria, angioedema, and local irritation for superficial drugs ■ Symptoms of hepatic toxicity—jaundice, dark urine, light-coloured stools, and pruritis ■ Nausea, vomiting, and diarrhea ■ Signs and symptoms of hypo- or hyperglycemia
■ Encourage adherence with instructions for taking oral antifungals (to increase medication effectiveness).	Instruct client to: ■ Swish the oral suspension to coat all mucous membrane, then swallow medication ■ Spit out medication instead of swallowing if GI irritation occurs ■ Allow troche to dissolve completely, rather than chewing or swallowing; it may take 30 minutes for it to completely dissolve ■ Avoid food or drink for 30 minutes following administration ■ Remove dentures prior to using the oral suspension ■ Take ketoconazole with water, fruit juice, coffee, or tea to enhance dissolution and absorption
■ Monitor topical application.	■ Instruct client to avoid wearing tight-fitting undergarments if using ointment in the vaginal or groin area.
■ Avoid occlusive dressings. (Dressings increase moisture in the infected area and encourage development of additional yeast infections.)	■ Instruct client to report any redness or skin rash.
■ Monitor for contact dermatitis with topical formulations. (This is related to the preservatives found in many of the formulations.) ■ Encourage infection control practices (to prevent the spread of infection).	Instruct client to: ■ Clean affected area daily ■ Apply medication with a glove ■ Wash hands properly before and after application ■ Change socks daily if rash is on feet

Evaluation of Outcome Criteria

Evaluate the effectiveness of drug therapy by confirming that client goals and expected outcomes have been met (see "Planning").

See Table 33.3, as well as the oral and topical systemic drugs in Table 33.2 (page 447), for a list of drugs to which these nursing actions apply.

conditions where sanitation and personal hygiene are poor and population density is high. In addition, protozoan infections often occur in clients who are immunocompro-mised, such as those in the advanced stages of AIDS. The most common protozoan disease in humans is malaria. Drugs for malarial infections are shown in Table 33.4.

TABLE 33.4   Drugs for Malaria

Drug	Route and Adult Dose)
atovaquone (Mepron)	PO; 750 mg bid for 21 d
hydroxychloroquine sulfate (Apo-Hydroxychloroquine, Plaquenil) (see page 666 for the Prototype Drug box)	PO; 620 mg initial dose, then 310 mg weekly
mefloquine (Apo-Mefloquine, Lariam)	PO; prevention: begin 250 mg once a week for 4 wk, then 250 mg every other week; treatment: 1250 mg as a single dose
primaquine	PO; 15 mg qd for 2 wk
atovaquone/proguanil (Malarone)	PO; atovaquone 250 mg plus proguanil 100 mg daily taken at least 24 hr before arrival in endemic area and 1 wk after leaving
pyrimethamine (Daraprim)	PO; 25 mg once per week for 10 wk
quinine (Apo-Quinine)	PO; 260–650 mg tid for 3 d; IV for severe malaria

33.7 Pharmacotherapy of Malaria

Drug therapy of protozoan infections is difficult due to the animals' complicated life cycles. When faced with adverse conditions, protozoans can form cysts that allow the animal to survive in harsh environments and infect other hosts. When cysts occur inside the host, the parasite is often resistant to pharmacotherapy. With few exceptions, antibiotics, antifungals, and antiviral drugs are ineffective against protozoans.

Malaria is caused by four species of the protozoan *Plasmodium*. Malaria is the second most common fatal infectious disease in the world, with 300 to 500 million cases occurring annually. Although an average of only 538 cases are treated per year in Canada, increased immigration and foreign travel have resulted in a gradual increase in cases.

Malaria begins with a bite from an infected female *Anopheles* mosquito. Once inside the human host, *Plasmodium* multiplies in the liver and transforms into progeny called **merozoites**. About 14 to 25 days after the initial infection, the merozoites are released into the blood. The merozoites infect red blood cells, which eventually rupture, releasing more merozoites and causing severe fever and chills. This is called the **erythrocytic stage** of the infection. *Plasmodium* can remain in body tissues for extended periods and cause relapses months, or even years, after the initial infection. The life cycle of *Plasmodium* is shown in Figure 33.1.

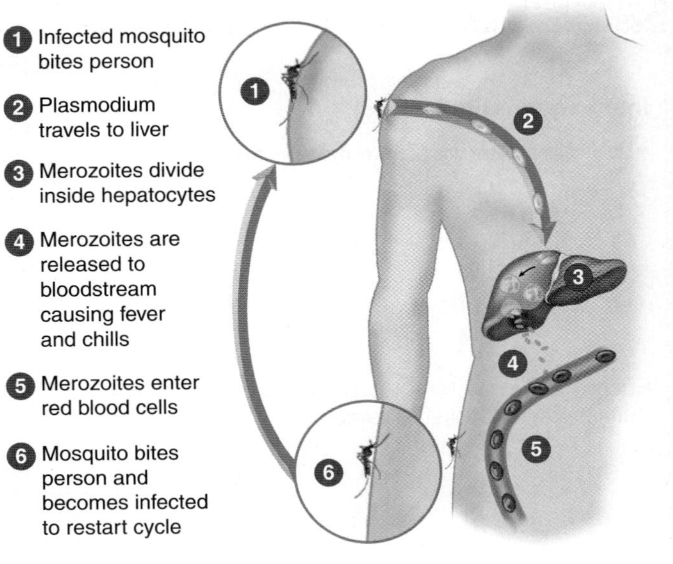

Pharmacotherapy of malaria attempts to interrupt the complex life cycle of *Plasmodium*. Although successful early in the course of the disease, therapy becomes increasingly difficult as the parasite enters different stages of its life cycle. Goals of antimalarial therapy include prevention of the disease, treatment of acute attacks, and prevention of relapses.

Prevention of malaria is the best therapeutic option because the disease is very difficult to treat after it has been acquired. Staying indoors from dusk to dawn when mosquitoes are biting most, wearing long-sleeved shirts and long pants, sleeping under a mosquito net, and using DEET-based insect repellents are recommended. Health Canada recommends that travellers to endemic areas receive prophylactic antimalarial drugs prior to and during their visit and for 1 to 4 weeks after leaving, depending on the specific drug. Because resistance has become a major problem in many regions of the world, in 2001 the World Health Organization (WHO) recommended the use of artemisinin-based combination therapies (ACTs) in order to ensure high cure rates of *Plasmodium falciparum* malaria and to reduce the spread of drug resistance. In 2005, WHO called on all countries to develop combination drug therapies and begin the process of withdrawing monotherapies. Atovaquone/proguanil (Malarone) is a combination of two antimalarial drugs that is taken daily. It recently became available in Canada for treatment of malaria and prevention of chloroquine-resistant malaria. It is useful for those making short trips into malaria risk areas.

During treatment of acute attacks, drugs are used to interrupt the erythrocytic stage and eliminate the merozoites

1. Infected mosquito bites person
2. Plasmodium travels to liver
3. Merozoites divide inside hepatocytes
4. Merozoites are released to bloodstream causing fever and chills
5. Merozoites enter red blood cells
6. Mosquito bites person and becomes infected to restart cycle

● **Figure 33.1** Life cycle of *Plasmodium*

from red blood cells. Treatment is most successful if begun immediately after symptoms are recognized. Parenteral quinine is the drug of choice in Canada for the treatment of severe and complicated malaria. The Canadian Malaria Network was established to provide 24-hour access to this life-saving drug for persons with severe malaria. It also gathers surveillance data to improve the prevention, diagnosis, and management of malaria in Canada.

In order to prevent relapse, drugs are given to eliminate the latent forms of *Plasmodium* residing in the liver. Primaquine phosphate is one of the few drugs able to affect a total cure.

NURSING CONSIDERATIONS

The role of the nurse in antimalarial therapy involves careful monitoring of the client's condition and providing education as it relates to the prescribed drug regimen. Prior to the initiation of drug therapy, the client's health history should be taken. Those with hematological disorders and severe skin disorders such as psoriasis and those who are pregnant should not take antimalarial drugs. These drugs should be used cautiously in clients with pre-existing cardiovascular disease and those who are lactating.

Initial lab work should include CBC, liver and renal function tests, and a test for G6PD deficiency. Chloroquine may precipitate anemia in those with G6PD deficiency; furthermore, it concentrates in the erythrocytes and leukocytes and may cause bone marrow depression. A baseline ECG should be taken because of potential cardiac complications associated with some antimalarial drugs. Other baseline information should include vital signs, especially temperature and blood pressure, and hearing and vision testing. All other medication taken by the client should be fully evaluated for compatibility with antimalarial medications as drug-drug interactions are common.

During treatment, all vital signs should be closely monitored and periodic ECGs and CBCs should be obtained. Especially monitor for GI side effects such as vomiting, diarrhea, and abdominal pain; oral antimalarial drugs can be given with food to reduce GI distress. Assess for signs of allergic reaction, such as flushing, rashes, edema, and pruritus. Monitor for signs of toxicity, which include ringing in the ears with quinine and severe cardiac complications and/or CNS complications such as seizures and blurred vision.

Client education as it relates to antimalarial drugs should include goals, reasons for obtaining baseline data, and possible side effects. Instruct the client and caregivers to do the following:

- Complete the full course of treatment.
- Take with food to decrease GI upset.
- Change position slowly to decrease postural hypotension.
- Use effective contraception measures to prevent pregnancy.
- Abstain from alcohol.
- Do not perform hazardous tasks until the effects of the drug are known.
- Report significant side effects such as flushing, rashes, edema, itching, ringing in the ears, blurred vision, and seizures.

33.8 Pharmacotherapy of Non-Malarial Protozoan Infections

Although infection by *Plasmodium* is the most significant protozoan disease worldwide, infections caused by other protozoans affect significant numbers of people in endemic areas. These infections include amebiasis, toxoplasmosis, giardiasis, cryptosporidiosis, trichomoniasis, trypanosomiasis, and leishmaniasis. Like *Plasmodium*, the non-malarial protozoan infections occur more frequently in areas where public sanitation is poor and population density is high. Several of these infections occur in severely immunocompromised clients. Each of the organisms has unique differences in its distribution pattern and physiology. Descriptions of common non-malarial protozoan infections are given in Table 33.5.

One such protozoan infection, amebiasis, affects over 50 million people and causes 100,000 deaths worldwide. Caused by the protozoan *Entamoeba histolytica*, amebiasis is common in Africa, Latin America, and Asia. Although primarily a disease of the large intestine, where it causes ulcers, *E. histolytica* can invade the liver and create abscesses. The primary symptom of amebiasis is amebic **dysentery**, a severe form of diarrhea. Drugs used to treat amebiasis include those that act directly on amebas in the intestine and those that are administered for their systemic effects on the liver and other organs. Drugs for non-malarial protozoan infections are shown in Table 33.6.

NURSING CONSIDERATIONS

The role of the nurse in non-malarial antiprotozoan therapy involves careful monitoring of the client's condition and providing education as it relates to the prescribed drug regimen. Prior to the initiation of drug therapy, the client's health history should be taken. Antiprotozoan therapy is contraindicated in clients with blood dyscrasias and active organic disease of the CNS and during the first month of pregnancy. These drugs are contraindicated in alcoholics; the medication is not administered until more than 24 hours after the client's last drink of alcohol. It should be used cautiously in clients with peripheral neuropathy or pre-existing liver disease. These drugs should be used cautiously in clients who have a history of bone marrow depression because of the possibility of leukopenia. Safety and efficacy have not been established in children.

Initial lab work should include CBC and thyroid and liver function tests. Baseline vital signs should be obtained. Evaluate all other drugs taken by the client for compatibility with antiprotozoan drugs. Closely monitor vital signs and thyroid function during therapy because serum iodine may increase and cause thyroid enlargement with iodoquinol.

TABLE 33.5 Non-Malarial Protozoan Infections

Name of Protozoan	Description of Disease
Cryptosporidium (various species)	cryptosporidiosis: primarily a disease of the intestines; often seen in immunocompromised clients
Entamoeba histolytica	amebiasis: primarily a disease of the large intestine that may cause liver abscesses; rarely travels to other organs such as the brain, lungs, or kidney
Giardia lamblia	giardiasis: primarily a disease of the intestines that may cause malabsorption, gas, and abdominal distension
Leishmania (various species)	leishmaniasis: affects various body systems including the skin, liver, spleen, or blood depending on the species
Pneumocystis carinii	pneumocystosis: primarily causes pneumonia in immunocompromised patients
Toxoplasma gondii	toxoplasmosis: causes a fatal encephalitis in immunocompromised patients
Trichomonas vaginalis	trichomoniasis: causes inflammation of the vagina and urethra and is spread through sexual contact
Trypanosoma brucei	trypanosomiasis: the African form, known as sleeping sickness, causes CNS depression in severe infections; the American form, known as Chagas disease, invades cardiac tissue

TABLE 33.6	Drugs for Non-Malarial Protozoan Infections
Drug	**Route and Adult Dose**
metronidazole (Apo-Metronidazole, Flagyl)	PO; 250–750 mg tid
pentamidine (Pentacarinat, Pneumopent)	IV; 4 mg/kg qd for 14–21 days; infuse over 60 min
tetracycline (Sumycin) and doxycycline (Vibramycin)	PO; 250–500 mg bid–qid (1–2 g/d) IM; 250 mg qd or 300 mg qd in two to three divided doses

MediaLink World Health Organization

Monitor for GI distress; oral medications can be given with food to decrease unpleasant effects. Clients taking metronidazole may complain of dryness of mouth and a metallic taste. Monitor for CNS toxicity such as seizures, paresthesia, nausea, and vomiting and for allergic responses such as urticaria and pruritus.

Client education as it relates to non-malarial antiprotozoan drug therapy should include goals, reasons for obtaining baseline data, and possible side effects. Instruct the client and caregivers to do the following:

- Complete the full course of treatment.
- Take with food to decrease GI upset.
- Use effective contraception measures to prevent pregnancy.
- Avoid using hepatotoxic drugs, including alcohol, which may cause an disulfiram-like reaction.
- Recognize that urine may turn reddish-brown as an effect of the medication.
- Have any sexual partners treated concurrently to prevent re-infection.

- Immediately report seizures, numbness in limbs, nausea, vomiting, hives, or itching.

SPECIAL CONSIDERATIONS

Parasitic Infections in Children

Many parasitic infections are common among children, with the national rates highest in children less than 5 years of age. In public health labs, the most commonly diagnosed intestinal parasite is giardiasis. These cases are usually associated with water-related activities such as swimming and possibly the use of diapers.

Children adopted from Asian countries, Central and South America, and Eastern Europe also have a high rate of parasitic infection. Up to 35% of foreign-born adopted children are reported to be infected with *Giardia lamblia*. Environments in which these children have been living, particularly those from orphanages, often provide favourable conditions for infectious disease. The Centers for Disease Control and Prevention (CDC) recommends that internationally adopted children undergo examination of at least one stool sample, and three stool samples if GI symptoms are present. Unfortunately, evidence has shown that in communities where helminthic infections are common, poor nutritional status, anemia, and impaired growth and learning in children result.

Pr PROTOTYPE DRUG | Metronidazole (Apo-Metronidazole, Flagyl)

ACTIONS AND USES

Metronidazole is the prototype drug for most forms of amebiasis, being effective against both the intestinal and hepatic stages of the disease. Resistant forms of *E. histolytica* have not yet emerged with metronidazole. The drug is unique among antiprotozoan drugs in that it also has antibiotic activity against anaerobic bacteria and thus is used to treat a number of respiratory, bone, skin, and CNS infections. Metronidazole is a drug of choice for two other protozoan infections: giardiasis and trichomoniasis. It is used for *Helicobacter pylori* infections of the stomach. It is also used prophylactically in colorectal surgery. Topical forms of this agent are used to treat rosacea, a disease characterized by skin reddening and hyperplasia of the sebaceous glands, particularly around the nose and face.

PHARMACOKINETICS

Metronidazole is about 80% absorbed after oral administration. It is widely distributed. It crosses the placenta and enters breast milk and the CSF. It is partially metabolized by the liver and partially excreted unchanged in urine and feces. Half-life is 6 to 12 hours.

ADMINISTRATION ALERTS

- Extended-release form must be swallowed whole.
- Metronidazole is contraindicated during the first trimester of pregnancy.
- Metronidazole is pregnancy category B.
- Abstain from using alcohol

ADVERSE EFFECTS AND INTERACTIONS

The most common side effects of metronidazole are anorexia, nausea, diarrhea, dizziness, and headache. Dryness of the mouth and an unpleasant metallic taste may be experienced. Although side effects are relatively common, most are not serious enough to cause discontinuation of therapy.

Metronidazole interacts with several drugs. For example, oral anticoagulants potentiate hypoprothrombinemia. In combination with alcohol, metronidazole may elicit a disulfiram-like reaction. This would include other medications that may contain alcohol. The drug also may elevate lithium levels.

 See the Companion Website for a Nursing Process Focus Chart specific to this drug.

NURSING PROCESS FOCUS Clients Receiving Metronidazole (Apo-Metronidazole, Flagyl)	
Assessment	**Potential Nursing Diagnoses/Identified Patterns**
Prior to administration: ■ Obtain complete health history including allergies, drug and herbal history, and possible drug interactions. ■ Obtain results from serological studies, stool samples, or cultures of the suspected area of infection to determine the need for therapy. ■ Obtain baseline vital signs, especially pulse and blood pressure. ■ Obtain complete blood count.	■ Nutritional adequacy ■ Risk for injury related to dizziness secondary to side effect of drug ■ Discomfort ■ Risk for dehydration and altered nutrition related to nausea and vomiting secondary to side effect of drug ■ Need for knowledge regarding drug therapy and adverse effects ■ Safety from injury related to side effects of drug therapy

Planning: Client Goals and Expected Outcomes
The client will: ■ Report decreased signs and symptoms of amebic or other infection ■ Demonstrate an understanding of the drug's action by accurately describing drug side effects and precautions ■ Immediately report effects such as seizures, numbness in limbs, nausea, vomiting, hives, or itching

Implementation	
Interventions (Rationales)	**Client Education/Discharge Planning**
■ Monitor complete blood count periodically. (The drug may cause leukopenia.) ■ Encourage treatment of sexual partner. (Asymptomatic trichomoniasis in the male is a frequent source of reinfection.) ■ Monitor use of alcohol. (Metronidazole interferes with the metabolism of alcohol.) ■ Monitor CNS toxicity. (High doses may cause seizures and peripheral neuropathy possibly related to the medication's distribution into the CSF.) ■ Monitor for allergic reactions. ■ Monitor for gastrointestinal distress. (This is the most common adverse effect.)	■ Instruct client to notify the healthcare provider of fever or other signs of infection. ■ Instruct client that simultaneous treatment of a sexual partner is necessary. Instruct client to: ■ Abstain from alcohol including any OTC medication that contains alcohol (liquid cough and cold products) ■ Report side effects such as cramping, vomiting, flushing, and headache, which may result with alcohol use ■ Instruct client to immediately report seizures, numbness of limbs, nausea, and vomiting. ■ Instruct client to immediately report hives and itching, rash, flushing, fever, and/or joint pain. Instruct client to: ■ Take medication with food to decrease gastrointestinal distress ■ Recognize that medication may cause a metallic taste in the mouth

Evaluation of Outcome Criteria
Evaluate the effectiveness of drug therapy by confirming that client goals and expected outcomes have been met (see "Planning").

DRUGS FOR HELMINTHIC INFECTIONS

Helminths consist of various species of parasitic worms that have more complex anatomy, physiology, and life cycles than the protozoans. Diseases due to these pathogens affect more than 2 billion people worldwide and are quite common in areas lacking high standards of sanitation. Helminthic infections in the United States and Canada are neither common nor fatal, although drug therapy may be indicated. Drugs for helminthic infections are shown in Table 33.7.

TABLE 33.7 Drugs for Helminthic Infections	
Drug	*Route and Adult Dose*
mebendazole (Vermox)	PO; 100 mg for one dose or 100 mg bid for 3 d
praziquantel (Biltricide)	PO; 5 mg/kg for one dose or 25 mg/kg tid
pyrantel (Antiminth)	PO; 11 mg/kg for one dose (max 1 g)

Prevention of Childhood Helminthic Infections

Pinworms and roundworms (helminths) are more commonly seen in children because many of their hygiene and play habits contribute to transmission and re-infestation. Instruct parents and family members about ways to prevent exposure to and spread of helminths. Teach children correct handwashing techniques, emphasizing cleaning under the nails and washing before eating, after using the toilet, and after playing with pets. Discourage placing the fingers in the mouth, biting nails, and scratching the anal area. Children should wear shoes when playing outside. Avoid use of sandboxes that are accessed by dogs or cats; keep sandboxes covered when not in use. Clean all fruits and vegetables before eating. Keep diapers and undergarments clean and dry.

33.9 Pharmacotherapy of Helminthic Infections

Helminths are classified as roundworms (nematodes), flukes (trematodes), or tapeworms (cestodes). The most common helminthic disease worldwide is caused by the roundworm *Ascaris lumbricoides*; however, infection by the pinworm *Enterobius vermicularis* is more common in North America. Drugs used to treat these infections are called anthelmintics.

Like protozoans, helminths have several stages in their life cycle, which includes immature and mature forms. Typically, the immature forms of helminths enter the body through the skin or digestive tract. Most attach to the human intestinal tract, although some form cysts in skeletal muscle or in organs such as the liver.

Pharmacotherapy is not indicated for all helminthic infections because the adult parasites often die without re-infecting the host. When the infestation is severe or complications occur, pharmacotherapy is initiated. Complications caused by extensive infections may include physical obstruction in the intestine, malabsorption, increased risk for secondary bacterial infections, and severe fatigue.

Pharmacotherapy is aimed at eradicating the parasites locally in the intestine and systemically in the tissues and organs they have invaded. Some anthelmintics are effective against multiple organisms, whereas others are specific for a certain species.

NURSING CONSIDERATIONS

The role of the nurse in anthelmintic therapy involves careful monitoring of the client's condition and providing education as it relates to the prescribed drug regimen. Prior to the initiation of drug therapy, the client's health history should be taken. Anthelmintic therapy should be used cautiously in clients who are pregnant or lactating, have pre-existing liver disease, or are under the age of 2 years.

Initial lab tests should include a CBC and liver function studies. A stool specimen is obtained for verification and identification of the parasite and to determine the need for therapy. Other baseline information should include vital signs. Evaluate all other medications taken by the client for compatibility with anthelmintic drugs.

Closely monitor lab results and vital signs during therapy. Cases of leukopenia, thrombocytopenia, and agranulocytosis have been associated with the use of albendazole. Assessment of the client's health habits and living conditions should be done to locate and treat others that may be exposed and to identify means to prevent re-infection.

Monitor for GI symptoms such as abdominal pain and distension and diarrhea because these symptoms may occur as worms die. Such side effects are likely to occur more frequently in clients with Crohn's disease and ulcerative colitis because of the inflammatory process in the intestine. The nurse must monitor for CNS side effects such as drowsiness with thiabendazole. Allergic responses include urticaria and pruritus.

Client education as it relates to anthelmintic drug therapy should include goals, reasons for obtaining baseline data,

---

Pr **PROTOTYPE DRUG** | Mebendazole (Vermox)

ACTIONS AND USES

Mebendazole is used in the treatment of a wide range of helminthic infections, including those caused by roundworm (*Ascaris*) and pinworm (*Enterobiasis*) species. As a broad-spectrum drug, it is particularly valuable in mixed helminthic infections. It is effective against both the adult and larval stages of these parasites.

PHARMACOKINETICS

Mebendazole is poorly absorbed after oral administration, which allows it to retain high concentrations in the intestine. For pinworm infections, a single dose is usually sufficient; other infections require 3 days of therapy. Half-life is 3 to 9 hours.

ADMINISTRATION ALERTS

- Drug is most effective when chewed and taken with a fatty meal.
- Mebendazole is pregnancy category C.

ADVERSE EFFECTS AND INTERACTIONS

Because so little of the drug is absorbed, mebendazole does not generally cause serious systemic side effects. As the worms die, some abdominal pain and distension and diarrhea may be experienced.

Carbamazepine and phenytoin can increase the metabolism of mebendazole.

 See the Companion Website for a Nursing Process Focus Chart specific to this drug.

and possible side effects. Instruct the client and caregivers to do the following:

- Complete the full course of treatment.
- Use effective contraception measures to prevent pregnancy during therapy.

- Avoid hazardous activities until the effects of the drug are known.
- Concurrently treat those having close contact with the client in order to prevent re-infection.
- Report significant side effects such as itching and hives.

NURSING PROCESS FOCUS Clients Receiving Mebendazole (Vermox)

Assessment	Potential Nursing Diagnoses/Identified Patterns
Prior to administration: ■ Obtain complete health history including allergies, drug history, and possible drug interactions. ■ Obtain a stool specimen for verification of parasite and need for therapy. ■ Obtain complete blood count. ■ Assess the client's living situation, including number of individuals in close contact with the client.	■ Abdominal pain related to side effect of drug ■ Risk for dehydration related to diarrhea secondary to drug therapy ■ Need for knowledge regarding drug therapy and adverse effects

Planning: Client Goals and Expected Outcomes

The client will:
- Report decreased signs and symptoms of parasitic infection
- Demonstrate an understanding of the drug's action by accurately describing drug side effects and precautions
- Immediately report effects such as itching, hives, diarrhea, and fever

Implementation

Interventions (Rationales)	Client Education/Discharge Planning
■ Monitor stools (to assess effectiveness of drug therapy). ■ Monitor for side effects. ■ Monitor complete blood count. (Thrombocytopenia, reversible neutropenia, and leukopenia may occur during therapy.) ■ Monitor for pregnancy. (Even one dose of this medication during the first trimester has been shown to cause fetal damage.) ■ Monitor self-administration of medication, including chewing tablets or crushing and mixing with fatty foods. (Drug is most effective when taken with fatty foods, which increase absorption.) ■ Evaluate health habits. (Lifestyle changes may be required to prevent the spread of infestation and prevent future infections.)	■ Instruct client to bring stool sample to lab for testing. ■ Instruct client to report transient abdominal pain, diarrhea, and fever. ■ Instruct client to report any bleeding or signs of infection. Instruct client to: ■ Use effective birth control during drug therapy ■ Notify healthcare provider of any signs or suspicion of pregnancy ■ Instruct client that tablets can be chewed, swallowed, or crushed and mixed with food, especially fatty foods such as cheese or ice cream. Instruct client: ■ That all family members should be treated at the same time to prevent re-infection ■ To wash all fruits and vegetables and to cook meat thoroughly ■ To carefully wash hands with soap and water before and after eating and toileting ■ To wash toilet seats with disinfectant ■ To keep nails clean and out of mouth ■ To wear tight underwear and change daily ■ To sleep alone and wash bedding ■ That it is extremely important to complete the entire course of drug therapy

Evaluation of Outcome Criteria

Evaluate the effectiveness of drug therapy by confirming that client goals and expected outcomes have been met (see "Planning").

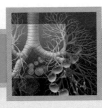

CHAPTER REVIEW

KEY CONCEPTS

The numbered key concepts provide a succinct summary of the important points from the corresponding numbered section within the chapter. If any of these points are not clear, refer to the numbered section within the chapter for review. Expanded versions can be found on the Companion Website.

33.1 Fungi are more complex than bacteria and require special classes of drugs because they are unaffected by antibiotics.

33.2 Fungal infections are classified as either superficial, affecting hair, skin, nails, and mucous membranes, or systemic, affecting internal organs.

33.3 Antifungal medications act by disrupting aspects of growth or metabolism that are unique to these organisms.

33.4 Amphotericin B is a drug of choice for serious fungal infections of internal organs. Systemic mycoses affect the internal organs and may require prolonged and aggressive drug therapy.

33.5 The azole drugs have become widely used in the pharmacotherapy of both systemic and superficial mycoses due to their favourable safety profile.

33.6 Antifungal drugs to treat superficial mycoses may be given topically or orally. They are safe and effective in treating infections of the skin, nails, and mucous membranes.

33.7 Malaria is the most common protozoal disease and requires multidrug therapy due to the complicated life cycle of the parasite and to reduce resistance.

33.8 Treatment of non-malarial protozoan disease generally requires a different set of medications than those used for malaria. Other common protozoal diseases that may be indications for pharmacotherapy include amebiasis, toxoplasmosis, giardiasis, cryptosporidiosis, trichomoniasis, trypanosomiasis, and leishmaniasis.

33.9 Helminths are parasitic worms that cause significant disease in certain regions of the world. The goals of pharmacotherapy are to kill the parasites locally and to disrupt their life cycle.

REVIEW QUESTIONS

1. Explain how antibacterial pharmacotherapy differs from antifungal and antiparasitic drug therapy.

2. How do most clients in Canada and the United States acquire protozoan infections?

3. Why is knowledge of a parasite's life cycle important to selecting the proper medication?

CRITICAL THINKING QUESTIONS

1. A nurse is caring for a severely immunosuppressed client who is on IV amphotericin B (Fungizone). The nurse understands that this medication is highly toxic to the client. What are three priority nursing assessment areas for clients on this medication?

2. A young female client has been given a prescription for metronidazole (Flagyl) for a vaginal yeast infection. What is a priority of teaching for this client?

3. A client is travelling to Africa for 3 months and is requesting a prescription for atovaquone (Mepron) to prevent malaria. What premedication assessment must be done for this client?

EXPLORE
MediaLink

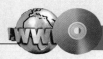 **www.pearsoned.ca/adams-king**

 MEDIALINK DVD-ROM
- **Audio Glossary**
- **CRNE Review**
- **Animation**
  Mechanism of Action: Fluconazole

 COMPANION WEBSITE
- **CRNE Review**
- **Case Study:** Client with oropharyngeal candidiasis treated with fluconazole
- **Dosage Calculations**

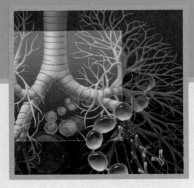

CHAPTER 34

Drugs for Viral Infections

DRUGS AT A GLANCE

AGENTS FOR HIV-AIDS

Nucleoside and nucleotide reverse transcriptase inhibitors

    zidovudine (Novo-AZT, Retrovir)

Non-nucleoside reverse transcriptase inhibitors

    nevirapine (Viramune)

Protease inhibitors

    saquinavir (Invirase)

Fusion inhibitors

AGENTS FOR HERPES VIRUSES

    acyclovir (Zovirax)

AGENTS FOR INFLUENZA

AGENTS FOR HEPATITIS

Interferons
Non-interferons

OBJECTIVES

After reading this chapter, the student should be able to do the following:

1. Identify drug classes used for treating viral diseases.
2. Explain the therapeutic action of each class of antiretroviral and antiviral drug in relation to the pathophysiology of viral diseases.
3. Explain the purpose and expected outcomes of HIV pharmacotherapy.
4. Explain the advantages of HAART in the pharmacotherapy of HIV infection.
5. Discuss the role of the nurse regarding the non-pharmacological management of viral diseases through client teaching.
6. Describe the nurse's role in the pharmacological management of clients receiving antiretroviral and antiviral drugs.
7. For each of the drug classes listed in Drugs at a Glance, identify a representative drug and explain its mechanism of action, therapeutic effects, and important adverse effects.
8. Describe and explain, based on pharmacological principles, the rationale for nursing assessment, planning, and interventions for clients receiving antiretroviral and antiviral drugs.
9. Use the nursing process to care for clients receiving antiretroviral and antiviral drugs.

MediaLink

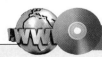

www.pearsoned.ca/adams-king

CRNE review, case studies, and other interactive resources for this chapter can be found on the Companion Website at **www.pearsoned.ca/adams-king.** Click on "Chapter 34" to select the activities for this chapter. For animations, more CRNE review questions, and an audio glossary, access the accompanying DVD-ROM in this textbook.

Viruses are microscopic infectious agents capable of causing disease in humans and other organisms. After infecting an organism, viruses use host enzymes and cellular structures to replicate. Although the number of antiviral drugs has increased dramatically in recent years due to research into the AIDS epidemic, antivirals remain the least effective of all the anti-infective drug classes.

PHARMFACTS

Viral Diseases

- In Canada, more than 28,000 new cases of sexually transmitted infections (STIs) are reported annually.
- Most STIs occur without symptoms.
- The most common STIs in Canada are chlamydia, genital herpes, human papillomavirus (HPV), and gonorrhea.
- The incidence of genital herpes is increasing worldwide. About 20% of adults of reproductive age are infected with genital herpes. Genital herpes is more common in women than in men and in African Canadians than other ethnic groups.
- About 59,000 Canadians are currently living with HIV infection.
- The number of people in Canada newly infected with HIV in 2005 was estimated to be 2300 to 4500. Roughly 70% of new HIV infections occur in men, with the largest risk category being men who have sex with other men.
- Of the new HIV infections in women, 75% are acquired through heterosexual contact.

Source: Public Health Agency of Canada; Society of Obstetricians and Gynecologists of Canada.

34.1 Characteristics of Viruses

Viruses are non-living agents that infect bacteria, plants, and animals. Viruses contain none of the cellular organelles necessary for self-survival that are present in living organisms. In fact, the structure of viruses is quite primitive, compared to even the simplest cell. Surrounded by a protein coat, or **capsid**, a virus possesses only a few dozen genes, either in the form of ribonucleic acid (RNA) or deoxyribonucleic acid (DNA), that contain the necessary information needed for viral replication. Some viruses also have a lipid envelope surrounding them. A mature infective particle is called a **virion**. Figure 34.1 shows the basic structure of the human immunodeficiency virus (HIV).

Although non-living and structurally simple, viruses are capable of remarkable feats. They infect their host by entering a target cell and then using the machinery inside that cell to replicate. Thus, viruses are **intracellular parasites**—they must be inside a host cell to cause infection. The viral host is often very specific; it may be a single species of plant, bacteria, or animal or even a single type of cell within that species. Most often viruses infect only one species, although cases have been documented where viruses can mutate and cross species, as is likely the case for HIV.

Many viral infections, such as the common cold caused by rhinoviruses, are self-limiting and require no medical intervention. Although symptoms may be annoying, the virus disappears in 7 to 10 days and causes no permanent effects if the client is otherwise healthy. Others, such as those caused by HIV and the hepatitis virus, can result in serious and even fatal consequences and require aggressive drug therapy. Antiviral pharmacotherapy can be extremely challenging due to the rapid mutation rate of viruses, which can quickly render drugs ineffective. Also complicating therapy is the intracellular nature of the virus, which makes it difficult for drugs to find their viral targets without giving excessively high doses that injure normal cells. Antiviral drugs have narrow spectrums of activity, usually limited to one specific virus.

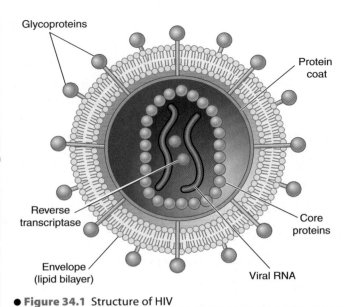

● **Figure 34.1** Structure of HIV

HIV-AIDS

Acquired immunodeficiency syndrome (AIDS) is characterized by profound immunosuppression that leads to opportunistic infections and malignancies not commonly found in clients with functioning immune defences. It results from infection with HIV. Antiretroviral drugs for **HIV-AIDS**

slow the growth of HIV by several different mechanisms. Resistance to these drugs is a major clinical problem, and a pharmacological cure for HIV-AIDS is not yet achievable.

34.2 Replication of HIV

Infection with HIV occurs by exposure to contaminated body fluids, most commonly blood or semen. Transmission may occur through sexual activity (oral, anal, or vaginal), contact of infected fluids with broken skin or mucous membranes, and needle sticks. Infants can receive the virus during birth or breastfeeding.

Shortly after entry into the body, the virus attaches to its preferred target—the **CD4 receptor** on T4 (helper) lymphocytes. After entering the host cell, HIV converts its RNA strands to DNA using the viral enzyme **reverse transcriptase**. The viral DNA enters the nucleus of the T4 lymphocyte where it becomes incorporated into the host's DNA. It may remain in the host's DNA for many years before it becomes activated to begin producing more viral particles. The new virions eventually bud from the host cell and enter the bloodstream. As a final step, the viral enzyme **protease** cleaves some of the proteins associated with the HIV DNA, enabling it to infect other T4 lymphocytes. Knowledge of the replication cycle of HIV, as shown in Figure 34.2, is critical to understanding the pharmacotherapy of HIV-AIDS.

Only a few viruses such as HIV are able to construct DNA from RNA using reverse transcriptase; no bacteria, plants,

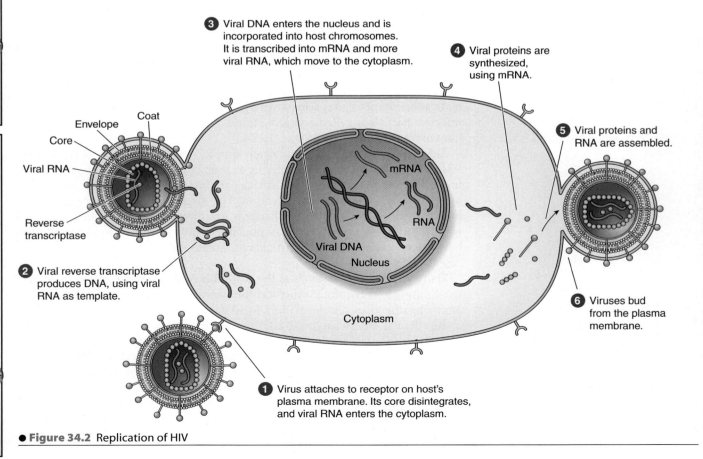

● **Figure 34.2** Replication of HIV

LIFESPAN CONSIDERATIONS

HIV in Pregnant, Pediatric, and Geriatric Populations

Optimal care and maximal viral suppression during pregnancy may reduce the risk of HIV transmission to the fetus/infant from 25% to less than 1%. Combination antiretroviral therapy is the standard treatment in pregnancy, regardless of viral load and CD4 count. However, the safety of these drugs in pregnancy has yet to be established. Until the fetus is born and becomes an independent neonate, the woman's legal right to make a therapeutic decision has priority under Canadian law.

The younger the age at which the child acquires HIV, the poorer the prognosis. Combination therapy is also used with children. Because children develop opportunistic infections, including serious respiratory infections, at a much more rapid rate than do adults, prophylactic treatment against *Pneumocystis carinii* pneumonia may also be started early. Nurses can assist the caregivers of the child to learn to manage the intense medication regimen and to identify the early symptoms of opportunistic diseases.

The diagnosis of the geriatric client may be delayed because HIV is often not suspected in this population. The geriatric client who has become infected with HIV may be reluctant to disclose activities that are considered high-risk behaviours. The geriatric client may have greater difficulty handling the rigorous regimen of the treatment. The physiological changes associated with aging increase the possibility of drug toxicity in this population. The social factors must also be considered because these clients may be living alone or even be the primary caretaker of a disabled spouse. The ability of a client to be sexually active is not determined by age; therefore, it is very important to stress sexual activity precautions to prevent spread of HIV.

Source: Burdge et al. and the Canadian HIV Trials Network Working Group on Vertical HIV Transmission. (2003). Canadian consensus guidelines for the management of pregnant HIV-positive women and their offspring. Canadian Medical Association Journal, 168, 1683–1688; Adams et al. (2008).

or animals are able to perform this unique metabolic function. All living organisms make RNA from DNA. Because of their "backward," or reverse, synthesis, these viruses are called retroviruses and drugs used to treat them are called **antiretrovirals**.

34.3 General Principles of HIV Pharmacotherapy

The widespread appearance of HIV infection in 1981 created enormous challenges for public health and an unprecedented need for the development of new antiviral drugs. HIV-AIDS is unlike any other infectious disease because it is sexually transmitted, uniformly fatal, and demands a continuous supply of new drugs for client survival. The challenges of HIV-AIDS have resulted in the development of over 18 new antiretroviral drugs, and many others are in various stages of clinical trials. Unfortunately, the initial hope of curing HIV-AIDS through antiretroviral therapy or vaccines has not been realized; none of these drugs produce a cure for this disease. HIV mutates extremely rapidly, and resistant strains develop so quickly that the creation of novel approaches to antiretroviral drug therapy must be an ongoing process.

While pharmacotherapy for HIV-AIDS has not produced a cure, it has resulted in a number of therapeutic successes.

For example, many clients with HIV infection are able to live symptom-free lives for a much longer time due to medications. Furthermore, the transmission of the virus from an HIV-infected mother to her newborn has been reduced dramatically due to intensive drug therapy of the mother prior to delivery and of the baby immediately following birth. These two factors have resulted in a significant decline in the death rate due to HIV-AIDS. Unfortunately, this decline has not been observed in African countries, where antiviral drugs are not as readily available, largely due to their high cost.

After HIV incorporates its viral DNA into the nucleus of the T4 lymphocyte, it may remain dormant for several months to many years. During this **latent phase of HIV infection**, clients are asymptomatic and may not even realize they are infected. Once diagnosis is established, a decision must be made as to when to begin pharmacotherapy. The advantage of beginning therapy during the asymptomatic (chronic) stage is that the viral load, or burden, can be reduced. Early treatment may delay the onset of acute symptoms and the development of AIDS.

The decision to begin treatment during the chronic phase has many negative consequences. Drugs for HIV-AIDS are expensive. These drugs produce a number of uncomfortable and potentially serious side effects. Therapy over many years promotes viral resistance: when the acute stage eventually develops, the drugs may no longer be effective. Two laboratory tests used to guide pharmacotherapy are measurement of the amount of HIV RNA in the plasma and the absolute CD4 lymphocyte count. In asymptomatic clients, initiation of therapy is based on laboratory criteria, primarily the viral load and secondly the CD4 lymphocyte count. A plasma viral load above 5000 to 10,000 HIV-1 RNA copies/mL, regardless of the CD4 count, is an indication for treatment. A CD4 count of less than $0.3 \times 109/L$ is an indication for treatment regardless of the plasma viral load, to prevent further damage to the immune system. These tests are performed every 3 to 6 months to assess the degree of success of drug therapy.

The decision to begin therapy during the acute phase when symptoms are present is a much easier decision. The severe symptoms of AIDS can rapidly progress to death. Thus, therapy is nearly always initiated during this phase.

The therapeutic goals for the pharmacotherapy of HIV-AIDS include the following:

- Evidence of reduction of HIV in the blood
- Increased lifespan
- Better quality of life

34.4 Classification of Drugs for HIV-AIDS

Antiretroviral drugs block phases of the HIV replication cycle. The standard pharmacotherapy for HIV-AIDS includes aggressive treatment with as many as four drugs

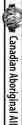

MediaLink   Canadian Aboriginal AIDS Network

MediaLink   HIV Medication Guide

TABLE 34.1 Antiretroviral Drugs for HIV-AIDS

Drug	Route and Adult Dose
Non-Nucleoside Reverse Transcriptase Inhibitors	
delavirdine (Rescriptor)	PO; 400 mg tid
efavirenz (Sustiva)	PO; 600 mg qd
nevirapine (Viramune)	PO; 200 mg qd for 14 d, then increase to bid
Nucleoside and Nucleotide Reverse Transcriptase Inhibitors	
abacavir (Ziagen)	PO; 300 mg bid
didanosine (Videx)	PO; 125–300 mg bid
emtricitabine (Emtriva)	PO; 200 mg once daily
lamivudine (3TC)	PO; 150 mg bid
stavudine (Zerit)	PO; 40 mg bid
tenofovir disoproxil fumarate (Viread)	PO; 300 mg once daily
zidovudine (Novo-AZT, Retrovir)	PO; 200 mg q4h (1200 mg/d), after 1 mo may reduce to 100 mg q4h (600 mg/d) IV; 1–2 mg/kg q4h (1200 mg/d)
Protease Inhibitors	
amprenavir (Agenerase)	PO; 150 mg bid
atazanavir (Reyataz)	PO; 400 mg qd
indinavir (Crixivan)	PO; 200–400 mg tid
nelfinavir (Viracept)	PO; 750 mg tid
ritonavir (Norvir)	PO; 80–100 mg bid
saquinavir (Invirase)	PO; 600 mg tid
Integrase Inhibitors	
enfuviride (Fuzeon)	SC; 90 mg bid
Raltegravir (Isentress)	PO; 400 mg bid

concurrently, a regimen called **highly active antiretroviral therapy (HAART)**. The goal of HAART is to reduce the plasma HIV RNA to its lowest possible level. It must be understood, however, that HIV is harboured in locations other than the blood, such as lymph nodes; therefore, elimination of the virus from the blood is not a cure. The simultaneous use of drugs from several classes also reduces the probability that the virus will become resistant to treatment. These drugs are shown in Table 34.1.

HIV-AIDS antiretroviral drugs are classified into the following six groups, based on their mechanism of activity:

- Nucleoside reverse transcriptase inhibitor (NRTI)
- Non-nucleoside reverse transcriptase inhibitor (NNRTI)
- Protease inhibitor
- Nucleotide reverse transcriptase inhibitor (RTI)
- Fusion inhibitor
- Integrase inhibitor

The last two classes include recently discovered agents that act by unique mechanisms. Tenofovir is a NRTI that is structurally similar to adenosine monophosphate (AMP). After metabolism, Tenofovir is incorporated into viral DNA in a manner similar to the NRTIs. Enfuvirtide blocks the fusion of the HIV virion to the CD4 receptor. Raltegravir blocks HIV integrase and prevents HIV from inserting its genes into uninfected DNA.

REVERSE TRANSCRIPTASE INHIBITORS

Drugs in the reverse transcriptase inhibitor class comprise agents that are structurally similar to nucleosides, the building blocks of DNA. This class includes non-nucleoside reverse transcriptase inhibitors, which bind directly to the viral enzyme reverse transcriptase and inhibit its function, and nucleotide reverse transcriptase inhibitors.

34.5 Pharmacotherapy with Reverse Transcriptase Inhibitors

One of the early steps in HIV infection is the synthesis of viral DNA from the viral RNA inside the T4 lymphocyte. The enzyme performing this step is reverse transcriptase. Because reverse transcriptase is a viral enzyme not found in animal cells, selective inhibition of viral replication is possible.

As viral DNA is synthesized, building blocks known as nucleosides are required. The NRTIs chemically resemble naturally occurring nucleosides. As reverse transcriptase uses these NRTIs to build the DNA, however, the viral DNA strand is prevented from lengthening. The prematurely terminated chain prevents the viral DNA from being inserted into the host chromosome.

Pr PROTOTYPE DRUG | Zidovudine (Novo-AZT, Retrovir)

ACTIONS AND USES

Zidovudine was discovered in the 1960s, and its antiviral activity was demonstrated prior to the AIDS epidemic. Structurally, it resembles thymidine, one of the four nucleoside building blocks of DNA. As the reverse transcriptase enzyme begins to synthesize viral DNA, it mistakenly uses zidovudine as one of the nucleosides, thus creating a defective DNA strand. Because of its widespread use since the emergence of AIDS, resistant HIV strains are common. It is used in combination with other antiretrovirals for symptomatic and asymptomatic HIV-infected clients, for reducing transmission of HIV from pregnant woman to fetus, and for post-exposure prophylaxis in healthcare workers and others.

PHARMACOKINETICS

Zidovudine is well absorbed after oral administration. It is widely distributed, crosses the placenta, and enters the CNS. It is mostly metabolized by the liver. Less than 20% is excreted unchanged in urine. Its half-life is about 1 hour.

ADMINISTRATION ALERTS

- Administer on an empty stomach, with water only.
- Avoid administering with fruit juice.
- Zidovudine is pregnancy category C.

ADVERSE EFFECTS AND INTERACTIONS

Zidovudine can result in severe toxicity to blood cells at high doses; anemia and neutropenia are common and may limit therapy. Many clients experience anorexia, nausea, and diarrhea. Clients may report fatigue and generalized weakness.

Zidovudine interacts with many drugs. Acetaminophen and ganciclovir may worsen bone marrow suppression. The following drugs may increase the risk of AZT toxicity: atovaquone, amphotericin B, ASA, doxorubicin, fluconazole, methadone, and valproic acid. Other antiretroviral agents may cause lactic acidosis and severe hepatomegaly with steatosis.

Use with caution with herbal supplements, such as St. John's wort, which may cause a decrease in antiretroviral activity.

 See the Companion Website for a Nursing Process Focus Chart specific to this drug.

Pr PROTOTYPE DRUG | Nevirapine (Viramune)

ACTIONS AND USES

Nevirapine is an NNRTI that binds directly to reverse transcriptase, disrupting the enzyme's active site. This inhibition prevents viral DNA from being synthesized from HIV RNA. It is readily absorbed following an oral dose. Since resistance develops rapidly when used as monotherapy, nevirapine is nearly always used in combination with other antivirals in HAART.

ADMINISTRATION ALERTS

- Administer with food to minimize gastric distress.
- Nevirapine is pregnancy category C.

PHARMACOKINETICS

Nevirapine is well absorbed after oral administration. It crosses the placenta and enters breast milk. It enters the CNS. It is mostly metabolized by the liver. A small amount is excreted unchanged in urine. Its half-life is 25 to 30 hours.

ADVERSE EFFECTS AND INTERACTIONS

Nevirapine increases the levels of metabolic enzymes in the liver; thus, it has the potential to interact with drugs metabolized by this organ. Therapy is sometimes contraindicated in clients with hepatic impairment. GI-related effects such as nausea, diarrhea, and abdominal pain are experienced by some clients. Skin rashes, fever, and fatigue are frequent side effects. Though rare, some clients acquire Stevens-Johnson syndrome, a sometimes fatal skin condition affecting mucous membranes and large areas of the body. Resistance can develop quite rapidly, which may extend to other NNRTIs.

Nevirapine interacts with several other drugs. For example, nevirapine may decrease plasma concentrations of protease inhibitors and oral contraceptives. It may also decrease methadone levels, inducing opiate withdrawal.

Use with caution with herbal supplements, such as St. John's wort, which may cause a decrease in antiretroviral activity.

 See the Companion Website for a Nursing Process Focus Chart specific to this drug.

A second mechanism for inhibiting reverse transcriptase is to affect the enzyme's function. Drugs in the NNRTI class act by binding near the active site of the enzyme, causing a structural change in the enzyme molecule. This causes a direct inhibition of enzyme function.

Although there are differences in their pharmacokinetic and toxicity profiles, no single NRTI or NNRTI offers a significant therapeutic advantage over any other. Choice of agent depends on client response and the experience of the healthcare provider. Because some of these drugs, such as zidovudine, have been used consistently for over 15 years, the potential for resistance must be considered when selecting the specific agent. The NRTIs and NNRTIs are nearly always used in multidrug combinations in HAART.

PROTEASE INHIBITORS

Drugs in the protease inhibitor class block the viral enzyme protease, which is responsible for the final assembly of the HIV virions.

Cultural and Psychosocial Issues with Antiretroviral Drug Adherence

One key to success of antiretroviral therapy is client adherence to the prescribed medication plan. Drug adherence is difficult for most people once they feel well; clients may not feel sick while taking the medications and be more prone to skip doses for various reasons. Many factors can enhance the probability that the client will adhere to treatment. For example, a multidisciplinary assessment can screen clients for depression, alcohol or drug abuse, or negative attitudes, and interventions can be initiated to minimize the impact on adherence. Cultural factors and personal beliefs may also influence adherence. Education at an appropriate level is essential so the client can understand the disease process as well as the role the medications play in securing a positive outcome. Agencies such as the Canadian Aboriginal AIDS Network and Canadian AIDS Society provide resources for clients. Developing trust and open communication between the client and healthcare provider is essential to improve the chances of drug adherence and to reach common therapeutic goals.

34.6 Pharmacotherapy with Protease Inhibitors

Near the end of its replication cycle, HIV has assembled all the necessary molecular components for the creation of new virions. Using the metabolic machinery of the host cell, HIV RNA has been synthesized using the viral DNA that was incorporated into the host's genome. The structural and regulatory proteins of HIV have been synthesized using this viral RNA as a template.

As the newly formed virions bud from the host cell and are released into the surrounding extracellular fluid, one final step remains before the HIV is mature: a long polypeptide chain must be cleaved to produce the final HIV proteins. The enzyme performing this step is HIV protease.

The protease inhibitors attach to the active site of the HIV protease enzyme and prevent the final maturation of the virions. When combined with other antiretroviral drug classes, the protease inhibitors are capable of lowering plasma HIV RNA to levels below the detectable range. The protease inhibitors are metabolized in the liver and have the potential to interact with many different drugs. In general, they are well tolerated, with GI complaints being the most common side effects. Various lipid abnormalities, or lipodystrophies, have been reported, including elevated cholesterol and triglyceride levels and abdominal obesity.

Of the six available protease inhibitors, all have equivalent efficacy and a similar range of adverse effects. Choice of protease inhibitor is generally based on clinical response and the experience of the healthcare provider. Cross-resistance among the various protease inhibitors has been reported.

NURSING CONSIDERATIONS

The following material provides a discussion of NRTIs, NNRTIs, and protease inhibitors. Because antiretrovirals are commonly prescribed for HIV infection, a Nursing Process Focus has been provided for them in this chapter.

Although NRTI, NNRTI, and protease inhibitors act by different mechanisms, the associated nursing care is similar. The role of the nurse involves careful monitoring of the client's condition and providing education as it relates to the prescribed drug regimen. The nurse is instrumental in providing client education, and psychosocial support will be crucial. Clients will experience tremendous emotional distress at various times during treatment. Denial and anger may be evident in the client's behaviour as he or she attempts to cope with the diagnosis.

Assess the client's understanding of the HIV disease process. Although drug therapies may slow the progression of the virus, they are not a cure. Prior to the administration of antiretroviral drugs, assess for symptoms of HIV and for any opportunistic infections. Plasma HIV RNA (viral load) assays, CD4 counts, complete blood count, liver and renal profiles, and blood glucose levels should also be monitored. These diagnostic values will determine the effectiveness as well as the toxicity of the drugs employed.

Verify the drug combination to determine potential side effects and precautions. All antiretroviral agents are contraindicated during pregnancy and lactation. The list of diseases and conditions that necessitate close observation is quite extensive for the antiretrovirals. Typically, agents classified as NTRI should be used cautiously in clients with pancreatitis, peripheral vascular disease, neuropathy, kidney disorders, liver disorders, cardiac disease, and alcohol abuse. NNTRI agents necessitate judicious use in clients with liver impairment and CNS diseases. Protease inhibitors are potentially problematic for clients suffering from sensitivity to sulfonamides, liver disorders, and renal insufficiency. It should be understood that in the acute stages of AIDS, treatment may proceed despite relative contraindications.

Some antiretroviral drugs vary in the way in which they should be taken. For example, clients taking an NRTI drug should be instructed to take the medication on an empty stomach. These drugs should always be taken with water only and never with fruit juice because acidic fruit juices interact with them. On the other hand, nevirapine and saquinavir mesylate should be taken with food to minimize gastric distress. With all antiretroviral drugs, it is critical that the client be instructed to consult with the healthcare provider before taking any OTC medication or herbal supplement to avoid drug interactions.

Many of the side effects of antiretrovirals can dramatically influence activities of daily living. Some of these drugs may cause dizziness or other troublesome CNS effects. When such side effects occur, the client may be instructed to take the medication just before sleep. The client should also be advised not to drive or perform hazardous activities until reaction to the medication is known. Specific side effects depend on the drugs used. The nurse must be vigilant in assessing for side effects and assisting clients to manage their therapeutic regimen.

Client education as it relates to antiretroviral drugs should include goals, reasons for obtaining baseline data such as vital signs and tests for cardiac and renal disorders, and possible side effects. Instruct the client to report adverse effects specific to the antiretroviral agent prescribed. For example, when teaching clients about NRTIs, instruct the client to report fever, skin rash, abdominal pain, nausea, vomiting, numbness, and burning of feet or hands. When teaching clients receiving NNRTIs, instruct the client to report fever, chills, rash, blistering of skin, reddening of skin, and muscle or joint pain to the healthcare provider. Clients taking protease inhibitors should report rash, abdominal pain, headache, insomnia, fever, constipation, cough, fainting, and visual changes.

The role of the nurse in teaching the client taking antiretroviral agents is critical and may enhance the quality of life of the individual. Because these clients are highly susceptible to infections, it is essential that the nurse describe the symptoms of infection, such as fever, chills, sore throat, and cough, and the importance of immediately seeking medical care should these signs develop. Additionally, the client should be taught methods to minimize exposure to infection. Frequent handwashing, as well as avoiding crowds and people with colds, flu, and other infections, will greatly reduce the client's likelihood of becoming infected. The client should also be instructed to take additional measures to reduce microbial infections, such as increasing fluid intake, emptying the bladder frequently, and coughing and deep breathing several times per day to expel invading organisms.

Nurses should also incorporate health promotional teaching to the client receiving these drugs. Because clients on antiretroviral agents typically have impaired immune systems, instruct them to engage in activities that support immune function. These activities include adequate rest and sleep, consuming a diet that provides essential vitamins and minerals, and drinking six to eight glasses of water per day.

NATURAL THERAPIES

Complementary and Alternative Medicine for HIV

With no cure and the available drugs producing numerous adverse effects, it is not surprising that many clients infected with HIV turn to complementary and alternative medicine (CAM). It is estimated that as many as 70% of HIV-AIDS clients use CAM during the course of their illness. Most clients use CAM in addition to antiretroviral therapy to control serious side effects, combat weight loss, and boost their immune system. Relieving stress and depression are also common reasons for seeking CAM. The most common herbal products reported by HIV-AIDS clients are garlic, ginseng, echinacea, and aloe. Unfortunately, few controlled studies have examined the safety or efficacy of CAM in HIV-AIDS clients.

Supportive education regarding the use of CAM should be provided. Although the use of these therapies should not be discouraged, clients must be strongly warned not to use CAM in place of conventional medical treatment. In addition, some herbs such as St. John's wort can increase the hepatic metabolism of antiretrovirals, resulting in an increased or decreased effect. Garlic coadministered with saquinavir has been shown to greatly reduce plasma levels of the antiretroviral. Urge the client to obtain CAM information from reliable sources and to always report the use of CAM therapies to the healthcare provider.

Another important factor in health teaching with these clients focuses on disease transmission. The client should be taught that antiretroviral agents may decrease the level of HIV infection in the blood but will not prevent the risk of transmission to other individuals. The nurse must discuss sensitive issues with the client, including abstinence, the use of barrier protection such as condoms during sexual activity, and the avoidance of sharing needles with other individuals. Open and honest dialogue will occur only if the nurse has developed a therapeutic rapport with the client based on trust and acceptance. Additional teaching points are discussed in "Nursing Process Focus: Clients Receiving Antiretroviral Agents."

Pr PROTOTYPE DRUG | Saquinavir (Invirase)

ACTIONS AND USES

Saquinavir was the first protease inhibitor approved by the FDA in 1995. By effectively inhibiting HIV protease, the final step in the assembly of an infectious HIV virion is prevented. The first formulation of saquinavir was a hard gelatin capsule that was poorly absorbed. The newer formulation is a soft gelatin capsule that gives a significantly higher absorption rate, particularly when taken with a high-fat, high-calorie meal. Because of its short half-life, it is usually taken every 8 hours.

PHARMACOKINETICS

Saquinavir undergoes rapid and extensive first-pass metabolism after oral administration. It is 98% bound to plasma proteins. A minor amount enters the CNS. It is mostly metabolized by the liver. Less than 1% is excreted unchanged in urine. Its half-life is 7 to 13 hours.

ADMINISTRATION ALERTS

- Administer with food to minimize gastric distress.
- Invirase and Fortovase are not equivalent and cannot be interchanged.
- Saquinavir is pregnancy category B.

ADVERSE EFFECTS AND INTERACTIONS

Saquinavir is well tolerated by most clients. The most frequently reported problems are GI related, such as nausea, vomiting, dyspepsia, and diarrhea. General fatigue and headache are possible. Though not common, reductions in platelets and erythrocytes have been reported. Resistance to saquinavir may develop with continued use and may include cross-resistance with other protease inhibitors.

Saquinavir interacts with several drugs, including rifampin and rifabutin, which significantly decrease saquinavir levels. Phenobarbital, phenytoin, and carbamazepine may also reduce saquinavir levels. Conversely, ketoconazole and ritonavir may increase levels.

Use with caution with herbal supplements, such as St. John's wort, which may cause a decrease in antiretroviral activity.

 See the Companion Website for a Nursing Process Focus Chart specific to this drug.

NURSING PROCESS FOCUS Clients Receiving Antiretroviral Agents

Assessment	Potential Nursing Diagnoses/Identified Patterns

Prior to administration:
■ Obtain complete health history including allergies, drug history, and possible drug interactions.
■ Obtain complete physical examination.
■ Assess for the presence/history of HIV infection.
■ Obtain the following laboratory studies:
  ■ HIV RNA assay / CD4 count
  ■ Complete blood count (CBC)
  ■ Liver function
  ■ Renal function
  ■ Blood glucose
	■ Need for knowledge regarding disease process, transmission, and drug therapy
	■ Safety from injury related to side effects of drugs therapy
	■ Risk for infection related to impaired immune system
	■ Fear related to HIV diagnosis

Planning: Client Goals and Expected Outcomes

The client will:
■ Exhibit a decrease in viral load and an increase in CD4 count
■ Demonstrate knowledge of disease process, transmission, and treatment
■ Demonstrate an understanding of the drug's action by accurately describing drug side effects and precautions
■ Complete full course of therapy and comply with follow-up care

Implementation

Interventions (Rationales)	Client Education/Discharge Planning
■ Monitor for symptoms of hypersensitivity reactions. (Zalcitabine may cause anaphylactic reaction.)	■ Instruct client to discontinue the medication and inform healthcare provider if symptoms of hypersensitivity reaction develop, such as wheezing; shortness of breath; swelling of face, tongue, or hands; itching or rash.
■ Monitor vital signs, especially temperature, and for symptoms of infection. Monitor white blood cell count. (Antiretroviral drugs such as delavirdine may cause neutropenia.)	Instruct client: ■ To report symptoms of infection, such as fever, chills, sore throat, and cough ■ On methods to minimize exposure to infections such as frequent handwashing; avoiding crowds and people with colds, flu, and other infections; limiting exposure to children and animals; increasing fluid intake; emptying bladder frequently; and coughing and deep breathing several times per day
■ Monitor client for signs of stomatitis. (Immunosuppression may result in the proliferation of oral bacteria.)	■ Advise client to be alert for mouth ulcers and to report their appearance.
■ Monitor blood pressure. (Antiviral agents such as abacavir may cause significant decrease in blood pressure.)	Instruct client to: ■ Rise slowly from lying or sitting position to minimize effects of postural hypotension. ■ Report changes in blood pressure
■ Monitor HIV RNA assay, CD4 count, liver function, kidney function, complete blood count, blood glucose, and serum amylase and triglyceride levels. (These will determine effectiveness and toxicity of drug.)	Instruct client: ■ On the purpose of required laboratory tests and scheduled follow-ups with healthcare provider ■ To monitor weight and presence of swelling ■ To keep all appointments for laboratory tests
■ Determine potential drug-drug and drug-food interactions. (Antiretroviral medications have multiple drug-drug interactions and must be taken as prescribed.)	Instruct client: ■ When to take the specific medication in relationship to food intake ■ About foods or beverages to avoid when taking medication; some antiretrovirals should not be taken with acidic fruit juice ■ To take medication exactly as directed; do not skip any doses ■ To consult with healthcare provider before taking any OTC medications or herbal supplements

continued

NURSING PROCESS FOCUS Clients Receiving Antiretroviral Agents *(Continued)*

Interventions (Rationales)	Client Education/Discharge Planning
■ Monitor for symptoms of pancreatitis including severe abdominal pain, nausea, vomiting, and abdominal distention. (Antiretroviral agents such as didanosine may cause pancreatitis.)	■ Instruct client to report the following immediately: fever, severe abdominal pain, nausea/vomiting, and abdominal distention
■ Monitor skin for rash; withhold medication and notify physician at first sign of rash. (Several antiretroviral drugs may cause Stevens-Johnson syndrome, which may be fatal.)	■ Advise client to check skin frequently and notify healthcare provider at first sign of any rash.
■ Establish therapeutic environment to ensure adequate rest, nutrition, hydration, and relaxation. (Support of the immune system is essential in HIV clients to minimize opportunistic infections.)	Teach client to incorporate the following health-enhancing activities: ■ Adequate rest and sleep ■ Proper nutrition that provides essential vitamins and nutrients ■ Intake of six to eight glasses of water/day
■ Monitor blood glucose levels. (Antiretroviral drugs may cause hyperglycemia, especially in clients with type 1 diabetes.)	■ Instruct client to report excessive thirst, hunger, and urination to healthcare provider. ■ Instruct diabetic clients to monitor blood glucose levels regularly.
■ Monitor for neurological side effects such as numbness and tingling of the extremities. (Many NRTI agents cause peripheral neuropathy.)	Instruct client to: ■ Report numbness and tingling of extremities ■ Use caution when in contact with heat and cold due to possible peripheral neuropathy
■ Determine the effect of the prescribed antiretroviral agents on oral contraceptives. (Many agents reduce the effectiveness of oral contraceptives.)	■ Instruct client to use an alternate form of birth control while taking antiretroviral medications.
■ Provide resources for medical and emotional support.	■ Advise client on community resources and support groups.
■ Assess client's knowledge level regarding use and effect of medication.	Advise client: ■ That medication may decrease the level of HIV infection in the blood but will not prevent transmitting the disease ■ To use barrier protection during sexual activity ■ To avoid sharing needles ■ To not donate blood

Evaluation of Outcome Criteria

Evaluate the effectiveness of drug therapy by confirming that client goals and expected outcomes have been met (see "Planning").

See Table 34.1 (page 466) for a list of drugs to which these nursing actions apply.

HERPES VIRUSES

Herpes simplex viruses (HSVs) are a family of DNA viruses that cause repeated, blister-like lesions on the skin, genitals, and other mucosal surfaces. Antiviral drugs can lower the frequency of acute herpes episodes and diminish the intensity of acute disease. These drugs are shown in Table 34.2.

TABLE 34.2 Drugs for Herpes Viruses

Drug	Route and Adult Dose
acyclovir (Zovirax)	PO; 400 mg tid
docosanol (Abreva)	Topical; 10% cream applied to cold sore up to five times/d for 10 d
famciclovir (Famvir)	PO; 500 mg tid for 7 d
ganciclovir (Cytovene)	IV; 5 mg/kg infused over 1 h bid
idoxuridine (Herplex)	Topical; one drop in each eye q1h during the day and q2h at night
penciclovir (Denavir)	Topical; apply q2h while awake for 4 d
trifluridine (Viroptic)	Topical; one drop in each eye q2h during waking hours (max nine drops/day)
valacyclovir (Valtrex)	PO; 1.0 g tid

34.7 Pharmacotherapy of Herpes Virus Infections

Herpes viruses are usually acquired through direct physical contact with an infected person. Herpes viruses can also be transmitted from infected mothers to their newborns, sometimes resulting in severe CNS disease. The herpes virus family includes the following:

- HSV-type 1 – primarily causes infections of the eye, mouth, and lips, although the incidence of genital infections is increasing
- HSV-type 2 – genital infections
- Cytomegalovirus (CMV) – affects multiple body systems in immunosuppressed clients
- Varicella-zoster virus (VZV) – shingles (zoster) and chicken pox (varicella)
- Epstein-Barr virus (EBV) – mononucleosis and a form of cancer known as Burkitt's lymphoma

Pharmacotherapy of initial HSV-1 and HSV-2 infections is usually accomplished through oral antiviral therapy for 7 to 10 days. Topical forms of several antivirals are available for local applications, though they are not as efficacious as the oral forms. In immunocompromised clients, IV acyclovir may be indicated.

Following its initial entrance into the client, HSV may remain in a latent, asymptomatic, non-replicating state in ganglia for many years. Immunosuppression, physical challenges, or emotional stress can promote active replication of the virus and the reappearance of characteristic lesions. Although recurrent herpes lesions are usually mild and often require no drug treatment, clients who experience frequent recurrences may benefit from low doses of prophylactic antiviral therapy. It should be noted that the antiviral drugs used to treat herpes viruses do not cure clients; the virus remains with them for their lifetime.

NURSING CONSIDERATIONS

The following material provides a discussion of the nursing considerations for clients receiving antiviral medications not associated with HIV infection.

The role of the nurse in antiviral therapy involves careful monitoring of the client's condition and providing education as it relates to the prescribed drug regimen. Because many of these viral infections are systemic and not localized, perform a complete physical assessment prior to drug administration. Once a baseline assessment, including vital signs, weight, and laboratory studies (CBC, viral cultures, liver and kidney function) is completed, focus on the presenting symptoms of the viral infection. For clients with pre-existing renal or hepatic disease, the drugs should be used with extreme caution. Although many antiviral medications are listed as pregnancy categories B or C, their judicious use is still warranted during pregnancy. Viral infections that can be treated with antiviral drugs include keratoconjunctivitis and infections resulting from herpes simplex viruses, CMV, Epstein-Barr virus, varicella-zoster virus, and respiratory syncytial virus.

Depending on the specific antiviral drug, these agents can be administered intravenously, orally, topically, and through inhalation. Instruct the client in the proper administration techniques. Additionally, it is important that the nurse emphasize adherence with antiviral therapy such as taking the exact dose around the clock even if sleep is interrupted. Many antiviral drugs cause GI distress and should be taken with food. Monitor the client for side effects throughout the course of the treatment and assist the client with managing

---

Pr PROTOTYPE DRUG | Acyclovir (Zovirax)

ACTIONS AND USES

Acyclovir was approved in 1982 as one of the first antiviral drugs. The activity of acyclovir is limited to the herpes viruses, for which it is a drug of choice. It is most effective against HSV-1 and HSV-2 and effective only at high doses against CMV and varicella-zoster. Acyclovir acts by inhibiting the viral enzyme thymidine kinase, thus preventing viral DNA synthesis. Acyclovir decreases the duration and severity of herpes episodes. When given for prophylaxis, it may decrease the frequency of herpes episodes, but it does not cure the client. It is available in topical form for direct treatment of active lesions, in oral form for prophylaxis, and in IV form for particularly severe episodes.

PHARMACOKINETICS

Acyclovir is about 75% absorbed after oral administration. Distribution is wide. It crosses the placenta and enters breast milk. It enters the CNS. It is about 25% protein bound. A small amount is metabolized by the liver. Over 90% is excreted unchanged in urine. Its half-life is 2.5 to 4 hours. Because of its short half-life, acyclovir may be administered orally up to five times a day.

ADMINISTRATION ALERTS

- When given IV, the drug may cause painful inflammation of vessels at the site of infusion.
- Administer around the clock, even if sleep is interrupted.
- Administer with food.
- Acyclovir is pregnancy category C.

ADVERSE EFFECTS AND INTERACTIONS

There are few adverse effects of acyclovir when administered topically or orally. Because nephrotoxicity is possible when the medication is given IV, frequent laboratory tests may be performed to monitor kidney function. Resistance has developed to the drug, particularly in clients with HIV-AIDS.

Acyclovir interacts with several drugs. For example, probenecid decreases acyclovir elimination, and zidovudine may cause increased drowsiness and lethargy.

 See the Companion Website for a Nursing Process Focus Chart specific to this drug.

antiviral-related problems. For example, because ganciclovir may cause bone marrow suppression, clients should be monitored for anemia, thrombocytopenia, and neutropenia. Because many antiviral drugs are nephrotoxic and hepatotoxic, monitor the client for dysfunction of the kidneys and liver.

Client education as it relates to antiviral drugs should include goals, reasons for obtaining baseline data such as vital signs and tests for cardiac and renal disorders, and possible side effects. Teach the client modes of transmission and methods to prevent spreading the disease, and advise the client that these drugs do not prevent transmission of the virus to other individuals.

Following are other important points to include when teaching clients regarding antiviral agents:

- Report the following symptoms immediately: blood in urine, bruising, yellowing of the skin, fever, chills, confusion, nervousness, dizziness, nausea, and vomiting.
- Take the medication for the full course of therapy and continue taking it, even if symptoms improve, until the full prescription has been taken.
- Keep all appointments for follow-up care.
- Take necessary safety precautions while taking the drug because some antivirals may cause dizziness and drowsiness.
- Do not drive or perform hazardous activities until the effects of the drug are known.
- Consult the healthcare provider before taking any OTC medications or herbal supplements because of potentially toxic drug-drug interactions.
- Apply topical preparations with an applicator or a glove to prevent the spread of the virus to other areas.
- Do not apply any other types of cream, ointment, or lotion to the infected sites.

INFLUENZA

Influenza is a viral infection characterized by acute symptoms that include sore throat, sneezing, coughing, fever, and chills. The infectious viral particles are easily spread via airborne droplets. In vulnerable and immunosuppressed clients, an influenza infection may be fatal. Influenza may be seasonal or pandemic. All of the influenza pandemics of the 20th century were avian in origin. In 1919, a worldwide outbreak of influenza killed approximately 20 million people. In China in 1997, the avian influenza virus A (H5N1 strain) was first transmitted from birds to humans. Since 2003, the virus has appeared in several different countries, causing deaths in humans. This is of global concern because sustained human-to-human transmission of the virus potentially may occur and result in a pandemic. Pandemics are caused by type A viruses. Seasonal influenza may be caused by type A or B. The RNA-containing influenza viruses should not be confused with *Haemophilus influenzae*, which is a bacterium that causes respiratory disease.

34.8 Pharmacotherapy of Influenza

The best approach to influenza infection is prevention through annual vaccination. Those who benefit greatly from vaccinations include residents of long-term care facilities, those with chronic cardiopulmonary disease, pregnant women in their second or third trimester during the peak flu season, and healthy adults over age 50. Depending on the stage of the disease, HIV-positive clients usually benefit from vaccination. Adequate immunity is achieved about 2 weeks after vaccination and lasts for several months up to a year. Additional details on vaccines are presented in Chapter 30.

Antivirals may be used to prevent influenza or decrease the severity of symptoms. The drug amantadine has been available to prevent and treat influenza for many years. Chemoprophylaxis with amantadine or rimantadine is indicated for unvaccinated individuals after a confirmed outbreak of influenza type A. Therapy with these antivirals is sometimes started concurrently with vaccination; the antiviral offers protection during the period before therapeutic antibody titres are achieved from the vaccine. These drugs are generally prescribed for clients who are at greatest risk of the severe complications of influenza. Antivirals for influenza are shown in Table 34.3.

A new class of drug, the neuraminidase inhibitors, was introduced in 1999 to treat active influenza infections. Because seasonal as well as H5N1 viruses develop rapid resistance to amantadine, the neuraminidase inhibitors are often first choice drugs if administered early in the disease. If given within 48 hours of the onset of symptoms, oseltamivir and zanamivir are reported to shorten the normal 7-day duration of influenza symptoms to 5 days. They may reduce complications of influenza such as bronchitis and pneumonia that could lead to death. Oseltamivir is given orally, whereas zanamivir is inhaled. Because these agents produce only

TABLE 34.3 Drugs for Influenza	
Drug	*Route and Adult Dose*
Influenza Prophylaxis	
amantadine (Symmetrel)	PO; 100 mg bid
Influenza Treatment: Neuraminidase Inhibitors	
oseltamivir (Tamiflu)	PO; 75 mg bid for 5 d
zanamivir (Relenza)	Inhalation; two inhalations for 5 d

modest effects on an active infection, prevention through vaccination remains the best alternative.

HEPATITIS

Viral **hepatitis** is a common infection caused by a number of different viruses. Although each virus has its own unique clinical features, they all cause inflammation and necrosis of liver cells. Symptoms of hepatitis may be acute or chronic. Acute symptoms include fever, chills, fatigue, anorexia, nausea, and vomiting. Chronic hepatitis may result in prolonged fatigue, jaundice, liver cirrhosis, and ultimately hepatic failure.

34.9 Pharmacotherapy of Hepatitis

Hepatitis A virus (HAV), sometimes called infectious hepatitis, is caused by an RNA virus. It is spread by the oral-fecal route primarily in regions of the world having poor sanitation. Hepatitis B virus (HBV), known as serum hepatitis, is caused by a DNA virus and is transmitted primarily through exposure to contaminated blood and body fluids. HBV has a much greater incidence of chronic hepatitis and a greater mortality rate than HAV. The hepatitis C, D, and E viruses are sometimes referred to as non A–non B viruses.

The best treatment for viral hepatitis is prevention through immunization, which is available for HAV and HBV. HAV vaccine is indicated for those living in communities with high infection rates and for travellers to countries with high endemic HAV infection. Immune globulin, a concentrated solution of antibodies, is sometimes administered to close personal contacts of infected clients to prevent transmission of HAV. The immunoglobulins induce passive protection and provide prophylaxis for about 3 months.

Traditionally, HBV vaccine has been indicated for healthcare workers and others who are routinely exposed to blood and body fluids. Because this vaccination protocol failed to address hepatitis B in early childhood, universal vaccination of all children is now recommended. Post-exposure treatment of hepatitis B may include hepatitis B immunoglobulins and an antiviral agent such as interferon alfa-2a or lamivudine. Adefovir is a recently approved therapy for chronic hepatitis B infections. Following metabolism, adefovir is incorporated into the growing viral DNA strand, causing it to terminate prematurely.

Most clients recover completely from HAV and HBV infection without drug therapy, though complete recovery may take many months. The overall mortality rate is less than 1%. Neonates and immunocompromised clients are at higher risk of developing chronic hepatitis.

Transmitted primarily through exposure to infected blood or body fluid, hepatitis C virus (HCV) is more common than HBV. Up to 50% of all HIV-AIDS clients are coinfected with HCV. A large percentage of clients infected with HCV proceed to chronic hepatitis; HCV is the most common cause of liver transplants. A specific vaccine is not available for hepatitis C. Current pharmacotherapy for chronic HCV infection includes treatment with Rebetron, a combination agent consisting of interferon alfa-2b and ribavirin. After 24 weeks of treatment with Rebetron, about 30% to 50% of clients will respond with increased liver function. If response is not attained, therapy may continue for as long as 12 to 18 months. Peginterferon alfa-2a and peginterferon alfa-2b are recently approved therapies for chronic hepatitis C. **Pegylation** is a process that attaches polyethylene glycol to the interferon to extend its pharmacological activity. This permits the interferon to remain in the body longer and exert prolonged activity. Drugs for hepatitis are shown in Table 34.4.

TABLE 34.4 Drugs for Hepatitis	
Drug	*Route and Adult Dose*
Interferons	
interferon alfa-2b (Intron A) (see page 394 for the Prototype Drug box)	IM/SC; 2 million U/m^2 three times/wk
peginterferon alfa-2a (Pegasys)	SC; 180 µg once weekly for 48 wk
Non-Interferons/Combinations	
adefovir dipivoxil (Hepsera)	PO; 10 mg qd
lamivudine (3TC)	PO; 150 mg bid
ribavirin/interferon alfa-2b (Pegetron/Intron A)	Adults more than 75 kg: Rebeton PO; 3 × 200 mg capsules in the AM and 3 × 200 mg capsules in the PM; Intron A SC; 3 million IU three times/wk

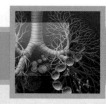

CHAPTER REVIEW

KEY CONCEPTS

The numbered key concepts provide a succinct summary of the important points from the corresponding numbered section within the chapter. If any of these points are not clear, refer to the numbered section within the chapter for review. Expanded versions can be found on the Companion Website.

34.1 Viruses are non-living intracellular parasites that require host machinery to replicate.

34.2 HIV attacks the T4 lymphocyte and uses reverse transcriptase to make viral DNA.

34.3 Antiretroviral drugs used in the treatment of HIV-AIDS do not cure the disease but do help many clients to live longer. Pharmacotherapy may be initiated in the acute (symptomatic) or chronic (asymptomatic) phase of HIV infection.

34.4 Drugs from five drug classes are combined in the pharmacotherapy of HIV-AIDS. The nucleotide reverse transcriptase inhibitors and the fusion inhibitors have been recently developed.

34.5 The reverse transcriptase inhibitors block HIV replication at the level of the reverse transcriptase enzyme.

34.6 The protease inhibitors inhibit the final assembly of the HIV virion.

34.7 Pharmacotherapy can lessen the severity of acute herpes simplex infections and prolong the latent period of the disease.

34.8 Drugs are available to prevent and to treat influenza infections. Vaccination is the best choice as drugs are relatively ineffective once symptoms appear.

34.9 Hepatitis A and B are best treated through immunization. Newer drugs for HBV and HBC have led to therapies for chronic hepatitis.

REVIEW QUESTIONS

1 What is the advantage of using combinations of agents to treat HIV infection?

2 Is it better to treat HIV before or after acute symptoms occur? What are the advantages and disadvantages of each?

3 From a pharmacological perspective, explain why is it better to prevent influenza than to treat it.

4 What are the therapeutic goals for the pharmacotherapy of clients with HAV or HBV?

CRITICAL THINKING QUESTIONS

1. A 72-year-old client lives in an assisted living residence where another resident has developed influenza A. The home health nurse advises the client that he is to receive amantadine therapy. What is the rationale supporting this therapy? How could the nurse assist the client to comply with amantadine therapy?

2. A newly diagnosed HIV-positive client has been put on zidovudine (Retrovir). What is a priority for the nurse to monitor in this client? What support and teaching will this client likely require?

3. A healthcare provider has ordered acyclovir (Zovirax) as an IV bolus to infuse over 15 minutes. The client is seriously ill with a systemic herpes virus infection, and the healthcare provider wants the client to have immediate access to the medication. What is the nurse's response?

EXPLORE
MediaLink

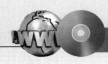

www.pearsoned.ca/adams-king

 MEDIALINK DVD-ROM
- **Audio Glossary**
- **CRNE Review**
- **Animations:**
  Mechanism of Action: Acyclovir
  Mechanism of Action: Saquinavir
  Mechanism of Action: Zidovudine

 COMPANION WEBSITE
- **CRNE Review**
- **Case Study:** HIV pharmacotherapy
- **Dosage Calculations**

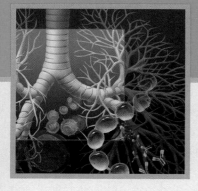

Drugs for Neoplasia

DRUGS AT A GLANCE

ALKYLATING AGENTS

Nitrogen mustards
- *cyclophosphamide (Cytoxan)*

Nitrosoureas

Miscellaneous alkylating agents

ANTIMETABOLITES

Folic acid antagonist
- *methotrexate (Apo-Methotrexate)*

Pyrimidine analogs

Purine analogs

ANTITUMOUR ANTIBIOTICS
- *doxorubicin (Adriamycin)*

PLANT-DERIVED ANTINEOPLASTIC AGENTS

Vinca alkaloids
- *vincristine (Oncovin)*

Taxoids

Topoisomerase inhibitors

HORMONES AND HORMONE ANTAGONISTS

Adrenocorticoids

Androgens and androgen antagonists

Estrogens and estrogen antagonists
- *tamoxifen (Apo-Tamox, Tamofen)*

Progestins

Other hormone agents

MISCELLANEOUS ANTINEOPLASTICS

Biological response modifiers

Other anticancer drugs

OBJECTIVES

After reading this chapter, the student should be able to do the following:

1. Identify the three primary therapies for cancer.
2. Explain the therapeutic action of each class of antineoplastic (anticancer) drug in relation to the differences between normal cells and cancer cells.
3. Explain the significance of growth fraction and the cell cycle to the success of chemotherapy.
4. Explain how combination therapy and special dosing protocols increase the effectiveness of chemotherapy.
5. Discuss the role of the nurse in reducing risk of cancer through client teaching.
6. For each of the drug classes listed in Drugs at a Glance, identify a representative drug and explain its mechanism of action, therapeutic effects, and important adverse effects.
7. Describe and explain, based on pharmacological principles, the rationale for nursing assessment, planning, and interventions for clients receiving drug therapy for cancer.
8. Discuss safety precautions when handling and administering antineoplastics.
9. Discuss interventions in the event of infiltration of vesicant drugs.
10. Use the nursing process to care for clients receiving drug therapy for cancer.

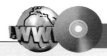

MediaLink

www.pearsoned.ca/adams-king

CRNE review, case studies, and other interactive resources for this chapter can be found on the Companion Website at **www.pearsoned.ca/adams-king.** Click on "Chapter 35" to select the activities for this chapter. For animations, more CRNE review questions, and an audio glossary, access the accompanying DVD-ROM in this textbook.

ancer is one of the most feared diseases in society for a number of valid reasons. It is often silent, producing no symptoms until it is too advanced to be cured. It sometimes requires painful and disfiguring surgery. It may strike at an early age, even during childhood, to deprive clients of a normal lifespan. Perhaps worst of all, the medical treatment of cancer often cannot offer a cure, and progression to death is sometimes slow, painful, and psychologically difficult for clients and their loved ones.

Many successes have been made in the diagnosis, understanding, and treatment of cancer. Some types of cancer are now curable, and therapies may give the client a longer, symptom-free life. This chapter examines the role of drugs in the treatment of cancer. Medications used to treat this disease are called anticancer drugs, antineoplastics, or cancer chemotherapy drugs.

35.1 Characteristics of Cancer: Uncontrolled Cell Growth

Cancer is a disease characterized by abnormal, uncontrolled cell division. Cell division is a normal process occurring extensively in most body tissues from conception to late childhood. Cells stop their rapid division by repressing genes responsible for cell growth. Genes controlling replication are turned back on when it becomes necessary to replace worn-out cells, as in the case of blood cells and the mucosa of the digestive tract.

Cancer is thought to result from damage to the genes controlling cell growth. Once damaged, the cell is no longer responsive to normal chemical signals checking its growth. The cancer cells lose their normal functions, divide rapidly, and invade surrounding cells. The abnormal cells often travel to distant sites where they populate new tumours, a process called **metastasis**. Figure 35.1 illustrates some characteristics of cancer cells.

Tumour is defined as a swelling, abnormal enlargement, or mass. **Neoplasm** is often used interchangeably with tumour. Tumours may be solid masses, such as lung and breast cancer, or they may be widely disseminated in the blood, such as leukemia. Tumours are named according to their tissue of origin, generally with the suffix -*oma*. Table 35.1 gives examples of various types of tumour.

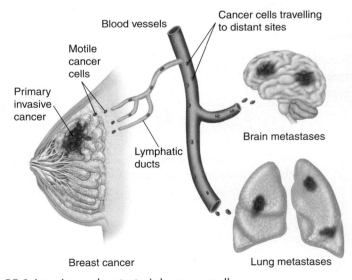

● **Figure 35.1** Invasion and metastasis by cancer cells

TABLE 35.1   Classification of Tumours

Name	Description	Examples
benign tumour	slow growing; does not metastasize and rarely requires drug treatment	adenoma, papilloma, lipoma, osteoma, meningioma
malignant tumour	grows rapidly larger; often becomes resistant to treatment and results in death if untreated	malignant melanoma
sarcoma	cancer of connective tissue; grows extremely rapidly and metastasizes early in the progression of the disease	osteogenic sarcoma, fibrosarcoma, Kaposi's sarcoma, angiosarcoma
carcinoma	cancer of epithelial tissue; most common type of malignant neoplasm; grows rapidly and metastasizes	malignant melanoma, renal cell carcinoma, adenocarcinoma, hepatocellular carcinoma
leukemia	cancer of the blood-forming cells in bone marrow; may be acute or chronic	myelocytic leukemia, granulocytic leukemia
lymphoma	cancer of lymphoid tissue	Hodgkin's disease, lymphoblastic lymphoma
glioma	cancer of glial (interstitial) cells in the brain, spinal cord, pineal gland, posterior pituitary gland, or retina	telangiectatic glioma, brainstem glioma

PHARMFACTS

Cancer in Canada

- Cancer is the second most frequent cause of death in Canada.
- It is estimated that 159,000 new cancer cases occur each year, with about 72,700 deaths.
- The most common cancers are lung, breast, prostate, colorectal, and non-Hodgkin lymphoma.
- Lung cancer rates in males have been declining by 2.8% per year since 1999. Lung cancer rates in females have been increasing by 1.4% per year since 1994.
- Breast cancer death rates have been declining since the mid-1980s, likely due to early detection, lifestyle modifications, and improved therapies following breast cancer surgery.
- Although the incidence of prostate cancer shows a gradual increase, death rates have declined by 2.7% per year since 1994.
- Mortality rates for colorectal cancer have been declining in both men and women since 1994, likely due to improved treatments.

Source: Canadian Cancer Society/National Cancer Institute of Canada. (2007). Canadian Cancer Statistics 2007. Toronto, ON: Canadian Cancer Society/National Cancer Institute of Canada.

35.2 Causes of Cancer

Numerous environmental factors have been found to cause cancer or to be associated with a higher risk of developing the disease. These factors are known as *carcinogens*. Many chemical carcinogens have been identified. Chemicals in tobacco smoke are thought to be responsible for about one-third of all cancers and 85% of all new cases of lung cancer in Canada. Chemicals such as asbestos and benzene have been associated with a higher incidence of cancer in the workplace. In some cases, the actual site of the cancer may be distant from the entry location, as with bladder cancer caused by the inhalation of certain industrial chemicals. Some known chemical carcinogens are listed in Table 35.2.

A number of physical factors are also associated with cancer. For example, exposure to large amounts of x-rays is associated with a higher risk of leukemia. Ultraviolet (UV) light from the sun is a known cause of skin cancer.

Viruses are associated with about 15% of all human cancers. Examples include herpes simplex types I and 2, Epstein-Barr virus, human papillomavirus (HPV), cytomegalovirus, and human T-lymphotrophic viruses. In February 2007, the National Advisory Committee on

TABLE 35.2   Common Chemical Carcinogens

Agent	Type of Cancer
alcohol	liver
arsenic	skin and lung
asbestos	lung
benzene	leukemia
nickel	lung and nasal
polycyclic aromatic hydrocarbons	lung and skin
tobacco substances	lung
vinyl chloride	liver

Immunization (NACI)—the expert committee that advises the Public Health Agency of Canada relating to immunization—recommended that females between 9 and 26 years of age be given the human papillomavirus (HPV) vaccine to prevent cervical cancer caused by HPV.

Factors that suppress the immune system, such as HIV or drugs given after transplant surgery, may encourage the growth of cancer cells.

Some cancers have a strong genetic component. The fact that close relatives may acquire the same type of cancer suggests that certain genes may predispose close relatives to the condition. These abnormal genes somehow interact with chemical, physical, and biological agents to promote cancer formation. **Oncogenes** normally promote cell growth. When mutated, they can lead to cancer. Other genes, called tumour suppressor genes, may inhibit the formation of tumours. If these suppressor genes contain a mutation, cancer may result. Damage to the tumour suppressor gene known as p53 is associated with cancers of the breast, lung, brain, colon, and bone.

Although the formation of cancer has a genetic component, it also has a strong environmental component. Adopting healthy lifestyle habits may reduce the risk of developing cancer. Proper nutrition, avoiding chemical and physical risks, and keeping regular health checkups can help prevent cancer from developing into a fatal disease. The following are lifestyle factors regarding cancer prevention or diagnosis to include when teaching clients about cancer prevention:

- Eliminate tobacco use and exposure to second-hand smoke.
- Limit or eliminate consumption of alcohol.
- Reduce fat in the diet, particularly from animal sources.
- Choose most foods from plant sources; increase fibre in the diet.
- Exercise regularly and keep body weight within recommended guidelines.
- Self-examine your body monthly for abnormal lumps and skin lesions.
- When exposed to direct sun, use skin lotions with the highest SPF (sun protection factor) value.
- Have periodic diagnostic testing performed at recommended intervals.
- Women should have periodic mammograms, as directed by their healthcare provider.
- Men should have a digital rectal prostate examination and a prostate-specific antigen test annually after age 50.
- Have a fecal occult blood test (FOBT) and flexible sigmoidoscopy performed at age 50, with FOBT annually after age 50.
- Women who are sexually active or have reached age 18 should have an annual Pap test and pelvic examination.
- Females between nine and 26 years of age may be given the human papillomavirus (HPV) vaccine to prevent cervical cancer caused by HPV.

NATURAL THERAPIES

Selenium's Role in Cancer Prevention

Selenium is an essential trace element that is necessary for healthy immune function. It is a vital antioxidant, especially when combined with vitamin E. It protects the immune system by preventing the formation of free radicals, which can damage cells.

Selenium can be found in meat and grains, Brazil nuts, brewer's yeast, broccoli, brown rice, dairy products, garlic, molasses, and onions. The amount of selenium in food, however, has a direct correlation to the selenium content of the soil. The soil of much Canadian farmland, except the southern halves of Alberta, Saskatchewan, and Manitoba, is low in selenium, resulting in selenium-deficient produce. Low dietary intake of selenium is associated with increased incidence of several cancers, including lung, colorectal, skin, and prostate. Selenium supplementation results in increased natural killer cell activity and may provide protection against some cancers.

35.3 Treatment of Cancer: Surgery, Radiation Therapy, and Chemotherapy

There is a much greater possibility of a cure if cancer is treated in its early stages, when the tumour is small and localized to a single area. Once the cancer has spread to distant sites, curing it is much more difficult; thus, it is important to diagnose the disease as early as possible. In an attempt to remove every cancer cell, three treatment approaches are utilized: surgery, radiation therapy, and chemotherapy.

Surgery is performed to remove a tumour that is localized to one area or when the tumour is pressing on nerves, the airway, or other vital tissues. Surgery lowers the number of cancer cells in the body so that radiation and pharmacotherapy can be more successful. Surgery is not an option for tumours of blood cells or when it would not be expected to extend a client's lifespan or to improve the quality of life.

Radiation therapy is an effective non-surgical way to kill tumour cells; approximately 50% of clients with cancer receive radiation therapy as part of their treatment. High doses of ionizing radiation are aimed directly at the tumour and are confined to this area to the maximum extent possible. Radiation treatments may follow surgery to kill any cancer cells left behind following the operation. Radiation is sometimes given as **palliation** for inoperable cancers to shrink the size of a tumour that may be pressing on vital organs or to relieve pain, difficulty breathing, or difficulty swallowing.

Pharmacotherapy of cancer is called **chemotherapy**. Because drugs are transported through the blood, they have the potential to reach cancer cells in virtually every location in the body. Some drugs can pass across the blood-brain barrier to treat brain tumours. Others are instilled directly into body cavities, such as the urinary bladder, to deliver the highest dose possible to the cancer cells without producing systemic side effects.

Anticancer drugs are sometimes given, in concert with surgery and radiation, to attempt a total cure or complete eradication of all tumour cells from the body. In other cases, the cancer is too advanced to expect a cure, and antineo-plastic agents are given for palliation to reduce the size of the tumour. Palliation eases the severity of pain or discomfort and may extend the client's lifespan or improve quality of life. In a few cases, drugs are given as prophylaxis, with the goal of preventing cancer from occurring in clients at high risk of developing tumours.

35.4 Growth Fraction and Success of Chemotherapy

Although most cancers are rapidly growing, not all cells in a tumour are replicating at any given time. Since antineoplastic agents are generally more effective against cells that are actively replicating, the percentage of tumour cells prolifer-ating at the time of chemotherapy is critical.

Both normal and cancerous cells go through a sequence of events known as the cell cycle, which is illustrated in Figure 35.2. Cells spend most of their lifetime in the G_0 phase. Although sometimes called the resting stage, the G_0 phase is when cells conduct their everyday activities such as metabolism, impulse conduction, contraction, or secretion. If the cell receives a signal to divide, it leaves G_0 to enter the G_1 phase, where it synthesizes the RNA, proteins, and other components needed to duplicate its DNA during the S phase. Following duplication of its DNA, it enters the premitotic phase, or G_2. Following mitosis in the M phase, the cell re-enters its resting G_0 phase where it may remain for extended periods depending on the specific tissue and surrounding cellular signals.

The actions of some antineoplastic agents are specific to certain phases of the cell cycle, while others are mostly independent of the cell cycle. For example, mitotic inhibitors such as vincristine affect the M phase. Antimetabolites such as fluorouracil are most effective during the S phase. The effects of alkylating agents such as cyclophosphamide are generally independent of the phase of the cell cycle. Some of these agents are shown in Figure 35.2.

The **growth fraction** is a measure of how many cells in a tumour are undergoing mitosis. It is a ratio of the number of replicating cells to the number of resting cells. Solid tumours such as breast and lung cancer generally have a low growth fraction, so they are less sensitive to antineoplastic agents. Certain leukemias and lymphomas have a higher growth fraction and exhibit a greater antineoplastic success rate. Some normal tissues, such as hair follicles, bone marrow, and the GI epithelium, also have a high growth fraction and are sensitive to the effects of these drugs.

35.5 Achieving a Total Cancer Cure

To cure a client, it is believed that every single cancer cell must be destroyed or removed from the body. Even one malignant cell could potentially produce enough daughter cells to kill a client. Unlike anti-infective therapy in which the client's immune system is an active partner in eliminat-ing large numbers of microorganisms, the immune system is able to eliminate only a small number of cancer cells.

As an example, consider that a small 1 cm breast tumour may already contain 1 billion cancer cells before it is detected.

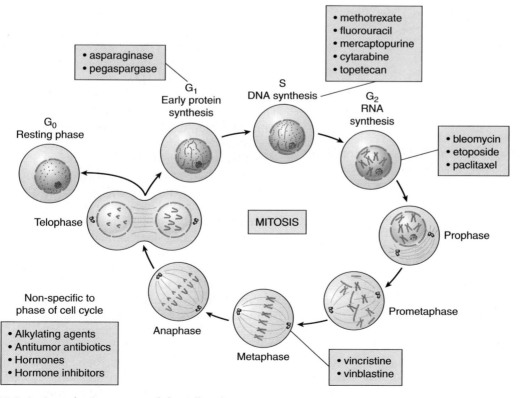

● **Figure 35.2** Antineoplastic agents and the cell cycle

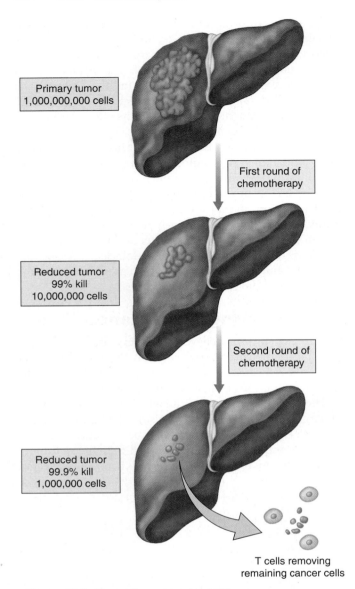

Primary tumor
1,000,000,000 cells

First round of
chemotherapy

Reduced tumor
99% kill
10,000,000 cells

Second round of
chemotherapy

Reduced tumor
99.9% kill
1,000,000 cells

T cells removing
remaining cancer cells

● **Figure 35.3** Chemotherapy and cell kill

A drug killing 99% of these cells would be considered a very effective drug, indeed. Yet even with this fantastic achievement, 10 million cancer cells would remain, any one of which could cause the tumour to return and kill the client. The relationship between chemotherapy and cell kill is shown in Figure 35.3. This example reinforces the need to diagnose and treat tumours at an early stage using several therapies such as drugs, radiation, and surgery when possible.

35.6 Special Pharmacotherapy Protocols and Strategies for Cancer Chemotherapy

While cancer cells are clearly abnormal in many ways, much of their physiology is identical to that of normal cells. It is thus difficult to kill cancer cells selectively without profoundly affecting normal cells. Complicating the chance of a pharmacological cure is the fact that cancer cells often develop resistance to antineoplastic drugs.

A number of treatment strategies have been found to increase the effectiveness of anticancer drugs. In most cases, multiple drugs from different antineoplastic classes are given during a course of chemotherapy. These multiple drugs affect different stages of the cancer cell's life cycle, attacking the tumour through several mechanisms of action, thus increasing the percentage of cell kill. Combination chemotherapy also allows the dosage of each individual agent to be lower, thus reducing toxicity and slowing the development of resistance. Examples of combination therapies include cyclophosphamide, methotrexate, fluorouracil (CMF) for breast cancer and cyclophosphamide, doxorubicin, vincristine (CDV) for lung cancer.

Specific dosing schedules, or protocols, have been found to increase the effectiveness of the antineoplastic agents. For example, some of the anticancer drugs are given as single doses or perhaps a couple of doses over a few days. Several weeks may pass before the next series of doses begins. This gives normal cells time to recover from the adverse effects of the drugs and allows tumour cells that may not have been replicating at the time of the first dose to begin dividing and become more sensitive to the next round of chemotherapy.

35.7 Toxicity of Antineoplastic Agents

All anticancer drugs have the potential to cause serious toxicity. These drugs are often pushed to their maximum possible dosages so that the greatest tumour kill can be obtained. Such high dosages always result in adverse effects in the client. Table 35.3 provides typical adverse effects of anticancer drugs.

Because these drugs primarily affect rapidly dividing cells, normal cells that are replicating are most susceptible to the adverse effects. Hair follicles are damaged, resulting in hair loss, or **alopecia**. The epithelial lining of the digestive tract is commonly affected, resulting in bleeding or severe diarrhea. The vomiting centre in the medulla is triggered by many antineoplastics, resulting in significant nausea and vomiting. Because of this effect, antineoplastics are sometimes classified by their emetic potential. Before starting therapy with the highest emetic potential agents, clients may be pretreated with antiemetic drugs such as prochlorperazine, metoclopramide, and lorazepam (see Chapter 37).

Stem cells in the bone marrow may be destroyed by antineoplastics, causing anemia, leukopenia, and thrombocytopenia. These side effects are the ones that most often cause discontinuation of chemotherapy. Efforts to restore bone marrow function may include stem cell transplant and therapy with growth factors such as granulocyte colony-stimulating factor (filgrastim) or granulocyte-macrophage colony-stimulating factor (sargramostim).

Each antineoplastic drug has a documented **nadir**, the lowest point to which the neutrophil count is depressed by the chemotherapeutic agent. The nurse can calculate the absolute neutrophil count (ANC) by multiplying the white blood cell count times the percentage of neutrophils. This

TABLE 35.3 Common Adverse Effects of Anticancer Drugs		
Changes to the Blood	**Changes to the GI Tract**	**Other Effects**
anemia (low red blood cells)	anorexia	alopecia
leukopenia or neutropenia (low white blood cells)	bleeding	fatigue
thrombocytopenia (low platelets)	diarrhea extreme nausea and vomiting	fetal death/birth defects opportunistic infections ulceration and bleeding of the lips and gums

can be obtained by reading the client's CBC with differential. In general, the drug should not be administered if the client is immunodeficient.

When possible, antineoplastics are given locally by topical application or through direct instillation into a tumour site to minimize systemic toxicity. Most antineoplastics, however, are given intravenously. Extravasation from an injection site can produce severe tissue and nerve damage, and even loss of a limb. Certain antineoplastics have specific antidotes for extravasation. For example, extravasation of carmustine is treated with injection of equal parts of sodium bicarbonate and normal saline into the extravasation site. Before administering an intravenous antineoplastic agent, the nurse should know the current guidelines for emergency treatment of extravasation for the particular agent. Central lines (subclavian vein) should be used with vesicants whenever possible.

Drugs used in cancer chemotherapy come from diverse pharmacological and chemical classes. Antineoplastics have been extracted from plants and bacteria, as well as being created entirely in the laboratory. Some of the drug classes attack vital cellular macromolecules, such as DNA and proteins, while others interfere with vital metabolic pathways of rapidly growing cells. The common theme among all the antineoplastic agents is that they kill or at least stop the growth of cancer cells.

Classification of the various antineoplastics is quite variable as some of these drugs kill cancer cells by several different mechanisms and have characteristics from more than one class of drug. Furthermore, the mechanisms by which some antineoplastics act are not completely understood. A simple method of classifying this complex group of drugs includes the following six categories:

1. Alkylating agents
2. Antimetabolites
3. Antitumour antibiotics
4. Hormones and hormone antagonists having antineoplastic activity
5. Natural products having antineoplastic activity
6. Miscellaneous anticancer drugs

ALKYLATING AGENTS

The first alkylating agents, the **nitrogen mustards**, were developed in secrecy as chemical warfare agents during World War II. Although the drugs in this class have quite different

chemical structures, all share the common characteristic of forming bonds, or linkages, with DNA, a process called **alkylation**. Figure 35.4 illustrates the process of alkylation.

35.8 Pharmacotherapy with Alkylating Agents

Alkylation changes the shape of the DNA double helix and prevents the nucleic acid from completing normal cell division. Each alkylating agent attaches to DNA in a different manner; however, they collectively have the effect of killing or at least slowing the replication of tumour cells. Although the process of alkylation occurs independently of the cell cycle, the killing action does not occur until the cell begins to divide. The alkylating agents have a broad spectrum and are used against many types of malignancies. They are some of the most widely used antineoplastic drugs. These agents are shown in Table 35.4.

Blood cells are particularly sensitive to alkylating agents, and bone marrow suppression is the most important adverse effect of this class. Within days after administration, declines in erythrocytes, leukocytes, and platelets may be measured. Damaging effects on the epithelial cells lining the GI tract are also common with alkylating agents.

NURSING CONSIDERATIONS

The role of the nurse in alkylating agent therapy involves careful monitoring of the client's condition and providing

MediaLink

Current Indications for Antineoplastics

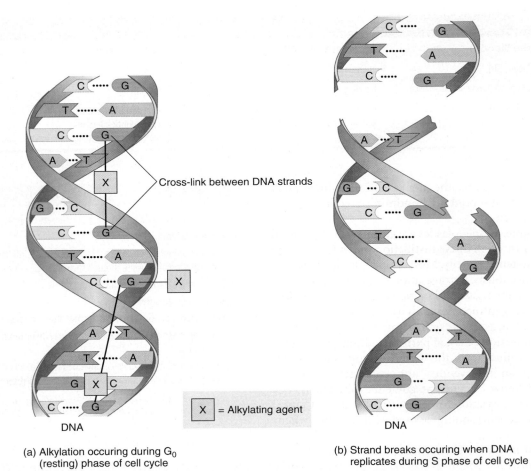

(a) Alkylation occuring during G_0 (resting) phase of cell cycle

(b) Strand breaks occuring when DNA replicates during S phase of cell cycle

● **Figure 35.4** Mechanism of action of the alkylating agents

TABLE 35.4	**Alkylating Agents**
Drug	*Route and Adult Dose*
Nitrogen Mustards	
chlorambucil (Leukeran)	PO; initial dose 0.1–0.2 mg/kg qd; maintenance dose 4–10 mg/d
cyclophosphamide (Cytoxan)	PO; initial dose 1–5 mg/qd; maintenance dose 1–5 mg/kg q7–10d
estramustine (Emcyt)	PO; 5 mg/kg tid–qid
ifosfamide (Ifex)	IV; 1.2 g/m^2 qd for 5 consecutive days
mechlorethamine (Mustargen)	IV; 6 mg/m^2 on day 1 and 8 of a 28-day cycle
melphalan (Alkeran)	PO; 6 mg qd for 2–3 wk
Nitrosoureas	
carmustine (BiCNU, Gliadel)	IV; 200 mg/m^2 q6wk
lomustine (CeeNU)	PO; 130 mg/m^2 as a single dose
streptozocin (Zanosar)	IV; 500 mg/m^2 for 5 consecutive days
Miscellaneous Alkylating Agents	
busulfan (Myleran)	PO; 4–8 mg/d
carboplatin (Paraplatin)	IV; 360 mg/m^2 once q4wk
cisplatin (Platinol)	IV; 20 mg/m^2 qd for 5 d
dacarbazine (DTIC)	IV; 2–4.5 mg/kg qd for 10 d
temozolomide (Temodar)	PO; 150 mg/m^2 qd for 5 consecutive days

education as it relates to the prescribed drug treatment. Before starting any form of chemotherapy, assess baseline vital signs, complete blood count, and the client's overall health status, including renal and liver function, intake and output, and body weight. Alkylating agents must be administered with caution to clients with hepatic or renal impairment, recent steroid therapy, leukopenia, or thrombocytopenia.

Alkylating agents are highly toxic to tissues with a rapid growth rate. Bone marrow depression occurs because these agents kill normal hematopoietic cells. These drugs may cause injury to the GI mucosa and hair follicles. Mustard agents may cause skin eruptions such as blistering. Alkylating agents may depress spermatogenesis and oocyte production, and secondary leukemias are frequently associated with this class of drugs. Platinum alkylating agents (e.g., cisplatin) may cause high-frequency hearing loss.

Remain alert to the possible development of blood dyscrasias by observing the client for signs and symptoms such as bruising or bleeding and by closely monitoring the CBC with differential and platelet count. Clients of childbearing age should be informed of the potential adverse impact on fertility. Cyclophosphamide also diminishes sex drive. Clients should be encouraged to frankly discuss sexual issues with the nurse, especially regarding options to preserve fertility.

Alkylating agents range from pregnancy category C (streptozocin, cyclophosphamide) to category X (estramustine). Both females and males should be counselled to abstain from coitus or to use reliable contraception during therapy and for 4 months thereafter. The nurse can assist the client in choosing an appropriate method for the client's cultural background, lifestyle, and health.

Client education as it relates to alkylating agents should include therapeutic goals; reasons for obtaining baseline data such as vital signs, blood work, and tests for cardiac and renal disorders; and possible side effects. Following are important points to include when teaching clients regarding alkylating agents:

- Sterility and amenorrhea may occur in clients on mechlorethamine or cyclophosphamide therapy, but these are reversible once therapy is discontinued.
- Obtain routine hearing screenings during therapy.
- Report any buzzing, ringing, or tingling sensation in the ears, or decreased hearing.
- Immediately report the following: tachycardia, fever, chills, sore throat, dyspnea, gout, kidney stones, skin rashes.

Please refer to "Nursing Process Focus: Clients Receiving Antineoplastic Therapy" (page 494) for additional teaching points.

ANTIMETABOLITES

Antimetabolites are drugs that are chemically similar to essential building blocks of the cell. They are structurally similar to certain critical cell molecules. They interfere with aspects of the nutrient or nucleic acid metabolism of rapidly growing tumour cells.

Pr PROTOTYPE DRUG | Cyclophosphamide (Cytoxan)

ACTIONS AND USES

Cyclophosphamide is a commonly prescribed nitrogen mustard. It is used alone, or in combination with other drugs, against a wide variety of cancers, including Hodgkin's disease, lymphoma, multiple myeloma, breast cancer, and ovarian cancer. Cyclophosphamide acts by attaching to DNA and disrupting replication, particularly in rapidly dividing cells. It is one of only a few anticancer drugs that are well absorbed when given orally. Because of its potent immunosuppressive properties, it has been used for certain non-neoplastic disorders such as prevention of transplant rejection and severe rheumatoid arthritis.

ADMINISTRATION ALERTS

- Dilute prior to IV administration.
- Monitor platelet count prior to IM administration; if low, hold dose.
- To avoid GI upset, take with meals or divide doses.
- Cyclophosphamide is pregnancy category C.

PHARMACOKINETICS

Cyclophosphamide is administered IV or PO. It is well absorbed from the GI tract. The inactive parent drug is metabolized into active drug in the liver. It is widely distributed, crosses the placenta, enters breast milk, and some drug crosses the blood-brain barrier. About 30% is excreted unchanged in urine. Half-life is 4 to 6.5 hours.

ADVERSE EFFECTS AND INTERACTIONS

The powerful immunosuppressant effects of cyclophosphamide peak 1 to 2 days after administration. Leukocyte counts sometimes serve as a guide to dosage adjustments during therapy. Thrombocytopenia is common, though less severe than with many other alkylating agents. Nausea, vomiting, anorexia, and diarrhea are frequently experienced. Cyclophosphamide damages hair follicles to cause alopecia, though this effect is usually reversible. Several metabolites of cyclophosphamide may cause hemorrhagic cystitis if the urine becomes concentrated; clients should be advised to maintain high fluid intake during therapy. Unlike other nitrogen mustards, cyclophosphamide exhibits little neurotoxicity.

Cyclophosphamide interacts with many drugs. For example, immunosuppressant agents used concurrently may increase risk of infections and further development of neoplasms. There is an increased chance of bone marrow toxicity if cyclophosphamide is used concurrently with allopurinol. If anticoagulants are used concurrently, increased anticoagulant effects may occur, leading to hemorrhage.

If used concurrently with digoxin, decreased serum levels of digoxin occur. Concurrent use with insulin may lead to increased hypoglycemia. Phenobarbital, phenytoin, or glucocorticoids used concurrently may lead to an increased rate of cyclophosphamide metabolism by the liver. Thiazide diuretics used concurrently lead to increased possibility of leukopenia.

Use with caution with herbal supplements, such as echinacea, which is an immune stimulator and may interfere with the drug's immunosuppressant effects.

 See the Companion Website for a Nursing Process Focus Chart specific to this drug.

35.9 Pharmacotherapy with Antimetabolites

Rapidly growing cancer cells require large quantities of nutrients and other chemicals to construct proteins and nucleic acids. When cancer cells treated with antimetabolites attempt to synthesize proteins, RNA, or DNA, they use the antimetabolites instead of normal cellular precursors. By disrupting metabolic pathways in this manner, antimetabolites can kill cancer cells or slow their growth. These agents are prescribed for leukemias and solid tumours and are shown in Table 35.5.

The purine and pyrimidine analogs resemble the natural precursors for nucleic acid biosynthesis. For example, the pyrimidine analog fluorouracil is able to block the formation of thymidylate, an essential chemical needed to make DNA; it is used in treating various solid tumours. After becoming activated and incorporated into DNA, cytarabine blocks DNA synthesis; it is an important drug in forcing remission of acute myelocytic leukemia. Figure 35.5 illustrates the structural similarities of some antimetabolites to their natural counterparts.

NURSING CONSIDERATIONS

The role of the nurse in antimetabolite therapy involves careful monitoring of the client's condition and providing education as it relates to the prescribed drug treatment. Before initiating chemotherapy, assess baseline vital signs, complete blood count, and the client's overall health status, including renal and liver function, intake and output, and body weight.

Many antimetabolites are contraindicated in pregnancy; for example, methotrexate is a category X drug and pregnancy should be avoided for at least 6 months following termination of therapy. Further contraindications include hepatic, cardiac, and renal insufficiency; myelosuppression; and blood dyscrasias. Clients with peptic ulcer, ulcerative colitis, or poor nutritional status should be monitored closely. Antimetabolites cause many of the adverse effects common to other antineoplastics, including alopecia, fatigue, nausea, vomiting, diarrhea, bone marrow depression, and blood dyscrasias. These drugs may also cause photosensitivity and idiosyncratic pneumonitis.

Observe the client for signs and symptoms of respiratory infection, including shortness of breath, cough, fever, and especially rash or chest pain (pleurisy). Viral infections such as those from herpes viruses, including varicella-zoster, can be especially virulent when experienced during antimetabolite therapy. Immunizations, especially attenuated vaccines, should be avoided during this time due to drug-induced impaired immunity. Clients should be encouraged to regularly practise deep breathing, if necessary, with the aid of an incentive spirometer.

Client education as it relates to antimetabolites should include goals of therapy; reasons for obtaining baseline data such as vital signs, tests for immune, lung, and renal disorders, and blood work; and possible side effects. Following are important points to include when teaching clients regarding antimetabolites:

- Avoid immunizations and people with active infections.
- Regularly practise deep breathing exercises.
- Eliminate or reduce respiratory irritants in the environment such as second-hand tobacco smoke and aerosol cosmetics (e.g., hair spray and deodorant).
- Immediately report the following: shortness of breath, chest pain, cough, fever, rash, dizziness, bruising, or bleeding.

Please refer to "Nursing Process Focus: Clients Receiving Antineoplastic Therapy" (page 494) for additional teaching points.

ANTITUMOUR ANTIBIOTICS

The antitumour antibiotics class of drug contains antibiotics, obtained from bacteria, that have the ability to kill cancer

TABLE 35.5 Antimetabolites

Drug	Route and Adult Dose
Folic Acid Antagonist	
methotrexate (Apo-Methotrexate)	PO; 10–30 mg/d for 5 days
Pyrimidine Analogs	
capecitabine (Xeloda)	PO; 2500 mg/m^2 qd for 2 wk
cytarabine (Cytosar, DepoCyt)	IV; 200 mg/m^2 as a continuous infusion over 24 hr
fluorouracil (Fluoroplex)	IV; 12 mg/kg qd for 4 consecutive days
gemcitabine (Gemzar)	IV; 1000 mg/m^2 once weekly for 7 wk
Purine Analogs	
cladribine (Leustatin)	IV; 0.09 mg/m^2 qd as a continuous infusion
fludarabine (Fludara)	IV; 25 mg/m^2 qd for 5 consecutive days
mercaptopurine (Purinethol)	PO; 2.5 mg/kg qd
thioguanine (Lanvis)	PO; 2 mg/kg qd

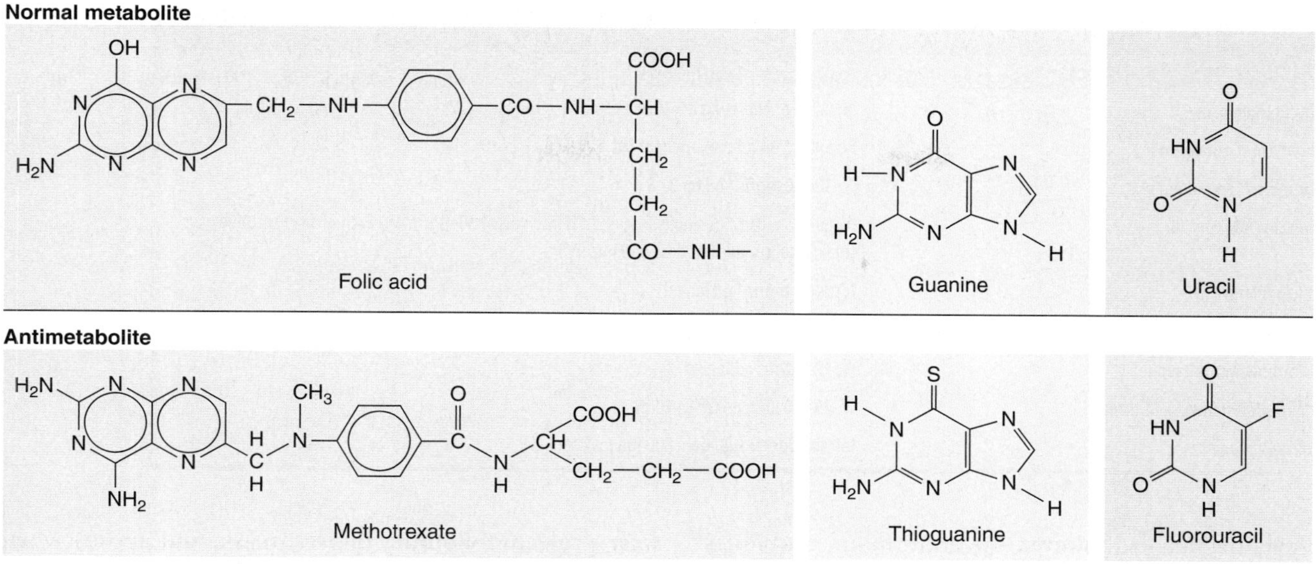

Normal metabolite

Folic acid

Guanine

Uracil

Antimetabolite

Methotrexate

Thioguanine

Fluorouracil

● **Figure 35.5** Structural similarities between antimetabolites and their natural counterparts

---

Pr PROTOTYPE DRUG | Methotrexate (Apo-Methotrexate)

ACTIONS AND USES

Methotrexate inhibits folic acid (vitamin B_9) metabolism. By blocking the synthesis of folic acid, methotrexate is able to inhibit replication, particularly in rapidly dividing cells. It is prescribed alone or in combination with other drugs for choriocarcinoma, osteogenic sarcoma, leukemias, head and neck cancers, breast carcinoma, and lung carcinoma. It is occasionally used to treat non-neoplastic disorders such as severe psoriasis and rheumatoid arthritis that have not responded to other medications.

ADMINISTRATION ALERTS

- Avoid skin exposure to drug. Avoid inhaling drug particles.
- Dilute prior to IV administration.
- Methotrexate is pregnancy category X.

PHARMACOKINETICS

Methotrexate is administered IV or PO. It is well absorbed from the GI tract. It is widely distributed, crosses the placenta, and enters breast milk. Sub-therapeutic amounts cross the blood-brain barrier. It is excreted mostly unchanged in urine. Half-life increases with dose and ranges from 3 to 15 hours.

ADVERSE EFFECTS AND INTERACTIONS

The adverse effects of methotrexate appear primarily in rapidly dividing tissues such as the GI epithelium and stem cells in the bone marrow. A potent immunosuppressant, methotrexate can result in fatal bone marrow toxicity at high doses. Leucovorin, a reduced form of folic acid, is sometimes administered with methotrexate to "rescue" normal cells or protect against severe bone marrow damage. Urine may be alkalinized to help protect the kidneys from toxicity. Hemorrhage and bruising are often observed due to low platelet counts. Nausea, vomiting, and anorexia are common. Although rare, pulmonary toxicity may develop and be quite serious.

Methotrexate interacts with several drugs. Bone marrow suppressants such as chemotherapeutic agents or radiation therapy may cause increased effects; the client will require a lower dose of methotrexate.

In concurrent use with NSAIDs, methotrexate may lead to severe methotrexate toxicity. ASA may interfere with excretion of methotrexate, leading to increased serum levels and toxicity. Concurrent administration with live oral vaccine may result in decreased antibody response and increased adverse reactions to the vaccine.

Use with caution with herbal supplements, such as echinacea, which may interfere with the drug's immunosuppressant effects.

 See the Companion Website for a Nursing Process Focus Chart specific to this drug.

---

cells. They are not widely used but are very effective against certain tumours.

35.10 Pharmacotherapy with Antitumour Antibiotics

Antitumour properties have been identified in a number of substances isolated from microorganisms. These chemicals are more cytotoxic than the traditional antibiotics, and their use is restricted to treating a few specific types of cancer. For example, the only indication for idarubicin is acute myelogenous leukemia. Testicular carcinoma is the only indication for plicamycin. The antitumour antibiotics are shown in Table 35.6.

The antitumour antibiotics bind to DNA and affect its function by a mechanism similar to that of the alkylating agents. Because of this, their general actions and side effects are similar to those of the alkylating agents. Unlike

TABLE 35.6 Antitumour Antibiotics	
Drug	**Route and Adult Dose**
bleomycin (Blenoxane)	IV; 0.25–0.5 units/kg q4–7d
dactinomycin (Cosmegen)	IV; 500 μg qd for maximum of 5 d
daunorubicin (Cerubidine)	IV; 30–60 mg/m² qd for 3–5 d
doxorubicin (Adriamycin)	IV; 60–75 mg/m² as single dose at 21-d intervals or 30 mg/m² on each of 3 consecutive days (max; total cumulative dose 550 mg/m²)
idarubicin (Idamycin)	IV; 8–12 mg/m² qd for 3 d
mitomycin (Mitamycin)	IV; 2 mg/m² as a single dose
mitoxantrone (Mitoxantrone)	IV; 12 mg/m² qd for 3 d
plicamycin (Mithramycin, Mithracin)	IV; 25–30 μ/kg qd for 8–10 d
valrubicin (Valtaxin)	Intrabladder instillation; 800 mg qwk for 6 wk

the alkylating agents, however, the antitumour antibiotics must be administered intravenously or through direct instillation via a catheter into a body cavity.

NURSING CONSIDERATIONS

The role of the nurse in antitumour antibiotic therapy involves careful monitoring of the client's condition and providing education as it relates to the prescribed drug treatment. Before initiating chemotherapy, assess the complete blood count and the client's overall health status, including renal and liver function, intake and output, and body weight. Interview the client regarding any history of allergy prior to initiating therapy. Vital signs, including auscultation of heart and chest sounds, and a baseline ECG should be obtained to rule out signs of cardiac abnormality or heart failure. Also assess for pregnancy and lactation as antitumour antibiotics range from pregnancy category C (dactinomycin, plicamycin, and valrubicin) to category D (bleomycin, daunorubicin, all others).

Antitumour antibiotics require cautious use in many clients. These drugs produce the same general cytotoxic effects as other antineoplastics, including alopecia, fatigue, nausea, vomiting, diarrhea, bone marrow suppression, and blood dyscrasias. As antibiotics, the risk of hypersensitivity reactions such as life-threatening angioedema exists. Antitumour antibiotics can be damaging to the myocardium; thus, they should be used with extreme caution, if at all, in clients with cardiac disease. Doxorubicin should be used cautiously if the client has received cyclophosphamide, pelvic radiation, or radiation therapy to areas surrounding the heart or has a history of atopic dermatitis. Other effects include hyperpigmentation of the mucosa and nail beds, particularly among African Canadians, and changes in the rectal mucosa. For this reason, suppositories and the taking of rectal temperature are contraindicated.

The nurse must be extremely cautious when administering antitumour antibiotics. Doxorubicin is easily absorbed through the skin and by inhalation and may cause fetal death or birth defects as well as liver disease. Therefore, wear protective clothing (gloves, mask, and apron) when preparing the drug.

Client education as it relates to antitumour antibiotics should include goals; reasons for obtaining baseline data such as vital signs, blood work, ECG, and other cardiac tests; and possible side effects. Following are important points to include when teaching clients regarding antitumour antibiotics:

- Proper attention to good oral hygiene is important. Changes in the colour of the mucosa can make it difficult to distinguish the degree of tissue oxygenation or the severity of mouth sores. Inform the dentist of antitumour antibiotic therapy.
- Avoid using OTC rectal drugs, such as for hemorrhoids, and taking rectal temperature.
- Seek emergency medical treatment for signs of severe allergic reaction or possible heart attack, such as shortness of breath, thick tongue, throat tightness or facial swelling, rash, palpitations, and chest, arm, or back pain.
- Immediately report headache, dizziness, or rectal bleeding.

Please refer to "Nursing Process Focus: Clients Receiving Antineoplastic Therapy" (page 494) for additional teaching points.

PLANT-DERIVED ANTINEOPLASTIC AGENTS

Plants have been a valuable source of antineoplastic agents. These agents act by preventing cell division.

35.11 Pharmacotherapy with Plant-Derived Antineoplastic Agents

Agents with antineoplastic activity have been isolated from a number of plants, including the common periwinkle (*Vinca rosea*), Pacific yew (*Taxus brevifolia*), mayapple (*Podophyllum peltatum*), and the Chinese tree *Camptotheca acuminata*. Although structurally different, medications in this class have the common ability to affect cell division; thus, some of them are called mitotic inhibitors. The plant-derived drugs are shown in Table 35.7.

Pr PROTOTYPE DRUG | Doxorubicin (Adriamycin)

ACTIONS AND USES

Doxorubicin attaches to DNA, distorting its double helical structure and preventing DNA synthesis. It is only administered by IV infusion. Doxorubicin is one of the broader spectrum cytotoxic antibiotics, prescribed for solid tumours of the lung, breast, ovary, and bladder and for various leukemias and lymphomas. It is structurally similar to daunorubicin.

A novel delivery method has been developed for both doxorubicin and daunorubicin. The drug is enclosed in small lipid sacs, or vesicles, called **liposomes**. The liposomal vesicle is designed to open and release the antitumour antibiotic when it reaches a cancer cell. The goal is to deliver a higher concentration of drug to the cancer cells, while sparing normal cells. An additional advantage is that liposomal doxorubicin has a half-life of 50 to 60 hours, which is about twice that of regular doxorubicin. The primary indication for this delivery method is AIDS-related Kaposi's sarcoma.

PHARMACOKINETICS

Since doxorubicin is administered IV, bioavailability is 100%. Doxorubicin is widely distributed but does not cross the blood-brain barrier. Tissue binding is extensive. It is mostly metabolized in the liver. Doxorubicin is mostly excreted in bile. Half-life is about 17 hours.

ADMINISTRATION ALERTS

- Extravasation from an injection site can cause severe pain and extensive tissue damage.
- For infants and children, verify concentration and rate of IV infusion with physician.
- Avoid skin contact with drug. If exposure occurs, wash thoroughly with soap and water.
- Doxorubicin is pregnancy category D.

ADVERSE EFFECTS AND INTERACTIONS

The most serious concern, which sometimes limits doxorubicin therapy, is cardiotoxicity. Acute effects include dysrhythmias; delayed effects may include irreversible heart failure. Like many of the anticancer drugs, doxorubicin may profoundly lower blood cell counts. Acute nausea and vomiting are common and often require antiemetic therapy. Complete, though reversible, hair loss occurs in most clients. It may cause the soles of feet, palms of hands, and nail beds to darken.

Doxorubicin interacts with many drugs. For example, if digoxin is taken concurrently, the client will have decreased serum digoxin levels. Phenobarbital taken concurrently leads to increased plasma clearance of doxorubicin and decreased effectiveness. Concurrent use of phenytoin may lead to decreased phenytoin level and possible seizure activity. Hepatotoxicity may occur if mercaptopurine is taken concurrently. Concurrent use of verapamil may increase serum doxorubicin levels, leading to doxorubicin toxicity.

Use with caution with herbal supplements. For example, green tea may enhance the antitumour activity of doxorubicin.

See the Companion Website for a Nursing Process Focus Chart specific to this drug.

TABLE 35.7 Plant-Derived Antineoplastic Agents

Drug	Route and Adult Dose
Vinca Alkaloids	
vinblastine sulfate (Velbe)	IV; 3.7–18.5 mg/m^2 qwk
vincristine sulfate (Oncovin)	IV; 1.4 mg/m^2 qwk (max 2 mg/m^2)
vinorelbine tartrate (Navelbine)	IV; 30 mg/m^2 qwk
Taxoids	
docetaxel (Taxotere)	IV; 60–100 mg/m^2 q3wk
paclitaxel (Taxol)	IV; 135–175 mg/m^2 q3wk
Topoisomerase Inhibitors	
etoposide (VePesid)	IV; 50–100 mg/m^2 qd for 5 d
teniposide (Vumon)	IV; 165 mg/m^2 q3–4d for 4 wk
irinotecan hydrochloride (Camptosar)	IV; 125 mg/m^2 qwk for 4 wk
topotecan hydrochloride (Hycamtin)	IV; 1.5 mg/m^2 qd for 5 d

The **vinca alkaloids** vincristine and vinblastine are older drugs derived from the periwinkle plant. Over 100 alkaloids have been isolated from the periwinkle, and their properties were described in folklore in several regions of the world long before their modern medical uses were discovered. Despite being derived from the same plant, vincristine, vinblastine, and the semisynthetic vinorelbine exhibit different effects and toxicity profiles.

The **taxoids**, which include paclitaxel and docetaxel, were originally isolated from the bark of the Pacific yew, which is an evergreen found in forests throughout the western United States. Over 19 different taxane alkaloids have been isolated from the tree and several are being investigated for potential antineoplastic activity. Paclitaxel is used for metastatic ovarian and breast cancer and for Kaposi's sarcoma. Unlabelled uses include many other cancers. A semisynthetic product of paclitaxel, docetaxel is claimed to have greater antitumour properties with lower toxicity. Bone marrow toxicity is usually the dose-limiting factor for the taxoids. Like the vinca alkaloids, the taxoids are mitotic inhibitors.

North American First Nations described uses of the mayapple (or wild mandrake) long before podophyllotoxin, the active ingredient in the plant, was isolated. As a botanical, podophyllum has been used as an antidote for snakebites, a cathartic, and a topical treatment for warts. Teniposide and etoposide are semisynthetic products of podophyllotoxin. These agents act by inhibiting **topoisomerase I**, an enzyme that helps repair DNA damage. By binding in a complex with topoisomerase and DNA, these antineoplastics cause strand breaks that accumulate and cause permanent damage to the DNA. Etoposide is used for refractory testicular carcinoma, small oat-cell carcinoma of the lung, and choriocarcinoma. Teniposide is used only for refractory acute lymphoblastic leukemia in children. Bone marrow toxicity is the primary dose-limiting side effect.

Other recently isolated topoisomerase I inhibitors include topotecan and irinotecan. These agents are called **camptothecins** because they were first isolated from *Camptotheca acuminata,* a tree native to China. The camptothecins are only administered intravenously, and their use is limited. Topotecan is used for metastatic ovarian cancer and small-cell lung cancer after failure of initial chemotherapy. Irinotecan is indicated for metastatic cancer of the colon or rectum. Like many other cytotoxic natural products, bone marrow suppression is the dose-limiting toxicity for the camptothecins.

NURSING CONSIDERATIONS

The role of the nurse in plant-derived antineoplastic therapy involves careful monitoring of the client's condition and providing education as it relates to the prescribed drug treatment. Before initiating chemotherapy, assess baseline vital signs, complete blood count, and client's overall health status, including renal and liver function, intake and output, and body weight.

Because natural plant extracts may produce allergic reactions in susceptible individuals, interview the client regarding any allergy to plants or flowers, including herbs and foods, which may provide clues to possible hypersensitivity to these drugs. Infusion hypersensitivity is an adverse reaction that may be ameliorated by steroid therapy. Vincristine may produce acute bronchospasm and skin rashes. Inquire regarding pregnancy and lactation as many of these agents are contraindicated in pregnancy. Vincristine is contraindicated in clients with obstructive jaundice and those with demyelinating forms of Charcot-Marie-Tooth disease.

These drugs produce many of the same cytotoxic effects as other antineoplastics, including alopecia, fatigue, nausea, vomiting, diarrhea, bone marrow suppression, and blood dyscrasias. Plant-derived antineoplastics should also be used cautiously in many pre-existing conditions, such as seizure disorders; vincristine may lower the seizure threshold. Vincristine should also be used cautiously in clients with leukopenia, neuromuscular disease, and hypertension. These agents may cause muscle weakness, peripheral neuropathy (including nerve pain), and paralytic ileus. Emphasize the need to establish a nutritional plan to combat constipation, including high fluid and fibre intake. Plant-derived antineoplastics can affect blood pressure, causing either hypotension or hypertension. Observe the client for symptoms such as headache, dizziness, and syncope. These drugs may produce severe mental depression; thus, remain alert to the possibility of suicidal ideation. Referrals for spiritual or emotional care such as a chaplain, mental health nurse, or social worker should be offered.

Client education as it relates to plant-derived antineoplastics should include goals; reasons for obtaining baseline data such as vital signs, blood work, and renal and liver function tests; and possible side effects. Following are important points to include when teaching clients regarding this class of drug:

- Seek emergency medical treatment for signs of severe allergic reaction: shortness of breath, thick tongue, throat tightness or difficulty swallowing, and rash.
- Seek medical treatment for severe convulsions or suicide risk, such as feelings of despair, verbalized suicide plan, or attempt.
- Immediately report the following: muscle weakness; difficulty walking or talking; visual disturbances; stomach, bone, or joint pain; swelling, especially in the legs or ankles; rectal bleeding; or significant changes in bowel habits.
- Avoid using OTC suppositories and taking rectal temperature.
- Avoid activities requiring physical stamina until effects of the drug are known.
- Obtain assistance with walking if weakness or staggering gait is a problem.
- Maintain good bowel habits including adequate fluid and fibre intake.

Please refer to "Nursing Process Focus: Clients Receiving Antineoplastic Therapy" (page 494) for additional teaching points.

ANTITUMOUR HORMONES AND HORMONE ANTAGONISTS

Hormones significantly affect the growth of some tumours. Use of natural or synthetic hormones or their antagonists as antineoplastic agents is a strategy used to slow the growth of hormone-dependent tumours.

Pr **PROTOTYPE DRUG** | Vincristine (Oncovin)

ACTIONS AND USES

Vincristine is a cell-cycle-specific agent that affects rapidly growing cells by preventing their ability to complete mitosis. It is thought to exert this action by inhibiting microtubule formation in the mitotic spindle. Although it must be given intravenously, a major advantage of vincristine is that it causes minimal immunosuppression. It has a wider spectrum of clinical activity than vinblastine and is usually prescribed in combination with other antineoplastics for the treatment of Hodgkin's disease, non-Hodgkin lymphomas, leukemias, Kaposi's sarcoma, Wilms' tumour, bladder carcinoma, and breast carcinoma.

ADMINISTRATION ALERTS

- Extravasation could result in serious tissue damage. Stop injection immediately if extravasation occurs. Apply local heat and inject hyaluronidase as ordered. No specific antidote is available. Observe site for sloughing.
- Avoid eye contact, which causes severe irritation and corneal changes.
- Vincristine is pregnancy category D.

PHARMACOKINETICS

Since vincristine is administered IV, bioavailability is 100%. It is widely and rapidly distributed. Tissue binding is extensive. Excretion is biliary with fecal elimination. Half-life is 10 to 38 hours.

ADVERSE EFFECTS AND INTERACTIONS

The most serious limiting adverse effects of vincristine relate to nervous system toxicity. Children are particularly susceptible. Symptoms include numbness and tingling in the limbs, muscular weakness, loss of neural reflexes, and pain. Paralytic ileus may occur in young children. Severe constipation is common. Reversible alopecia occurs in most clients.

Vincristine interacts with many drugs. For example, asparaginase used concurrently with or before vincristine may cause increased neurotoxicity secondary to decreased hepatic clearance of vincristine. Doxorubicin or prednisone may increase bone marrow depression. Calcium channel blockers may increase vincristine accumulation in cells. Concurrent use of digoxin may decrease digoxin levels, so the client may need an increased digoxin dose. When vincristine is given with methotrexate, the client may need lower doses of methotrexate. Vincristine may decrease serum phenytoin levels, leading to increased seizure activity.

 See the Companion Website for a Nursing Process Focus Chart specific to this drug.

35.12 Pharmacotherapy with Antitumour Hormones and Hormone Antagonists

A number of hormones are used in cancer chemotherapy, including glucocorticoids, estrogens, and androgens. In addition, several hormone antagonists have been found to exhibit antitumour activity. The mechanism of hormone antineoplastic activity is largely unknown. It is likely, however, that these antitumour properties are independent of their normal hormone mechanisms since the doses utilized in cancer chemotherapy are magnitudes larger than the amount normally present in the body. Only the antitumour properties of these hormones are discussed in this section; for other indications and actions, the student should refer to other chapters in this text. The antitumour hormones and hormone antagonists are shown in Table 35.8.

In general, the hormones and hormone antagonists act by blocking substances needed for tumour growth. Because these agents are not cytotoxic, they produce few of the debilitating side effects seen with other antineoplastics. They can, however, produce significant side effects when given at high doses for prolonged periods. Because they rarely cure the cancer when used singly, they are normally given for palliation.

The primary adrenocortical hormones used in chemotherapy are dexamethasone and prednisone. Because of their natural ability to suppress lymphocytes, the principal value of the glucocorticoids is in the treatment of lymphomas, Hodgkin's disease, and leukemias. They are sometimes given to reduce the nausea, weight loss, and tissue inflammation caused by other antineoplastics. Prolonged use can result in symptoms of Cushing's disease.

The sex hormones are used to treat tumours that contain specific hormone receptors. Two androgens, fluoxymesterone and testolactone, are used for breast cancer in postmenopausal women. The estrogens ethinyl estradiol and diethylstilbestrol (DES) are used to treat metastatic breast cancer and prostate cancer. The progestins medroxyprogesterone and megestrol (Megace) are used to treat endometrial cancer.

Hormone inhibitors include the antiandrogens bicalutamide, nilutamide, and flutamide, which are prescribed for advanced prostate cancer. Antiestrogens include tamoxifen and anastrozole, which are indicated for breast cancer. Anastrozole, letrozole, and exemestane are called **aromatase inhibitors** because they block the enzyme aromatase, which normally converts adrenal androgen to estradiol. Aromatase inhibitors can reduce plasma estrogen levels by as much as 95%, and they are used in postmenopausal women with advanced breast cancer whose disease has progressed beyond tamoxifen therapy.

NURSING CONSIDERATIONS

The role of the nurse in antitumour hormone and hormone antagonist therapy involves careful monitoring of the client's condition and providing education as it relates to the prescribed drug treatment. Before initiating chemotherapy, assess baseline vital signs, complete blood count, and the

TABLE 35.8   Hormone and Hormone Antagonists Used for Neoplasia

Drug	Route and Adult Dose
Hormones	
dexamethasone (ApO-Dexamethasone)	PO; 0.25–4 mg bid–qid
diethylstilbestrol (Stilbestrol)	PO/IV; 500 mg qd (max. 1 g qd); for pallation:1–15 mg qd
ethinyl estradiol (PMS-Estradiol)	PO; for treatment of breast cancer: 1 mg tid for 2–3 months; for palliation of prostate cancer: 0.15–3 mg/day
medroxyprogesterone (Provera, Depo-Provera) (see page 595 for the Prototype Drug box)	IM; 400–1000 mg qwk
megestrol (Megace)	PO; 40–160 mg bid–qid
prednisone (Apo-Prednisone) (see page 407 for the Prototype Drug box)	PO; 20–100 mg/m^2 qd
testosterone (Depo-Testosterone) (see page 606 for the Prototype Drug box)	IM; 200–400 mg q2–4wks
Hormone Antagonists	
anastrozole (Arimidex)	PO; 1 mg qd
bicalutamide (Casodex)	PO; 50 mg qd
exemestane (Aromasin)	PO; 25 mg qd after a meal
flutamide (Apo-Flutamide, Euflex)	PO; 250 mg tid
fulvestrant (Faslodex)	IM; 250 mg once
goserelin (Zoladex)	SC; 3.6 mg q28d
letrozole (Femara)	PO; 2.5 mg qd
leuprolide (Eligard, Lupron)	SC; 1 mg qd
nilutamide (Anandron)	PO; 300 mg/d for 30 days, then 150 mg qd
ⓟ tamoxifen citrate (Apo-Tamox, Tamofen)	PO; 10–20 mg 1–2 times/d (morning and evening)

client's overall health status, including renal and liver function, intake and output, and body weight. Assess for pregnancy and breastfeeding as both are contraindicated with the antitumour hormones and hormone antagonists.

Therapy using hormones other than tamoxifen may be palliative rather than curative; it is important that both the client and family understand this limitation before beginning chemotherapy. They must understand that while the client may appear to be improving, the cancer is likely continuing to worsen.

One of the most common yet distressing side effects of sex hormone therapy is the development of cross-gender secondary sexual characteristics, such as gynecomastia in males and hirsutism in females. Fertility is sometimes affected. Discuss these effects frankly with the client and offer support and simple interventions to increase self-esteem. The nurse may discuss clothing options to disguise gynecomastia or methods of facial hair removal, such as waxes or depilatories.

The use of glucocorticoids may increase the risk of sexually transmitted infections and other infections by suppressing the immune response. Glucocorticoid therapy may cause swelling, weight gain, redistribution of body fat (Cushing's syndrome), and hyperglycemia. Discuss body image concerns and nutritional strategies to increase energy and limit weight gain. Weight gain remains a concern for a number of cancer clients—especially in the early phases of

the disease. In some cases, cancer clients who are experiencing cachexia may benefit from glucocorticoid-induced weight gain. Glucocorticoids should be administered with caution to clients with diabetes mellitus. Obtain results of laboratory blood tests, including serum glucose, hormone levels, and electrolytes.

Client education as it relates to hormone therapy for cancer should include therapeutic goals; reasons for obtaining baseline data such as vital signs and tests for cardiac, renal, and endocrine function; and possible side effects. Instruct the diabetic client to monitor blood glucose more frequently; the client may need adjustments in antidiabetic medications. Instruct the client to report serum blood glucose readings as ordered by the healthcare provider (e.g., "less than 4 mmol/L or more than 11 mmol/L").

Following are other important points to include when teaching clients regarding hormonal therapy for cancer:

- Immediately report the following: shortness of breath, chest pain, difficulty with urination (too much, too little, pain, or irritation), excessive thirst, bleeding or injuries, sore throat, fever, and other signs of infection.

- Avoid persons with active infections.

- Practise excellent oral hygiene and skin care.

Please refer to "Nursing Process Focus: Clients Receiving Antineoplastic Therapy" (page 494) for additional teaching points.

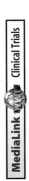
MediaLink   Clinical Trials

Pr PROTOTYPE DRUG | Tamoxifen (Apo-Tamox, Tamofen)

ACTIONS AND USES

Tamoxifen is given orally and is a drug of choice for treating metastatic breast cancer. It is sometimes classified as a selective estrogen receptor modulator (SERM). Tamoxifen is effective against breast tumours that require estrogen for their growth. These susceptible cancer cells are known as estrogen receptor (ER) positive. While it blocks estrogen receptors on breast cancer cells, tamoxifen actually activates estrogen receptors in other parts of the body. This results in typical estrogen-like effects such as reduced low-density lipoprotein (LDL) levels and increased bone mineral density. The drug is unique among antineoplastics because it is given not only to clients with breast cancer but also to high-risk clients to prevent the disease. Few if any other antineoplastics are given prophylactically, due to their toxicity.

PHARMACOKINETICS

Tamoxifen is well absorbed after oral administration. It is widely distributed. It is mostly metabolized by the liver and mostly excreted in feces. Half-life is 7days.

ADMINISTRATION ALERTS

- Give with food or fluids to decrease GI irritation.
- Do not crush or chew drug.
- Avoid antacid for 1 to 2 hours following PO dosage of tamoxifen.
- Tamoxifen is pregnancy category D.

ADVERSE EFFECTS AND INTERACTIONS

Other than nausea and vomiting, tamoxifen produces little of the serious toxicity observed with other antineoplastics. Of concern, however, is the association of tamoxifen therapy with an increased risk of endometrial cancer and thromboembolic disease. Hot flashes, fluid retention, and vaginal discharge are relatively common. Clients experiencing abnormal vaginal bleeding or menstrual irregularities during therapy should be evaluated promptly. Tamoxifen causes initial "tumour flare"—an idiosyncratic increase in tumour size—but this is an expected therapeutic event.

Tamoxifen interacts with several other drugs. For example, anticoagulants taken concurrently may increase the risk of bleeding. Concurrent use with cytotoxic agents may increase the risk of thromboembolism.

 See the Companion Website for a Nursing Process Focus Chart specific to this drug.

BIOLOGICAL RESPONSE MODIFIERS AND MISCELLANEOUS ANTINEOPLASTICS

Biological response modifiers approach cancer treatment from a different perspective than other chemotherapeutic agents. Rather than being cytotoxic to cancer cells, they stimulate the client's own immune system to fight the cancer.

35.13 Pharmacotherapy with Biological Response Modifiers and Miscellaneous Antineoplastics

Certain anticancer drugs act through mechanisms other than those previously described. For example, asparaginase deprives cancer cells of asparagine, an essential amino acid; it is used for acute lymphocytic leukemia. Mitotane (Lysodren), similar to the insecticide DDT, poisons cancer cells by forming links to proteins; it is used for advanced adrenocortical cancer. One of the newest antineoplastics, imatinib (Gleevec), inhibits the enzyme tyrosine kinase; it is currently used in chronic myeloid leukemia and shows promise for treating other cancers. These agents are shown in Table 35.9.

Biological response modifiers are a relatively new class of medications that do not kill tumour cells directly but instead stimulate the body's immune system. When given concurrently with other antineoplastics, biological response modifiers help to limit the severe immunosuppressive effects caused by other agents. Refer to Chapter 30 for additional information on the biological response modifiers and the Prototype Drug box for interferon alfa-2 (page 394).

LIFESPAN CONSIDERATIONS

Chemotherapy in Older Adults

Older adults have a higher incidence of most types of cancer. This could be a result of a greater accumulation of carcinogenic effects over time and age-related reduction in immune system function.

Due to age-related changes, such as decreasing mobility of the myeloid cells from the bone marrow to bloodstream, elderly clients with cancer are not likely to respond as effectively to stress that would normally trigger hematopoiesis. This results in greater susceptibility to bone marrow suppression. Client teaching of older adults and their caregivers should include the following:

- Elderly clients receiving chemotherapy drugs may experience toxic effects from the binding of the drugs to red blood cells at a higher rate due to normal age-related factors of fewer circulating red blood cells. Inform the client to report and monitor any bleeding or bruising and to avoid all ASA products.

- For reduction of neutropenia and prevention of infection, instruct the client in the importance of monitoring temperature daily and avoiding antipyretics to reduce fever before calling healthcare provider. Instruct the client to avoid crowds and people with respiratory infections. The client and caregivers should be instructed to use frequent handwashing to prevent the transmission of pathogens.

- Because older adults often have deficient nutritional intake, teach the client and caregivers regarding healthy food choices and assess for the client's ability to swallow food and medications.

- Because constipation may occur, encourage the client to obtain adequate fluid intake and to increase dietary fibre by eating whole grains and leafy vegetables.

TABLE 35.9 Biological Response Modifiers and Miscellaneous Antineoplastics

Drug	Route and Adult Dose
alemtuzumab (Mabcampath)	IV; 3–30 mg qd
altretamine (Hexalen)	PO; 65 mg/m^2 qd
arsenic trioxide (Trisenox)	IV; 0.15 mg/kg qd (max 60 doses)
asparaginase (Kidrolase)	IV; 200 IU/kg qd
bortezomib (Velcade)	IV; 1.3 mg/m^3 as bolus twice weekly for 2 weeks
gefitinib (Iressa)	PO; 250–500 mg qd
hydroxyurea (Apo-Hydroxyurea, Hydrea)	PO; 20–30 mg/kg qd
imatinib mesylate (Gleevec)	PO; 400–600 mg qd
interferon alfa-2 (Intron A) (see page 394 for the Prototype Drug box)	SC/IM; 2–3 million units qd for leukemia; increase to 36 million units qd for Kaposi's sarcoma
levamisole (Ergamisol)	PO; 50 mg tid for 3 d
mitotane (Lysodren)	PO; 1-6 g/day given in 3-4 divided doses (max 10 g/day)
procarbazine (Matulane)	PO; 2–4 mg/kg qd
rituximab (Rituxan)	IV; 375 mg/m^2 qd as a continuous infusion
trastuzumab (Herceptin)	IV; 4 mg/kg as a single dose, then 2 mg/kg qwk
tositumomab (Bexxar)	IV; 450 mg over 60 minutes
zoledronic acid (Zometa)	IV; 4 mg over at least 15 minutes

NURSING PROCESS FOCUS   Clients Receiving Antineoplastic Therapy

Assessment	Potential Nursing Diagnoses/Identified Patterns
Prior to administration: ■ Obtain complete health history including lab values such as platelets, Hct, leukocyte count, liver and kidney function tests, and serum electrolytes. ■ Obtain drug history to determine possible drug interactions and allergies. ■ Assess neurological status including mood and/or sensory impairment. ■ Assess for history or presence of herpes zoster or chickenpox. (Immuno-suppressive effects of cyclophosphamide and vincristine can cause life-threatening exacerbations.)	■ Need for knowledge regarding drug therapy and adverse effects ■ Risk for inadequate nutrition related to drug side effects ■ Risk for tissue injury related to extravasation ■ Risk for infection related to impaired immune system ■ Fatigue related to side effects of drug ■ Emotional needs related to cancer diagnosis and treatment

Planning: Client Goals and Expected Outcomes

The client will:
■ Experience a reduction in tumour mass and/or progression of abnormal cell growth
■ Experience a safe environment with no evidence of physical injury
■ Demonstrate an understanding of the drug's action by accurately describing drug side effects, precautions, and therapeutic goals

Implementation

Interventions (Rationales)	Client Education/Discharge Planning
■ Monitor hematological/immune status. ■ Observe for signs and symptoms of myelosuppression. (This could be indicative of overdose.) ■ Monitor complete blood count and temperature. ■ Collect stool samples for guaiac testing of occult blood. (Antineoplastics may cause anemia.)	Instruct client to: ■ Immediately report profound fatigue, fever, sore throat, epigastric pain, coffee-grounds vomit, bruising, tarry stools, or frank bleeding ■ Abstain from taking ASA unless prescribed ■ Avoid persons with active infections ■ Monitor vital signs (especially temperature) daily, ensuring proper use of home equipment ■ Anticipate fatigue and balance daily activities to prevent exhaustion ■ Avoid activities requiring mental alertness and physical strength until effects of the drug are known

continued

NURSING PROCESS FOCUS   Clients Receiving Antineoplastic Therapy   *(Continued)*

Interventions (Rationales)	**Client Education/Discharge Planning**
▪ Monitor cardiorespiratory status. ▪ Monitor vital signs and chest/heart sounds. (Cyclophosphamide may cause myopericarditis and lung fibrosis. Doxorubicin may cause sinus tachycardia, cardiac depression, and delayed onset CHF.) ▪ Observe ECG for T-wave flattening, ST depression, and voltage reduction. ▪ Monitor for shortness of breath and pitting edema.	Instruct client: ▪ To immediately report dyspnea; chest, arm, neck, or back pain; tachycardia; cough; frothy sputum; swelling; or activity intolerance ▪ To maintain a regular schedule of ECGs as advised by the healthcare provider ▪ That heart changes may be a sign of drug toxicity; HF may not appear for up to 6 months after completion of doxorubicin therapy
▪ Monitor renal status, urinary output, intake and output, and daily weights. (Cyclophosphamide may cause renal toxicity and/or hemorrhagic cystitis. Vincristine and methotrexate increase uric acid levels, contributing to renal calculi and gout. Vincristine may also cause water retention and highly concentrated urine.)	Instruct client: ▪ To immediately report the following: changes in thirst or the colour, quantity, and character of urine (e.g., "cloudy," with odour or sediment); joint, abdominal, flank, or lower back pain; difficult urination; and weight gain ▪ That doxorubicin will turn urine red-brown for 1 to 2 days after administration; blood in the urine may occur several months after cyclophosphamide has been discontinued ▪ To consume 3 L of fluid on the day before treatment and daily for 72 hr after (when client has no prescribed fluid restriction)
▪ Monitor GI status and nutrition. Administer antiemetics 30 to 45 minutes prior to antineoplastic administration or at the first sign of nausea. (Profound nausea, dry heaves, and/or vomiting are common with antineoplastic therapy. Dry mouth can also occur.)	Instruct client to: ▪ Report loss of appetite, nausea/vomiting, diarrhea, mouth redness, soreness, or ulcers ▪ Consume frequent small meals, drink plenty of cold liquids; avoid strong odours and spicy foods to control nausea ▪ Examine mouth daily for changes ▪ Use a soft toothbrush; avoid toothpicks
▪ Monitor for constipation. (Ileus or constipation and fecal impaction may occur with vincristine use, especially among older adults.)	Instruct client to: ▪ Report changes in bowel habits ▪ Increase activity, fibre, and fluids to reduce constipation
▪ Monitor neurological/sensory status. (Antineoplastics may cause peripheral neuropathy and mental depression. Vincristine may cause ataxia and hand/foot drop. Tamoxifen may cause photophobia and decreased vision. Such neurological changes may be irreversible.)	Instruct client to: ▪ Report changes in skin colour, vision, and hearing; numbness or tingling; staggering gait; or depressed mood; obtain no-self-harm contract ▪ Limit sun exposure; wear sunscreen, sunglasses, and long sleeves when outdoors
▪ Monitor genitourinary status. (Antineoplastic agents, including hormones, and especially tamoxifen, may alter menstrual cycles in women and may produce impotence in men. Tamoxifen increases the risk of endometrial cancer.) ▪ Monitor for hypersensitivity and other adverse reactions.	Instruct client to: ▪ Report changes in menstruation, sexual functioning, and/or vaginal discharge ▪ Recognize the risk of endometrial cancer before giving tamoxifen ▪ Instruct client to immediately report chest or throat tightness, difficulty swallowing, swelling (especially facial), abdominal pain, headache, or dizziness
▪ Monitor hair and skin status. (Alopecia is associated with most chemotherapy and may be a sign of overdosage. Methotrexate can cause a variety of skin eruptions.)	Instruct client to: ▪ Immediately report desquamation of skin on hands and feet, rash, pruritus, acne, or boils ▪ Wear a cold gel cap during chemotherapy to minimize hair loss
▪ Monitor for conjunctivitis. (Doxorubicin may cause conjunctivitis.)	▪ Instruct client or caregiver to immediately report eye redness, stickiness, pain, or weeping.
▪ Monitor liver function tests. (Antineoplastics are metabolized by the liver, increasing the risk of hepatotoxicity.)	Instruct client to: ▪ Report jaundice, abdominal pain, tenderness or bloating, or change in stool colour ▪ Adhere to laboratory testing for serum blood level tests of liver enzymes as directed
▪ Administer with caution to clients with diabetes mellitus. (Hypoglycemia may occur secondary to combination of cyclophosphamide and insulin.)	Instruct client to: ▪ Report signs and symptoms of hypoglycemia (e.g., sudden weakness, tremors) ▪ Monitor blood glucose daily; consult the healthcare provider regarding reportable results (e.g., less than 70 mg/dL)

Evaluation of Outcome Criteria

Evaluate the effectiveness of drug therapy by confirming that client goals and expected outcomes have been met (see "Planning").

See Tables 35.2 through 35.8 (pages 479–492) for lists of drugs to which these nursing actions apply.

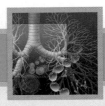

CHAPTER REVIEW

KEY CONCEPTS

The numbered key concepts provide a succinct summary of the important points from the corresponding numbered section within the chapter. If any of these points are not clear, refer to the numbered section within the chapter for review. Expanded versions can be found on the Companion Website.

35.1 Cancer is characterized by the rapid, uncontrolled growth of cells that invade normal tissues and eventually metastasize. Benign neoplasms are slow growing and rarely result in death; however, malignant neoplasms are fast growing and often fatal.

35.2 The causes of cancer may be chemical, physical, or biological.

35.3 Cancer may be treated using surgery, radiation therapy, and chemotherapy.

35.4 The growth fraction, the percentage of cancer cells undergoing mitosis at any given time, is a major factor determining success of chemotherapy.

35.5 To achieve a total cure, every malignant cell must be removed or killed through surgery, radiation, drugs, or by the client's own immune system.

35.6 Use of multiple drugs and special dosing protocols are strategies that allow for lower doses, fewer side effects, and greater success of chemotherapy.

35.7 Serious toxicity, including thrombocytopenia, anemia, leukopenia, alopecia, and severe nausea, vomiting, and diarrhea, limits therapy with most antineoplastic agents.

35.8 Alkylating agents act by changing the structure of DNA in cancer cells. Some have a very broad spectrum of clinical activity.

35.9 Antimetabolites act by disrupting critical pathways in cancer cells, such as folate or DNA metabolism.

35.10 Due to their cytotoxicity, a few antibiotics are used to treat cancer by inhibiting cell growth. They have a narrow spectrum of clinical activity.

35.11 Some plant extracts have been isolated that kill cancer cells by preventing cell division.

35.12 Some hormones and hormone antagonists are non-cytotoxic agents that are effective against reproductive-related tumours such as breast, prostate, and uterine. They are less cytotoxic than other antineoplastics.

35.13 Biological response modifiers have been found to be effective against tumours by stimulating the client's immune system.

REVIEW QUESTIONS

1 What is the fundamental feature that makes a cancer cell different from a normal cell?

2 Why is it important to kill or remove 100% of the cancer cells to effect a cure?

3 Why is combination therapy with antineoplastics more successful than monotherapy?

CRITICAL THINKING QUESTIONS

1. A client is newly diagnosed with cancer and is about to start chemotherapy. What would be the priority teaching for this client?

2. The chemotherapy medications often cause neutropenia in the client with cancer. What would be a priority for the nurse to teach a client who is a mother with three young children ages 3 to 7 years and who will receive chemotherapy at home?

3. A nurse is taking chemotherapy IV medication to a client's room and the IV bag suddenly leaks solution (approximately 50 mL) on the floor. What action should the nurse take?

EXPLORE MediaLink

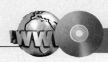 www.pearsoned.ca/adams-king

 MEDIALINK DVD-ROM
- Audio Glossary
- CRNE Review
- Animations
  Mechanism of Action: Cyclophosphamide
  Mechanism of Action: Methotrexate

 COMPANION WEBSITE
- CRNE Review
- **Case Study:** Client taking antineoplastic agents
- **Dosage Calculations**

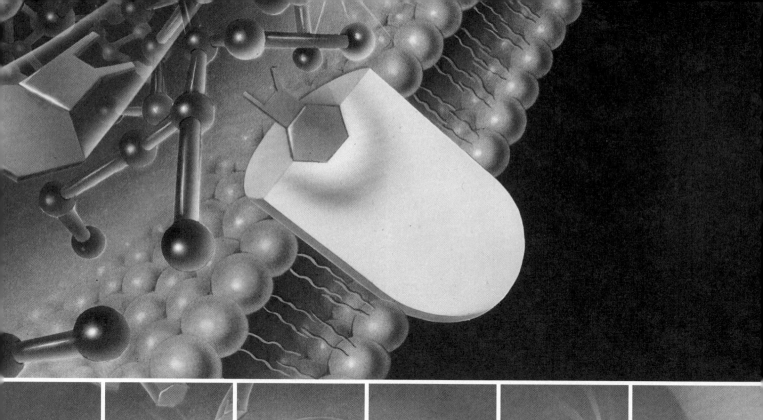

Unit 7

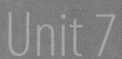

The Gastrointestinal System

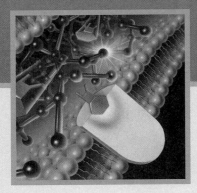

CHAPTER 36

Drugs for Peptic Ulcer Disease

DRUGS AT A GLANCE

H₂-RECEPTOR ANTAGONISTS
   ranitidine (Zantac)

PROTON PUMP INHIBITORS
   omeprazole (Losec)

ANTACIDS
   aluminum hydroxide (Amphojel, others)

ANTIBIOTICS

MISCELLANEOUS AGENTS

OBJECTIVES

After reading this chapter, the student should be able to do the following:

1. Identify drug classes used to treat peptic ulcer disease.
2. Explain the therapeutic action of each drug class in relation to the pathophysiology of peptic ulcer disease.
3. Explain why two or more antibiotics are used concurrently in the treatment of *Helicobacter pylori*.
4. Describe the nurse's role in the pharmacological management of clients receiving drugs for peptic ulcer disease.
5. For each of the drug classes listed in Drugs at a Glance, identify a representative drug and explain its mechanism of action, therapeutic effects, and important adverse effects.
6. Describe and explain, based on pharmacological principles, the rationale for nursing assessment, planning, and interventions for clients with peptic ulcer disease.
7. Use the nursing process to care for clients receiving drug therapy for peptic ulcer disease.

MediaLink

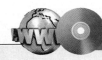

www.pearsoned.ca/adams-king

CRNE review, case studies, and other interactive resources for this chapter can be found on the Companion Website at **www.pearsoned.ca/adams-king.** Click on "Chapter 36" to select the activities for this chapter. For animations, more CRNE review questions, and an audio glossary, access the accompanying DVD-ROM in this textbook.

KEY TERMS

Very little of the food we eat is directly available to body cells. Food must be broken down, absorbed, and chemically modified before it is in a form useful to cells. The digestive system performs these functions, and more. Some disorders of the digestive system are mechanical in nature, slowing or accelerating the transit of food through the gastrointestinal tract. Others are metabolic, affecting the secretion of digestive fluids or the absorption of essential nutrients. Many signs and symptoms are non-specific and may be caused by any number of different disorders. This chapter will examine the pharmacotherapy of common diseases of the upper digestive system.

PHARMFACTS

Peptic Ulcer Disease

- About 5% to 10% of the world's population suffers at least once from peptic ulcers.
- The *Helicobacter pylori* bacterium is the most common cause of peptic ulcer disease.
- Of the 20% to 40% of Canadians who harbour *H. pylori*, most have no symptoms and only about 15% will develop a peptic ulcer.
- Foods and substances that reduce gastric acidity may help to relieve the pain.
- Milk may provide temporary relief until its digestion increases acid production.
- Smoking and foods that contain caffeine, such as coffee, tea, and soft drinks, may stimulate gastric acid production and worsen pain.
- OTC drugs are available to help reduce gastric acidity and promote comfort.
- Pharmacotherapy with prescription drugs is often required to eliminate *H. pylori* and promote healing.

36.1 Normal Digestive Processes

The digestive system consists of two basic anatomical divisions: the alimentary canal and the accessory organs. The **alimentary canal**, or gastrointestinal (GI) tract, is a long, continuous, hollow tube that extends from the mouth to the anus. The accessory organs of digestion include the salivary glands, liver, gallbladder, and pancreas. Major structures of the digestive system are illustrated in Figure 36.1.

Digestion is the process by which ingested food is broken down to small molecules that can be absorbed. The primary functions of the GI tract are to physically transport ingested food and to provide the necessary enzymes and surface area for chemical digestion and absorption.

The inner lining of the alimentary canal is the **mucosa**, from which mucus and the various acids, bases, and enzymes that break down food are secreted. In many parts of the alimentary canal, the mucosa is folded and contains deep grooves and pits. The small intestine is lined with tiny projections called villi (which have microvilli) that provide a huge surface area for the absorption of food and medications.

Substances are propelled along the GI tract by **peristalsis**, the rhythmic contractions of layers of smooth muscle. The speed at which substances move through the GI tract is critical to the absorption of nutrients and water and the removal of wastes. If peristalsis is too fast, nutrients and drugs will not have sufficient contact with the mucosa to be absorbed. In addition, the large intestine will not have enough time to absorb water, and diarrhea may result. Abnormally slow transit may result in constipation or even obstructions in the small or large intestine. Disorders of the large intestine are discussed in Chapter 37.

To chemically break down ingested food, a large number of enzymes and other substances are required. Digestive enzymes are secreted by the salivary glands,

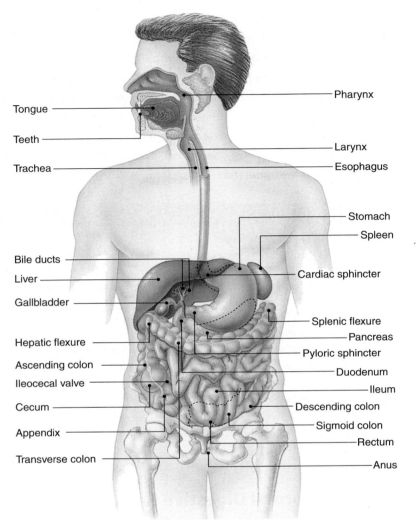

● **Figure 36.1** The digestive system
Source: Pearson Education/PH College.

stomach, small intestine, and pancreas. The liver makes bile, which is stored in the gallbladder, until needed for lipid digestion.

Because these digestive substances are not common targets for drug therapy, their discussion in this chapter is limited, and the student should refer to anatomy and physiology texts for additional information.

36.2 Acid Production by the Stomach

Food passes from the esophagus to the stomach by travelling through the cardiac (lower esophageal) sphincter. This ring of smooth muscle usually prevents the stomach contents from moving back up the esophagus, a condition known as **esophageal reflux**. A second ring of smooth muscle, the pyloric sphincter, is located at the entrance to the small intestine. This sphincter regulates the flow of substances leaving the stomach.

The stomach thoroughly mixes ingested food and secretes substances that promote the process of chemical digestion. Gastric glands extending deep into the mucosa of

the stomach contain several cell types critical to digestion and the pharmacotherapy of digestive disorders. **Chief cells** secrete pepsinogen, an inactive form of the enzyme pepsin that chemically breaks down proteins. **Parietal cells** secrete 1 to 3 L of hydrochloric acid each day. This strong acid helps to break down food, activates pepsinogen, and kills microbes that may have been ingested. Parietal cells also secrete **intrinsic factor**, which is essential for the absorption of vitamin B_{12} (see Chapter 38).

The combined secretions of the chief cells and parietal cells form gastric juice, which is the most acidic fluid in the body, having a pH of 1.5 to 3.5. A number of natural defences protect the stomach mucosa against this extremely acidic fluid. Certain cells lining the surface of the stomach secrete a thick, protective mucous layer and bicarbonate ions to neutralize the acid. These form such an effective protective layer that the pH at the mucosal surface is nearly neutral. Once reaching the duodenum, the stomach contents are further neutralized by bicarbonate from pancreatic and biliary secretions. These natural defences are shown in Figure 36.2.

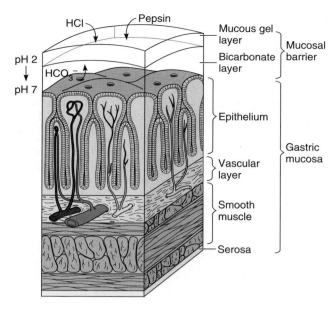

● **Figure 36.2** Natural defences against stomach acid

36.3 Pathogenesis of Peptic Ulcer Disease

An ulcer is an erosion of the mucosal layer of the GI tract, usually associated with acute inflammation. Although ulcers may occur in any portion of the alimentary canal, the duodenum is the most common site. A **peptic ulcer** is a lesion located in either the stomach (gastric ulcer) or small intestine (duodenal ulcer). Peptic ulcer disease (PUD) is associated with the following risk factors:

- Close family history of peptic ulcer disease
- Blood group O
- Smoking tobacco
- Beverages and food containing caffeine
- Drugs, particularly glucocorticoids, ASA, and NSAIDs
- Excessive psychological stress
- Infection with *Helicobacter pylori*

The primary cause of PUD is infection by the gram-negative bacterium **Helicobacter pylori**. In non-infected clients, duodenal ulcers are commonly caused by drug therapy with NSAIDs. Secondary factors that contribute to the ulcer and its subsequent inflammation include hyper-secretion of gastric acid and hyposecretion of adequate mucus for protection. Figure 36.3 illustrates the mechanism of peptic ulcer formation.

The characteristic symptom of a duodenal ulcer is a gnawing or burning, upper abdominal pain that occurs 1 to 3 hours after a meal. The pain disappears upon ingestion of food, and nighttime pain, nausea, and vomiting are uncommon. If the erosion progresses deeper into the mucosa, bleeding occurs and may be evident as either bright red blood in vomit or black, tarry stools. Many duodenal ulcers heal spontaneously, although they frequently recur

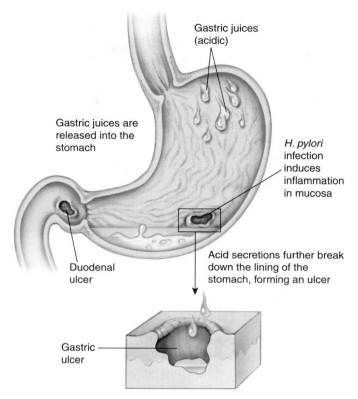

● **Figure 36.3** Mechanism of peptic ulcer formation
Source: Pearson Education/PH College.

after months of remission. Long-term medical follow-up is usually not necessary.

Gastric ulcers are less common than the duodenal type and have different symptoms. Although relieved by food, pain may continue even after a meal. Loss of appetite, known as anorexia, as well as weight loss and vomiting are more common. Remissions may be infrequent or absent. Medical follow-up of gastric ulcers should continue for several years because a small percentage of the erosions become cancerous. The most severe ulcers may penetrate through the wall of the stomach and cause death. Whereas duodenal ulcers occur most frequently in the 30- to 50-year age group, gastric ulcers are more common after age 60.

Ulceration in the lower small intestine is known as Crohn's disease, and ulceration in the large intestine is ulcerative colitis. These diseases, together categorized as inflammatory bowel disease, are discussed in Chapter 37.

LIFESPAN CONSIDERATIONS

Ulcers

- Peptic ulcers affect both men and women.
- Ulcers occur most frequently in early middle age onward.
- Duodenal ulcers are the most common type of ulcer.
- Gastric ulcers occur most often in older adults.
- The frequent use of NSAIDs by teenage girls and young women to control menstrual cramps may contribute to the development of ulcers in this population.

36.4 Pathogenesis of Gastroesophageal Reflux Disease

Gastroesophageal reflux disease (GERD) is a common condition in which the acidic contents of the stomach move upward into the esophagus. This causes an intense burning (heartburn) and may lead to ulcers in the esophagus.

The cause of GERD is usually a weakening of the lower esophageal sphincter. The sphincter may no longer close tightly, allowing the contents of the stomach to move upward when the stomach contracts. GERD is associated with obesity, and losing weight may eliminate the symptoms. Many of the drugs prescribed for peptic ulcers are also used to treat GERD, with the goal being to reduce gastric acid secretion. Because drugs provide only symptomatic relief, surgery may become necessary to eliminate the cause of GERD.

36.5 Pharmacotherapy of Peptic Ulcer Disease

Before initiating pharmacotherapy, clients are usually advised to change lifestyle factors that contribute to PUD or GERD. For example, eliminating tobacco and alcohol use, and perhaps reducing stress, may cause an ulcer to go into remission.

For clients requiring pharmacotherapy, a wide variety of both prescription and OTC drugs are available. These drugs fall into four primary classes, plus one miscellaneous group:

- H_2-receptor antagonists
- Proton pump inhibitors
- Antacids
- Antibiotics
- Miscellaneous drugs

The goals of pharmacotherapy are to provide immediate relief from symptoms, promote healing of the ulcer, and prevent future recurrence of the disease. The choice of medi-

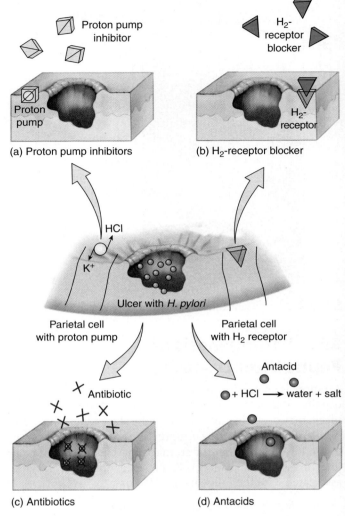

(a) Proton pump inhibitors

(b) H_2-receptor blocker

(c) Antibiotics

(d) Antacids

● **Figure 36.4** Mechanisms of action of antiulcer drugs

cation depends on the source of the disease (infectious versus inflammatory), the severity of symptoms, and the convenience of OTC versus prescription drugs. The mechanisms of action of the four major drug classes for PUD are shown in Figure 36.4.

H_2-RECEPTOR ANTAGONISTS

The discovery of the H_2-receptor antagonists in the 1970s marked a major breakthrough in the treatment of PUD. Since then, they have become available OTC and are often drugs of choice in the treatment of peptic ulcer disease. These agents are shown in Table 36.1.

36.6 Pharmacotherapy with H_2-Receptor Antagonists

Histamine has two types of receptors: H_1 and H_2. Activation of H_1-receptors produces the classic symptoms of allergy, whereas the H_2-receptors are responsible for increasing acid secretion in the stomach. Cimetidine, the first **H_2-receptor antagonist**, and other drugs in this class are quite effective

---

NATURAL THERAPIES

Ginger's Tonic Effects on the GI Tract

The use of ginger (*Zingiber officinalis*) for medicinal purposes dates back to antiquity in India and China. The active ingredients of ginger, and those that create its spicy flavour and pungent odour, are located in its roots (rhizomes). It is sometimes standardized according to its active substances, gingerols and shogaols. It is sold in pharmacies as dried ginger root powder, at a dose of 250 to 1000 mg, and it is readily available at most grocery stores for home cooking. Ginger is one of the best studied herbs, and it appears to be useful for a number of digestive-related conditions. Perhaps its widest use is for treating nausea, including that caused from motion sickness, pregnancy morning sickness, and postoperative procedures. It has been shown to stimulate appetite, promote gastric secretions, and increase peristalsis. Its effects appear to be from direct action on the GI tract rather than on the CNS. Ginger has no toxicity when used at recommended doses. Overdoses may lead to CNS depression, inhibition of platelet aggregation, and cardiotonic effects.

TABLE 36.1 H₂-Receptor Antagonists

Drug	Route and Adult Dose
cimetidine (Apo-Cimetidine, Tagamet)	PO; 300–400 mg bid–qd or 800 mg at hs for active ulcers; 300 mg bid or 400 mg at hs for ulcer prophylaxis
famotidine (Apo-Famotidine, Pepcid)	PO; 20 mg bid or 40 mg at hs for active ulcers; 20 mg at hs for ulcer prophylaxis
nizatidine (Apo-Nizatidine, Axid)	PO; 300 mg at hs for active ulcers; 150 mg at hs for ulcer prophylaxis
ⓟ ranitidine (Zantac)	PO; 100–150 mg bid or 300 mg at hs for active ulcer; 150 mg at hs for ulcer prophylaxis

at suppressing the volume and acidity of stomach acid. These drugs are used to treat the symptoms of both PUD and GERD, and several agents in this class are available OTC for the treatment of heartburn. Side effects of the H₂-receptor blockers are minor and rarely cause discontinuation of therapy.

NURSING CONSIDERATIONS

The role of the nurse in H₂-receptor antagonist therapy involves careful monitoring of the client's condition and providing education as it relates to the prescribed drug regimen. Because some H₂-receptor blockers are available without prescription, assess the client's use of OTC formulations to avoid duplication of doses. If using OTC formulations, clients should be advised to seek medical attention if symptoms persist or recur. Persistent pain or heartburn may be symptoms of more serious disease that requires medical treatment. Drugs in this class are usually well tolerated. Cimetidine is used less frequently than other H₂-receptor antagonists because of numerous drug-drug interactions (it inhibits hepatic drug-metabolizing enzymes) and because it must be taken up to four times a day. Safety

during pregnancy and lactation for drugs in this class has not been established (pregnancy category B).

IV preparations of H₂-receptor antagonists are occasionally utilized. Because dysrhythmias and hypotension have occurred with IV cimetidine, ranitidine or famotidine is utilized if the IV route is necessary.

CNS side effects such as dizziness, drowsiness, confusion, and headache are more likely to occur in elderly clients. Assess for kidney and liver function. These drugs are mainly excreted via the kidneys. Clients with diminished kidney function require smaller dosages and are more likely to experience adverse effects due to the accumulation of the drug in the blood. Although rare, these medications can cause hepatotoxicity. Long-term use of H₂-receptor antagonists may lead to vitamin B₁₂ deficiency because they decrease absorption of the vitamin. Iron supplements may be needed as this mineral is best absorbed in an acidic environment. Monitor CBC for possible anemia with long-term use.

Client education as it relates to H₂-receptor antagonists should include goals, reasons for obtaining baseline data such as vital signs and tests for cardiac and renal disorders, and possible side effects. See "Nursing Process Focus: Clients Receiving H₂-Receptor Antagonist Therapy" for specific teaching points.

ⓟ PROTOTYPE DRUG | Ranitidine (Zantac)

ACTIONS AND USES

Ranitidine acts by blocking H₂-receptors in the stomach to decrease acid production. It has a higher potency than cimetidine that allows it to be administered once daily, usually at bedtime. Adequate healing of the ulcer takes approximately 4 to 8 weeks, although those at high risk of PUD may continue on drug maintenance for prolonged periods to prevent recurrence. Gastric ulcers heal more slowly than duodenal ulcers, and thus require longer therapy. IV and IM forms are available for the treatment of stress-induced bleeding in acute situations.

PHARMACOKINETICS

Ranitidine has a duration of action of 8 to 12 hours. Oral drug is metabolized in the liver on first pass. About 50% is absorbed, and 30% is excreted unchanged in the urine. The half-life is 1.7 to 3 hours.

ADMINISTRATION ALERT

- Ranitidine may cause an increase in serum creatinine, AST, ALT, alkaline phosphatase, and total bilirubin.
- Ranitidine is pregnancy category B.

ADVERSE EFFECTS AND INTERACTIONS

Ranitidine does not cross the blood-brain barrier to any appreciable extent, so the confusion and CNS depression observed with cimetidine are not expected with ranitidine. Although rare, severe reductions in the number of red and white blood cells and platelets are possible; thus, periodic blood counts may be performed. High doses may result in impotence or a loss of libido in men.

Although ranitidine has fewer drug-drug interactions than cimetidine, it interacts with several drugs. For example, ranitidine may reduce the absorption of cefpodoxime, ketoconazole, and itraconazole.

 See the Companion Website for a Nursing Process Focus chart specific to this drug.

H₂-Receptor Antagonists and Vitamin B₁₂ in Older Adults

H_2-receptor blockers decrease the secretion of hydrochloric acid in the stomach. However, gastric acid is essential for releasing vitamin B_{12} from food, in which it is bound in a protein matrix. By affecting stomach acidity, these drugs can affect the absorption of this essential vitamin.

H_2-receptor blockers are frequently prescribed for older adults, who are more likely to have pre-existing lower vitamin B_{12} reserves or even deficiencies. With aging, the ability to produce adequate amounts of hydrochloric acid, intrinsic factor, and digestive enzymes progressively diminishes. These losses can lead to lower absorption rates, depletion of reserves, and eventual B_{12} deficiency. The nurse must educate older adults taking these drugs on the importance of including plenty of foods rich in vitamin B_{12} in their diets, including red meat, poultry, fish, and eggs.

PROTON PUMP INHIBITORS

Proton pump inhibitors act by blocking the enzyme responsible for the secretion of hydrochloric acid in the stomach. They are widely used in the short-term therapy of peptic ulcer disease. These agents are shown in Table 36.2.

36.7 Pharmacotherapy with Proton Pump Inhibitors

Proton pump inhibitors are relatively new drugs that have become widely used for the treatment of PUD and GERD. Drugs in this class reduce acid secretion in the stomach by binding irreversibly to the enzyme H^+, K^+-ATPase. In the parietal cells of the stomach, H^+, K^+-**ATPase** acts as a pump

---

NURSING PROCESS FOCUS   Client Receiving H₂-Receptor Antagonist Therapy

Assessment	Potential Nursing Diagnoses/Identified Patterns
Prior to administration: ■ Obtain a complete health history including allergies, drug history, and possible drug interactions. ■ Assess client for signs of GI bleeding. ■ Obtain baseline vital signs. ■ Assess level of consciousness. ■ Obtain results of CBC and liver and renal function tests.	■ Risk for falls related to adverse effect of drug ■ Need for knowledge regarding drug therapy ■ Acute pain related to gastric irritation from ineffective drug therapy ■ Nutrition imbalance related to adverse effects of drug

Planning: Client Goals and Expected Outcomes

The client will:
- Report episodes of drowsiness, dizziness
- Report recurrence of abdominal pain or discomfort during drug therapy
- Accurately describe the drug's intended effects, side effects, and precautions

Implementation

Interventions (Rationales)	Client Education/Discharge Planning
■ Monitor use of OTC drugs to avoid drug interactions, especially with cimetidine therapy. ■ Monitor level of abdominal pain or discomfort to assess effectiveness of drug therapy. ■ Monitor client use of alcohol. (Alcohol can increase gastric irritation.) ■ Discuss possible drug interactions. (Antacids can decrease the effectiveness of other drugs taken concurrently.) ■ Institute effective safety measures regarding falls. (Drugs may cause drowsiness or dizziness.) ■ Explain need for lifestyle changes. (Smoking and certain foods increase gastric acid secretion.) ■ Observe client for signs of GI bleeding.	■ Instruct client to consult with healthcare provider before taking other medications or herbal products. ■ Advise client that pain relief may not occur for several days after beginning therapy. ■ Instruct client to avoid alcohol use. ■ Instruct client to take H₂-receptor antagonists and other medications at least 1 hour before antacids. ■ Instruct client to avoid driving or performing hazardous activities until drug effects are known. Encourage client to: ■ Stop smoking; provide information on smoke cessation programs ■ Avoid alcohol and foods that cause stomach discomfort ■ Instruct client to immediately report episodes of blood in stool or vomitus or increase in abdominal discomfort.

Evaluation of Outcome Criteria

Evaluate the effectiveness of drug therapy by confirming that client goals and expected outcomes have been met (see "Planning").

See Table 36.1 for a list of drugs to which these nursing actions apply.

TABLE 36.2 Proton Pump Inhibitors	
Drug	**Route and Adult Dose**
esomeprazole (Nexium)	PO; 20–40 mg qd
lansoprazole (Prevacid)	PO; 15–60 mg qd
omeprazole (Losec)	PO; 10–40 mg qd–bid
pantoprazole (Pantololoc)	PO; 20–40 mg qd
rabeprazole (Pariet EC)	PO; 10–20 mg qd

to release acid (also called hydrogen ions [H$^+$] or protons) onto the surface of the GI mucosa. The proton pump inhibitors reduce acid secretion to a greater extent than the H$_2$-receptor antagonists and have a longer duration of action. All agents in this class have similar efficacy and side effects. The side effects of proton pump inhibitors are generally infrequent and minor. The newer agents esomeprazole and pantoprazole offer the convenience of once-a-day dosing.

NURSING CONSIDERATIONS

The role of the nurse in proton pump inhibitor therapy involves careful monitoring of the client's condition and providing education as it relates to the prescribed drug regimen. Proton pump inhibitors are usually well tolerated for short-term use. With long-term use, liver function should be periodically monitored as well as serum gastrin because oversecretion of gastrin occurs with constant acid suppression. Generally, proton pump inhibitors are not used during pregnancy and lactation; they range from pregnancy category B (rabeprazole) to C (omeprazole and lansoprazole). The nurse should assess for drug-drug interactions. Proton pump inhibitors will affect the absorption of medications,

vitamins, and minerals that need an acidic environment in the stomach. The nurse should obtain the client's history of smoking because smoking increases stomach acid production.

These drugs should be taken 30 minutes prior to eating, usually before breakfast. Proton pump inhibitors are unstable in an acidic environment and are enteric coated to be absorbed in the small intestine. These drugs may be administered at the same time as antacids. Proton pump inhibitors are usually administered in combination with clarithromycin for the treatment of *H. pylori*.

The nurse should monitor for adverse effects such as diarrhea, headache, and dizziness. Proton pump inhibitors are a relatively new class of drug; therefore, the long-term effects have not been fully determined.

Client education as it relates to proton pump inhibitors should include goals; reasons for obtaining baseline data, such as vital signs, diagnostic procedures, and laboratory tests; and possible side effects. Following are important points to include when teaching clients regarding proton pump inhibitors:

- Take medication before meals.
- Inform healthcare provider of significant diarrhea.

Pr PROTOTYPE DRUG | Omeprazole (Losec)

ACTIONS AND USES

Omeprazole was the first proton pump inhibitor to be approved for peptic ulcer disease. It reduces acid secretion in the stomach by binding irreversibly to the enzyme H$^+$, K$^+$-ATPase. Although this agent can take 2 hours to reach therapeutic levels, its effects may last 72 hours. It is used for the short-term therapy (4 to 8 weeks) of peptic ulcers and GERD. Most clients are symptom free after 2 weeks of therapy. It is used for longer periods in clients who have chronic hypersecretion of gastric acid, a condition known as **Zollinger-Ellison syndrome**. It is the most effective drug for this syndrome. Omeprazole is only available in oral form.

PHARMACOKINETICS

Omeprazole is rapidly absorbed and 95% protein bound. It is metabolized by the liver and is excreted by the kidneys. The half-life is 0.5 to 1 hour.

ADMINISTRATION ALERTS

- Administer before meals.
- Tablets should not be chewed, divided, or crushed.
- Drug may be administered with antacids.
- Omeprazole is pregnancy category C.

ADVERSE EFFECTS AND INTERACTIONS

Adverse effects are generally minor and include headache, nausea, diarrhea, rash, and abdominal pain. The main concern with proton pump inhibitors is that long-term use has been associated with an increased risk of gastric cancer in laboratory animals. Because of this possibility, therapy is generally limited to 2 months.

Omeprazole interacts with several drugs. For example, concurrent use of diazepam, phenytoin, and CNS depressants will cause increased blood levels of these drugs. Concurrent use of warfarin may increase the likelihood of bleeding.

 See the Companion Website for a Nursing Process Focus chart specific to this drug.

TABLE 36.3 Antacids

Drug	Route and Adult Dose
aluminum hydroxide (Amphojel, others)	PO; 600 mg tid or qid
calcium carbonate (Caltrate, Tums)	PO; 1–2 g bid–tid
calcium carbonate with magnesium hydroxide (Mylanta, Rolaids)	PO; 2–4 capsules or tablets PRN (max 12 tablets/day)
magnesium hydroxide (Milk of Magnesia)	PO; 2.4–4.8 g (30–60 mL)/d in 1 or more divided doses
magnesium hydroxide and aluminum hydroxide (Almajel, Diovol, Gellusil, Maalox)	PO; 2–4 tablets PRN (max 16 tablets/day)
magnesium hydroxide and aluminum hydroxide with simethicone (Mylanta, Maalox Plus, others)	PO; 10–20 mL PRN (max 120 mL/day) or 2–4 tablets PRN (max 24 tablets/day)
sodium bicarbonate (Alka-Seltzer) (see page 638 for the Prototype Drug box)	PO; 0.3–2.0 g qd–qid or 1/2 tsp of powder in glass of water

- Do not crush, break, or chew the medication.
- Avoid smoking, alcohol, and foods that cause gastric discomfort.
- Report GI bleeding, abdominal pain, and heartburn.
- Eat foods with beneficial bacteria, such as yogurt, or take *Acidophilus* to replace "friendly" bacteria.
- Sleep with head elevated 30 degrees. A foam wedge under the top end of the mattress or risers under the top end of the bed frame may be used to keep the head elevated.

ANTACIDS

Antacids are alkaline substances that have been used to neutralize stomach acid for hundreds of years. These agents, shown in Table 36.3, are readily available as OTC drugs.

36.8 Pharmacotherapy with Antacids

Prior to the development of H_2-receptor antagonists and proton pump inhibitors, antacids were the mainstay of peptic ulcer and GERD pharmacotherapy. Indeed, many clients still use these inexpensive and readily available OTC drugs. Antacids, however, are no longer recommended as the sole drug class for peptic ulcer disease.

Antacids are alkaline, inorganic compounds of aluminum, magnesium, sodium, or calcium. The most common are combinations of aluminum hydroxide and magnesium hydroxide, which are bases capable of rapidly neutralizing stomach acid. Chewable tablets and liquid formulations are available. Simethicone is sometimes added to antacid preparations because it reduces gas bubbles that cause bloating and discomfort. A few products combine antacids and H_2-receptor blockers into a single tablet; for example, Pepcid Complete contains calcium carbonate, magnesium hydroxide, and famotidine.

Unless taken in extremely large amounts, antacids are very safe. Antacids containing sodium, calcium, or magnesium can result in absorption of these minerals into the general circulation. This absorption is generally not a problem unless the client is on a sodium-restricted diet or has other conditions such as diminished renal function that could result in accumulation of these minerals. In fact, some manufacturers advertise their antacid products as calcium supplements. Clients should follow the label instructions carefully and not take more than the recommended dosage.

NURSING CONSIDERATIONS

The role of the nurse in antacid therapy involves careful monitoring of the client's condition and providing education as it relates to the prescribed drug regimen. Antacids are for occasional use only, and clients should seek medical attention if symptoms persist or recur. The nurse should obtain a medical history, including the use of OTC and prescription drugs. The nurse should assess the client for signs of renal insufficiency; magnesium-containing antacids should be used with caution in these clients. Hypermagnesemia may occur because the kidneys are unable to excrete excess magnesium.

When used according to label directions, antacids have few side effects. Magnesium- and aluminum-based products may cause diarrhea, and those with calcium may cause constipation.

Client education as it relates to antacids should include goals, reasons for obtaining baseline data, and possible side effects. Following are important points the nurse should include when teaching clients regarding antacids:

- Clients with renal failure should avoid magnesium-based antacids.
- Clients with heart failure or hypertension should be advised to avoid sodium-based antacids.
- Take antacids at least 2 hours before or 2 hours after other oral medications. Antacids directly affect the acidity of the stomach and may interfere with drug absorption.
- Note the number and consistency of stools since antacids may alter bowel activity.
- Medication may make stools appear white.
- Shake liquid preparations thoroughly before dispensing.

PROTOTYPE DRUG | Aluminum Hydroxide (Amphojel, others)

ACTIONS AND USES

Aluminum hydroxide is an inorganic agent used alone or in combination with other antacids such as magnesium hydroxide. Unlike calcium-based antacids that can be absorbed and cause systemic effects, aluminum compounds have minimal absorption. Their primary action is to neutralize stomach acid by raising the pH of the stomach contents. Unlike H_2-receptor antagonists and proton pump inhibitors, aluminum antacids do not reduce the volume of acid secretion. They are most effectively used in combination with other antiulcer agents for the symptomatic relief of heartburn due to PUD or GERD.

PHARMACOKINETICS

Aluminum hydroxide has an onset of action of 20 to 40 minutes. The duration of action is 2 hours when taken with food and 3 hours when taken 1 to 2 hours after food. It has an unknown half-life, is minimally absorbed, and is mostly excreted in the feces.

ADMINISTRATION ALERTS

- Aluminum antacids should be administered at least 2 hours before or after other drugs because drug absorption could be affected.
- There is no specific treatment for overdose.
- Aluminum hydroxide is pregnancy category C.

ADVERSE EFFECTS AND INTERACTIONS

When given in high doses, aluminum compounds may interfere with phosphate metabolism and cause constipation. They are often combined with magnesium compounds, which counteract the constipation. Like many other antacids, aluminum compounds should not be taken with other medications as they may interfere with their absorption. Sodium polystyrene sulfonate may cause systemic alkalosis. Excessive or chronic use may lead to hypophosphatemia.

 See the Companion Website for a Nursing Process Focus chart specific to this drug.

ANTIBIOTICS

The gram-negative bacterium *H. pylori* is associated with 90% of all duodenal ulcers and 75% of all gastric ulcers. It is also strongly associated with gastric cancer. In order to more rapidly and completely eliminate peptic ulcers, several antibiotics are used to eradicate this bacterium.

36.9 Pharmacotherapy with Combination Antibiotic Therapy

H. pylori has adapted well as a human pathogen by devising ways to neutralize the high acidity surrounding it and by making chemicals called adhesins that allow it to stick tightly to the GI mucosa. *H. pylori* infections can remain active for life if not treated appropriately. Elimination of this organism causes ulcers to heal more rapidly and to remain in remission longer. The following antibiotics are commonly used for this purpose:

- Amoxicillin (Amoxil, others)
- Clarithromycin (Biaxin)
- Metronidazole (Flagyl)
- Tetracycline (Apo-Tetra, others)
- Bismuth subsalicylate (Pepto-Bismol)

Two or more antibiotics are given concurrently to increase the effectiveness of therapy and to lower the potential for bacterial resistance. The antibiotics are also combined with a proton pump inhibitor or an H_2-receptor antagonist. Bismuth compounds are sometimes added to the antibiotic regimen. Although technically not antibiotics, bismuth compounds inhibit bacterial growth and prevent *H. pylori*

from adhering to the gastric mucosa. Antibiotic therapy generally continues for 7 to 14 days. Additional information on antibacterial agents can be found in Chapter 32.

36.10 Miscellaneous Drugs for Peptic Ulcer Disease

Several additional drugs are beneficial in treating peptic ulcer disease. Sucralfate consists of sucrose (a sugar) plus aluminum hydroxide (an antacid). The drug produces a thick, gel-like substance that coats the ulcer, protecting it against further erosion and promoting healing. It does not affect the secretion of gastric acid. Little of the drug is absorbed from the GI tract. Other than constipation, side effects are minimal.

Misoprostol is a prostaglandin-like substance that acts by inhibiting gastric acid secretion and stimulating the production of protective mucus. Its primary use is for the prevention of peptic ulcers in clients taking high doses of NSAIDs or glucocorticoids. Diarrhea and abdominal cramping are relatively common. Classified as a pregnancy category X drug, misoprostol is contraindicated in pregnant clients. In fact, misoprostol is sometimes used to terminate pregnancies, as discussed in Chapter 41.

Prior to the discovery of safer and more effective drugs, anticholinergics such as atropine were used to treat peptic ulcers. Pirenzepine is a cholinergic blocker (muscarinic) available in Canada that inhibits the autonomic receptors responsible for gastric acid secretion. Although the action of pirenzepine is somewhat selective to the stomach, other anticholinergic effects such as dry mouth and constipation are possible. It is rare to find anticholinergics used for treating peptic ulcer today.

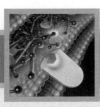

CHAPTER REVIEW

KEY CONCEPTS

The numbered key concepts provide a succinct summary of the important points from the corresponding numbered section within the chapter. If any of these points are not clear, refer to the numbered section within the chapter for review. Expanded versions can be found on the Companion Website.

36.1 The digestive system is responsible for breaking down food, absorbing nutrients, and eliminating wastes. Transit time through the GI tract can affect drug action.

36.2 The stomach secretes enzymes and acid that accelerate the process of chemical digestion.

36.3 Peptic ulcer disease (PUD) is caused by an erosion of the mucosal layer of the stomach or duodenum. Gastric ulcers are more commonly associated with cancer and require longer follow-up.

36.4 Gastroesophageal reflux disease (GERD) is caused by acidic stomach contents entering the esophagus. GERD and PUD are treated with similar medications.

36.5 Peptic ulcer disease is best treated by a combination of lifestyle changes and pharmacotherapy.

36.6 H_2-receptor blockers slow acid secretion by the stomach and are often drugs of choice in treating PUD and GERD.

36.7 Proton pump inhibitors block the enzyme H^+, K^+-ATPase and are effective at reducing gastric acid secretion.

36.8 Antacids are effective at neutralizing stomach acid and are inexpensive OTC therapy for PUD and GERD.

36.9 Combinations of antibiotics are administered to eliminate *H. pylori*, the cause of many peptic ulcers.

36.10 Several miscellaneous drugs, including sucralfate, misoprostol, and pirenzepine, are also beneficial in treating PUD.

REVIEW QUESTIONS

1 Many common antacids are combinations of salts containing aluminum and magnesium. For which population of clients are such antacids contraindicated? What products should be used instead?

2 Before starting drug therapy for PUD, the client should attempt to make changes to lifestyle factors that are associated with this disorder. What is the nurse's role in assisting the client to initiate such changes?

3 Explain the following statement: All H_2-receptor antagonists are antihistamines, but not all antihistamines are H_2-receptor antagonists.

4 The use of amoxicillin (Amoxil) and clarithromycin (Biaxin) in treating PUD is to eliminate *H. pylori* from the GI tract. Why, even though the client is feeling better midway through the treatment regimen, is it important to comply with the directions on the prescription bottle to take all of the medication?

CRITICAL THINKING QUESTIONS

1. A client with chronic hyperacidity of the stomach takes aluminum hydroxide (Amphojel) on a regular basis. The client presents to the clinic with complaints of increasing weakness. What may the nurse's assessment find as the cause of this weakness? What interventions are needed?

2. Nurses who work at night are at higher risk for developing peptic ulcer disease. Why is this?

3. A client who is on ranitidine (Zantac) for PUD smokes and drinks alcohol daily. Will the ranitidine be effective for this client? Why or why not?

EXPLORE
MediaLink

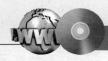

www.pearsoned.ca/adams-king

MEDIALINK DVD-ROM
- **Audio Glossary**
- **CRNE Review**
- **Animations**
  Mechanism of Action: Omeprazole
  Mechanism of Action: Ranitidine

COMPANION WEBSITE
- **CRNE Review**
- **Case Study:** Client with peptic ulcer disease
- **Dosage Calculations**

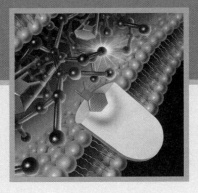

CHAPTER 37

Drugs for Gastrointestinal Disorders

DRUGS AT A GLANCE

DRUGS FOR CONSTIPATION: LAXATIVES

Bulk-forming agents
> *psyllium mucilloid (Metamucil, Psyllium)*

Stool softeners / surfactants

Stimulants

Saline and osmotic agents

Miscellaneous agents

DRUGS FOR DIARRHEA: ANTIDIARRHEALS

Opioids
> *diphenoxylate with atropine (Lomotil)*

Miscellaneous agents

DRUGS FOR NAUSEA AND VOMITING

Anticholinergics

Antihistamines

Benzodiazepines

Cannabinoids

Glucocorticoids

Phenothiazines and phenothiazine-like agents
> *prochlorperazine (PMS-Prochlorperazine, Stemetil)*

Serotonin receptor antagonists

DRUGS FOR WEIGHT LOSS
> *sibutramine (Meridia)*

DRUGS FOR PANCREATITIS
> *pancrelipase (Lipancreatin, Pancrease)*

OBJECTIVES

After reading this chapter, the student should be able to do the following:

1. Identify drug classes used for treating bowel disorders, nausea, vomiting, obesity, and pancreatitis.

2. Explain the therapeutic action of each class of drugs used to treat bowel disorders, nausea, vomiting, obesity, and pancreatitis in relation to the pathophysiology of these conditions.

3. Discuss the role of the nurse regarding the non-pharmacological management of constipation.

4. Describe the nurse's role in the pharmacological management of clients receiving drugs for the management of bowel disorders, nausea, vomiting, obesity, and pancreatitis.

5. For each of the drug classes listed in Drugs at a Glance, identify a representative drug and explain its mechanism of action, therapeutic effects, and important adverse effects.

6. Describe and explain, based on pharmacological principles, the rationale for nursing assessment, planning, and interventions for clients with bowel disorders, nausea, vomiting, obesity, and pancreatitis.

7. Use the nursing process to care for clients receiving drug therapy for bowel disorders, nausea, vomiting, obesity, and pancreatitis.

MediaLink

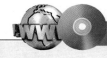 www.pearsoned.ca/adams-king

CRNE review, case studies, and other interactive resources for this chapter can be found on the Companion Website at **www.pearsoned.ca/adams-king.** Click on "Chapter 37" to select the activities for this chapter. For animations, more CRNE review questions, and an audio glossary, access the accompanying DVD-ROM in this textbook.

Bowel disorders, nausea, and vomiting are among the most common complaints for which clients seek medical consultation. These non-specific symptoms may be caused by any number of infectious, metabolic, inflammatory, neoplastic, or neuropsychological disorders. In addition, nausea, vomiting, constipation, and diarrhea are the most common side effects of oral medications. Symptoms often resolve without the need for pharmacotherapy. When severe or prolonged, however, bowel disorders, nausea, and vomiting may lead to serious consequences unless drug therapy is initiated. Pancreatitis is a less common and more serious disorder that requires pharmacotherapy. This chapter will examine the pharmacotherapy of these conditions associated with the gastrointestinal (GI) tract.

PHARMFACTS

Gastrointestinal Symptoms and Disorders

- Digestive symptoms are among the most frequently experienced symptoms in adults; the incidence increases with age.
- At least 11% of all hospitalizations are related to digestive disorders.
- Approximately 3% of deaths in persons over age 65 years are the result of colorectal cancer.
- Irritable bowel syndrome affects 10% to 20% of adults.
- The incidence of vomiting associated with motion sickness peaks during ages 4 to 10, then begins to decline.
- A variety of OTC and prescription drugs are available for relief of digestive symptoms.

37.1 Normal Function of the Lower Digestive Tract

The lower portion of the GI tract consists of the small and large intestines, as shown in Figure 37.1. The first 25 cm of the small intestine, the **duodenum**, is the site where partially digested food from the stomach, known as **chyme**, mixes with bile from the gallbladder and digestive enzymes from the pancreas. The duodenum is sometimes considered part of the upper GI tract because of its close proximity to the stomach. The most common disorder of the duodenum, peptic ulcer, is discussed in Chapter 36.

The remainder of the small intestine consists of the jejunum and ileum. The **jejunum** is the site where most nutrient absorption occurs. The **ileum** empties its contents into the large intestine through the ileocecal valve. Peristalsis through the intestines is controlled by the autonomic nervous system. Activation of the parasympathetic division will increase peristalsis and speed materials through the intestine; the sympathetic division has the opposite effect. Travel time for chyme through the entire small intestine varies from 3 to 6 hours.

The large intestine, or colon, receives chyme from the ileum in a fluid state. The major function of the colon is to reabsorb water from the chyme and to excrete the remaining material from the body. The colon harbours a substantial number of bacteria and fungi, which are called the host flora. These organisms serve a useful purpose by synthesizing B complex vitamins and vitamin K. Disruption of the host flora in the colon can lead to diarrhea. With few exceptions, little absorption of nutrients occurs during the 12- to 24-hour journey through the colon.

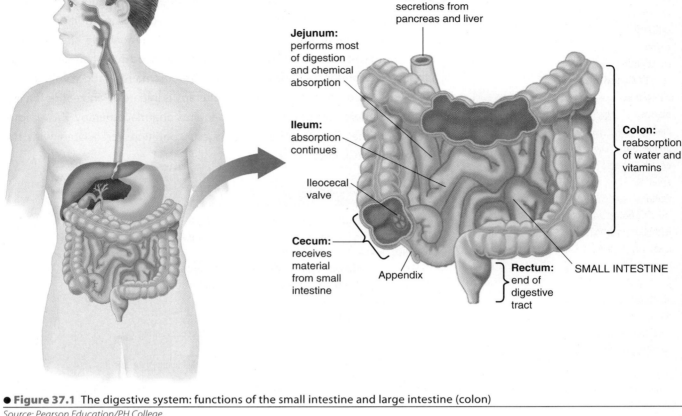

● **Figure 37.1** The digestive system: functions of the small intestine and large intestine (colon)

Source: Pearson Education/PH College.

CONSTIPATION

Constipation is identified by a decrease in the frequency and number of bowel movements. Stools may become dry, hard, and difficult to evacuate from the rectum.

37.2 Pathophysiology of Constipation

As waste material travels through the large intestine, water is reabsorbed. Reabsorption of the proper amount of water results in stools of a normal, soft consistency. If the waste material remains in the colon for an extended period, however, too much water will be reabsorbed, leading to small, hard stools. Constipation may cause abdominal distention and discomfort, and flatulence.

The etiology of constipation may be related to a lack of exercise, insufficient food intake (especially insoluble **dietary fibre**), diminished fluid intake, or a medication regimen that includes drugs that reduce intestinal motility. Lifestyle modifications that incorporate positive dietary changes and physical activity should be considered before drugs are utilized. Foods that can cause constipation include alcoholic beverages, products with a high content of refined white flour, dairy products, and chocolate. The normal frequency of bowel movements varies widely among individuals, from two to three per day to as few as one per week.

Occasional constipation is common and does not require drug therapy. Chronic constipation experienced as infrequent and painful bowel movements, accompanied by severe straining, may justify initiation of treatment. In its most severe form, constipation can lead to a fecal impaction and complete obstruction of the bowel. Constipation occurs more frequently in older adults because fecal transit time through the colon slows with aging; this population also exercises less and has a higher frequency of chronic disorders that cause constipation. Laxatives are drugs that promote bowel movements. Many are available OTC for the self-treatment of simple constipation. Laxatives are identified in Table 37.1.

LAXATIVES

37.3 Pharmacotherapy with Laxatives

Laxatives are drugs that promote evacuation of the large bowel, or **defecation**. **Cathartic** implies a stronger and more complete bowel emptying. A variety of prescription and OTC formulations are available, including tablets, liquids, and suppositories, to treat existing constipation or to prevent this disorder.

Prophylactic laxative pharmacotherapy is appropriate postoperatively. Such treatment is indicated to preclude straining or bearing down during defecation—a situation

TABLE 37.1   Laxatives and Cathartics

Drug	Route and Adult Dose
Bulk-Forming Agents	
calcium polycarbophil (Prodiem, Equalactin)	PO; 1 g qd prn
methylcellulose (Entrocel)	PO; 5–20 mL tid in 8–10 oz water
psyllium mucilloid (Metamucil, Psyllium)	PO; 1–2 tsp in 8 oz water qd prn
Saline and Osmotic Agents	
magnesium hydroxide (Milk of Magnesia)	PO; 20–60 mL qd prn
polyethylene glycol (Prolax)	PO; 17g in 8 oz of liquid qd for 2–4 days
sodium biphosphate (Fleet Phospho-Soda)	PO; 15–30 mL mixed in water qd prn
Stimulants	
bisacodyl (Dulcolax)	PO; 10–15 mg qd prn
castor oil	PO; 15–60 mL qd prn
phenolphthalein (Ex-Lax, Feen-a-Mint, Correctol)	PO; 60–240 mg qd prn
Stool Softeners/Surfactants	
docusate (Colace, Soflax, others)	PO; 50–500 mg qd
Miscellaneous Agents	
mineral oil	PO; 45 mL bid

that has the potential to precipitate increased intra-abdominal and intraocular pressure and blood pressure. Drugs, in conjunction with enemas, are often given to cleanse the bowel prior to diagnostic or surgical procedures of the colon or genitourinary tract. Cathartics are usually the drug of choice preceding diagnostic procedures of the colon, such as colonoscopy and barium enema.

When taken in prescribed amounts, laxatives have few side effects. These drugs are often classified into four primary groups and a miscellaneous category:

- Bulk-forming agents absorb water, thus adding size to the fecal mass. They are often taken prophylactically to prevent constipation.
- Stool softeners (surfactants) reduce surface tension by causing more water and fat to be absorbed into the stool. They are often used in clients who have undergone recent surgery.
- Stimulants irritate the bowel to increase peristalsis; they may cause cramping in clients.
- Osmotic laxatives such as saline are not absorbed in the intestine; they pull water into the fecal mass to create a more watery stool.
- Miscellaneous agents include mineral oil, which acts within the intestine by lubricating the stool and the colon mucosa.

NURSING CONSIDERATIONS

The role of the nurse in laxative therapy involves careful monitoring of the client's condition and providing education as it relates to the prescribed drug. Prior to pharma-cotherapy with laxatives, the nurse must assess the abdomen for distention and bowel sounds. If there is absence of bowel sounds, peristalsis must be restored prior to laxative therapy. Assess bowel patterns. A client with a sudden, unexplained change in bowel patterns should be evaluated as it could indicate a serious condition such as colon cancer. Also assess for esophageal obstruction, intestinal obstruction, fecal impaction, and undiagnosed abdominal pain. Laxatives are contraindicated in all of these conditions due to the risk of causing bowel perforation. If diarrhea occurs, laxative use should be discontinued. There are many products to prevent and treat constipation. Because most are OTC medications, there is a risk for misuse and overuse.

Bulk-forming laxatives are pregnancy category C and should be used with caution during pregnancy and lactation. Because fibre absorbs water and expands to provide "bulk," these agents must be taken with plenty of water. These laxatives will not be effective unless taken with one to two glasses of water. Assess the client's ability to swallow as obstruction can occur if the product does not clear the esophagus or if a stricture exists. Bulk-forming products may take 24 to 48 hours to be effective and may be taken on a regular basis to prevent constipation.

Stool softeners are generally prescribed for clients who have experienced a sudden change in lifestyle that puts them at risk for constipation, such as a surgery, injury, or conditions such as MI where straining during defecation should be avoided. They are contraindicated during pregnancy and lactation (pregnancy category C). Assess for the development of diarrhea and cramping; if diarrhea develops, the medication should be withheld. Docusate is contraindicated in clients with abdominal pain accompanied by nausea and vomiting, with fecal impaction, and with intestinal obstruction or perforation. Docusate sodium should not be given to clients on sodium restriction. Docusate potassium should not be given to clients with renal impairment. Docusate increases systemic absorption of mineral oil, so these two medications should not be given concurrently. Docusate should not be taken with certain herbal products such as senna, cascara, rhubarb, and aloe as it will increase their absorption and the risk of liver toxicity.

Stimulant laxatives act as irritants to the bowel and increase peristalsis. They are the quickest acting and most likely to cause diarrhea and cramping. Bowel rupture could occur if obstruction is present. Stimulant laxatives are not used during pregnancy and lactation (pregnancy category C). Because of their rapid and potent effects, the nurse must pay particular attention to responding to the client's need to use a bedpan or quickly get to the bathroom. These products are also used as a "bowel prep" prior to bowel exams or surgeries, sometimes in combination with osmotic laxatives and enemas. As the client will be NPO prior to the procedure, it is important to assess for signs of dehydration and changes in vital signs. It may be necessary to initiate IV fluids. Herbal stimulant laxatives, such as cascara and senna, are common components of OTC weight-loss products, and clients taking them may experience rebound, severe constipation if these medications are abruptly withdrawn.

Saline or osmotic laxatives pull water into the GI tract. Most are pregnancy category B. Dehydration may result when these medications are taken frequently or in excess if the client has inadequate fluid intake. Osmotic laxatives are highly potent, work within hours, and are often a part of bowel prep.

Lactulose relieves constipation by increasing stool water content and acidity. Lactulose is a disaccharide that reaches the colon mostly unchanged, increasing osmotic pressure and water content. In the colon, bacteria act on lactulose to produce lactic acid and draw ammonia ions from the bloodstream. The acidification of colonic contents helps to increase stool volume and frequency. Reducing the dose usually controls abdominal cramping and diarrhea should they occur. Lactulose should not be taken within 2 hours of another medication because the desired effect of the other medication may be reduced. Lactulose should not be used in the presence of abdominal pain, nausea, fever, or vomiting. It is contraindicated in diabetes and is pregnancy category B.

Client education as it relates to these medications should include goals, reasons for obtaining baseline data such as vital signs and abdominal assessment, and possible side effects. Following are other important points to include when teaching clients regarding laxatives:

- Follow label instructions carefully, and do not take more than the recommended dose.
- If changes in bowel patterns persist or become more severe, seek medical attention.
- Take bulk-forming agents at a different time than other medications to ensure proper absorption.

See "Nursing Process Focus: Clients Receiving Laxative Therapy" for additional teaching points.

DIARRHEA

Diarrhea is an increase in the frequency and fluidity of bowel movements. Diarrhea is not a disease; it is a symptom of an underlying disorder.

Pr PROTOTYPE DRUG | Psyllium Mucilloid (Metamucil, Psyllium)

ACTIONS AND USES

Psyllium is derived from the seeds of the plantain plant. Like other bulk-forming laxatives, psyllium is an insoluble fibre that is indigestible and not absorbed from the GI tract. When taken with a sufficient quantity of water, psyllium swells and increases the size of the fecal mass. The larger the fecal mass, the more the defecation reflex will be stimulated, thus promoting the passage of stool. Several doses of psyllium may be needed to produce a therapeutic effect. Frequent use of psyllium may effect a small reduction in blood cholesterol level.

PHARMACOKINETICS

Psyllium is not absorbed and has an onset of action of 12 to 24 hours.

ADMINISTRATION ALERTS

- Mix with 250 mL of water, fruit juice, or milk, and administer immediately.
- Follow each dose with an additional 250 mL of liquid.
- Observe elderly clients closely for possible aspiration.
- Psyllium is pregnancy category C.

ADVERSE EFFECTS AND INTERACTIONS

Psyllium rarely produces side effects. It generally causes less cramping than the stimulant-type laxatives and results in a more natural bowel movement. If taken with insufficient water, it may cause obstructions in the esophagus or intestine. Psyllium should not be administered to clients with undiagnosed abdominal pain.

Psyllium may decrease the absorption and effects of warfarin, digoxin, nitrofurantoin, antibiotics, and salicylates.

 See the Companion Website for a Nursing Process Focus chart specific to this drug.

NURSING PROCESS FOCUS   Clients Receiving Laxative Therapy

Assessment	Potential Nursing Diagnoses/Identified Patterns
Prior to administration: ■ Obtain complete health history including allergies, drug history, and possible drug interactions. ■ Assess bowel elimination pattern. ■ Assess bowel sounds.	■ Risk for injury (intestinal obstruction) related to adverse effects from drug therapy ■ Constipation ■ Fluid and electrolyte imbalance

Planning: Client Goals and Expected Outcomes

The client will:
■ Report relief from constipation
■ Demonstrate an understanding of the drug's action by accurately describing drug side effects and precautions
■ Immediately report effects such as nausea, vomiting, diarrhea, abdominal pain, and lack of bowel movement

Implementation

Interventions (Rationales)	Client Education/Discharge Planning
■ Monitor frequency, volume, and consistency of bowel movements. (Changes in bowel habits can indicate a serious condition.)	Advise client to: ■ Discontinue laxative use if diarrhea occurs ■ Notify healthcare provider if constipation continues ■ Take medication as prescribed ■ Increase fluids and dietary fibre, such as whole grains, fibrous fruits, and vegetables ■ Expect results from medication within 2 to 3 days after initial dose
■ Monitor client's ability to swallow. (Bulk laxatives can swell and cause obstruction in the esophagus.)	■ Instruct client to discontinue medication and notify healthcare provider if having difficulty swallowing.
■ Monitor client's fluid intake. (Esophageal or intestinal obstruction may result if the client does not take adequate amounts of fluid with the medication.)	Instruct client to: ■ Drink six 250 mL glasses of fluid per day ■ Mix medication in 250 mL of liquid ■ Drink at least 250 mL of additional fluid

Evaluation of Outcome Criteria

Evaluate the effectiveness of drug therapy by confirming that client goals and expected outcomes have been met (see "Planning").

See Table 37.1 for a list of drugs to which these nursing actions apply.

37.4 Pathophysiology of Diarrhea

Occasionally, the large intestine does not reabsorb enough water from the fecal mass and stools become watery. Like constipation, occasional diarrhea is a common disorder that does not warrant drug therapy. When prolonged or severe, especially in children, diarrhea can result in significant loss of body fluids and pharmacotherapy is indicated. Prolonged diarrhea may lead to acid-base or electrolyte disorders (see Chapter 44).

Diarrhea may be caused by certain medications, infections of the bowel, and substances such as lactose. Antibiotics often cause diarrhea by killing normal intestinal flora, thus giving rise to an overgrowth of opportunistic pathogenic organisms. It is vital to assess and treat the etiology of the diarrhea. Assessing the client's recent travels, dietary habits, immune system competence, and recent drug history may provide information about the etiology of the diarrhea. Critically ill clients with a reduced immune response who are exposed to many antibiotics may have diarrhea related to pseudomembranous colitis, a condition that may lead to shock and death.

Ulceration in the distal portion of the small intestine, called **Crohn's disease**, and erosions in the large intestine, called **ulcerative colitis**, are common causes of diarrhea. Together these diseases are categorized as inflammatory bowel disease and are treated with anti-inflammatory medications (see Chapter 31). Particularly severe cases of inflammatory bowel disease may require immunosuppressant drugs such as cyclosporine or methotrexate.

Irritable bowel syndrome (IBS), also known as spastic colon or mucous colitis, is a common disorder of the lower GI tract. Symptoms include abdominal pain, bloating, excessive gas, and colicky cramping. Bowel habits are frequently

TABLE 37.2 Antidiarrheals

Drug	Route and Adult Dose
Opioids	
belladonna with opium	Rectal; 1 suppository bid–qid prn
diphenoxylate with atropine (Lomotil)	PO; 1–2 tabs or 5–10 mL tid–qid
loperamide (Imodium)	PO; 4 mg as a single dose, then 2 mg after each diarrhea episode (max 16 mg/d)
Miscellaneous Agents	
bismuth subsalicylate (Pepto-Bismol)	PO; 2 tabs or 30 mL regular strength after each diarrhea episode (max 4.2 g/d)
bismuth subsalicylate with kaolin-pectin (Kaopectate)	PO; 2 tabs or 30 mL regular strength after each diarrhea episode (max 4.2 g/d)

affected, with diarrhea alternating with constipation, and there may be mucus in the stool. IBS is considered a functional bowel disorder, meaning that the normal operation of the digestive tract is impaired without the presence of detectable organic disease. It is not a precursor of more serious disease. Stress is often a precipitating factor along with dietary factors. Treatment is supportive with drug therapy targeted at symptomatic treatment.

ANTIDIARRHEALS

For occasional, mild cases of diarrhea, OTC products are effective at returning elimination patterns to normal. For chronic or severe cases, the opioids are the most efficacious of the antidiarrheal agents. The antidiarrheals are shown in Table 37.2.

37.5 Pharmacotherapy with Antidiarrheals

Pharmacotherapy related to diarrhea depends on the severity of the condition and identifiable etiological factors. If the cause is an infectious disease, then an antibiotic or antiparasitic drug is indicated. Should the etiology be inflammatory in nature, anti-inflammatory drugs are warranted. When the cause appears to be due to a side effect of pharmacotherapy, the healthcare provider may discontinue the offending medication, lower the dose, or substitute an alternative drug.

The most effective drugs for the symptomatic treatment of diarrhea are the opioids. They slow peristalsis in the colon, with only a slight risk of dependence. The most common opioid antidiarrheals are codeine and diphenoxylate with atropine. Diphenoxylate is a Schedule V agent that acts directly on the intestine to slow peristalsis, thereby allowing for more fluid and electrolyte absorption in the large intestine. The opioids cause CNS depression at high doses and are generally reserved for more severe cases due to the potential for dependence.

OTC drugs for diarrhea act by a number of different mechanisms. Loperamide is an analog of meperidine, although it has no narcotic effects and is not classified as a controlled substance. Low-dose loperamide is available OTC; higher doses are available by prescription. Other OTC treatments include bismuth subsalicylate, which acts to bind and absorb toxins. The psyllium and pectin preparations may also slow diarrhea since they tend to absorb large amounts of fluid and form bulkier stools. Intestinal flora modifiers are supplements that help to correct the altered GI flora; a good source of healthy bacteria is yogurt with active cultures.

NURSING CONSIDERATIONS

The role of the nurse in antidiarrheal therapy involves careful monitoring of the client's condition and providing education as it relates to the prescribed drug regimen. Antidiarrheal drugs should be given for symptomatic relief of diarrhea while the underlying etiology is treated. Because diarrhea can cause a loss of fluid and electrolytes, hydration status and serum potassium, magnesium, and bicarbonate should be assessed. Assess for blood in the stool. The nurse needs to be especially observant of infants, children, and older adults because diarrhea can quickly lead to dehydration and electrolyte imbalance in these clients. Because antidiarrheals are excreted in the liver and kidneys, hepatic and renal function should be assessed.

Antidiarrheals are generally not used during pregnancy and lactation. They should not be used in conditions where constipation should be avoided, such as pseudomembranous colitis or severe ulcerative colitis, because the drugs could worsen or mask these conditions. Toxic megacolon has occurred in clients with ulcerative colitis taking loperamide (Imodium). Because drowsiness may occur with opioids, assess the client's ability to get out of bed safely. Antidiarrheals are contraindicated in clients with severe dehydration, electrolyte imbalance, liver and renal disorders, and glaucoma. Opioid antidiarrheals should be used with caution in clients with a history of drug abuse. Adverse reactions occur more frequently in children, especially those with Down syndrome.

Client education as it relates to these drugs should include goals, reasons for obtaining baseline data such as vital signs and abdominal assessment, and possible side effects. Following are other important points to include when teaching clients regarding antidiarrheals:

- Seek medical care for diarrhea that does not resolve within 2 days, or if a fever develops or dehydration

SPECIAL CONSIDERATIONS

Cultural Remedies for Diarrhea

Because diarrhea is an age-old malady that affects all populations, different cultures have adopted tried-and-true symptomatic remedies for the condition. One preparation, used by people in many regions of the world, is cornstarch (a heaping teaspoonful) in a glass of tepid water. For centuries, mothers have boiled rice and given the diluted rice water to babies with diarrhea. The rationale behind these two therapies is that they work by absorbing excess water in the intestines, thus stopping the diarrhea. Although a rationale was not related in earlier times, people of many cultures found that eating grated apple that had turned brown alleviated symptoms. This apparently evolved into what is known today as the ABCs of diarrhea treatment: apples, bananas (just barely ripe), and carrots. The underlying principle is that the pectin present in these foods oxidizes, producing the same ingredient found in many OTC diarrhea medicines. Packets of oral rehydration salts (ORS) that include sodium, potassium, and glucose to be mixed in water (245 mOsm/L) are recommended by the World Health Organization for home management of diarrhea. Current recommendations can be found on its website.

occurs. (Infants, children, and older adults are at greatest risk and may need medical attention sooner.)

- Discontinue medication once frequent or watery stools have stopped.
- Seek medical care if the presence of blood is found in the stool.

See "Nursing Process Focus: Clients Receiving Antidiarrheal Therapy" for additional teaching points.

NAUSEA AND VOMITING

Nausea is an unpleasant, subjective sensation that usually occurs in the midepigastrium and is accompanied by weakness, diaphoresis, and hyperproduction of saliva. It is sometimes accompanied by dizziness. Intense nausea often leads

LIFESPAN CONSIDERATIONS

Management of Diarrhea

- Infants, children, and older adults with diarrhea are at risk for rapidly occurring dehydration and electrolyte imbalance.
- Rehydration and electrolyte replacement are important components of treatment.
- Antidiarrheals are not generally used during pregnancy and lactation.
- Clients of all ages should be advised to seek medical care if diarrhea does not resolve within two days or if fever or dehydration occurs.
- Elderly clients are at increased risk for falls related to the drowsiness that may occur with dehydration and opioid antidiarrheals.

SPECIAL CONSIDERATIONS

Treatment for Watery Diarrhea in Infants and Children

- Oral rehydration solutions should be used routinely for watery diarrhea and dehydration.
- Feeding should be continued through rehydration to maintain nutrition.
- Antimotility drugs (e.g., loperamide and Lomotil) should not be used due to safety considerations.
- Acetorphan (not yet available in Canada) is a safe and effective antisecretory drug that can be used routinely.
- Bismuth subsalicylate is an effective and generally safe antisecretory drug; it should not be given in the presence of chicken pox or influenza because of the danger of Reye's syndrome.
- Kaolin-pectin, fibre, and activated charcoal should not be used.
- Some *Lactobacillus* species may be used to modify intestinal flora.
- Folic acid and vitamin A are indicated only in cases of overt deficiency.
- Antibiotics should be used sparingly except in cases of severe bacterial diarrhea.
- Zinc therapy may be useful in malnourished children.

Source: Recommendations of the Canadian Paediatric Society's Nutrition Committee, February 2006, "http://www.cps.ca/".

Pr PROTOTYPE DRUG | Diphenoxylate with Atropine (Lomotil)

ACTIONS AND USES

The primary antidiarrheal ingredient in Lomotil is diphenoxylate. Like other opioids, diphenoxylate slows peristalsis, allowing time for additional water reabsorption from the colon and formation of more-solid stools. It acts within 45 to 60 minutes. It is effective for moderate to severe diarrhea, but it is not recommended for children. The atropine in Lomotil is not added for its anticholinergic effect, but to discourage clients from taking too much of the drug.

PHARMACOKINETICS

Diphenoxylate is well absorbed, enters breast milk, and is mostly metabolized by the liver. It has a half-life of 2.5 hours.

ADMINISTRATION ALERT

- Diphenoxylate is pregnancy category C.

ADVERSE EFFECTS AND INTERACTIONS

Unlike most opioids, diphenoxylate has no analgesic properties and has an extremely low potential for abuse. Some clients experience dizziness or drowsiness, and care should be taken not to drive or operate machinery until the effects of the drug are known.

Diphenoxylate with atropine interacts with several other drugs. For example, other CNS depressants, including alcohol, will add to its CNS depressant effect. At higher doses, the anticholinergic effects of atropine may be observed, which include drowsiness, dry mouth, and tachycardia. When taken with MAO inhibitors, diphenoxylate may cause hypertensive crisis.

 See the Companion Website for a Nursing Process Focus chart specific to this drug.

NURSING PROCESS FOCUS Clients Receiving Antidiarrheal Therapy

Assessment	Potential Nursing Diagnoses/Identified Patterns
Prior to administration: ■ Obtain complete health history including allergies, drug history, and possible drug interactions. ■ Assess sodium, chloride, and potassium levels. ■ Evaluate results of stool culture. ■ Assess for presence of dehydration. ■ Obtain vital signs and ECG.	■ Risk for fluid volume: deficit related to fluid loss from diarrhea ■ Risk for injury (falls) related to drowsiness, a side effect of drug therapy

Planning: Client Goals and Expected Outcomes

The client will:
■ Report relief of diarrhea
■ Demonstrate an understanding of the drug's action by accurately describing drug side effects and precautions
■ Immediately report effects such as persistent diarrhea, constipation, abdominal pain, blood in stool, confusion, dizziness, or fever

Implementation

Interventions (Rationales)	Client Education/Discharge Planning
■ Monitor frequency, volume, and consistency of stools. (This will determine the effectiveness of drug therapy.)	Advise client to: ■ Record the frequency of stools ■ Note if any blood is present in stools ■ Report immediately any abdominal pain or abdominal distention
■ Minimize the risk of dehydration and electrolyte imbalance. (These may occur secondary to diarrhea.)	■ Instruct client to increase fluid intake and drink electrolyte-enriched fluids. ■ Instruct client to include foods that will minimize diarrhea, such as yogurt, bland foods and foods high in pectin (apples, bananas and citrus fruits).
■ Prevent accidental overdosage.	■ Advise client who is using liquid preparations to use the dropper included to measure medication dosage. Do not use household measurements.
■ Monitor for dry mouth. (This is a side effect of the medications.)	■ Advise client to suck on ice or sour candy or to chew gum to relieve sensation of dry mouth.
■ Initiate safety measures to prevent falls. (These medications may cause drowsiness.)	Advise client to: ■ Refrain from driving or performing hazardous activities until the effects of drug are known ■ Abstain from using alcohol and other CNS depressants
■ Monitor electrolyte levels.	Advise client to: ■ Keep all laboratory appointments ■ Report weakness and muscle cramping

Evaluation of Outcome Criteria

Evaluate the effectiveness of drug therapy by confirming that client goals and expected outcomes have been met (see "Planning").

See Table 37.2 for a list of drugs to which these nursing actions apply.

to vomiting, or **emesis**, in which the stomach contents are forced upward into the esophagus and out the mouth.

37.6 Pathophysiology of Nausea and Vomiting

Vomiting is a defence mechanism used by the body to rid itself of toxic substances. Vomiting is a reflex primarily controlled by a portion of the medulla of the brain known as the **vomiting centre**, which receives sensory signals from the digestive tract, the inner ear, and the cerebral cortex. Interestingly, the vomiting centre is not protected by the blood-brain barrier, as is the vast majority of the brain. These neurons can directly sense the presence of toxic substances in the blood. Once the vomiting reflex is triggered, wavelike contractions of the stomach quickly propel its contents up and out of the body.

Nausea and vomiting are common symptoms associated with a wide variety of conditions such as GI infections, food poisoning, stress, nervousness, emotional imbalances, changes in body position (motion sickness), and extreme pain. Other conditions that promote nausea and vomiting are general anesthetic agents, migraine headache, trauma to the head or abdominal organs, inner ear disorders, and diabetes. Psychological factors play a significant role as clients often become nauseated during periods of extreme stress or when confronted with unpleasant sights, smells, or sounds.

The nausea and vomiting experienced by many women during the first trimester of pregnancy is referred to as morning sickness. Should this become acute, with continual vomiting, this condition may lead to hyperemesis gravidarum, a situation in which the health and safety of the mother and developing baby can become severely compromised. Pharmacotherapy is only initiated after other antinausea measures have been ineffective.

Many drugs, by their chemical nature, bring about nausea or vomiting as a side effect. The most extreme example of this occurs with the antineoplastic drugs, most of which cause intense nausea and vomiting.

The foremost problem secondary to nausea and vomiting is dehydration. When large amounts of fluids are vomited, water in the plasma moves from the blood to other body tissues, resulting in dehydration. Because the contents lost from the stomach are strongly acidic, vomiting may cause a change in the pH of the blood, resulting in metabolic alkalosis. With excessive loss, severe acid-base disturbances can lead to vascular collapse that results in death if medical intervention is not initiated. Dehydration is exceptionally dangerous for infants, small children, and older adults and is evidenced by dry mouth, sticky saliva, and reduced urine output with urine that is dark yellow-orange to brown.

Nausea and vomiting may be prevented or alleviated with natural remedies or by the use of drugs from several different classes. The treatment goal for nausea or vomiting is removal of the cause, when feasible.

ANTIEMETICS

Drugs from at least eight different classes are used to prevent nausea and vomiting. Many of these act by inhibiting dopamine or serotonin receptors in the brain. The antiemetics are shown in Table 37.3.

TABLE 37.3 Select Antiemetics

Drug	Route and Adult Dose
Anticholinergics	
scopolamine (Buscopan, Hyoscine, Transderm-V)	PO; 10 mg q4–6h Transdermal; 0.5 mg q72h
Antihistamines	
dimenhydrinate (Apo-Dimenhydrinate, others)	PO; 50–100 mg q4–6h (max 400 mg/day)
diphenhydramine (Benadryl, Gravol, others) (see page 412 for the Prototype Drug box)	PO; 25–50 mg tid–qid (max 300 mg/day)
hydroxyzine (Apo-, PMS-Hydroxyzine, Atarax)	PO; 10–50 mg tid or qid
Benzodiazepines	
diazepam (Apo-Diazepam, Valium) (see page 162 for the Prototype Drug box)	IV/IM; 5–10 mg, repeat if needed at 10–15 min intervals up to 30 mg, then repeat if needed q2–4h
lorazepam (Ativan) (see page 149 for the Prototype Drug box)	IV; 1.0–1.5 mg prior to chemotherapy
Cannabinoids	
cannabidiol (Sativex)	Buccal; 1 spray q4h prn (max 4 per day)
Glucocorticoids	
dexamethasone (Apo-Dexamethasone, Decadron)	PO; 0.25–4 mg bid–qid
methylprednisolone (Solu-Medrol, others)	PO; 4–48 mg/d in divided doses IV; 40–250 mg q4–6h
Phenothiazines and Phenothiazine-Like Agents	
metoclopramide (Apo-Metoclop, Maxeran)	PO; 2 mg/kg 1 h prior to chemotherapy
perphenazine (Apo-, PMS-Perphenazine)	PO; 8–16 mg bid–qid
prochlorperazine (PMS-Prochlorperazine, Stemetil)	PO; 5–10 mg tid or qid
promethazine (Histanil, Phenergan, others)	PO; 12.5–25 mg q4h–qid
Serotonin Receptor Antagonists	
dolasetron (Anzemet)	PO; 100 mg 1 h prior to chemotherapy
granisetron (Kytril)	IV; 10 µg/kg 30 minutes prior to chemotherapy
ondansetron (Apo-, Novo-Ondansetron, Zofran)	PO; 4 mg tid prn

37.7 Pharmacotherapy with Antiemetics

A large number of **antiemetics** are available to treat nausea and vomiting, and selection of a particular agent depends on the experience of the healthcare provider and the cause of the nausea. For example, nausea due to motion sickness is effectively treated with anticholinergics or antihistamines. Nausea and vomiting associated with antineoplastic agents is often treated with the phenothiazines, glucocorticoids, or serotonin receptor blockers. Aprepitant is the first of a new class of antiemetic, the neurokinin receptor antagonists, used to prevent nausea and vomiting following antineoplastic therapy. To prevent loss of the medication due to vomiting, many antiemetics are administered through the IM, IV, or suppository routes.

Clients receiving antineoplastic drugs may receive three or more antiemetics to reduce the nausea and vomiting from chemotherapy. In fact, therapy with antineoplastic drugs is one of the most common reasons why antiemetic drugs are prescribed.

Motion sickness is a disorder affecting a portion of the inner ear known as the **vestibular apparatus** that is associated with significant nausea. The most common drug used for motion sickness is scopolamine, which is usually administered as a transdermal patch. Antihistamines such as dimenhydrinate and meclizine are also effective but may cause significant drowsiness in some clients. Drugs used to treat motion sickness are most effective when taken 20 to 60 minutes before travel is expected.

On some occasions, it is desirable to *stimulate* the vomiting reflex with drugs called **emetics**. Indications for emetics include ingestion of poisons and overdoses of oral drugs. Ipecac syrup, given orally, or apomorphine, given SC, will induce vomiting in about 15 minutes.

NURSING CONSIDERATIONS

The role of the nurse in antiemetic therapy involves careful monitoring of the client's condition and providing education as it relates to the prescribed drug regimen. Assess symptoms that precipitated the vomiting or that are occurring concurrently. If a client becomes sedated and continues to vomit, a nasogastric tube insertion with suction may be indicated. Antiemetics are contraindicated in clients who are hypersensitive to the drugs, have bone marrow depression, are comatose, or experience vomiting of unknown etiology. These drugs are used with caution in clients with breast cancer. Client safety is a concern as drowsiness is a frequent side effect of antiemetics. Clients may be at risk for falls because of medication side effects and sensation of weakness from vomiting. Orthostatic hypotension is a side effect of some antiemetics.

Drugs used to stimulate emesis should only be used in emergency situations under the direction of a healthcare provider. They are used only when the client is alert, due to the risk of aspiration. When the client is comatose, a gastric lavage tube is placed and attached to suction to empty gastric contents.

Client education as it relates to antiemetics should include goals, reasons for obtaining baseline data such as vital signs and abdominal assessment, and possible side effects. Following are important points to include when teaching clients regarding antiemetics:

- Use assistance to get out of bed until effects of medication are known.
- Avoid driving and performing hazardous tasks.
- If blood is vomited, or if the vomiting is associated with severe abdominal pain, notify the healthcare provider immediately.
- Do not use OTC antiemetics for prolonged periods; vomiting may be a symptom of a serious disorder that requires medical attention.
- Before inducing vomiting with an OTC emetic, check with the healthcare provider; some poisons and caustic chemicals should not be vomited.

WEIGHT LOSS

Hunger occurs when the hypothalamus recognizes the levels of certain chemicals (glucose) or hormones (insulin) in the blood. Hunger is a normal physiological response that drives people to seek nourishment. Appetite is somewhat different from hunger. Appetite is a psychological response that drives food intake based on associations and memory. For example, people often eat not because they are experiencing hunger, but because it is a particular time of day or they find the act of eating pleasurable or social.

DRUGS FOR WEIGHT LOSS

Despite the public's desire for effective drugs to induce weight loss, there are few such drugs on the market. The approved agents are used for the treatment of obesity, although they produce only modest effects.

NATURAL THERAPIES

Probiotics for Diarrhea

Lactobacillus acidophilus is a probiotic bacterium normally found in the human alimentary canal and the vagina. It is considered to be protective, inhibiting the growth of potentially pathogenic species such as *Escherichia coli*, *Candida albicans*, *Campylobacter pylori*, and *Gardnerella vaginalis*. One mechanism used by *L. acidophilus* to limit the growth of other bacterial species is the generation of hydrogen peroxide, which is toxic to most cells.

The primary use of *L. acidophilus* is to restore the normal flora of the intestine following diarrhea, particularly from antibiotic therapy. This probiotic may also help to restore normal microflora in the vagina, although the evidence for this effect is not conclusive. *L. acidophilus* may be obtained by drinking *L. acidophilus* milk or by eating yogurt or kefir containing live (or active) cultures. Those wishing to obtain *L. acidophilus* from yogurt should read the labels carefully because not all products contain active cultures; frozen yogurt contains no active cultures. Supplements include capsules, tablets, and granules. Doses are not standardized, and tablet doses range from 50 to 500 mg.

Pr PROTOTYPE DRUG | Prochlorperazine (PMS-Prochlorperazine, Stemetil)

ACTIONS AND USES

Prochlorperazine is a phenothiazine, a class of drug usually prescribed for psychoses (see Chapter 17). The phenothiazines are the largest group of drugs prescribed for severe nausea and vomiting, and prochlorperazine is the most frequently prescribed antiemetic in its class. Prochlorperazine acts by blocking dopamine receptors in the brain, which inhibits signals to the vomiting centre in the medulla.

PHARMACOKINETICS

Prochlorperazine is frequently given IM or rectally, whereby absorption is more consistent than when given orally. It is widely distributed and is about 90% protein bound. It is highly metabolized by the liver. Its half-life is unknown.

ADMINISTRATION ALERTS

- Administer oral dosage 2 hours before or after antacids and antidiarrheals.
- Prochlorperazine is pregnancy category C.

ADVERSE EFFECTS AND INTERACTIONS

Prochlorperazine produces dose-related anticholinergic side effects such as dry mouth, sedation, constipation, orthostatic hypotension, and tachycardia. When used for prolonged periods at higher doses, extrapyramidal symptoms resembling those of Parkinson's disease are a serious concern.

Prochlorperazine interacts with alcohol to increase CNS depression. Antacids and antidiarrheals inhibit absorption of prochlorperazine. When taken with phenobarbital, metabolism of prochlorperazine is increased.

 See the Companion Website for a Nursing Process Focus chart specific to this drug.

37.8 Pharmacotherapy with Drugs for Weight Loss

Obesity may be defined as being more than 20% above the ideal body weight. Because of the prevalence of obesity in society and the difficulty most clients experience when following weight reduction plans for extended periods of time, drug manufacturers have long sought to develop safe drugs that induce weight loss. In the 1970s, amphetamine and dextroamphetamine (Dexedrine) were widely prescribed as **anorexiants** to reduce appetite; however, these drugs are addictive and are rarely prescribed for this purpose today. In the 1990s, the combination of fenfluramine and phentermine (Fen-Phen) was widely prescribed until fenfluramine was removed from the market for causing heart valve defects.

Attempts to produce drugs that promote safer weight loss by blocking lipid absorption resulted in orlistat (Xenical). Orlistat blocks the absorption of about 30% of dietary fat in the GI tract by inhibiting gastrointestinal lipases that are required for the systemic absorption of dietary triglycerides. Because orlistat may decrease absorption of other substances, including fat-soluble vitamins and some drugs, vitamin supplements and monitoring are often required. GI side effects such as flatus, oily fecal spotting, and abdominal discomfort can be avoided by restricting fat intake. GI side effects often diminish after 4 weeks of therapy. When combined with a reduced-calorie diet and moderate exercise, orlistat produces a gradual weight loss of about 10% of initial body weight over a period of a year.

Sibutramine, a serotonin and norepinephrine reuptake inhibitor, is the most widely prescribed appetite suppressant for short-term use in the control of obesity. Sibutramine is generally well tolerated with common side effects of dry mouth, insomnia, and headache. It may have significant interactions with other medications, which are usually related to increased serotonin and norepinephrine action. The client should not take any OTC cold, cough, decongestant, or allergy medicine without notifying the healthcare provider as these drugs commonly contain adrenergics and may increase heart rate and blood pressure. Weight-loss drugs are prescribed for clients with a body mass index (BMI) of at least 30 or greater, or a BMI of 27 or greater with other risk factors for disease such as hypertension, hyperlipidemia, or diabetes.

NURSING CONSIDERATIONS

The role of the nurse in weight-loss therapy involves careful monitoring of the client's condition and providing education as it relates to the prescribed drug regimen. With weight-loss drugs, encourage lifestyle changes that will have a greater effect on weight reduction in the long term. Drugs for weight loss have limited effectiveness, and some have serious side effects.

Amphetamine and other stimulant-type anorexiants can be dangerous due to cardiovascular side effects such as hypertension, tachycardia, and dysrhythmias and due to their potential for dependence. Use of these drugs must be closely monitored. These drugs should not be used during pregnancy or lactation.

Orlistat is contraindicated in pregnancy and lactation (pregnancy category B), malabsorption syndrome, cholestasis, and obesity due to organic causes. Blood glucose levels should be monitored in clients with diabetes mellitus. Orlistat is used with caution in clients with frequent diarrhea and those with known deficiencies of fat-soluble vitamins. A fat-soluble vitamin supplement should be taken at least 2 hours before or after a dose of orlistat. Clients should be advised to take orlistat during or immediately following a meal containing fat.

Sibutramine should not be used during pregnancy or lactation (pregnancy category C). It is contraindicated in clients with cardiac conditions such as dysrhythmias, coronary artery disease, heart failure, and poorly controlled hypertension. It should not be administered concurrently with other serotonin reuptake inhibitors such as fluoxetine. Sibutramine is used with caution in clients with a history of hypertension, seizures, and narrow-angle glaucoma. Prior to and during administration, liver function tests, bilirubin levels, alkaline phosphatase levels, and lipid profiles should be obtained. Heart rate and blood pressure should be monitored and sustained increases reported immediately.

Client education as it relates to these drugs should include goals, reasons for obtaining baseline data such as vital signs, and possible side effects. Following are important points to include when teaching clients regarding weight-loss drugs:

- Lifestyle modifications are necessary for sustained weight loss to occur; client should be encouraged to seek support groups for long-term weight management.
- Maintain close medical follow-up with amphetamine medications.
- Do not take any OTC or herbal medications without healthcare provider approval.
- Advise clients taking orlistat of the following:
  - Take a multivitamin each day.
  - Dose may be omitted if there is no fat present in the meal or the meal is skipped.
  - Excessive flatus and fecal leakage may occur when a high-fat meal is consumed.

PANCREATITIS

The pancreas secretes essential digestive enzymes. The enzymatic portion of pancreatic juice contains carboxypeptidase, chymotrypsin, and trypsin, which are converted to their active forms once they reach the small intestine. Three other pancreatic enzymes—lipase, amylase, and nuclease—are secreted in their active form but require the presence of bile for optimum activity. Because lack of secretion can result in malabsorption disorders, replacement therapy is sometimes required.

Pancreatitis results when amylase and lipase remain in the pancreas rather than being released into the duodenum. The enzymes escape into the surrounding tissue, causing inflammation in the pancreas, or pancreatitis. Pancreatitis can be either acute or chronic.

37.9 Pharmacotherapy of Pancreatitis

Acute pancreatitis usually occurs in middle-aged adults and is often associated with gallstones in women and alcoholism in men. Symptoms of acute pancreatitis present suddenly, often after eating a fatty meal or consuming excessive amounts of alcohol. The most common symptom is a continuous, severe pain in the epigastric area that often radiates to the back. Lab reports may reveal elevated serum amylase and lipase as well as hypocalcemia. Most clients recover from the illness and regain normal pancreatic function. Some clients have recurrent attacks and progress to chronic pancreatitis.

Many clients with acute pancreatitis require only bedrest and withholding of food and fluids by mouth for a few days for the symptoms to subside. For clients with acute pain, meperidine (Demerol) brings effective relief. To reduce or neutralize gastric secretions, H_2-blockers, such as cimetidine, or proton pump inhibitors, such as omeprazole, may be prescribed. To decrease the amount of pancreatic enzymes secreted, carbonic anhydrase inhibitors, such as acetazolamide, or antispasmodics, such as dicyclomine, may be prescribed. In particularly severe cases, IV fluids and total parenteral nutrition (TPN) may be necessary.

Most cases of chronic pancreatitis are associated with alcoholism. Alcohol is thought to promote the formation of insoluble proteins that occlude the pancreatic duct. Pancreatic juice is prevented from flowing into the duodenum and remains in the pancreas to damage cells and cause inflammation. Other causes include spasms of the hepatopancreatic sphincter and strictures or stones in the pancreatic duct system. Symptoms include chronic epigastric or left upper quadrant pain, anorexia, nausea, vomiting, and weight loss. **Steatorrhea**, the passing of bulky, foul-smelling, fatty stools, occurs late in the course of the disease.

Pr PROTOTYPE DRUG | Sibutramine (Meridia)

ACTIONS AND USES

Sibutramine is a selective serotonin reuptake inhibitor (SSRI) that is widely prescribed as an appetite suppressant for the short-term control of obesity. When combined with a reduced-calorie diet, sibutramine may produce a gradual weight loss of at least 10% of initial body weight over a period of a year. Sibutramine therapy is not recommended for longer than 1 year.

PHARMACOKINETICS

As a result of first-pass metabolism, sibutramine is converted to active metabolites M1 and M2. Following wide distribution, the active metabolites are metabolized to inactive compounds that are excreted mostly by the kidneys. The half-life of M1 is 14 hours and M2 is 16 hours.

ADMINISTRATION ALERTS

- Allow at least 2 weeks between discontinuing MAO inhibitors and starting sibutramine.
- Sibutramine is pregnancy category C.

ADVERSE EFFECTS AND INTERACTIONS

Headache is the most common complaint reported during sibutramine therapy, although insomnia and dry mouth are also possible. It should be used with great care in clients with cardiac disorders as it may cause tachycardia and raise blood pressure. It is a Schedule IV drug with low potential for dependence.

Sibutramine interacts with several other drugs. For example, decongestant, cough, and allergy medications may cause elevated blood pressure. Ketoconazole and erythromycin may inhibit the metabolism of sibutramine. Concurrent use with a MAO inhibitor or SSRI may cause serotonin syndrome.

 See the Companion Website for a Nursing Process Focus chart specific to this drug.

Drugs prescribed for the treatment of acute pancreatitis may also be prescribed in cases of chronic pancreatitis. In addition, the client with chronic pancreatitis may require insulin and is likely to need antiemetics and a pancreatic enzyme supplement such as pancrelipase or pancreatin to digest fats, proteins, and complex carbohydrates because chronic pancreatitis eventually leads to pancreatic insufficiency.

NURSING CONSIDERATIONS

The role of the nurse in pancreatic enzyme replacement therapy involves careful monitoring of the client's condition and providing education as it relates to the prescribed drug regimen. Assessment of the client with acute or chronic pancreatitis should include a complete assessment, physical examination, health history, psychosocial history, and lifestyle history. Obtain information about alcohol use and other drugs, tobacco use, and dietary habits. Spicy foods, gas-forming foods, cola drinks, coffee, and tea stimulate gastric and pancreatic secretions; assess the client for intake of these foods.

Assess and monitor the presence, amount, and type of pain as well as breathing patterns, which may be rapid and shallow due to pain. Assess the symmetry of the chest wall and the movement of the chest and diaphragm since the client with pancreatitis is at risk for atelectasis and can develop pleural effusion as a result of ineffective breathing patterns. Monitor blood gases as hypoventilation can result in hypercapnia. The client may have other abnormal findings such as elevated serum and urinary amylase, and elevated serum bilirubin. Monitor the client's nutritional status and hydration status, which may be impaired due to nausea and vomiting. Assess for signs of infection. Contraindications include a history of allergy to pork protein or enzymes because the drug has a porcine (pork) origin. Safety in pregnancy and lactation has not been established.

Client education as it relates to pancreatic enzymes should include goals, reasons for obtaining baseline data such as vital signs and tests for cardiac and renal disorders, and possible side effects. Explain the importance of bedrest and a calm environment in decreasing metabolic rate, pain, and pancreatic secretions. Following are other important points to include when teaching clients regarding pancreatic enzyme replacement:

- Eliminate all alcohol, smoking, spicy foods, gas-forming foods, cola drinks, coffee, and tea.
- Restrict fat intake and eat smaller and more frequent meals.
- Take pancreatic enzymes with meals or snacks.
- Weigh self and report significant changes to the healthcare provider.
- Report pain and seek relief before it becomes intense.
- Report episodes of nausea and vomiting.
- Sitting up, leaning forward, or curling in a fetal position may help decrease pain.
- Observe stools for colour, frequency, and consistency and report abnormalities.

SPECIAL CONSIDERATIONS

Psychosocial and Community Impacts of Alcohol-Related Pancreatitis

Clients with acute pancreatitis are most often middle-aged; those with chronic pancreatitis are most often in their 50s or 60s. Clients whose pancreatitis is associated with gallstones may receive a different type and amount of support from significant others, the community, and even from nurses compared with those who have pancreatitis associated with alcoholism. Nurses need to examine their feelings and attitudes related to alcoholism in general and to clients with alcoholism-associated pancreatitis in particular and will need to adopt attitudes to help the client attain treatment goals.

Clients who abuse alcohol often need referral to community agencies to manage their addiction and/or to remain in recovery. Family members may also need referral to community agencies for help in dealing with altered family processes due to the client's drinking and any role they may have played in enabling the client to abuse alcohol.

Pr PROTOTYPE DRUG | Pancrelipase (Lipancreatin, Pancrease)

ACTIONS AND USES

Pancrelipase contains lipase, protease, and amylase of porcine origin. This agent facilitates the breakdown and conversion of lipids into glycerol and fatty acids, starches into dextrin and sugars, and proteins into peptides. It is used as replacement therapy for clients with insufficient pancreatic exocrine secretions. Pancrelipase is available in powder, tablet, and delayed-release capsule formulations. On an equal-weight basis, pancrelipase is more potent than pancreatin, with 12 times the lipolytic activity. It also contains at least four times as much trypsin and amylase.

PHARMACOKINETICS

Pancrelipase is given orally and acts locally in the GI tract. It is not absorbed and is excreted in the feces.

ADMINISTRATION ALERTS

- Do not crush or open enteric-coated tablets.
- Powder forms may be sprinkled on food.
- Give the drug with meals or 1 to 2 hours before meals, or as directed by the healthcare provider.
- Pancrelipase is pregnancy category C.

ADVERSE EFFECTS AND INTERACTIONS

Side effects of pancrelipase are uncommon since the enzymes are not absorbed. The most common side effects are GI symptoms of nausea, vomiting, and/or diarrhea. The drug can cause metabolic symptoms of hyperuricosuria.

Pancrelipase interacts with iron, which may result in decreased absorption of iron.

 See the Companion Website for a Nursing Process Focus chart specific to this drug.

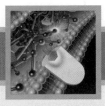

CHAPTER REVIEW

KEY CONCEPTS

The numbered key concepts provide a succinct summary of the important points from the corresponding numbered section within the chapter. If any of these points are not clear, refer to the numbered section within the chapter for review. Expanded versions can be found on the Companion Website.

37.1 The small intestine is the location for most nutrient and drug absorption. The large intestine is responsible for the reabsorption of water.

37.2 Constipation, the infrequent passage of hard, small stools, is a common disorder caused by slow motility of material through the large intestine.

37.3 Laxatives are drugs given to promote emptying of the large intestine by stimulating peristalsis, lubricating the fecal mass, or adding more bulk to the colon contents.

37.4 Diarrhea is an increase in the fluidity of feces that occurs when the colon fails to reabsorb enough water.

37.5 For simple diarrhea, OTC medications are effective. Opioids are the most effective drugs for controlling severe diarrhea.

37.6 Vomiting is a defence mechanism used by the body to rid itself of toxic substances. Nausea is an uncomfortable feeling that may precede vomiting.

37.7 Symptomatic treatment of nausea and vomiting includes drugs from many different classes, including phenothiazines, antihistamines, cannabinoids, corticosteroids, benzodiazepines, and serotonin receptor antagonists.

37.8 Weight-loss drugs are used for the short-term management of obesity, but these drugs produce only modest effects.

37.9 Pancreatitis results when pancreatic enzymes are trapped in the pancreas and are not released into the duodenum. Pharmacotherapy includes replacement enzymes and supportive drugs for pain relief and gastric acid reduction.

REVIEW QUESTIONS

1 Bismuth compounds are used to treat several digestive disorders. What are they?

2 What type of teaching plan, including dietary modifications and pharmacological products, might be developed to "wean" a person off chronic laxative use?

3 There are various classifications of drugs employed in the treatment of nausea and vomiting. Which class is considered to be of greatest benefit?

4 Anorexiants, used to treat obesity, are seldom effective for long-term weight loss. Why, then, are they prescribed?

CRITICAL THINKING QUESTIONS

1. The client has been taking diphenoxylate (Lomotil) for diarrhea for the past 3 days. The client has had diarrhea five times today. What are the priorities for nursing care?

2. The healthcare provider has ordered morphine and prochlorperazine for a client with postoperative pain. The client insists that she is "needle phobic" and wants all the medication in one syringe. What is the nurse's response?

3. A client comes to the clinic complaining of no bowel movement for 4 days (other than small amounts of liquid stool). The client has been taking psyllium mucilloid (Metamucil) for his constipation and wants to know why this is not working. What is the nurse's response?

EXPLORE
MediaLink

  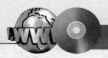

www.pearsoned.ca/adams-king

MEDIALINK DVD-ROM
- Audio Glossary
- CRNE Review
- Animation
  Mechanism of Action: Tegaserod

COMPANION WEBSITE
- CRNE Review
- **Case Study:** Constipation and diarrhea
- Dosage Calculations

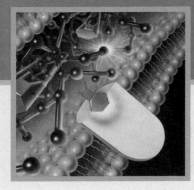

CHAPTER 38

Drugs for Nutritional Disorders

DRUGS AT A GLANCE

VITAMINS
Lipid soluble
> ℗ vitamin A (Arovit A)

Water soluble
> ℗ folic acid (Apo-Folic)

MINERALS
Macrominerals
> ℗ magnesium sulfate (Epsom Salts)

Microminerals

NUTRITIONAL SUPPLEMENTS
Enteral nutrition
Parenteral nutrition

OBJECTIVES

After reading this chapter, the student should be able to do the following:

1. Identify drug classes used for treating nutritional disorders.
2. Explain the therapeutic action of common vitamins and minerals and conditions for which they may be beneficial.
3. Compare and contrast the properties of water-soluble and fat-soluble vitamins.
4. Compare and contrast the properties of macrominerals and trace minerals.
5. Compare and contrast enteral and parenteral methods of providing nutrition.
6. Identify differences among oligomeric, polymeric, modular, and specialized formulations for enteral nutrition.
7. For each of the drug classes listed in Drugs at a Glance, identify a representative drug and explain its mechanism of action, therapeutic effects, and important adverse effects.
8. Describe and explain, based on pharmacological principles, the rationale for nursing assessment, planning, and interventions for clients with nutritional disorders.
9. Use the nursing process to care for clients receiving pharmacotherapy for nutritional disorders.

MediaLink

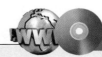 www.pearsoned.ca/adams-king

CRNE review, case studies, and other interactive resources for this chapter can be found on the Companion Website at **www.pearsoned.ca/adams-king**. Click on "Chapter 38" to select the activities for this chapter. For animations, more CRNE review questions, and an audio glossary, access the accompanying DVD-ROM in this textbook.

The nutritional supplement business is a multibillion-dollar industry. Although clever marketing often leads clients to believe that vitamin and dietary supplements are essential to maintain health, most people obtain all the necessary nutrients through a balanced diet. Once the body has obtained the amounts of vitamins, minerals, and nutrients it needs to carry on metabolism, the excess is simply excreted or stored. In certain conditions, however, dietary supplementation is necessary and will benefit the client's health. This chapter focuses on these conditions and explores the role of vitamins, minerals, and nutritional supplements in pharmacology.

PharmFacts

Vitamins, Minerals, and Nutritional Supplements

- Over 40% of Canadians take vitamin supplements daily.
- There is no difference between the chemical structure of a natural vitamin and a synthetic vitamin, yet consumers pay much more for the natural type. However, natural forms of vitamin E may be used more efficiently by the body.
- Vitamin B_{12} is only present in animal products. Vegetarians may find adequate amounts in fortified cereals, nutritional supplements, and yeast.
- Clients who never go outside or are rarely exposed to the sun may need vitamin D supplements.
- Vitamins technically cannot increase a client's energy level. Energy can only be provided by adding calories in carbohydrates, proteins, and lipids.
- Socioeconomic and geographic factors may influence access to fresh produce and the incidence of vitamin and nutrient deficiencies.
- The incidence of vitamin deficiencies is greater in some northern Aboriginal populations.
- Ethnic variations in diet may influence nutrient balance.

LIFESPAN CONSIDERATIONS

Vitamins, Minerals, and Other Nutrients

- Vitamin and mineral requirements change across the lifespan.
- Infants, children, and clients who are pregnant or lactating have different nutritional needs than the average adult.
- Administration of folic acid during pregnancy has been found to reduce birth defects in the nervous system of the baby.
- Heavy menstrual periods may result in significant iron loss.
- Perimenopausal women and older adults may benefit from calcium and vitamin D supplements to prevent osteoporosis.
- Adults over age 50 years absorb less vitamin B_{12} from food and may require fortified foods or a supplement.

VITAMINS

Vitamins are essential substances needed in very small amounts to maintain homeostasis. Clients with a low or unbalanced dietary intake, those who are pregnant, or those experiencing a chronic disease may benefit from vitamin therapy.

38.1 Role of Vitamins in Maintaining Health

Vitamins are organic compounds required by the body in very small amounts for growth and for the maintenance of normal metabolic processes. Since the discovery of thiamine in 1911, over a dozen vitamins have been identified. Because scientists did not know the chemical structures of the vitamins when they were discovered, they assigned letters and numbers such as A, B_{12}, and C. These names are still widely used today.

An important characteristic of vitamins, with the exception of vitamin D, is that human cells cannot synthesize them. Vitamins, or their precursors known as **provitamins**, must be supplied in the diet. A second important characteristic is that if the vitamin is not present in adequate amounts, then the body's metabolism will be disrupted and disease will result. Furthermore, the symptoms of the deficiency can be reversed by the administration of the missing vitamin.

Vitamins serve diverse and important roles. For example, the B complex vitamins are coenzymes essential to many metabolic pathways. Vitamin A is a precursor of retinal, a pigment needed for vision. Calcium metabolism is regulated by a hormone that is derived from vitamin D. Without vitamin K, abnormal prothrombin is produced and blood clotting is affected.

38.2 Classification of Vitamins

A simple way to classify vitamins is by their ability to mix with water. Those that dissolve easily in water are called water-soluble vitamins. Examples include vitamin C and the B vitamins. Those that dissolve in lipids are called fat- or lipid-soluble and include vitamins A, D, E, and K.

The difference in solubility affects the way the vitamins are absorbed by the GI tract and stored in the body. The water-soluble vitamins are absorbed with water in the digestive tract and readily dissolve in blood and body fluids. When excess water-soluble vitamins are absorbed, they cannot be stored for later use and are simply excreted in the urine. Because they are not stored to any significant degree, they must be ingested daily; otherwise, deficiencies will quickly develop.

Fat-soluble vitamins, on the other hand, cannot be absorbed in sufficient quantity in the small intestine unless they are ingested with lipids. These vitamins can be stored in large quantities in the liver and adipose tissue. Should the client not ingest sufficient amounts, fat-soluble vitamins are removed from storage depots in the body, as needed. Unfortunately, storage may lead to dangerously high levels of these vitamins if they are taken in excessive amounts.

38.3 Recommended Dietary Reference Intakes

Scientists in Canada and the United States have been working together to establish nutrient recommendations based on the latest scientific research. These recommendations for the dietary intake of vitamins and other nutrients are called the **dietary reference intakes (DRIs)**. The DRI values represent the *average* amount of vitamin or other nutrient needed daily to prevent a deficiency in a healthy adult. The DRIs are revised periodically to reflect the latest scientific research. Current DRIs for vitamins are shown in Table 38.1.

TABLE 38.1	Vitamins				
		RDI			
Vitamin	**Function**	**Men**	**Women**	**Common Cause of Deficiency**	
A	visual pigments, epithelial cells	900 µg (3000 IU)	700 µg (2333 IU)	prolonged dietary deprivation, particularly when rice is the main food source; pancreatic disease; cirrhosis	
B complex: biotin	coenzyme in metabolic reactions	30 µg	30 µg	deficiencies are rare	
cyanocobalamin, B_{12}	coenzyme in nucleic acid metabolism	2.4 µg	2.4 µg	lack of intrinsic factor; inadequate intake of foods of animal origin	
folate (B_9)	coenzyme in amino acid and nucleic acid metabolism	400 µg	400 µg	pregnancy; alcoholism; cancer; oral contraceptive use	
niacin, B_3	coenzyme in metabolic reactions	16 mg	14 mg	prolonged dietary deprivation, particularly when corn (maize) or millet is the main food source; chronic diarrhea; liver disease; alcoholism	
pantothenic acid (B_5)	coenzyme in metabolic reactions	5 mg	5 mg	deficiencies are rare	
pyridoxine, B_6	coenzyme in amino acid metabolism	1.3 mg	1.3 mg	alcoholism; oral contraceptive use; malabsorption diseases	
riboflavin, B_2	coenzyme in metabolic reactions	1.3 mg	1.1 mg	inadequate consumption of milk or animal products; chronic diarrhea; liver disease; alcoholism	
thiamine, B_1	coenzyme in metabolic reactions	1.2 mg	1.1 mg	prolonged dietary deprivation, particularly when rice is the main food source; hyperthyroidism; pregnancy; liver disease; alcoholism	
C (ascorbic acid)	coenzyme and antioxidant			90 mg	75 mg	inadequate intake of fruits and vegetables; pregnancy; chronic inflammatory disease; burns; diarrhea; alcoholism
D	calcium and phosphate metabolism	5–15 µg* (200–600 IU)	5–15 µg* (200–600 IU)	low dietary intake; inadequate exposure to sunlight *Several sources now recommend 25 µg (1000 IU)/day.	
E	antioxidant	15 mg	15 mg	premature birth; malabsorption diseases	
K	cofactor in blood clotting	120 µg	95 µg	newborns; liver disease; long-term parenteral nutrition; certain drugs such as cephalosporins and salicylates	

The need for certain vitamins and minerals varies widely. Infants, children, and clients who are pregnant, have chronic disease, or exercise vigorously have different nutritional needs than the average adult. Recognizing and adjusting for these nutritional differences is essential to maintaining good health.

Vitamin, mineral, or herbal supplements should never substitute for a balanced diet. Sufficient intake of proteins, carbohydrates, and lipids is needed for proper health. Furthermore, although the label on a vitamin supplement may indicate that it contains 100% of the DRI for a particular vitamin, the body may absorb as little as 10% to 15% of the amount ingested. With the exception of vitamins A and D, it is not harmful for most clients to consume two to three times the recommended level.

Health Canada, under the Food and Drugs Act, regulates labelling of food products. In order to help consumers select foods based on nutritional requirements, standardized Nutrition Facts tables are mandatory on most food products. As shown in Figure 38.1, the Nutrition Facts table lists the amount of calories and 13 core nutrients per serving of the product as well as the "% Daily Value" based on DRIs.

38.4 Indications for Vitamin Pharmacotherapy

Most clients who eat a normal, balanced diet are able to obtain all the necessary nutrients they need without vitamin supplementation. Indeed, megavitamin therapy is not only expensive, but also harmful to health if taken for prolonged periods. **Hypervitaminosis**, or toxic levels of vitamins, has been reported for vitamins A, C, D, E, B_6, niacin, and folic acid. In North America, syndromes of vitamin excess may actually be more common than those of vitamin deficiency.

Vitamin deficiencies follow certain patterns. The following are general characteristics of vitamin deficiency disorders:

- Clients more commonly present with multiple vitamin deficiencies than with a single vitamin deficiency.

- Symptoms of deficiency are non-specific and often do not appear until the deficiency has been present for a prolonged period.

- Deficiencies in North Americans are most often the result of poverty, fad diets, chronic alcohol or drug abuse, or prolonged parenteral feeding.

Certain clients and conditions require higher levels of vitamins. Infancy and childhood are times of potential deficiency due to the high growth demands placed on the body. In addition, requirements for all nutrients are increased during pregnancy and lactation. With normal aging, the absorption of food diminishes and the quantity of ingested food is often reduced, leading to a higher risk of vitamin deficiencies in elderly clients. Vitamin deficiencies in clients with chronic liver and kidney disease are well documented.

Certain drugs affect vitamin metabolism. Alcohol is known for its ability to inhibit the absorption of thiamine and folic acid: alcohol abuse is the most common cause of thiamine deficiency in North America. Folic acid levels may be reduced in clients taking phenothiazines, oral contraceptives, phenytoin, or barbiturates. Vitamin D deficiency can be caused by therapy with certain anticonvulsants. Inhibition of vitamin B_{12} absorption has been reported with a number of drugs, including trifluoperazine, alcohol, and oral contraceptives. The nurse must be aware of these drug interactions and recommend vitamin therapy when appropriate.

LIPID-SOLUBLE VITAMINS

The lipid-soluble vitamins are abundant in both plant and animal foods and are relatively stable during cooking.

38.5 Pharmacotherapy with Lipid-Soluble Vitamins

Lipid-soluble vitamins are absorbed from the intestine with dietary lipids and are stored primarily in the liver. When consumed in high amounts, these vitamins can accumulate to toxic levels and produce hypervitaminosis. Because these are OTC agents, clients must be strongly advised to carefully follow the instructions of the healthcare provider, or the label directions, for proper dosage. It is not unusual to find some OTC preparations that contain 200% to 400% of the DRI. Lipid-soluble vitamins for treating nutritional deficiency are given in Table 38.2.

Vitamin A, also known as retinol, is obtained from foods containing **carotenes**, which are precursors to vitamin A that are converted to retinol in the wall of the small intestine following absorption. The most abundant and biologically active carotene is beta carotene. During metabolism, each molecule of beta carotene yields two molecules of vitamin A. Good sources of dietary vitamin A include yellow and dark leafy vegetables, butter, eggs, whole milk, and liver.

Vitamin D is actually a group of chemicals sharing similar activity. Vitamin D_2, also known as **ergocalciferol**, is obtained from fortified milk, margarine, and other dairy

Nutrition Facts

Per 125 mL (87 g)

Amount	% Daily Value
Calories 80	
Fat 0.5 g	1 %
Saturated 0 g + Trans 0 g	0 %
Cholesterol 0 mg	
Sodium 0 mg	0 %
Carbohydrate 18 g	6 %
Fibre 2 g	8 %
Sugars 2 g	
Protein 3 g	
Vitamin A 2% Vitamin C 10 %	
Calcium 0% Iron 2 %	

● **Figure 38.1** Nutrition Facts table

TABLE 38.2 Lipid-Soluble Vitamins for Treating Nutritional Disorders	
Drug	**Route and Adult Dose**
vitamin A (Arovit A)	PO; 500,000 IU/day for 3 d followed by 50,000 IU/d for 2 wk, then 10,000–20,000 IU d for 2 mo
	IM; 100,000 IU/d for 3 d followed by 50,000 IU/d for 2 wk
vitamin D: calcitriol (Calcijex, Rocaltrol)	PO; 0.25 µg/d, may be increased by 0.25 µg/day q4–8wk for dialysis clients or q2–4wk for hypoparathyroid clients if necessary
	IV; 0.5 µg three times/wk at the end of dialysis, may need up to 3 µg three times/wk
vitamin E: tocopherol (Aquasol E, Pro E, others)	PO/IM; 60–75 IU/d
vitamin K: phytonadione (AquaMEPHYTON)	PO/SC/IM; 2.5–10 mg (up to 25 mg), may be repeated after 6–8 hr if needed

products. Vitamin D_3 is formed in the skin by a chemical reaction requiring ultraviolet radiation. The pharmacology of the D vitamins and a Prototype Drug for the active form of vitamin D (page 659) are detailed in Chapter 46.

Vitamin E consists of about eight chemicals, called **tocopherols**, having similar activity. Alpha-tocopherol comprises 90% of the tocopherols and is the only one of pharmacological importance. Dosage is sometimes reported as milligrams of alpha-tocopherol equivalents (TE). Vitamin E is found in plant seed oils, whole-grain cereals, eggs, and certain organ meats such as liver, pancreas, and heart. It is considered a primary antioxidant, preventing the formation of free radicals that damage cell membranes and cellular structures. Deficiency in adults has only been observed with severe malabsorption disorders; however, deficiency in premature neonates may lead to hemolytic anemia. Clients may self-administer vitamin E because it is thought to be useful in preventing heart disease and increasing sexual prowess. Unlike most other vitamins, therapeutic doses of vitamin E have not been clearly established, although supplements available OTC suggest doses of 100 to 400 units per day. In addition to oral and IM preparations, a topical form is available to treat dry, cracked skin.

Vitamin K is also a mixture of several chemicals. Vitamin K_1 is found in plant sources, particularly green leafy vegetables, tomatoes, cauliflower, egg yolks, liver, and cheese. Vitamin K_2 is synthesized by microbial flora in the colon. Deficiency states, caused by inadequate intake or by antibiotic destruction of normal intestinal flora, may result in delayed hemostasis. The body does not have large stores of vitamin K, and a deficiency may occur in only 1 to 2 weeks. Certain clotting factors (II, VII, IX, and X) are dependent on vitamin K for their biosynthesis. Vitamin K is used as a treatment for clients with clotting disorders and is the antidote for warfarin (Coumadin) overdose. It is also given to infants at birth to promote blood clotting. Administration of vitamin K completely reverses deficiency symptoms.

NURSING CONSIDERATIONS

The role of the nurse in drug therapy with fat-soluble vitamins involves careful monitoring of the client's condition and providing education as it relates to the prescribed drug regimen. The nurse is responsible for assessing, counselling, and monitoring clients taking fat-soluble vitamins. Because these vitamins are available OTC, clients consider them relatively harmless. The nurse should teach clients that excessive vitamin intake can be harmful.

For all fat-soluble vitamins, the nurse should begin with assessment for deficiency. The symptoms of inadequate supply or storage of fat-soluble vitamins are dependent on the specific nutrient. For example, clients deficient in vitamin A frequently report problems with night vision, skin lesions, or mucous membrane dysfunction. A baseline visual acuity exam should be performed. In severe vitamin D deficiency, clients experience skeletal abnormalities, such as rickets in children and osteomalacia in adults. The nurse should assess laboratory tests for serum levels of calcium, phosphorus, magnesium, alkaline phosphatase, and creatinine to determine electrolyte and mineral balance. An insufficient level of vitamin E has no obvious effects, but the vitamin is believed to protect cellular components from oxidation. Bleeding tendencies are characteristic of vitamin K deficiency. Clients should be assessed for impaired liver function, because fat-soluble vitamins are stored in the liver, and for malabsorption disorders that could prevent the absorption of the vitamins.

The nurse should also assess the client's dietary intake. Clients should be instructed about foods that may supply the necessary fat-soluble vitamins essential for good health. When performing dietary counselling, it is critical that the nurse consider the socioeconomic status and culture of the client when recommending foods that may be used to treat deficiency. The nurse should suggest foods that the client can afford and would eat.

Fat-soluble vitamins stored in the liver can accumulate to toxic levels, causing accidental hypervitaminosis. Chronic overdose will affect many organs, including the liver. Excessive vitamin A intake during pregnancy can result in severe birth defects. Intravenous infusion of vitamin K is only used in emergency situations because it may cause bronchospasm and respiratory or cardiac arrest. Large doses of vitamin E appear to be non-toxic; however, the nurse should monitor clients concurrently taking warfarin for increased risk of bleeding.

Client education as it relates to fat-soluble vitamins should include goals, reasons for obtaining baseline data such as lab

Pr PROTOTYPE DRUG | Vitamin A (Arovit A)

ACTIONS AND USES

Vitamin A is essential for general growth and development, particularly of the bones, teeth, and epithelial membranes. It is necessary for proper wound healing, essential for the biosynthesis of steroids, and is one of the pigments required for night vision. Vitamin A is indicated in deficiency states and during periods of increased need such as pregnancy, lactation, or debilitated states. Night blindness and slow wound healing can be effectively treated with as little as 30,000 IU of vitamin A given daily over a week. It is also prescribed for GI disorders when absorption in the small intestine is diminished or absent. Topical forms are available for acne, psoriasis, and other skin disorders. Doses of vitamin A are sometimes measured in retinoid equivalents (RE). In severe deficiency states, up to 500,000 IU may be given per day for 3 days, gradually tapering off to 10,000 to 20,000 IU/day.

PHARMACOKINETICS

Vitamin A is metabolized in the liver and GI tract and is excreted in urine and feces. It has a variable half-life.

ADMINISTRATION ALERTS

- Vitamin A is pregnancy category A at low doses.
- Vitamin A is pregnancy category X at doses above the RDA.

ADVERSE EFFECTS AND INTERACTIONS

Adverse effects are not observed with low doses of vitamin A. Acute ingestion produces serious CNS toxicity, including headache, irritability, drowsiness, delirium, and possible coma. Long-term ingestion of high amounts causes drying and scaling of the skin, alopecia, fatigue, anorexia, vomiting, and leukopenia.

People taking vitamin A should avoid taking mineral oil and cholestyramine as both may decrease the absorption of vitamin A.

---

tests for liver function and CBC, and possible side effects. Following are important points the nurse should include when teaching clients about fat-soluble vitamins:

- Take vitamins only as prescribed or as directed on the label. Do not double the dosage.
- Discontinue using the vitamin and notify the healthcare provider immediately if toxicity symptoms occur.
- Consult the healthcare provider before taking OTC drugs; they might contain additional fat-soluble vitamins and lead to toxicity.
- Include vitamin-rich foods in your diet to decrease the need for vitamin supplements.

WATER-SOLUBLE VITAMINS

The water-soluble vitamins consist of the B complex vitamins and vitamin C.

SPECIAL CONSIDERATIONS

Vitamin Supplements and Client Communication

In the current culture, many people take vitamin supplements. Product advertising promotes vitamin supplements as a means to maintain optimal health. If taken in recommended dosages, vitamin toxicity is not a concern in healthy people; however, some vitamin supplements should be taken with caution as they can interact with prescribed medications. Some food products are fortified with vitamins or minerals. For example, certain manufacturers claim that their cereals and juices have 100% of the DRI for particular vitamins and minerals. People who take supplements may not consider these fortified foods as vitamin sources, and accidental overdosage can result.

Healthcare providers should adopt a non-judgmental attitude that promotes trust and honest communication with the client. In this way, the client will be open about the use of vitamin and nutritional supplements. Acceptance and understanding are necessary to assist clients to take vitamins in a responsible way that does not compromise clinical drug treatment.

NURSING PROCESS FOCUS   Clients Receiving Vitamin A (Arovit A) **Pr**

Assessment	Potential Nursing Diagnoses/Identified Patterns
Prior to administration: ■ Obtain complete health history including allergies, drug history, and possible drug interactions. ■ Obtain complete physical examination. ■ Assess for the presence/history of vitamin A deficiency such as inadequate dietary intake, malabsorption diseases, and impaired liver function. ■ Obtain baseline vision acuity examination. ■ Assess integrity of skin and mucous membranes. ■ Obtain the following laboratory studies: serum vitamin A level, CBC, liver function profile, and serum protein/albumin levels.	■ Nutritional deficiency ■ Disturbed sensory perception related to vitamin A deficiency ■ Risk for impaired skin integrity ■ Deficient knowledge regarding drug therapy

continued

NURSING PROCESS FOCUS Clients Receiving Vitamin A (Arovit A) *(Continued)*	

Planning: Client Goals and Expected Outcomes

The client will:
- Exhibit improvement in serum vitamin A level
- Demonstrate an understanding of the drug's action by accurately describing drug side effects and precautions
- Immediately report side effects such as increased nausea, vomiting, headache, loss of hair, lethargy, and malaise

Implementation

Interventions (Rationales)	Client Education/Discharge Planning
■ Monitor client's diet to determine intake of vitamin A foods. (Deficiency state may be caused by poor dietary habits.)	Instruct client to: ■ Maintain a dietary log for 48 hours ■ Eat foods rich in vitamin A such as egg yolks, butter, milk, liver, dark leafy vegetables, and orange fruits and vegetables
■ Periodically monitor visual acuity. (Vitamin A may cause miosis, papilledema, and nystagmus.)	■ Advise client to report any changes in vision.
■ Monitor for symptoms of vitamin A toxicity. (Storage of excess vitamin A can lead to hypervitaminosis.)	Instruct client to: ■ Watch for signs and symptoms of vitamin A overdose such as nausea, vomiting, anorexia, dry skin and lips, headache, and loss of hair ■ Immediately stop taking medication if signs of toxicity are noted
■ Monitor for signs of intracranial pressure. (Vitamin A may cause increased intracranial pressure if taken in large doses.)	Instruct client to: ■ Follow dosage directions given by the healthcare provider or on the label ■ Immediately report any changes in neurological status such as increased sleepiness, headaches, lethargy, and malaise
■ Assess for use of mineral oil. (Mineral oil inhibits the absorption of vitamin A.)	■ Advise client to avoid laxatives that contain mineral oil.
■ Monitor for drug interactions with oral contraceptives. (Concurrent use of vitamin A and oral contraceptives can cause toxic levels of vitamin A.)	Instruct client to: ■ Adhere to medication schedule and avoid double doses of the vitamin ■ Keep appointments for follow-up laboratory studies if taking oral contraceptives

Evaluation of Outcome Criteria

Evaluate the effectiveness of drug therapy by confirming that client goals and expected outcomes have been met (see "Planning").

38.6 Pharmacotherapy with Water-Soluble Vitamins

The B-complex group is composed of 12 different vitamins that are grouped together because they were originally derived from yeast and foods that counteracted the disease beriberi. They have very different chemical structures and serve different metabolic functions. The B vitamins are known by their chemical name as well as their vitamin number. For example, vitamin B_{12} is also called cyanocobalamin. Water-soluble vitamins for treating nutritional deficiencies are given in Table 38.3.

Vitamin B_1, or thiamine, is a precursor of an enzyme responsible for several steps in the oxidation of carbohydrates. It is abundant in both plant and animal products, especially whole-grain foods, dried beans, and peanuts. Because of its abundance, thiamine deficiency in North America is not common, except in alcoholics and in clients with chronic liver disease. Thiamine deficiency, or **beriberi**, is characterized by neurological signs such as paresthesia, neuralgia, and progressive loss of feeling and reflexes. Chronic deficiency can result in heart failure. Severe deficiencies may require parenteral thiamine up to 100 mg/day. With pharmacotherapy, symptoms can be completely reversed in the early stages of the disease; however, permanent disability can result in clients with prolonged deficiency.

Vitamin B_2, or riboflavin, is a component of coenzymes that participate in a number of different oxidation-reduction reactions. Riboflavin is abundantly found in plant and animal products, including wheat germ, eggs, cheese, fish, nuts, and leafy vegetables. Like thiamine, deficiency of riboflavin is most commonly observed in alcoholics. Signs of deficiency include corneal vascularization and anemia, as well as skin abnormalities such as dermatitis and cheilosis. Most symptoms are resolved by administering 25 to 100 mg/day until improvement is noted.

TABLE 38.3   Water-Soluble Vitamins for Treating Nutritional Disorders

Drug	Route and Adult Dose
vitamin B_1: thiamine hydrochloride (Betaxin)	PO; 5–30 mg/d IV/IM; 50–100 mg tid
vitamin B_2: riboflavin	PO; 5–10 mg/d
vitamin B_3: niacin (Novo-Niacin, others)	PO; 10–20 mg/d IV/IM/SC; 25–100 mg two to five times/d
vitamin B_6: pyridoxine hydrochloride	PO/IM/IV; 2.5–10 mg/d times 3 wk, then may reduce to 2.5–5 mg/d
vitamin B_9: folic acid (Apo-Folic)	PO/IM/SC/IV; ≤ 1 mg/d
vitamin B_{12}: cyanocobalamin	IM/Deep SC; 30 μg/d for 5–10 d, then 100–200 μg/mo
vitamin C: ascorbic acid (Activa C, Apo-C, Bio-C, others)	PO/IV/IM/SC; 150–500 mg/d in one to two doses

Vitamin B_3, or niacin, is a key component of nicotinamide adenine dinucleotide (NAD) and nicotinamide adenine dinucleotide phosphate (NADP), two coenzymes that are essential for oxidative metabolism. Niacin is synthesized from the amino acid tryptophan and is widely distributed in both animal and plant foods, including beans, wheat germ, meats, nuts, and whole-grain breads. Niacin deficiency, or **pellagra**, is most commonly seen in alcoholics and in areas of the world where corn is the primary food source. Early symptoms include fatigue, anorexia, and drying of the skin. Advanced symptoms include three classic signs: dermatitis, diarrhea, and dementia. Deficiency is treated with niacin at dosages ranging from 10 to 25 mg/day. When used to treat hyperlipidemia, niacin is given as nicotinic acid and doses are much higher—up to 3 g/day (see Chapter 22).

Vitamin B_6, or pyridoxine, consists of several closely related compounds, including pyridoxine itself, pyridoxal, and pyridoxamine. Vitamin B_6 is essential for the synthesis of heme and is a primary coenzyme involved in the metabolism of amino acids. It is also needed for the synthesis of the neurotransmitter gamma-aminobutyric acid (GABA). Deficiency states can be the result of alcoholism, uremia, hypothyroidism, or heart failure. Certain drugs can cause vitamin B_6 deficiency, including isoniazid, cycloserine, hydralazine, oral contraceptives, and pyrazinamide. Clients receiving these drugs may routinely receive B_6 supplements. Deficiency symptoms include skin abnormalities, cheilosis, fatigue, and irritability. Symptoms reverse after administration of about 10 to 20 mg/day for several weeks.

Vitamin B_9, more commonly known as folate or folic acid, is metabolized to tetrahydrofolate, which is essential for normal DNA synthesis and for erythropoiesis. Folic acid is widely distributed in plant products, especially green leafy vegetables and citrus fruits. This vitamin is highlighted as a Prototype Drug on the next page.

Vitamin B_{12}, or cyanocobalamin, is folate of a cobalt-containing vitamin that is a required coenzyme for a number of metabolic pathways. It also has important roles in cell replication, erythrocyte maturation, and myelin synthesis. Sources include lean meat, seafood, liver, and milk. Deficiency of vitamin B_{12} results in **pernicious (megaloblastic) anemia**. This vitamin is featured as a Prototype Drug in Chapter 28 (page 364).

Vitamin C, or ascorbic acid, is the most commonly purchased OTC vitamin. It is a potent antioxidant and serves many functions, including collagen synthesis, tissue healing, and maintenance of bone, teeth, and epithelial tissue. Many consumers purchase the vitamin for its ability to prevent the common cold, a function that has not been definitively proven. Deficiency of vitamin C, or **scurvy,** is caused by diets deficient in fruits and vegetables. Alcoholics, cigarette smokers, cancer clients, and those with renal failure are at highest risk of vitamin C deficiency. Symptoms include fatigue, bleeding gums and other hemorrhages, gingivitis, and poor wound healing. Symptoms can normally be reversed by the administration of 300 to 1000 mg/day of vitamin C for several weeks.

NURSING CONSIDERATIONS

The role of the nurse in water-soluble vitamin therapy involves careful monitoring of the client's condition and providing education as it relates to the prescribed drug regimen. Water-soluble vitamins are used for multiple reasons in healthcare. The nurse should determine the reason for the specific vitamin therapy being prescribed and assess for the presence or absence of the associated symptoms.

Thiamine is often administered to hospitalized clients who have severe liver disease. If thiamine deficiency is not corrected in these clients, irreversible brain damage may occur. There are no known adverse effects from oral administration of thiamine, and parenteral administration rarely causes any type of adverse effect. Niacin may be administered in the treatment of niacin deficiency or as an adjunct in cholesterol-lowering therapy. Pyridoxine deficiency is associated with poor nutritional status, chronic debilitating diseases, and alcohol abuse. Both niacin and pyridoxine may cause severe flushing. The nurse should inform the client that this is an expected reaction and will not cause permanent harm. Most clients tolerate therapy with B vitamins with few adverse effects.

Vitamin C, readily available as an OTC nutritional supplement, may cause diarrhea, nausea, vomiting, abdominal pain, and hyperuricemia in high doses. Clients with a history of kidney stones should be cautioned against using vitamin C unless directed by a healthcare provider because excessive intake may promote renal calculi formation. Clients taking vitamin C should be advised to increase fluid intake. Most clients are able to take vitamin C without experiencing serious side effects.

Client education as it relates to water-soluble vitamins should include goals, reasons for obtaining baseline data such as CBC and lab tests for liver function, and possible side effects. Following are the important points the nurse should include when teaching clients about water-soluble vitamins:

- Niacin and pyridoxine may cause a feeling of warmth and flushing of skin, but this will diminish with continued therapy.
- Include vitamin-rich foods (whole grains, fresh vegetables, fresh fruits, lean meats, and dairy products) in the diet to decrease the need for vitamin supplements.
- Water-soluble vitamins are not stored in the body and must be replenished daily.
- Take vitamins only as prescribed or as directed on the label. Do not double the dosage.

NATURAL THERAPIES

Vitamin C and the Common Cold

Although there is a great deal of anecdotal evidence that vitamin C helps to fend off a cold, the claims are unsubstantiated; however, vitamin C may be useful as an immune stimulator and modulator in some circumstances. Several studies have shown that vitamin C can significantly reduce the duration and severity of colds in some people and reduce the incidence in others. It is thought that this is due, at least in part, to the antihistamine activity of vitamin C. The best results were obtained with doses of 2 g/day (or greater). Preliminary evidence also suggests that vitamin C can be useful in improving respiratory infections.

Pr PROTOTYPE DRUG | Folic Acid (Apo-Folic)

ACTIONS AND USES

Folic acid is administered to reverse symptoms of deficiency, which most commonly occurs in clients with inadequate intake, such as with chronic alcohol abuse. Because this vitamin is destroyed by high temperatures, people who overcook their food may experience folate deficiency. Pregnancy markedly increases the need for dietary folic acid; folic acid is given during pregnancy to promote normal fetal growth. Because insufficient vitamin B_{12} creates a lack of activated folic acid, deficiency symptoms resemble those of vitamin B_{12} deficiency. The megaloblastic anemia observed in folate-deficient clients, however, does not include the severe nervous system symptoms seen in clients with B_{12} deficiency. Administration of 1 mg/day of oral folic acid often reverses the deficiency symptoms within 5 to 7 days.

PHARMACOKINETICS

Folic acid is well absorbed and widely distributed. It peaks in 30 to 60 minutes. It is metabolized in the liver to its active metabolite, dihydrofolate reductase. Excess folic acid is excreted by the kidneys.

ADMINISTRATION ALERT

- Folic acid is pregnancy category A.

ADVERSE EFFECTS AND INTERACTIONS

Side effects during folic acid therapy are uncommon. Clients may feel flushed following IV injections. Allergies to folic acid are possible.

Folic acid interacts with many drugs. For example, phenytoin, trimethoprim-sulfisoxazole, and other medications may interfere with the absorption of folic acid. Chloramphenicol may antagonize effects of folate therapy. Oral contraceptives, alcohol, barbiturates, methotrexate, and primidone may cause folate deficiency.

NURSING PROCESS FOCUS   Clients Receiving Folic Acid (Apo-Folic)

Assessment	Potential Nursing Diagnoses/Identified Patterns
Prior to administration: - Obtain complete health history including allergies, drug history, and possible drug interactions. - Obtain complete physical examination with special attention to symptoms related to anemic states such as pallor, fatigue, weakness, tachycardia, and shortness of breath. - Obtain the following laboratory studies: folic acid levels, hemoglobin, hematocrit, and reticulocyte counts. - Obtain CBC to determine the type of anemia present. (Folic acid is not beneficial in normocytic anemia, refractory anemia, and aplastic anemia.)	- Nutritional deficiency - Deficient knowledge regarding drug therapy

continued

NURSING PROCESS FOCUS   Clients Receiving Folic Acid (Apo-Folic)   *(Continued)*

Planning: Client Goals and Expected Outcomes
The client will: ■ Exhibit improvement in serum folic acid level ■ Demonstrate an understanding of the drug's action by accurately describing drug side effects and precautions ■ Immediately report side effects such as continued weakness and fatigue

Implementation	
Interventions (Rationales)	**Client Education/Discharge Planning**
■ Monitor client's dietary intake of folic acid–containing foods. (Deficiency state may be caused by poor dietary habits.)	Instruct client to: ■ Eat foods high in folic acid such as vegetables, fruits, and organ meats ■ Consult with healthcare provider concerning amount of folic acid that should be in the diet
■ Encourage client to conserve energy. (Anemia, caused by folic acid deficiency, may lead to weakness and fatigue.)	Advise client to: ■ Rest when tired and not to overexert ■ Plan activities to avoid fatigue
■ Encourage client to take medication appropriately.	Instruct client to: ■ Avoid use of alcohol because it increases folic acid requirements ■ Take only the amount of the drug prescribed

Evaluation of Outcome Criteria
Evaluate the effectiveness of drug therapy by confirming that client goals and expected outcomes have been met (see "Planning").

MINERALS

Minerals are inorganic substances needed in small amounts to maintain homeostasis. Minerals are classified as macrominerals or microminerals; the macrominerals must be ingested in larger amounts. A normal, balanced diet will provide the proper amounts of the required minerals for most clients. The primary minerals used in pharmacotherapy are shown in Table 38.4.

38.7 Pharmacotherapy with Minerals

Minerals are essential substances that constitute about 4% of the body weight and serve many diverse functions. Some are present primarily as essential ions or electrolytes in body fluids; others are bound to organic molecules such as hemoglobin, phospholipids, or metabolic enzymes. Those minerals that function as critical electrolytes in the body, most notably sodium and potassium, are covered in more detail in Chapter 44. Sodium chloride and potassium chloride are featured as Prototype Drugs (pages 635 and 636).

Because minerals are needed in very small amounts for human metabolism, a normal balanced diet will supply the necessary quantities for most clients. Like vitamins, excess amounts of minerals can lead to toxicity, and clients should be advised not to exceed recommended doses. Mineral supplements, however, are indicated for certain disorders. Iron-deficiency anemia is the most common nutritional deficiency in the world and is a common indication for iron supplements. Women at high risk of osteoporosis are advised

to consume extra calcium, either in their diet or as a dietary supplement.

Certain drugs affect normal mineral metabolism. Clients taking loop or thiazide diuretics can have significant potassium loss. Corticosteroids and oral contraceptives are among several classes of drug that can promote sodium retention. The uptake of iodine by the thyroid gland can be impaired by certain oral hypoglycemics and lithium carbonate. Oral contraceptives have been reported to lower the plasma levels of zinc and to increase those of copper. Changes to mineral intake may be required when these drugs are used.

38.8 Pharmacotherapy with Macrominerals

Macrominerals (major minerals) are inorganic substances that must be obtained daily from dietary sources in amounts of 100 mg or higher. The macrominerals include calcium, chlorine, magnesium, phosphorous, potassium, sodium, and sulfur. As bone salts, calcium and phosphorous comprise approximately 75% of the total mineral content in the body. Recommended DRIs have been established for each of the macrominerals except sulfur, as listed in Table 38.5.

Calcium is essential for nerve conduction, muscular contraction, and hemostasis. Much of the body's calcium is bound in the bony matrix of the skeleton. Hypocalcemia occurs when serum calcium falls below 4.5 mEq/L and may be caused by inadequate intake of calcium-containing foods,

TABLE 38.4 Minerals for Treating Nutritional Disorders

Drug	Route and Adult Dose
sodium bicarbonate (see page 638 for the Prototype Drug box)	PO; 0.3–2.0 g qd–qid or 1 tsp of powder in glass of water
potassium chloride (K-Dur, Riva-K, Slow K, others) (see page 636 for the Prototype Drug box)	PO; 10–100 mEq/h in divided doses IV; 10–40 mEq/h diluted to at least 10–20 mEq/100 mL of solution (max 200–400 mEq/d)
Calcium Salts	
calcium carbonate (Caltrate, Calcite, Calsan, others)	PO; 1–2 g bid–tid
calcium chloride (Calciject, Calcitrans, others)	IV; 0.5–1.0 g qd–q3d
calcium citrate (Citracal)	PO; 1–2 g bid–tid
calcium phosphate tribasic	PO; 1–2 g bid–tid
calcium gluconate (Calciforte) (see page 657 for the Prototype Drug box)	PO; 1–2 g bid–qid
calcium lactate	PO; 325 mg–1.3 g tid with meals
Iron Salts	
ferrous fumarate (Palafer)	PO; 200 mg tid–qid
ferrous gluconate (Apo-Ferrous Gluconate)	PO; 325–600 mg qid, may be gradually increased to 650 mg qid as needed and tolerated
ferrous sulfate (Apo-Ferrous Sulfate) (see page 366 for the Prototype Drug box)	PO; 750–1500 mg qd in one to three divided doses
iron dextran (Dextran)	IM/IV; dose is individualized and determined from a table of correlations between client's weight and hemoglobin per package insert (max 100 mg [2 mL] of iron dextran within 24 hr)
iron sucrose injection (Venofer)	IV; 1 mL (20 mg) injected in dialysis line at rate of 1 mL/min up to 5 mL (100 mg), or infuse 100 mg in NS over 15 min one to three times/wk
Magnesium	
magnesium chloride (Magnolex)	PO; 270–400 mg qd
magnesium oxide	PO; 400–1200 mg/d in divided doses
magnesium sulfate (Epsom Salt)	IV/IM; 0.5–3.0 g qd
Phosphorous	
monobasic potassium phosphate	PO; 1 g qid
monobasic potassium and sodium phosphates	PO; 250 mg qid (max 2 g phosphorous/d)
potassium phosphate	PO; 1.45 g qid IV; 10 mmol phosphorous/d
potassium and sodium phosphates	PO; 250 mg phosphorous qid
Zinc	
zinc acetate (Zincum Aceticum)	PO; 50 mg tid
zinc gluconate	PO; 20–100 mg (20 mg lozenges may be taken to a max of six lozenges/d)
zinc sulfate	PO; 15–220 mg qd

lack of vitamin D, chronic diarrhea, or decreased secretion of parathyroid hormone. Symptoms of hypocalcemia involve the nervous and muscular systems. The client often becomes irritable and restless, and muscular twitches, cramps, spasms, and cardiac abnormalities are common. Long-term hypocalcemia may lead to fractures. Pharmacotherapy includes calcium compounds, which are available in many oral formulations including calcium carbonate, calcium citrate, calcium gluconate, and calcium lactate. In severe cases, IV preparations are administered. Calcium gluconate is featured as a Prototype Drug in Chapter 46 (page 657).

Phosphorous is an essential mineral that is often bound to calcium in the form of calcium phosphate in bones. In addition to its role in bone formation, phosphorous is a component of ATP and nucleic acids. Phosphate (PO_4^{-2}) is an important buffer in the blood. Because of its close relationship to phosphate, phosphorous balance is normally considered the same as phosphate balance. Symptoms of hypophosphatemia include weakness, muscle tremor, anorexia, weak pulse, and bleeding abnormalities. When serum phosphorous falls below 1.5 mEq/L, phosphate therapy is usually administered. Sodium phosphate and potassium phosphate are available for phosphorous deficiencies.

Magnesium is the second most abundant intracellular cation. Like potassium, it is necessary for proper neuromus-

TABLE 38.5 Macrominerals

Mineral	DRI	Function
calcium	1000–1200 mg	forms bone matrix; regulates nerve conduction and muscle contraction
chloride	1800–2300 mg	major anion in body fluids; part of gastric acid secretion
Iron	men: 8 mg women: 8–18 mg	prevention of iron-deficiency anemia
magnesium	men: 400–420 mg women: 310–320 mg	cofactor for many enzymes; necessary for normal nerve conduction and muscle contraction
phosphorous	700 mg	forms bone matrix; part of ATP and nucleic acids
potassium	4700 g	necessary for normal nerve conduction and muscle contraction; principal cation in intracellular fluid; essential for acid-base and electrolyte balance
sodium	1200–1500 mg	necessary for normal nerve conduction and muscle contraction; principal cation in extracellular fluid; essential for acid-base and electrolyte balance
sulfur	not established	component of proteins, B vitamins, and other critical molecules

cular function. Magnesium serves a metabolic role in activating certain enzymes in the breakdown of carbohydrates and proteins. Hypomagnesemia is generally asymptomatic until serum magnesium falls below 1.0 mEq/L. Because it produces few symptoms in its early stages, it is sometimes described as the most common undiagnosed electrolyte abnormality. Clients may experience general weakness, dysrhythmias, hypertension, loss of deep tendon reflexes, and respiratory depression. These symptoms are sometimes mistaken for hypokalemia. Pharmacotherapy with magnesium sulfate can quickly reverse symptoms of hypomagnesemia. Magnesium sulfate is a CNS depressant and is sometimes given to either prevent or terminate seizures associated with eclampsia. Magnesium salts have additional applications as cathartics and antacids (magnesium citrate,

magnesium hydroxide, and magnesium oxide) and as analgesics (magnesium salicylate).

NURSING CONSIDERATIONS

The role of the nurse in macromineral therapy involves careful monitoring of the client's condition and providing education as it relates to the prescribed drug regimen. Macrominerals are used for multiple reasons in healthcare. The nurse should determine the reason for the specific macromineral therapy being prescribed and assess for the presence or absence of the associated symptoms.

Although minerals cause no harm in small amounts, larger doses can cause life-threatening adverse effects. Calcium is

Pr PROTOTYPE DRUG | Magnesium Sulfate

ACTIONS AND USES

Severe hypomagnesemia can be rapidly reversed by the administration of IM or IV magnesium sulfate. Hypomagnesemia has a number of causes, including loss of body fluids due to diarrhea, diuretics, and nasogastric suctioning; and prolonged parenteral feeding with magnesium-free solutions. Oral forms of magnesium sulfate are used as cathartics when complete evacuation of the colon is desired. Its action as a CNS depressant has led to its occasional use as an anticonvulsant.

PHARMACOKINETICS

Magnesium sulfate is well absorbed, widely distributed, and excreted mainly by the kidneys. Its onset of action is 1 to 2 hours. It has an unknown half-life.

ADMINISTRATION ALERTS

- Continuously monitor client during IV infusion for early signs of decreased cardiac function.
- Monitor serum magnesium levels every 6 hours during parenteral infusion.
- When giving IV infusion, give required dose over 4 hours.
- Magnesium sulfate is pregnancy category A.

ADVERSE EFFECTS AND INTERACTIONS

IV infusions of magnesium sulfate require careful observation to avoid toxicity. Early signs of magnesium overdose include flushing of the skin, sedation, confusion, intense thirst, and muscle weakness. Extreme levels cause neuromuscular blockade with resultant respiratory paralysis and heart block and may cause circulatory collapse, complete heart block, and respiratory failure. Plasma magnesium levels should be monitored frequently. Clients receiving CNS depressants may experience increased sedation. Because of these potentially fatal adverse effects, the use of magnesium sulfate is restricted to severe magnesium deficiency. Mild to moderate hypomagnesemia is treated with oral forms of magnesium such as magnesium gluconate or magnesium hydroxide.

Administration of neuromuscular blocking agents with magnesium sulfate may increase respiratory depression and apnea.

one of the most common minerals in use. To prevent and treat osteoporosis, it is recommended that adult women take 1200 mg/day of calcium. Common side effects include mild GI distress and constipation. Prolonged therapy with calcium may increase the risk of hypercalcemia, especially in clients with decreased liver and renal function. Symptoms of hypercalcemia include nausea, vomiting, constipation, frequent urination, lethargy, and depression. Since calcium interacts with many drugs, such as glucocorticoids, thiazide diuretics, and tetracyclines, the client should inform the healthcare provider when using calcium supplements. The client should also be advised to avoid zinc-rich foods such as legumes, nuts, sprouts, and soy that impair calcium absorption.

Phosphorous is a mineral sometimes used as a dietary supplement. Clients who are on a sodium- or potassium-restricted diet should not use phosphorous supplements. Most adverse effects of excess phosphate are mild and include GI distress, diarrhea, and dizziness. The client should stop taking phosphorous at the first sign of seizure activity as excess phosphorous can promote seizures. Antacids should be avoided because they may decrease serum phosphorous levels.

Magnesium sulfate is given to correct hypomagnesemia, evacuate the bowel in preparation for diagnostic examinations, and treat seizures associated with eclampsia of pregnancy. The medication is given orally to replace magnesium and by the IM or IV routes to prevent or terminate eclamptic seizures. When given IV, it is important for the nurse to assess the neurological status of the client because overdose can lead to reduced reflexes and muscle weakness. The nurse should monitor for loss of consciousness (LOC) changes, deep tendon reflexes, thirst, and confusion. Because of its effects on muscles and the heart, it is contraindicated in clients with myocardial damage, heart block, and recent cardiac arrest. It has a laxative effect when given orally, so it should not be given to clients with abdominal pain, nausea, vomiting, or intestinal obstruction. Magnesium sulfate should be used with caution in clients with impaired kidney function and those on cardiac glycosides.

Client education as it relates to macromineral therapy should include goals, reasons for obtaining baseline data such as CBC and lab tests for liver function, and possible side effects. Following are the important points the nurse should include when teaching clients about minerals:

- Take minerals only as prescribed or as directed on the label. Overdose may lead to toxicity.
- Discontinue using the medication and notify the healthcare provider immediately if toxicity symptoms occur.
- Consult the healthcare provider before taking OTC drugs; they might contain additional minerals and lead to toxicity.
- Eat a well-balanced diet to eliminate or reduce the need for mineral supplements.

NURSING PROCESS FOCUS	Clients Receiving Magnesium Sulfate (Pr)	
Assessment	**Potential Nursing Diagnoses/Identified Patterns**
Prior to administration: - Obtain complete health history including allergies, drug history, and possible drug interactions. - Obtain complete physical examination with special attention to respiratory status and deep tendon reflexes. - Assess for the presence/history of malnutrition, hypomagnesia, seizure activity, preeclampsia, and kidney disease. - Obtain serum magnesium level and renal profile.	- Deficient knowledge regarding drug therapy - Risk for injury related to disease conditions and adverse effects of drug
Planning: Client Goals and Expected Outcomes	
The client will: - Exhibit improvement in serum magnesium level - Accurately describe the drug's intended effects, side effects, and precautions - Immediately report side effects such as lowered pulse, dizziness, difficulty breathing, and weakness	
Implementation	
Interventions (Rationales)	**Client Education/Discharge Planning**
- Assess magnesium level to determine deficiency. (The therapeutic range is very narrow; toxic levels may develop quickly.)	- Instruct client that magnesium sulfate should only be taken on the advice of a healthcare provider.
- Monitor vital signs frequently throughout intravenous infusion. (Magnesium sulfate depresses respirations, pulse rate, and rhythm.)	- Instruct client to report any difficulty breathing, low pulse rate, or dizziness.
- Report urine output of <100 mL/hr to healthcare provider. (Clients who have impaired renal function will have decreased renal clearance, leading to toxicity.)	- Instruct client to report any problems with urination or edema.

continued

NURSING PROCESS FOCUS Clients Receiving Magnesium Sulfate *(Continued)*	
Interventions (Rationales)	**Client Education/Discharge Planning**
▪ Observe newborns for signs and symptoms of magnesium toxicity if the mother received magnesium sulfate during labour. (The neonate may have received some amount of magnesium that could cause skeletal muscle and cardiac muscle depression.)	▪ Advise labouring mothers who are receiving magnesium sulfate that the newborn will be monitored closely after birth.
Evaluation of Outcome Criteria	
Evaluate the effectiveness of drug therapy by confirming that client goals and expected outcomes have been met (see "Planning").	

38.9 Pharmacotherapy with Microminerals

The nine **microminerals**, commonly called **trace minerals**, are required daily in amounts of 20 mg or less. The fact that they are needed in such small amounts does not diminish their role in human health; deficiencies in some of the trace minerals can result in profound illness. The functions of some of the trace minerals, such iron and iodine, are well established; the roles of others are less completely understood. The DRI for each of the microminerals is shown in Table 38.6.

Iron is an essential micromineral most commonly associated with hemoglobin. Excellent sources of dietary iron include meat, shellfish, nuts, and legumes. Excess iron in the body results in hemochromatosis, whereas lack of iron results in iron-deficiency anemia. The pharmacology of iron supplements is presented in Chapter 28, where ferrous sulfate is featured as a Prototype Drug (page 366).

Iodine is a trace mineral needed to synthesize thyroid hormone. The most common source of dietary iodine is iodized salt. When dietary intake of iodine is low, hypothyroidism occurs and enlargement of the thyroid gland (goiter) results. At high concentrations, iodine suppresses thyroid function. Lugol's solution, a mixture containing 5% elemental iodine and 10% potassium iodide, is given to hyperthyroid clients prior to thyroidectomy or during a thyrotoxic crisis. Sodium iodide acts by rapidly suppressing the secretion of thyroid hormone and is indicated for clients having an acute thyroid crisis. Radioactive iodine (I-131) is given to destroy overactive thyroid glands. Pharmacotherapeutic uses of iodine as a drug extend beyond the treatment of thyroid disease. Iodine is an effective topical antiseptic that can be found in creams, tinctures, and solutions. Iodine molecules such as iothalamate and diatrizoate are very dense and serve as diagnostic contrast agents in radiological procedures of the urinary and cardiovascular systems. The role of potassium iodide in protecting the thyroid gland during acute radiation exposure is discussed in Chapter 3.

Fluorine is a trace mineral found abundantly in nature and is best known for its effects on bones and teeth. Research has validated that adding fluoride to the water supply in very small amounts (1 part per billion) can reduce the incidence of dental caries. This effect is more pronounced in children as fluoride is incorporated into the enamel of growing teeth.

TABLE 38.6 Microminerals		
Trace Mineral	**DRI**	**Function**
chromium	0.05–2.0 mg	potentiates insulin and promotes normal protein, fat, and carbohydrate
cobalt	0.1 μg	cofactor for vitamin B_{12} and several oxidative enzymes
copper	1.5–3.0 mg	cofactor for hemoglobin synthesis
fluorine	1.5–4.0 mg	influences tooth structure and has possible effects on growth
iodine	150 μg	component of thyroid hormones
iron	men: 10–12 mg women: 10–15 mg	component of hemoglobin and some enzymes of oxidative phosphorylation
manganese	2–5 mg	cofactor in some enzymes of lipid, carbohydrate, and protein metabolism
molybdenum	75–250 mg	cofactor for certain enzymes
selenium	men: 50–70 μg women: 50–55 μg	antioxidant cofactor for certain enzymes
zinc	12–15 mg	cofactor of certain enzymes, including carbonic anhydrase; needed for proper protein structure, normal growth, and wound healing

Concentrated fluoride solutions can also be applied topically by dental professionals. Sodium fluoride and stannous fluoride are components of most toothpastes and oral rinses. Because high amounts of fluoride can be quite toxic, the use of fluoride-containing products should be closely monitored in children.

Zinc is a component of at least 100 enzymes, including alcohol dehydrogenase, carbonic anhydrase, and alkaline phosphatase. This trace mineral has a regulatory function in enzymes controlling nucleic acid synthesis and has been implicated in wound healing, male fertility, bone formation, and cell-mediated immunity. Zinc sulfate, zinc acetate, and zinc gluconate are available to prevent and treat deficiency states. In addition, lozenges containing zinc are available OTC for treating sore throats and symptoms of the common cold.

NUTRITIONAL SUPPLEMENTS

The nurse will encounter a large number of clients who are undernourished. Major goals in resolving nutritional deficiencies are to identify the specific type of deficiency and supply the missing nutrient. Nutritional supplements may be needed for short-term therapy or for the remainder of the client's life.

38.10 Etiology of Undernutrition

When the client is taking in or absorbing fewer nutrients than required for normal body growth and maintenance, **undernutrition** occurs. Successful pharmacotherapy relies on the skills of the nurse in identifying the symptoms and causes of the client's undernutrition.

Causes of undernutrition range from the simple to the complex and include the following:

- Aging
- HIV-AIDS
- Alcoholism
- Burns
- Cancer
- Chronic inflammatory bowel disease
- Eating disorders
- Gastrointestinal disorders
- Chronic neurological disease such as progressive dysphagia and multiple sclerosis
- Short-bowel syndrome
- Surgery
- Trauma

The most obvious cause for undernutrition is low dietary intake, although reasons for the inadequate intake must be assessed. Clients may have no resources to purchase food and may be suffering from starvation. Clinical depression leads many clients to shun food. Elderly clients may have poor-fitting dentures or difficulty chewing or swallowing after a stroke. In terminal disease, clients may be comatose or otherwise unable to take food orally. Although the etiologies differ, clients with insufficient intake will exhibit a similar pattern of general weakness, muscle wasting, and loss of subcutaneous fat.

When the undernutrition is caused by lack of one specific nutrient, vitamin, or mineral, the disorder is more difficult to diagnose. Clients may be on a fad diet lacking only protein or only fat. Certain digestive disorders may lead to malabsorption of specific nutrients or vitamins. Clients may simply avoid certain foods such as green leafy vegetables, dairy products, or meat products, which can lead to specific nutritional deficiencies. Proper pharmacotherapy requires the expert knowledge and assessment skills of the nurse so that the correct treatment can be administered.

38.11 Enteral Nutrition

A large number of nutritional supplements are available. A common method of classifying these agents is by their route of administration. When products are administered via the gastrointestinal tract, either orally or through a feeding tube, this is classified as **enteral nutrition**. Administration by means of IV infusion is called **parenteral nutrition.**

When the client's condition permits, enteral nutrition is best provided by oral consumption. Oral feeding allows natural digestive processes to occur and requires less intense nursing care. It does, however, rely on client adherence since it is not feasible for the healthcare provider to observe the client at every meal.

Tube feeding, or enteral tube alimentation, is necessary when the client has difficulty swallowing or is otherwise unable to take meals orally. Various tube feeding routes are possible, including nasogastric, nasoduodenal, nasojejunal, gastrostomy, or jejunostomy. An advantage of tube feeding is that the nurse can precisely measure and record the amount of enteral nutrition the client is receiving.

The particular enteral product is chosen to address the specific nutritional needs of the client. Because of the wide diversity in their formulas, it is difficult to categorize enteral products, and several different methods are used. A simple method is to classify enteral products as oligomeric, polymeric, modular, or specialized formulations.

Oligomeric formulations are agents containing varying amounts of free amino acids and peptide combinations. Indications include partial bowel obstruction, irritable bowel syndrome, radiation enteritis, bowel fistulas, and short-bowel syndrome. Sample products include Vivonex T.E.N. and Tolerex.

Polymeric formulations are the most common enteral preparations. These products contain various mixtures of proteins, carbohydrates, and lipids. Indications include general undernutrition, although the client must have a fully functioning GI tract. Sample products include Isosource, Resource, and Ensure-Plus.

Modular formulations contain a single nutrient, protein, lipid, or carbohydrate. Indications include a single nutrient deficiency. They may be added to other formulations to provide more specific nutrient needs. Sample products include ProMod, Polycose, Resource GlutaSolve, and MCT Oil.

Specialized formulations are products that contain a specific nutrient combination for a particular condition. Indications include a specific disease state such as hepatic failure, renal failure, or a specific genetic enzyme deficiency. Sample products include Citrotein, Pulmocare, and Suplena.

Clients sometimes exhibit GI intolerance to enteral nutrition, usually expressed as vomiting, nausea, or diarrhea. Therapy is often started slowly, with small quantities, so that side effects can be assessed. The nurse must be observant for drug interactions that occasionally occur when drugs are given along with enteral nutrition.

38.12 Total Parenteral Nutrition

When a client's metabolic needs are unable to be met through enteral nutrition, **total parenteral nutrition (TPN)**, or hyperalimentation, is indicated. For short-term therapy, peripheral vein TPN may be utilized. Because of the risk of phlebitis, however, long-term therapy often requires central vein TPN. Clients who have undergone major surgery or trauma and those who are severely undernourished are candidates for central vein TPN. Because the GI tract is not being utilized, clients with severe malabsorption disease may be treated successfully with TPN.

TPN is able to provide all of a client's nutritional needs in a hypertonic solution containing amino acids, lipid emulsions, carbohydrates (as dextrose), electrolytes, vitamins, and minerals. The particular formulation may be specific to the disease state, such as renal failure or hepatic failure. TPN should be administered through an infusion pump so that nutrition can be precisely monitored. Clients in various settings such as acute care, long-term care, and home health care often benefit from TPN therapy. See "Nursing Process Focus: Clients Receiving Total Parenteral Nutrition" for more information.

NURSING PROCESS FOCUS   Clients Receiving Total Parenteral Nutrition

Assessment	Potential Nursing Diagnoses/Identified Patterns
Prior to administration: ■ Obtain complete health history including allergies, drug history, and possible drug interactions. ■ Obtain complete physical examination. ■ Assess for the presence/history of nutritional deficit such as inadequate oral intake, gastrointestinal disease, and increased metabolic need. ■ Obtain the following laboratory studies: total protein/albumin levels, creatinine/BUN, CBC, electrolytes, lipid profile, and serum iron levels.	■ Nutritional deficiency ■ Knowledge regarding drug therapy may be inadeqate ■ R isk for infection ■ Risk for fluid imbalance

Planning: Client Goals and Expected Outcomes

The client will:
- Exhibit improvement or stabilization of nutritional status
- Accurately describe the drug's intended effects, side effects, and precautions
- Immediately report side effects such as symptoms of hypoglycemia or hyperglycemia, fever, chills, cough, or malaise

Implementation

Interventions (Rationales)	Client Education/Discharge Planning
■ Monitor vital signs, observing for signs of infection such as elevated temperature. (Bacteria may grow in high glucose and high protein solutions.)	■ Instruct client to report fever, chills, soreness or drainage of the infusion site, cough, and malaise.
■ Take extraordinary precautions to prevent infection. ■ Use strict aseptic technique with IV tubing, dressing changes, and TPN solution. ■ Refrigerate solution until 30 min before using. ■ Comply with healthcare facility protocol for tubing and filter changes.	■ Instruct client that the infusion site is at high risk for infection and stress the need for sterile dressings and aseptic technique with solutions and tubing.
■ Monitor blood glucose levels. Observe for signs of hyper- or hypoglycemia and administer insulin as directed. (Blood glucose levels may be affected if TPN is turned off, the rate is reduced, or if excess levels of insulin are added to the solution.)	Instruct client to report symptoms of: ■ Hyperglycemia (excessive thirst, copious urination, and insatiable hunger) ■ Hypoglycemia (nervousness, irritability, and dizziness)
■ Monitor for signs of fluid overload. (TPN is a hypertonic solution and can create intravascular shifting of extracellular fluid.)	■ Instruct client to report shortness of breath, heart palpitations, swelling, or decreased urine output.

continued

NURSING PROCESS FOCUS	Clients Receiving Total Parenteral Nutrition *(Continued)*
Interventions (Rationales)	**Client Education/Discharge Planning**
■ Monitor renal status, including intake and output ratio, daily weight, and laboratory studies such as serum creatinine and BUN.	Instruct client to: ■ Weigh self daily ■ Monitor intake and output ■ Report sudden increases in weight or decreased urinary output ■ Keep all appointments for follow-up care and laboratory testing
■ Maintain accurate infusion rate with infusion pump. ■ Make rate changes gradually and never discontinue TPN abruptly. ■ Increase or decrease flow rate by no more than 10% to prevent fluctuation in blood glucose levels.	Instruct client: ■ About the importance of maintaining the prescribed rate of infusion ■ To never stop the TPN solution abruptly unless instructed by the healthcare provider
Evaluation of Outcome Criteria	
Evaluate the effectiveness of drug therapy by confirming that client goals and expected outcomes have been met (see "Planning").	

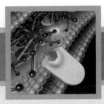

CHAPTER REVIEW

KEY CONCEPTS

The numbered key concepts provide a succinct summary of the important points from the corresponding numbered section within the chapter. If any of these points are not clear, refer to the numbered section within the chapter for review. Expanded versions can be found on the Companion Website.

38.1 Vitamins are organic substances that are needed in small amounts to promote growth and maintain health. Deficiency of a vitamin will result in disease.

38.2 Vitamins are classified as lipid soluble (A, D, E, and K) or water soluble (C and B complex).

38.3 Failure to meet the recommended dietary reference intake (DRI) for vitamins may result in deficiency disorders.

38.4 Vitamin therapy is indicated for conditions such as poor nutritional intake, pregnancy, and chronic disease states.

38.5 Deficiencies of vitamins A, D, E, or K are indications for pharmacotherapy with lipid-soluble vitamins.

38.6 Deficiencies of vitamin C, thiamine, niacin, riboflavin, folic acid, cyanocobalamin, or pyridoxine are indications for pharmacotherapy with water-soluble vitamins.

38.7 Minerals are inorganic substances needed in very small amounts to maintain normal body metabolism.

38.8 Pharmacotherapy with macrominerals includes agents containing calcium, magnesium, potassium, or phosphorous.

38.9 Pharmacotherapy with microminerals includes agents containing iron, iodine, fluorine, or zinc.

38.10 Undernutrition may be caused by low dietary intake, malabsorption disorders, fad diets, or wasting disorders such as cancer or AIDS.

38.11 Enteral nutrition, provided orally or through a feeding tube, is a means of meeting a client's complete nutritional needs.

38.12 Total parenteral nutrition (TPN) is a means of supplying nutrition to clients via a peripheral vein (short term) or central vein (long term).

REVIEW QUESTIONS

1 What are some client conditions in which the DRI for a vitamin may not be sufficient?

2 What is the difference between a vitamin and a mineral?

3 Under what conditions might a client be switched from enteral nutrition to TPN?

CRITICAL THINKING QUESTIONS

1. A client has been self-medicating with vitamin B_3 (niacin) for an elevated cholesterol level. The client comes to the clinic with a severe case of redness and flushing and is concerned about an allergic reaction. What is the nurse's response?

2. A client complains of a constant headache for the past several days. The only supplements the client has been taking are megadoses of vitamins A, C, and E. What would be a priority for the nurse with this client?

3. A client presents to the healthcare provider with complaints of severe flank pain. This client has a history of renal calculi. The only medication the client takes is a multivitamin daily as well as vitamin C. What is the potential problem?

EXPLORE
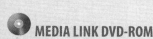
MediaLink

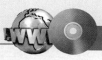

www.pearsoned.ca/adams-king

MEDIA LINK DVD-ROM
- Audio Glossary
- CRNE Review

COMPANION WEBSITE
- CRNE Review
- Case Study: Vitamin pharmacotherapy
- Dosage Calculations

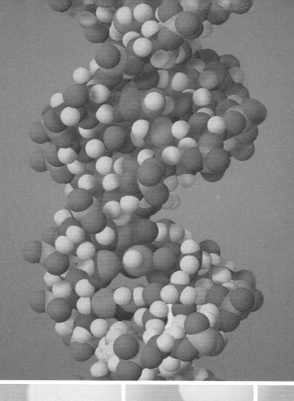

Unit 8

The Endocrine and Genitourinary Systems

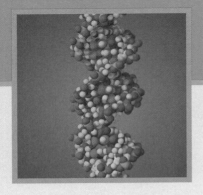

CHAPTER 39

Drugs for Pituitary, Thyroid, and Adrenal Disorders

DRUGS AT A GLANCE

HYPOTHALAMIC AND PITUITARY DRUGS

Hypothalamic agents

Anterior pituitary agents
- *vasopressin (Pressyn AR)*

THYROID DRUGS

Thyroid agents
- *levothyroxine (Levothyroxine, others)*

Antithyroid agents
- *propylthiouracil (Propyl-Thyracil)*

ADRENAL DRUGS

Glucocorticoids
- *hydrocortisone (Hydrocortisone)*

Antiadrenal agents

OBJECTIVES

After reading this chapter, the student should be able to do the following:

1. Explain the concept of negative feedback in the endocrine system.
2. Describe the clinical uses of the hypothalamic and pituitary hormones.
3. Explain the pharmacotherapy of diabetes insipidus.
4. Explain the therapeutic actions of drugs used to treat hypothyroidism and hyperthyroidism in relation to the underlying pathophysiology and signs and symptoms.
5. Describe the signs and symptoms of Addison's disease and Cushing's syndrome.
6. Explain the pharmacotherapy of adrenal gland disorders.
7. For each of the drug classes listed in Drugs at a Glance, identify a representative drug and explain its mechanism of action, therapeutic effects, and important adverse effects.
8. Describe and explain, based on pharmacological principles, the rationale for nursing assessment, planning, interventions, and outcomes evaluation for clients with pituitary, thyroid, and adrenal disorders.
9. Use the nursing process to care for clients who are receiving drug therapy for pituitary, thyroid, and adrenal disorders.

MediaLink

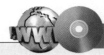

www.pearsoned.ca/adams-king

CRNE review, case studies, and other interactive resources for this chapter can be found on the Companion Website at **www.pearsoned.ca/adams-king**. Click on "Chapter 39" to select the activities for this chapter. For animations, more CRNE review questions, and an audio glossary, access the accompanying DVD-ROM in this textbook.

ike the nervous system, the endocrine system is a major controller of homeostasis. Whereas a nerve exerts instantaneous control over a single muscle fibre or gland, a hormone from the endocrine system may affect all body cells and take as long as several days to produce an optimum response. Small amounts of hormones may produce profound effects on the body. Conversely, deficiencies of small quantities may produce equally profound physiological changes. This chapter examines common endocrine disorders and their pharmacotherapy. The reproductive hormones are covered in Chapters 41 and 42.

39.1 The Endocrine System and Homeostasis

The endocrine system consists of various glands that secrete **hormones**, which are chemical messengers released in response to a change in the body's internal environment. The hormone attempts to return the body to homeostasis. For example, when the level of glucose in the blood rises above normal, the pancreas secretes insulin to return glucose levels to normal. The various endocrine glands and their hormones are illustrated in Figure 39.1.

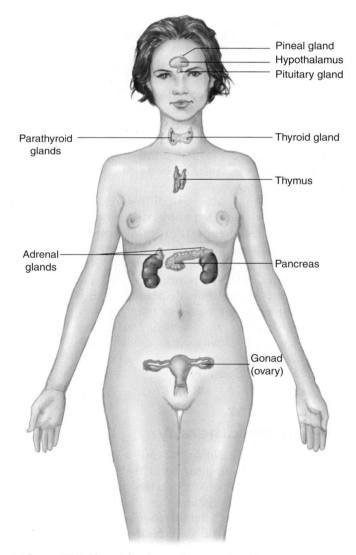

● **Figure 39.1** The endocrine system

Source: Pearson Education/PH College.

After secretion, hormones enter the blood and are transported throughout the body. Some, such as insulin and thyroid hormone, have receptors on nearly every cell in the body. Others, such as parathyroid hormone (PTH) and oxytocin, have receptors on only a few specific types of cell.

In the endocrine system, it is common for one hormone to control the secretion of another. In addition, it is common for the last hormone secreted in the pathway to provide feedback to turn off the secretion of the first hormone. For example, as serum calcium falls, PTH is released; PTH causes an increase in serum calcium, which provides feedback to the parathyroid glands to shut off PTH secretion. This common feature of endocrine homeostasis is known as **negative feedback.**

39.2 The Hypothalamus and Pituitary Gland

Two endocrine structures in the brain deserve special recognition because they control many other endocrine glands. The hypothalamus secretes **releasing hormones** that travel via blood vessels a short distance to the anterior pituitary gland. These releasing hormones signal to the pituitary which hormone is to be released. After secretion from the pituitary, the hormone travels to its target tissues to cause its effects. For example, the hypothalamus secretes thyrotropin-releasing hormone (TRH) that travels to the pituitary gland with the message to secrete thyroid-stimulating hormone (TSH). TSH then travels to its target organ, the thyroid gland, to stimulate the release of thyroid hormone. Although the pituitary is often called the master gland, the pituitary and hypothalamus are best visualized as an integrated unit.

The pituitary gland is composed of two distinct regions. The anterior pituitary, or **adenohypophysis**, consists of glandular tissue and secretes adrenocorticotropic hormone (ACTH), thyroid-stimulating hormone (TSH), growth hormone, prolactin, follicle-stimulating hormone (FSH), and luteinizing hormone (LH). The posterior pituitary, or **neurohypophysis**, contains nervous tissue rather than glandular tissue. Neurons in the posterior pituitary store antidiuretic hormone (ADH) and oxytocin, which are released in response to nerve impulses from the hypothalamus. Hormones associated with the hypothalamus and pituitary gland are shown in Figure 39.2.

39.3 Indications for Hormone Pharmacotherapy

The goals of hormone pharmacotherapy vary widely. In many cases, the hormone is administered as replacement therapy for clients who are unable to secrete sufficient quantities of their own endogenous hormones. Examples of replacement therapy include the administration of thyroid hormone after the thyroid gland has been surgically removed and supplying insulin to clients whose pancreas is not functioning. Replacement therapy usually supplies the

physiological, low level of the hormone that would normally be present in the body. A summary of select endocrine disorders and their drug therapy is shown in Table 39.1.

Some hormones are used in cancer chemotherapy. Examples include testosterone for breast cancer and estrogen for testicular cancer. The antineoplastic mechanism of action of these hormones is not known. When used as antineoplastics, the doses of the hormones far exceed the levels normally present in the body. Hormones are nearly always used in combination with other antineoplastic medications, as discussed in Chapter 35.

Another goal of pharmacotherapy may be to produce an exaggerated response that is part of the normal action of the hormone in order to achieve some therapeutic advantage. Supplying hydrocortisone to suppress inflammation is an example of taking advantage of the normal action of the glucocorticoids, but the hormone is given in higher amounts than would normally be present in the body. Supplying small amounts of estrogen or progesterone at specific times during the menstrual cycle can prevent ovulation and pregnancy. In this example, the client is given natural hormones; however, they are taken at a time when levels in the body are normally low.

DISORDERS OF THE HYPOTHALAMUS AND PITUITARY GLAND

Because of its critical role in controlling other endocrine tissues, lack of adequate pituitary secretion can have multiple, profound effects on body function. Hypopituitarism can be caused by various tumours of the pituitary (and associated brain regions), trauma, autoimmune disorders, or stroke. Pharmacotherapy involves administration of the missing hormone, perhaps for the life of the client.

39.4 Pharmacotherapy with Pituitary and Hypothalamic Hormones

Of the 15 different hormones secreted by the pituitary and hypothalamus, only a few are used in pharmacotherapy, as listed in Table 39.2. There are several reasons why they are not widely utilized. Some of these hormones can only be obtained from natural sources and can be quite expensive when used in therapeutic quantities. Furthermore, it is usually more effective to give drugs that directly affect secretion at the target organs. Two pituitary hormones, prolactin and oxytocin, affect the female reproductive system and are discussed in Chapter 41. Corticotropin affects the adrenal gland and is discussed later in this chapter. Of those remaining, growth hormone and antidiuretic hormone have the most clinical utility.

GROWTH HORMONE

Growth hormone, or **somatotropin**, stimulates the growth and metabolism of nearly every cell in the body. Deficiency

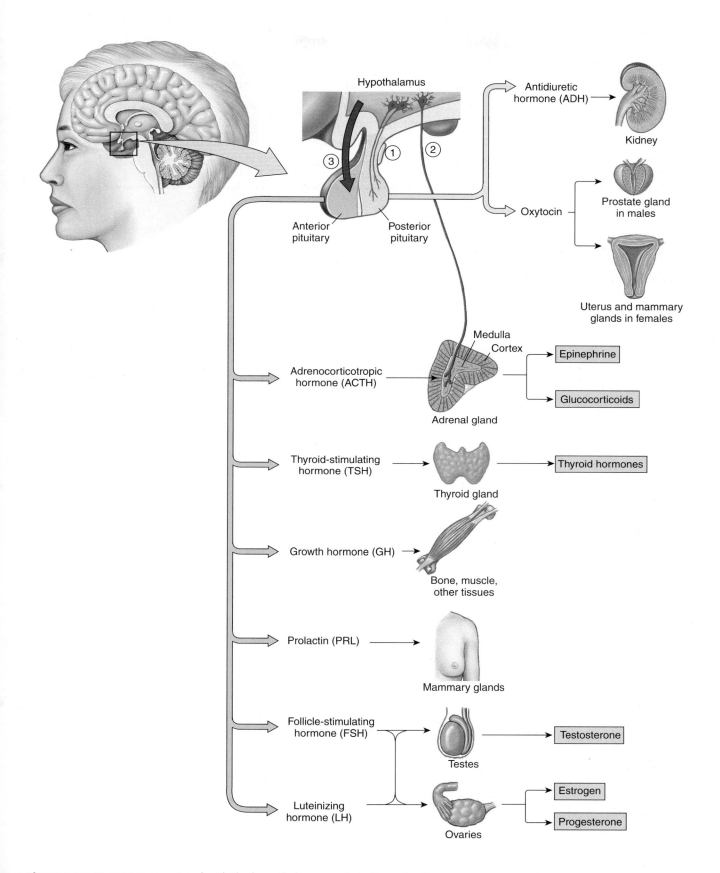

● **Figure 39.2** Hormones associated with the hypothalamus and pituitary gland
Source: Pearson Education/PH College.

TABLE 39.1 Select Endocrine Disorders and Their Drug Treatment

Gland	Hormone	Disorder	Drugs
adrenal cortex	glucocorticoids	hypersecretion: Cushing's syndrome	antiadrenal agents
		hyposecretion: Addison's disease	glucocorticoids
pituitary	growth hormone	hyposecretion: dwarfism	somatrem and somatropin
	antidiuretic hormone	hyposecretion: diabetes insipidus	vasopressin, desmopressin, and lypressin
thyroid	thyroid hormone (T_3 and T_4)	hypersecretion: Grave's disease	propylthiouracil, methimazole, and I-131
		hyposecretion: myxedema (adults) and cretinism (children)	thyroid hormone

of this hormone in children results in dwarfism; however, it does not cause the profound mental impairment seen in clients lacking thyroid hormone. Somatrem and somatropin are preparations of human growth hormone made by recombinant DNA techniques that are available for replacement therapy in children. If therapy is begun early in life, as much as 15 cm of growth may be achieved. In addition to treatment of growth hormone deficiency in children, growth hormone therapy is approved for adult replacement therapy and for treatment in girls with short stature due to Turner Syndrome. Somatropin is pregnancy category C and is contraindicated in clients after the epiphyses have closed. This drug has many potential side effects, and clients must undergo regular assessment of glucose tolerance and thyroid function during pharmacotherapy. All of the growth hormone preparations are administered by the parenteral route.

Octreotide is a synthetic growth hormone antagonist structurally related to **somatostatin** (growth hormone–inhibiting hormone). In addition to inhibiting growth hormone, octreotide promotes fluid and electrolyte reabsorption from the GI tract and prolongs intestinal transit time. It has limited applications in treating growth hormone excess in adults (acromegaly) and in treating the severe diarrhea sometimes associated with metastatic carcinoid tumours. Acromegaly may also be treated with pegvisomant, which is a growth hormone receptor antagonist.

TABLE 39.2 Hypothalamic and Pituitary Agents

Drug	Route and Adult Dose
Hypothalamic Agents	
gonadorelin acetate (Lutrepulse)	SC/IV; 100 mcg
gonadorelin hydrochloride (Factrel)	SC/IV; 100 mcg administered in women during the early phase of menstrual cycle (days 1 to 7) if it can be determined
nafarelin (Synarel)	Inhalation; two inhalations/d (200 μg/inhalation), one in each nostril beginning between days 2 and 4 of menstrual cycle (max 800 μg/d)
octreotide (Sandostatin)	SC; 100–600 μg/d in two to four divided doses; may switch to IM depot injection after 2 wk at 20 mg q4wk for 2 mo
protirelin (Relefact TRH)	IV; 500 μg bolus over a period of 15–30 sec
Anterior Pituitary Agents	
corticotropin (ACTH)	IV; 10–25 U in 500 mL D5W infused over 8 hr
cosyntropin (Cortrosyn)	IM/IV; 0.25 mg injected over 2 min
menotropins (Pergonal, Menopur)	IM; 75–150 IU daily for the first 5 days of treatment; subsequent doses adjusted to individual response
somatropin (Humatrope)	SC (Child); Humatrope 0.18 mg/kg/wk divided into equal doses on three alternate days
thyrotropin (Thyrogen)	IM/SC; 10 U daily for 1–3 d
Posterior Pituitary Agents	
desmopressin acetate (Apo-Desmopressin, DDAVP)	IV; 0.3 mcg/kg in 2 divided doses; intranasal: 0.1 mL (10 mcg) in 1–3 divided doses
oxytocin (Oxytocin) (see page 598 for the Prototype Drug box)	IV; 1 mU/min, may increase by 1 mU/min q15min (max 20 mU/min)
vasopressin (Pressyn AR)	IM/SC; 5–10 U aqueous solution bid–qid (5–60 U/d) or 1.25–2.5 U in oil q2–3d

ANTIDIURETIC HORMONE

As its name implies, antidiuretic hormone (ADH) conserves water in the body. ADH is secreted from the posterior pituitary gland when the hypothalamus senses that plasma volume has decreased or that the osmolality of the blood has become too high. ADH acts on the collecting ducts in the kidney to increase water reabsorption. **Diabetes insipidus** is a rare disease caused by a deficiency of ADH. Clients with this disorder have an intense thirst and produce very dilute urine due to the large volume of water lost by the kidneys. ADH is also called vasopressin because it has the capability to raise blood pressure when secreted in large amounts. Vasopressin is available as a drug for the treatment of diabetes insipidus.

Desmopressin (DDAVP) is the most common form of ADH in use. It has a duration of action of 8 to 20 hours, whereas vasopressin and lypressin have durations of only 2 to 8 hours. Desmopressin is available as a nasal spray and is easily self-administered; vasopressin must be administered IM or SC. The client may also more easily increase or decrease the dosage of desmopressin depending on urine output. Desmopressin is also available in subcutaneous, intravenous, and oral forms. Desmopressin and lypressin do not have the intense vasoconstricting effects of vasopressin.

NURSING CONSIDERATIONS

The role of the nurse in antidiuretic hormone therapy involves careful monitoring of the client's condition and providing education as it relates to the prescribed drug treatment. The therapeutic goal for clients receiving antidiuretic hormone therapy is focused on maintaining fluid and electrolyte status. For clients taking antidiuretic hormones, assess for fluid and electrolyte imbalances and assess urine specific gravity prior to administration. A low specific gravity indicates lack of urine concentration and suggests ADH deficiency. Periodically assess urine specific gravity during pharmacotherapy to determine if the therapeutic effect is being achieved. Closely monitor the client's vital signs, especially pulse and blood pressure, as antidiuretic hormone can affect plasma volume and is a potent vasoconstrictor.

Body weight, intake, and output must be monitored because these drugs may cause excess water retention. Also monitor the neurological status of the client. Symptoms of water intoxication may first present as headache accompanied by confusion and drowsiness. The use of vasopressin is contraindicated in clients with pre-existing heart disease. Furthermore, it should be used cautiously in elderly clients because of the possibility of undiagnosed heart disease.

Client education as it relates to antidiuretic hormone should include goals, reasons for obtaining baseline data such as vital signs and tests for cardiac and renal function, and possible side effects. The client should be instructed to check weight at least two times per week and report significant changes to the healthcare provider. See "Nursing Process Focus: Clients Receiving Antidiuretic Hormone Therapy" for additional points to include when teaching about this class of drug.

MediaLink   Human Growth Foundation

Pr   PROTOTYPE DRUG | Vasopressin (Pressyn AR)

ACTIONS AND USES

Two ADH preparations are available for the treatment of diabetes insipidus: vasopressin (Pressyn AR) and desmopressin (Apo-Desmopressin, DDAVP). Vasopressin is a synthetic hormone that has a structure identical to that of human ADH. It acts on the renal collecting tubules to increase their permeability to water, thus enhancing water reabsorption. Although it acts within minutes, vasopressin has a short half-life that requires it to be administered three to four times per day. Vasopressin tannate is formulated in peanut oil to increase its duration of action. Vasopressin is usually given IM or IV, although an intranasal form is available for mild diabetes insipidus. Desmopressin has a longer duration of action than vasopressin and results in fewer serious adverse effects. Desmopressin is occasionally used by the intranasal route for enuresis (bedwetting).

PHARMACOKINETICS

Vasopressin is widely distributed in extracellular fluid. It is rapidly metabolized by the liver and kidneys. Its half-life is 10 to 20 minutes.

ADMINISTRATION ALERTS

- Vasopressin tannate should never be administered IV because it is an oil.
- Vasopressin aqueous injection may be given by continuous IV infusion after it is diluted in normal saline or D5W.
- Vasopressin is pregnancy category X.

ADVERSE EFFECTS AND INTERACTIONS

Vasopressin has a strong vasoconstrictor action that is unrelated to its antidiuretic properties, thus hypertension is possible. The drug can precipitate angina episodes and myocardial infarction in clients with coronary artery disease. Excessive fluid retention can cause water intoxication, including symptoms of headache, restlessness, drowsiness, and coma. Water intoxication can usually be avoided by teaching the client to decrease water intake during vasopressin therapy.

Vasopressin injection interacts with several other drugs. For example, alcohol, epinephrine, heparin, lithium, and phenytoin may decrease the antidiuretic effects of vasopressin. Neostigmine may increase vasopressor actions. Carbamazepine and thiazide diuretics may increase antidiuretic activity.

 See the Companion Website for a Nursing Process Focus chart specific to this drug.

NURSING PROCESS FOCUS	Clients Receiving Antidiuretic Hormone Therapy

Assessment	Potential Nursing Diagnoses/Identified Patterns
Prior to administration: <ul><li>Obtain complete health history including allergies, drug history, and possible drug interactions.</li><li>Obtain complete physical examination.</li><li>Assess for the presence/history of neurosurgery, pituitary tumours, head injury, and nocturia.</li><li>Obtain laboratory studies including urine specific gravity, urine/serum osmolarity, and serum electrolytes.</li></ul>	<ul><li>Safety from injury related to side effects of drug therapy</li><li>Risk for fluid imbalance</li><li>Risk for sleep disturbances related to effects of drug therapy and frequent nocturia</li><li>Need for knowledge regarding drug therapy and adverse afffects</li></ul>

Planning: Client Goals and Expected Outcomes

The client will:
- Exhibit normal fluid and electrolyte balance
- Report uninterrupted sleep patterns
- Identify and report side effects to healthcare provider
- Demonstrate an understanding of the drug's action

Implementation

Interventions (Rationales)	Client Education/Discharge Planning
<ul><li>Monitor vital signs. (Changes may indicate alterations in body fluid status such as hyper- or hypovolemia.)</li></ul>	<ul><li>Instruct the client to report irregular heartbeat, shortness of breath, dizziness, or headache.</li></ul>
<ul><li>Monitor cardiovascular status such as peripheral pulses, heart sounds, skin temperature and colour, and ECG. (ADH has potent vasoconstriction properties and may cause hypertension and dysrhythmias.)</li></ul>	<ul><li>Instruct the client in the importance of follow-up care and to take medication exactly as prescribed.</li></ul>
<ul><li>Administer fluid replacement as directed. (IV infusions should be regulated to maintain body fluid balance.)</li><li>Encourage oral fluid intake to satisfy thirst only. (Excessive fluid intake may trigger a diabetes insipidus episode.)</li></ul>	Instruct client to: <ul><li>Monitor fluid balance and report vomiting, diarrhea, perfuse sweating, and frequent urination</li><li>Consume fluid to satisfy thirst and to report excessive unquenchable thirst</li></ul>
<ul><li>Monitor intake/output ratio and weigh client daily. (ADH may result in fluid retention that can lead to water intoxication. Daily weight is an indicator of fluid retention.)</li></ul>	Instruct client: <ul><li>To weigh self daily and report excessive gains or losses</li><li>In titration techniques based on urinary output</li></ul>
<ul><li>Monitor for presence of nocturia or nocturnal enuresis. Determine the client's ability to satisfy physiological sleep needs. (Less frequent nighttime urination is an indication of the effectiveness of ADH therapy.)</li></ul>	Instruct client to: <ul><li>Keep a sleep log, recording the number of times per night he or she is awakened to urinate</li><li>Avoid potentially hazardous activities due to possible drowsiness until therapeutic effect of drug is achieved and drownsiness is no longer a risk</li><li>Have frequent rest periods or daytime naps if sleep deprivation is present until therapeutic effect is achieved</li></ul>
<ul><li>Monitor for symptoms of fluid volume overload such as headache, restlessness, shortness of breath, tachycardia, hypertension, and low urinary output. (These are signs of water intoxication.)</li></ul>	<ul><li>Instruct client to report headaches, shortness of breath, palpitations, and low urine output.</li></ul>
<ul><li>Monitor status of nasal mucous membranes if nasal preparations are pre-scribed. (Intranasal use can cause changes in the nasal mucosa, resulting in unpredictable drug absorption.)</li></ul>	Instruct client: <ul><li>To report worsening of condition since route of administration may need to be changed</li><li>To report drainage or irritation of the nasal mucosa if taking nasal preparation</li><li>In subcutaneous injection methods, as appropriate</li></ul>

continued

NURSING PROCESS FOCUS Clients Receiving Antidiuretic Hormone Therapy *(Continued)*	
Interventions (Rationales)	**Client Education/Discharge Planning**
■ Monitor laboratory studies, including urine and serum osmolarity, urine specific gravity, and serum electrolytes. (These assess fluid volume status.)	Instruct client: ■ To measure urine specific gravity ■ In the importance of keeping all laboratory appointments

Evaluation of Outcome Criteria
Evaluate the effectiveness of drug therapy by confirming that client goals and expected outcomes have been met (see "Planning").
See Table 39.2, under the heading "Posterior Pituitary Agents," for a list of drugs to which these nursing actions apply.

THYROID GLAND DISORDERS

39.5 Normal Function of the Thyroid Gland

The thyroid gland secretes hormones that affect nearly every cell in the body. By stimulating the enzymes involved with glucose oxidation, thyroid gland hormones regulate **basal metabolic rate**, the baseline speed by which cells perform their functions. By increasing cellular metabolism, thyroid hormone increases body temperature. The gland also helps to maintain blood pressure and regulate growth and development.

The thyroid gland has two basic cell types that secrete different hormones. **Parafollicular cells** secrete calcitonin, a hormone that is involved with calcium homeostasis (see Chapter 46). **Follicular cells** in the gland secrete thyroid hormone, which is actually a combination of two different hormones: thyroxine (T_4) and triiodothyronine (T_3). Iodine is essential for the synthesis of these hormones and is provided through the dietary intake of common iodized salt. The names of these hormones refer to the number of bound iodine atoms in each molecule, either three (T_3) or four (T_4).

Thyroxine is the major hormone secreted by the thyroid gland. At the target tissues, however, thyroxine is converted to T_3 through the enzymatic cleavage of one iodine atom. T_3 is thought to enter the target cells, where it binds to intracellular receptors within the nucleus.

Thyroid function is regulated through multiple levels of hormonal control. Falling thyroxine levels in the blood signal the hypothalamus to secrete thyroid-releasing hormone (TRH), or thyrotropin. TRH stimulates the pituitary gland to secrete thyroid-stimulating hormone (TSH), which then stimulates the thyroid gland to release thyroid hormone. Rising levels of thyroid hormone in the blood trigger a negative feedback response to shut off secretion of TRH and TSH. The negative feedback mechanism for the thyroid gland is shown in Figure 39.3.

THYROID AGENTS

Thyroid disorders are common and drug therapy is often indicated. The correct dose of thyroid drug is highly individualized

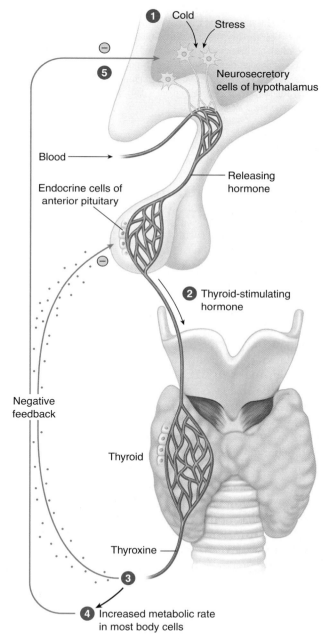

● **Figure 39.3** Feedback mechanisms of the thyroid gland: (1) stimulus; (2) release of TSH; (3) release of thyroid hormone; (4) increased basal metabolic rate; (5) negative feedback

NATURAL THERAPIES

Treatments for Thyroid Disease

Thyroid disease is a serious condition that usually requires medical attention. As a preventive measure, one can consume substances that contain precursors to thyroid hormone. Since T_3 and T_4 both require iodine, dietary intake of this mineral must be sufficient. Iodized salt usually contains enough iodine for proper thyroid function; however, kelp and seafood, particularly shellfish, are additional, natural sources of iodine. T_3 and T_4 also contain the amino acid tyrosine, which is usually obtained from protein sources such as meat or eggs. Other rich sources of tyrosine include avocados, bananas, lima beans, and various seeds. Supplementation with L-tyrosine is usually not necessary.

A number of natural therapies have been used to treat overactive thyroid glands. Lemon balm (*Melissa officinalis*) is a beautiful perennial plant that has a slight lemon odour when the leaves are crushed. Although native to the Mediterranean region, it is widely cultivated in Europe, Asia, and North America. The leaves have traditional medicinal use as a sedative and antispasmodic, which has been reported for hundreds of years. It has been shown to block the antibodies responsible for destroying the thyroid gland in Grave's disease, although this effect has yet to be confirmed in clinical studies. Lemon balm is usually taken as a tea, several times daily, although capsules, extracts, and tinctures are available.

and requires careful, periodic adjustment. The medications used to treat thyroid disease are shown in Table 39.3.

39.6 Pharmacotherapy of Hypothyroidism

Hypothyroidism may result from either a poorly functioning thyroid gland or low secretion of TSH by the pituitary gland. Early symptoms of hypothyroidism in adults, or **myxedema**, include fatigue, general weakness, muscle cramps, and dry skin. More severe symptoms include slurred speech, bradycardia, weight gain, decreased sense of taste and smell, and intolerance to cold environments. The etiology of myxedema may include autoimmune disease, surgical removal of the thyroid gland, or aggressive treatment with antithyroid drugs. The most common cause of hypothyroidism in Canada is chronic autoimmune thyroiditis, known as Hashimoto's disease. At high doses, the antidysrhythmic drug amiodarone can induce hypothyroidism in clients due to its high iodine content. Enlargement of the thyroid gland, or goiter, may be absent or present, depending on the cause of the disease. Hypothyroidism usually responds well to pharmacotherapy with natural or synthetic thyroid hormone.

NURSING CONSIDERATIONS

The role of the nurse in thyroid hormone therapy involves careful monitoring of the client's condition and providing education as it relates to the prescribed drug treatment. Assess the client for signs and symptoms of thyroid disease. Also assess and monitor the client's vital signs as cardiovascular complications may occur as a result of drug therapy.

Levothyroxine (Synthroid) is a commonly used thyroid hormone replacement. Thoroughly assess cardiovascular function because this drug may cause cardiovascular collapse in clients with undiagnosed heart disease due to an increase in basal metabolic rate. This action may precipitate dysrhythmias in clients with undiagnosed heart disease, especially in elderly clients. The drug should also be used with caution in clients with impaired renal function because the increased metabolic rate increases the workload of the kidney. Clients with diabetes mellitus, diabetes insipidus, or Addison's disease experience a worsening of symptoms because of the initial increase in basal metabolism. The drug is contraindicated in clients with adrenal insufficiency.

Desiccated thyroid is made of dried beef and pork thyroid glands. It is used less frequently than levothyroxine because it does not produce reliable results. Desiccated thyroid will cause the same cardiac complications as levothyroxine. Liothyronine sodium is a short-acting synthetic form of the natural thyroid hormone that can be administered IV to individuals with myxedema coma. The short duration of action allows for rapid dosage adjustments in critically ill clients.

Thyroid hormones have their optimum effect when taken on an empty stomach. Clients should be taught the signs and symptoms of hyperthyroidism such as nervousness, weight loss, diarrhea, and intolerance to heat. The client should notify the healthcare provider at the first sign of any of these symptoms.

Client education as it relates to thyroid hormones should include goals, reasons for obtaining baseline data such as vital signs and tests for cardiac and renal function, and possible side effects. See "Nursing Process Focus: Clients Receiving Thyroid Hormone Replacement" for specific teaching points.

TABLE 39.3 Thyroid and Antithyroid Drugs

Drug	Route and Adult Dose
Thyroid Agents	
levothyroxine (Levothyroxine, Synthroid, others)	PO; 75–125 µg qd /d (1.5 µg/kg/day)
liothyronine (Cytomel)	PO; 25–75 µg qd
thyroid (Thyroid, Thyrodinum)	PO; 60–100 mg qd
Antithyroid Agents	
potassium iodide and iodine (Lugol's solution, Thyro-Block)	PO; 50–250 mg tid 10–14 days before surgery
propylthiouracil (Propyl-Thyracil)	PO; 100–150 mg tid
radioactive iodide (Iodotope)	PO; 0.8–150 mCi (curies are units of radioactivity)

Pr **PROTOTYPE DRUG** | Levothyroxine (Levothyroxine, others)

ACTIONS AND USES

Levothyroxine is a synthetic form of thyroxine (T_4) used for replacement therapy in clients with low thyroid function. Actions are those of thyroid hormone and include loss of weight, improved tolerance to environmental temperature, increased activity, and increased pulse rate. Doses are highly individualized. Therapy may take 3 weeks or longer before T_4 levels stabilize. Doses may require periodic adjustments for several months. Serum TSH levels are monitored to determine whether the client is receiving sufficient levothyroxine—low TSH levels usually indicate that the dosage of T_4 needs to be increased.

PHARMACOKINETICS

Levothyroxine is variable absorbed. It is metabolized by the liver and excreted in the bile and feces. Its half-life is 6 to 7 days.

ADMINISTRATION ALERT

- Administer medication at the same time every day, preferably in the morning to decrease incidence of drug-related insomnia.
- Levothyroxine is pregnancy category A.

ADVERSE EFFECTS AND INTERACTIONS

The difference between a therapeutic dose of levothyroxine and one that produces adverse effects is narrow. Care must be taken to avoid over-treatment with this drug. Adverse effects are those of hyperthyroidism and include palpitations, dysrhythmias, anxiety, insomnia, weight loss, and heat intolerance. Menstrual irregularities may occur in females, and long-term use of levothyroxine has been associated with osteoporosis in women.

Levothyroxine interacts with many other drugs; for example, cholestyramine and colestipol decrease absorption of levothyroxine. Concurrent administration of epinephrine and norepinephrine increases risk of cardiac insufficiency. Oral anticoagulants may potentiate hypoprothrombinemia.

Use with caution with herbal supplements, such as lemon balm, which may interfere with thyroid hormone action.

 See the Companion Website for a Nursing Process Focus chart specific to this drug.

NURSING PROCESS FOCUS   Clients Receiving Thyroid Hormone Replacement

Assessment	Potential Nursing Diagnoses/Identified Patterns
Prior to administration: ■ Obtain complete health history including allergies, drug history, and possible drug interactions. ■ Obtain complete physical examination. ■ Assess for the presence/history of symptoms of hypothyroidism. ■ Obtain ECG and laboratory studies including T_4, T_3, and serum TSH levels.	■ Activity intolerance related to disease process ■ Fatigue related to impaired metabolic status ■ Need for knowledge regarding drug therapy and adverse effects ■ Risk for altered body image related to side effects of drug therapy

Planning: Client Goals and Expected Outcomes

The client will:
- Demonstrate an understanding of the drug's action by accurately describing drug side effects and precautions
- Exhibit normal thyroid hormone levels
- Report a decrease in hypothyroid symptoms
- Experience no significant adverse effects from drug therapy
- Demonstrate an understanding of hypothyroidism and the need for life-long therapy

Implementation

Interventions (Rationales)	Client Education/Discharge Planning
■ Monitor vital signs. (Changes in metabolic rate will be manifested as changes in blood pressure, pulse, and body temperature.)	■ Instruct client to report dizziness, palpitations, and intolerance to temperature changes.
■ Monitor for decreasing symptoms related to hypothyroidism such as fatigue, constipation, cold intolerance, lethargy, depression, and menstrual irregularities. (Decreasing symptoms will determine that drug is achieving therapeutic affect.)	■ Instruct client about the signs of hypothyroidism and to report symptoms.
■ Monitor for symptoms related to hyperthyroidism such as nervousness, insomnia, tachycardia, dysrhythmias, heat intolerance, chest pain, and diarrhea. (Symptoms of hyperthyroidism indicate the drug is at a toxic level.)	■ Instruct client about the signs of hyperthyroidism and to report symptoms.
■ Monitor T_3, T_4, and TSH levels. (This helps to determine the effectiveness of pharmacotherapy.)	■ Instruct client about the importance of ongoing monitoring of thyroid hormone levels and to keep all laboratory appointments.

continued

NURSING PROCESS FOCUS	Clients Receiving Thyroid Hormone Replacement *(Continued)*
Interventions (Rationales)	**Client Education/Discharge Planning**
▪ Monitor blood glucose levels, especially in individuals with diabetes mellitus. (Thyroid hormone increases metabolic rate, and glucose utilization may be altered.)	▪ Instruct the diabetic client to monitor blood glucose levels and adjust insulin doses as directed by the healthcare provider.
▪ Provide supportive nursing care to cope with symptoms of hypothyroidism, such as constipation, cold intolerance, and fatigue, until drug has achieved therapeutic effect.	Instruct client to: ▪ Increase activity and fluid and fibre intake to reduce constipation ▪ Wear additional clothing and maintain a comfortable room environment for cold intolerance ▪ Plan activities and include rest periods to avoid fatigue
▪ Monitor weight at least weekly. (Weight loss is expected due to increased metabolic rate. Weight changes help to determine the effectiveness of drug therapy.)	▪ Instruct client to weigh weekly and to report significant changes.
▪ Monitor client for signs of decreased adherence with therapeutic treatment.	▪ Instruct client about the disease and the importance of life-long therapy and follow-up care.

Evaluation of Outcome Criteria
Evaluate the effectiveness of drug therapy by confirming that client goals and expected outcomes have been met (see "Planning").

See Table 39.3, under the heading "Thyroid Agents," for a list of drugs to which these nursing actions apply.

PHARMFACTS

Thyroid Disorders

- One in every 20 Canadians has some type of thyroid disorder.
- Hypothyroidism is 10 times more common in women; hyperthyroidism is 5 to 10 times more common in women.
- The two most common thyroid diseases, Grave's disease and Hashimoto's thyroiditis, are autoimmune diseases, and they may have a genetic link.
- One out of of every 4000 babies is born without a working thyroid gland.
- About 15,000 new cases of thyroid cancer are diagnosed each year.
- One out of every five women over age 75 has Hashimoto's thyroiditis.
- Postpartum thyroiditis occurs in 5% to 9% of women after giving birth and may recur in future pregnancies.
- Both hyperthyroidism and hypothyroidism can affect a woman's ability to become pregnant and can cause miscarriages.

SPECIAL CONSIDERATIONS

Shift Workers, Hypothyroidism, and Drug Adherence

Many body processes such as temperature, blood pressure, certain hormone levels, biochemical processes, and alertness fluctuate on a 24-hour schedule known as the circadian rhythm. Circadian processes are thought to be triggered by daylight. Normal circadian cycles may be interrupted in those people who work varied shifts. Likewise, medications that must be given at a specified time to enhance their potential effect can be a concern for shift workers.

Thyroid medication is best given at the same time each day; however, this can be a challenge for shift workers, especially if they rotate shifts. These drugs are best given after awakening in the morning as they can disturb sleep patterns. For a shift worker, the time of awakening may vary depending on the shift worked. It is essential that the client be aware of this challenge and work with the healthcare provider to reach a medication schedule that allows optimization of the drug effects.

ANTITHYROID AGENTS

Medications are often used to treat the cause of hyperthyroidism or to relieve its distressing symptoms. The goal of antithyroid therapy is to lower the activity of the thyroid gland.

39.7 Pharmacotherapy of Hyperthyroidism

Hypersecretion of thyroid hormone results in symptoms that are the opposite of hypothyroidism: increased body metabolism, tachycardia, weight loss, elevated body temperature, and anxiety. The most common type of hyperthyroidism is called **Grave's disease**. Considered an autoimmune disease in which the body develops antibodies against its own thyroid gland, Grave's disease is four to eight times more common in women and most often occurs between the ages of 30 and 40 years. Other causes of hyperthyroidism are adenomas of the thyroid, pituitary tumours, and pregnancy. If the cause of the hypersecretion is found to be a tumour, or if the disease cannot be controlled through pharmacotherapy, removal of the thyroid gland is indicated.

The two most common drugs for hyperthyroidism, propylthiouracil (PTU) and methimazole, are called thioamides. These agents act by inhibiting the incorporation of iodine atoms into T_3 and T_4. Methimazole has a much longer half-life that offers the advantage of less frequent dosing, although side effects can be more severe. Although both thioamides are pregnancy category D agents, methimazole crosses the placenta more readily than propylthiouracil and is contraindicated in pregnant clients.

A third antithyroid drug, sodium iodide-131, is a radioisotope used to destroy overactive thyroid glands by emitting ionizing radiation. Shortly after oral administration, I-131 accumulates in the thyroid gland, where it destroys follicular cells. The goal of pharmacotherapy with I-131 is to destroy just enough of the thyroid gland so that thyroid function returns to normal levels. Full benefits may take several months. Although most clients require only a single dose, others may need additional treatments. Small diagnostic doses of I-131 are used in nuclear medicine to determine the degree of iodide uptake in the various parts of the thyroid gland.

Non-radioactive sodium iodide is used to treat other thyroid conditions. Lugol's solution is a mixture of 5% elemental iodine and 10% potassium iodide that is used to suppress thyroid function 10 to 15 days prior to thyroidectomy. Sodium iodide is administered IV (along with propylthiouracil) to manage an acute, life-threatening form of hyperthyroidism known as **thyrotoxic crisis**, or **thyroid storm**. Potassium iodide is administered to protect the thyroid from radiation damage following a nuclear exposure.

NURSING CONSIDERATIONS

The role of the nurse in antithyroid therapy involves careful monitoring of the client's condition and providing education as it relates to the prescribed treatment. Assess the client for signs of hypothyroidism such as weight gain, hypotension, bradycardia, fatigue, depression, sensitivity to cold environments, hair loss, and dry skin. Assess for complications and adverse effects specific to the antithyroid medication prescribed for the client.

For clients receiving propylthiouracil (PTU), monitor white blood cell count periodically because PTU may cause agranulocytosis, which puts the client at risk for infection. Assess for signs of jaundice and monitor liver enzymes because PTU is metabolized by the liver. Carefully monitor bleeding times for clients receiving anticoagulants because propylthiouracil causes an increase in bleeding.

Methimazole is similar in structure to propylthiouracil but is more toxic. Assess for blood dyscrasias such as agranulocytosis and jaundice. These adverse effects usually disappear when the drug is discontinued.

Radioactive iodine (I-131) is used to permanently decrease thyroid function. Monitor thyroid function tests because this medication often requires adjustments to achieve a therapeutic dose that achieves a euthyroid state. Inform the client about signs and symptoms of hypothyroidism. Because the client emits radiation after receiving this drug, contact with children and pregnant women should be avoided for the week following administration; close contact with others should be limited for a few days.

I-131 is contraindicated in clients who are pregnant or breastfeeding. Women who are receiving this agent should take precautions to avoid pregnancy. If a woman suspects she is pregnant, she should contact her healthcare provider immediately. Women who will be receiving this treatment should stop breastfeeding for the duration of therapy and discuss alternative feeding methods with their healthcare provider.

Client education as it relates to antithyroid agents should include goals; reasons for obtaining baseline data such as vital signs and liver, renal, and cardiac function tests; and possible drug side effects. Include the following points when teaching clients about antithyroid agents:

- Keep all scheduled laboratory visits for testing.
- Do not breastfeed.
- Practise reliable contraception and notify the healthcare provider if pregnancy is planned or suspected.
- Immediately report nervousness, palpitations, and heat intolerance because these may indicate that the dose is too low.
- Immediately report excess fatigue, slow speech, hoarseness, and slow pulse because these may indicate that the dose is too high.
- Inform the healthcare provider if you are taking any of the following medications because they are contraindicated with antithyroid agents: aminophylline, heparin, and digoxin.

See "Nursing Process Focus: Clients Receiving Antithyroid Therapy" for specific teaching points.

Pr PROTOTYPE DRUG | Propylthiouracil (Propyl-Thyracil)

ACTIONS AND USES

Propylthiouracil (PTU) is administered to clients with hyperthyroidism. It acts by interfering with the synthesis of T_3 and T_4 in the thyroid gland. It also prevents the conversion of T_4 to T_3 in the target tissues. Its action may be delayed from several days to as long as 6 to 12 weeks. Effects include a return to normal thyroid function, resulting in weight gain, reduced anxiety, less insomnia, and slower pulse rate. Due to its short half-life, PTU is usually administered several times a day.

PHARMACOKINETICS

PTU is variably absorbed from the GI tract. It is widely distributed, crosses the placenta, and enters breast milk. It is metabolized by the liver. Its half-life is 1 to 2 hours.

ADMINISTRATION ALERTS

- Administer with meals to reduce GI distress.
- Propylthiouracil is pregnancy category D.

ADVERSE EFFECTS AND INTERACTIONS

Overtreatment with PTU produces symptoms of hypothyroidism. Rash is the most common side effect. A small percentage of clients experience agranulocytosis, which is the drug's most serious adverse effect. Periodic laboratory blood counts and TSH values are necessary to establish proper dosage.

Antithyroid medications interact with many other drugs. For example, PTU can reverse the efficacy of drugs such as aminophylline, anticoagulants, and cardiac glycosides.

 See the Companion Website for a Nursing Process Focus chart specific to this drug.

NURSING PROCESS FOCUS Clients Receiving Antithyroid Therapy

Assessment	Potential Nursing Diagnoses/Identified Patterns
Prior to administration: ■ Obtain complete health history including allergies, drug history, and possible drug interactions. ■ Obtain complete physical examination. ■ Assess for the presence/history of hyperthyroidism. ■ Obtain laboratory studies including T_3/T_4 levels, TSH level, ECG, and CBC.	■ Risk for injury related to side effects of drug therapy ■ Risk for infection related to drug-induced agranulocytosis ■ Need for knowledge regarding drug therapy and adverse effects ■ Risk for altered body image related to side effects of drug therapy

Planning: Client Goals and Expected Outcomes

The client will:
■ Demonstrate an understanding of the drug's action by accurately describing drug side effects and precautions
■ Exhibit a decrease in the symptoms of hyperthyroidism
■ Exhibit normal thyroid hormone levels
■ Exhibit no drug adverse effects such as agranulocytosis or gastrointestinal distress
■ Demonstrate an understanding of the disease process and health maintenance strategies

Implementation

Interventions (Rationales)	Client Education/Discharge Planning
■ Monitor vital signs. (Changes in metabolic rate will be manifested as changes in blood pressure, pulse, and body temperature.)	Instruct client: ■ To count pulse for a full minute and record pulse with every dose ■ In pulse rate parameters that require notification of the healthcare provider (pulse rate more than . . . ; pulse rate greater than . . .) ■ To report dizziness, palpitations, and intolerance to temperature changes
■ Monitor thyroid function tests. (This is used to determine the effectiveness of the drug therapy.)	■ Instruct client in the importance of follow-up care and to keep all laboratory appointments.
■ Monitor for signs of infection, including CBC and WBC count. (Antithyroid drug may cause agranulocytosis.)	Instruct client: ■ That antithyroid medication may affect the body's ability to defend against bacteria and viruses ■ To report sore throat, fever, chills, malaise, and weakness
■ Monitor weight at least weekly. (As a result of slower metabolism, weight gain is expected.)	■ Instruct client to weigh weekly and to report significant changes.
■ Monitor for drowsiness. Ensure safe environment. (Antithyroid medications may cause drowsiness.)	■ Instruct client that medication may cause drowsiness and to avoid hazardous activities until the effects of the drug are known.
■ Monitor for gastrointestinal distress. (Antithyroid medications may cause nausea/vomiting.)	■ Instruct client to take antithyroid medication with food.
■ Monitor for a decrease in symptoms related to hyperthyroidism such as nervousness, insomnia, tachycardia, dysrhythmias, heat intolerance, chest pain, and diarrhea. (This will determine if drug is at a therapeutic level.)	■ Instruct client about the signs of hyperthyroidism and to report them to the healthcare provider.
■ Monitor for symptoms related to hypothyroidism such as fatigue, constipation, cold intolerance, lethargy, depression, and menstrual irregularities. (These symptoms indicate drug is at a toxic level.)	■ Instruct client about the signs of hypothyroidism and to report them to the healthcare provider.
■ Monitor for activity intolerance. (Hyperthyroidism results in protein catabolism, overactivity, and increased metabolism, leading to exhaustion.)	■ Instruct client to schedule rest periods while performing activities of daily living until medication has achieved therapeutic effect.
■ Monitor dietary intake. Avoid foods with high iodine content such as soy, tofu, turnips, iodized salt, and some breads, as directed. (Iodine increases the production of thyroid hormones, which is not desirable in these clients.)	■ Instruct client about the use of iodized salt, shellfish, and OTC medications.
■ Monitor client's response to drug therapy.	■ Instruct client to keep a log of responses to medication including pulse, tolerance to heat/cold, weight, mood status, and energy level. Inform client that stabilization of thyroid hormone levels may take several months.

Evaluation of Outcome Criteria

Evaluate the effectiveness of drug therapy by confirming that client goals and expected outcomes have been met (see "Planning").

See Table 39.3 (page 556), under the heading "Antithyroid Agents," for a list of drugs to which these nursing actions apply.

ADRENAL GLAND DISORDERS

Though small in size, the adrenal glands secrete hormones that affect every body tissue. Adrenal disorders range from excess hormone secretion to deficient hormone secretion. The specific pharmacotherapy depends on which portion of the adrenal gland is responsible for the abnormal secretion.

39.8 Normal Function of the Adrenal Gland

The adrenal glands secrete three essential classes of steroid hormone: **glucocorticoids**, mineralocorticoids, and gonadocorticoids. Collectively, the glucocorticoids and mineralocorticoids are called corticosteroids, or adrenocortical hormones. The terms *corticosteroid* and *glucocorticoid* are sometimes used interchangeably in clinical practice. However, the term *corticosteroid* implies a drug has both glucocorticoid and mineralocorticoid activity.

The gonadocorticoids secreted by the adrenal cortex are mostly androgens, though small amounts of estrogens are also produced. The amounts of these adrenal sex hormones are normally far less than the levels secreted by the testes or ovaries. It is believed that gonadocorticoids contribute to the onset of puberty. The adrenal glands also are the primary source of endogenous estrogen in postmenopausal women. Hypersecretion of gonadocorticoids, such as that caused by a tumour of the adrenal cortex, results in hirsutism and masculinization. The physiological effects of androgens are detailed in Chapter 42.

Aldosterone accounts for over 95% of the mineralocorticoids secreted by the adrenals. The primary function of aldosterone is to promote sodium reabsorption and potassium excretion by the renal tubule, thus regulating plasma volume. When plasma volume falls, the kidney secretes renin, which results in the production of angiotensin II. Angiotensin II then causes aldosterone secretion, which promotes sodium and water retention. Certain adrenal tumours cause excessive secretion of aldosterone, a condition known as hyperaldosteronism, which is characterized by hypertension and hypokalemia.

More than 30 glucocorticoids are secreted from the adrenal cortex, including cortisol, corticosterone, and cortisone. Cortisol, also called hydrocortisone, is secreted in the highest amount and is the most important pharmacologically. Glucocorticoids affect the metabolism of nearly every cell and prepare the body for long-term stress. The effects of glucocorticoids are diverse and include the following:

- Increase the level of blood glucose (hyperglycemic effect) by inhibiting insulin secretion and promoting gluconeogenesis, which is the synthesis of carbohydrates from lipid and protein sources
- Increase the breakdown of proteins and lipids and their utilization as energy sources
- Suppress the immune and inflammatory responses (Chapters 30 and 31)
- Increase the sensitivity of vascular smooth muscle to norepinephrine and angiotensin II
- Influence the CNS by affecting mood and maintaining normal brain excitability

39.9 Control of Glucocorticoid Secretion

Control of glucocorticoid levels in the blood begins with corticotropin-releasing factor (CRF), which is secreted by the hypothalamus. CRF travels to the pituitary where it causes the release of **adrenocorticotropic hormone (ACTH)**. ACTH then travels through the blood and reaches the adrenal cortex, causing it to release glucocorticoids. When the level of cortisol in the blood rises, it provides negative feedback to the hypothalamus and pituitary to shut off further release of glucocorticoids. This negative feedback mechanism is shown in Figure 39.4.

ACTH, also known as corticotropin, is available as a medication in three different preparations: corticotropin injection, repository corticotropin, and corticotropin zinc hydroxide. A fourth drug, cosyntropin, closely resembles ACTH. Although these preparations stimulate the adrenal gland to produce glucocorticoids, they are rarely used to

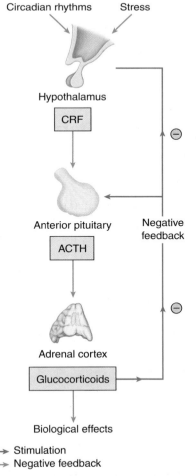

● **Figure 39.4** Feedback control of the adrenal cortex

TABLE 39.4	Select Glucocorticoids	
Drug	**Route and Adult Dose**	
Short Acting		
cortisone (Cortistan, Cortone)	PO; 20–300 mg qd	
ⓟ hydrocortisone (Hydrocortisone)	PO; 2–80 mg tid–qid	
Intermediate Acting		
methylprednisolone (Medrol)	PO; 2–60 mg qd–qid	
prednisolone (Dioptimyd)	PO; 5–60 mg qd–qid	
prednisone (Apo-Prednisone) (see page 407 for the Prototype Drug box)	PO; 5–60 mg qd–qid	
triamcinolone (Aristocort)	PO; 4–48 mg qd–bid	
Long Acting		
betamethasone (Celestone)	PO; 0.6–7.2 mg qd	
dexamethasone (Dexamethasone)	PO; 0.25–4.0 mg bid–qid	

correct corticosteroid deficiency. The ACTH agents cannot be given by the oral route, and they produce numerous side effects. The primary use of these agents is to diagnose adrenal disorders. After administration of cosyntropin, plasma levels of cortisol are measured to determine if the adrenal glands responded to the ACTH stimulation.

GLUCOCORTICOIDS

The glucocorticoids are used as replacement therapy for clients with adrenocortical insufficiency and to dampen inflammatory and immune responses. The glucocorticoids, listed in Table 39.4, are one of the most widely prescribed drug classes.

39.10 Pharmacotherapy with Glucocorticoids

Lack of adequate corticosteroid production, known as adrenocortical insufficiency, may be caused by hyposecretion of the adrenal cortex or by inadequate secretion of ACTH from the pituitary. Symptoms include hypoglycemia, fatigue, hypotension, increased skin pigmentation, and GI disturbances such as anorexia, vomiting, and diarrhea. Low plasma cortisol, accompanied by high plasma ACTH levels, is diagnostic because this indicates that the adrenal gland is not responding to ACTH stimulation. Primary adrenocortical insufficiency, known as **Addison's disease**, is quite rare and includes a deficiency of both glucocorticoids and mineralocorticoids. Autoimmune destruction of both adrenal glands is the most common cause of Addison's disease. Secondary adrenocortical insufficiency is more common and responds to glucocorticoid pharmacotherapy.

Acute adrenocortical insufficiency may result when glucocorticoids are abruptly withdrawn from a client who has been on long-term glucocorticoid therapy. When glucocorticoids are taken as medications for prolonged periods, they provide negative feedback to the pituitary to stop secreting ACTH. Without stimulation by ACTH, the adrenal cortex shrinks and stops secreting endogenous glucocorticoids, a condition known as adrenal atrophy. If the glucocorticoid medication is abruptly withdrawn, the shrunken adrenal glands will not be able to secrete sufficient glucocorticoids and symptoms of acute adrenocortical insufficiency will appear. Symptoms include nausea, vomiting, lethargy, confusion, and coma. Immediate administration of IV therapy with hydrocortisone is essential as shock may quickly result if the symptoms remain untreated. Other possible causes of acute adrenocortical insufficiency include infection, trauma, and cancer.

For chronic corticosteroid insufficiency, replacement therapy with glucocorticoids is indicated. The goal of replacement therapy is to achieve the same physiological level of hormones in the blood that would be present if the adrenal glands were functioning properly. Clients requiring replacement therapy usually need to take glucocorticoids their entire lifetime. Clients with adrenal insufficiency may also need a mineralocorticoid, such as fludrocortisone.

Glucocorticoids are prescribed for a large number of other disorders in addition to acute and chronic adrenal insufficiency. Their ability to quickly and effectively suppress the inflammatory and immune responses gives them tremendous therapeutic utility to treat a diverse set of conditions. Following are the indications for pharmacotherapy with glucocorticoids:

- Adrenal insufficiency
- Allergies, including seasonal rhinitis (Chapter 31)
- Asthma (Chapter 29)
- Chronic inflammatory bowel disease, including ulcerative colitis and Crohn's disease (Chapter 37)
- Hepatic, neurological, and renal disorders characterized by edema
- Neoplastic disease, including Hodgkin's disease, leukemias, and lymphomas (Chapter 35)
- Post-transplant rejection (Chapter 30)

- Rheumatic disorders, including rheumatoid arthritis, ankylosing spondylitis, and bursitis (Chapter 46)
- Shock (Chapter 27)
- Skin disorders, including contact dermatitis and rashes (Chapter 47)

More than 20 glucocorticoids are available as medications, and the choice of a particular agent depends primarily on the pharmacokinetic properties of the drug. The duration of action, which is often used to classify these agents, ranges from short to long. Some, such as hydrocortisone, have mineralocorticoid activity that causes sodium and fluid retention; others, such as prednisone, have no such effect. Some glucocorticoids are available by only one route.

Glucocorticoids interact with many drugs. Their hyperglycemic effects may decrease the effectiveness of antidiabetic agents. Combining glucocorticoids with other ulcerogenic drugs such as ASA and other NSAIDs markedly increases the risk of peptic ulcer. Administration with non-potassium-sparing diuretics may lead to hypocalcemia and hypokalemia. The following strategies are used to decrease the incidence of serious adverse effects from glucocorticoids:

- Keep doses to the lowest possible amount that will achieve a therapeutic effect.
- Administer glucocorticoids every other day (alternate-day dosing) to limit adrenal atrophy.
- For acute conditions, give clients large amounts for a few days and then gradually decrease the drug dose until it is discontinued.
- Give the drugs locally by inhalation, intra-articular injection, or topical application to the skin, eyes, or ears, when feasible, to diminish the possibility of systemic effects.

NURSING CONSIDERATIONS

The role of the nurse in glucocorticoid therapy involves careful monitoring of the client's condition and providing education as it relates to the prescribed drug treatment. There are many glucocorticoid drugs available, including prednisone, methylprednisolone, dexamethasone, and the inhaled and topical glucocorticoid preparations. Assess vital signs for temperature and blood pressure elevations because glucocorticoid therapy may predispose the client to infection and raises blood pressure. Monitor potassium, T_3, and T_4 levels because they may be decreased when taking glucocorticoids. Monitor glucose levels because glucocorticoids may cause hyperglycemia and immunosuppression, which delays wound healing. Monitor clients on long-term glucocorticoid therapy for osteoporosis and elevated serum cholesterol levels. Long-term administration of glucocorticoids may cause Cushing's syndrome. Assess for signs and symptoms of Cushing's syndrome, such as moon face, buffalo hump, and mood and personality disorders. Individuals with medical conditions such as asthma, COPD, chronic renal failure, Crohn's disease, ulcerative colitis, rheumatoid arthritis, and lupus typically receive long-term glucocorticoid therapy in times of stress or exacerbation of their condition to suppress the inflammatory response. These individuals should be taught the importance of and rationale for adherence to the prescribed medication administration and the importance of gradual dosage reductions.

Systemic glucocorticoid therapy is generally contraindicated for pregnant and lactating women. Animal studies have demonstrated that high doses of systemic glucocorticoids consistently cause cleft palate, although human data are less clear. Use of a systemic glucocorticoid during pregnancy must be carefully weighed against the severity of maternal disease. If pharmacotherapy is necessary, hydrocortisone, cortisone, prednisone, and methylprednisolone are suggested since they are more readily inactivated by placental enzymes, as opposed to dexamethasone and betamethasone, which are more likely to reach the fetus in the active state.

Client education as it relates to glucocorticoid therapy includes goals, reasons for obtaining baseline data such as vital signs and tests for thyroid hormone levels, and possible drug side effects. Include the following points when teaching clients about glucocorticoid therapy:

- Report unusual changes in mood or personality, moon face, and buffalo hump because these are signs of overdosage (Cushing's syndrome).
- Practise reliable contraception, and notify the healthcare provider if pregnancy is planned or suspected.
- Do not breastfeed while taking these medications.
- Report wounds that are unusually slow to heal.
- Keep all scheduled appointments and laboratory visits for testing.
- Report fever, which may indicate an underlying infection.

See "Nursing Process Focus: Clients Receiving Systemic Glucocorticoid Therapy" for specific teaching points.

Cushing's syndrome occurs when high levels of glucocorticoids are present in the body over a prolonged period. Although hypersecretion of these hormones can occur due to pituitary or adrenal tumours, the most common cause of Cushing's syndrome is long-term therapy with high doses of systemic glucocorticoid medications. Signs and symptoms include adrenal atrophy, osteoporosis, increased risk of infection, delayed wound healing, acne, peptic ulcers, and a redistribution of fat around the face (moon face), shoulders, and neck (buffalo hump). Mood and personality changes may occur, and the client may become psychologically dependent on the drug. Some glucocorticoids, including hydrocortisone, also have mineralocorticoid activity and can cause retention of sodium and water. Because of their anti-inflammatory properties, glucocorticoids may mask signs of infection with a resulting delay in antibiotic therapy.

Pr PROTOTYPE DRUG | Hydrocortisone (Hydrocortisone)

ACTIONS AND USES

Structurally identical to the natural hormone cortisol, hydrocortisone is a synthetic corticosteroid that is the drug of choice for treating adrenocortical insufficiency. When used for replacement therapy, it is given at physiological doses. Once proper dosing is achieved, its therapeutic effects should mimic those of endogenous corticosteroids. Hydrocortisone is also available for the treatment of inflammation, allergic disorders, and many other conditions. Intra-articular injections may be given to decrease severe inflammation in affected joints.

Hydrocortisone is available in six different formulations. Hydrocortisone base (Aeroseb-HC, Alphaderm, Cetacort, others) and hydrocortisone acetate (Anusol HC, Cortaid, Cortef Acetate) are available as oral preparations, creams, and ointments. Hydrocortisone cypionate (Cortef Fluid) is an oral suspension. Hydrocortisone sodium phosphate (Hydrocortone Phosphate) and hydrocortisone sodium succinate (A-Hydrocort, Solu-Cortef) are for parenteral use only. Hydrocortisone valerate (Westcort) is only for topical applications.

PHARMACOKINETICS

Hydrocortisone is well absorbed after oral administration. It is widely distributed, crosses the placenta, and enters breast milk. It is metabolized by the liver. Its half-life in plasma is 1.5 to 2 hours and in tissue, 8 to 12 hours. Adrenal suppression lasts 1.5 days.

ADMINISTRATION ALERTS

- Administer exactly as prescribed and at the same time every day.
- Administer oral formulations with food.
- Hydrocortisone is pregnancy category C.

ADVERSE EFFECTS AND INTERACTIONS

When used at physiological doses for replacement therapy, adverse effects of hydrocortisone should not be evident. The client and nurse must be vigilant, however, in observing for signs of Cushing's syndrome, which can develop with over-treatment. If taken for longer than 2 weeks, hydrocortisone should be discontinued gradually. Hydrocortisone possesses some mineralocorticoid activity, so sodium and fluid retention may be noted. A wide range of CNS effects have been reported, including insomnia, anxiety, headache, vertigo, confusion, and depression. Cardiovascular effects may include hypertension and tachycardia. Long-term therapy may result in peptic ulcer disease.

Hydrocortisone interacts with many drugs; for example, barbiturates, phenytoin, and rifampin may increase hepatic metabolism, thus decreasing hydrocortisone levels. Estrogens potentiate the effects of hydrocortisone. NSAIDs compound ulcerogenic effects. Cholestyramine and colestipol decrease hydrocortisone absorption. Diuretics and amphotericin B exacerbate hypokalemia. Anticholinesterase agents may produce severe weakness. Hydrocortisone may cause a decrease in immune response to vaccines and toxoids.

Use with caution with herbal supplements, such as aloe and buckthorn (a laxative), which may create a potassium deficiency with chronic use or abuse.

 See the Companion Website for a Nursing Process Focus chart specific to this drug.

39.11 Pharmacotherapy of Cushing's Syndrome

Cushing's syndrome has a high mortality rate, and the therapeutic goal is to identify and treat the cause of the excess glucocorticoid secretion. If the cause is over-treatment with glucocorticoid drugs, a gradual reduction in dose is sufficient to reverse the syndrome. When the cause of the hypersecretion is an adrenal tumour or perhaps an ectopic tumour secreting ACTH, surgical removal is indicated. Clients with severe disease will receive drug therapy to quickly lower serum glucocorticoid levels. Combination therapy with aminoglutethimide and metyrapone is sometimes used. Aminoglutethimide suppresses adrenal function within 3 to 5 days; however, therapy is usually limited to 3 months because of its ineffectiveness over time. The antifungal drug ketoconazole has been found to be a safer therapy for long-term use. Most antiadrenal agents inhibit the metabolic conversion of cholesterol to adrenal corticosteroids. They are not curative; their use is temporary until the tumour can be removed or otherwise treated with radiation or antineoplastics.

NURSING CONSIDERATIONS

The role of the nurse in antiadrenal therapy for Cushing's syndrome involves careful monitoring of the client's condition and providing education as it relates to the prescribed drug treatment. Assess and monitor lab values, including platelet count, bilirubin, and prothrombin. Assess for jaundice, bruising, and bleeding because antiadrenal therapy may cause leukopenia and thrombocytopenia. Monitor for orthostatic hypotension because the drugs cause decreased aldosterone production. Monitor for dizziness and assist with ambulation. Caution the client to change positions slowly. Ketoconazole administered at high levels is an effective corticosteroid inhibitor. This medication is metabolized in the liver; therefore, hepatic function must be assessed prior to administration and monitored during therapy. Ketoconazole is contraindicated in those with liver dysfunction and those who abuse alcohol. Obtain a thorough history to assess for alcohol intake or possible HIV infection because these medications are contraindicated in these clients.

Client education as it relates to antiadrenal drugs should include goals, reasons for obtaining baseline data such as

NURSING PROCESS FOCUS   Clients Receiving Systemic Glucocorticoid Therapy

Assessment	Potential Nursing Diagnoses/Identified Patterns
Prior to administration: ■ Obtain complete health history including allergies, drug history, and possible drug interactions. ■ Obtain complete physical examination, focusing on presenting symptoms. ■ Determine the reason the medication is being administered. ■ Obtain laboratory studies (long-term therapy) including serum sodium and potassium levels, hematocrit and hemoglobin levels, blood glucose level, and BUN.	■ Risk for injury related to side effects of drug therapy ■ Risk for infection related to immunosuppression ■ Need for knowledge regarding drug therapy and adverse effects ■ Risk for altered body image related to side effects of drug therapy

Planning: Client Goals and Expected Outcomes

The client will:

■ Demonstrate an understanding of the drug's action by accurately describing drug side effects and precautions

■ Exhibit a decrease in the symptoms for which the drug is being given

■ Exhibit no symptoms of infection

■ Adhere to the treatment plan

Implementation

Interventions (Rationales)	Client Education/Discharge Planning
■ Monitor vital signs. (Blood pressure may increase because of increased blood volume and potential vasoconstriction effect.)	■ Instruct client to report dizziness, palpitations, or headaches.
■ Monitor for infection. Protect client from potential infections. (Glucocorticoids increase susceptibility to infections by suppressing the immune response.)	Instruct client to: ■ Avoid people with infection ■ Report fever, cough, sore throat, joint pain, increase weakness, and malaise ■ Consult with the healthcare provider before getting any immunizations
■ Monitor client's adherence with drug treatment. (Sudden discontinuation of these agents can precipitate an adrenal crisis.)	Instruct client: ■ To never suddenly stop taking the medication ■ In proper use of self-administering tapering dose pack ■ To take oral medications with food
■ Monitor for symptoms of Cushing's syndrome such as moon face, "buffalo hump" contour of shoulders, weight gain, muscle wasting, increased deposits of fat in the trunk. (Symptoms may indicate excessive use of glucocorticoids.)	Instruct client: ■ To weigh self daily ■ That initial weight gain is expected; provide the client with weight gain parameters that warrant reporting ■ That there are multiple side effects of therapy and that changes in health status should be reported
■ Monitor blood glucose levels. (Glucocorticoids cause an increase in gluconeo-genesis and reduce glucose utilization.)	Instruct client to: ■ Report symptoms of hyperglycemia such as excessive thirst, copious urination, and insatiable appetite ■ Adjust insulin dose based on blood glucose level, as directed by the health-care provider
■ Monitor skin and mucous membranes for lacerations, abrasions, or breaks in integrity. (Glucocorticoids impair wound healing.)	Instruct client to: ■ Examine skin daily for cuts and scrapes and to cover any injuries with sterile bandage ■ Watch for symptoms of skin infection such as redness, swelling, and drainage ■ Notify the healthcare provider of any non-healing wound or symptoms of infection
■ Monitor gastrointestinal status for peptic ulcer development. (Glucocorticoids decrease gastric mucus production and predispose client to peptic ulcers.)	■ Instruct client to report GI side effects such as heartburn, abdominal pain, or tarry stools.

continued

NURSING PROCESS FOCUS Clients Receiving Systemic Glucocorticoid Therapy   (*Continued*)

Interventions (Rationales)	Client Education/Discharge Planning
■ Monitor serum electrolytes. (Glucocorticoids cause hypernatremia and hypokalemia.)	Instruct client to: ■ Consume a diet high in protein, calcium, and potassium but low in fat and concentrated simple carbohydrates ■ Keep all laboratory appointments
■ Monitor changes in musculoskeletal system. (Glucocorticoids decrease bone density and strength and cause muscle atrophy and weakness.)	Instruct client: ■ To participate in exercise or physical activity to help maintain bone and muscle strength ■ That the drug may cause weakness in bones and muscles and to avoid strenuous activity that may cause injury
■ Monitor emotional stability. (Glucocorticoids may produce mood and behaviour changes such as depression or feeling of invulnerability.)	■ Instruct client that mood changes may be expected and to report mental status changes to the healthcare provider.

Evaluation of Outcome Criteria

Evaluate the effectiveness of drug therapy by confirming that client goals and expected outcomes have been met (see "Planning").

See Table 39.4 (page 562) for a list of drugs to which these nursing actions apply.

vital signs and the existence of underlying hematological disorders, and possible drug side effects. Include the following points when teaching clients about anti-adrenal drugs:

- Immediately report unusual bleeding, change in colour of stool or urine, or yellowing of eyes or skin.
- Monitor temperature and report fever.
- Change positions slowly to avoid dizziness.
- Take medication with fruit juice or water to enhance absorption.
- Avoid alcohol use.
- Practise reliable contraception and notify the healthcare provider if pregnancy is planned or suspected.
- Keep all scheduled appointments and laboratory visits for testing.

- Practise relaxation techniques because increased stress may cause adverse effects of the drug.

LIFESPAN CONSIDERATIONS

Treatment of Cushing's Syndrome during Pregnancy

Aminoglutethimide is contraindicated during pregnancy. In animal studies, the drug has been shown to prevent fetal implantation and increase the potential for fetal death. Also, in pregnant animals, the drug causes an unusual condition known as pseudohermaphrodism, in which an individual has the internal reproductive organs of only one gender but exhibits both male and female external genitalia.

Ketoconazole, in high doses, has also been shown to be teratogenic and embryotoxic in animals.

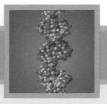

CHAPTER REVIEW

KEY CONCEPTS

The numbered key concepts provide a succinct summary of the important points from the corresponding numbered section within the chapter. If any of these points are not clear, refer to the numbered section within the chapter for review. Expanded versions can be found on the Companion Website.

39.1 The endocrine system maintains homeostasis by using hormones as chemical messengers that are secreted in response to changes in the internal environment.

39.2 The hypothalamus secretes releasing hormones, which direct the anterior pituitary gland as to which hormones should be released.

39.3 Hormones are used as replacement therapy, as antineoplastics, and for their natural therapeutic effects such as their suppression of body defences.

39.4 Only a few pituitary and hypothalamic hormones, including growth hormone and ACTH, have clinical applications as drugs.

39.5 The thyroid gland secretes thyroxine and triiodothyronine, which control the basal metabolic rate and affect every cell in the body.

39.6 Hypothyroidism may be treated by administering thyroid hormone.

39.7 Hyperthyroidism is treated by administering agents that decrease the activity of the thyroid gland or that kill overactive thyroid cells.

39.8 The adrenal cortex secretes glucocorticoids, gonadotropins, and mineralocorticoids. The glucocorticoids mobilize the body for long-term stress and influence carbohydrate, lipid, and protein metabolism in most cells.

39.9 Glucocorticoid release is controlled by ACTH from the pituitary.

39.10 Adrenocortical insufficiency may be acute or chronic. Glucocorticoids are prescribed for adrenocortical insufficiency and a wide variety of other conditions.

39.11 Antiadrenal drugs may be used to treat Cushing's syndrome by inhibiting corticosteroid synthesis. Their use is usually limited to 3 months of therapy.

REVIEW QUESTIONS

1 Why are hypothalamic and pituitary hormones not widely used in pharmacotherapeutics?

2 If thyroid hormone is secreted by the thyroid gland, how can a deficiency in this hormone be caused by disease in the hypothalamus or pituitary?

3 Why does administration of glucocorticoids for extended periods result in adrenal atrophy, and what strategies can be used to lessen the risk of adrenal atrophy?

CRITICAL THINKING QUESTIONS

1. A 5-year-old girl requires treatment for diabetes insipidus acquired following a case of meningitis. The child has suffered serious complications including blindness and mental retardation. Her diabetes insipidus is being treated with intranasal desmopressin, and the child's mother has been asked to help evaluate the drug's effectiveness using urine volumes and urine specific gravity. Discuss the changes that would indicate that the drug is effective.

2. A 17-year-old boy with a history of severe asthma is admitted to the intensive care unit. He is comatose, appears much younger than his listed age, and has a short stature. The nurse notes that the asthma has been managed with prednisone for 15 days, until 3 days ago. The client's father is extremely anxious and says that he was unable to refill his son's prescription until he got his pay. What is the nurse's role in this situation?

3. A 9-year-old boy has been diagnosed with growth hormone deficiency. His parents have decided to proceed with a prescribed treatment of somatropin (Humatrope). Outline the basic information the parents need to know regarding treatment, side effects, and evaluation of effectiveness.

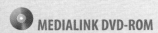

EXPLORE
MediaLink

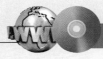

www.pearsoned.ca/adams-king

MEDIALINK DVD-ROM
- **Audio Glossary**
- **CRNE Review**

COMPANION WEBSITE
- **CRNE Review**
- **Case Study:** Client with diabetes incipitus
- **Dosage Calculations**

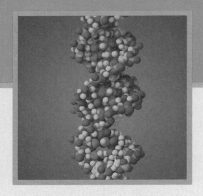

CHAPTER 40

Drugs for Diabetes Mellitus

DRUGS AT A GLANCE

INSULINS

regular insulin (Humulin-R, Novolin ge Toronto, Hypurin-R)

ORAL ANTIHYPERGLYCEMICS

glyburide (Apo-Glyburide)

OBJECTIVES

After reading this chapter, the student should be able to do the following:

1. Describe the endocrine and exocrine functions of the pancreas.
2. Compare and contrast type 1 and type 2 diabetes mellitus in relation to their pathophysiology and treatment.
3. Compare and contrast types of insulin.
4. Describe the signs and symptoms of insulin overdose and underdose.
5. Compare and contrast drug classes used to treat type 2 diabetes mellitus.
6. Describe the nurse's role in the pharmacological management of diabetes mellitus.
7. For each of the drug classes listed in Drugs at a Glance, identify a representative drug and explain its mechanism of action, therapeutic effects, and important adverse effects.
8. Use the nursing process to care for clients receiving drug therapy for diabetes mellitus.

MediaLink

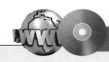 www.pearsoned.ca/adams-king

CRNE review, case studies, and other interactive resources for this chapter can be found on the Companion Website at **www.pearsoned.ca/adams-king**. Click on "Chapter 40" to select the activities for this chapter. For animations, more CRNE review questions, and an audio glossary, access the accompanying DVD-ROM in this textbook.

The pancreas serves unique and vital functions by supplying essential digestive enzymes while also secreting the hormones responsible for glucose homeostasis. From a pharmacological perspective, the most important disorder associated with the pancreas is diabetes mellitus. Millions of people have diabetes, a disease caused by genetic and environmental factors that impairs the cellular utilization of glucose. Because glucose is essential to every cell in the body, the effects of diabetes are widespread. Diabetes merits special consideration in pharmacology because the nurse will encounter many clients with this disorder.

40.1 Normal Functions of the Pancreas

Located behind the stomach and between the duodenum and spleen, the pancreas is an essential organ to both the digestive and endocrine systems. It is responsible for the secretion of several enzymes into the duodenum that assist in the chemical digestion of nutrients. This is its **exocrine** function. Clusters of cells in the pancreas, called **islets of Langerhans**, are responsible for its endocrine function: the secretion of glucagon and insulin. Alpha cells secrete glucagon, and beta cells secrete insulin, as illustrated in Figure 40.1. As with other endocrine organs, the pancreas secretes these hormones directly into blood capillaries, where they are available for transport to body tissues. Insulin and glucagon play key roles in keeping glucose levels within a normal range in the blood.

Insulin secretion is regulated by a number of chemical, hormonal, and neural factors. One important regulator is the level of glucose in the blood. After a meal, when blood glucose levels rise, the islets of Langerhans are stimulated to secrete insulin, which causes glucose to leave the blood and enter cells. High insulin levels and falling blood glucose levels provide negative feedback to the pancreas to stop secreting insulin.

Insulin affects carbohydrate, lipid, and protein metabolism in most cells of the body. One of its most important actions is to assist in glucose transport: without insulin, glucose cannot enter cells. Activation of insulin receptors leads to internal cellular mechanisms that directly affect glucose uptake by regulating the number and operation of protein molecules in the cell membrane that transport glucose into the cell. A cell may be literally swimming in glucose, but glucose cannot enter and be used as an energy source by the cell without insulin present. Insulin is said to have a **hypoglycemic effect** because its presence causes glucose to *leave* the blood and serum glucose to *fall*. The brain is an important exception because it does not require insulin for glucose transport.

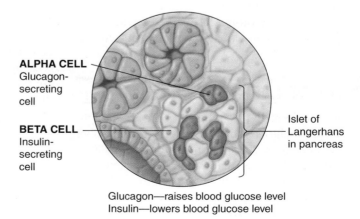

ALPHA CELL
Glucagon-
secreting
cell

BETA CELL
Insulin-
secreting
cell

Islet of
Langerhans
in pancreas

Glucagon—raises blood glucose level
Insulin—lowers blood glucose level

● **Figure 40.1** Glucagon- and insulin-secreting cells in the islets of Langerhans

Source: Pearson Education/PH College.

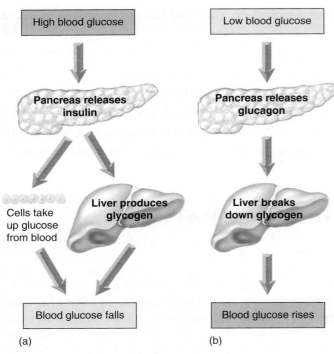

● **Figure 40.2** Relationship among insulin, glucagon, and blood glucose

Islet cells in the pancreas also secrete glucagon. Glucagon is an antagonist to insulin. When levels of glucose are low, glucagon is secreted. Its primary function is to maintain adequate blood glucose levels between meals. Glucagon has a **hyperglycemic effect** because its presence causes blood glucose to rise. Figure 40.2 illustrates the relationship among blood glucose, insulin, and glucagon.

Blood glucose levels are usually kept within a normal range by insulin and glucagon; however, other hormones and drugs can affect glucose metabolism. Hyperglycemic hormones include epinephrine, thyroid hormones, growth hormone, and corticosteroids. Common drugs that can raise blood glucose levels include phenytoin, NSAIDs, and diuretics. Drugs with a hypoglycemic effect include alcohol, lithium, angiotensin-converting enzyme (ACE) inhibitors (ACEIs), and beta-adrenergic blockers. Blood glucose levels should be periodically monitored in clients receiving medications that exhibit hypoglycemia or hypoglycemic effects.

DIABETES MELLITUS

Worldwide, approximately 135 million people are thought to have diabetes mellitus (DM); by 2025, this number is expected to increase to 300 million (Hjelm et al., 2003). The etiology of DM includes a combination of genetic and environmental factors. The recent increase in the frequency of the disease is probably the result of trends toward more sedentary and stressful lifestyles, increased consumption of highly caloric foods with resultant obesity, and increased longevity.

Diabetes mellitus is a group of metabolic diseases in which there is deficient insulin secretion or decreased sensitivity of insulin receptors on target cells, resulting in hyperglycemia. DM includes type 1, type 2, gestational diabetes, and other specific types such as those found in Cushing's syndrome or that are chemically induced. Discussion in this chapter is limited to type 1 and type 2 DM.

40.2 Etiology and Characteristics of Type 1 Diabetes Mellitus

Type 1 DM was previously called *juvenile-onset diabetes* because it is often diagnosed between the ages of 11 and 13 years. Because the symptoms of type 1 DM can occur for the first time in adulthood, this was not the most accurate name for this disorder. This type of diabetes is also referred to as insulin-dependent DM. Type 1 DM accounts for 10% of all cases of diabetes and is one of the most common diseases of childhood. **Type I DM** results from autoimmune destruction of pancreatic beta cells, causing an absolute lack of insulin secretion. The disease is thought to be an interaction of genetic, immunological, and environmental factors. Children and siblings of those with DM have a higher risk of developing the disorder. The signs and symptoms of type 1 DM are consistent from client to client, with the most diagnostic sign being sustained hyperglycemia. Following are the typical signs and symptoms:

- Hyperglycemia – fasting blood glucose greater than 7.0 mmol/L on at least two separate occasions
- Polyuria – excessive urination
- Polyphagia – increased hunger
- Polydipsia – increased thirst
- Glucosuria – high levels of glucose in the urine
- Weight loss
- Fatigue

Untreated DM produces long-term damage to arteries, which leads to heart disease, stroke, kidney disease, and blindness. Lack of adequate circulation to the feet may cause gangrene of the toes, which may require amputation. Nerve degeneration is common and produces symptoms ranging from tingling in the fingers or toes to complete loss of sensation of a limb. Because glucose is unable to enter cells, lipids are utilized as an energy source and **keto acids** are produced as waste products. These keto acids can give the client's breath an acetone-like, fruity odour. More important, high levels of keto acids lower the pH of the blood, causing **diabetic ketoacidosis (DKA)**, which may progress to coma and possible death if untreated.

INSULIN

Insulin was discovered in 1921/22 by Canadian researchers Frederick Banting and Charles Best. Prior to that time, type 1 diabetics were unable to adequately maintain normal blood glucose, experienced many complications, and

PHARMFACTS

Diabetes Mellitus

- More than 2 million Canadians have diabetes.
- Healthcare costs for diabetes and its complications are about $9 billion per year.
- The risk of developing diabetes increases with age:
  - 7.1% of all Canadians 20 years and older have diabetes.
  - 18% of all Canadians 60 years and older have diabetes.
- Diabetes is the seventh leading cause of death (death rates per 100,000 persons are 4.6 for men and 7.1 for women).
- Diabetes is the leading cause of blindness and end-stage renal disease.
- Diabetes is responsible for 50% of non-traumatic lower limb amputations.
- Type 2 DM accounts for 90% of all cases of diabetes.
- Risk factors for type 2 DM include the following:
  - Age 40 and over
  - Being related to a person with diabetes
  - Aboriginal, Hispanic, South Asian, or African ancestry
  - Overweight or obesity
  - The prevalence of type 2 DM in Aboriginals is three to five times higher than in the general Canadian population.

Source: Public Health Agency of Canada, using National Diabetes Surveillance System (NDSS) data files contributed by all provinces and territories, as of October 31, 2007.

usually died at a young age. Increased insulin availability and improvements in insulin products, personal blood glucose monitoring devices, and the insulin pump have made it possible for clients to maintain better control of their blood glucose levels. The level of glycosylated hemoglobin (A1C) in the blood may be assessed periodically to estimate overall glucose control across a 3-month period. A1C levels indicate the percentage of hemoglobin to which glucose has become bound, a process referred to as glycosylation. Higher levels of A1C are found in people with persistently

LIFESPAN CONSIDERATIONS

Gestational Diabetes

Gestational diabetes mellitus (GDM) is a condition that is diagnosed during pregnancy and usually is not present after the postpartum period, approximately 6 weeks after delivery. Placental lactogen and destruction of maternal insulin by the placenta contribute to GDM by increasing insulin resistance in the mother. The incidence of GDM has been on the rise in the past decade, and many healthcare providers recommend performing glucose tests at about 24 to 28 weeks' gestation to rule out GDM. Following diagnosis of GDM, changes in dietary and exercise habits are implemented. If these changes are ineffective in controlling blood glucose level, the client will be prescribed a regimen of insulin injections. Educate clients about the potential problems to the fetus and to themselves during the pregnancy, labour, birth, and postpartum period if the treatment prescribed by the healthcare provider is not followed. A child born to a mother diagnosed with GDM has a 40% chance of being obese and developing type 2 DM in later life. The mother has increased potential for developing GDM in future pregnancies. Oral antihyperglycemic agents are contraindicated during pregnancy because of their potential teratogenic effects on the fetus.

LIFESPAN CONSIDERATIONS

Diabetes in the Geriatric Population

The geriatric population also presents with specific problems with regard to maintaining a normal blood glucose level. If geriatric clients have been diabetic for most of their life, they may choose to ignore their recommended therapy because they feel it will make little difference at this time in their life. Also, elderly clients frequently display cognitive impairment that distorts their judgment and their desire to maintain their prescribed diet. Monitor these clients closely, because diet is a major factor in the control of blood glucose levels.

elevated blood glucose. As exposure to glucose in the blood increases, the percentage of A1C increases. A target A1C of less than 7% is desirable to prevent complications.

40.3 Pharmacotherapy with Insulin

Because clients with type 1 DM have a total lack of endogenous insulin secretion, replacement therapy with insulin is required. Insulin requirements vary in response to fluctuations in blood glucose that occur with daily activities such as exercise, eating, and sleep. The goal of insulin therapy is to prevent long-term complications of diabetes by keeping blood glucose levels within the target range, shown in Table 40.1. Therefore, insulin administration is planned in conjunction with current blood glucose level, nutrient intake, and exercise. The fundamental principle of insulin pharmacotherapy is that the right amount of insulin must be available to cells when glucose is present in the blood. Without insulin present, glucose from a meal can build up to high levels in the blood, a condition called hyperglycemia. This situation may occur when a client forgets to administer insulin in conjunction with a meal. Administering insulin when glucose is not available can lead to hypoglycemia and coma. For this reason, insulin is normally withheld when clients are fasting for laboratory tests. Clients are counselled that they must consume food once they have received their insulin. Regular, moderate exercise increases the cellular responsiveness to insulin, lowering the amount of insulin needed to maintain normal blood glucose levels. During heavy prolonged exercise, such as in competitive sports, individuals may become hypoglycemic and need to consume food or drink to raise their blood glucose to normal levels. Those regularly engaging in strenuous activities should eat food or consume a sports drink just prior to commencing the activity, as a preventive measure. Nurses play an important role in educating clients about managing and adhering to their insulin therapy.

Several types of insulin are available, differing in their source, onset, and duration of action. Until the 1980s, the source of all insulin was beef or pork pancreas. Almost all insulin today, however, is human insulin obtained through recombinant DNA technology. Human insulin can be modified to alter its pharmacokinetics, such as a more rapid onset of action (lispro) or a more prolonged duration of action (glargine). Human insulin is more effective, causes

TABLE 40.1	Target Blood Glucose and A1C Levels	
Adults and Adolescents	**Normal Range**[*]	**Target Goals**[†]
A1C	4–6%	< 7%
Fasting or before meal	4.0–6.0 mmol/L	4.0–7.0 mmol/L
2 hours after meal	5.0–8.0 mmol/L	5.0–10.0 mmol/L
Children with Type 1 DM (12 and under)	**Age < 5 Years**	**Age 5–12 Years**
Fasting or before meal	6.0–12.0 mmol/L	4.0–10.0 mmol/L
A1C	≤ 9.0%	≤ 8.0%
Pregnancy and Gestational Diabetes		
Fasting or before meal	3.8–5.2 mmol/L	
1 hour after meal	5.5–7.7 mmol/L	
2 hours after meal	5.0–6.6 mmol/L	
A1C	≤ 6.0% (normal)	

[*]Normal range should be considered if it can be achieved safely.
[†]Target goals should be tailored to individual needs.
Source: Canadian Diabetes Association. (2003). Clinical practice guidelines for the prevention and management of diabetes in Canada. Canadian Journal of Diabetes, 27, 1–163.

fewer allergies, and has a lower incidence of resistance than animal-source insulin. However, a small number of clients may still use pork insulin (or beef insulin, through a special access program) because they experience hypoglycemia without clearly recognizable symptoms and wide and sudden swings in blood glucose levels when using human insulin. Health Canada monitors adverse effects associated with taking insulin.

Doses and routes of insulin are highly individualized for each client. Some clients may need two or more doses daily. The most common route of administration for insulin is SC injection. Some clients have an insulin pump that is programmed to deliver small doses of insulin at predetermined intervals, with larger boluses programmed manually at mealtimes. The pump delivers insulin through a small pliable catheter that is anchored in the subcutaneous tissue of the abdomen. Dry powder insulin for inhalation is now available. Bolus doses are delivered through a special inhalation device. Inhaled insulin may be used as an adjunct to subcutaneous or oral antihyperglycemic therapy. The inhalation route is contraindicated in clients with lung disorders. Common insulin preparations are listed in Table 40.2.

The primary adverse effect of insulin therapy is hypoglycemia. Symptoms of hypoglycemia occur when a client with type 1 DM has more insulin in the blood than is needed for the amount of circulating blood glucose. This may occur when the insulin level peaks, during exercise, when the client receives too much insulin owing to a medication error, or when the client skips a meal. Some of the symptoms of hypoglycemia are the same as those of diabetic ketoacidosis. Those symptoms that differ and help in determining if a client is hypoglycemic include pale, cool, and moist skin, with blood glucose less than 4 mmol/L and

a sudden onset of symptoms. Left untreated, severe hypoglycemia may result in death.

Other adverse effects of insulin include localized allergic reactions at the injection site, generalized urticaria, and swollen lymph glands. Some clients will experience **Somogyi phenomenon**. This is a rapid decrease in blood glucose, usually during the night, that stimulates the release of hormones that elevate blood glucose (epinephrine, cortisol, and glucagon), resulting in an elevated morning blood glucose level. Additional insulin above the client's normal dose may produce a rapid rebound hypoglycemia.

The hormone glucagon may be administered as an emergency replacement therapy for diabetic clients when they are in a hypoglycemic state and have impaired glucagon secretion. Glucagon (1 mg) may be given IV, IM, or SC to reverse hypoglycemic symptoms in 20 minutes or less, depending on the route. Pre-filled 50 mL syringes of D50W for IV infusion are commonly available to treat hypoglycemia in hospitalized clients. Agency guidelines for D50W infusion must be followed.

NURSING CONSIDERATIONS

The role of the nurse in insulin therapy involves careful monitoring of the client's condition and providing education as it relates to the prescribed drug treatment. Be familiar with the onset, peak, and duration of action of the prescribed insulin (refer to Table 40.2) as well as any other important aspects of the specific insulin, and convey this information to the client.

Assess the client for signs and symptoms of hypoglycemia as well as the adequacy of glucose monitoring. Hypoglycemia is most likely to occur when insulin reaches its

TABLE 40.2	Insulin Preparations				
Type	**Trade Name**	**Onset**	**Peak Action**	**Duration**
Rapid-acting analog (clear)	Humalog (insulin lispro) NovoRapid (insulin aspart)	10–15 minutes	60–90 minutes	4–5 hours
Regular/fast-acting (clear)	Humulin-R Novolin ge Toronto Hypurin-R	30–60 minutes	2–4 hours	5–8 hours
Intermediate-acting (cloudy)	Humulin-N Humulin-L Hypurin-N Novolin ge NPH	1–3 hours	5–8 hours	up to 18 hours
Long-acting (cloudy)	Humulin-U	3–4 hours	8–15 hours	22–26 hours
Extended long-acting analog	Lantus (insulin glargine)	90 minutes	—	24 hours
Pre-mixed (cloudy); a single vial or cartridge contains a fixed ratio of insulin (% rapid- or fast-acting to % intermediate-acting insulin)	Humalog Mix25 TM Humulin (20/80, 30/70) Novolin ge (10/90, 20/80, 30/70, 40/60, 50/50)	5–15 minutes	0.75–2.5 hours	18–24 hours

peak effect or during exercise or acute illness. Obtain food for the client and determine that the client is ready to eat before administering insulin. Insulin is normally withheld when clients are fasting for tests or procedures. Assess the client's level of understanding of the symptoms of insulin reaction, hypoglycemia, and diabetic ketoacidosis. Teach the client to recognize key symptoms and what action to take in response to them. Contraindications to insulin include sensitivity to an ingredient in the formulation and hypoglycemia that would be worsened by administration of insulin. Use with caution in pregnant clients and in those with severe stress or infection. Clients with these conditions usually have increased insulin requirements and must be monitored more carefully.

Two of the most frequently prescribed types of insulin are NPH and regular insulin. Intermediate or NPH insulin is used to provide a longer acting source of insulin compared with regular insulin and other types of short-acting insulin. NPH insulin is normally administered 30 minutes before the first meal of the day, but in some instances a second, smaller dose is taken before the evening meal or at bedtime. Some clients are prescribed insulin that is pre-mixed, such as 70% NPH with 30% regular or rapid acting. If the client is prescribed a pre-mixed insulin solution, it is important that proper instruction be given, especially if the client will be using additional regular or rapid-acting insulin on a sliding scale.

Under some circumstances, regular insulin may be given IV, but other types of insulin, including NPH, are to be given only as SC injections. Intermediate insulin cannot be given IV. Rapid-acting insulin lispro is being used more frequently. The onset of action is 10 to 15 minutes, which is much faster than the onset of 30 to 60 minutes associated with regular insulin. The peak effect of rapid-acting insulin lispro occurs in 30 to 60 minutes, and its duration of action is 5 hours or less. It is often used with insulin infusion pumps.

Insulin glargine is a newer agent that is a recombinant human insulin analog. It must not be mixed in the syringe with any other insulin and must be administered subcutaneously. Insulin glargine exhibits a constant, long-duration hypoglycemic effect with no defined peak. It is prescribed once daily, at bedtime.

Long-acting insulin is prescribed for some clients. Protamine zinc (PZI) has an onset of 4 to 8 hours, a peak of 14 to 24 hours, and a duration of 36 hours. Extended insulin zinc suspension has an onset of 4 to 6 hours, a peak of 10 to 30 hours, and a duration of 36 hours. A pre-mixed insulin, Novolin Mix (70% N and 30% R) has an onset of 4 to 8 hours, a peak of 16 to 18 hours, and duration greater than 36 hours. Insulins available in Canada are listed with their onset of action, peak effects, and duration of action in Table 40.2.

When administering insulin, ensure that the units on the syringe match the units on the insulin vial. For example, when U100 insulin is ordered, the vial must be U100 and the syringe must also be calibrated for U100. Although U100 is the most often used strength of insulin, U500 is available for clients who have developed insulin resistance and need a much higher dose to manage blood glucose. When U500 insulin is given, a syringe calibrated for U500 is necessary. It is also imperative to understand that not all types of insulin are compatible and may not be mixed together in a single syringe. Clear insulin must be drawn into the syringe first to reduce the possible contamination of the clear insulin by an insulin containing a suspension.

Client education at it relates to insulin therapy should include goals, reasons for obtaining baseline data such as vital signs and the existence of underlying hypoglycemic disorders, and possible drug side effects. Include the following points when teaching clients about insulin therapy:

- Closely monitor blood glucose before each meal and before insulin administration, as directed by the healthcare provider.

- Always carry a source of simple sugar in case of hypoglycemic reactions. If blood glucose is less than 4 mmol/L, take a fast-acting carbohydrate (15 g glucose tablets, 3 tsp. sugar, or 1/2 cup orange juice). Repeat in 15 minutes if blood glucose level is still less than 4 mmol/L. If there is more than 1 hour until the next meal, eat a snack of a starch and protein (cheese and 6 crackers, or half of a peanut butter sandwich).

- Immediately report nervousness, confusion, excessive sweating, rapid pulse, or tremors because these are signs of overdosage (hypoglycemia).

- Immediately report increased thirst or urine output, decreased appetite, or excessive fatigue because these are signs of underdosage (hyperglycemia).

- When in doubt about whether symptoms indicate hypoglycemia or hyperglycemia, treat for hypoglycemia. Hypoglycemia progresses rapidly, whereas hyperglycemia progresses slowly.

- Rotate insulin sites to prevent lipodystrophy.

- Do not inject insulin into areas that are raised, swollen, dimpled, or itching.

- Keep insulin vials that are currently in use at room temperature because insulin at that temperature is less irritating to skin and helps to prevent lipodystrophy.

- When not needed, refrigerate insulin to keep it stable.

- Strictly follow the prescribed diet (e.g., calorie restrictions, food exchanges, carbohydrate counting) unless otherwise instructed.

- Wear a MedicAlert bracelet to alert emergency personnel of DM. Notify caregivers, co-workers, and others who may be able to render assistance.

- Use only an insulin syringe calibrated to the same strength as the insulin.

- Use only the type of insulin prescribed by the healthcare provider.

Pr PROTOTYPE DRUG | Regular Insulin (Humulin-R, Novolin ge Toronto, Hypurin-R)

ACTIONS AND USES

Regular insulin is prepared from pork pancreas or as human insulin through recombinant DNA technology. It is classified as short-acting insulin, with an onset of 30 to 60 minutes, a peak effect in 2 to 3 hours, and a duration of 5 to 7 hours. Its primary action is to promote the entry of glucose into cells. For the emergency treatment of acute ketoacidosis, it may be given SC or IV. Regular insulin is also available as Humulin 70/30 (a mixture of 30% regular insulin and 70% isophane insulin) or as Humulin 50/50 (a mixture of 50% of both regular and isophane insulin).

ADMINISTRATION ALERTS

- Hypoglycemic reactions may occur quickly if regular insulin is not supported by sufficient food or is given when the client is hypoglycemic.
- Regular insulin is the only type of insulin that may be used for IV injection.
- Injection sites must be rotated. When the client is hospitalized, use sites not normally used while the client is at home.
- Administer approximately 30 minutes before meals so insulin will be absorbed and available when the client begins to eat.
- Regular insulin is pregnancy category B.

PHARMACOKINETICS

Regular insulin is rapidly absorbed from SC tissue. It is widely distributed. It is metabolized in the liver, spleen, kidney, and muscle. Half-life in diabetes is 1.5 hours.

ADVERSE EFFECTS AND INTERACTIONS

The most serious adverse effect of insulin therapy is hypoglycemia. Hypoglycemia may result from taking too much insulin, not properly timing the insulin injection with food intake, or skipping a meal. Dietary carbohydrates must have reached the blood when insulin is injected; otherwise, the drug will remove too much glucose and signs of hypoglycemia—tachycardia, confusion, sweating, and drowsiness—will ensue. If severe hypoglycemia is not quickly treated with glucose, convulsions, coma, and death may follow.

Regular insulin interacts with many drugs. For example, the following substances may potentiate hypoglycemic effects: alcohol, salicylates, MAO inhibitors, anabolic steroids, and guanethidine. The following substances may antagonize hypoglycemic effects: corticosteroids, thyroid hormones, and epinephrine. Serum glucose levels may be increased with furosemide or thiazide diuretics. Symptoms of hypoglycemic reaction may be masked with beta-adrenergic blockers.

Use with caution with herbal supplements, such as garlic and ginseng, which may potentiate the hypoglycemic effects of insulin.

See the Companion Website for a Nursing Process Focus chart specific to this drug.

LIFESPAN CONSIDERATIONS

Psychosocial Impacts on the Young Diabetic

For the child or adolescent who has diabetes, there are psychosocial and cultural considerations of adherence to medication and dietary regimens. Even if diagnosed early in life (with learned behaviours regarding the disease parameters), the elementary school years can be difficult for some children with diabetes. Social events such as birthday parties, field trips, and after-school snack time, where sweet treats are the norm, serve as a physical and psychological temptation. During adolescence, when the teen wants to fit in with a peer group, the diabetic treatment can become more difficult. It is during this time that failure to take insulin or to follow dietary guidelines becomes an issue that may negatively affect present and future health. Some teens may have insulin pumps and can more easily take extra insulin to cover foods not usually on their diet. The ability to do this helps teens feel less different from peers, but carried to excess, this practice can also lead to problems. The nurse plays a vital role in educating the client and family and in making referrals to community agencies that may assist in helping the young person keep blood sugar in control while preserving self-esteem.

SPECIAL CONSIDERATIONS

Carbohydrate Counting: Flexible Carbohydrate Plan

Carbohydrate counting provides meal flexibility while improving Hb A1C levels. In carbohydrate counting, the insulin dose is adjusted based on carbohydrate content—the more carbohydrates, the more rapid the absorption rate, the more insulin that will be required. The client is prescribed an insulin-to-carbohydrate ratio. At every meal, the client counts carbohydrates and adjusts the dose. For example, if the client is having 2 slices of bread, and 1 slice of bread is 15 g of carbohydrate requiring 1 unit of insulin, 2 units of rapid-acting insulin is required.

The client is also prescribed a *correction factor*. Clients with diabetes do not always achieve their before-meal target glucose level of 6 mmol/L. If blood glucose is 12 mmol/L before one meal, for example, the correction factor is applied. If the prescribed correction factor is to increase the insulin dose by 1 unit for every 3 mmol/L above the target glucose level, the client would inject an additional 2 units of insulin for that mealtime.

NURSING PROCESS FOCUS   Clients Receiving Insulin Therapy

Assessment	Potential Nursing Diagnoses/Identified Patterns
Prior to administration: ■ Obtain complete health history including allergies, drug history, and possible drug interactions. ■ Assess vital signs. If the client has a fever or elevated pulse, assess further to determine the cause as infection can alter the amount of insulin required. ■ Assess blood glucose level. ■ Assess appetite and presence of symptoms that indicate the client may not be able to consume or retain the next meal. ■ Assess subcutaneous areas for potential insulin injection sites. ■ Assess knowledge of insulin and ability to self-administer insulin.	■ Impaired sensory perception (neuropathy) related to complications of diabetes ■ Risk for impaired skin integrity ■ Need for knowledge regarding drug therapy ■ Risk for fluid imbalance ■ Risk for infection related to blood glucose elevations and impaired circulation ■ Risk for injury (hypoglycemia) related to adverse effects of drug therapy ■ Need for knowledge and skills for self-injection ■ Need for knowledge related to dietary modifications (e.g., carbohydrate counting)

Planning: Client Goals and Expected Outcomes

The client will:
- Immediately report irritability, dizziness, diaphoresis, hunger, behaviour changes, and changes in LOC
- Demonstrate ability to self-administer insulin
- Demonstrate ability an understanding of lifestyle and dietary modifications necessary for successful maintenance of drug therapy
- Describe management of emergencies (hypoglycemia and hyperglycemia)

Implementation

Interventions (Rationales)	Client Education/Discharge Planning
■ Increase frequency of blood glucose monitoring if the client is experiencing fever, nausea, vomiting, or diarrhea. (Illness usually requires adjustments in insulin doses.)	■ Instruct client to increase blood glucose monitoring when experiencing fever, nausea, vomiting, or diarrhea.
■ Check urine for ketones if blood glucose is over 14 mmol/L. (Ketones will spill into the urine at this glucose level and provide an early sign of diabetic ketoacidosis.)	Teach client: ■ When and how to check urine for glucose and ketones ■ That ketoacidosis normally develops slowly but is a serious problem that needs to be corrected
■ Monitor weight on a routine basis. (Changes in weight will alter insulin needs.)	■ Instruct client to weigh self on a routine basis at the same time each day, and to report significant changes.
■ Monitor vital signs. (Increased pulse and blood pressure are early signs of hypoglycemia. Clients with diabetes may have circulatory problems and/or impaired kidney function that can increase blood pressure.)	■ Teach client how to take blood pressure and pulse and to report significant changes, such as the first sign of heart irregularity.

continued

MediaLink   Health Canada: Diabetes

MediaLink   Public Health Agency of Canada: Diabetes

NURSING PROCESS FOCUS Clients Receiving Insulin Therapy *(Continued)*	
Interventions (Rationales)	**Client Education/Discharge Planning**
■ Monitor potassium level. (Insulin causes potassium to move into the cell and may cause hypokalemia.) ■ Check blood glucose and feed client some form of simple sugar at the first sign of hypoglycemia. (Using a simple sugar will raise blood sugar immediately.)	■ Instruct client to report the first sign of heart irregularity. Advise client: ■ To check blood glucose and eat a simple sugar at the first sign of hypoglycemia; if symptoms do not improve, call 911 ■ Not to skip meals and to follow a diet specified by the healthcare provider ■ That exercise may increase insulin needs ■ To check blood glucose before and after exercise and to keep a simple sugar on their person while exercising ■ Before strenuous exercise, to eat some form of simple sugar or complex carbohydrate as a prophylaxis against hypoglycemia
Evaluation of Outcome Criteria	
Evaluate the effectiveness of drug therapy by confirming that client goals and expected outcomes have been met (see "Planning").	

See Table 40.2 for a list of drugs to which these nursing actions apply.

40.4 Etiology and Characteristics of Type 2 Diabetes Mellitus

There are a number of differences between type 1 and type 2 DM. Because type 2 DM usually begins in middle age, it has been referred to as maturity-onset diabetes. This is an inaccurate description of this disorder, however, because increasing numbers of children are being diagnosed with type 2 DM (see Lifespan Considerations: Pediatric Type 2 Diabetes). Approximately 90% of all diabetics are type 2. Adults and children who develop type 2 DM are most often overweight and sedentary. Aboriginal children are in a high-risk group for type 2 DM, perhaps because their diets are high in carbohydrates and fats and they may experience higher stress levels.

Unlike in type 1 DM, the pancreas in type 2 DM is capable of secreting insulin, although the amount may be deficient in some clients. The fundamental problem in **type 2 DM** is that insulin receptors in the target tissues have become insensitive to the hormone. This phenomenon is referred to as **insulin resistance**. Thus, the insulin secreted does not bind to its receptors as efficiently, and less effect is achieved.

Another important difference is that proper diet and exercise can sometimes increase the sensitivity of insulin receptors to the point that drug therapy is unnecessary for type 2 DM. Many clients with type 2 DM are obese and will need a medically supervised plan to reduce weight gradually and exercise safely. This is an important lifestyle change for such clients; they will need to maintain these changes for a lifetime. Clients with poorly managed type 2 DM often suffer from the same complications as clients with type 1 DM (e.g., retinopathy, neuropathy, and nephropathy).

ORAL ANTIHYPERGLYCEMICS

Type 2 DM is often controlled with oral antihyperglycemic agents, which are prescribed after diet and exercise have failed to reduce blood glucose to normal levels. Insulin may also be necessary for type 2 diabetics who are unable to take or are unresponsive to oral agents. Insulin is commonly required temporarily by type 2 diabetics at times of increased stress such as surgery, illness, or loss.

40.5 Pharmacotherapy with Oral Antihyperglycemics

All oral antihyperglycemics have the common action of lowering blood glucose levels when taken on a regular basis. Antihyperglycemics are sometimes referred to as oral hypoglycemics, although this term is less accurate because the goal of therapy is to lower glucose to normal levels, never to induce hypoglycemia. Many antihyperglycemics have the potential to cause hypoglycemia; thus, periodic laboratory tests are conducted to monitor blood glucose levels. Oral antihyperglycemics are not effective for type 1 DM. The oral antihyperglycemics are listed in Table 40.3.

Classification of oral antihyperglycemic drugs is based on their chemical structure and mechanism of action. The five classes of oral antihyperglycemic medications used for type 2 DM are sulfonylureas, biguanides, thiazolidinediones, alpha-glucosidase inhibitors, and meglitinides. Therapy is usually initiated with a single agent. If therapeutic goals are not achieved with monotherapy, two agents are administered concurrently. Failure to achieve normal blood glucose levels with two oral antihyperglycemics usually indicates a need for insulin.

Type 2 diabetics may be advised to maintain a preprandial blood glucose level at or just below 6.0 mmol/L. In healthy persons, the beta cells secrete insulin in response to small increases in blood glucose, which is referred to as an *acute insulin response*. This response is diminished at 6.4 mmol/L, and the higher the glucose level the less likely it is that the beta cells will respond by secreting insulin. Because

TABLE 40.3   Oral Antihyperglycemics

Drug	Route and Adult Dose
Alpha-Glucosidase Inhibitors	
acarbose (Glucobay)	PO; 25–100 mg tid (max 300 mg/d)
miglitol (Glyset)	PO; 25–100 mg tid (max 300 mg/d)
Biguanides	
metformin HCl (Glucophage)	PO; 500 mg qd–tid (max 3 g/d)
Meglitinides	
nateglinide (Starlix)	PO; 60–120 mg tid
repaglinide (Gluconorm)	PO; 0.5–4.0 mg bid–qid
Sulfonylureas, First Generation	
acetohexamide (Dimelor, Dymelor)	PO; 250 mg qd (max 1500 mg/d)
chlorpropamide (Apo-Chlorpropamide)	PO; 100–250 mg qd (max 750 mg/d)
tolazamide (Tolamide, Tolinase)	PO; 100–500 mg qd–bid (max 1 g/d)
tolbutamide (Apo-Tolbutamide)	PO; 250–1500 mg qd–bid (max 3 g/d)
Sulfonylureas, Second Generation	
glimepiride (Amaryl)	PO; 1–4 mg qd (max 8 mg/d)
glipizide (Glucotrol)	PO; 2.5–20 mg qd–bid (max 40 mg/d)
glyburide (Apo-Glyburide)	PO; 1.25–10 mg qd–bid (max 20 mg/d)
Thiazolidinediones	
pioglitazone (Actos)	PO; 15–30 mg qd (max 45 mg/d)
rosiglitazone (Avandia)	PO; 2–4 mg qd–bid (max 8 mg/d)
Combination Drugs	
glipizide/metformin (Metaglip)	PO; 2.5 mg/250 mg qd (max 10 mg glipizide and 2000 mg metformin/d)
glyburide/metformin (Glucovance)	PO; 1.25 mg/250 mg qd–bid (max 20 mg glyburide and 2000 mg metformin/d)
rosiglitazone/metformin (Avandamet)	PO; variable dose (max 8 mg rosiglitazone and 1000 mg metformin/d)

clients with type 2 diabetes need to secrete some insulin, keeping the blood glucose level below 6.0 mmol/L before meals optimizes secretion of insulin.

Clients with type 2 DM need to recognize the symptoms of **hyperosmolar non-ketotic coma (HNKC)**, which is a life-threatening emergency. As with the onset of diabetic ketoacidosis in those with type 1 DM, HNKC develops slowly and is caused by insufficient circulating insulin. It is seen most often in older adults. The skin appears flushed, dry, and warm, like in diabetic ketoacidosis. Unlike diabetic ketoacidosis, HNKC does not affect breathing. Blood glucose levels may rise over 50 mmol/L and reach 100 mmol/L. HNKC has a higher mortality rate than DKA.

Sulfonylureas The sulfonylureas were the first oral anti-hyperglycemics available, and they are divided into first and second generation categories. Although drugs from both generations are equally effective at lowering blood glucose, the second generation drugs exhibit fewer drug-drug interactions. The sulfonylureas act by stimulating the release of insulin from pancreatic islet cells and by increasing the sensitivity of insulin receptors on target cells. The most common adverse effect of sulfonylureas is hypoglycemia, which

is usually caused by taking too much medication or not eating enough food. Persistent hypoglycemia from these agents may be prolonged and require administration of dextrose to return glucose to normal levels. Other side effects include weight gain, hypersensitivity reactions, GI distress, and hepatotoxicity. When alcohol is taken with these agents, some clients experience a disulfiram-like reaction, with flushing, palpitations, and nausea.

Biguanides Metformin, the only drug in this class, acts by decreasing the hepatic production of glucose (gluconeogenesis) and reducing insulin resistance. It does not promote insulin release from the pancreas. Most side effects are minor and GI related, such as anorexia, nausea, and diarrhea. Unlike the sulfonylureas, metformin does not cause hypoglycemia or weight gain. Rarely, metformin has been reported to cause lactic acidosis in clients with impaired liver function, owing to accumulation of medication in the liver.

Alpha-Glucosidase Inhibitors The alpha-glucosidase inhibitors, such as acarbose, act by blocking enzymes in the small intestine responsible for breaking down complex carbohydrates into monosaccharides. Because carbohydrates must be in the monosaccharide form to be absorbed, digestion of glucose is delayed. These agents are usually well tolerated and have minimal side effects. The most common side effects are GI related, such as abdominal cramping, diarrhea, and flatulence. Liver function should be monitored as a small incidence of liver impairment has been reported. Although alpha-glucosidase inhibitors do not produce hypoglycemia when used alone, hypoglycemia may occur when these agents are combined with insulin or a sulfonylurea. Concurrent use of garlic and ginseng may increase the hypoglycemic action of alpha-glucosidase inhibitors.

Thiazolidinediones The thiazolidinediones, or glitazones, reduce blood glucose by decreasing insulin resistance and inhibiting hepatic gluconeogenesis. Optimal lowering of blood glucose may take 3 to 4 months of therapy. The most common adverse effects are fluid retention, headache, and weight gain. Hypoglycemia does not occur with drugs in this class. Liver function should be monitored because thiazolidinediones may be hepatotoxic. One such drug, troglitazone, was withdrawn from the market because of drug-related deaths due to hepatic failure. Because of their tendency to promote fluid retention, thiazolidinediones are contraindicated in clients with serious heart failure or pulmonary edema. Rosiglitazone has been associated with a significant increase in heart attack and cardiovascular death.

Meglitinides The meglitinides are a newer class of oral antihyperglycemic that act by stimulating the release of insulin from pancreatic islet cells in a manner similar to that of the sulfonylureas. Both agents in this class have a short a duration of action of 2–4 hours. Their efficacy is equal to that of the sulfonylureas, and they are well tolerated. Hypoglycemia is the most common adverse effect.

Newer Agents Several new drugs have been developed that act by affecting the incretin-glucose control mechanism. Incretins are hormones secreted by the intestine following a meal, when blood glucose is elevated. Incretins signal the pancreas to increase insulin secretion and the liver to stop producing glucagon. Both of these actions lower blood glucose levels. Diabetic clients are unable to secrete incretins in adequate amounts, thus disrupting an important glucose control mechanism. Drugs may be used to modify the incretin system in diabetics in two ways: by mimicking the actions of incretins, or by reducing their destruction.

Another class of agents is the dipeptidyl peptidase-4 (DPP-4) inhibitors. The normal function of the DDP-4 enzyme is to break down incretins. These agents inhibit DPP-4, thereby reducing the destruction of incretins. Levels of incretin hormones increase, thus decreasing blood glucose levels in clients with type 2 diabetes.

Pramlintide is a new injectable drug for type 1 and type 2 DM that resembles human amylin, a hormone produced by the pancreas after meals that helps the body regulate blood glucose. Pramlintide slows absorption of glucose and inhibits the action of glucagon. Pramlintide lowers blood glucose levels and promotes weight loss.

Sibutramine, a drug that blocks serotonin and norepinephrine reuptake, is approved in Canada for use as an antidiabetic agent. Sibutramine increases satiety, decreases food consumption, and promotes weight loss. Because various oral antihyperglycemics work by different mechanisms to lower blood sugar and have different pharmacokinetic properties, combinations of antidiabetic agents have been developed to maximize the therapeutic effects and minimize adverse effects. One such combination drug is glyburide/metformin. The nurse can monitor the Drug Product Information Database and MedEffect on Health Canada's website to identify drugs in these classes that have been approved, received warnings, or withdrawn from the market.

NURSING CONSIDERATIONS

The role of the nurse in oral antihyperglycemic therapy involves careful assessment and monitoring of the client's condition and providing education as it relates to the prescribed drug treatment. The assessment of the client with type 2 diabetes includes a physical examination, health history, psychosocial history, and lifestyle history. A thorough assessment is needed because diabetes can affect multiple body systems. Psychosocial factors and lifestyle, as well as the knowledge base regarding diabetes, can affect the client's ability to keep his or her blood glucose within the normal range. Lifestyle factors and health history help to determine the type of drug to be prescribed.

Provide clients with information about the importance of keeping blood glucose levels within the target range. Target blood levels are shown in Table 40.1. Blood glucose should be monitored daily. Urinary ketones should be monitored during periods of acute illness and when blood glucose is over 14.0 mmol/L. Urine ketone test strips remain the most commonly used method for ketone testing; however, this method may provide false positive or false negative results. Monitor intake and output and review lab studies for liver function abnormalities. Monitor the client for signs and symptoms of illness or infection as illness can affect the client's medication needs. These drugs should be used cautiously in those with impaired renal and hepatic function and in those who are malnourished because these conditions interfere with absorption and metabolism of the oral antihyperglycemics. Caution should be exercised in clients with pituitary or adrenal disorders due to hormones from these sources affecting blood glucose levels. Oral antihyperglycemics are contraindicated in hypersensitivity, ketoacidosis, and diabetic coma. They are also contraindicated in clients who are pregnant or lactating as safety has not been established and these drugs may be secreted in breast milk.

Oral antihyperglycemics should be taken as directed by the prescriber. Some oral antidiabetic drugs are given 30 minutes before breakfast so that the drug will have reached the plasma when the client begins to eat. Others such as acarbose and miglitol are given with each meal.

Client education as it relates to oral antihyperglycemic drugs should include goals, importance of diet and exercise, reasons for obtaining baseline data such as vital signs and cardiac and renal function tests, and the recognition of symptoms of hypoglycemia. Include the following points when teaching clients about oral antihyperglycemics:

- Always carry a source of simple sugar in case of hypoglycemic reactions. If blood glucose is less than 4 mmol/L, take a fast-acting carbohydrate (15 g glucose tablets, 1/2 cup orange juice). Repeat in 15 minutes if blood glucose levels are still less than 4 mmol/L. If there is more than 1 hour until the next meal, eat a snack of a starch and protein (cheese and 6 crackers, half of a peanut butter sandwich).

- Wear a MedicAlert bracelet to alert emergency personnel of the diabetes. Notify caregivers, co-workers, and others who may be able to render assistance.

- Avoid the use of alcohol to avoid a disulfiram-like reaction.

- Maintain a specified diet and exercise plan while on antidiabetic drugs.

- Swallow tablets whole and do not crush sustained-release tablets.

- Take medication 30 minutes before breakfast, or as directed by the healthcare provider.

- Immediately report nervousness, confusion, excessive sweating, rapid pulse, or tremors because these are signs of overdosage (hypoglycemia).

- Immediately report increased thirst or urine output, decreased appetite, or excessive fatigue because these are signs of underdosage (hyperglycemia).

LIFESPAN CONSIDERATIONS

Pediatric Type 2 Diabetes

The rapid rise in the incidence of type 2 DM in children is a growing concern for healthcare providers. The disease is reaching epidemic proportions, especially in certain ethnic groups such as Aboriginals and those of African, Hispanic, and Asian descent. Children who develop type 2 diabetes are most often overweight and sedentary. Although insulin and metformin are the two drugs commonly used for treating pediatric type 2 DM, other drugs are sometimes prescribed. Insulin is the most effective agent, although children often respond negatively to daily injections. Metformin has been shown to be safe and effective in children, although drugs from other classes may need to be added to the regimen over time. The guidelines for pharmacotherapy of pediatric type 2 DM will likely change as research determines the best therapies for this age group.

NATURAL THERAPIES

Stevia for Hyperglycemia

Stevia (*Stevia rebaudiana*) is an herb indigenous to Paraguay that may be helpful to diabetics. The powdered extract is readily available as a food supplement and can be used in place of sugar. Its sweetening power is 300 times that of sugar, but it does not appear to have a negative effect on blood glucose or insulin secretion. In animal experiments, stevia significantly elevated the glucose clearance, an effect that may be beneficial to diabetics. Encourage all diabetic clients to discuss this supplement and other herbal products with a healthcare provider before taking them.

Pr PROTOTYPE DRUG | Glyburide (Apo-Glyburide)

ACTIONS AND USES

Glyburide is a second generation sulfonylurea offering advantages of higher potency, once-a-day dosing, fewer side effects, and fewer drug-drug interactions than some of the first generation drugs in this class. Glyburide stimulates the pancreas to secrete more insulin and also increases the sensitivity of insulin receptors at target tissues. Some degree of pancreatic function is required for glyburide to lower blood glucose. Maximum effects are achieved if the drug is taken 30 minutes prior to the first meal of the day.

ADMINISTRATION ALERTS

- Sustained-release tablets must be swallowed whole and not crushed or chewed.
- Sulfonylureas, including glyburide, should not be given after the last meal of the day.
- Administer medication as directed by the healthcare provider.
- Glyburide is pregnancy category C.

PHARMACOKINETICS

Glyburide is well absorbed after oral administration. It is widely distributed and crosses the placenta. It is 99% plasma protein bound. It is metabolized by the liver. Its half-life is about 10 hours.

ADVERSE EFFECTS AND INTERACTIONS

Hypoglycemia is less frequent with glyburide than with first generation sulfonylureas. Elderly clients are prone to hypoglycemia because many have decreased renal and hepatic function, which can cause an increase in the amount of medication circulating in the blood. For this reason, elderly clients are often prescribed a reduced dosage.

Clients should stay out of direct sunlight since rashes and photosensitivity are possible. Some clients experience mild, GI-related effects such as nausea, vomiting, or loss of appetite. Glyburide and other sulfonylureas have the potential to interact with a number of drugs; thus, the client should always consult with a healthcare provider before adding a new medication or herbal supplement. Ingestion of alcohol will result in distressing symptoms that include headache, flushing, nausea, and abdominal cramping.

Glyburide interacts with several drugs. For example, there is a cross-sensitivity with sulfonamides and thiazide diuretics. Oral anticoagulants, chloramphenicol, clofibrate, and MAO inhibitors may potentiate the hypoglycemic actions of glyburide.

Use with caution with herbal supplements, such as ginseng and garlic, which may increase hypoglycemic effects.

NURSING PROCESS FOCUS	Clients Receiving Oral Antihyperglycemic Therapy

Assessment Data	Potential Nursing Diagnoses/Identified Patterns
Prior to administration: ■ Obtain complete health history including allergies, drug history, and possible drug interactions. ■ Assess for pain location and level. ■ Assess knowledge of drug. ■ Assess ability to conduct blood glucose testing.	■ Risk for impaired skin integrity and infection related to blood glucose elevations and impaired circulation ■ Need for knowledge regarding drug therapy ■ Need for knowledge regarding glucose testing ■ Risk for hypoglycemia related to adverse effects of drug therapy ■ Need for knowledge related to lifestyle and dietary modifications

Planning: Client Goals and Expected Outcomes

The client will:
■ Demonstrate an understanding of the drug's action by accurately describing drug side effects and precautions
■ Describe signs and symptoms that should be reported immediately, including nausea, diarrhea, jaundice, rash, headache, anorexia, abdominal pain, tachycardia, seizures, and confusion
■ Demonstrate an ability to accurately self-monitor blood glucose; maintain blood glucose within a normal range

Implementation

Interventions (Rationales)	Client Education/Discharge Planning
■ Monitor blood glucose at least daily and monitor urinary ketones if blood glucose is over 14 mmol/L. (Ketones will spill into the urine at high blood glucose levels and provide an early sign of diabetic ketoacidosis.)	■ Teach client how to monitor blood glucose and test urine for ketones, especially when ill.
■ Monitor for signs of lactic acidosis if client is receiving a biguanide. (Mitochondrial oxidation of lactic acid is inhibited, and lactic acidosis may result.)	■ Instruct client to report signs of lactic acidosis such as hyperventilation, muscle pain, fatigue, increased sleeping.
■ Review lab tests for any abnormalities in liver function. (These drugs are metabolized in the liver and may cause elevations in AST and LDH. Metformin decreases absorption of vitamin B_{12} and folic acid, which may result in deficiencies of these substances.)	■ Instruct client to report the first sign of yellow skin, pale stools, or dark urine.
■ Obtain accurate history of alcohol use, especially if client is receiving a sulfonylurea or biguanide. (These drugs may cause a didulfiram-like reaction.)	■ Advise client to abstain from alcohol and to avoid liquid OTC medications, which may contain alcohol.
■ Monitor for signs and symptoms of increased stress, illness or infection. (These symptoms may increase blood glucose levels.)	■ Instruct client to report the first signs of fatigue, muscle weakness, and nausea. ■ Discuss importance of adequate rest and healthy routines.
■ Monitor blood glucose frequently, especially at the beginning of therapy and in elderly clients. ■ Monitor clients carefully who also take a beta-blocker because early signs of hypoglycemia may not be apparent.	Teach client: ■ Signs and symptoms of hypoglycemia, such as hunger, irritability, sweating ■ At first sign of hypoglycemia, to check blood glucose and eat a simple sugar; if symptoms do not improve, call 911 ■ To monitor blood glucose before breakfast and supper ■ Not to skip meals and to follow a diet specified by the healthcare provider
■ Monitor weight, weighing at the same time of day each time. (Changes in weight will impact the amount of drug needed to control blood glucose.)	■ Instruct client to weigh each week, at the same time of day, and report any significant loss or gain.
■ Monitor vital signs. (Increased pulse and blood pressure are early signs of hypoglycemia.)	■ Teach client how to take accurate blood pressure, temperature, and pulse.
■ Monitor skin for rashes and itching. (These are signs of an allergic reaction to the drug.)	■ Advise client of the importance of immediately reporting skin rashes and itching that is unaccounted for by dry skin.
■ Monitor activity level. (Dose may require adjustment with change in physical activity.)	■ Advise client to increase activity level, which will help lower blood glucose. ■ Advise client to closely monitor blood glucose when involved in vigorous physical activity.

Evaluation of Outcome Criteria

Evaluate the effectiveness of drug therapy by confirming that client goals and expected outcomes have been met (see "Planning").

See Table 40.3 for a list of drugs to which these nursing actions apply.

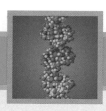

CHAPTER REVIEW

KEY CONCEPTS

The numbered key concepts provide a succinct summary of the important points from the corresponding numbered section within the chapter. If any of these points are not clear, refer to the numbered section within the chapter for review. Expanded versions can be found on the Companion Website.

40.1 The pancreas is both an endocrine and an exocrine gland. Insulin is released when blood glucose increases, and glucagon is released when blood glucose decreases.

40.2 Type 1 diabetes mellitus (DM) is caused by a lack of insulin secretion and is characterized by serious, chronic conditions affecting the cardiovascular and nervous systems.

40.3 Type 1 DM is treated by dietary restrictions, exercise, and insulin injections. The many types of insulin preparations

vary as to their onset of action, time to peak effect, and duration.

40.4 Type 2 DM is caused by a lack of sensitivity of insulin receptors at the target cells and a deficiency in insulin secretion. If untreated, the same chronic conditions result as in type 1 DM.

40.5 Type 2 DM is controlled through lifestyle changes and oral antihyperglycemic drugs.

REVIEW QUESTIONS

1 What are the major differences between types 1 and 2 DM?

2 Why are oral antihyperglycemic drugs ineffective at treating type 1 DM?

3 What nursing actions help to prevent lipodystrophy in diabetic clients?

CRITICAL THINKING QUESTIONS

1. A 28-year-old woman who is pregnant with her first child is diagnosed with gestational DM. She is concerned about the fact that she might have to take "shots." She tells the nurse at the public health clinic that she doesn't think she can self-administer an injection and asks if there is a pill that will control her blood sugar. She has heard her grandfather talk about his pills to control his "sugar." What should the nurse explain to this client?

2. When reviewing a client's insulin administration record, the nurse notes that the client is routinely rotating injection sites from arm to leg to abdomen. The nurse also notes that the client continues to have fluctuations in his blood

glucose levels despite receiving the same amount of insulin. What factors may be influencing the blood glucose fluctuations? What does the nurse need to explain to this client about site rotation?

3. A 16-year-old Aboriginal boy is newly diagnosed with type 2 diabetes. Discuss some of the risk factors for diabetes in this population. What treatment options are available for children? Develop a culturally sensitive teaching plan for this boy and his parents. Health Canada has a webpage specifically designed for Aboriginal Peoples with diabetes. What other resources may provide useful information for you (nurse) and your clients?

EXPLORE

MediaLink

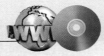

www.pearsoned.ca/adams-king

 MEDIALINK DVD-ROM
- Audio Glossary
- CRNE Review
- Animation
  Mechanism of Action: Glipizide

COMPANION WEBSITE
- CRNE Review
- Dosage Calculations
- **Case Study:** Diabetes and insulin

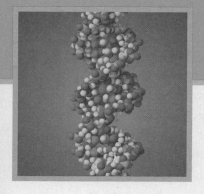

CHAPTER 41

Drugs for Disorders and Conditions of the Female Reproductive System

DRUGS AT A GLANCE

ORAL CONTRACEPTIVES

Estrogen-progestin combinations

> *ethinyl estradiol with norethindrone (Ortho-Novum 1/35)*

Progestin-only agents

DRUGS FOR EMERGENCY CONTRACEPTION AND PHARMACOLOGICAL ABORTION

HORMONE REPLACEMENT THERAPY

Estrogens and estrogen/ progestin combinations

> *conjugated estrogens (Premarin) and conjugated estrogens with medroxyprogesterone (Premplus)*

DRUGS FOR DYSFUNCTIONAL UTERINE BLEEDING

Progestins

> *medroxyprogesterone (Provera, Cycrin)*

UTERINE STIMULANTS AND RELAXANTS

Oxytocics (stimulants)

> *oxytocin (Syntocinon)*

Ergot alkaloids

Prostaglandins

Tocolytics (relaxants)

Beta₂-adrenergic agonists

Other tocolytics

DRUGS FOR FEMALE INFERTILITY AND ENDOMETRIOSIS

OBJECTIVES

After reading this chapter, the student should be able to do the following:

1. Describe the roles of the hypothalamus, pituitary, and ovaries in maintaining female reproductive function.
2. Explain the mechanisms by which estrogens and progestins prevent conception.
3. Explain how drugs may be used to provide emergency contraception and to terminate early pregnancy.
4. Describe the role of drug therapy in the treatment of menopausal and postmenopausal symptoms.
5. Identify the role of the female sex hormones in the treatment of cancer.
6. Discuss the uses of progestins in the therapy of dysfunctional uterine bleeding.
7. Compare and contrast the use of uterine stimulants and relaxants in the treatment of antepartum and postpartum clients.
8. Explain how drug therapy may be used to treat female infertility.
9. For each of the drug classes listed in Drugs at a Glance, identify a representative drug and explain its mechanism of action, therapeutic effects, and important adverse effects.
10. Describe and explain, based on pharmacological principles, the rationale for nursing assessment, planning, and interventions for clients with conditions of the female reproductive system.
11. Use the nursing process to care for clients who are receiving drug therapy for disorders and conditions of the female reproductive system.

MediaLink

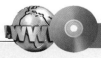 www.pearsoned.ca/adams-king

CRNE review, case studies, and other interactive resources for this chapter can be found on the Companion Website at **www.pearsoned.ca/adams-king**. Click on "Chapter 41" to select the activities for this chapter. For animations, more CRNE review questions, and an audio glossary, access the accompanying DVD-ROM in this textbook.

Hormones from the pituitary gland and gonads provide for the growth and maintenance of the female reproductive organs. Endogenous hormones can be supplemented with natural or synthetic hormones to achieve a variety of therapeutic goals, ranging from replacement therapy, to prevention of pregnancy, to milk production. This chapter examines drugs used to treat disorders and conditions associated with the female reproductive system.

41.1 Hypothalamic and Pituitary Regulation of Female Reproductive Function

Regulation of the female reproductive system is achieved by hormones from the hypothalamus, pituitary gland, and ovary. The hypothalamus secretes **gonadotropin-releasing hormone (GnRH)**, which travels a short distance to the pituitary to stimulate the secretion of **follicle-stimulating hormone (FSH)** and **luteinizing hormone (LH)**. Both of these pituitary hormones act on the ovary and cause immature ovarian follicles to begin developing. The rising and falling levels of pituitary hormones create two interrelated cycles that occur on a periodic, monthly basis—the ovarian and uterine cycles. The hormonal changes that occur during the ovarian and uterine cycles are illustrated in Figure 41.1.

Under the influence of FSH and LH, several ovarian follicles begin the maturation process each month during a woman's reproductive years. On approximately day 14 of the ovarian cycle, a surge of LH secretion causes one follicle to expel its oocyte, a process called **ovulation**. The ruptured follicle, minus its oocyte, remains in the ovary and is transformed into the hormone-secreting **corpus luteum**. The oocyte, on the other hand, begins its journey through the fallopian tube and eventually reaches the uterus. If conception does not occur, the outer lining of the uterus degenerates and is shed during menstruation.

41.2 Ovarian Control of Female Reproductive Function

As ovarian follicles mature they secrete the female sex hormones **estrogen** and **progesterone**. Estrogen is actually a generic term for three different hormones: estradiol, estrone, and estriol. Estrogen is responsible for the maturation of the female reproductive organs and for the appearance of the secondary sex

PHARMFACTS

Female Reproductive Conditions

- There is a wide range of ages when women reach menopause: 8 of 100 women will stop menstruating before age 40, and 5 of 100 women will continue menstruating beyond age 60.
- About half of the cases of dysfunctional uterine bleeding are diagnosed in women over 45 years of age; however, 20% of cases occur under the age of 20.
- The most common reason why a woman may become pregnant while on oral contraceptives is skipping a dose.
- A non-smoking woman aged 25 to 29 has a 2 in 100,000 chance of dying from complications due to oral contraceptives. The risk of a woman in this age group dying in an automobile accident is 74 in 100,000.
- Oral contraceptives have more benefits than just contraception. It is estimated that each year they prevent the following:
  - 51,000 cases of pelvic inflammatory disease
  - 9,900 hospitalizations for ectopic pregnancy
  - 27,000 cases of iron deficiency anemia
  - 20,000 hospitalizations for certain types of non-malignant breast disease

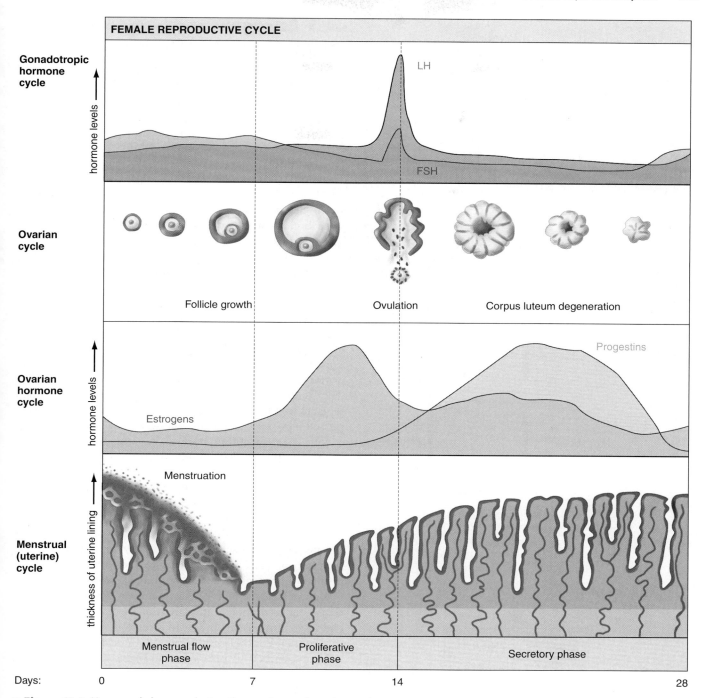

● **Figure 41.1** Hormonal changes during the ovarian and uterine cycles

Source: Pearson Education/PH College.

characteristics. In addition, estrogen has numerous metabolic effects on non-reproductive tissues, including the brain, kidneys, blood vessels, and skin. For example, estrogen helps to maintain low blood cholesterol levels and facilitates calcium uptake by bones to help maintain proper bone density (see Chapter 46). When women enter menopause at about age 50 to 55, the ovaries stop secreting estrogen.

In the last half of the ovarian cycle, the corpus luteum secretes a class of hormones called progestins, the most abundant of which is progesterone. In combination with estrogen, progesterone promotes breast development and regulates the monthly changes of the uterine cycle. Under the influence of estrogen and progesterone, the uterine endometrium becomes vascular and thickens in preparation for receiving a fertilized egg. High progesterone and estrogen levels in the final third of the uterine cycle provide negative feedback to shut off GnRH, FSH, and LH secretion. This negative feedback loop is illustrated in Figure 41.2. Without stimulation from FSH and LH, estrogen and progesterone levels fall sharply, the endometrium is shed, and menstrual bleeding begins.

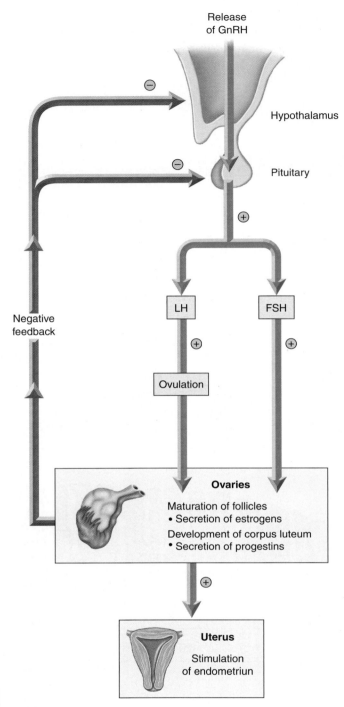

● **Figure 41.2** Negative feedback control of the female reproductive hormones

CONTRACEPTION

ORAL CONTRACEPTIVES

Oral contraceptives are drugs used to prevent pregnancy. Most oral contraceptives are a combination of estrogens and progestins. In small doses, they prevent fertilization by inhibiting ovulation. Select oral contraceptives are shown in Table 41.1.

41.3 Estrogens and Progestins as Oral Contraceptives

The most widespread pharmacological use of the female sex hormones is to prevent pregnancy. When used appropriately, they are nearly 100% effective. Most oral contraceptives contain a combination of estrogen and progestin; a few preparations contain only progestin. The most common estrogen used for contraception is ethinyl estradiol, and the most common progestin is norethindrone.

A large number of oral contraceptive preparations are available, differing in dose and type of estrogen and progestin. Selection of a specific formulation is individualized to each client and is determined by which drug gives the best contraceptive protection with the fewest side effects. Daily doses of estrogen in oral contraceptives have declined from 150 μg, 40 years ago, to about 35 μg in modern formulations. This reduction has resulted in a decrease in estrogen-related adverse effects.

Typically, drug administration of an oral contraceptive begins on day 5 of the ovarian cycle and continues for 21 days. During the other 7 days of the month, the client takes a placebo. While the placebo serves no pharmacological purpose, it does encourage the client to take the pills on a daily basis. Some of these placebos contain iron, which replaces iron lost from menstrual bleeding. If a daily dose is missed, two pills taken the following day usually provide adequate contraception. If more than one day is missed, the client should observe other contraceptive precautions, such as using condoms, until the oral contraceptive doses can be resumed at the beginning of the next monthly cycle. Figure 41.3 shows a typical monthly oral contraceptive packet with the 28 pills.

The estrogen-progestin oral contraceptives act by providing negative feedback to the pituitary to shut down the secretion of LH and FSH. Without the influence of these pituitary hormones, the ovarian follicle cannot mature and ovulation is prevented. The estrogen-progestin agents also reduce the likelihood of implantation by making the uterine endometrium less favourable to receive an embryo. In addition to their contraceptive function, these agents are sometimes prescribed to promote timely and regular monthly cycles and to reduce the incidence of dysmenorrhea.

The three types of estrogen-progestin formulations are monophasic, biphasic, and triphasic. The most common is monophasic, which delivers a constant amount of estrogen and progestin throughout the menstrual cycle. In biphasic agents, the amount of estrogen in each pill remains constant, but the amount of progestin is increased toward the end of the menstrual cycle to better nourish the uterine lining. In triphasic formulations, the amounts of both estrogen and progestin vary in three distinct phases during the 28-day cycle.

The progestin-only oral contraceptives, sometimes called minipills, prevent pregnancy primarily by producing thick, viscous mucus at the entrance to the uterus that discourages penetration by sperm. They also tend to inhibit implantation of a fertilized egg. Minipills are less effective than estrogen-

TABLE 41.1   Select Oral Contraceptives

Trade Name	Type	Estrogen	Progestin
Alesse	monophasic	ethinyl estradiol; 20 μg	levonorgestrel; 0.1 mg
Desogen	monophasic	ethinyl estradiol; 30 μg	desogestrel; 0.15 mg
Loestrin 1.5/30 Fe	monophasic	ethinyl estradiol; 30 μg	norethindrone; 1.5 mg
Lo/Ovral	monophasic	ethinyl estradiol; 30 μg	norgestrel; 0.3 mg
Ortho-Cyclen	monophasic	ethinyl estradiol; 35 μg	norgestimate; 0.25 mg
Yasmin	monophasic	ethinyl estradiol; 30 μg	drospirenone; 3 mg
Ortho-Novum 10/11	biphasic	ethinyl estradiol; 35 μg	norethindrone; 0.5 mg (phase 1)
		ethinyl estradiol; 35 μg	norethindrone; 1.0 mg (phase 2)
Ortho-Novum 7/7/7	triphasic	ethinyl estradiol; 35 μg	norethindrone; 0.5 mg (phase 1)
		ethinyl estradiol; 35 μg	norethindrone; 0.75 mg (phase 2)
		ethinyl estradiol; 35 μg	norethindrone; 1.0 mg (phase 3)
Ortho Tri-Cyclen	triphasic	ethinyl estradiol; 35 μg	norgestimate; 0.5 mg (phase 1)
		ethinyl estradiol; 35 μg	norgestimate; 0.75 mg (phase 2)
		ethinyl estradiol; 35 μg	norgestimate; 1.0 mg (phase 3)
Tri-Levlen	triphasic	ethinyl estradiol; 35 μg	levonorgestrel; 0.05 mg (phase 1)
		ethinyl estradiol; 40 μg	levonorgestrel; 0.075 mg (phase 2)
		ethinyl estradiol; 30 μg	levonorgestrel; 0.125 mg (phase 3)
Triphasil	triphasic	ethinyl estradiol; 30 μg	norgestrel; 0.05 mg (phase 1)
		ethinyl estradiol; 40 μg	norgestrel; 0.075 mg (phase 2)
		ethinyl estradiol; 30 μg	norgestrel; 1.25 mg (phase 3)
Micronor	progestin only	none	norethindrone; 0.35 mg
Nor-Q.D.	progestin only	none	norethindrone; 0.35 mg
Ovrette	progestin only	none	norgestrel; 0.075 mg

progestin combinations, having a failure rate of 1% to 4%. Their use also results in a higher incidence of menstrual irregularities such as amenorrhea, prolonged bleeding, and breakthrough spotting. They are generally reserved for clients who are at high risk of side effects from estrogen.

Several long-term formulations of oral contraceptives are available. A deep IM injection of medroxyprogesterone acetate (Depo-Provera) provides 3 months of contraceptive protection. Ortho-Evra is a transdermal patch containing ethinyl estradiol and norelgestromin that is worn on the skin. The patch is changed every 7 days for the first 3 weeks, followed by no patch during week 4. NovaRing is a small ring containing estrogen and progestin that is inserted into the vagina to provide 3 weeks of contraceptive protection. The ring is removed during week 4, and a new ring is inserted during the first week of the next menstrual cycle. Merena consists of a polyethylene cylinder that is placed in the uterus and releases levonorgestrel. This drug acts locally to prevent conception over 5 years. The efficacy of these long-term formulations is similar to that of oral contraceptives. They offer a major advantage for women who are likely to forget their daily pill or who prefer greater ease of use.

The "extended regimen" oral contraceptives are newer contraceptive drugs. Seasonale consists of tablets containing levonorgestrel and ethinyl estradiol that are taken for 84 consecutive days, followed by 7 inert tablets (without hormones). This allows for continuous contraceptive protection while extending the time between menses; only four periods are experienced per year. Seasonique is similar, but instead of inert tablets for 7 days, the client takes low-dose estrogen tablets. Seasonique is claimed by the manufacturer to have a lower incidence of bloating and breakthrough bleeding.

Although oral contraceptives are safe for the large majority of women, there are some potentially serious adverse effects. As with other medications, the higher the dose of estrogen or progesterone, the more likely the risk of side effects. With oral contraceptives, however, some side effects are more prominent at *lower* doses. Thus, physicians try to prescribe the oral contraceptive with the lowest dose of hormones that will achieve the therapeutic goal of pregnancy prevention with minimal side effects.

Numerous drug-drug interactions are possible with estrogen and with progesterone. Several anticonvulsants and antibiotics can reduce the effectiveness of oral contraceptives, thus increasing a woman's risk of pregnancy. Because oral contraceptives can reduce the effectiveness of warfarin, insulin, and certain oral antihyperglycemic agents, dosage adjustment may be necessary.

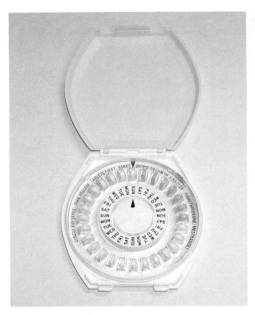

● **Figure 41.3** An oral contraceptive packet showing the daily doses and the different formulation taken in the last 7 days of the 28-day cycle

The risk of cancer following long-term oral contraceptive use has been extensively studied. Because some studies have shown a small increase in breast cancer incidence, oral contraceptives are contraindicated in clients with known or suspected breast cancer. The incidences of endometrial cancer and ovarian cancer, however, are significantly reduced

after long-term oral contraceptive administration. It is likely that the relationship between the long-term use of these drugs and cancer will continue to be a controversial and frequently researched topic.

NURSING CONSIDERATIONS

The role of the nurse in oral contraceptive therapy involves careful monitoring of the client's condition and providing education as it relates to the prescribed drug treatment. Oral contraception is the most effective form of birth control, and there are many products available. Oral contraception is contraindicated for women with a history of stroke, MI, coronary artery disease, thromboembolic disorders, or estrogen-dependent tumours because of increases in estrogen levels and risk of thrombus formation. Assess for pregnancy before initiating oral contraceptive therapy. Obtain a complete health history including personal and family history of breast cancer, liver tumours, and hemorrhagic disorders because these conditions are contraindications to the use of oral contraceptives. Risks and adverse effects are greater for women who smoke and are older than 35 years of age. Oral contraceptives should be used with caution in clients with hypertension, deep vein thrombosis, cardiac or renal disease, liver dysfunction, diabetes, gallbladder disease, and a history of depression.

Blood pressure should be monitored as oral contraceptives can cause mild to moderate hypertension. Monitor for symptoms of thrombophlebitis, such as pain, redness, and tenderness of the calves. Oral contraceptives can mimic cer-

---

Pr PROTOTYPE DRUG | Ethinyl Estradiol with Norethindrone (Ortho-Novum 1/35)

ACTIONS AND USES

Ortho-Novum is typical of the monophasic oral contraceptives, containing fixed amounts of estrogen (0.035 mg) and progesterone (1 mg) for 21 days followed by placebo tablets for 7 days. It is nearly 100% effective at preventing conception. Ortho-Novum is also available in biphasic and triphasic preparations. All preparations prevent ovulation by negative feedback control targeted at the hypothalamic-pituitary axis. When the right combination of estrogens and progestins is present in the bloodstream, the release of FSH and LH is inhibited, thus preventing ovulation. Non-contraceptive benefits of Ortho-Novum include improvement in menstrual cycle regularity and decreased incidence of dysmenorrhea.

PHARMACOKINETICS

Estradiol is well absorbed after oral administration. It is widely distributed, crosses the placenta and enters breast milk. It is metabolized by the liver. Its half-life is unknown.

ADMINISTRATION ALERTS

- Tablets must be taken exactly as directed.
- If dose is missed, take as soon as remembered, or take two tablets the next day.
- Ethinyl estradiol with norethindrone is pregnancy category X.

ADVERSE EFFECTS AND INTERACTIONS

Common side effects include edema, unexplained loss of vision, diplopia, intolerance to contact lenses, gallbladder disease, nausea, abdominal cramps, changes in urinary function, dysmenorrhea, breast fullness, fatigue, skin rash, acne, headache, weight gain, mid-cycle breakthrough bleeding, vaginal candidiasis, photosensitivity, and changes in urinary patterns. Cardiovascular side effects may include hypertension and thromboembolic disorders.

Ethinyl estradiol interacts with many drugs. For example, rifampin, some antibiotics, barbiturates, anticonvulsants, and antifungals decrease the efficacy of oral contraceptives, so increased risk of breakthrough bleeding and increased risk of pregnancy may occur. Ortho-Novum may also decrease the effects of oral anticoagulants.

Use with caution with herbal supplements. For example, breakthrough bleeding has been reported with concurrent use of St. John's wort.

 See the Companion Website for a Nursing Process Focus chart specific to this drug.

tain symptoms of pregnancy, including breast tenderness, nausea, bloating, and chloasma. Reassure the client that these side effects do not indicate pregnancy. Oral contraceptives may increase the risk of certain types of breast cancer; therefore, teach clients how to perform breast self-exams and provide information on the routine scheduling of mammograms appropriate for their age bracket.

Client education as it relates to oral contraceptives should include goals, reasons for baseline assessment of vital signs and cardiovascular status, and possible drug side effects. Include the following points when teaching the client about oral contraceptives:

- Take medications as directed by the healthcare provider.
- Follow instructions for missed doses.
- Immediately report calf pain or redness, dyspnea, and chest pain.
- Monitor blood pressure regularly and report elevations.

- Avoid smoking.
- Perform monthly self-examination of breasts.
- Seek professional help if symptoms of depression occur.

See "Nursing Process Focus: Clients Receiving Oral Contraceptive Therapy" for specific teaching points.

EMERGENCY CONTRACEPTION AND PHARMACOLOGICAL ABORTION

Emergency contraception is the prevention of implantation following unprotected intercourse. Pharmacological abortion is the removal of an embryo by the use of drugs, after implantation has occurred. The treatment goal is to provide effective, immediate prevention or termination of pregnancy. Agents used for these purposes are shown in Table 41.2.

MediaLink Mechanism of Action: Ortho-Novum

NURSING PROCESS FOCUS   Clients Receiving Oral Contraceptive Therapy

Assessment	Potential Nursing Diagnoses/Identified Patterns
Prior to administration: ■ Obtain health history including cigarette smoking and personal/family history of breast cancer. ■ Obtain drug history to determine possible drug interactions and allergies. ■ Assess cardiovascular status including hypertension, history of MI, CVA, and thromboembolic disease. ■ Determine if client is pregnant or lactating.	■ Risk for fluid and electrolyte imbalance ■ Need for knowledge regarding drug therapy and adverse effects ■ Need for knowledge regarding importance of adherence to dosing schedule and management of a missed dose

Planning: Client Goals and Expected Outcomes

The client will:
- Report effective birth control
- Demonstrate an understanding of the drug's action by accurately describing drug side effects and precautions
- Take medication exactly as ordered to prevent pregnancy
- Immediately report effects such as symptoms of thrombophlebitis, difficulty breathing, visual disturbances, and severe headache

Implementation

Interventions (Rationales)	Client Education/Discharge Planning
■ Monitor for the development of breast or other estrogen-dependent tumours. (Estrogen may cause tumour growth or proliferation.)	■ Instruct client to immediately report if first-degree relative is diagnosed with any estrogen-dependent tumour.
■ Monitor for thrombophlebitis or other thromboembolic disease. (Estrogen predisposes to thromboembolic disorders by increasing levels of clotting factors.)	■ Instruct client to immediately report pain in calves, limited movement in legs, dyspnea, sudden severe chest pain, headache, seizures, anxiety, or fear.
■ Monitor for cardiac disorders and hypertension. (These drugs increase blood levels of angiotensin and aldosterone, which increases blood pressure.)	Instruct client to: ■ Report immediately signs of possible cardiac problems such as chest pain, dyspnea, edema, tachycardia or bradycardia, and palpitations ■ Monitor blood pressure regularly ■ Report symptoms of hypertension such as headache, flushing, fatigue, dizziness, palpitations, tachycardia, nosebleeds
■ Encourage client not to smoke. (Smoking increases risk of thromboembolic disease.)	Instruct client to: ■ Be aware that the combination of oral contraceptives and smoking greatly increases risk of cardiovascular disease, especially MI ■ Be aware that the risk increases with age (>35) and with number of cigarettes smoked (15 or more/day)

continued

NURSING PROCESS FOCUS   Clients Receiving Oral Contraceptive Therapy   *(Continued)*

Interventions (Rationales)	Client Education/Discharge Planning
■ Monitor blood and urine glucose levels. (These drugs increase serum glucose levels.) ■ Monitor client's knowledge level of proper administration. (Incorrect use may lead to pregnancy.) ■ Encourage compliance with follow-up treatment. (Follow-up is necessary to avoid serious adverse effects.)	■ Instruct client to monitor urine and blood glucose regularly and contact healthcare provider if hyperglycemia or hypoglycemia occur. Instruct client to: ■ Discontinue medication and notify healthcare provider if significant bleeding occurs at mid-cycle ■ Take missed dose as soon as remembered or take two tablets the next day. Use an alternate form of contraception for the remainder of the cycle. If three consecutive tablets are missed, begin a new compact of tablets, starting 7 days after last tablet was taken ■ Contact healthcare provider if two consecutive periods are missed, as pregnancy may have occurred Instruct client to: ■ Schedule annual Pap smears ■ Perform self-breast exams monthly and obtain routine mammograms as recommended by the healthcare provider
Evaluation of Outcome Criteria	
Evaluate the effectiveness of drug therapy by confirming that client goals and expected outcomes have been met (see "Planning").	

See Table 41.1 (page 587) for a list of drugs to which these nursing actions apply.

41.4 Drugs for Emergency Contraception and Termination of Early Pregnancy

Over half of pregnancies in North America are unplanned. Some of these occur due to the inconsistent use or failure of contraceptive devices; even oral contraceptives have a failure rate of 0.3% to 1%. Emergency contraception following unprotected intercourse offers a means of protecting against unwanted pregnancies. The goal is to prevent implantation of a fertilized ovum.

Emergency contraception can be accomplished pharmacologically by the administration of various doses and combinations of estrogen and progestins. These drugs should be administered as soon as possible after unprotected intercourse; if taken more than 72 hours later, they become less effective. After 7 days, they are no longer effective. When used this way, these drugs act by preventing ovulation or implantation; they do not induce abortion. Taking 0.75 mg of levonorgestrel in two doses, 12 hours apart, has been shown to prevent conception. A combination of ethinyl estradiol and levonorgestrel is also effective, though nausea and vomiting are common and an antiemetic drug may be indicated to reduce these unpleasant side effects.

Once the ovum has been fertilized, several pharmacological choices are available to terminate the pregnancy. A single dose of mifepristone followed 36 to 48 hours later

TABLE 41.2 Agents for Emergency Contraception and Pharmacological Abortion	
Drug	**Route and Adult Dose**
Agents for Emergency Contraception	
ethinyl estradiol (Estinyl, Feminore)	PO; 5 mg/d for 5 consecutive days beginning within 72 h of intercourse
ethinyl estradiol and levonorgestrel (Preven)	PO; 1 tablet (0.25 mg levonorgestrel and 0.05 mg ethinyl estradiol) taken as soon as possible but within 72 h of unprotected intercourse, followed by two pills 12 h later
levonorgestrel	PO; 2 tablets within 72 h of unprotected intercourse, 2 tablets 12 h later
Agents for Pharmacological Abortion	
carboprost tromethamine (Hemabate)	IM; initial: 250 µg (1 mL) repeated at 1.5- to 3.5-hour intervals if indicated by uterine response; dosage may be increased to 500 µg (2 mL) if uterine contractility is inadequate after several doses of 250 µg (1 mL); not to exceed total dose of 12 mg or continuous administration for more than 2 d
dinoprostone (Cervidil, Prepidil, Prostin E_2)	Intravaginal; insert suppository high in vagina, repeat q2–5h until abortion occurs or membranes rupture (max total dose 240 mg)
methotrexate with misoprostol	IM; methotrexate (50 mg/m^2) followed 5 days later by intravaginal 800 µg of misoprostol
mifepristone (Mifeprix) with misoprostol	PO; day one: 600 mg of mifepristone; day three (if abortion has not occurred): 400 µg of misoprostol

by a single dose of misoprostol is a frequently used treatment. Mifepristone is a synthetic steroid that blocks progesterone receptors in the uterus. If given within 3 days of intercourse, mifepristone alone is almost 100% effective at preventing pregnancy. Given up to 9 weeks after conception, mifepristone aborts the implanted embryo. Misoprostol is a prostaglandin that causes uterine contractions, thus increasing the effectiveness of the pharmacological abortion.

Although mifepristone-misoprostol should never be substituted for effective means of contraception, such as oral contraceptives, these medications do offer women a safer alternative to surgical abortion. The primary adverse effect is cramping that occurs soon after taking misoprostol. The most serious adverse effect is prolonged bleeding, which may continue for 1 to 2 weeks after dosing.

A few other agents may be used to promote pharmacological abortion. Methotrexate, an antineoplastic agent, combined with intravaginal misoprostol usually induces abortion within 24 hours. The prostaglandins carboprost and dinoprostone induce strong uterine contractions that can expel an implanted embryo up to the second trimester.

MENOPAUSE

Menopause is characterized by a progressive decrease in estrogen secretion by the ovaries, resulting in the permanent cessation of menses. Menopause is neither a disease nor a disorder but is a natural consequence of aging that is often accompanied by a number of unpleasant symptoms. Some of these symptoms respond well to pharmacotherapy.

41.5 Hormone Replacement Therapy

Over the past 30 years, healthcare providers have commonly prescribed hormone replacement therapy to treat unpleasant symptoms of menopause and to prevent the long-term consequences of estrogen loss listed in Table 41.3. Select estrogens and progestins and their dosages are shown in Table 41.4

Hormone replacement therapy (HRT) refers to replacement of both estrogen and progesterone, whereas **estrogen replacement therapy (ERT)** refers to the replacement of estrogen alone. In 2002, the results of a large clinical study by the Women's Health Initiative (WHI) regarding the effects of HRT and ERT were analyzed. Data from the WHI research suggest that clients receiving HRT (Premplus) experienced a small, though significant, increased risk of serious adverse effects such as coronary artery disease, stroke, breast cancer, dementia, and venous thromboembolism. The risks were higher in women older than age 60; women aged 50 to 59 actually experienced a slight *decrease* in cardiovascular side effects. The potential adverse effects documented in the WHI study, and others, were significant enough to suggest that the potential benefits of long-term HRT may not outweigh the risks for many women. However, the results of this study remain controversial.

Women in the WHI study who took estrogen alone (Premarin) experienced a slightly increased risk of stroke, but no increased risk of breast cancer or heart disease. Estrogen has been shown to prevent osteoporosis and reduce incidence of fractures. The use of estrogen alone (ERT) is considered appropriate only for women who have had hysterectomies since it increases the risk of uterine cancer.

Although there is consensus that HRT does offer relief from immediate, distressing menopausal symptoms, as of 2008, it was recommended that women *not* undergo HRT to prevent coronary heart disease. In addition, although HRT appears to prevent osteoporotic bone fractures, women are encouraged to discuss alternatives with their healthcare provider. Undoubtedly, research will continue to provide valuable information on the long-term effects of HRT. Until then, the choice of HRT to treat menopausal symptoms remains a highly individualized one, between the client and her healthcare provider.

In addition to their use in treating menopausal symptoms, estrogens are used for female hypogonadism, primary

TABLE 41.3	Potential Consequences of Estrogen Loss Related to Menopause
Stage	**Symptoms/Conditions**
early menopause	mood disturbances, depression, irritability
	insomnia
	hot flashes
	irregular menstrual cycles
	headaches
mid-menopause	vaginal atrophy, increased infections, painful intercourse
	skin atrophy
	stress urinary incontinence
	sexual disinterest
postmenopause	cardiovascular disease
	osteoporosis
	Alzheimer's-like dementia
	colon cancer

TABLE 41.4 Select Estrogens and Progestins

Drug	Route and Adult Dose
Estrogens	
estradiol (Estraderm, Estrace)	PO; 1–2 mg qd
estradiol cypionate (Dep-Gynogen, Depogen)	IM; 1–5 mg q3–4wk
estradiol valerate (Delestrogen, Duragen-10, Valergen)	IM; 10–20 mg q4wk
estrogen, conjugated (Premarin)	PO; 0.3–1.25 mg qd for 21 days each month
estropipate (Ogen)	PO; 0.75–6 mg qd for 21 days each month
ethinyl estradiol (Estinyl, Feminone)	PO; 0.02–0.05 mg qd for 21 days each month
Progestins	
medroxyprogesterone (Provera, Cycrin)	PO; 5–10 mg qd on days 1–12 of menstrual cycle
norethindrone acetate (Norlutate)	PO; 5 mg qd for 2 weeks; increase by 2.5 mg/d q2wk (max 15 mg/d)
norethindrone (Micronor, Nor-Q.D.)	PO; 0.35 mg qd beginning on day 1 of menstrual cycle
progesterone micronized (Prometrium)	PO; 400 mg at hs for 10 days
Estrogen-Progestin Combinations	
conjugated estrogens, equine/medroxyprogesterone acetate (Premplus)	PO; 0.625 mg/d continuously or in 25-day cycles
estradiol/norgestimate (Ortho-Prefest)	PO; 1 tablet of 1 mg estradiol for 3 days, followed by 1 tablet of 1 mg estradiol combined with 0.09 mg norgestimate for 3 days; regimen is repeated continuously without interruption
ethinyl estradiol/norethindrone acetate (FemHRT)	PO; 5 µg (1 tablet) qd

ovarian failure, and as replacement therapy following surgical removal of the ovaries, usually combined with a progestin. The purpose of the progestin is to counteract some of the adverse effects of estrogen on the uterus. When used alone, estrogen increases the risk of uterine cancer.

High doses of estrogens are used to treat prostate and breast cancer. Prostate cancer is usually dependent on androgens for growth; administration of estrogens suppresses androgen secretion. As an antineoplastic hormone, estrogen is rarely used alone. It is one of many agents used in combination for the chemotherapy of cancer.

NURSING CONSIDERATIONS

For the use of estrogen-containing products as oral contraceptives, refer to "Nursing Process Focus: Clients Receiving Oral Contraceptive Therapy (page 589)."

The role of the nurse in HRT involves careful monitoring of the client's condition and providing education as it relates to the prescribed drug treatment. Conjugated estrogens are contraindicated for use in breast cancer (except in clients being treated for metastatic disease) and any suspected estrogen-dependent cancer. These conditions put the client at a higher risk for developing another cancer. Assess for pregnancy; conjugated estrogen is contraindicated in pregnancy and for use in women who intend to become pregnant in the immediate future because it can cause fetal harm. Assess for a history of thromboembolic disease because of potential side effects of the drug. Obtain a complete health history, including family history of breast and genital cancer. Cautious use of estrogen therapy must be exercised in a client whose first-degree relative has a history of breast or genital cancer. Estrogen monotherapy places the woman at higher risk for cancer of the female reproductive organs. Obtain a history of CAD, hypertension, cerebrovascular disease, fibrocystic breast disease, breast nodules, and abnormal mammograms. Because of the risk of thromboembolism, monitor the client closely for signs and symptoms of thrombus or embolus, such as pain in calves, limited movement in legs, dyspnea, sudden severe chest pain, or anxiety. Encourage the client to report signs of depression, decreased libido, headache, fatigue, and weight gain. Because controversy surrounds the long-term use of these drugs as HRT, it is imperative for women to be aware of current research and discuss treatment alternatives with their healthcare provider before beginning pharmacotherapy. When using these drugs to treat male clients, inform them that secondary female characteristics, such as higher voice, sparse body hair, and increased breast size, may develop. Inform the client that impotence may also occur.

Client education as it relates to HRT should include goals, reasons for obtaining baseline data such as vital signs and the existence of underlying cardiovascular disorders, and possible drug side effects. Include the following points when teaching clients about hormone replacement therapy:

- Immediately report calf tenderness, chest pain, or dyspnea.
- Take with food if GI upset occurs.
- Schedule an annual Pap smear and breast examination.
- Perform monthly self-examinations of breasts.
- Do not take other prescribed drugs, OTC medications, herbal remedies, or dietary supplements without notifying the healthcare provider.

See "Nursing Process Focus: Clients Receiving Hormone Replacement Therapy" for specific teaching points.

MediaLink Menopause

Pr PROTOTYPE DRUG | Conjugated Estrogens (Premarin) and Conjugated Estrogens with Medroxyprogesterone (Premplus)

ACTIONS AND USES

Premarin contains a mixture of different estrogens. It exerts several positive metabolic effects, including an increase in bone density and a reduction in LDL cholesterol. It may also lower the risk of coronary artery disease and colon cancer in some clients. When used as postmenopausal hormone replacement therapy, estrogen is typically combined with a progestin, as in Premplus. Conjugated estrogens may be administered by the IM or IV route for abnormal uterine bleeding due to hormonal imbalance.

ADMINISTRATION ALERTS

- Use a calibrated dosage applicator for administration of vaginal cream.
- For IM or IV administration of conjugated estrogens, reconstitute by first removing approximately 5 mL of air from the dry powder vial and then slowly injecting the diluent into the vial, aiming it at the side of the vial. Gently agitate to dissolve; do not shake.
- Administer IV push slowly, at a rate of 5 mg/min.
- Premarin and Premplus are pregnancy category X.

PHARMACOKINETICS

Premarin is well absorbed after oral administration. It is widely distributed, crosses the placenta, and enters breast milk. It is metabolized by the liver. Its half-life is unknown.

ADVERSE EFFECTS AND INTERACTIONS

Adverse effects of Premplus or Premarin include nausea, fluid retention, edema, breast tenderness, abdominal cramps and bloating, acute pancreatitis, appetite changes, skin eruptions, mental depression, decreased libido, headache, fatigue, nervousness, and weight gain. Effects are dose dependent. Estrogens, when used alone, have been associated with a higher risk of uterine cancer. Although adding a progestin may exert a protective effect by lowering the risk of uterine cancer, recent studies suggest that the progestin may increase the risk of breast cancer following long-term use. The risk of adverse effects increases in clients over age 35.

Drug interactions include a decreased effect of tamoxifen, enhanced corticosteroid effects, and decreased effects of anticoagulants, especially warfarin. The effects of estrogen may be decreased if taken with barbiturates or rifampin, and there is a possible increased effect of tricyclic antidepressants if taken with estrogens.

Use with caution with herbal supplements. For example, red clover and black cohosh may interfere with estrogen therapy. Effects of estrogen may be enhanced if combined with ginseng.

 See the Companion Website for a Nursing Process Focus chart specific to this drug.

NURSING PROCESS FOCUS   Clients Receiving Hormone Replacement Therapy

Assessment	Potential Nursing Diagnoses/Identified Patterns
Prior to administration: - Obtain complete health history including personal or familial history of breast cancer, gall bladder disease, diabetes mellitus, liver or kidney disease. - Obtain drug history to determine possible drug interactions and allergies. - Assess cardiovascular status including hypertension, history of MI, CVA, and thromboembolic disease. - Determine if client is pregnant or lactating.	- Risk for fluid excess related to side effect of drug - Need for knowledge regarding drug therapy and possible adverse effects such as thrombophlebitis and pulmonary or cerebral embolism - Need for knowledge regarding importance of adherence to dosing schedule and management of a missed dose

Planning: Client Goals and Expected Outcomes

The client will:
- Report relief from symptoms of menopause
- Demonstrate an understanding of the drug's action by accurately describing drug side effects and precautions
- Immediately report such effects as symptoms of thrombophlebitis, difficulty breathing, visual disturbances, severe headache, and seizure activity

Implementation

Interventions (Rationales)	Client Education/Discharge Planning
- Monitor for thromboembolic disease. (Estrogen increases risk for thromboembolism.) - Monitor for abnormal uterine bleeding. (If undiagnosed tumour is present, these drugs can increase its size and cause uterine bleeding.) - Monitor breast health. (Estrogens promote the growth of certain breast cancers.)	- Instruct client to report shortness of breath, feeling of heaviness, chest pain, severe headache, warmth, or swelling in affected part, usually the legs or pelvis. - Instruct client to report excessive uterine bleeding or that which occurs between menstruations. - Instruct client to have regular breast exams, perform monthly BSE and obtain routine mammograms, as recommended by healthcare provider.

continued

NURSING PROCESS FOCUS   Clients Receiving Hormone Replacement Therapy   *(Continued)*

Interventions (Rationales)	Client Education/Discharge Planning
■ Monitor for vision changes. (These drugs may worsen myopia or astigmatism and cause intolerance of contact lenses.)	Instruct client to: ■ Obtain regular eye exams during HRT ■ Report changes in vision ■ Report any difficulty in wearing contact lenses
■ Encourage client not to smoke. (Smoking increases risk of cardiovascular disease.)	■ Instruct client to avoid smoking and participate in smoking cessation programs, if necessary.
■ Encourage client to avoid caffeine. (Estrogens and caffeine may lead to increased CNS stimulation.)	Instruct client to: ■ Restrict caffeine consumption ■ Recognize common foods that contain caffeine: coffee, tea, carbonated beverages, chocolate, certain OTC medications ■ Report unusual nervousness, anxiety, and insomnia
■ Monitor glucose levels. (Estrogens may increase blood glucose levels.)	Instruct client to: ■ Monitor blood and urine glucose frequently, if diabetic ■ Report any consistent changes in blood glucose
■ Monitor for seizure activity. (Estrogen-induced fluid retention may increase risk of seizures.)	■ Instruct client to be alert for possibility of seizures, even at night, and report any seizure-type symptoms
■ Monitor client's understanding and proper self-administration. (Improper administration may increase incidence of adverse effects.)	Instruct client to: ■ Administer proper dose, form, and frequency of medication ■ Take with food to decrease GI irritation ■ Take daily dose at HS to decrease occurrence of side effects ■ Document menstruation and any problems that occur

Evaluation of Outcome Criteria

Evaluate the effectiveness of drug therapy by confirming that client goals and expected outcomes have been met (see "Planning").

See Table 41.4 (page 592), under the heading "Estrogens," for a list of drugs to which these nursing actions apply.

SPECIAL CONSIDERATIONS

Estrogen Use and Psychosocial Issues

Because undesirable side effects may occur with estrogen use, communicate these prior to implementation of drug therapy. The nurse can explore the client's reaction to these potential risks. An assessment of the client's emotional support system should also be made before initiating drug therapy. Hirsutism, loss of hair, or a deepening of the voice can occur in the female client. The male client may develop secondary female characteristics such as a higher voice, lack of body hair, and increased breast size. Impotence may also develop and is viewed as a concern by most men.

Clients should be taught that these adverse effects are reversible and may subside with adjustment of dosage or discontinuation of estrogen therapy. This knowledge may allow both male and female clients to remain compliant when adverse effects occur. During therapy, clients may need emotional support to assist in dealing with these body image issues. The nurse can encourage this support, discuss these issues with family members, and refer clients for counselling. For the female client, the nurse can refer to an esthetician for hair removal or wig fitting. The male client and his sexual partner may need a referral to deal with issues surrounding impotence and its effect on their relationship.

NATURAL THERAPIES

Chaste Berry for PMS and Menopause

The chaste tree (*Vitex agnus-castus*) is a shrub common to river banks in the southern Mediterranean region. The dried berries have been used for thousands of years, with recorded references dating to the time of Hippocrates.

Chaste berries contain a number of active substances that increase dopamine action and also affect the pituitary gland. Inhibition of FSH release leads to effects similar to progesterone. Extracts have a physiological effect on premenstrual syndrome (PMS), as well as the unpleasant symptoms of menopause. Many women who take the herbal remedy report reduction in PMS symptoms such as bloating, breast fullness, headache, irritability, mood swings, and anger. There is better regulation of the menstrual cycle and less bleeding. When used during menopause, it may help to reverse vaginal changes and diminished libido. It is reported to decrease prolactin levels and milk production in lactating women. Adverse effects are minor and include GI upset, rash, and headaches.

UTERINE ABNORMALITIES

Dysfunctional uterine bleeding is a condition in which hemorrhage occurs on a non-cyclic basis or in abnormal amounts. It is the health problem most frequently reported by women and a common reason for hysterectomy. Progestins are the drugs of choice for treating uterine abnormalities.

41.6 Pharmacotherapy with Progestins

Secreted by the corpus luteum, the function of endogenous progesterone is to prepare the uterus for implantation of the embryo and pregnancy. If implantation does not occur, levels of progesterone fall dramatically and menses begins. If pregnancy occurs, the ovary will continue to secrete progesterone to maintain a healthy endometrium until the placenta develops sufficiently to begin producing the hormone. Whereas the function of estrogen is to cause proliferation of the endometrium, progesterone limits and stabilizes endometrial growth.

Dysfunctional uterine bleeding can have a number of causes, including early abortion, pelvic neoplasms, thyroid disorders, pregnancy, and infection. Types of dysfunctional uterine bleeding include the following:

• Amenorrhea – absence of menstruation

• Oligomenorrhea – infrequent menstruation

• Menorrhagia – prolonged or excessive menstruation

• Breakthrough bleeding – hemorrhage between menstrual periods

• Postmenopausal bleeding – hemorrhage following menopause

Dysfunctional uterine bleeding is often caused by a hormonal imbalance between estrogen and progesterone. Although estrogen increases the thickness of the endometrium, bleeding occurs sporadically unless balanced by an adequate amount of progesterone secretion. Administration of a progestin in a pattern starting 5 days after the onset of menses and continuing for the next 20 days can sometimes help to re-establish a normal, monthly cyclic pattern. Oral contraceptives may also be prescribed for this disorder.

In cases of heavy bleeding, high doses of conjugated estrogens may be administered for 3 weeks prior to adding medroxyprogesterone for the last 10 days of therapy. Treatment with NSAIDs sometimes helps to reduce bleeding and ease painful menstrual flow. If aggressive hormonal therapy fails to stop the heavy bleeding, dilation and curettage (D&C) may be necessary.

Progestins are occasionally prescribed for the treatment of metastatic endometrial carcinoma. In these cases, they are used for palliation, usually in combination with other antineoplastics. Select progestins and their dosages are shown in Table 41.4 (page 592).

NURSING CONSIDERATIONS

The role of the nurse in progestin therapy involves careful monitoring of the client's condition and providing education as it relates to the prescribed drug treatment. Before administering progesterone, obtain baseline data including blood pressure, weight, and pulse. Laboratory tests including CBC, liver function, serum glucose, and an electrolyte profile should be obtained. Progestin is contraindicated for use in clients with a personal or close family history of breast or genital malignancies, thromboembolic disorders, impaired liver function, and undiagnosed vaginal bleeding. It is also contraindicated in pregnancy or lactation. Clients with allergies to peanuts should avoid the use of Prometrium because the oral capsules contain peanut oil. Progestin must be used with caution in women with a history of depression, anemia, diabetes, asthma, seizure disorders, cardiac or kidney disorders, migraine headaches, previous ectopic pregnancies, history of sexually transmitted infections, unresolved abnormal Pap smears, or previous pelvic surgeries.

Pr PROTOTYPE DRUG | Medroxyprogesterone (Provera, Cycrin)

ACTIONS AND USES

Medroxyprogesterone is a synthetic progestin with a prolonged duration of action. Like its natural counterpart, the primary target tissue for medroxyprogesterone is the endometrium of the uterus. It inhibits the effect of estrogen on the uterus, thus restoring normal hormonal balance. Applications include dysfunctional uterine bleeding and secondary amenorrhea. Medroxyprogesterone may also be given IM for the palliation of metastatic uterine or renal carcinoma.

PHARMACOKINETICS

Medroxyprogesterone is well absorbed after oral administration. It is widely distributed and enters breast milk. It is metabolized by the liver. Its half-life is about 14.5 hours.

ADMINISTRATION ALERTS

■ Give PO with meals to avoid gastric distress.

■ Observe IM sites for abscess: presence of lump and discoloration of tissue.

■ Medroxyprogesterone is pregnancy category X.

ADVERSE EFFECTS AND INTERACTIONS

The most common side effects are breakthrough bleeding and breast tenderness. Weight gain, depression, hypertension, nausea, vomiting, dysmenorrheal and vaginal candidiasis may also occur. The most serious side effects relate to increased risk for thromboembolic disease.

Serum levels of medroxyprogesterone are decreased by aminoglutethimide, barbiturates, primidone, rifampin, rifabutin, and topiramate.

Use with caution with herbal supplements. For example, St. John's wort may cause intermenstrual bleeding and loss of efficacy.

 See the Companion Website for a Nursing Process Focus chart specific to this drug.

Monitor the client for side effects of these hormones. Susceptible clients may experience acute intermittent porphyria as a reaction to progesterone, so assess the client for severe, colicky abdominal pain, vomiting, distention, diarrhea, and constipation. Common side effects of progesterone include breakthrough bleeding, nausea, abdominal cramps, dizziness, edema, and weight gain. Monitor also for amenorrhea; sudden, severe headache; and signs of pulmonary embolism such as sudden severe chest pain and dyspnea; report such symptoms to the healthcare provider immediately. Because progesterone can cause photosensitivity and phototoxicity, monitor for pruritus, sensitivity to light, acne, rash, and alopecia. Phototoxic reactions cause serious sunburn within 5 to 18 hours of sun exposure.

Client education as it relates to progestins should include goals, reasons for assessing cardiovascular status, and possible side effects. See "Nursing Process Focus: Clients Receiving Progestin Therapy" for specific teaching points.

LABOUR AND BREASTFEEDING

OXYTOCICS AND TOCOLYTICS

Oxytocics are agents that stimulate uterine contractions to promote the induction of labour. **Tocolytics** are used to inhibit uterine contractions during premature labour. These agents are shown in Table 41.5.

41.7 Pharmacological Management of Uterine Contractions

The most widely used oxytocic is the natural hormone oxytocin, which is secreted by the posterior portion of the pitu-

---

NURSING PROCESS FOCUS Clients Receiving Progestin Therapy

Assessment	Potential Nursing Diagnoses/Identified Patterns
Prior to administration: ■ Obtain complete health history including personal and familial history of breast, endometrial, or renal cancer; liver or kidney disease; dysfunctional uterine bleeding; endometrial hyperplasia. ■ Obtain drug history to determine possible drug interactions and allergies. ■ Assess cardiovascular status including history of thromboembolic disease.	■ Risk for fluid excess related to side effect of drug ■ Need for knowledge regarding drug therapy and adverse effects ■ Need for knowledge regarding importance of adherence to dosing schedule

Planning: Client Goals and Expected Outcomes
The client will: ■ Report relief from dysfunctional uterine bleeding or amenorrhea ■ Demonstrate an understanding of the drug's action by accurately describing drug side effects and precautions ■ Immediately report effects such as signs of embolism; sudden, severe headache; edema; vision changes; and phototoxicity

Implementation	
Interventions (Rationales)	**Client Education/Discharge Planning**
■ Monitor lab tests including liver function, blood glucose, and sodium and chloride levels. (Progestins can affect electrolyte balance and liver function.)	■ Instruct client to obtain periodic lab tests and to monitor glucose levels closely if diabetic.
■ Monitor for vision changes. (Progestins may cause retinal emboli or cerebrovascular thrombosis.)	■ Instruct client to report unexplained partial or complete loss of vision, ptosis, or diplopia.
■ Monitor for fluid imbalance. (Progestins cause fluid retention and weight gain.)	■ Instruct client to monitor for edema or weight gain by weighing self weekly and recording, especially clients who have asthma, seizure disorders, cardiac or kidney impairment, or migraines.
■ Monitor for integumentary effects of medication. (Progestins have multiple effects on the skin and associated structures.)	Instruct client to: ■ Report itching, photosensitivity, acne, rash, and hair overgrowth or loss ■ Avoid exposure to UV light and prolonged periods of time in the sun ■ Use sunscreen (> SPF 12) when outdoors ■ Recognize that these changes are temporary and will improve upon discontinuation of this medication

Evaluation of Outcome Criteria
Evaluate the effectiveness of drug therapy by confirming that client goals and expected outcomes have been met (see "Planning").

See Table 41.4 (page 592), under the heading "Progestins," for a list of drugs to which these nursing actions apply.

TABLE 41.5   Uterine Stimulants and Relaxants

Drug	Route and Adult Dose
Stimulants (Oxytocics)	
oxytocin (Syntocinon)	IV (antepartum); 1 mU/min starting dose to a maximum of 20 mU/min
Ergot Alkaloids	
ergonovine maleate (Ergotrate Maleate)	PO; 1 tablet (0.2 mg) tid–qid after childbirth for a maximum of 1 week
methylergonovine maleate (Methergine)	PO; 0.2–0.4 mg bid–qid
Prostaglandins	
carboprost tromethamine (Hemabate)	IM; initial:250 µg (1 mL) repeated at 1.5- to 3.5-hour intervals if indicated by uterine response
dinoprostone (Cervidil, Prepidil, Prostin E$_2$)	Intravaginal; 10 mg
misoprostol (Cytotec)	PO; 400 µg as a single dose
Relaxants (Tocolytics)	
Beta$_2$-Adrenergic Agonists	
ritodrine hydrochloride (Yutopar)	IV; 50–100 µg/min starting dose, increased by 50 µg/min q10min
Other Tocolytics	
magnesium sulfate (see p. 539 for the Prototype Drug box)	IV; 1–4 g in 5% dextrose by slow infusion
nifedipine (Adalat) (see p. 261 for the Prototype Drug box)	PO; 10 mg as a single dose

itary gland. The target organs for oxytocin are the uterus and the breast. It is secreted in increasingly larger amounts as the growing fetus distends the uterus. As blood levels of oxytocin rise, the uterus is stimulated to contract, thus promoting labour and the delivery of the baby and the placenta. As pregnancy progresses, the number of oxytocin receptors in the uterus increases, making the uterus more sensitive to the effects of the hormone. Parenteral oxytocin may be given to initiate labour. Doses in an IV infusion are increased gradually, every 15 to 60 minutes, until a normal labour pattern is established. After delivery, an IV infusion of oxytocin may be given to control postpartum uterine bleeding by temporarily impeding blood flow to this organ.

In postpartum clients, oxytocin is released in response to suckling, causing milk to be ejected (let down) from the mammary glands. Oxytocin does not increase the volume of milk production. This function is provided by the pituitary hormone prolactin, which increases the synthesis of milk. The actions of oxytocin during breastfeeding are illustrated in Figure 41.4. When given for milk letdown, oxytocin is given intranasally several minutes before breastfeeding or pumping is anticipated.

Several prostaglandins are also used as uterine stimulants. Unlike most hormones that travel through the blood to affect distant tissues, **prostaglandins** are local hormones that act directly at the site where they are secreted. Although the body makes dozens of different prostaglandins, only a few have clinical utility. Dinoprostone, prostaglandin E$_2$, is used to initiate labour, to prepare the cervix for labour, or to expel a fetus that has died. Mifepristone, a synthetic analog of prostaglandin E$_1$, is used for emergency contraception and for pharmacological abortion, as described earlier in

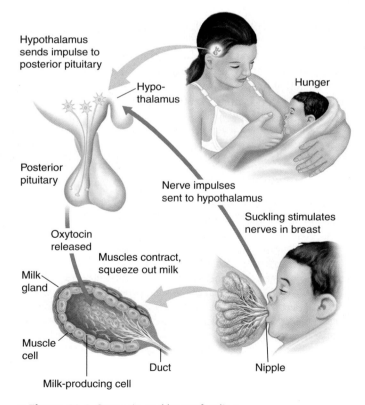

● **Figure 41.4** Oxytocin and breastfeeding

this chapter. Carboprost, 15-methylprostaglandin F$_2$ alpha, can induce pharmacological abortion and may be indicated to control postpartum bleeding.

Tocolytics are uterine relaxants prescribed to *inhibit* the uterine contractions experienced during premature labour. Suppressing labour allows additional time for the fetus to develop and may permit the pregnancy to reach normal term. Premature birth is a leading cause of infant death. Typically, the mother is hooked up to a monitor with a sensor that records uterine contractions and this information is used to determine the doses and timing of tocolytic medications.

Two beta$_2$-adrenergic agonists are used as uterine relaxants. Ritodrine may be given by the oral or IV route to suppress labour contractions. It is more effective when administered before labour intensifies, and its use normally results in only a 1- to 2-day prolongation of pregnancy. Terbutaline is another beta$_2$-agonist that may be used for uterine relaxation, though it is not approved for this purpose. The benefits of tocolytics must be carefully weighed against their potential adverse effects, which include tachycardia in both the mother and the fetus.

NURSING CONSIDERATIONS

The role of the nurse in uterine stimulant therapy involves careful monitoring of both the client and fetus and providing education as it relates to the administered drug. The healthcare provider must evaluate the client for fetal presentation, especially for the presence of cephalopelvic disproportion.

To safely administer oxytocin, the fetus must be viable and vaginal delivery must be possible. If invasive cervical cancer, active herpes genitalis, or cord prolapse exists, oxytocin is contraindicated. Oxytocin is also contraindicated in clients with a history of previous uterine or cervical surgery, including cesarean section. This drug is not used if the client is a grand multipara, is older than 35 years of age, or has a history of uterine sepsis or traumatic birth. Previous sensitivity or allergic reaction to an ergot derivative contraindicates the use of oxytocin. Dinoprostone use is contraindicated in clients with active cardiac, pulmonary, renal, or hepatic disease. These medications must be used cautiously with vasoconstrictive drugs.

Monitor the client for side effects of these hormone-based medications. Because oxytocin increases the frequency and force of uterine contractions, the client in labour must be assessed frequently for elevations in blood pressure, heart rate, and fetal heart rate. The infusion must be discontinued if fetal distress is detected in order to prevent fetal anoxia. The nurse should administer oxygen and have the client change position to improve fetal oxygenation. Hypertensive crisis may occur if local or regional anesthesia is used in combination with oxytocin.

Uterine hyperstimulation is characterized by contractions that are less than 2 minutes apart, with force greater than 50 mm Hg or that last longer than 90 seconds. Oxytocin should be discontinued immediately if hyperstimulation occurs. Monitor fluid balance because prolonged IV infusion of oxytocin may cause water intoxication. Symptoms of water intoxication must be assessed and reported immediately and include drowsiness, listlessness, headache, confusion, anuria, and weight gain. Side effects of oxytocin include anxiety, maternal dyspnea, hypotension or hypertension, nausea, vomiting, neonatal jaundice, and maternal or fetal dysrhythmias.

See "Nursing Process Focus: Clients Receiving Oxytocin" for specific teaching points regarding this Prototype Drug.

Pr **PROTOTYPE DRUG** | Oxytocin (Syntocinon)

ACTIONS AND USES

Oxytocin is a natural hormone secreted by the posterior pituitary that is a drug of choice for inducing labour. Oxytocin is given by several different routes depending on its intended action. Given by IV infusion antepartum, oxytocin induces labour by increasing the frequency and force of contractions of uterine smooth muscle. It is timed to the final stage of pregnancy, after the cervix is dilated, membranes have ruptured, and presentation of the fetus has occurred. Oxytocin may also be administered postpartum to reduce hemorrhage after expulsion of the placenta and to aid in returning normal muscular tone to the uterus. A second route of administration is intranasally to promote the ejection of milk from the mammary glands. Milk letdown occurs within minutes after applying spray or drops to the nostril during breastfeeding.

PHARMACOKINETICS

Oxytocin is well absorbed and widely distributed. It is rapidly metabolized by the liver. Its half-life is 3 to 9 minutes.

ADMINISTRATION ALERTS

- Dilute 10 U oxytocin in 1000 mL IV fluid prior to administration. For postpartum administration, up to 40 U may be added to 1000 mL of IV fluid.
- Incidence of allergic reactions is higher when given by IM or IV injection, rather than IV infusion.
- Oxytocin is pregnancy category X.

ADVERSE EFFECTS AND INTERACTIONS

When given IV, vital signs of the fetus and client are monitored continuously to avoid complications in the fetus, such as dysrhythmias or intracranial hemorrhage. Serious complications in the client may include uterine rupture, seizures, or coma. The risk of uterine rupture increases in women who have delivered five or more children. Though experience has shown the use of oxytocin to be quite safe, labour should only be induced by this drug when there are demonstrated risks to the mother or fetus in continuing the pregnancy.

Oxytocin interacts with several drugs. For example, vasoconstrictors used concurrently with oxytocin cause severe hypertension.

Use with caution with herbal supplements. For example, ephedra or ma huang used with oxytocin may lead to hypertension.

NURSING PROCESS FOCUS   Clients Receiving Oxytocin

Assessment	Potential Nursing Diagnoses/Identified Patterns
Prior to administration: ■ Obtain complete health history including past and present gynecologic and obstetric history. ■ Obtain drug history to determine possible drug interactions and allergies.	■ Risk for fluid excess related to ADH side effect of drug ■ Need for knowledge regarding drug therapy and possible adverse effects such as thrombophlebitis and pulmonary or cerebral embolism ■ Need for knowledge regarding importance of adherence to dosing schedule and management of a missed dose ■ Risk for injury to fetus related to strong uterine contractions

Planning: Client Goals and Expected Outcomes

The client will:
■ Report increase in force and frequency of uterine contractions and/or letdown of milk for breastfeeding
■ Demonstrate an understanding of the drug's action by accurately describing drug side effects and precautions
■ Immediately report effects such as listlessness, headache, confusion, anuria, hypotension, nausea, vomiting, and weight gain

Implementation

Interventions (Rationales)	Client Education/Discharge Planning
■ Monitor fetal heart rate. (Increase in force and frequency of uterine contractions may cause fetal distress.)	■ Instruct client about the purpose and importance of fetal monitoring.
■ Monitor maternal status including blood pressure, pulse, and frequency, duration, and intensity of contractions.	■ Instruct client about the importance of monitoring maternal status.
■ Monitor fluid balance. (Prolonged IV infusion may cause water intoxication.)	■ Instruct client to report drowsiness, listlessness, headache, confusion, anuria, weight gain.
■ Monitor for postpartum/postabortion hemorrhage. (Oxytocin can be used to control postpartum bleeding.)	Instruct client: ■ About the importance of being monitored frequently after delivery or after abortion ■ To report severe vaginal bleeding or increase in lochia
■ Monitor lactation status. (Oxytocin causes milk ejection within minutes after administration.)	Instruct client: ■ That oxytocin does not increase milk production ■ To monitor for decreased breast pain, redness, hardness, if taking oxytocin to decrease breast engorgement

Evaluation of Outcome Criteria

Evaluate the effectiveness of drug therapy by confirming that client goals and expected outcomes have been met (see "Planning").

FEMALE INFERTILITY

Infertility is defined as the inability to become pregnant after at least 1 year of frequent, unprotected intercourse. Infertility is a common disorder, with as many as 25% of couples experiencing difficulty in conceiving children at some point during their reproductive lifetimes. It is estimated that females contribute to approximately 60% of the infertility disorders. Agents used to treat infertility are shown in Table 41.6.

41.8 Pharmacotherapy of Female Fertility

Causes of female infertility are varied and include lack of ovulation, pelvic infection, and physical obstruction of the fallopian tubes. Extensive testing is often necessary to determine the exact cause of the infertility. For women whose infertility has been determined to have an endocrine etiology, pharmacotherapy may be of value. Endocrine disruption of reproductive function can occur at the level of the hypothalamus, pituitary, or ovary, and pharmacotherapy is targeted to the specific cause of the dysfunction.

Lack of regular ovulation is a cause of infertility that can be successfully treated with drug therapy. Clomiphene is a drug of choice for female infertility that acts as an antiestrogen. Clomiphene stimulates the release of LH, resulting in the maturation of more ovarian follicles than would normally occur. The rise in LH level is sufficient to induce ovulation in about 90% of treated clients. The pregnancy rate of clients taking clomiphene is high, and twins occur in about 5% of treated clients. Therapy is usually begun with a

TABLE 41.6   Agents for Female Infertility

Drug	Mechanism
bromocriptine mesylate (Parlodel)	reduces high prolactin levels
clomiphene (Clomid, Serophene)	promotes follicle maturation and ovulation
danazol (Danocrine)	controls endometriosis
Human FSH (purified from the urine of postmenopausal women) urofollitropin (Fertinex, Metrodin)	promotes follicle maturation and ovulation
Recombinant FSH follitropin alfa (Gonal-F) follitropin beta (Follistim)	promotes follicle maturation and ovulation
GnRH and GnRH Analogs cetrorelix acetate (Cetrotide) leuprolide acetate (Lupron, Lupron Depot) nafarelin acetate (Synarel) ganirelix acetate (Antagon) gonadorelin acetate (Lutrepulse) goserelin acetate (Zoladex)	promotes follicle maturation and ovulation or control of endometriosis
human chorionic gonadotropin (A.P.L., Chorex, Choron 10, Profasi HP, Pregnyl)	promotes follicle maturation and ovulation
human menopausal gonadotropin (Pergonal, Humegon, Repronex)	promotes follicle maturation and ovulation

low dose of 50 mg for 5 days, following menses. If ovulation does not occur, the dose is increased to 100 mg for 5 days, then to 150 mg. If ovulation still is not induced, human chorionic gonadotropin (HCG) is added to the treatment. Made by the placenta during pregnancy, HCG is similar to LH and can mimic the LH surge that normally causes ovulation. The use of clomiphene assumes that the pituitary gland is able to respond by secreting LH and that the ovaries are responsive to LH. If either of these assumptions is false, other treatment options should be considered.

If the endocrine disruption is at the pituitary level, therapy with human menopausal gonadotropin (HMG) or gonadotropin-releasing hormone (GnRH) may be indicated. These therapies are generally indicated only after clomiphene has failed to induce ovulation. HMG is a combination of FSH and LH extracted from the urine of postmenopausal women, who secrete large amounts of these hormones. Also called menotropins, HMG acts on the ovaries to increase follicle maturation and results in a 25% incidence of multiple pregnancies. Successful therapy with HMG assumes that the ovaries are responsive to LH and FSH. Newer formulations use recombinant DNA technology to synthesize gonadotropins containing nearly pure FSH, rather than extracting the FSH-LH mixture from urine.

Given IV, gonadorelin is a synthetic analog of GnRH that is prescribed for clients unresponsive to clomiphene. GnRH analogs take over the function of the hypothalamus and attempt to restart normal hormonal rhythms. Other medications used to stimulate ovulation are bromocriptine and HCG.

Endometriosis, a common cause of infertility, is characterized by the presence of endometrial tissue in non-uterine locations such as the pelvis and ovaries. Being responsive to hormonal stimuli, this abnormal tissue can cause pain, dysfunctional bleeding, and dysmenorrhea. Leuprolide is a GnRH agonist that produces an initial release of LH and FSH, followed by suppression due to the negative feedback effect on the pituitary. Many women experience relief from the symptoms of endometriosis after 3 to 6 months of leuprolide therapy, and the benefits may extend well beyond the treatment period. Leuprolide is also indicated for the palliative therapy of prostate cancer. As an alternative choice, danazol is an anabolic steroid that suppresses FSH production, which in turn shuts down both ectopic and normal endometrial activity. While leuprolide is only given by the parenteral route, danazol is given orally.

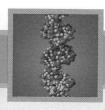

CHAPTER REVIEW

KEY CONCEPTS

The numbered key concepts provide a succinct summary of the important points from the corresponding numbered section within the chapter. If any of the points are not clear, refer to the numbered section within the chapter for review. Expanded versions can be found on the Companion Website.

41.1 Female reproductive function is controlled by GnRH from the hypothalamus and by FSH and LH from the pituitary.

41.2 Estrogens are secreted by ovarian follicles and are responsible for the secondary sex characteristics of the female. Progestins are secreted by the corpus luteum and prepare the endometrium for implantation.

41.3 Low doses of estrogens and progestins prevent conception by blocking ovulation.

41.4 Drugs for emergency contraception may be administered within 72 hours of unprotected sex to prevent implantation of the fertilized egg. Other agents may be given to stimulate uterine contractions to expel the implanted embryo.

41.5 Estrogen-progestin combinations are used for hormone replacement therapy during and after menopause; however, their long-term use may have serious adverse effects.

41.6 Progestins are prescribed for dysfunctional uterine bleeding. High doses of progestins are also used as antineoplastics.

41.7 Oxytocics are drugs that stimulate uterine contractions and induce labour. Tocolytics slow uterine contractions to delay labour.

41.8 Medications may be administered to stimulate ovulation in order to increase female fertility.

REVIEW QUESTIONS

1 Why is a progestin usually prescribed along with estrogen in oral contraceptives and when treating postmenopausal symptoms?

2 What is the difference between the effects of prolactin and oxytocin on the breast?

3 Explain why lack of sufficient pituitary secretion can cause female infertility. Describe several pharmacological approaches to treating infertility due to pituitary hyposecretion.

CRITICAL THINKING QUESTIONS

1. A 28-year-old female has a 3-year history of pelvic pain, dyspareunia, and infertility. She has been diagnosed with endometriosis and is prescribed leuprolide once a month by IM injection. Discuss the mechanism of action of leuprolide in managing the client's endometriosis.

2. A labour and delivery nurse places one-fourth of a tablet (crushed) of misoprostol on the cervix of a client who is being induced because she is 2 weeks past her due date. After several hours, the client begins to have contractions and the nurse notes late decelerations on the monitor. The nurse flushes the drug out of the client's vagina with saline as per hospital protocol. Is it possible that the misoprostol stimulated these uterine contractions? Why or why not?

3. A nurse is assessing a 32-year-old postpartum client and notes 2+ pitting edema of the ankles and pre-tibial area. The client denied having "swelling" prior to delivery. The nurse reviews the client's chart and notes that she was induced with oxytocin over a 23-hour period. Is there any relationship between this drug treatment and the client's current presentation? What additional assessments should be made?

EXPLORE
MediaLink
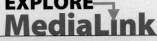
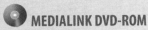

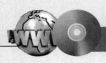

www.pearsoned.ca/adams-king

MEDIALINK DVD-ROM
- **CRNE Review**
- **Audio Glossary**
- **Video**
  Preeclampsia
- **Animation**
  Mechanism of Action: Estradiol

COMPANION WEBSITE
- **CRNE Review**
- **Dosage Calculations**
- **Case Study:** Client taking hormone replacement therapy

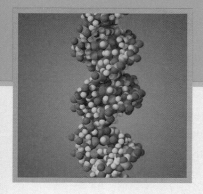
Drugs for Disorders and Conditions of the Male Reproductive System

DRUGS AT A GLANCE

AGENTS FOR MALE HYPOGONADISM

Androgens
   Ⓟ *testosterone base (Andro 100, others)*

AGENTS FOR MALE INFERTILITY

AGENTS FOR ERECTILE DYSFUNCTION

Phosphodiesterase-5 inhibitors
   Ⓟ *sildenafil (Viagra)*

AGENTS FOR BENIGN PROSTATIC HYPERPLASIA

Alpha₁-adrenergic blockers

5-alpha reductase inhibitors
   Ⓟ *finasteride (Proscar)*

OBJECTIVES

After reading this chapter, the student should be able to do the following:

1. Identify drug classes used for treating disorders of the male reproductive system.
2. Explain the therapeutic action of each class of drug in relation to the pathophysiology of the disorder being treated.
3. Explain the role of androgens in the treatment of male hypogonadism.
4. Describe the misuse and dangers associated with the use of anabolic steroids to enhance athletic performance.
5. Discuss the use of androgens as antineoplastic agents.
6. Explain the limited role of drugs in the therapy of male infertility.
7. Describe the role of drug therapy in the treatment of erectile dysfunction.
8. Describe the role of drug therapy in the treatment of benign prostatic hyperplasia (BPH).
9. For each of the drug classes listed in Drugs at a Glance, identify a representative drug and explain its mechanism of action, therapeutic effects, and important adverse effects.
10. Describe and explain, based on pharmacological principles, the rationale for nursing assessment, planning, and interventions for clients receiving pharmacological therapy for disorders and conditions of the male reproductive system.
11. Use the nursing process to care for clients who are receiving drug therapy for disorders and conditions of the male reproductive system.

MediaLink

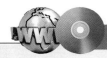 www.pearsoned.ca/adams-king

CRNE review, case studies, and other interactive resources for this chapter can be found on the Companion Website at **www.pearsoned.ca/adams-king**. Click on "Chapter 42" to select the activities for this chapter. For animations, more CRNE review questions, and an audio glossary, access the accompanying DVD-ROM in this textbook.

KEY TERMS

like in the female, male reproductive function is regulated by a small number of hormones from the hypothalamus, pituitary, and gonads. Because hormonal secretion in the male is regular throughout the adult lifespan, pharmacological treatment of reproductive disorders in the male is less complex, and more limited, than in the female. This chapter examines drugs used to treat disorders and conditions of the male reproductive system.

PHARMFACTS

Male Reproductive Conditions and Disorders

- Erectile dysfunction affects about 1 in 4 men over age 65.
- Benign prostatic hyperplasia (BPH) affects 50% of men over age 60, and 90% of men over age 80.
- BPH is the most common benign neoplasm affecting middle-aged and elderly men.
- Approximately 30% of men are subfertile, and at least 2% of men are totally infertile.
- Smoking over 20 cigarettes a day has been shown to reduce both sperm count and sperm motility.

42.1 Hypothalamic and Pituitary Regulation of Male Reproductive Function

The same pituitary hormones that control reproductive function in the female (Chapter 41) also affect the male. Although the name follicle-stimulating hormone (FSH) applies to its target in the female ovary, this same hormone regulates sperm production in the male. In males, luteinizing hormone (LH), sometimes called interstitial cell-stimulating hormone (ICSH), regulates the production of testosterone.

Although secreted in small amounts by the adrenal glands in females, **androgens** are considered male sex hormones. The testes secrete testosterone, the primary androgen responsible for maturation of the male sex organs and the secondary sex characteristics of the male. Unlike the cyclic secretion of estrogen and progesterone in the female, the secretion of testosterone is relatively constant in the adult male. Should the level of testosterone in the blood rise above normal, negative feedback is provided to the pituitary to shut off the secretion of LH and FSH. The relationship between the hypothalamus, pituitary, and the male reproductive hormones is illustrated in Figure 42.1.

Like estrogen, testosterone has metabolic effects in tissues outside the reproductive system. Of particular note is its ability to build muscle mass, which contributes to the differences in muscle strength and body composition between males and females.

MALE HYPOGONADISM

ANDROGENS

Androgens include testosterone and related hormones that control many aspects of male reproductive function. Therapeutically they are used to treat hypogonadism and certain cancers. These agents are shown in Table 42.1.

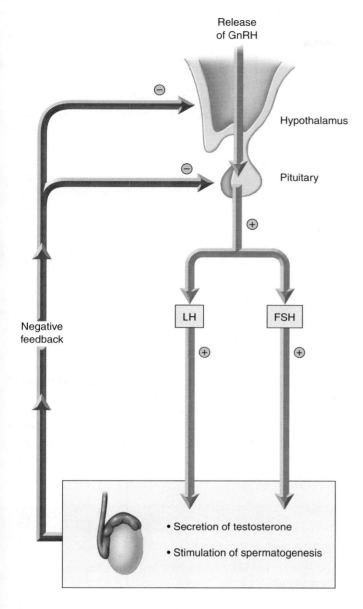

● Figure 42.1 Hormonal control of the male reproductive hormones

42.2 Pharmacotherapy with Androgens

Lack of sufficient testosterone secretion by the testes can result in male **hypogonadism**. Insufficient testosterone secretion may be caused by disorders of the pituitary or the testes. Deficiency in FSH and LH secretion by the pituitary will result in a lack of stimulus to the testes to produce androgens. Lack of FSH and LH secretion may have a number of causes, including Cushing's syndrome, thyroid disorders, estrogen-secreting tumours, and therapy with GnRH agonists such as leuprolide. Hypogonadism may be congenital or acquired later in life.

Hypogonadism may also occur in clients with normal pituitary function if the testes are diseased or otherwise unresponsive to FSH-LH. Examples of conditions that may cause testicular failure include mumps, testicular trauma or inflammation, and certain autoimmune disorders.

Symptoms of male hypogonadism include diminished appearance of the secondary male sex characteristics: sparse axillary, facial, and pubic hair; increase in subcutaneous fat; and small testicular size. In adult males, lack of testosterone can lead to erectile dysfunction, low sperm counts, and decreased **libido** (interest in intercourse). Non-specific complaints may include fatigue, depression, and reduced muscle mass. In young males, lack of sufficient testosterone secretion may lead to delayed puberty.

Pharmacotherapy for male hypogonadism includes replacement therapy with testosterone or other androgens. Androgen therapy promotes normal gonadal development and often restores normal reproductive function. Secondary male sex characteristics reappear, a condition called masculinization or **virilization.**

Testosterone is available in a number of different formulations. Testosterone cypionate and testosterone enanthate are slowly absorbed after IM injections, which are given every 2 to 4 weeks. Testosterone pellets are implanted SC and last 3 to 6 months. Several skin patch products are available, which release testosterone over a 24-hour period. Testoderm patches are applied to the scrotal area, whereas Testoderm TTS and Androderm patches are applied to the

TABLE 42.1 Select Androgens	
Drug	**Route and Adult Dose**
danazol (Danocrine)	PO; 200–400 mg bid for 3–6 months
fluoxymesterone (Halotestin)	PO; 2.5–20 mg qd for replacement therapy
methyltestosterone (Android, Testred)	PO; 10–50 mg qd
nandrolone phenpropionate (Durabolin, Hybolin)	IM; 50–100 mg qwk
testolactone (Teslac)	PO; 250 mg qid
testosterone (Andro 100, Histerone, Testoderm)	PO; 10–25 mg q2–3d
testosterone cypionate (Depotest, Andro-Cyp, Depo-Testosterone)	IM; 50–400 mg q2–4wk; Topical: 4–6 mg qd applied to scrotum
testosterone enanthate (Andro L.A., Delatest, Delatestryl)	IM; 50–400 mg q2–4wk

arm, back, or upper buttocks. Two gel systems are available as Testim and Androgel, which are applied to the shoulders, upper arm, or abdomen. The alcohol-based gels dry quickly, and the testosterone is absorbed into the skin and released slowly to the blood. Buccal tablets adhere to the buccal mucosa in the small depression in the mouth where the gum meets the upper lip above the incisor teeth, and from there the drug is released and absorbed directly into the bloodstream over a 12-hour period.

Androgens have important physiological effects outside the reproductive system. Testosterone promotes the synthesis of erythropoietin, which explains why males usually have a slightly higher hematocrit than females. Testosterone has a profound anabolic effect on skeletal muscle, which is the rationale for giving this drug to debilitated clients who have muscle wasting disease.

Anabolic steroids are testosterone-like compounds with hormonal activity that are taken inappropriately by athletes who hope to build muscle mass and strength, thereby obtaining a competitive edge. When taken in large doses for prolonged periods, anabolic steroids can produce significant adverse effects, some of which may persist for months after discontinuation of the drug. These agents tend to raise cholesterol levels and may cause low sperm counts and impotence in men. In female athletes, menstrual irregularities are likely, with an obvious increase in masculine appearance. Permanent liver damage may result. Behavioural changes include aggression and psychological dependence. The use of anabolic steroids to improve athletic performance is illegal and strongly discouraged by healthcare providers and athletic associations. Most androgens are classified as Schedule III drugs due to their abuse potential.

High doses of androgens are occasionally used as a palliative measure to treat certain types of breast cancer, in combination with other antineoplastics. Because most prostate carcinomas are testosterone dependent, androgens should not be prescribed for older males unless the possibility of prostate cancer has been ruled out. Clients with prostate carcinoma are sometimes given a GnRH agonist such as leuprolide to reduce circulating testosterone levels.

NURSING CONSIDERATIONS

The role of the nurse in androgen therapy involves careful monitoring of the client's condition and providing education as it relates to the prescribed drug regimen. Conduct a physical assessment for evidence of decreased hormone production, such as decreased or absent body hair, small testes, impaired sexual functioning, or delayed signs of puberty. Also assess the client's emotional status as depression and mood swings may be symptoms of decreased hormone secretion. Monitor lab results, especially liver enzymes, if the client has a history of anabolic steroid use. Contraindications to androgen therapy include prostatic or male breast cancer, renal disease, cardiac and liver dysfunction, hypercalcemia, benign prostatic hyperplasia (BPH), and hypertension. Androgens must be used cautiously in prepubertal males, older adults, and in acute intermittent porphyria. Monitor for side effects such as acne, skin irritation, edema, and increased libido in male clients taking androgens. Some

---

Pr PROTOTYPE DRUG | Testosterone Base (Andro 100, others)

ACTIONS AND USES

The primary therapeutic use of testosterone is for the treatment of hypogonadism in males by promoting virilization, including enlargement of the sexual organs, growth of facial hair, and a deepening of the voice. In adult males, testosterone administration will increase libido and restore masculine characteristics that may be deficient. Testosterone base acts by stimulating RNA synthesis and protein metabolism. High doses may suppress spermatogenesis.

PHARMACOKINETICS

Testosterone is well absorbed after buccal, transdermal, or IM administration. It is widely distributed, crosses the placenta, and enters breast milk. Testosterone is metabolized by the liver. Its half-life in plasma is less than 2 hours.

ADMINISTRATION ALERTS

- Place patch on hair-free, dry skin of the abdomen, back, thigh, upper arm, or as directed.
- Change patch site within an anatomical region every 24 hours and rotate to a different anatomical region every 7 days.
- Give IM injection into gluteal muscles.
- Testosterone is pregnancy category X.

ADVERSE EFFECTS AND INTERACTIONS

An obvious side effect of testosterone therapy is virilization, which is usually only of concern when the drug is taken by female clients. Increased libido may also occur. Salt and water are often retained, causing edema, and a diuretic may be indicated. Liver damage is rare, although it is a potentially serious adverse effect with some of the orally administered androgens. Acne and skin irritation is common during therapy.

Testosterone base interacts with several drugs. For example, when taken concurrently with oral anticoagulants, testosterone base may potentiate hypoprothrombinemia.

Use with caution with herbal supplements. Insulin requirements may decrease, and the risk of hepatotoxicity may increase when used with echinacea.

 See the Companion Website for a Nursing Process Focus chart specific to this drug.

adverse reactions found to occur in females as a result of androgen use include deepening of the voice, increased acne or oily skin, increased hair growth, enlarged clitoris, and irregular menses.

Client education as it relates to androgen therapy should include goals; reasons for obtaining baseline data such as vital signs and tests for cardiac, liver, and renal function; and possible side effects. See "Nursing Process Focus: Clients Receiving Androgen Therapy" for specific teaching points.

MALE INFERTILITY

It is estimated that 30% to 40% of couples' infertility is caused by difficulties with the male reproductive system. Male infertility may have psychological etiology, which must be ruled out before pharmacotherapy is considered.

SPECIAL CONSIDERATIONS

Androgen Abuse by Athletes

A serious problem with androgens is their abuse by athletes. The drugs have been used and abused to increase weight, muscle mass, and muscle strength. What began as a movement by weightlifters to enhance muscle mass in the early 1960s has progressed to most competitive sports and all age groups. Teen use has been increasing, and not just among athletes; some report taking the drugs simply to look better.

Anabolic steroids may be taken orally or IM. The oral forms are absorbed rapidly; they are sometimes preferred since they are excreted quickly and thus are less likely to be detected on drug screening. The IM injections may be water or oil based, with the oil forms having a prolonged duration and being more detectable. Most professional sport associations in Canada prohibit the use of androgens for these purposes, and any athlete proven to use them is banned from participation. Further encouraging their use is the fact that the serious effects of anabolic steroids are long term but not readily observable.

MediaLink   Resources for Male Infertility

NURSING PROCESS FOCUS   Clients Receiving Androgen Therapy

Assessment	Potential Nursing Diagnoses/Identified Patterns
Prior to administration: ■ Obtain complete health history including male breast or prostatic cancer; BPH; cardiac, kidney, or liver disease; diabetes; and hypercalcemia. ■ Obtain lab results, including renal function tests, BUN, creatinine, and PSA. ■ Obtain drug history to determine possible drug interactions and allergies.	■ Risk for sexual dysfunction related to effects of drug therapy or decreased hormone function ■ Risk for sleep disturbances related to effects of drug therapy ■ Need for knowledge regarding drug therapy and adverse effects ■ Risk for altered body image related to side effects of drug therapy

Planning: Client Goals and Expected Outcomes

The client will:
■ Demonstrate improvement of the underlying condition for which testosterone was ordered
■ Demonstrate an understanding of the drug's action by accurately describing drug side effects and precautions and importance of follow-up care

Implementation

Interventions (Rationales)	Client Education/Discharge Planning
■ Monitor serum cholesterol levels. (Elevated cholesterol levels secondary to testosterone administration may increase client's risk of cardiovascular disease.)	Instruct client to: ■ Have cholesterol levels measured periodically during therapy ■ Implement changes that may lower risk of hypercholesterolemia: decrease fat in the diet, increase exercise, decrease consumption of red meat
■ Monitor calcium levels. (Testosterone can cause hypercalcemia.)	Instruct client to: ■ Have calcium levels checked during therapy ■ Recognize and report symptoms of increased serum calcium, including deep bone and flank pain, anorexia, nausea/vomiting, thirst, constipation, lethargy, and psychoses
■ Monitor bone growth in children and adolescents. (Premature epiphyseal closing may occur, leading to growth retardation.)	■ Instruct pediatric caregiver to have bone age determinations on the child every 6 months.
■ Monitor input, output, and client weight. (Testosterone can cause retention of salt and water, leading to edema.)	■ Instruct client to check weight twice weekly and report increases, particularly if accompanied by dependent edema.
■ Monitor blood glucose, especially in diabetics. (Testosterone therapy may change glucose tolerance.)	Instruct client to: ■ Monitor blood glucose daily and report significant changes to healthcare provider ■ Recognize that adjustments may need to be made in hypoglycemic medications and diet

continued

NURSING PROCESS FOCUS Clients Receiving Androgen Therapy *(Continued)*	
Interventions (Rationales)	**Client Education/Discharge Planning**
▪ Monitor proper self-administration.	Instruct client to: ▪ Mark calendar so medication can be taken/given at appropriate intervals ▪ Apply transdermal patch to dry, clean scrotal skin that has been dry shaved and not to use chemical depilatories ▪ Notify female partner of transdermal patch; there is a chance of absorbing testosterone, resulting in mild virilization ▪ Avoid showering or swimming for at least 1 hour after gel application
Evaluation of Outcome Criteria	
Evaluate the effectiveness of drug therapy by confirming that client goals and expected outcomes have been met (see "Planning").	

See Table 42.1 (page 605) for a list of drugs to which these nursing actions apply.

42.3 Pharmacotherapy of Male Infertility

Like female infertility, male infertility may have a number of complex causes. **Oligospermia**, the presence of less than 20 million sperm per millilitre of ejaculate is considered abnormal. **Azoospermia**, the complete absence of sperm in ejaculate, may indicate an obstruction of the vas deferens or ejaculatory duct, which can be corrected surgically. Infections such as mumps, chronic tuberculosis, and sexually transmitted infections can contribute to infertility. The possibility of erectile dysfunction must be considered and treated as discussed in Section 42.4. Infertility may occur with or without signs of hypogonadism.

The goal of endocrine pharmacotherapy of male infertility is to increase sperm production. Therapy often begins with IM injections of human chorionic gonadotropin (HCG), three times per week over 1 year. Although secreted by the placenta, the effects of HCG in the male are identical to those of LH: increasing testosterone secretion and stimulating spermatogenesis. Sperm counts are conducted periodically to assess therapeutic progress. If HCG is unsuccessful, therapy with menotropins may be attempted. Menotropins consist of a mixture of purified FSH and LH. For infertile clients exhibiting signs of hypogonadism, testosterone therapy also may be indicated.

Other pharmacological approaches to treating male infertility have been attempted. Antiestrogens such as tamoxifen and clomiphene have been used to block the negative feedback of estrogen (from the adrenal glands) to the pituitary and hypothalamus, thus increasing the levels of FSH and LH. Testolactone, an aromatase inhibitor, has been administered to block the metabolic conversion of testosterone to estrogen. Various nutritional supplements, such as zinc to improve sperm production, L-arginine to improve sperm motility, and vitamins C and E as antioxidants to reduce reactive intermediates, have been tested. Unfortunately, these and other attempts have not been conclusively shown to have any positive effect on male infertility.

Drug therapy for infertility is not as successful for males as it is for females because only about 5% of infertile males have a disorder with an endocrine etiology. Many years of therapy may be required. Because of the expense and the large number of injections needed, other means of conception may be explored, such as in vitro fertilization or intrauterine insemination.

ERECTILE DYSFUNCTION

Erectile dysfunction, or **impotence**, is a common disorder in men. The defining characteristic of this condition is the consistent inability to either obtain an erection or to sustain an erection long enough to achieve successful intercourse.

42.4 Pharmacotherapy of Erectile Dysfunction

The incidence of erectile dysfunction increases with advancing age, although it may occur in a male adult of any age. Certain diseases, most notably atherosclerosis, diabetes, stroke, and hypertension, are associated with a higher incidence of the condition. Psychogenic causes may include depression, fatigue, guilt, or fear of sexual failure. A number of common drugs cause impotence as a side effect in some men, including thiazide diuretics, phenothiazines, serotonin reuptake inhibitors, tricyclic antidepressants, propranolol, and diazepam. Loss of libido may be due to low testosterone secretion.

Penile erection has both neuromuscular and vascular components. Autonomic nerves dilate arterioles leading to the major erectile tissues of the penis, called the **corpora cavernosa** (singular: corpus cavernosum). The corpora have vascular spaces that fill with blood to cause rigidity. The vasoconstriction of veins draining blood from the corpora allows the penis to remain rigid long enough for successful penetration. After ejaculation, the veins dilate, blood leaves the corpora, and the penis quickly loses its rigidity. Organic causes of erectile dysfunction may include damage to the nerves or blood vessels involved in the erection reflex.

The marketing of sildenafil, an inhibitor of the enzyme phosphodiesterase-5, has revolutionized the medical therapy of erectile dysfunction. When sildenafil was approved as the first pharmacological treatment for erectile dysfunction in 1998, it set a record for pharmaceutical sales for any new drug in US history. Prior to the discovery of sildenafil, rigid or inflatable penile prostheses were implanted into the corpora. As an alternative to prostheses, drugs such as alprostadil or the combination of papaverine plus phentolamine were injected directly into the corpora cavernosa just prior to intercourse. Injections caused pain in many clients and reduced the spontaneity associated with pleasurable intercourse. These alternative therapies are rare today, though they may be used for clients in whom sildenafil is contraindicated.

The nurse should be aware that sildenafil does not cause an erection; it merely enhances the erection caused by physical contact or other sexual stimuli. In addition, sildenafil is not as effective in promoting erections in men who do not have erectile dysfunction. Despite considerable research interest, no effects of sildenafil have been shown on female sexual function, and this drug is not approved for use by women.

Another phosphodiesterase-5 inhibitor, vardenafil, acts by the same mechanism as sildenafil but has a faster onset and slightly longer duration of action. The two drugs exhibit similar types of side effects. Tadalafil is a third phosphodiesterase-5 inhibitor that acts within 30 minutes and is reported to have a prolonged duration lasting from 24 to 36 hours.

NURSING CONSIDERATIONS

The role of the nurse in pharmacotherapy with erectile dysfunction agents involves careful monitoring of the client's condition and providing education as it relates to the prescribed drug regimen. Obtain a complete physical examination including history of impaired sexual function, cardiovascular disease, and presence of emotional disturbances. Obtain and monitor results of lab tests related to liver function. Sildenafil and vardenafil are contraindicated with the use of organic nitrates and nitroglycerin because they potentiate the effect of nitrates, leading to severe hypotension. Nitrates are also found in recreational drugs, including amyl nitrate and nitrite, commonly called "poppers." Coadministration of vardenafil and alpha-adrenergic blockers can also lead to profound hypotension. These agents are contraindicated in clients with severe cardiovascular disease and in the presence of anatomical deformities of the penis.

Use cautiously in the client with hepatic dysfunction because these drugs are metabolized in the liver and drug accumulation may lead to toxicity. Clients with cirrhosis or severe decreased liver function should start with lower doses. Leukemia, sickle cell anemia, multiple myeloma, ulcer, and retinitis pigmentosa clients should also use sildenafil cautiously.

Monitor for side effects of the drug. Monitor for vision changes such as blurred vision, being unable to differentiate between green and blue, objects having a blue tinge, and photophobia. Also observe safety precautions until it is known if sensory-perceptual alterations will occur, so falls and other accidents can be avoided. The client should be monitored for presence of headache, dizziness, flushing, rash, nasal congestion, diarrhea, dyspepsia, urinary tract infection (UTI), chest pain, and indigestion.

Client education as it relates to erectile dysfunction agents should include goals, reasons for obtaining baseline data such as vital signs and tests for liver and cardiac function, and possible side effects. For clients receiving sildenafil

---

Pr PROTOTYPE DRUG | Sildenafil (Viagra)

ACTIONS AND USES

Sildenafil acts by relaxing smooth muscle in the corpus cavernosum, thus allowing increased blood flow into the penis. The increased blood flow results in a firmer and longer-lasting erection in about 70% of men taking the drug. The onset of action is relatively rapid, less than 1 hour, and its effects last 2 to 4 hours. Sildenafil blocks the enzyme phosphodiesterase-5.

PHARMACOKINETICS

Sildenafil is rapidly absorbed after oral administration. It is widely distributed, but little enters semen. Sildenafil is 96% plasma protein bound. It is mostly metabolized by the liver. It is mostly excreted in feces with a small amount excreted in urine. Half-life is 4 hours.

ADMINISTRATION ALERTS

- Avoid administration of sildenafil with meals, especially high-fat meals, because absorption is decreased.
- Avoid grapefruit juice when administering sildenafil.

ADVERSE EFFECTS AND INTERACTIONS

The most serious adverse effect, hypotension, occurs in clients concurrently taking organic nitrates for angina. Common side effects include headache, dizziness, flushing, rash, nasal congestion, diarrhea, dyspepsia, UTI, chest pain, and indigestion. Priapism, a sustained erection lasting longer than 6 hours, has been reported with sildenafil use and may lead to permanent damage to penile tissues.

Sildenafil interacts with many drugs. Cimetidine, erythromycin, and ketoconazole will increase serum levels of sildenafil and necessitate lower drug doses. Protease inhibitors will cause increased sildenafil levels, which may lead to toxicity. Rifampin may decrease sildenafil levels, leading to decreased effectiveness.

 See the Companion Website for a Nursing Process Focus chart specific to this drug.

or vardenafil, the following are the important teaching points:

- Do not take more than one dose in a 24-hour period.
- Have vital signs, including blood pressure, checked routinely.
- Take sildenafil 1 hour prior to sexual activity and vardenafil 25 to 40 minutes prior to sexual activity.
- If taking nitrates or alpha-blockers, do not use erectile dysfunction agents.
- Do not share medication.
- Do not take more than the recommended dose as this increases the risk of side effects.

BENIGN PROSTATIC HYPERPLASIA

Benign prostatic hyperplasia (BPH) is an enlargement of the prostate gland that occurs in most men of advanced age. It is a non-malignant disorder that progressively decreases the outflow of urine by obstructing the urethra, causing difficult urination. BPH is not considered to be a precursor to prostate carcinoma.

BPH is characterized by increased urinary frequency (usually with small amounts of urine), increased urgency to urinate, post-void leakage, excessive nighttime urination, decreased force of the urine stream, and a sensation that the bladder did not empty completely. The urinary outlet obstruction can lead to serious complications such as urinary infections or uremia. In severe cases, a surgical procedure called transurethral resection is needed to restore the patency of the urethra. BPH is illustrated in Figure 42.2.

ANTIPROSTATIC AGENTS

Only a few drugs are available for the pharmacotherapy of BPH. Early in the course of the disease, drug therapy may be of benefit. These agents are shown in Table 42.2.

42.5 Pharmacotherapy of Benign Prostatic Hyperplasia

Although most of the symptoms of BPH are caused by static pressure of the enlarged prostate on the urethra, approximately 40% of the pressure has a functional component caused by increased smooth muscle tone in the region. Alpha$_1$-adrenergic receptors are located in smooth muscle cells in the neck of the urinary bladder and in the prostate gland. The role of these receptors in normal physiology is not completely understood. When activated, however, the alpha$_1$-adrenergic receptors provide resistance to urine outflow from the bladder and inhibit the micturition reflex.

Only a few drugs are available to treat benign enlargement of the prostate. Although the drugs have limited efficacy, they have some value in treating mild disease, as an

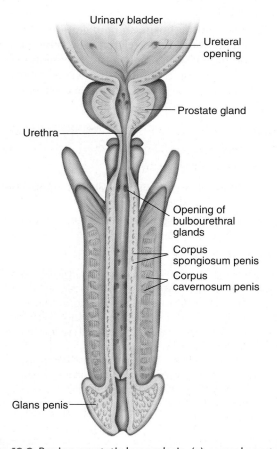

(a)

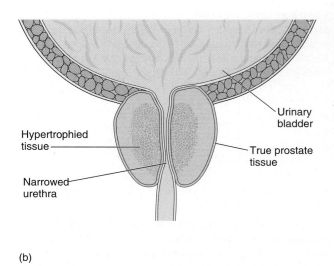

(b)

● **Figure 42.2** Benign prostatic hyperplasia: (a) normal prostate and penis; (b) benign prostatic hyperplasia

Source: Pearson Education/PH College.

TABLE 42.2   Agents for Benign Prostatic Hyperplasia

Drug	Route and Adult Dose
Alpha-Adrenergic Blockers	
doxazosin (Cardura) (see page 268 for the Protoype Drug box)	PO; 1–8 mg qd
prazosin (Minipress)	PO; 1 mg qid or bid
tamsulosin (Novo-Tamsulosin)	PO; 0.4 mg qd 30 min after a meal 0.8 mg qd (max 0.8 mg/d)
terazosin (Apo-Terazosin)	PO; start with 1 mg hs, then 1–5 mg/d (max 20 mg/d)
5-Alpha Reductase Inhibitors	
finasteride (Proscar)	PO; 5 mg qd

alternative to surgery. Because pharmacotherapy alleviates the symptoms but does not cure the disease, these medications must be taken the remainder of the client's life or until surgery is indicated. The most common drug for BPH is finasteride, a 5-alpha-reductase inhibitor.

Although primarily used for hypertension, several alpha$_1$-adrenergic blockers have been approved for BPH. The selective alpha$_1$-blockers relax smooth muscle in the prostate gland, bladder neck, and urethra, thus easing the urinary obstruction. Doxazosin and terazosin are of particular value to clients who have both hypertension and BPH; these two disorders occur concurrently in about 25% of men over age 60. A third alpha$_1$-blocker, tamsulosin, has no effect on blood pressure and its only indication is BPH. Drugs in this class improve urine flow and reduce other bothersome symptoms of BPH within 1 to 2 weeks after start of therapy. Primary adverse effects include headache, fatigue, and dizziness. Doxazosin and terazosin are not associated with an increased risk of sexual dysfunction, but ejaculatory dysfunction has been reported with tamsulosin. Reflex tachycardia due to stimulation of baroreceptors is common with alpha-blockers. Additional information on the alpha-blockers is presented in Chapter 21.

NURSING CONSIDERATIONS

The role of the nurse in drug therapy with antiprostatic agents involves careful monitoring of the client's condition and providing education as it relates to the prescribed drug regimen. Obtain a complete physical examination including history of cardiovascular disease and sexual dysfunction. Also assess changes in urinary elimination including urinary retention, nocturia, dribbling, difficulty starting urinary stream, frequency, and urgency. If the client is prescribed alpha-blockers for treatment of prostatic hypertrophy, the client's vital signs should be assessed, especially blood pressure and heart rate. The client may experience hypotension with the first few doses, and orthostatic hypotension may persist throughout treatment. The first-dose phenomenon, especially syncope, can occur. Monitor the client for evidence of orthostatic hypotension, dizziness, and GI disturbances. Older adults are especially prone to the hypotensive and hypothermic effects related to vasodilation caused

by these drugs. Alpha-blockers should be used cautiously in clients with asthma or heart failure because they cause bradycardia and bronchoconstriction.

Exercise caution in clients with decreased hepatic function because the drugs are metabolized in the liver. Clients with obstructive uropathy should use finasteride cautiously. Monitor the emotional status of clients taking alpha-blockers as depression is a common side effect. Inform the client that it may take 6 to 12 months of treatment before the drug relieves symptoms of BPH. Improvement will last only as long as the medication is continued.

Monitor for side effects of the antiprostatic agent. Side effects include impotence, decreased volume of ejaculate, and decreased libido. Inform the client to report these occurrences to the healthcare provider.

Client education related to antiprostatic agents should include goals, reasons for obtaining baseline data such as vital signs and tests for cardiac and renal function, and possible side effects. For clients receiving an alpha-blocker, the following are the important teaching points:

- Report increased difficulty with urinary voiding.
- Report significant side effects.
- Take medication at bedtime, and take the first dose immediately before getting into bed.
- Always arise slowly, avoiding sudden posture changes.

NATURAL THERAPIES

Saw Palmetto

Saw palmetto *(Serona repens)* is a bushy palm that grows in the coastal regions of the southern United States. The portion having medicinal properties is the berries of the plant. Like finasteride, saw palmetto is thought to help stop a cascade of prostate-damaging enzymes that may lead to BPH. It also occupies binding sites on the prostate that are typically occupied by dihydrotestosterone (DHT), an enzyme that may trigger BPH. It may reduce prostate swelling and inflammation by blocking estradiol, a type of estrogen that can cause prostate cells to multiply. Several clinical studies have suggested that saw palmetto is as effective as finasteride at treating mild to moderate BPH and produces fewer side effects.

Saw palmetto contains a variety of sterols and free fatty acids that are thought to be responsible for its beneficial actions, although the sterol beta-sitosterol has recently been proposed as the major active ingredient. Doses range from 160 to 320 mg/day of standardized extract or 2 to 3 mg/day of dried berries.

Pr PROTOTYPE DRUG | Finasteride (Proscar)

ACTIONS AND USES

Finasteride acts by inhibiting 5-alpha-reductase, the enzyme responsible for converting testosterone to one of its metabolites, 5-alpha-dihydrotestosterone. This metabolite causes proliferation of prostate cells and promotes enlargement of the gland. Because it inhibits the metabolism of testosterone, finasteride is sometimes called an antiandrogen. Finasteride promotes shrinkage of an enlarged prostate and subsequently helps to restore urinary function. It is most effective in clients with larger prostates. This drug is also marketed as Propecia, which is prescribed to promote hair regrowth in clients with male-pattern baldness. Doses of finasteride are five times higher when prescribed for BPH than when prescribed for baldness.

PHARMACOKINETICS

Finasteride is well absorbed after oral administration. It is widely distributed, crosses the blood-brain barrier, and enters prostate tissue. Finasteride is 90% plasma protein bound. It is mostly metabolized by the liver. The drug is mostly excreted in feces with a lesser amount excreted in urine. Half-life is 6 hours.

ADMINISTRATION ALERTS

- Tablets may be crushed for oral administration.
- The pregnant nurse should avoid handling crushed medication as it may be absorbed through the skin and cause harm to a male fetus.

ADVERSE EFFECTS AND INTERACTIONS

Finasteride causes various types of sexual dysfunction in up to 16% of clients, including impotence, diminished libido, and ejaculatory dysfunction.
No clinically significant drug interactions have been established.
Use with caution with herbal supplements. For example, saw palmetto may potentiate the effects of finasteride.

NURSING PROCESS FOCUS   Clients Receiving Finasteride (Proscar)

Assessment	Potential Nursing Diagnoses/Identified Patterns
Prior to administration: ■ Obtain complete health history including liver disease and altered urinary functioning. ■ Obtain drug history to determine possible drug interactions and allergies. ■ Determine if client has a female partner who is pregnant or who is planning to become pregnant.	■ Risk for sexual dysfunction related to effects of drug therapy or decreased hormone production ■ Non-adherence related to side effects of drug therapy ■ Need for knowledge regarding drug therapy and adverse effects

Planning: Client Goals and Expected Outcomes

The client will:
- Experience a decreased size of enlarged prostate gland
- Demonstrate an understanding of the drug's action by accurately describing drug side effects and precautions and importance of follow-up care

Implementation

Interventions (Rationales)	Client Education/Discharge Planning
■ Monitor urinary function. (Finasteride may interfere with PSA test results.)	Instruct client to: ■ Schedule a digital rectal exam and PSA test periodically during therapy ■ Recognize and report symptoms of BPH: urinary retention, hesitancy, difficulty starting stream, decreased diameter of stream, nocturia, dribbling, frequency ■ Avoid all fluids in evenings, especially caffeine-containing fluids and alcohol, to avoid nocturia ■ Drink adequate fluids early in day to decrease chances of kidney stones and UTI
■ Monitor female partner for pregnancy. (Finasteride is teratogenic to the male fetus.)	Instruct client and/or female partner to: ■ Avoid semen of man using finasteride ■ Avoid touching crushed tablets of finasteride to prevent transdermal absorption and the transfer of medication through placenta to fetus ■ Use a reliable barrier contraceptive during therapy

continued

NURSING PROCESS FOCUS Clients Receiving Finasteride (Proscar) *(Continued)*	
Interventions (Rationales)	**Client Education/Discharge Planning**
■ Monitor client's commitment to the medication regimen. (Maximum therapeutic effects may take several months.)	Instruct client and/or female partner to: ■ Continue medication even if no decrease in symptoms for 6 to 12 months, or no increase in hair growth for 3 months ■ Recognize that life-long therapy may be necessary to control symptoms of BPH
■ Monitor for adverse reactions.	■ Instruct client and/or female partner to report impotence, decreased volume of ejaculate, or decreased libido.
Evaluation of Outcome Criteria	
Evaluate the effectiveness of drug therapy by confirming that client goals and expected outcomes have been met (see "Planning").	

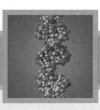

CHAPTER REVIEW

KEY CONCEPTS

The numbered key concepts provide a succinct summary of the important points from the corresponding numbered section within the chapter. If any of these points are not clear, refer to the numbered section within the chapter for review. Expanded versions can be found on the Companion Website.

42.1 FSH and LH from the pituitary regulate the secretion of testosterone, the primary hormone contributing to the growth, health, and maintenance of the male reproductive system.

42.2 Androgens are used to treat hypogonadism in males and breast cancer in females. Anabolic steroids are frequently abused by athletes and can result in serious adverse effects with long-term use.

42.3 Male infertility is difficult to treat pharmacologically; medications include HCG, menotropins, testolactone, and antiestrogens.

42.4 Erectile dysfunction is a common disorder that may be successfully treated with sildenafil, an inhibitor of the enzyme phosphodiesterase-5.

42.5 In its early stages, benign prostatic hyperplasia may be treated successfully with drug therapy, including finasteride and alpha$_1$-adrenergic blockers.

REVIEW QUESTIONS

1 Why is sildenafil used to treat erectile dysfunction rather than testosterone?

2 Why is the treatment of male infertility less successful than the treatment of female infertility?

3 Why is treatment with alpha$_1$-adrenergic blockers more successful at alleviating symptoms of BPH than 5-alpha-reductase inhibitors in men with only slightly enlarged prostates?

CRITICAL THINKING QUESTIONS

1. A 78-year-old widower has come to see his healthcare provider. The nurse practitioner interviews the client about his past medical history and current health concerns. The client states that he is planning to marry "a very nice lady" but is concerned about his sexual performance. He asks about a prescription for sildenafil. What additional historical data does the nurse need to collect given this client's age?

2. A 16-year-old male goes out for the football team. He is immediately impressed with the size of several junior and senior linemen. One older student offers to "hook him up" with a source of androstenedione (Andro). From a developmental perspective, explain why this young man may be susceptible to anabolic steroid abuse. How might anabolic steroid abuse impact his body and health? What is the role of the nurse in regard to anabolic steroid abuse?

3. A 68-year-old man has been diagnosed with benign prostatic hyperplasia (BPH). As the nurse prepares to educate him about his prescription for finasteride, he says that he has been hearing about the benefits of saw palmetto, an herbal preparation. Discuss the mechanism of action of finasteride and compare it to that of saw palmetto.

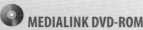

EXPLORE MediaLink

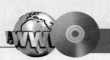

www.pearsoned.ca/adams-king

MEDIALINK DVD-ROM
- Audio Glossary
- CRNE Review
- Animation
  Mechanism of Action: Sildenafil

 COMPANION WEBSITE
- CRNE Review
- Case Study: Client taking male hormones
- Dosage Calculations

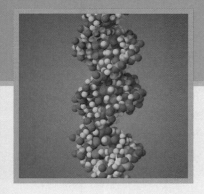

CHAPTER 43

Drugs for Renal Disorders and Diuretic Therapy

DRUGS AT A GLANCE

LOOP (HIGH-CEILING) DIURETICS

THIAZIDE AND THIAZIDE-LIKE DIURETICS
  chlorothiazide (Diuril)

POTASSIUM-SPARING DIURETICS
  spironolactone (Aldactone)

MISCELLANEOUS AGENTS
Carbonic anhydrase inhibitors
Osmotic diuretics

OBJECTIVES

After reading this chapter, the student should be able to do the following:

1. Identify drug classes used for treating renal disorders and fluid excess.
2. Explain the therapeutic action of each class of diuretic in relation to underlying pathophysiology.
3. Compare and contrast the loop, thiazide, and potassium-sparing diuretics in terms of action and indications for their use.
4. Discuss the role of the nurse regarding non-pharmacological care and client teaching.
5. Describe the nurse's role in the pharmacological management of clients receiving diuretics and other therapies for renal disorders.
6. Describe the adjustments in pharmacotherapy that must be considered in clients with renal failure.
7. For each of the drug classes listed in Drugs at a Glance, identify a representative drug and explain its mechanism of action, therapeutic effects, and important adverse effects.
8. Describe and explain, based on pharmacological principles, the rationale for nursing assessment, planning, and interventions for clients receiving diuretics.
9. Use the nursing process to care for clients receiving therapy for fluid excess and renal disorders.

MediaLink

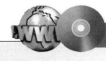

www.pearsoned.ca/adams-king

CRNE review, case studies, and other interactive resources for this chapter can be found on the Companion Website at **www.pearsoned.ca/adams-king**. Click on "Chapter 43" to select the activities for this chapter. For animations, more CRNE review questions, and an audio glossary, access the accompanying DVD-ROM in this textbook.

KEY TERMS

The kidneys serve an amazing role in maintaining proper homeostasis. By filtering a volume equivalent to all the body's extracellular fluid every 100 minutes, the kidneys are able to make immediate adjustments to fluid volume, electrolyte composition, and acid-base balance. The purpose of this chapter is to examine agents that influence kidney function by increasing urine output. Chapter 44 will cover agents that more specifically affect fluid, electrolyte, and acid-base imbalances.

PHARMFACTS

Renal Disorders

- Kidney disease can strike anyone at any age.
- It is estimated that 2 million Canadians have chronic kidney disease.
- Each day, an average of 14 Canadians learn that their kidneys have failed.
- The three leading causes of kidney failure in are type 2 diabetes, hypertension, and glomerulonephritis.
- If kidney failure is not treated, the person dies within days or weeks.
- Annually, almost 20,000 Canadians are on dialysis.
- Over 1000 kidney transplants are performed annually in Canada.
- Of the 4240 Canadians on the waiting list for a transplant (as of December 2006), 3075 were awaiting a kidney transplant.
- The sale and purchase of organs for transplant is illegal in Canada.

Source: The Kidney Foundation of Canada, "http://www.kidney.sk.ca/ prevention/statistics/canada.html".

MediaLink   Animation: Basic Function of the Kidney

MediaLink   Nephrology Channel

43.1 Functions of the Kidneys

When most people think of the kidneys, they think of excretion. Although this is certainly true, the kidneys have many other homeostatic functions. The kidneys are the primary organs for regulating fluid balance, electrolyte composition, and acid-base balance of body fluids. They also secrete the enzyme renin, which helps to regulate blood pressure (Chapter 21), and erythropoietin, a hormone that stimulates red blood cell production (Chapter 28). In addition, the kidneys are responsible for the production of calcitriol, the active form of vitamin D, which helps maintain bone homeostasis (Chapter 46). It is not surprising that the overall health of the client is strongly dependent on proper functioning of the kidneys.

The urinary system consists of two kidneys, two ureters, one urinary bladder, and a urethra. Each kidney contains over 1 million **nephrons**, the functional units of the kidney. As blood enters a nephron, it is filtered through a semipermeable membrane known as **Bowman's capsule**. Water and other small molecules readily pass through Bowman's capsule and enter the first section of the nephron, the **proximal tubule**. Once in the nephron, the fluid is called **filtrate**. After leaving the proximal tubule, the filtrate travels through the **loop of Henle** and, subsequently, the **distal tubule**. Nephrons empty their filtrate into common collecting ducts, which empty into larger collecting structures inside the kidney. Fluid leaving the collecting ducts and entering subsequent portions of the kidney is called urine. Parts of the nephron are illustrated in Figure 43.1.

43.2 Renal Reabsorption and Secretion

When filtrate passes through Bowman's capsule, its composition is the same as plasma minus large proteins, such as albumin, that are too large to pass through the filter. As the filtrate travels through the nephron, its composition changes dramatically. Some substances in the filtrate pass across the walls of the nephron

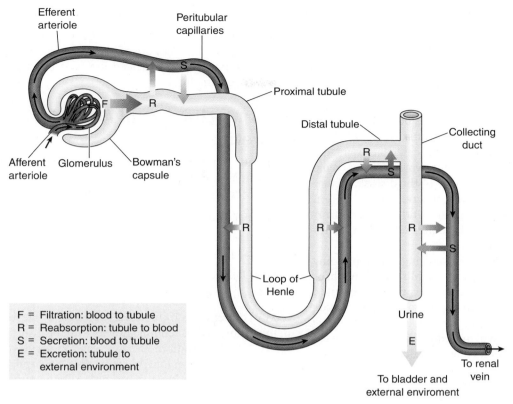

F = Filtration: blood to tubule
R = Reabsorption: tubule to blood
S = Secretion: blood to tubule
E = Excretion: tubule to
    external environment

● **Figure 43.1** The nephron

to re-enter the blood, a process known as **reabsorption**. Water is the most important molecule reabsorbed in the tubule. For every 178 L of water entering the filtrate each day, 172 L are reabsorbed, leaving only 1.5 L to be excreted in the urine. Glucose, amino acids, and essential ions such as sodium, chloride, calcium, and bicarbonate are also reabsorbed.

Certain ions and molecules too large to pass through Bowman's capsule may still enter the urine by crossing from the blood to the filtrate by a process known as **secretion**. Potassium, phosphate, hydrogen, ammonium ions, and many organic acids enter the filtrate through this mechanism.

Reabsorption and secretion are critical to the pharmacokinetics of many drugs. Some drugs are reabsorbed, whereas others are secreted into the filtrate. For example, approximately 90% of a dose of penicillin G enters the urine through secretion. The processes of reabsorption and secretion are shown in Figure 43.1.

RENAL FAILURE

Renal failure is a decrease in kidney function resulting in an inability to maintain electrolyte and fluid balance and excrete nitrogenous waste products. Renal failure may be acute or chronic and may result from disorders of other body systems or be intrinsic to the kidney itself. The primary treatment goal is to maintain blood flow through the kidney and adequate urine output.

43.3 Pharmacotherapy of Renal Failure

Before pharmacotherapy may be considered in a client with renal failure, an accurate diagnosis of the kidney impairment is necessary. The basic diagnostic test is a **urinalysis**, which examines urine for the presence of blood cells, proteins, pH, specific gravity, ketones, glucose, and microorganisms. Although it is easy to perform, the urinalysis is non-specific and does not identify the etiology of the kidney disease. Many diseases can cause abnormal urinalysis values. To provide a more definitive diagnosis, diagnostic imaging such as computed tomography, sonography, or magnetic resonance imaging may be necessary. Renal biopsy may be performed to obtain a more specific diagnosis.

Renal failure is classified as acute or chronic. Acute renal failure requires immediate treatment because retention of nitrogenous waste products in the body such as urea and creatinine, known as **azotemia**, can result in death if untreated. The most common cause of acute renal failure is renal hypoperfusion—lack of sufficient blood flowing through the kidneys. Hypoperfusion can lead to permanent damage to kidney cells. To correct this type of renal failure, the cause of the hypoperfusion must be quickly identified and corrected. Potential causes include heart failure, dysrhythmias, hemorrhage, and dehydration.

Chronic renal failure occurs over a period of months or years. Over half of the cases of chronic renal failure occur in clients with long-standing hypertension or diabetes mellitus.

Due to its long development and non-specific symptoms, chronic renal failure may go undiagnosed for many years, until the impairment becomes irreversible. In end-stage renal disease, dialysis and kidney transplantation become treatment alternatives.

Pharmacotherapy of renal failure attempts to treat the cause of the dysfunction. Diuretics are given to increase urine output as long as renal function is possible, and cardiovascular drugs are commonly administered to treat underlying hypertension or heart failure. Dietary management is often necessary to prevent worsening of renal impairment. Depending on the stage of the disease, dietary management may include protein restriction and reduction of sodium, potassium, phosphorous, and magnesium. A summary of the pharmacological agents used to treat kidney failure is given in Table 43.1.

The nurse serves a key role in recognizing and responding to renal failure. Once a diagnosis is established, all nephrotoxic medications should be either discontinued or used with extreme caution. Common nephrotoxic drugs include NSAIDs, aminoglycoside antibiotics, amphotericin B, many antineoplastic agents, and ACE inhibitors in volume-depleted clients. Because the kidneys excrete most drugs, medications will require a significant dosage reduction in clients with moderate to severe renal failure. The importance of this cannot be overemphasized: administering the "average" dose to a client in severe renal failure can have fatal consequences.

NATURAL THERAPIES

Cranberry for Urinary Tract Infections

Since the mid-1800s, cranberry has been used for the prevention of urinary tract infections. Cranberry causes an increase in the urine acidity, which discourages the growth of pathogenic microorganisms. A component in cranberries stops bacteria from adhering to bladder walls. Well-controlled studies have yet to clearly demonstrate that cranberry juice can lower the pH enough to actually kill organisms; however, anecdotal evidence remains strong in support of the treatment. The only reported adverse effect from cranberry is increased diarrhea when large quantities are ingested. If a juice form is used, unsweetened juices are preferred over sweetened. Dehydrated extracts of cranberries and blueberries are also available in capsule or tablet form.

DIURETICS

Diuretics are drugs that adjust the volume and/or composition of body fluids. They are of particular value in the treatment of renal failure, hypertension, and heart failure (by removing edema fluid).

43.4 Mechanism of Action of Diuretics

A **diuretic** is a drug that increases urine output. Mobilizing excess fluid in the body for the purpose of excretion is particularly desirable in the following conditions:

- Hypertension
- Heart failure
- Kidney failure
- Liver failure or cirrhosis
- Pulmonary edema

Most diuretics act by blocking sodium (Na^+) reabsorption in the nephron, thus sending more Na^+ to the urine. Chloride ion (Cl^-) follows sodium. Because water molecules also tend to travel with sodium ions, blocking the reabsorption of Na^+ will increase the volume of urination, known as diuresis. Some drugs, such as furosemide, act by preventing the reabsorption of sodium in the loop of Henle. Because of the abundance of sodium in the filtrate within the loop of Henle, furosemide is capable of producing large increases in urine output. Other drugs, such as the thiazides, act on the distal tubule. Because most Na^+ has already been reabsorbed from the filtrate by the time it reaches the distal tubule, the thiazides produce less diuresis than furosemide. The sites in the nephron at which the various diuretics act are shown in Figure 43.2.

It is common practice to combine two or more drugs in the pharmacotherapy of hypertension and fluid retention disorders. The primary rationales for combination therapy are that the incidence of side effects is decreased and the pharmacological effect may be enhanced. For client convenience, some of these drugs are combined in single tablet

TABLE 43.1 Pharmacological Management of Renal Failure

Complication	Pathogenesis	Treatment
anemia	hypoperfusion of kidneys results in less erythropoietin synthesis	erythropoietin (epoetin alfa, Procrit, Epogen)
hyperkalemia	kidneys are unable to adequately excrete potassium	dietary restriction of potassium; polystyrene sulfate (Kayexalate) with sorbitol
hyperphosphatemia	kidneys are unable to adequately excrete phosphate	dietary restriction of phosphate; phosphate binders such as calcium carbonate (Os-Cal 500, others), calcium acetate (PhosLo), or sevelamer HCl (Renagel)
hypervolemia	hypoperfusion of kidneys leads to water retention	dietary restriction of sodium; loop diuretics in acute conditions, thiazide diuretics in mild conditions
hypocalcemia	hyperphosphatemia leads to loss of calcium	usually corrected by reversing the hyperphosphatemia but additional calcium supplements may be necessary
metabolic acidosis	kidneys are unable to adequately excrete metabolic acids	sodium bicarbonate or sodium citrate

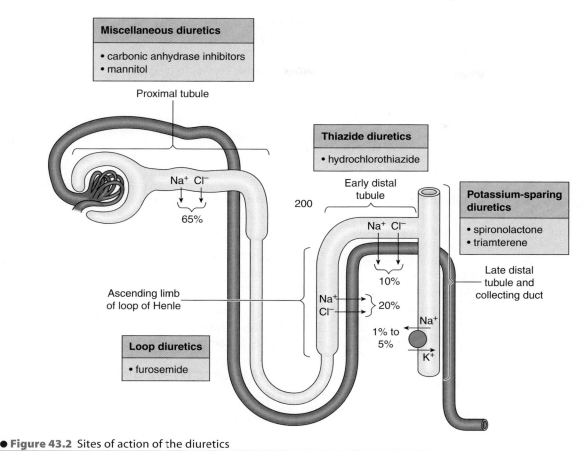

Miscellaneous diuretics

- carbonic anhydrase inhibitors
- mannitol

Proximal tubule

Thiazide diuretics

- hydrochlorothiazide

Na⁺ Cl⁻

65%

200

Early distal tubule

Potassium-sparing diuretics

- spironolactone
- triamterene

Na⁺ Cl⁻

10%

Ascending limb of loop of Henle

Na⁺ Cl⁻

20%

Late distal tubule and collecting duct

1% to 5%

Na⁺

Loop diuretics

- furosemide

Na⁺

K⁺

● **Figure 43.2** Sites of action of the diuretics

formulations. Examples of single tablet diuretic combinations include the following:

- Aldactazide: hydrochlorothiazide and spironolactone
- Apresazide: hydrochlorothiazide and hydralazine
- Dyazide: hydrochlorothiazide and triamterene
- Maxzide: hydrochlorothiazide and triamterene

43.5 Pharmacotherapy with Loop Diuretics

The most effective diuretics are called loop (high-ceiling) diuretics. Drugs in this class act by blocking the reabsorption of sodium and chloride in the loop of Henle. When given IV, they have the ability to cause large amounts of fluid to be excreted by the kidney in a very short time. Loop diuretics are used to reduce the edema associated with heart failure, hepatic cirrhosis, or chronic renal failure. Furosemide and torsemide are also approved for hypertension. The loop diuretics are shown in Table 43.2.

Furosemide is the most commonly prescribed loop diuretic. A Prototype Drug profile for furosemide is provided in Chapter 24 (page 314). Unlike the thiazide diuretics, furosemide is able to increase urine output even when blood flow to the kidneys is diminished, which makes it of particular value in clients with renal failure. Torsemide has a longer half-life than furosemide, which offers the advantage

of once-a-day dosing. Bumetanide is 40 times more potent than furosemide but has a shorter duration of action.

The rapid excretion of large amounts of water has the potential to produce serious adverse effects such as dehydration and electrolyte imbalances. Signs of dehydration include thirst, dry mouth, weight loss, and headache. Hypotension, dizziness, and fainting can result from the fluid loss. Excess potassium loss may result in dysrhythmias; potassium supplements may be indicated to prevent **hypokalemia**. Potassium loss is of particular concern to clients who are also taking digoxin. Although rare, ototoxicity is possible and other ototoxic drugs such as the aminoglycoside antibiotics should be avoided during loop diuretic therapy. Because of the potential for serious side effects, the loop diuretics are normally reserved for clients with moderate to severe fluid retention or when other diuretics have failed to achieve therapeutic goals.

NURSING CONSIDERATIONS

The role of the nurse in loop diuretic therapy involves careful monitoring of the client's condition and providing education as it relates to the prescribed drug regimen. Prior to initiation of therapy, obtain baseline values for weight, blood pressure (sitting and supine), pulse, respiration, and electrolytes. Any sites of edema, and its extent, should be recorded. Measure the abdominal girth of clients with fluid

TABLE 43.2 Loop Diuretics

Drug	Route and Adult Dose
bumetanide (Burinex)	PO; 0.5–2 mg qd; may repeat at 4–5 h intervals if needed (max 10 mg/d) IV/IM; 0.5–1 mg over 1–2 min, repeated q2–3h prn (max 10 mg/d)
ethacrynic acid (Edecrin)	PO; 50–100 mg qd–bid, may increase by 25–50 mg prn (max 400 mg/d) IV; 0.5–1 mg/kg or 50 mg up to 100 mg; may repeat if necessary
furosemide (Lasix) (see page 314 for the Prototype Drug box)	PO; 20–80 mg in 1 or more divided doses (max 600 mg/d) IV/IM; 20–40 mg in 1 or more divided doses (max 600 mg/d)

in the abdomen (ascites). Loop diuretics should be used with caution in clients with cardiovascular disease, renal impairment, diabetes mellitus, or a history of gout. They should also be used with caution in clients who are pregnant or who are concurrently taking digoxin, lithium, ototoxic drugs, NSAIDs, or other antihypertensives.

Blood pressure and pulse rate should be monitored regularly. Should a substantial drop in blood pressure occur, the medication should be withheld and the pressure reported to the physician. Intake and output should be monitored, including weighing the client daily and evaluating for decreased edema. Potassium levels should be monitored closely as loop diuretics cause potassium depletion. Closely observe elderly clients for weakness, hypotension, and confusion. Monitor lab results for electrolyte imbalance, elevated BUN, hyperglycemia, and anemia, which can be side effects of diuretics. Monitor vital signs and intake and output carefully to establish effectiveness of the medication. Rapid and excessive diuresis can result in dehydration, hypovolemia, and circulatory collapse.

Client education as it relates to loop diuretics should include goals, reasons for obtaining baseline data such as vital signs and tests for renal disorders, and possible side effects. Following are important points to include when teaching clients regarding loop diuretics:

- Weigh self daily, preferably in the morning before eating.
- Maintain a weight record.
- Monitor blood pressure and report substantial pressure drops.

LIFESPAN CONSIDERATIONS

Diuretic Therapy in Older Adult Clients

Diuretic therapy is commonly used to treat older adults with chronic diseases such as heart failure. The target goal for diuretic therapy is removal of excess fluid to reduce the cardiac workload. This can be a problem for older adults for several reasons. Diuretics can cause frequent urination, which can be inconvenient and increase the likelihood of incontinence in an elderly person. With the threat of this embarrassment, the older adult may opt for less participation in activities, resulting in social isolation. Depression may result. In addition to these risks, diuretics can cause electrolyte imbalances, making older adults susceptible to faintness, dizziness, and falls. Again, fear of these adverse effects can promote isolation. Nurses must assess for these concerns and work with older adults to help them maintain diuretic therapy and maintain the quality of their lives.

- Make position changes slowly because diuretics in combination with other drugs can cause dizziness.
- Report any hearing loss.
- Monitor blood glucose diligently (for diabetic clients).
- Report tenderness or swelling in joints, which may indicate gout.

See "Nursing Process Focus: Clients Receiving Diuretic Therapy" in this chapter (page 624) for the complete nursing process applied to caring for clients receiving diuretic therapy.

43.6 Pharmacotherapy with Thiazide Diuretics

The thiazides comprise the largest, most commonly prescribed class of diuretics. These drugs act on the distal tubule to block Na^+ reabsorption and increase potassium and water excretion. Their primary use is for the treatment of mild to moderate hypertension; however, they are also indicated for edema due to mild to moderate heart failure, liver failure, or renal failure. They are less efficacious than the loop diuretics and are not effective in clients with severe renal failure. The thiazide diuretics are shown in Table 43.3.

All the thiazide diuretics have equivalent efficacy and safety profiles. They differ, however, in their potency and duration of action. Four drugs, chlorthalidone, indapamide, metolazone, and quinethazone, are not true thiazides, but they are included with this drug class because they have similar actions and side effects.

Other than lack of ototoxicity, the side effects of the thiazides are identical to those of the loop diuretics, though their frequency is less. Diabetic clients should be made aware that thiazide diuretics sometimes raise blood glucose levels.

NURSING CONSIDERATIONS

The role of the nurse in thiazide diuretic therapy involves careful monitoring of the client's condition and providing education as it relates to the prescribed drug regimen. Prior to administering diuretics, assess for hypotension and withhold the medication if low blood pressure is present. Assess for hypersensitivity to thiazides or sulfonamides, anuria, and hypokalemia because thiazides are contraindicated in clients with these conditions. They should be used with

TABLE 43.3	Thiazide and Thiazide-Like Diuretics
Drug	*Route and Adult Dose*
Short Acting	
℗ chlorothiazide (Diuril)	PO; 250 mg–1 g/d in 1–2 divided doses IV; 250 mg–1 g/d in 1–2 divided doses
hydrochlorothiazide (HCTZ, Urozide) (see page 258 for the Prototype Drug box)	PO; 25–200 mg/d in 1–3 divided doses
Intermediate Acting	
hydroflumethiazide (Diucardin, Saluron)	PO; 25 mg–200 mg/d in 1–2 divided doses
metolazone (Zaroxolyn, Mykrox)	PO; 5–20 mg qd
quinethazone (Hydromox)	PO; 50–100 mg qd
Long Acting	
chlorthalidone (Apo-Chlorthalidone)	PO; 50–100 mg qd
indapamide (Lozide)	PO; 2.5–5 mg qd
methyclothiazide (Aquatensen, Enduron)	PO; 2.5–10 mg qd
polythiazide (Renese)	PO; 1–4 mg qd

caution in clients who are allergic to sulfa, are diabetic, or have impaired renal or hepatic function. Baseline lab tests such as CBC, electrolytes, BUN, creatinine, uric acid, and blood glucose should be obtained. All diuretics, including thiazide diuretics, reduce circulating blood volume that may cause orthostatic hypotension and changes in serum electrolyte levels. Examine the skin and mucous membranes for turgor and moisture because diuretics are notorious for causing dehydration. Monitor vital signs, especially blood pressure, when caring for clients taking thiazides. The "Nursing Process Focus: Patients Receiving Diuretic Therapy" in Chapter 21 (page 258) provides a quick guide to the care of all individuals receiving diuretic therapy.

Because the effectiveness of diuretic therapy is measured in weight loss and fluid output, the client should be weighed at the same time of day, wearing the same type of clothing. A weight gain of more than 1 kg should be reported as it may indicate fluid retention. The nurse must carefully monitor intake and output to determine hydration status and effectiveness of the medication. Conditions such as diarrhea, vomiting, or profuse sweating will increase fluid loss and put the client at greater risk for dehydration.

Assess for signs and symptoms of dehydration and excessive loss of sodium, potassium, and chloride ions. Concurrent therapy with digoxin requires careful monitoring to avoid excessive potassium loss. Like loop diuretics, the thiazides cause potassium depletion, so clients should be monitored for signs of hypokalemia. Dietary intake of high-sodium foods may negate the effects of thiazide diuretics in reducing blood pressure or relieving excessive fluid volume.

Some thiazide diuretics may cause hyperglycemia and glycosuria in diabetic clients. Blood glucose levels should be monitored closely and dosage adjustments of hypoglycemic drugs may be indicated. Also, some clients with gout may experience hyperuricemia secondary to the thiazide's inter-ference with uric acid excretion. Monitor uric acid levels and assess for symptoms of gout such as pain, swelling, and redness in the joints.

Client education as it relates to thiazides should include goals, reasons for obtaining baseline data such as vital signs and lab work, and possible side effects. Following are important points to include when teaching clients regarding thiazide diuretics:

- Monitor blood pressure on a regular basis; withhold medication and report a blood pressure below specific written parameters.
- Weigh self every morning before breakfast, wearing the same weight of clothing.
- Consume foods that are high in potassium content such as oranges, peaches, bananas, dried apricots, potatoes, tomatoes, and broccoli.
- Avoid foods high in sodium content, such as canned foods, "fast" foods, and frozen dinners.
- Protect skin from exposure to direct sunlight because these medications can cause photosensitivity.
- Take thiazide diuretics in the morning, when possible, to prevent the need to get up through the night to urinate.
- Keep a symptom log during the initial phase of therapy to assist the healthcare provider in tailoring dosage as needed.
- Use additional health promotional activities, in addition to diuretics, to help reduce blood pressure, such as smoking cessation, exercise, weight control, stress management, and moderate consumption of alcohol, if any.

See "Nursing Process Focus: Clients Receiving Diuretic Therapy" in this chapter (page 624) for the complete nursing process applied to caring for clients receiving diuretic therapy.

Pr PROTOTYPE DRUG | Chlorothiazide (Diuril)

ACTIONS AND USES

The most common indication for chlorothiazide is mild to moderate hypertension. It may be combined with other antihypertensives in the multidrug therapy of severe hypertension. It is also prescribed to treat fluid retention due to heart failure, liver disease, and corticosteroid or estrogen therapy.

ADMINISTRATION ALERTS

- Give oral doses in the morning to avoid interrupted sleep due to nocturia.
- Give IV at a rate of 0.5 g over 5 minutes when administering intermittently.
- When administering IV, take special care to avoid extravasation as this drug is highly irritating to tissues.
- Chlorothiazide is pregnancy category C.

PHARMACOKINETICS

Chlorothiazide is well absorbed after oral administration. When given orally, it may take as long as 4 weeks to obtain the optimum therapeutic effect. When given IV, results are seen in 15 to 30 minutes. It is widely distributed, crosses the placenta, and enters breast milk. It is excreted mainly unchanged in urine. Its half-life is 1.5 hours.

ADVERSE EFFECTS AND INTERACTIONS

Excess loss of water and electrolytes can occur during chlorothiazide pharmacotherapy. Symptoms include thirst, weakness, lethargy, muscle cramping, hypotension, and tachycardia. Due to the potentially serious consequences of hypokalemia, clients concurrently taking digoxin should be carefully monitored. The intake of potassium-rich foods should be increased, and potassium supplements may be indicated.

Chlorothiazide interacts with several drugs. For example, when administered with amphotericin B or corticosteroids, hypokalemic effects are increased. Antidiabetic medications such as sulfonylureas and insulin may be less effective when taken with chlorothiazide. Cholestyramine and colestipol decrease absorption of chlorothiazide. Concurrent administration with digoxin may cause digitoxin toxicity due to increased potassium and magnesium loss. Alcohol potentiates the hypotensive action of some thiazide diuretics, and caffeine may increase diuresis.

Use with caution with herbal supplements, such as licorice, which, in large amounts, will create an additive effect of hypokalemia. Aloe may increase potassium loss.

 See the Companion Website for a Nursing Process Focus chart specific to this drug.

43.7 Pharmacotherapy with Potassium-Sparing Diuretics

Hypokalemia is one of the most serious adverse effects of the thiazide and loop diuretics. The therapeutic advantage of the potassium-sparing diuretics is that mild diuresis can be obtained without affecting blood potassium levels. The potassium-sparing diuretics are shown in Table 43.4.

Normally, sodium and potassium are exchanged in the distal tubule: Na^+ is reabsorbed back into the body, and K^+ is secreted into the tubule. Potassium-sparing diuretics block this exchange, causing sodium to stay in the tubule and ultimately leave through the urine. When sodium is blocked, the body retains more K^+. Because most of the sodium has already been removed before the filtrate reaches the distal tubule, potassium-sparing diuretics produce only mild diuresis. Their primary use is in combination with thiazide or loop diuretics, to minimize potassium loss.

Unlike the loop and thiazide diuretics, clients taking potassium-sparing diuretics should not take potassium supplements or be advised to add potassium-rich foods to their diet. Intake of excess potassium when taking these medications may lead to hyperkalemia.

NURSING CONSIDERATIONS

The role of the nurse in potassium-sparing diuretic therapy involves careful monitoring of the client's condition and providing education as it relates to the prescribed drug regimen. The nurse must constantly monitor the client for signs of hyperkalemia, such as irritability, anxiety, abdominal cramping, and irregularities in pulse, because these diuretics prevent potassium from being excreted. Also assess for anuria, acute renal insufficiency, and impaired kidney function because potassium-sparing diuretics are contraindicated in these conditions. They should be used with caution in clients who have a BUN of 40 mg/dL or greater and in clients with liver disease. As with thiazide diuretics, monitor blood pressure before administering these drugs as they cause a reduction in circulating blood volume and decreased blood pressure. Electrolyte levels, especially potassium and sodium, and renal function tests should be obtained before initiating therapy and frequently during early therapy. Also assess for signs of hypersensitivity reaction, such as fever, sore throat, malaise, joint pain, ecchymoses, profound fatigue, shortness of breath, and pallor.

TABLE 43.4 Potassium-Sparing Diuretics	
Drug	*Route and Adult Dose*
amiloride (Midamor)	PO; 5 mg qd (max 20 mg/d)
spironolactone (Aldactone)	PO; 25–400 mg qd–bid
triamterene (Apo-Triazide)	PO; 100 mg bid (max 300 mg/d)

Some potassium-sparing diuretics cause dizziness when first prescribed, so the nurse must be careful to ensure client safety when the client is changing position and ambulating. The client should be instructed to continue taking the medication even though he or she may be feeling well.

Clients taking potassium-sparing diuretics may experience decreased libido. Additional hormonal side effects that may occur with these diuretics include hirsutism, irregular menses, amenorrhea, and postmenopausal bleeding in females and gynecomastia and impotence in males. Report these side effects to the healthcare provider immediately, and provide emotional support.

Follow-up care is critical with clients taking potassium-sparing diuretics. The client should have weekly blood pressure monitoring and ECG tests as directed by the healthcare provider, especially if therapy is prolonged.

Client education as it relates to potassium-sparing diuretics should include goals, reasons for obtaining baseline data such as vital signs and lab tests for electrolytes, and possible side effects. Following are important points to include when teaching clients regarding potassium-sparing diuretics:

- Report signs of hyperkalemia immediately, including irritability, anxiety, abdominal cramping, and irregular heart beat.
- Avoid using salt substitutes that are potassium based.
- Avoid eating excess amounts of foods high in potassium such as oranges, peaches, potatoes, tomatoes, broccoli, bananas, and dried apricots.
- Avoid performing tasks that require mental alertness until effects of medication are known.

- Do not abruptly discontinue taking the diuretic unless recommended by the healthcare provider.
- Take medication exactly as ordered and keep all appointments for follow-up care.
- Keep a symptom log during the initial phase of therapy to assist the healthcare provider in tailoring dosage as needed.
- Use additional health promotional activities to help reduce blood pressure, such as smoking cessation, exercise, weigh control, stress management, and moderate consumption of alcohol, if any.

See "Nursing Process Focus: Clients Receiving Diuretic Therapy" on the next page for the complete nursing process applied to caring for clients receiving diuretic therapy.

43.8 Miscellaneous Diuretics for Specific Indications

A few diuretics, shown in Table 43.5, cannot be classified as loop, thiazide, or potassium-sparing agents. These diuretics have limited and specific indications. Three of these drugs inhibit **carbonic anhydrase**, an enzyme that affects acid-base balance by its ability to form carbonic acid from water and carbon dioxide. For example, acetazolamide is a carbonic anhydrase inhibitor used to decrease intraocular fluid pressure in clients with open-angle glaucoma (see Chapter 48). Unrelated to its diuretic effect, acetazolamide also has applications as an anticonvulsant and in treating motion sickness.

The osmotic diuretics also have very specific applications. For example, mannitol is used to maintain urine flow in

---

Pr PROTOTYPE DRUG | Spironolactone (Aldactone)

ACTIONS AND USES

Spironolactone acts by blocking sodium reabsorption in the distal tubule. It accomplishes this by inhibiting aldosterone, the hormone secreted by the adrenal cortex that is responsible for increasing the renal reabsorption of sodium in exchange for potassium, thus causing water retention. When blocked by spironolactone, sodium and water excretion is increased and the body retains more potassium. The other two potassium-sparing diuretics do not exert an antialdosterone effect, but instead act by directly inhibiting the sodium-potassium exchange mechanism in the renal tubule.

PHARMACOKINETICS

Spironolactone is well absorbed after oral administration. It is widely distributed, crosses the placenta, and enters breast milk. It is mostly metabolized by the liver to canrenone, its active diuretic compound. Its half-life is 13 to 24 hours.

ADMINISTRATION ALERTS

- Give with food to increase absorption of drug.
- Do not give potassium supplements.
- Spironolactone is pregnancy category D.

ADVERSE EFFECTS AND INTERACTIONS

Spironolactone does such an efficient job of retaining potassium that **hyperkalemia** may develop. The probability of hyperkalemia is increased if the client takes potassium supplements or is concurrently taking ACE inhibitors. Signs and symptoms of hyperkalemia include muscle weakness, ventricular tachycardia, and fibrillation. When serum potassium levels are monitored carefully and maintained within normal values, side effects of spironolactone are uncommon.

Spironolactone interacts with several drugs. For example, when combined with ammonium chloride, acidosis may occur. ASA and other salicylates may decrease the diuretic effect of the medication. Concurrent use of spironolactone and digoxin may decrease the effects of digoxin. When taken with potassium supplements, ACE inhibitors, and ARBs, hyperkalemia may result.

 See the Companion Website for a Nursing Process Focus chart specific to this drug.

TABLE 43.5	Miscellaneous Diuretics
Drug	**Route and Adult Dose**
Carbonic Anhydrase Inhibitors	
acetazolamide (Diamox)	PO; 250–375 mg qd
dichlorphenamide (Daranide, Oratrol)	PO; 25–50 mg qd–tid
methazolamide (Neptazane)	PO; 50–100 mg bid–tid
Osmotic Type	
mannitol (Osmitrol)	IV; 100 g infused over 2–6 h
urea (Apo-Hydroxyurea)	IV; 1.0–1.5 g/kg over 1–2.5 h

clients with acute renal failure or during prolonged surgery. Since this agent is not reabsorbed in the tubule, it is able to maintain the flow of filtrate even in cases of severe renal hypoperfusion. Mannitol can also be used to lower intraocular pressure in certain types of glaucoma. It is a highly potent diuretic that is only given by the IV route. Unlike other diuretics that draw excess fluid away from tissue spaces, mannitol can worsen edema and thus must be used with caution in clients with pre-existing heart failure or pulmonary edema.

NURSING PROCESS FOCUS   Clients Receiving Diuretic Therapy

Assessment	Potential Nursing Diagnoses/Identified Patterns
Prior to administration: ■ Obtain complete health history (mental and physical), including data on recent surgeries or trauma. ■ Obtain vital signs; assess in context of client's baseline values. ■ Obtain client's medication history, including nicotine and alcohol consumption to determine possible drug allergies and/or interactions. ■ Obtain blood and urine specimens for laboratory analysis.	■ Risk for fluid and electrolyte imbalance ■ Risk for deficient fluid volume related to excess diuresis ■ Need for knowledge regarding drug therapy and adverse effects ■ Safety from injury related to side effects of drug therapy

Planning: Client Goals and Expected Outcomes

The client will:
■ Exhibit normal fluid balance and maintain electrolyte levels within normal limits during drug therapy
■ Demonstrate an understanding of the drug's action by accurately describing drug side effects and precautions
■ Immediately report effects such as symptoms of hyperkalemia or hypokalemia and hypersensitivity

Implementation

Interventions (Rationales)	Client Education/Discharge Planning
■ Monitor laboratory values. (Diuretics can cause electrolyte imbalances.)	■ Instruct client to inform laboratory personnel of diuretic therapy when providing blood or urine samples.
■ Monitor vital signs, especially blood pressure. (Diuretics reduce blood volume, resulting in lowered blood pressure.)	Instruct client to: ■ Monitor blood pressure as specified by the healthcare provider, and ensure proper use of home equipment ■ Withhold medication for severe hypotensive readings as specified by the healthcare provider (e.g., "hold for levels below 88/50")
■ Observe for changes in level of consciousness, dizziness, fatigue, and postural hypotension. (Reduction in blood volume due to diuretic therapy may produce changes in LOC or syncope.)	Instruct client to: ■ Immediately report any change in consciousness, especially feeling faint ■ Avoid abrupt changes in posture; rise slowly from prolonged periods of sitting/lying down ■ Obtain blood pressure readings in sitting, standing, and supine positions

continued

NURSING PROCESS FOCUS   Clients Receiving Diuretic Therapy   *(Continued)*

Interventions (Rationales)	Client Education/Discharge Planning
▪ Monitor for fluid overload by measuring intake, output, and daily weight. (Intake, output, and daily body weight are indications of the effectiveness of diuretic therapy.)	Instruct client to: ▪ Immediately report any severe shortness of breath, frothy sputum, profound fatigue and edema in extremities, potential signs of heart failure, or pulmonary edema ▪ Accurately measure intake, output, and body weight and report weight gain of 1 kg or more within 2 days or a decrease in output ▪ Avoid excessive heat, which contributes to fluid loss through perspiration ▪ Consume adequate amounts of *plain water*
▪ Monitor potassium intake. (Potassium is vital to maintaining proper electrolyte balance and can become depleted with thiazide or loop diuretics.)	For clients receiving loop or thiazide diuretics, encourage foods high in potassium. For clients receiving potassium-sparing diuretics: ▪ Instruct client to avoid foods high in potassium ▪ Consult with healthcare provider before using vitamin/mineral supplements or electrolyte-fortified sports drinks
▪ Observe for signs of hypersensitivity reaction.	Instruct client or caregiver to report: ▪ Difficulty breathing, throat tightness, hives or rash, and bleeding ▪ Flu-like symptoms: shortness of breath, fever, sore throat, malaise, joint pain, profound fatigue
▪ Monitor hearing and vision. (Loop diuretics are ototoxic. Thiazide diuretics increase serum digitalis levels; elevated levels produce visual changes.)	▪ Instruct client to report any changes in hearing or vision such as ringing or buzzing in the ears, becoming "hard of hearing," experiencing dimness of sight, seeing halos, or having "yellow vision."
▪ Monitor reactivity to light exposure. (Some diuretics cause photosensitivity.)	Instruct client to: ▪ Limit exposure to the sun ▪ Wear dark glasses and light-coloured, loose-fitting clothes when outdoors

Evaluation of Outcome Criteria

Evaluate the effectiveness of drug therapy by confirming that client goals and expected outcomes have been met (see "Planning").

See Tables 43.2 through 43.5 (pages 620–624) for lists of drugs to which these nursing actions apply.

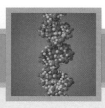

CHAPTER REVIEW

KEY CONCEPTS

The numbered key concepts provide a succinct summary of the important points from the corresponding numbered section within the chapter. If any of these points are not clear, refer to the numbered section within the chapter for review. Expanded versions can be found on the Companion Website.

43.1 The kidneys regulate fluid volume, electrolytes, and acid–base balance.

43.2 As filtrate travels through the nephron, its composition changes dramatically as a result of the processes of reabsorption and secretion.

43.3 The dosage levels for most medications must be adjusted in clients with renal failure. Diuretics may be used to maintain urine output while the cause of the hypoperfusion is treated.

43.4 Diuretics are drugs that increase urine output, usually by blocking sodium reabsorption.

43.5 The most efficacious diuretics are the loop (high-ceiling) agents that block the reabsorption of sodium in the loop of Henle.

43.6 The thiazides act by blocking sodium reabsorption in the distal tubule of the nephron, and they are the most widely prescribed class of diuretics.

43.7 Though less efficacious than the loop diuretics, potassium-sparing diuretics are used in combination with other agents and help to prevent hypokalemia.

43.8 Several less commonly prescribed classes such as the osmotic diuretics and the carbonic anhydrase inhibitors have specific indications in reducing intraocular fluid pressure (acetazolamide) or reversing severe renal hypoperfusion (mannitol).

REVIEW QUESTIONS

1 How does the composition of filtrate differ from that of blood?

2 Why are drugs that block sodium reabsorption at the loop of Henle more efficacious than those that act on the distal tubule?

3 Explain why hypokalemia is a common side effect of hydrochlorothiazide, yet hyperkalemia is more common with spironolactone. What advice should the client be given to avoid potassium imbalances?

CRITICAL THINKING QUESTIONS

1. A 43-year-old male is diagnosed with hypertension following an annual physical examination. The client is thin and states that he engages in fairly regular exercise but describes his job as highly stressful. He also has a positive family history of hypertension and stroke. The healthcare provider initiates therapy with losartan. After 2 months, the client has noted no appreciable difference in blood pressure values. The healthcare provider switches the client to Hyzaar, which proves to be very effective. Why is the new therapy more effective?

2. A 78-year-old female is admitted to the ICU with a diagnosis of heart failure. The nurse administers furosemide 40 mg IV push. What assessments should the nurse make to determine the effectiveness of this therapy?

3. A 17-year-old male is admitted to the ICU following a car-train collision. The client sustained a depressed skull fracture and is on a ventilator. Two days after surgery, there are obvious signs of increasing intracranial pressure. The nurse administers 32g of 15% mannitol solution per IV over 30 minutes. The client's mother asks the nurse to explain why her son needs this drug. What explanation should the nurse offer?

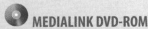
EXPLORE MediaLink

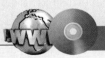
www.pearsoned.ca/adams-king

MEDIALINK DVD-ROM
- **Audio Glossary**
- **CRNE Review**
- **Video:** Renal Function
- **Animation**
  Mechanism in Action: Spironolactone

COMPANION WEBSITE
- **CRNE Review**
- **Case Study:** Client taking diuretics
- **Dosage Calculations**

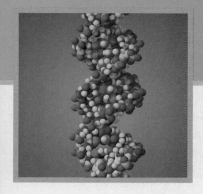

CHAPTER 44

Drugs for Fluid, Electrolyte, and Acid-Base Disorders

DRUGS AT A GLANCE

FLUID REPLACEMENT AGENTS

Colloids
   dextran 40 (Rheomacrodex)

Crystalloids

ELECTROLYTES
   sodium chloride
   potassium chloride (K-Dur, others)

ACID-BASE AGENTS
   sodium bicarbonate
   ammonium chloride

OBJECTIVES

After reading this chapter, the student should be able to do the following:

1. Explain how changes in the osmolality or tonicity of a fluid can cause water to move to a different compartment.
2. Compare and contrast colloids and crystalloids used in IV therapy.
3. Explain the importance of electrolyte balance in the body.
4. Discuss causes of sodium imbalance and the medications used to treat this condition.
5. Discuss causes of potassium imbalance and the medications used to treat this condition.
6. Discuss common causes of alkalosis and acidosis and the medications used to treat these disorders.
7. Describe the nurse's role in the pharmacological management of clients receiving drugs for fluid, electrolyte, and acid-base disorders.
8. For each of the drug classes listed in Drugs at a Glance, identify a representative drug and explain its mechanism of action, therapeutic effects, and important adverse effects.
9. Describe and explain, based on pharmacological principles, the rationale for nursing assessment, planning, and interventions for clients with fluid, electrolyte, and acid-base disorders.
10. Use the nursing process to care for clients who are receiving drug therapy for fluid, electrolyte, and acid-base disorders.

MediaLink

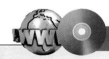

www.pearsoned.ca/adams-king

CRNE review, case studies, and other interactive resources for this chapter can be found on the Companion Website at **www.pearsoned.ca/adams-king**. Click on "Chapter 44" to select the activities for this chapter. For animations, more CRNE review questions, and an audio glossary, access the accompanying DVD-ROM in this textbook.

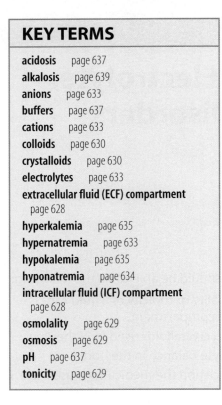

MediaLink   Animation: Fluid Balance

The maintenance of normal fluid volume, electrolyte composition, and acid-base balance is essential to life. Conditions such as hemorrhage and dehydration must be quickly treated; otherwise fluids and electrolytes will be rapidly depleted. Disorders of acid-base balance may be acute, as in diabetic ketoacidosis, or they may proceed more slowly, over a period of months. Fortunately, safe and effective drugs are available to quickly reverse most symptoms of fluid volume, electrolyte, and acid-base imbalance.

FLUID BALANCE

Body fluids travel between compartments, which are separated by semipermeable membranes. Control of water balance in the various compartments is essential to homeostasis. Fluid imbalances are frequent indications for pharmacotherapy.

44.1 Body Fluid Compartments

The bulk of body fluid consists of water, which serves as the universal solvent in which most of the body's nutrients, electrolytes, and minerals are dissolved. Water alone is responsible for about 60% of the total body weight.

In a simple model, water in the body can be located in one of two places, or compartments. The **intracellular fluid (ICF) compartment**, which contains water that is *inside* cells, accounts for about two-thirds of the total body water. The remaining one-third of body fluid resides *outside* cells in the **extracellular fluid (ECF) compartment**. The ECF compartment is further divided into two parts: fluid in the *plasma* and fluid in the *interstitial spaces* between cells. The relationship between these fluid compartments is illustrated in Figure 44.1.

A continuous exchange and mixing of fluids occurs between the compartments, which are separated by membranes. The plasma membranes of the cells separate the ICF from the ECF. The capillary membranes separate plasma from the interstitial fluid. Although water travels freely among the compartments, the movement of large molecules and those with electrical charges are governed by processes of diffusion and active transport. Movement of ions and drugs across membranes is a primary concern of pharmacokinetics (see Chapter 4).

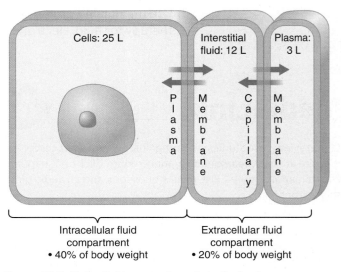

● **Figure 44.1** Major fluid compartments in the body

44.2 Osmolality, Tonicity, and the Movement of Body Fluids

Osmolality and *tonicity* are two related terms central to understanding fluid balance in the body. Large changes in the osmolality or tonicity of a body fluid can cause significant shifts in water balance between compartments. The nurse will often administer IV fluids to compensate for these changes.

The **osmolality** of a fluid is determined by the number of dissolved particles, or solutes, in 1 kg (1 L) of water. In most body fluids, three solutes determine the osmolality: sodium, glucose, and urea. Sodium is the greatest contributor to osmolality due to its abundance in most body fluids. The normal osmolality of body fluids ranges from 275 to 295 milliosmoles per kilogram (mOsm/kg).

The term *tonicity* is sometimes used interchangeably with osmolality, although they are somewhat different. Whereas osmolality is a laboratory value that can be precisely measured, **tonicity** is a general term used to describe the *relative* concentration of IV fluids. Tonicity is the ability of a solution to cause a change in water movement across a membrane due to osmotic forces. The tonicity of the plasma is used as the reference point when administering IV solutions: normal plasma is considered isotonic. Solutions that are isotonic have the same concentration of solutes (same osmolality) as the blood. Hypertonic solutions have a greater concentration of solutes than plasma, whereas hypotonic solutions have a lesser concentration of solutes than plasma.

Through **osmosis**, water moves from areas of low solute concentration (low osmolality), to areas of high solute concentration (high osmolality). If a hypertonic (hyperosmolar) IV solution is administered, the plasma gains more solutes than the interstitial fluid. Water will move, by osmosis, from the interstitial fluid to the plasma. Water will move in the opposite direction, from plasma to interstitial fluid, if a hypotonic solution is administered. Isotonic solutions will produce no net fluid shift. These movements are illustrated in Figure 44.2.

44.3 Regulation of Fluid Intake and Output

The average adult has a water intake of approximately 2500 mL/day from food and beverages. Water output is achieved through the kidneys, lungs, skin, feces, and sweat. To maintain water balance, water intake must equal water output. Gains or losses of water can be estimated by changes in total body weight.

The most important physiological regulator of fluid intake is the thirst mechanism. The sensation of thirst occurs when osmoreceptors in the hypothalamus sense a hypertonic ECF. As saliva secretion diminishes and the mouth dries, the individual is driven to ingest liquid. As the ingested water is absorbed, the osmolality of the ECF falls and the thirst centre in the hypothalamus is no longer stimulated.

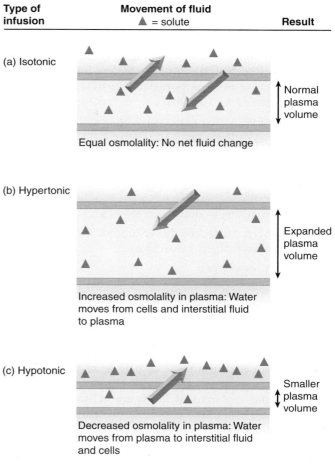

● **Figure 44.2** Movement of fluids and solution tonicity

The kidneys are the primary regulators of fluid output. Through the renin-angiotensin mechanism (see Chapter 21), the hormone aldosterone is secreted by the adrenal cortex. Aldosterone causes the kidneys to retain sodium and water, thus increasing the osmolality of the ECF. A second hormone, antidiuretic hormone (ADH), is released during periods of high plasma osmolality. ADH acts directly on the distal tubules of the kidney to increase water reabsorption.

Failure to properly balance intake with output can result in fluid volume disorders that are indications for pharmacological intervention. Fluid deficit disorders can cause dehydration or shock, which are treated by administering oral or intravenous fluids. Fluid excess disorders are treated with diuretics (see Chapter 43). When treating fluid volume disorders, the ultimate goal is to diagnose and correct the *cause* of the disorder, while administering supporting fluids and medications to stabilize the client.

FLUID REPLACEMENT AGENTS

Loss of fluids from the body can result in dehydration and shock. Fluid replacement solutions are used to maintain blood volume and support blood pressure.

44.4 Intravenous Therapy with Crystalloids and Colloids

When fluid output exceeds fluid intake, volume deficits may result. Shock, dehydration, or electrolyte loss may occur; large deficits are fatal unless treated. The following are some common reasons for fluid loss:

- Loss of GI fluids due to vomiting, diarrhea, chronic laxative use, or GI suctioning
- Excessive sweating during hot weather, athletic activity, or prolonged fever
- Severe burns
- Trauma resulting in significant blood loss
- Excessive renal fluid loss due to diuretic therapy or uncontrolled diabetic ketoacidosis
- Surgical procedures

The immediate goal in treating a volume deficit disorder is to replace the missing fluid. In non-acute circumstances, this may be achieved by administering fluids via the oral route or through a nasogastric tube. In acute situations, intravenous fluid therapy is indicated. Regardless of the route, careful attention must be paid to restoring normal levels of electrolytes as well as fluid volume.

Intravenous replacement fluids are of two basic types: colloids and crystalloids. **Colloids** are proteins or other large molecules that remain in the blood for a long time because they are too large to cross the capillary membrane. While circulating, they draw water molecules from the cells and tissues into the plasma through their ability to increase plasma osmolality and osmotic pressure. These agents are sometimes called plasma volume expanders. They are particularly important in treating hypovolemic shock due to burns, hemorrhage, or surgery. Several of these products contain dextran, a synthetic polysaccharide. Dextran infusions can double the plasma volume within a few minutes, though its effects last only about 12 hours. Plasma protein fraction contains 83% albumin and 17% plasma globulins. Plasma protein fraction and albumin are also indicated in clients with hypoproteinemia. Select colloid solutions are given in Table 44.1.

Crystalloids are IV solutions that contain electrolytes and other agents that are used to replace lost fluids and to promote urine output. Unlike colloids, crystalloid solutions are capable of quickly diffusing across membranes, leaving the plasma and entering the interstitial fluid and ICF. Isotonic, hypotonic, and hypertonic solutions are available. Some crystalloids contain dextrose, a form of glucose, commonly in concentrations of 2.5%, 5%, or 10%. Dextrose is added to provide nutritional value: 1 L of 5% dextrose supplies 170 calories. In addition, water is formed during the metabolism of dextrose, adding to the rehydration of the client.

Infusion of crystalloids will increase total fluid volume in the body, but the compartment that is most expanded depends on the solute (sodium) concentration. Infusion of hypertonic crystalloids will draw water from the cells and tissues and expand plasma volume. Hypotonic crystalloids will cause water to move out of the plasma to the tissues and cells; thus, these solutions are not considered efficient plasma volume expanders. Select crystalloid solutions are given in Table 44.2.

NURSING CONSIDERATIONS

The role of the nurse in fluid replacement therapy involves careful monitoring of the client's condition and providing education as it relates to the prescribed drug regimen. Prior to administration of colloids (plasma volume expanders), obtain a complete health history, drug history, and a physical examination. Lab tests, including CBC, serum electrolytes, BUN, and creatinine, should be obtained. Evaluate the client's fluid balance before initiating therapy. Administration of colloid solutions to dehydrated clients can lead to renal failure.

Colloidal solutions are contraindicated in clients with renal failure, hypervolemic conditions, severe heart failure, thrombocytopenia, and those with clotting abnormalities. They should be used with caution in clients with active hemorrhage, severe dehydration, chronic liver disease, or impaired renal function. Carefully monitor vital signs and observe the client for the first 30 minutes of the infusion for hypersensitivity reactions. The nurse should stop the infusion at the first sign of hypersensitivity.

Some colloidal solutions decrease platelet adhesion and lead to decreased coagulation. Plasma expanders will lower hematocrit and hemoglobin levels because of increased intravascular volume. Immediately report a hematocrit below 30% to the physician.

The primary nursing responsibility when caring for the client receiving plasma volume expanders is monitoring

TABLE 44.1 Select Colloid IV Solutions (Plasma Volume Expanders)	
Solution	*Tonicity*
5% albumin	isotonic
dextran 40 in normal saline	isotonic
dextran 40 in D5W	isotonic
dextran 70 in normal saline	isotonic
hetastarch 6% in normal saline	isotonic
plasma protein fraction	isotonic

TABLE 44.2	Select Crystalloid IV Solutions
Solution	**Tonicity**
normal saline (0.9% NaCl)	isotonic
hypertonic saline (3% NaCl)	hypertonic
hypotonic saline (0.45% NaCl)	hypotonic
lactated Ringer's	isotonic
Plasma-Lyte 148	isotonic
Plasma-Lyte 56	hypotonic
Dextrose Solutions	
5% dextrose in water (D5W)	hypotonic/isotonic[*]
5% dextrose in normal saline	hypertonic
5% dextrose in 0.2% saline	isotonic
5% dextrose in lactated Ringer's	hypertonic
5% dextrose in Plasma-Lyte 56	hypertonic

[*]Because dextrose is metabolized quickly, the solution is sometimes considered hypotonic.

fluid volume status. The client should be closely monitored for both fluid volume deficit and fluid volume excess. Vital signs and hemodynamic status should be monitored frequently during the infusion, until the client's condition stabilizes. The client's neurological status and urinary output should also be closely assessed as these two systems are critically dependent on proper fluid balance. The infusion of the solutions can create a multitude of problems for the critically ill client.

These medications are most often used to treat shock, so the client may not be alert. However, caregivers may need emotional support from the nurse, including updates about the client's condition and psychosocial support.

Client education as it relates to colloidal solutions should include goals, reasons for obtaining baseline data such as vital signs and lab tests, and possible side effects. Following are important points to include when teaching clients and families about colloidal solutions:

- Immediately report any signs of bleeding such as easy bruising, blood in the urine, or dark, tarry stools.
- Immediately report flushing, shortness of breath, or itching, which could indicate hypersensitivity to the medication.
- Immediately report shortness of breath, cough, chest congestion, or heart palpitations, which could indicate circulatory overload.

Pr PROTOTYPE DRUG | Dextran 40 (Rheomacrodex)

ACTIONS AND USES

Dextran 40 is a polysaccharide that is too large to pass through capillary walls. It is identical to dextran 70, except dextran 40 has a lower molecular weight. Dextran 40 acts by raising the osmotic pressure of the blood, thereby causing fluid to move from the tissues to the vascular spaces. Cardiovascular responses include increased blood pressure, increased cardiac output, and improved venous return to the heart. Indications include fluid replacement for clients experiencing hypovolemic shock due to hemorrhage, surgery, or severe burns. When given for acute shock, it is infused as rapidly as possible until blood volume is restored.

Dextran 40 also reduces platelet adhesiveness and improves blood flow through its ability to reduce blood viscosity. These properties have led to its use in preventing deep vein thromboses and pulmonary emboli.

PHARMACOKINETICS

Given as an IV infusion, it has the capability of expanding plasma volume within minutes after administration. Dextran 40 is excreted rapidly by the kidneys.

ADMINISTRATION ALERTS

- Emergency administration may be given at a rate of 1.2 to 2.4 g/min.
- Non-emergency administration should be infused no faster than 240 mg/min.
- Once opened, discard unused portion because dextran contains no preservatives.
- Dextran 40 is pregnancy category C.

ADVERSE EFFECTS

Vital signs should be monitored continuously to avoid hypertension caused by the plasma volume expansion. Signs of fluid overload such as tachycardia, peripheral edema, distended neck veins, dyspnea, or cough should be reported immediately. Because of its extensive renal excretion, dextran 40 is contraindicated in clients with renal failure. Due to its ability to quickly draw water from tissues, it is also contraindicated in clients with severe dehydration. A small percentage of clients are allergic to dextran 40, with urticaria being the most common sign.

There are no clinically significant interactions.

 See the Companion Website for a Nursing Process Focus chart specific to this drug.

NURSING PROCESS FOCUS Clients Receiving Fluid Replacement Therapy

Assessment	Potential Nursing Diagnoses/Identified Patterns
Prior to administration: ■ Obtain complete health history including allergies, drug history, and possible drug interactions. ■ Obtain complete physical examination. ■ Assess for the presence of fluid volume deficit. ■ Obtain the following laboratory studies: CBC, serum electrolytes, renal function (BUN and serum creatinine).	■ Risk for infection at IV site ■ Risk for fluid imbalance ■ Need for knowledge regarding drug therapy and adverse effects ■ Safety from injury related to side effects of drug therapy

Planning: Client Goals and Expected Outcomes

The client will:
■ Exhibit signs of normal fluid volume such as stable blood pressure and adequate urinary output
■ Demonstrate an understanding of the drug by accurately describing the drug's purpose, action, side effects, and precautions
■ Immediately report effects such as itching, shortness of breath, flushing, cough, and heart palpitations

Implementation

Interventions (Rationales)	Client Education/Discharge Planning
■ Monitor hemodynamic status every 15 to 60 min, including blood pressure, urinary output, and invasive pressure monitoring devices. (Plasma volume expanders cause rapid movement of water into the circulatory system.) ■ Monitor for hypersensitivity reactions such as urticaria, pruritus, dyspnea, flushing, and anaphylaxis. ■ Monitor for signs of circulatory overload such as dyspnea, cyanosis, cough, crackles, wheezes, and neck vein distention. (Medication may cause fluid overload quickly.) ■ Monitor for changes in CBC results. (Plasma volume expanders can inhibit coagulation and lower hematocrit and hemoglobin levels. Report reduction of hematocrit below 30%.)	Instruct client about: ■ Why vital signs and other assessments are being monitored frequently ■ Expected outcomes of plasma volume expansion therapy ■ Instruct client to report itching, shortness of breath, or flushing as symptoms occur. ■ Instruct client to report shortness of breath, cough, or heart palpitation as soon as such symptoms occur. ■ Instruct client of the need for frequent laboratory studies.

Evaluation of Outcome Criteria

Evaluate the effectiveness of drug therapy by confirming that client goals and expected outcomes have been met (see "Planning").

See Table 44.1 (page 630) for a list of drugs to which these nursing actions apply.

ELECTROLYTES

Electrolytes are small, charged molecules essential to homeostasis. Too little or too much of an electrolyte may result in serious disease and must be quickly corrected. Table 44.3 lists inorganic substances and their electrolytes that are important to human physiology.

44.5 Normal Functions of Electrolytes

Chapter 38 discusses the role of minerals in health and wellness. In certain body fluids, some of these minerals become ions and possess a charge. Small, inorganic molecules pos-

TABLE 44.3	Electrolytes Important to Human Physiology		
Compound	Formula	Cation	Anion
calcium chloride	$CaCl_2$	Ca^{+2}	Cl^-
disodium phosphate	Na_2HPO_4	Na^+	HPO_4^{-2}
potassium chloride	KCl	K^+	Cl^-
sodium bicarbonate	$NaHCO_3$	Na^+	HCO_3^-
sodium chloride	$NaCl$	Na^+	Cl^-
sodium sulfate	Na_2SO_4	Na^+	SO_4^{-2}

TABLE 44.4	Electrolyte Imbalances		
Ion	**Condition**	**Abnormal Serum Value (mEq/L)**	**Supportive Treatment***
calcium	hypercalcemia	>11	hypotonic fluid or calcitonin
	hypocalcemia	<4	calcium supplements or vitamin D
chloride	hyperchloremia	>112	hypotonic fluid
	hypochloremia	<95	hypertonic salt solution
magnesium	hypermagnesemia	>4	hypotonic fluid
	hypomagnesemia	<0.8	magnesium supplements
phosphate	hyperphosphatemia	>6	dietary phosphate restriction
	hypophosphatemia	<1	phosphate supplements
potassium	hyperkalemia	>5	hypotonic fluid, buffers, or dietary potassium restriction
	hypokalemia	<3.5	potassium supplements
sodium	hypernatremia	>145	hypotonic fluid or dietary sodium restriction
	hyponatremia	<135	hypertonic salt solution or sodium supplement

*For all electrolyte imbalances, the primary therapeutic goal is to identify and correct the *cause* of the imbalance.

sessing a positive or negative charge are called **electrolytes**. Positively charged electrolytes are called **cations**; those with a negative charge are **anions**.

Inorganic compounds are held together by ionic bonds. When placed in aqueous solution, these bonds break and the compound undergoes dissociation, or ionization. The resulting ions have charges and are able to conduct electricity, hence the name *electrolyte*. Electrolyte levels are measured in milliequivalents per litre (mEq/L).

Electrolytes are essential to many body functions, including nerve conduction, membrane permeability, muscle contraction, water balance, and bone growth and remodelling. Levels of electrolytes in body fluids must be maintained within narrow ranges. As electrolytes are lost due to normal excretory functions, they must be compensated by adequate intake, otherwise electrolyte imbalances can result. The major electrolyte imbalance states are shown in Table 44.4. Calcium, phosphorous, and magnesium imbalances are discussed in Chapter 38; the role of calcium in bone homeostasis is presented in Chapter 46.

44.6 Pharmacotherapy of Sodium Imbalances

Sodium is the major electrolyte in extracellular fluid. Due to sodium's central roles in neuromuscular function, acid-base balance, and overall fluid distribution, sodium imbalances can have serious consequences. Although definite sodium monitors or sensors have yet to be discovered in the body, the regulation of sodium balance is well understood.

Sodium balance and water balance are intimately connected. As sodium levels increase in a body fluid, solute particles accumulate, and the osmolality increases. Water will move toward this area of relatively high osmolality. In simplest terms, water travels toward or with sodium. The physiological consequences of this relationship cannot be overstated: as water content of the plasma increases, so does blood volume and blood pressure. Thus, sodium movement provides an important link between water retention, blood volume, and blood pressure.

In healthy individuals, sodium intake is equal to sodium output, which is under the regulation of the kidneys. High levels of aldosterone secreted by the adrenal cortex promote sodium and water retention by the kidneys. Inhibition of aldosterone promotes sodium and water excretion. When a client ingests high amounts of sodium, aldosterone secretion decreases and more sodium enters the urine. This relationship is illustrated in Figure 44.3.

Sodium excess, or **hypernatremia**, is a serum sodium level greater than 145 mEq/L. The most common cause of hypernatremia is kidney disease resulting in decreased sodium excretion. Hypernatremia may also be caused by excessive intake of sodium, either through dietary consumption or by overtreatment with IV fluids containing sodium chloride or sodium bicarbonate. Another cause of hypernatremia is high net water loss, such as that occurring from inadequate water intake, watery diarrhea, fever, or burns. In addition, high doses of glucocorticoids or estrogens promote sodium retention.

A high serum sodium level increases the osmolality of the plasma and draws fluid from interstitial spaces and cells, thus causing cellular dehydration. Manifestations of hypernatremia include thirst, fatigue, weakness, muscle twitching, convulsions, weight gain, and dyspnea. For minor hypernatremia, a low-salt diet may be effective in returning serum sodium to normal levels. In clients with acute hypernatremia, however, treatment goals are to rapidly return the osmolality of the plasma to normal and to excrete the excess sodium. If the client is hypovolemic, the administration of hypotonic fluids such as D5W or 0.45% NaCl will increase plasma volume while at the same time reducing plasma osmolality. For the client who is hypervolemic, diuretics may be used to remove sodium from the body.

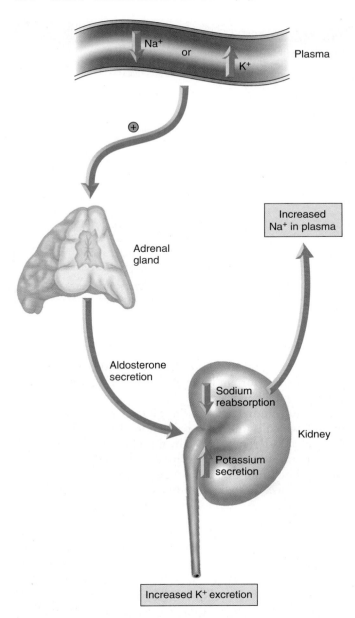

● **Figure 44.3** Renal regulation of sodium and potassium balance

Sodium deficiency, or **hyponatremia**, is a serum sodium level less than 135 mEq/L. Hyponatremia may occur through excessive dilution of the plasma or by increased sodium loss due to disorders of the skin, GI tract, or kidneys. Excessive ADH secretion or administration of hypotonic IV solutions can increase plasma volume and lead to hyponatremia. Significant loss of sodium by the skin may occur in burn clients and in those with excessive sweating or prolonged fever. Gastrointestinal losses occur from vomiting, diarrhea, or GI suctioning, and renal sodium loss may occur with diuretic use and in certain advanced kidney disorders. Early symptoms of hyponatremia include nausea, vomiting, anorexia, and abdominal cramping. Later signs include altered neurological function such as confusion, lethargy, convulsions, and muscle twitching or tremors. Tachycardia, hypotension, and dry skin and mucous membranes may also occur. Hyponatremia is usually treated with solutions of sodium chloride.

NURSING CONSIDERATIONS

The role of the nurse in sodium replacement therapy involves careful monitoring of the client's condition and providing education as it relates to the prescribed drug regimen. Because sodium and body water are so closely related, the nurse's primary role when caring for clients with sodium imbalances is monitoring fluid balance. Hyponatremia is seldom caused from inadequate dietary intake; however, in rare instances, this may occur in individuals following sodium-restricted diets or receiving diuretic therapy. In most cases, infusion of 0.45% or 0.9% sodium solutions are used to restore extracellular fluid balance.

Prior to and during administration of sodium solutions, assess sodium and electrolyte balance. When assessing for hyponatremia, observe for signs of nausea, vomiting, muscle cramps, tachycardia, dry mucous membranes, and headache. The nurse must also be alert for signs indicating hypernatremia, such as weakness, restlessness, irritability, seizures, coma, hypertension, tachycardia, fluid accumulation, pulmonary edema, and respiratory arrest.

Serum sodium levels, urine specific gravity, and serum and urine osmolarity should be monitored closely when administering hypertonic solutions. The client should be taught to report any symptoms that may relate to fluid overload during infusion of hypertonic saline solutions. The symptoms of this condition include shortness of breath, palpitation, headache, and restlessness.

Side effects of sodium chloride when given as an electrolyte replacement are rare. Some clients have self-induced hypernatremia by taking salt tablets, believing that they will replace sodium lost due to sweating. Those who sweat profusely due to working outdoors or exercising can avoid heat-related problems if they consume adequate amounts of water or balanced electrolyte solutions contained in sports drinks. The client should only consume salt tablets when instructed by the healthcare provider.

Client education as it relates to sodium replacement should include goals, reasons for obtaining baseline data such as vital signs and tests for cardiac and renal function, and possible side effects. Following are the important points to include when teaching clients regarding sodium replacements:

- Avoid taking sodium chloride (salt) tablets to replace sodium lost through perspiration.
- Drink adequate amounts of water or balanced sports drinks to replenish lost fluids and electrolytes.
- Immediately report symptoms of low sodium such as nausea, vomiting, muscle cramps, rapid heart rate, and headache.
- Immediately report symptoms of high sodium such as weakness, restlessness, irritability, seizures, hypertension, and fluid retention.

Pr PROTOTYPE DRUG | Sodium Chloride

ACTIONS AND USES

Sodium chloride (NaCl) is administered during periods of hyponatremia when serum levels fall below 130 mEq/L. Sodium chloride is available in several concentrations to treat different levels of hyponatremia. Normal saline consists of 0.9% NaCl and is used to treat mild hyponatremia. When serum sodium falls below 115 mEq/L, a 3% NaCl solution may be infused. Other concentrations include 0.45% and 0.22%, and both hypotonic and isotonic solutions are available. The decision about which NaCl concentration to administer is driven by the severity of the sodium deficiency. Infusions of high concentrations of NaCl are contraindicated in clients with heart failure or with impaired renal function.

PHARMACOKINETICS

Sodium chloride is well absorbed after oral administration. It is widely distributed. It is excreted by the kidneys.

ADMINISTRATION ALERT

- Sodium chloride is pregnancy category C.

ADVERSE EFFECTS

Clients receiving NaCl infusions must be monitored frequently to avoid symptoms of hypernatremia. Symptoms of excessive sodium include lethargy, confusion, muscle tremor or rigidity, hypotension, and restlessness. Because some of these symptoms are also common to hyponatremia, the healthcare provider must rely on periodic lab assessments to be certain sodium values lie within the normal range. When infusing 3% NaCl solutions, continuously check for signs of pulmonary edema.

There are no clinically significant drug interactions.

 See the Companion Website for a Nursing Process Focus chart specific to this drug.

44.7 Pharmacotherapy of Potassium Imbalances

Potassium is the most abundant intracellular cation and serves important roles in regulating intracellular osmolality and in maintaining acid-base balance. Potassium levels must be carefully balanced between adequate dietary intake and renal excretion. Like sodium, potassium excretion is influenced by the effect of aldosterone on the kidney. In fact, the renal excretion of sodium and potassium ions is closely linked—for every sodium ion that is reabsorbed, one potassium ion is secreted into the renal tubules. Serum potassium levels must be maintained within narrow limits; excess or deficiency states can be serious or fatal.

Hyperkalemia is a serum potassium level greater than 5 mEq/L, which may be caused by high consumption of potassium-rich foods or dietary supplements, particularly when clients are taking potassium-sparing diuretics such as spironolactone (see Chapter 43). Excess potassium may also accumulate when renal excretion is diminished due to kidney pathology. The most serious consequences of hyperkalemia are related to cardiac function: dysrhythmias and heart block are possible. Other symptoms are muscle twitching, fatigue, paresthesias, dyspnea, cramping, and diarrhea.

In mild cases of hyperkalemia, potassium levels may be returned to normal by restricting major dietary sources of potassium such as bananas, dried fruits, peanut butter, broccoli, and green leafy vegetables. If the client is taking a potassium-sparing diuretic, the dose must be lowered or an alternate drug may be considered. In severe cases, serum potassium levels may be temporarily lowered by administering glucose and insulin, which cause potassium to leave the extracellular fluid and enter cells. Calcium gluconate or calcium chloride may be administered on an emergency basis to counteract potential potassium toxicity on the heart. Sodium bicarbonate is sometimes infused to correct any acidosis that may be concurrent with the hyperkalemia. Elimination of excess potassium may be enhanced by giving polystyrene sulfonate orally or rectally. This agent, which exchanges sodium ion for potassium ion in the intestine, is given concurrently with a laxative such as sorbitol to promote rapid evacuation of the potassium.

Hypokalemia occurs when the serum potassium level falls below 3.5 mEq/L. Hypokalemia is a relatively common adverse effect resulting from high doses of loop diuretics such as furosemide (Lasix). In addition, strenuous muscular activity and severe vomiting or diarrhea can result in significant potassium loss. Because the body does not have large stores of potassium, adequate daily intake is necessary. Neurons and muscle fibres are most sensitive to potassium loss, and muscle weakness, lethargy, anorexia, dysrhythmias, and cardiac arrest are possible consequences. Mild hypokalemia is treated by increasing the dietary intake of potassium-rich foods, whereas more severe deficiencies require higher doses of oral or parenteral potassium supplements.

NURSING CONSIDERATIONS

The role of the nurse in potassium replacement therapy involves careful monitoring of the client's condition and providing education as it relates to the prescribed drug regimen. Potassium imbalances are probably the most common electrolyte disturbance that clients experience. Quick recognition of potassium imbalance will prevent life-threatening complications such as dysrhythmias, heart blocks, and cardiac arrest.

Potassium supplements are contraindicated in conditions that predispose the client to hyperkalemia, such as severe renal impairment and use of potassium-sparing diuretics. Potassium supplements are also contraindicated in acute dehydration, heat cramps, and in clients with digitalis intoxication with AV node disturbance. They should be used with caution in clients with kidney disease, cardiac disease, and systemic acidosis.

Oral potassium administration is used for the prevention and treatment of mild deficiency. Oral forms, especially tablets and capsules, which can produce high local concentrations of potassium, are irritating to the GI tract and may cause peptic ulcers. This is less likely with the use of tablets and capsules that contain microencapsulated particles. To minimize GI irritation, instruct the client to administer oral forms with meals. Prior to oral or IV administration of potassium chloride, serum potassium levels should be measured. Check for the most recent potassium level before administering any form of potassium. Too much potassium can be just as dangerous for the client as too little. In either case, the consequences can be fatal.

Intravenous potassium administration is used for clients with severe deficiency or for those who cannot tolerate oral forms. Monitor serum potassium levels throughout treatment to reduce the risk of hyperkalemia. Assess renal function prior to and during treatment and, if renal failure develops, the infusion should be stopped immediately. Monitor for ECG changes, which can be an early indication of developing hyperkalemia. Clients who experience potassium imbalances must be taught to avoid the underlying problems, comply with the medication regimen, and use dietary interventions to correct and maintain normal electrolyte balance.

Client education as it relates to potassium replacement should include goals, reasons for obtaining baseline data such as vital signs and tests for cardiac and renal function, and possible side effects. Following are important points to include when teaching clients regarding potassium replacements:

- Report symptoms of hypokalemia such as weakness, fatigue, lethargy, or anorexia.
- Report symptoms of hyperkalemia such as nausea, abdominal cramping, oliguria, weakness, changes in heart rate, and numbness or tingling of arms or legs.
- Report decreased urinary output since this can lead to hyperkalemia.
- Keep all lab appointments to assess serum potassium level.
- If taking a potassium supplement, avoid potassium-rich foods and salt substitutes that are potassium based.
- Take potassium supplements with food to decrease GI distress.

ACID-BASE BALANCE

Unless quickly corrected, acidosis and alkalosis can have serious and even fatal consequences. Acidic and basic agents may be given to rapidly correct pH imbalances in body fluids.

Pr PROTOTYPE DRUG | Potassium Chloride (K-Dur, others)

ACTIONS AND USES

Potassium chloride (KCl) is the drug of choice for treating or preventing hypokalemia. It is also used to treat mild forms of alkalosis. Oral formulations include tablets, powders, and liquids, usually heavily flavoured due to the unpleasant taste of the drug. Because the drug can cause peptic ulcers, the supplement should be diluted with plenty of water. When given IV, potassium preparations must be administered slowly since bolus injections can overload the heart and cause cardiac arrest. Because pharmacotherapy with loop or thiazide diuretics is the most common cause of potassium loss, clients taking these diuretics are usually instructed to take oral potassium supplements to prevent hypokalemia.

PHARMACOKINETICS

Potassium chloride is well absorbed after oral administration. It is widely distributed. It is excreted by the kidneys.

ADMINISTRATION ALERTS

- Always give oral medication while client is upright in order to avoid esophagitis.
- Tablets should not be crushed or chewed.
- Dilute liquid forms before giving through a nasogastric tube.
- Never administer IV push or in concentrated amounts.
- Be extremely careful to avoid extravasation and infiltration.
- Potassium chloride is pregnancy category A.

ADVERSE EFFECTS AND INTERACTIONS

Nausea and vomiting are common because potassium chloride irritates the GI mucosa. The drug may be taken with meals or antacids to lessen gastric distress. The most serious side effects of potassium chloride are related to the possible accumulation of potassium. Hyperkalemia may occur if the client takes potassium supplements concurrently with potassium-sparing diuretics. Kidney function should be assessed periodically. Since the kidneys perform over 90% of the body's potassium excretion, reduced renal function can rapidly lead to hyperkalemia, particularly in clients taking potassium supplements.

Potassium supplements interact with potassium-sparing diuretics and ACE inhibitors to increase the risk of hyperkalemia.

 See the Companion Website for a Nursing Process Focus chart specific to this drug.

Laxatives and Fluid-Electrolyte Balance

With aging, peristalsis slows, food intake diminishes, and physical activity declines; these factors can change bowel movement regularity. Many older adults believe they must have a bowel movement every day, and so they take daily laxatives. Chronic use of laxatives may result in fluid depletion and hyperkalemia. Stimulant laxatives, in particular, are the most frequently prescribed class of laxatives, and these agents alter electrolyte transport in the intestinal mucosa. Older adults are especially susceptible to fluid and electrolyte depletion with chronic laxative use. Teach the client to drink plenty of fluids when taking a laxative and that overuse of laxatives can result in adverse side effects, so they should be used only as directed. Recommend that older clients increase exercise (as tolerated) and add insoluble fibre to the diet to maintain elimination regularity.

44.8 Buffers and the Maintenance of Body pH

The degree of acidity or alkalinity of a solution is measured by its **pH**. A pH of 7.0 is defined as neutral; above 7.0 is basic or alkaline, and below 7.0 is acidic. To maintain homeostasis, the pH of plasma and most body fluids must be kept within the narrow range of 7.35 to 7.45. Nearly all proteins and enzymes in the body function optimally within this narrow range of pH. A few enzymes, most notably those in the digestive tract, require pH values outside the 7.35 to 7.45 range to function properly. The correction of acid-base imbalance is illustrated in Figure 44.4.

The body generates significant amounts of acid during normal metabolic processes. Without sophisticated means of neutralizing these metabolic acids, the overall pH of body fluids would quickly fall below the normal range. **Buffers** are chemicals that help maintain normal body pH by neutralizing strong acids and bases. The two primary buffers the body uses to keep pH within normal limits are bicarbonate ions and phosphate ions.

The body uses two mechanisms to remove acid. The CO_2 produced during body metabolism is efficiently removed by the lungs during exhalation. The kidneys remove excess acid in the form of hydrogen ion (H^+) by excreting it in the urine. If retained in the body, CO_2 and/or H^+ would lower body pH. Thus, the lung and the kidneys collaborate in the removal of acids to maintain normal acid-base balance.

44.9 Pharmacotherapy of Acidosis

Acidosis occurs when the pH of the plasma falls below 7.35, which is confirmed by measuring arterial pH, partial pressure of carbon dioxide (Pco_2), and plasma bicarbonate levels. Diagnosis must differentiate between respiratory etiology and metabolic (renal) etiology. Occasionally, the cause has mixed respiratory and metabolic components. The most profound symptoms of acidosis affect the central nervous system and include lethargy, confusion, and CNS depression leading to coma. A deep, rapid respiration rate indicates an attempt by the lungs to rid the body of excess acid. Common causes of acidosis are shown in Table 44.5.

NURSING CONSIDERATIONS

The role of the nurse in drug therapy of acidosis involves careful monitoring of the client's condition and providing education as it relates to the prescribed drug regimen. The focus of nursing care is directed toward correction and maintenance of acid-base status. Assess the arterial blood gas analysis, which reports pH, carbon dioxide levels (Pco_2), bicarbonate levels (HCO_3^-), and oxygenation status (Po_2 and O_2 saturation). Also assess the client for symptoms associated with acidosis, such as sleepiness, coma, disorientation, dizziness, headache, seizures, and hypoventilation. The nurse will further assess the client for causative factors that could produce acidosis, such as diabetes mellitus, shock,

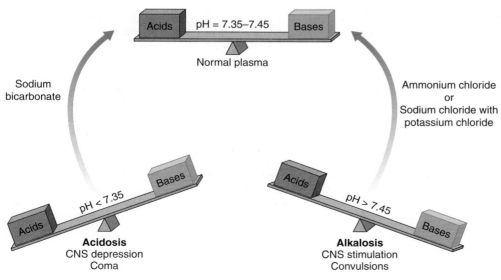

● **Figure 44.4** Acid-base imbalances

TABLE 44.5   Causes of Alkalosis and Acidosis

Acidosis	Alkalosis
Respiratory Origins	**Respiratory Origin**
• hypoventilation or shallow breathing	• hyperventilation due to asthma, anxiety, or high altitude
• airway constriction	
• damage to respiratory centre in medulla	
Metabolic Origins	**Metabolic Origins**
• severe diarrhea	• constipation for prolonged periods
• kidney failure	• ingestion of excess sodium bicarbonate
• diabetes mellitus	• diuretics that cause potassium depletion
• excess alcohol ingestion	• severe vomiting
• starvation	

diarrhea, and vomiting. Acidosis is frequently corrected when the underlying disease condition is successfully managed.

The client receiving sodium bicarbonate is prone to alkalosis, especially if an excessive amount has been administered. Monitor the client for symptoms of alkalosis such as irritability, confusion, cyanosis, slow respirations, irregular pulse, and muscle twitching. These symptoms would warrant withholding the medication and notifying the healthcare provider.

There are several contraindications and precautions related to the administration of sodium bicarbonate. Clients who have lost chloride due to vomiting or continuous GI suctioning and clients receiving diuretic therapy that may cause hypochloremia should not be given sodium bicarbonate. Clients who have hypocalcemia should not receive sodium bicarbonate because it may produce alkalosis. Due to the sodium content of this drug, it should be used judiciously in clients with cardiac disease and renal impairment.

Sodium bicarbonate may also be used to alkalinize the urine. This process is useful in the treatment of overdoses of certain acidic medications such as ASA and phenobarbital. When IV sodium bicarbonate is given, it causes the urine to become more alkaline. Less acid is reabsorbed in the renal tubules, so more acid and acidic medicine is excreted. This process is known as ion trapping. Closely monitor the client's acid-base status and report symptoms of imbalance to the healthcare provider. Provide care directed toward supporting critical body functions such as cardiovascular, respiratory, and neurological status that may be impaired secondary to the drug overdose.

Sodium bicarbonate (baking soda) is used as a home remedy to neutralize gastric acid in order to relieve heartburn or sour stomach. Although occasional use is acceptable, be aware that clients may misinterpret cardiac symptoms as heartburn and may overuse sodium bicarbonate, leading to systemic alkalosis.

Pr **PROTOTYPE DRUG** | Sodium Bicarbonate

ACTIONS AND USES

Sodium bicarbonate is the drug of choice for correcting acidosis. After dissociation, the bicarbonate ion acts by directly raising the pH of body fluids. Sodium bicarbonate may be given orally, if acidosis is mild, or IV in cases of acute disease. Although sodium bicarbonate neutralizes gastric acid, it is rarely used to treat peptic ulcers due to its tendency to cause uncomfortable gastric distension. After absorption, sodium bicarbonate makes the urine more alkaline, which aids in the renal excretion of acidic drugs such as barbiturates and salicylates.

ADMINISTRATION ALERTS

- Do not add oral preparation to calcium-containing solutions.
- Sodium bicarbonate is pregnancy category C.

PHARMACOKINETICS

Sodium bicarbonate is readily absorbed. It is widely distributed in extracellular fluid. It is excreted in urine. The half-life is unknown.

ADVERSE EFFECTS AND INTERACTIONS

Most of the side effects of sodium bicarbonate therapy are the result of metabolic alkalosis caused by too much bicarbonate ion. Symptoms may include confusion, irritability, slow respiration rate, and vomiting. Simply discontinuing the sodium bicarbonate infusion often reverses these symptoms; however, potassium chloride or ammonium chloride may be administered to reverse the alkalosis. During sodium bicarbonate infusions, serum electrolytes should be carefully monitored as sodium levels may give rise to hypernatremia and fluid retention. In addition, high levels of bicarbonate ion passing through the kidney tubules increase potassium secretion, and hypokalemia is possible.

Sodium bicarbonate interacts with several drugs. For example, it may decrease absorption of ketoconazole and may decrease elimination of dextroamphetamine, ephedrine, pseudoephedrine, and quinidine. Sodium bicarbonate may increase elimination of lithium, salicylates, and tetracyclines.

 See the Companion Website for a Nursing Process Focus chart specific to this drug.

NATURAL THERAPIES

Sea Vegetables for Acidosis

Sea vegetables, or seaweeds, are a form of marine alga that grows in the upper levels of the ocean, where sunlight can penetrate. Examples of these edible seaweeds include kelp, arame, and nori, which are used a great deal in Japanese cooking. Sea vegetables are found in coastal locations throughout the world. Kelp (*Laminaria*) is found in the cold waters of the North Atlantic and Pacific oceans.

Sea vegetables contain a multitude of vitamins, as well as protein. Their most notable nutritional aspect, however, is their mineral content. Plants from the sea contain more minerals than most other food sources, including calcium, magnesium, phosphorous, iron, potassium, and all essential trace elements. Because they are so rich in minerals, seaweeds act as alkalizers of the blood, helping to rid the body of acidic conditions (acidosis). Kelp is a particularly rich source of iron.

Client education as it relates to sodium bicarbonate should include goals, reasons for obtaining baseline data such as vital signs and electrolyte levels, and possible side effects. Following are important points to include when teaching clients regarding sodium bicarbonate:

• Contact a healthcare provider immediately if gastric discomfort continues or is accompanied by chest pain, dyspnea, or diaphoresis.

• Use non–sodium bicarbonate OTC antacids to prevent the problem of excess sodium or bicarbonate being absorbed into systemic circulation.

• Do not use any antacid, including sodium bicarbonate, for longer than 2 weeks without consulting the healthcare provider.

44.10 Pharmacotherapy of Alkalosis

At plasma pH values above 7.45, **alkalosis** develops. Like acidosis, alkalosis may have both respiratory and metabolic causes, as shown in Table 44.5. Also like acidosis, the CNS is greatly affected. Symptoms of CNS stimulation include nervousness, hyperactive reflexes, and convulsions. Slow, shallow breathing indicates that the body is attempting to retain acid and lower internal pH. In mild cases, alkalosis may be corrected by administering sodium chloride combined with potassium chloride. This combination increases the renal excretion of bicarbonate ion, which indirectly increases the acidity of the blood. More severe alkalosis may be treated with infusions of ammonium chloride.

NURSING CONSIDERATIONS

The role of the nurse in drug therapy with ammonium chloride involves careful monitoring of the client's condition and providing education as it relates to the prescribed drug regimen. The major treatment for both metabolic alkalosis and respiratory alkalosis is to first attempt to correct the underlying disease condition creating the imbalance. The administration of ammonium chloride is only used in clinical practice when the alkalosis is so severe that the pH must be restored quickly to prevent life-threatening consequences. This drug is contraindicated in the presence of liver disease since its acidifying action depends on proper liver functioning to convert ammonium ions to urea.

During the IV infusion of ammonium chloride, the nurse must continually assess for metabolic acidosis and ammonium toxicity. Symptoms of toxic levels of ammonium include pallor, sweating, irregular breathing, retching, bradycardia, twitching, and convulsions. If the client exhibits any of these symptoms, the nurse should immediately stop the infusion and contact the healthcare provider.

The nurse must also closely monitor the client's renal status during the administration of ammonium chloride because the excretion of this drug depends on normal kidney function. Monitor intake and output ratio, body weight, electrolyte status, and renal function studies for any sign of renal impairment.

When ammonium chloride is administered IV, closely monitor the intravenous infusion site because this drug is extremely irritating to veins and may cause severe inflammation. The drug must be infused slowly, no more than 5 mL/min, to prevent ammonia toxicity.

Like sodium bicarbonate, ammonium chloride is used as an ionic trapping agent in the treatment of drug overdoses. Ammonium chloride acidifies urine, which increases the excretion of alkaline substances such as amphetamines, phencyclidine (PCP/angel dust), and other basic substances. Overdoses of alkaline substances can greatly compromise the cardiovascular, respiratory, and neurological status, and the nursing role in these situations will be directed toward monitoring the client's acid-base status and supporting critical body functions.

Client education as it relates to ammonium chloride should include goals, reasons for obtaining baseline data such as vital signs and renal status, and possible side effects. Following are the important points to include when teaching clients and families regarding ammonium chloride:

• Report pain at IV site.

• If medication is taken orally, report anorexia, nausea, vomiting, and thirst.

• If medication is given parenterally, report rash, headache, bradycardia, drowsiness, confusion, depression, and excitement alternating with coma.

• Take ammonium chloride tablets for no longer than 6 days.

• Report severe GI upset, fever, chills, and changes in urine or stool colour.

• Take medication after meals or use enteric-coated tablets to decrease GI upset; swallow tablets whole.

Pr PROTOTYPE DRUG | Ammonium Chloride

ACTIONS AND USES

Severe alkalosis may be reversed by the administration of acidic agents such as ammonium chloride. During the hepatic conversion of ammonium chloride to urea, Cl^- and H^+ are formed, and the pH of body fluids decreases. Ammonium chloride acidifies the urine, which is beneficial in treating certain urinary tract infections. Historically, it has been used as a diuretic, though safer and more efficacious agents have made its use for this indication obsolete. By acidifying the urine, ammonium chloride promotes the excretion of alkaline drugs such as amphetamines. When given for acidosis, the IM or IV route is preferred.

PHARMACOKINETICS

Ammonium chloride is administered PO or IV. Ammonium chloride is rapidly absorbed. It is mostly metabolized in the liver. Excretion is by the kidneys.

ADMINISTRATION ALERTS

- IV solution should be infused slowly (no faster than 5 mL/min) to prevent ammonia toxicity.
- Ammonium chloride is pregnancy category B.

ADVERSE EFFECTS AND INTERACTIONS

Ammonium chloride is generally infused slowly to minimize the potential for producing acidosis. Observe for signs of CNS depression characteristic of acidosis. Ammonium chloride may interact with several drugs; for example, it may cause crystalluria when taken with aminosalicylic acid. Ammonium chloride increases excretion of amphetamines, flecainide, mexiletine, methadone, ephedrine, and pseudoephedrine and decreases urinary excretion of sulfonylureas and salicylates.

 See the Companion Website for a Nursing Process Focus chart specific to this drug.

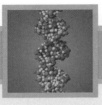

CHAPTER REVIEW

KEY CONCEPTS

The numbered key concepts provide a succinct summary of the important points from the corresponding numbered section within the chapter. If any of these points are not clear, refer to the numbered section within the chapter for review. Expanded versions can be found on the Companion Website.

44.1 There is a continuous exchange of fluids across membranes separating the intracellular and extracellular fluid compartments. Large molecules and those that are ionized are less able to cross membranes.

44.2 Changes in the osmolality of body fluids can cause water to move to different compartments.

44.3 Water balance is achieved through complex mechanisms that regulate fluid intake and output. The greatest contributor to osmolality is sodium, although glucose and urea also contribute.

44.4 Intravenous fluid therapy using crystalloids and colloids is used to replace lost fluids. Colloids such as dextran have the ability to rapidly expand plasma volume.

44.5 Electrolytes are charged substances that are essential to nerve conduction, membrane permeability, water balance, and other critical body functions.

44.6 Sodium is essential to maintain osmolality, water balance, and acid-base balance. Hypernatremia may be corrected with hypotonic IV fluids or diuretics, and hyponatremia is corrected with infusions of sodium chloride.

44.7 Potassium is essential for proper nervous and muscle function, as well as maintaining acid-base balance. Hyperkalemia may be treated with glucose and insulin or by administration of polystyrene sulfonate.

44.8 The body uses buffers to maintain overall pH within narrow limits.

44.9 Pharmacotherapy of acidosis, a plasma pH below 7.35, includes the administration of sodium bicarbonate.

44.10 Pharmacotherapy of alkalosis, a plasma pH above 7.45, includes the administration of ammonium chloride, or sodium chloride with potassium chloride.

REVIEW QUESTIONS

1 How does a colloid IV fluid differ from a crystalloid?

2 Do the terms *osmolality* and *tonicity* have the same meaning? Explain by using examples of how each term is properly used.

3 Compare and contrast the typical symptoms of hypernatremia and hyponatremia. How are they treated pharmacologically?

4 Compare and contrast the typical symptoms of hyperkalemia and hypokalemia. How are they treated pharmacologically?

5 Compare and contrast the typical symptoms of acidosis and alkalosis. How are they treated pharmacologically?

CRITICAL THINKING QUESTIONS

1. A 72-year-old male with a history of heart failure presents to the emergency room complaining of weakness and "palpitations." The client has been managed on furosemide (Lasix) and Lanoxin at home. His current ECG reveals atrial fibrillation, and serum electrolytes reveal a potassium level of 2.5 mEq/L. The physician orders an IV solution of 1000 cc Ringer's lactate with 40 mEq KCl to infuse over 8 hours. What are the issues the nurse must consider to safely administer this drug?

2. An 18-year-old woman with a blood pressure of 186/108 mm Hg is admitted to the labour and delivery unit for observation. She has 3–4⁺ pitting edema of the lower extremities and states that her hands and face are "swollen." The CBC reveals an elevated hemoglobin and hematocrit. The certified nurse midwife diagnoses the client with pregnancy-induced hypertension and orders an IV of D5LR. In addition, she requests that the nurse "push oral fluids." The nurse considers whether the midwife's order should be questioned. Discuss the appropriateness of this order.

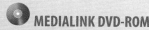

EXPLORE
MediaLink

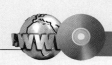

www.pearsoned.ca/adams-king

MEDIALINK DVD-ROM
- **Audio Glossary**
- **CRNE Review**
- **Animations**
  Acid-Base Balance
  Fluids

COMPANION WEBSITE
- **CRNE Review**
- **Case Study:** Client with fluid loss
- **Dosage Calculations**

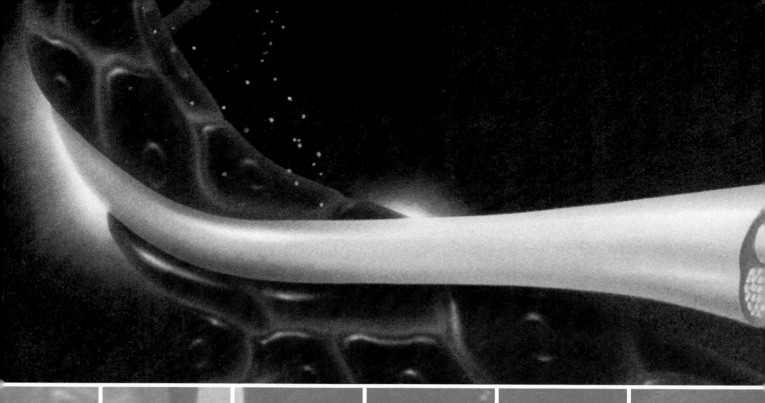

Unit 9 | The Musculoskeletal System, Integumentary System, and Eyes/Ears

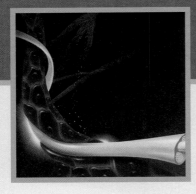

CHAPTER 45

Drugs for Muscle Spasms and Spasticity

DRUGS AT A GLANCE

CENTRALLY ACTING MUSCLE RELAXANTS
 cyclobenzaprine (Cycoflex, Flexeril)

DIRECT-ACTING ANTISPASMOTICS
 dantrolene sodium (Dantrium)

OBJECTIVES

After reading this chapter, the student should be able to do the following:

1. Discuss non-pharmacological therapies used to treat muscle spasms and spasticity.
2. Explain the therapeutic actions of centrally acting skeletal muscle relaxants and direct-acting antispasmodics in relation to the pathophysiology of muscle spasms and spasticity.
3. Discuss the nurse's role in the pharmacological and non-pharmacological treatment of clients with muscle spasms and spasticity.
4. For each of the drug classes listed in Drugs at a Glance, identify a representative drug and explain its mechanism of action, therapeutic effects, and important adverse effects.
5. Describe and explain, based on pharmacological principles, the rationale for nursing assessment, planning, and interventions for clients with muscle spasms and spasticity.
6. Use the nursing process to care for clients receiving therapy for muscle spasms.

MediaLink

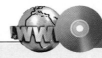

www.pearsoned.ca/adams-king

CRNE review, case studies, and other interactive resources for this chapter can be found on the Companion Website at **www.pearsoned.ca/adams-king**. Click on "Chapter 45" to select the activities for this chapter. For animations, more CRNE review questions, and an audio glossary, access the accompanying DVD-ROM in this textbook.

KEY TERMS

Disorders associated with movement are some of the most difficult conditions to treat because their underlying mechanisms may span at least four important systems in the body: nervous, muscular, endocrine, and skeletal systems. Proper body movement depends not only on intact neural pathways, but also on proper functioning of muscles, which, in turn, depends on the levels of minerals such as sodium, potassium, and calcium in the bloodstream. This chapter focuses on the pharmacotherapy of muscular disorders associated with muscle spasms and spasticity. Many of the drugs used to treat muscle spasms are distinct from those used for spasticity.

MUSCLE SPASMS

Muscle spasms are involuntary contractions of a muscle or group of muscles. The muscles become tightened, develop a fixed pattern of resistance, and exhibit a diminished level of functioning.

45.1 Causes of Muscle Injury and Spasms

Muscle spasms are a common condition usually associated with excessive use of and local injury to the skeletal muscle. Other causes of muscle spasms include epilepsy, hypocalcemia, pain, debilitating neurological disorders, genetic susceptibilities, and drug toxicities. Drug-induced muscle injury may lead to symptoms of muscle weakness or spasms that emerge over time. Causative agents may include lipid-lowering agents (such as statins), penicillamine, antimalarials, colchicine, corticosteroids, antipsychotic drugs, alcohol, and cocaine.

Clients with muscle spasms may experience inflammation, edema, and pain at the affected muscle, loss of coordination, and reduced mobility. When a muscle goes into spasm, it freezes in a contracted state. A **tonic spasm** is a single, prolonged contraction, whereas a **clonic spasm** is multiple, rapidly repeated contractions. Treatment of muscle spasms involves both non-pharmacological and pharmacological therapies.

PHARMFACTS

Conditions Associated with Muscle Spasms

- Over 12 million people worldwide have muscle spasms.
- Muscle spasms severe enough to warrant drug therapy are often found in clients who have had other debilitating disorders such as stroke, injury, neurodegenerative diseases, and cerebral palsy.
- Cerebral palsy is usually associated with events that occur before or during birth, but it may be acquired during the first few months or years of life as the result of head trauma or infection.
- Dystonia is the third most common movement disorder, following essential tremor and Parkinson's disease.
- Researchers have recognized multiple forms of inheritable dystonia and identified at least 10 genes or chromosomal locations responsible for the various manifestations.

45.2 Pharmacological and Non-Pharmacological Treatment of Muscle Spasms

Treating a client with complaints of muscle spasms requires a thorough history and physical exam to determine the etiology. After a determination has been made, non-pharmacological therapies are normally used in conjunction with

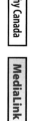

MediaLink ::: Muscular Dystrophy Canada

MediaLink ::: Institute of Musculoskeletal Health and Arthritis medications. Non-pharmacological measures may include immobilization of the affected muscle, application of heat or cold, hydrotherapy, ultrasound, supervised exercises, massage, and manipulation.

Pharmacotherapy for muscle spasms may include combinations of analgesics, anti-inflammatory agents, and centrally acting skeletal muscle relaxants. Most skeletal muscle relaxants relieve symptoms of muscular stiffness and rigidity resulting from muscular injury. They help to improve mobility in cases when clients have restricted movement. The therapeutic goals are to minimize pain and discomfort, increase range of motion, and improve the client's ability to function independently.

CENTRALLY ACTING SKELETAL MUSCLE RELAXANTS

The origin of action of many drugs used to treat muscle spasms is within the CNS. They inhibit motor neurons in the brain and spinal cord, causing muscles to relax.

45.3 Treating Muscle Spasms at the Level of the Central Nervous System

Skeletal muscle relaxants act at various levels within the CNS. Although their exact mechanisms are not fully known, it is believed that they generate their effects within the brain and/or spinal cord by inhibiting upper motor neuron activity, causing CNS depression or altering simple reflexes.

Antispasmodic drugs are used to treat local spasms resulting from muscular injury and may be prescribed alone or in combination with other medications to reduce pain and increase range of motion. Commonly used centrally acting medications include baclofen, cyclobenzaprine, tizanidine, and benzodiazepines such as diazepam, clonazepam, and lorazepam, as summarized in Table 45.1. All of the centrally acting agents have the potential to cause sedation.

Baclofen, structurally similar to the inhibitory neurotransmitter GABA, produces its effect by a mechanism that is not fully known. It inhibits neuronal activity within the brain and possibly the spinal cord, although there is some question as to whether the spinal effects of baclofen are associated with GABA. It may be used to reduce muscle spasms in clients with multiple sclerosis, cerebral palsy, or spinal cord injury. Common side effects of baclofen are drowsiness, dizziness, weakness, and fatigue. Baclofen is often a drug of first choice due to its wide safety margin.

Tizanidine is a centrally acting alpha$_2$-adrenergic agonist inhibiting motor neurons mainly at the spinal cord level. Clients receiving high doses report drowsiness; thus, it also affects some neural activity in the brain. Though uncommon, one adverse effect of tizanidine is hallucinations. The most frequent side effects are dry mouth, fatigue, dizziness, and sleepiness. Tizanidine is as effective as baclofen and is considered by some to be a drug of first choice.

As discussed in Chapter 14, benzodiazepines inhibit both sensory and motor neuron activity by enhancing the effects of GABA. Common adverse side effects include drowsiness and ataxia (loss of coordination). Benzodiazepines are usually prescribed for muscle relaxation when baclofen and tizanidine fail to produce adequate relief.

NATURAL THERAPIES

Cayenne for Muscular Tension

Several herbals are claimed to have muscle relaxant properties. These include celery seed, chamomile, goldenrod, rosemary, saw palmetto, wild yam, yarrow, and cayenne.

Cayenne (*Capsicum annum*), also known as chili pepper, paprika, or red pepper, has been used as a remedy for muscle tension. Applied in a cream base, it is commonly used to relieve muscle spasms in the shoulder and arm. Capsaicin, the active ingredient in cayenne, diminishes the chemical messengers that travel through the sensory nerves, therefore decreasing the sensation of pain (Nelson et al., 2004). Because its effects accumulate over time, creams containing capsaicin (0.025% to 0.075%) need to be applied regularly, up to four times daily, to be effective. Although no known medical condition exists that would prevent the use of cayenne, it should never be applied over broken skin. Topical use of full-strength cayenne should be limited to no more than 2 days because it may cause skin inflammation, blisters, and ulcers. It also needs to be kept away from eyes and mucous membranes to avoid burns. Hands must be washed thoroughly after use. Cayenne is also available in capsules (30 to 120 mg), taken three times daily, or as a tea.

MediaLink   Mechanism of Action: Cyclobenzaprine

TABLE 45.1 Centrally Acting Skeletal Muscle Relaxants

Drug	Route and Adult Dose
baclofen (Lioresal, Apo-. PMS-Baclofen)	PO; 5 mg tid (max 80 mg/d)
cyclobenzaprine hydrochloride (Cycoflex, Flexeril)	PO; 10–20 mg bid–qid (max 60 mg/d)
chlorzoxazone (Paraflex, Parafon Forte)	PO; 250–500 mg tid–qid (max 3 g/d)
clonazepam (Apo-, DOM-Clonazepam, Klonopin)	PO; 0.5 mg tid (max 20 mg/d)
diazepam (Valium, Apo-, PMS-Diazepam) (see page 162 for the Prototype Drug Box)	PO; 4–10 mg bid–qid IM/IV; 2–10 mg, repeat if needed in 3–4 h; IV pump; administer emulsion at 5 mg/min
lorazepam (Ativan, Apo-, DOM, PMS-Lorazepam) (see page 149 for the Prototype Drug Box)	PO; 1–2 mg bid–tid (max 10 mg/d) IV; up to 5. μg/kg (not to exceed 4 mg)
methocarbamol (Robaxin, PMS-Methocarbamol)	PO; 1.5 g qid for 2–3 d, then reduce to 1 g qid
orphenadrine (Disipal)	PO; 100 mg bid
tizanidine (Apo-Tizanidine)	PO; 4–8 mg tid–qid (max 36 mg/d)

Pr **PROTOTYPE DRUG** | Cyclobenzaprine (Cycoflex, Flexeril)

ACTIONS AND USES

Cyclobenzaprine relieves muscle spasms of local origin without interfering with general muscle function. This drug acts by depressing motor activity primarily in the brainstem but with limited effects occurring also in the spinal cord. It increases circulating levels of norepinephrine by blocking presynaptic uptake. Its mechanism of action is similar to the tricyclic antidepressants (see Chapter 16). It causes muscle relaxation in cases of acute muscle spasticity, but it is not effective in cases of cerebral palsy or diseases of the brain and spinal cord. This medication is meant to provide therapy for only 2 to 3 weeks.

PHARMACOKINETICS

Cyclobenzaprine is well absorbed from the GI tract. It has an onset of action of 1 hour and peaks in 3 to 8 hours. It is 93% protein bound and is metabolized by the liver. The half-life is 1 to 3 days.

ADMINISTRATION ALERTS

- The drug is not recommended for pediatric use.
- Maximum effects may take 1 to 2 weeks.
- Cyclobenzaprine is pregnancy category B.

ADVERSE EFFECTS AND INTERACTIONS

Adverse reactions to cyclobenzaprine include drowsiness, blurred vision, dizziness, dry mouth, rash, and tachycardia. One reaction, although rare, is swelling of the tongue. Alcohol, phenothiazines, and other CNS depressants may cause additive sedation. Cyclobenzaprine should not be used within 2 weeks of an MAO inhibitor since hyperpyretic crisis and convulsions may occur. It should be used with caution in clients with MI, dysrhythmias, or severe cardiovascular disease.

TREATMENT OF OVERDOSE

The intravenous administration of 1 to 3 mg of physostigmine salicylate is reported to reverse symptoms of poisoning by drugs with anticholinergic activity. Physostigmine may be helpful in the treatment of cyclobenzaprine overdose.

See the Companion Website for a Nursing Process Focus chart specific to this drug.

SPASTICITY

Spasticity is a condition in which certain muscle groups remain in a continuous state of contraction, usually as a result of damage to the CNS. The contracted muscles become stiff with increased muscle tone. Other signs and symptoms may include mild to severe pain, exaggerated deep tendon reflexes, muscle spasms, scissoring (involuntary crossing of the legs), and fixed joints.

45.4 Causes and Treatment of Spasticity

Spasticity usually results from damage to the motor area of the cerebral cortex that controls muscle movement. Etiologies most commonly associated with this condition include neurological disorders such as cerebral palsy, severe head injury, spinal cord injury or lesions, and stroke. **Dystonia**, a chronic neurological disorder, is characterized by involuntary muscle contraction that forces body parts into abnormal, occasionally painful movements or postures. It affects the muscle tone of the arms, legs, trunk, neck, eyelids, face, and vocal cords. Spasticity can be very distressing and can have a negative impact on a client's quality of life, whether the condition is short or long term. In addition to causing pain, impaired physical mobility reduces the ability to perform activities of daily living (ADL) and diminishes the client's sense of independence.

Effective treatment for spasticity includes both physical therapy and medications. Medications alone are not adequate in reducing the complications of spasticity. Regular and consistent physical therapy exercises have been shown to decrease the severity of symptoms. Types of treatment include muscle stretching to help prevent contractures, muscle group strengthening exercises, and repetitive motion exercises for improving accuracy. In extreme cases, surgery for tendon release or to sever the nerve-muscle pathway is occasionally used. Drugs effective in the treatment of spasticity include several classifications of antispasmodics that act in the CNS, at neuromuscular junctions, or in muscle tissue.

DIRECT-ACTING ANTISPASMODICS

45.5 Treating Muscle Spasms Directly at the Muscle Tissue

Drugs effective in the treatment of spasticity include two centrally acting drugs, baclofen and diazepam, and a direct-acting drug, dantrolene. The direct-acting drugs produce an antispasmodic effect at the level of the neuromuscular junction, as shown in Figure 45.1.

Dantrolene relieves spasticity by interfering with the release of calcium ions in skeletal muscle. Other direct-acting drugs include botulinum toxin type A and type B, used to offer significant relief of symptoms to people with dystonia, and quinine sulfate, used to treat leg cramps. Direct-acting drugs are summarized in Table 45.2.

Botulinum toxin is an unusual drug because, in higher quantities, it acts as a poison. *Clostridium botulinum* is the bacterium responsible for producing the toxin that causes the food poisoning known as botulism. At lower doses, however, botulinum toxin is safe and effective as a muscle relaxant for clients with dystonia. For example, it is used to

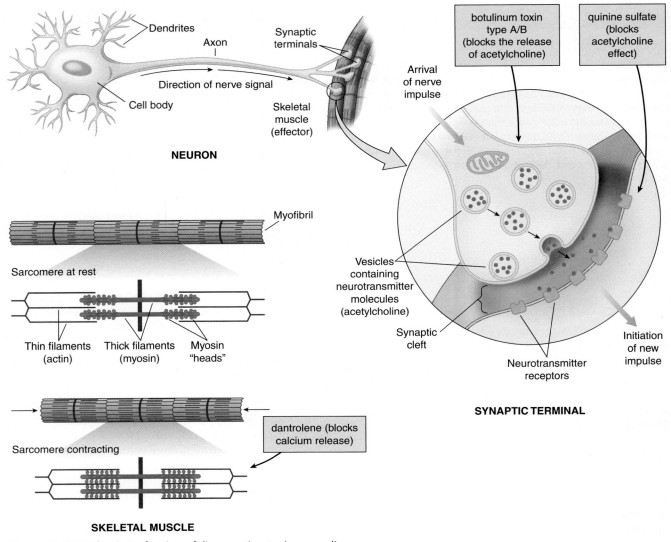

● **Figure 45.1** Mechanism of action of direct-acting antispasmodics

reduce spasticity, such as a clenched fist or bent elbow that can occur after a stroke or due to cerebral palsy, and for excessive blinking, crossed-eyes, and eyelid tics. It produces its effect by blocking the release of acetylcholine from cholinergic nerve terminals (Chapter 13).

In 2001, Health Canada approved botulinum toxin type A (Botox Cosmetic) injections for temporary improvement in the appearance of moderate to severe frown lines (vertical lines between the brows) in adult clients. It works to relax frown muscles by blocking nerve impulses that trigger

wrinkle-causing muscle contractions, creating a smooth appearance between the brows. Administered in a few tiny injections of purified protein, this minimally invasive treatment is simple and quick and delivers dramatic results with minimal discomfort. Results can be seen in as soon as 24 to 48 hours, and the effect lasts up to 4 months. Injections should not be repeated more than once every 3 months. Side effects include headache, nausea, flu-like symptoms, temporary eyelid drooping, mild pain, erythema at the injection site, and muscle weakness.

TABLE 45.2 Direct-Acting Antispasmodic Drugs

Drug	Route and Adult Dose
botulinum toxin type A (Botox, Cosmetic, Botox PWS)	25 U injected directly into target muscle (max 30-day dose should not exceed 200 U)
botulinum toxin type B	2500–5000 U/dose injected directly into target muscle; doses should be divided among muscle groups
⊙ dantrolene sodium (Dantrium)	PO; 25 mg qd; increase to 25 mg bid–qid; may increase every 4–7 d up to 100 mg bid–tid
quinine (Apo-, Novo-Quinine)	PO; 260–300 mg at hs

Pr PROTOTYPE DRUG | Dantrolene Sodium (Dantrium)

ACTIONS AND USES

Dantrolene is often used for spasticity, especially for spasms of the head and neck. It directly relaxes muscle spasms by interfering with the release of calcium ions from storage areas inside skeletal muscle cells. It does not affect cardiac or smooth muscle. Dantrolene is especially useful for muscle spasms when they occur after spinal cord injury or stroke and in cases of cerebral palsy, multiple sclerosis, and occasionally for the treatment of muscle pain after heavy exercise. It is also used for the treatment of malignant hyperthermia.

PHARMACOKINETICS

Taken orally, dantrolene is 35% absorbed, has an onset of action of 1 hour, peaks in 5 to 12 hours, and has a variable duration of action. It is metabolized by the liver. Its half-life is 9 hours.

ADMINISTRATION ALERTS

- Use the oral suspension within several days as it does not contain a preservative.
- IV solution has a high pH and therefore is extremely irritating to tissue.
- Dantrolene is pregnancy category C.

ADVERSE EFFECTS AND INTERACTIONS

Adverse effects include muscle weakness, drowsiness, dry mouth, dizziness, nausea, diarrhea, tachycardia, erratic blood pressure, photosensitivity, and urinary retention.

Dantrolene interacts with many other drugs. For example, it should not be taken with OTC cough preparations and antihistamines, alcohol, or other CNS depressants. Verapamil and other calcium channel blockers taken with dantrolene increase the risk of ventricular fibrillation and cardiovascular collapse. Clients with impaired cardiac or pulmonary function or hepatic disease should not take this drug.

 See the Companion Website for a Nursing Process Focus chart specific to this drug.

Because of the extreme weakness associated with botulinum, therapies may be needed to improve muscle strength. To circumvent major problems with mobility or posture, botulinum toxin is often applied to small muscle groups. Sometimes this drug is administered with centrally acting oral medications to increase functional use of a range of muscle groups.

Drawbacks to botulinum therapy are its delayed and limited effects. The treatment is mostly effective within 6 weeks and lasts for only 3 to 6 months. Another drawback is pain; botulinum is injected directly into the muscle. Pain associated with injections is usually blocked by a local anesthetic.

NURSING CONSIDERATIONS

The role of the nurse in antispasmodic therapy involves careful monitoring of the client's condition and providing education as it relates to the prescribed drug regimen. Assess adherence with drug use, side effects, and expected outcomes. Centrally acting drugs such as cyclobenzaprine and chlorzoxazone should be avoided in clients with liver disease. All centrally acting drugs cause CNS depression as evidenced by drowsiness and dizziness; therefore, clients should be advised to avoid hazardous activities such as driving until the effects of the drug are known. Clients should also be advised to avoid alcohol, benzodiazepines, opioids, and antihistamines as they can intensify the CNS depressant effects of the drugs. Clients should be warned against abrupt discontinuation of treatment because this may result in seizures.

Although dantrolene is a direct-acting muscle relaxant, it has similar effects and precautions as centrally acting drugs and is contraindicated in clients with liver disease, compromised pulmonary function, or cardiac dysfunction. The nurse should also be aware that a client with spasticity may not be able to self-medicate and caregiver assistance may be required.

Client education as it relates to centrally and direct-acting antispasmodics should include goals, reasons for obtaining baseline data such as health history and blood work, and possible side effects and interactions. See "Nursing Process Focus: Clients Receiving Drugs for Muscle Spasms or Spasticity" for specific points the nurse should include when teaching clients regarding this class of drug.

NURSING PROCESS FOCUS Clients Receiving Drugs for Muscle Spasms or Spasticity

Assessment	Potential Nursing Diagnoses/Identified Patterns
Prior to administration: ■ Obtain complete health history including allergies, drug history, and possible drug interactions. ■ Obtain complete physical examination. ■ Establish baseline level of consciousness, vital signs, muscle tone, range of motion, and degree of muscle spasm.	■ Pain (acute/chronic) related to muscle spasms ■ Mobility impairment related to acute/chronic pain and spasms ■ Risk for injury and discomfort related to drug side effects ■ Need for knowledge regarding to drug therapy and supportive therapies

continued

NURSING PROCESS FOCUS Clients Receiving Drugs for Muscle Spasms or Spasticity *(Continued)*

Planning: Client Goals and Expected Outcomes

The client will:
- Report a decrease in pain, increase in range of motion, and reduction of muscle spasm
- Exhibit no adverse effects from the therapeutic regimen
- Demonstrate an understanding of the therapeutic regime
- Demonstrate an understanding of the drug by accurately describing the drug's purpose, action, side effects, and precautions

Implementation

Interventions (Rationales)	Client Education/Discharge Planning
■ Monitor LOC and vital signs. (Some skeletal muscle relaxants alter the client's LOC. Others within this class may alter blood pressure and heart rate.)	Instruct client to: ■ Avoid driving and other activities requiring mental alertness until effects of the medication are known ■ Report any significant change in sensorium, such as slurred speech, confusion, hallucinations, or extreme lethargy ■ Report palpitations, chest pain, dyspnea, unusual fatigue, weakness, and visual disturbances ■ Avoid using other CNS depressants such as alcohol that will intensify sedation
■ Monitor pain. ■ Determine location, duration, and precipitating factors of the client's pain. (Drugs should diminish client's pain.)	Instruct client to: ■ Report the development of new sites of muscle pain ■ Use relaxation techniques, deep breathing, and meditation methods to facilitate relaxation and reduce pain
■ Monitor for withdrawal reactions. (Abrupt withdrawal of baclofen may cause visual hallucinations, paranoid ideation, and seizures.)	■ Advise client to avoid abrupt discontinuation of treatment.
■ Monitor muscle tone, range of motion, and degree of muscle spasm. (This will determine effectiveness of drug therapy.)	■ Instruct client to perform gentle range of motion exercises, only to the point of mild physical discomfort, throughout the day.
■ Provide additional pain relief measures such as positional support, gentle massage, and moist heat or ice packs. (Drugs alone may not be sufficient in providing pain relief.)	■ Instruct client to use complementary pain interventions such as positioning, gentle massage, and the application of heat or cold to the painful area.
■ Monitor for side effects such as drowsiness, dry mouth, dizziness, nausea, vomiting, faintness, headache, nervousness, diplopia, and urinary retention (cyclobenzaprine).	Instruct client to: ■ Report side effects ■ Take medication with food to decrease GI upset ■ Report signs of urinary retention such as a feeling of urinary bladder fullness, distended abdomen, and discomfort
■ Monitor for side effects such as muscle weakness, dry mouth, dizziness, nausea, diarrhea, tachycardia, erratic blood pressure, photosensitivity, and urinary retention. (These adverse effects occur with certain drugs in this class.)	Instruct client: ■ To use mouth rinses, sips of water, or sugarless candy or gum to help with dry mouth ■ That medication may cause a decrease in muscle strength and dosage may need to be reduced ■ To use sunscreen and protective clothing when outdoors

Evaluation of Outcome Criteria

Evaluate the effectiveness of drug therapy by confirming that client goals and expected outcomes have been met (see "Planning").

See Tables 45.1 (page 646) and 45.2 (page 648) for lists of drugs to which these nursing actions apply.

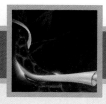

CHAPTER REVIEW

KEY CONCEPTS

The numbered key concepts provide a succinct summary of the important points from the corresponding numbered section within the chapter. If any of these points are not clear, refer to the numbered section within the chapter for review. Expanded versions can be found on the Companion Website.

45.1 Muscle spasms, involuntary contractions of a muscle or group of muscles, most commonly occur because of localized trauma to skeletal muscle.

45.2 Muscle spasms can be treated with non-pharmacological and pharmacological therapies.

45.3 Many muscle relaxants treat muscle spasms at the level of the CNS, generating their effect within the brain and/or spinal cord, usually by inhibiting upper motor neuron activity, causing sedation, or by altering simple reflexes.

45.4 Spasticity, a condition in which selected muscles are continuously contracted, results from damage to the CNS. Effective treatment for spasticity includes both physical therapy and medications.

45.5 Some antispasmodic drugs used for spasticity act directly on muscle tissue, relieving spasticity by interfering with the release of calcium ions.

REVIEW QUESTIONS

1 Compare and contrast the cause of localized muscle spasms and spasticity. What is the main goal of antispasmodic therapy for each condition?

2 Compare and contrast the two modes of action by which antispasmodic drugs relieve muscle spasms and symptoms of spasticity.

3 What can the nurse do to promote the therapeutic effects and minimize the side effects of antispasmodics?

CRITICAL THINKING QUESTIONS

1. A 46-year-old male quadriplegic has been experiencing severe spasticity in the lower extremities, making it difficult for him to maintain position in his electric wheelchair. Prior to the episodes of spasticity, the client was able to maintain a sitting posture. The risks and benefits of therapy with dantrolene (Dantrium) have been explained to him, and he has decided that the benefits outweigh the risks. What assessments should the nurse make to determine whether the treatment is beneficial?

2. A 52-year-old breast cancer survivor is taking tamoxifen and has experienced leg and foot cramps "almost nightly." She states that these cramps have markedly decreased the quality of her sleep and that she is ready to "just stop taking" the tamoxifen in order to end the leg cramps. The nurse is aware that tamoxifen is considered important in the chemoprevention of breast cancer. What treatment modalities can be offered to this client to promote her comfort and decrease the chance that she will stop therapy?

3. A 32-year-old wheat farmer injured his lower back while unloading a truck at a farm cooperative. His healthcare provider started him on cyclobenzaprine (Flexeril) 10 mg tid for 7 days and referred him to outpatient physical therapy. After 4 days, the client reports back to the office nurse that he is constipated and having trouble emptying his bladder. Discuss the cause of these side effects. What nursing actions are required?

EXPLORE
MediaLink
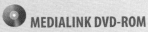

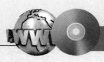
www.pearsoned.ca/adams-king

MEDIALINK DVD-ROM
- Audio Glossary
- CRNE Review
- Animation
  Mechanism of Action: Cyclobenzaprine

COMPANION WEBSITE
- CRNE Review
- Case Study: Treating muscle spasms
- Dosage Calculations

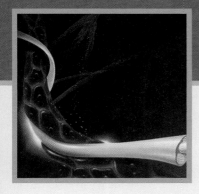
Drugs for Bone and Joint Disorders

DRUGS AT A GLANCE

CALCIUM SUPPLEMENTS AND VITAMIN D THERAPY
- calcium gluconate (Calciforte)
- calcitriol (Calcijex, Rocaltrol)

BONE RESORPTION INHIBITORS
Hormonal agents
- raloxifene (Evista)

Bisphosphonates
- etidronate disodium (Didronel)

DISEASE-MODIFYING DRUGS OF IMPORTANCE FOR RHEUMATOID ARTHRITIS
- hydroxychloroquine sulfate (Gen-Hydroxy-chloroquine)

URIC ACID INHIBITORS
- colchicine

OBJECTIVES

After reading this chapter, the student should be able to do the following:

1. Identify important signs and symptoms of disorders associated with an imbalance of calcium, vitamin D, parathyroid hormone, and calcitonin.
2. Explain the therapeutic action of each class of drug used for bone and joint disorders in relation to the pathophysiology of the disorder.
3. Describe the nurse's role in the pharmacological management of disorders caused by calcium and vitamin D deficiency.
4. Describe the nurse's role, including client teaching, regarding the use of non-pharmacological therapies to prevent and treat bone and joint disorders.
5. For each of the drug classes listed in Drugs at a Glance, identify a representative drug and explain its mechanism of action, therapeutic effects, and important adverse effects.
6. Describe and explain, based on pharmacological principles, the rationale for nursing assessment, planning, and interventions for clients with bone and joint disorders.
7. Use the nursing process to care for clients receiving drug therapy for bone and joint disorders.

MediaLink

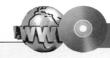 www.pearsoned.ca/adams-king

CRNE review, case studies, and other interactive resources for this chapter can be found on the Companion Website at **www.pearsoned.ca/adams-king**. Click on "Chapter 46" to select the activities for this chapter. For animations, more CRNE review questions, and an audio glossary, access the accompanying DVD-ROM in this textbook.

The skeletal system and joints are at the core of body movement. Disorders associated with bones and joints may affect a client's ability to fulfill daily activities and lead to immobility. In addition, the skeletal system serves as the primary repository of calcium, one of the body's most important minerals. This chapter focuses on the pharmacotherapy of important skeletal disorders such as osteomalacia, osteoporosis, arthritis, and gout. The importance of calcium balance and the action of vitamin D are stressed as they relate to the proper structure and function of bones.

LIFESPAN CONSIDERATIONS

Bone Health across the Lifespan

- The bone matrix, which is formed through a cyclic process of bone formation and resorption, becomes more brittle with age.
- About 1.4 million Canadians have osteoarthritis—one in four women and one in eight men.
- Postmenopausal women are at increased risk of osteoporosis. By age 65, one in every two women has osteoarthritis. By age 75, one in two will have an osteoporotic fracture. By age 90, one in three will have a hip fracture. About 25% die within a year of a hip fracture due to complications such as pulmonary embolism or stroke.
- The Osteoporosis Society of Canada recommends that Canadians aged 19 to 50, including pregnant or lactating women, receive 400 international units (IU) of vitamin D_3 per day.
- Adults over 50 should receive 800 IU of vitamin D_3 per day.
- Children and adolescents have the greatest need for calcium for strong bones and teeth and require adequate vitamin D in order to use the calcium.
- Regular physical activity is important for bone health at all ages.

Source: Bureau of Nutritional Sciences, Health Canada; The Osteoporosis Society of Canada, "http://www.osteoporosis.ca/english/About%20Osteoporosis/ Nutrition/Vitamin%20"; L'Abbe, M. R., Whiting, S. J., & Hanley, D. A. (2004). The Canadian health claim for calcium, vitamin D and osteoporosis. Journal of the American College of Nutrition, 23, 303–308.

46.1 Normal Calcium Physiology and Vitamin D

One of the most important minerals in the body responsible for bone formation is calcium. Levels of calcium in the blood are controlled by two endocrine glands: the parathyroid glands, which secrete parathyroid hormone (PTH), and the thyroid gland, which secretes calcitonin, as shown in Figure 46.1.

PTH stimulates bone cells called osteoclasts. These cells accelerate the process of **bone resorption**, a demineralization process that breaks down bone into its mineral components. Once bone is broken down, or resorbed, calcium becomes available to be transported and used elsewhere in the body. The opposite of this process is **bone deposition**, which is bone building. This process, which removes calcium from the blood, is stimulated by the hormone calcitonin.

PTH and calcitonin control calcium homeostasis in the body by influencing three major targets: bones, kidneys, and GI tract. The GI tract is mainly influenced by PTH and vitamin D. Vitamin D and calcium metabolism are intimately related: calcium disorders are often associated with vitamin D disorders.

Vitamin D is unique among vitamins in that the body is able to synthesize it from precursor molecules. In the skin, the inactive form of vitamin D, called **cholecalciferol**, is synthesized from cholesterol. Exposure of the skin to ultraviolet (UV) light increases the level of cholecalciferol in the blood. Sunlight exposure during Canadian winters is not adequate to prevent the occurrence of vitamin D deficiency, as evidenced by the high incidence of childhood rickets seen prior to

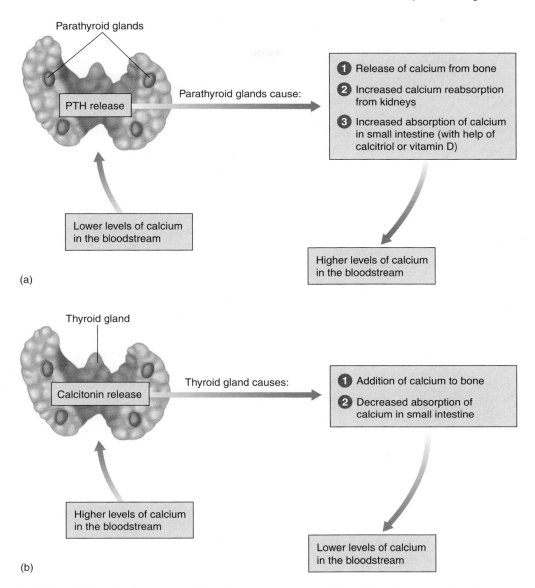

Parathyroid glands

Parathyroid glands cause:

1 Release of calcium from bone

2 Increased calcium reabsorption from kidneys

3 Increased absorption of calcium in small intestine (with help of calcitriol or vitamin D)

PTH release

Lower levels of calcium in the bloodstream

Higher levels of calcium in the bloodstream

(a)

Thyroid gland

Thyroid gland causes:

1 Addition of calcium to bone

2 Decreased absorption of calcium in small intestine

Calcitonin release

Higher levels of calcium in the bloodstream

Lower levels of calcium in the bloodstream

(b)

● **Figure 46.1** Regulation of calcium in the bloodstream: (a) parathyroid glands release parathyroid hormone (PTH); (b) thyroid gland releases calcitonin

the introduction of mandatory fortification of milk with vitamin D. Recent reports suggest that vitamin D levels in Canadians are still less than optimal (see References for this chapter for additional information). Cholecalciferol can be obtained from dietary products such as milk and other foods fortified with vitamin D. Figure 46.2 illustrates the metabolism of vitamin D.

Following its absorption or formation, cholecalciferol is converted to an intermediate vitamin form called **calcifediol**. Enzymes in the kidneys metabolize calcifediol to **calcitriol**, the active form of vitamin D. PTH stimulates the formation of calcitriol at the level of the kidneys. Clients with extensive kidney disease are unable to adequately synthesize calcitriol.

The primary function of calcitriol is to increase calcium absorption from the GI tract. Dietary calcium is absorbed more efficiently in the presence of active vitamin D and PTH, resulting in higher serum levels of calcium. Calcium is then transported from the blood to bone, muscle, and other tissues.

The importance of proper calcium balance in the body cannot be overstated. Calcium ion influences the excitability of all neurons. When calcium concentrations are too high (hypercalcemia), sodium permeability decreases across cell membranes. This is a dangerous state because nerve conduction depends on the proper influx of sodium into cells. When calcium levels in the bloodstream are too low (hypocalcemia), cell membranes become hyperexcitable. If this situation becomes severe, convulsions or muscle spasms may result. Calcium is also important for the normal functioning of other body processes such as blood coagulation and muscle contraction.

Sources of Vitamin D

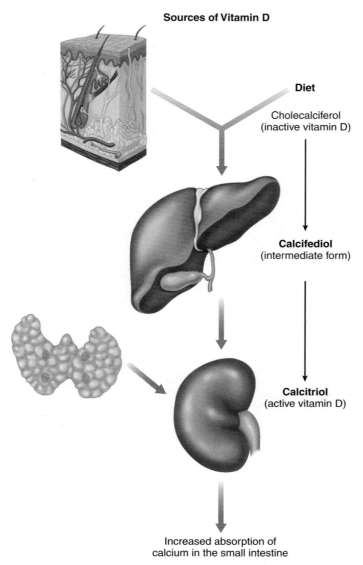

Diet

Cholecalciferol
(inactive vitamin D)

Calcifediol
(intermediate form)

Calcitriol
(active vitamin D)

Increased absorption of
calcium in the small intestine

● **Figure 46.2** Pathway of vitamin D activation and action

PHARMFACTS

Vitamin D and Calcium

- Vitamin D_3 increases calcium absorption by as much as 30% to 80%.
- Vitamin D is often added to calcium supplements.
- Seasonal differences in hours of sunlight may alter the requirement for vitamin D supplements, with higher doses required in Canadian winters.
- Increased use of sunscreen and hats to prevent skin cancer may contribute to vitamin D deficiency.
- It is difficult to get enough vitamin D from foods alone.
- In Canada, vitamin D fortification of milk (min 8.8 µg/L, max 11.7 µg/L) and margarine (13.25 µg/100 g) provides the major dietary sources of vitamin D.
- Multivitamins often provide from 125 to 400 IU of vitamin D and variable amounts of calcium. (Note: 1 µg of vitamin D equals 40 IU.)
- Calcium from "natural" sources such as oyster shells is not "refined" and may contain lead.

Source: Bureau of Nutritional Sciences, Health Canada); L'Abbe, M. R., Whiting, S. J., & Hanley, D. A. (2004). The Canadian health claim for calcium, vitamin D and osteoporosis. Journal of the American College of Nutrition, 23, 303–308.

CALCIUM-RELATED DISORDERS

Diseases and conditions of calcium and vitamin D metabolism include hypocalcemia, osteomalacia, osteoporosis, and Paget's disease. Therapies for calcium disorders include calcium supplements, vitamin D supplements, bisphosphonates, and several miscellaneous agents.

46.2 Pharmacotherapy of Hypocalcemia

Hypocalcemia is not a disease, but a sign of underlying pathology; therefore, diagnosis of the cause of hypocalcemia is essential. One common etiology is hyposecretion of PTH, as occurs when the thyroid and parathyroid glands are diseased or surgically removed. Digestive-related malabsorption disorders and vitamin D deficiencies also result in hypocalcemia. When taking a medical history, the nurse should assess for inadequate intake of calcium-containing foods.

Symptoms of hypocalcemia are those of nerve and muscle excitability. Muscle twitching, tremor, or cramping may be evident. Numbness and tingling of the extremities may occur, and convulsions are possible. Confusion and abnormal behaviour may be observed. Severe hypocalcemia requires IV administration of calcium salts, whereas less severe hypocalcemia can often be reversed with dietary modification or calcium supplements.

Increasing the consumption of calcium-rich foods, especially dairy products, fortified orange juice, cereals, and green leafy vegetables, may be sufficient to restore calcium balance when hypocalcemia is mild and non-life-threatening. If dietary modification is not practical or adequate, calcium supplements are available OTC or by prescription. Calcium supplements often contain vitamin D to increase absorption.

The two major forms of calcium are complexed and elemental. Most calcium supplements are in the form of complexed calcium. These products are often compared on the basis of their ability to release elemental calcium into the bloodstream. The greater the ability of complexed calcium to release elemental calcium, the more potent the supplement.

NURSING CONSIDERATIONS

The role of the nurse in calcium supplement therapy involves careful monitoring of the client's condition and providing education as it relates to the prescribed drug treatment. Assess for signs and symptoms of calcium imbalance. For hypercalcemia, assess for drowsiness, lethargy, weakness, headache, anorexia, nausea, vomiting, thirst, and increased urination. Hypocalcemia signs and symptoms to assess for include facial twitching, muscle spasms, paresthesias, and seizures. Obtain baseline and periodic vital signs, serum calcium levels, and ECG to determine the effectiveness of the medication. Obtain a thorough health history, including

Pr PROTOTYPE DRUG | Calcium Gluconate (Calciforte)

ACTIONS AND USES

Calcium gluconate and other calcium compounds are used to correct hypocalcemia and treat osteoporosis and Paget's disease. The objective of calcium therapy is to return serum calcium levels to normal. People at high risk for developing these conditions include postmenopausal women, those with little physical activity over a prolonged period, and clients taking certain medications such as corticosteroids, immunosuppressive drugs, and some antiseizure medications. Calcium gluconate is available in tablets, powder, or as a 10% solution for IV injection.

PHARMACOKINETICS

Calcium gluconate is mostly excreted in the feces. It has an unknown half-life.

ADMINISTRATION ALERTS

- Give oral calcium supplements with meals or within 1 hour following meals.
- If administering IV, inject slowly to avoid cardiac abnormalities.
- Calcium gluconate is pregnancy category B.

ADVERSE EFFECTS AND INTERACTIONS

The most common adverse effect of calcium gluconate is hypercalcemia, brought on by taking too much of this supplement. Symptoms include drowsiness, lethargy, weakness, headache, anorexia, nausea and vomiting, increased urination, and thirst. IV administration of calcium may cause hypotension, bradycardia, dysrhythmias, and cardiac arrest.

Concurrent use of cardiac glycosides increases the risk of dysrhythmia. Magnesium may compete for GI absorption. Calcium decreases the absorption of tetracyclines.

 See the Companion Website for a Nursing Process Focus chart specific to this drug.

---

dietary patterns, exercise patterns, bone health, pregnancy, medical conditions, and OTC, herbal, and prescribed medications. Calcium supplements are contraindicated in clients with hypercalcemia, digitalis toxicity, dysrhythmias, or renal calculi.

Client education as it relates to calcium supplements should include goals, reasons for obtaining baseline data, and possible side effects. Following are important points the nurse should include when teaching clients and caregivers about these supplements:

- Report signs or symptoms of hypercalcemia: drowsiness, lethargy, weakness, headache, anorexia, nausea and vomiting, increased urination, and thirst.
- Report signs or symptoms of hypocalcemia: seizures, muscle spasms, facial twitching, or paresthesias.

- Report side effects of medication such as nausea, vomiting, constipation, and difficulty urinating.
- Take safety precautions to prevent falling and fractures.
- Participate in active and passive range of motion exercises, as tolerated.
- Consume calcium-rich foods, including milk and dairy products, dark green vegetables, soy beans, and canned fish with bones, such as salmon.
- Avoid excessive intake of zinc-rich foods, such as nuts, legumes, seeds, sprouts, and tofu, as zinc decreases calcium absorption.
- Avoid taking antacids that contain calcium and avoid consuming calcium-fortified juices or foods without first notifying the healthcare provider.

NURSING PROCESS FOCUS   Clients Receiving Calcium Supplements

Assessment	Potential Nursing Diagnoses/Identified Patterns
Prior to administration: ■ Obtain complete health history including allergies, drug history, and possible drug interactions. ■ Assess baseline ECG. ■ Assess baseline vital signs, especially apical pulse for rate and rhythm, and blood pressure. ■ Assess lab work, including CBC and electrolytes, especially calcium.	■ Risk for injury related to loss of bone mass and side effects of drug ■ Need for knowledge regarding drug therapy ■ Need for knowledge regarding sources of calcium and vitamin D

Planning: Client Goals and Expected Outcomes

The client will:
- Have normal serum calcium levels (adult: 2.05–2.55 mmol/L; children: 2.10–2.75 mmol/L, depending on specific age)
- Demonstrate an understanding of the drug's action by accurately describing drug side effects and precautions and measures to take to decrease any side effects
- Immediately report side effects and adverse reactions

continued

NURSING PROCESS FOCUS   Clients Receiving Calcium Supplements   *(Continued)*

Implementation

Interventions (Rationales)	Client Education/Discharge Planning
▪ Monitor electrolytes throughout therapy. (Calcium and phosphorus levels tend to vary inversely. Low magnesium levels tend to coexist with low calcium levels.)	▪ Teach client importance of routine lab studies, so deviations from normal can be corrected immediately.
▪ Monitor for signs and symptoms of hypercalcemia. (Over-treatment may lead to excessive serum calcium levels.)	▪ Instruct client to report signs or symptoms of hypercalcemia: drowsiness, lethargy, weakness, headache, anorexia, nausea and vomiting, increased urination, and thirst.
▪ Initiate seizure precautions for clients at risk for hypocalcemia. (Low calcium levels may cause seizures.)	▪ Teach client to be aware of signs of hypocalcemia, such as seizures, muscle spasms, facial twitching, and paresthesias.
▪ Monitor for musculoskeletal difficulties. (Calcium gluconate is used to treat osteoporosis, rickets, osteomalacia.)	Instruct client to: ▪ Take special precautions to prevent fractures ▪ Report episodes of sudden pain, joints out of alignment, inability to assume normal positioning
▪ Monitor intake and output. Use cautiously in client with renal insufficiency. (Calcium is excreted by the kidneys.)	▪ Instruct client to report any difficulty in urination and to measure intake and output.
▪ Monitor cardiac functioning. (Possible side effects may include short QT wave, heart block, hypotension, dysrhythmia, or cardiac arrest with IV administration.)	▪ Inform client to recognize and report palpitations or shortness of breath to healthcare provider.
▪ Monitor injection site during intravenous administration for infiltration. (Extravasation may lead to necrosis.)	▪ Instruct client to report any pain at IV site.
▪ Monitor diet. (Consuming calcium-rich foods may increase effect of drug. Consuming foods rich in zinc may decrease calcium absorption.)	▪ Advise client to consume calcium-rich foods and avoid zinc-rich foods

Evaluation of Outcome Criteria

Evaluate the effectiveness of drug therapy by confirming that client goals and expected outcomes have been met (see "Planning").

46.3 Pharmacotherapy of Osteomalacia

Osteomalacia, referred to as rickets in children, is a disorder characterized by softening of bones without alteration of basic bone structure. The cause of osteomalacia and rickets is a lack of vitamin D and calcium in the diet, usually as a result of kidney failure or malabsorption of calcium from the GI tract. Signs and symptoms include hypocalcemia, muscle weakness, muscle spasms, and diffuse bone pain, especially in the hip area. Clients may also experience pain in the arms, legs, and spinal column. Classic signs of rickets in children include bowlegs and a pigeon breast. Children may also develop a slight fever and become restless at night.

Tests performed to verify osteomalacia include bone biopsy, bone radiographs, computed tomography (CT) scan of the vertebral column, and determination of serum calcium, phosphate, and vitamin D levels. Many of these tests are routine for bone disorders and are performed as needed to determine the extent of bone health.

In extreme cases, surgical correction of disfigured limbs may be required. Drug therapy for children and adults con-

sists of calcium supplements and vitamin D. A summary of drugs used for these conditions is provided in Table 46.1.

Inactive, intermediate, and active forms of vitamin D are also available as medications. The biological activity of 40 IU of vitamin D equals that of 1 μg of ergocalciferol or cholecalciferol. The amount of vitamin D a client needs will often vary depending on the amount of sunlight exposure. Growing children and adolescents require adequate calcium and vitamin D for strong bones and teeth. After age 70, the average recommended intake of vitamin D increases from 400 to 800 IU/day. Because vitamin D is needed to absorb calcium from the GI tract, many supplements combine vitamin D and calcium into a single tablet.

NURSING CONSIDERATIONS

The role of the nurse in vitamin D therapy involves careful monitoring of the client's condition and providing education as it relates to the prescribed drug regimen. Obtain a history of current medications and fat-soluble vitamin intake. Liver function should be assessed because liver impairment can lead to accumulation of this lipid-soluble

TABLE 46.1 Calcium Supplements and Vitamin D Therapy	
Drug	*Route and Adult Dose*
Calcium Supplements (all doses in terms of elemental calcium)	
calcium acetate	PO; 1–2 g bid–tid
calcium carbonate (Calsan, Caltrate, others)	PO; 1–2 g bid–tid
calcium chloride	IV; 0.5–1 g qd–q3d
calcium citrate (Citracal)	PO; 1–2 g bid–tid
calcium gluceptate	IV; 1.1–4.4 g qd IM; 0.5–1.1 g–qd
calcium gluconate (Calciforte)	PO; 1–2 g bid–qid IV; 4.5–16 mEq
calcium lactate	PO; 325 mg–1.3 g tid with meals
calcium phosphate tribasic	PO; 1 mL bid–tid
Vitamin D Supplements	
calcitriol (Calcijex, Rocaltrol)	PO; 0.25 μg qd
cholecalciferol (Vitamin D$_3$)	PD; 10–25 μg (400–1000 IU) per day
ergocalciferol (Vitamin D$_2$)	PO/IM; 25–125 μg/d for 6–12 wk

vitamin and toxicity. Assess sclera, skin pigment, bowel movements, and lab results for evidence of liver dysfunction. Because high levels of vitamin D may cause renal impairment, urinalysis and renal test results should be monitored. Calcium, phosphate, and magnesium levels may be altered by vitamin D therapy and also should be monitored. Assess for adverse effects of vitamin D therapy, such as hypercalcemia, headache, weakness, dry mouth, thirst, increased urination, and muscle or bone pain.

Client education as it relates to vitamin D supplements should include goals, reasons for obtaining baseline data, and possible side effects. Following are important points to include when teaching clients and caregivers about vitamin D:

• Consume dietary sources of vitamin D such as fortified milk. Children and pregnant women often require extra dietary vitamin D.

• Take vitamin D exactly as directed because too much may cause toxic levels.

• Report signs of excess vitamin D, such as fatigue, weakness, nausea, vomiting, and changes in colour or amount of urine.

• Exposure to sunlight for 20 minutes a day may supply enough vitamin D to prevent disease.

• Avoid alcohol and other hepatotoxic drugs.

• Report any changes in medications or supplements to the healthcare provider.

46.4 Pharmacotherapy of Osteoporosis

Osteoporosis is the most common metabolic bone disease, affecting about 1.4 million Canadians. This disorder is usually

---

Pr PROTOTYPE DRUG | Calcitriol (Calcijex, Rocaltrol)

ACTIONS AND USES

Calcitriol is the active form of vitamin D, available in both oral and IV formulations. It promotes the intestinal absorption of calcium and elevates serum levels of calcium. This medication is used in cases when clients have impaired kidney function or have hypoparathyroidism. Calcitriol reduces bone resorption and is useful in treating rickets. The effectiveness of calcitriol depends on the client receiving an adequate amount of calcium; therefore, it is usually prescribed in combination with calcium supplements.

PHARMACOKINETICS

Calcitriol has an onset of action of 2 to 6 hours, a peak action in 10 to 12 hours, and a duration of action of 3 to 5 days. It is excreted mainly in feces. Its half-life is 3 to 6 hours.

ADMINISTRATION ALERTS

- Protect capsules from light and heat.
- Withhold calcitriol and calcium supplement and notify the healthcare provider if hypercalcemia develops.
- Calcitriol is pregnancy category C.

ADVERSE EFFECTS AND INTERACTIONS

Common side effects include hypercalcemia, headache, weakness, dry mouth, thirst, increased urination, and muscle or bone pain. Thiazide diuretics may enhance effects of vitamin D, causing hypercalcemia. Too much vitamin D may cause dysrhythmia in clients receiving cardiac glycosides. Magnesium supplements should not be given concurrently due to increased risk of hypermagnesemia.

 See the Companion Website for a Nursing Process Focus chart specific to this drug.

asymptomatic until the bones become brittle enough to fracture or for a vertebra to collapse. In some cases, a lack of dietary calcium and vitamin D contribute to bone deterioration. In other cases, osteoporosis is due to disrupted bone homeostasis. Simply stated, bone resorption outpaces bone deposition, and clients develop weak bones. The following are risk factors for osteoporosis:

- Postmenopause
- Testosterone deficiency
- High alcohol or caffeine consumption
- Inadequate intake of vitamin D or calcium
- Anorexia nervosa
- Tobacco use
- Physical inactivity
- Drugs that lower serum calcium levels, such as some anticonvulsants

The most common risk factor associated with the development of osteoporosis is the onset of menopause. When women reach menopause, estrogen secretion declines and bones become weak and fragile. One theory to explain this occurrence is that normal levels of estrogen may limit the lifespan of osteoclasts, the bone cells that resorb bone. When estrogen levels decrease, osteoclast activity is no longer controlled, and bone demineralization is accelerated, resulting in loss of bone density. In women with osteoporosis, fractures often occur in the hips, wrists, forearms, or spine. The metabolism of calcium in osteoporosis is illustrated in Figure 46.3.

Many drug therapies are available for osteoporosis. These include calcium and vitamin D therapy, estrogen replacement therapy, estrogen receptor modulators, statins, slow-release sodium fluoride, bisphosphonates, and calcitonin. Many of these drug classes are also used for other bone disorders or conditions unrelated to the skeletal system. Select drugs for osteoporosis are listed in Table 46.2.

Hormone Replacement Therapy Until recently, hormone replacement therapy (HRT) with estrogen was one of the most common treatments for osteoporosis in post-

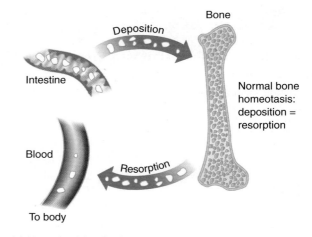

(a) Normal calcium intake

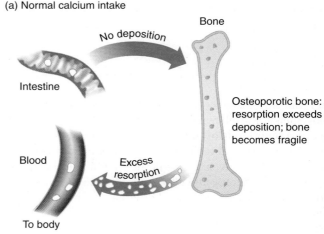

(b) Low calcium intake

● **Figure 46.3** Calcium metabolism in osteoporosis

menopausal women. HRT is very effective at preventing fractures due to osteoporosis. Because of increased risks of uterine cancer, thromboembolic disease, breast cancer, and other chronic disorders associated with estrogen and progesterone in combination, the use of HRT in treating osteoporosis is no longer recommended. Additional information on HRT and the effects of estrogen may be found in Chapter 41.

TABLE 46.2 Bone Resorption Inhibitor Drugs	
Drug	***Route and Adult Dose***
Hormonal Agents	
calcitonin—human (Apo-Calcitonin)	Paget's disease: SC; 0.5 mg qd
calcitonin—salmon (Calciman, Miacalcin)	Hypercalcemia: nasal spray; 200 IU/spray; SC/IM; 4 IU/kg bid, Paget's disease: SC/IM; 100 IU qd
raloxifene hydrochloride (Evista)	PO; 60 mg qd
Bisphosphonates	
alendronate sodium (Fosamax)	Osteoporosis treatment: PO; 10 mg qd; osteoporosis prevention: PO; 5 mg qd; Paget's disease: PO; 40 mg qd for 6 mo
etidronate disodium (Didronel)	PO; 5–10 mg/kg qd for 6 mo or 11–20 mg/kg qd for 3 mo
pamidronate disodium (Aredia)	IV; 15–90 mg in 1000 ml NS or D5W over 4–24 h
risedronate sodium (Actonel)	PO; 30 mg qd at least 30 min before the first drink or meal of the day for 2 mo

Calcitonin **Calcitonin** is a hormone secreted by the thyroid gland in response to elevated serum calcium. As a drug, it is approved for the treatment of osteoporosis in women who are more than 5 years postmenopause. It is available by nasal spray or subcutaneous injection. Calcitonin increases bone density and reduces the risk of vertebral fractures. Side effects are generally minor; the nasal formulation may irritate the nasal mucosa, and allergies are possible. Parenteral forms are rarely used because they may produce nausea and vomiting. In addition to treating osteoporosis, calcitonin is indicated for Paget's disease and hypercalcemia. Because calcitonin is less effective for osteoporosis than other therapies, it is considered a second-line treatment.

Selective Estrogen Receptor Modulators **Selective estrogen receptor modulators (SERMs)** are a relatively new class of drug used in the prevention and treatment of osteoporosis. SERMs bind to estrogen receptors and may be estrogen agonists or antagonists, depending on the specific drug and the tissue involved. For example, raloxifene blocks estrogen receptors in the uterus and breast; thus, it has no estrogen-like proliferative effects on these tissues that might promote cancer. Raloxifene does, however, decrease bone resorption, thus increasing bone density and reducing risk of fractures. Like estrogen, it has a cholesterol-lowering effect. Another SERM, tamoxifen, is used to treat breast cancer (see Chapter 35).

NURSING CONSIDERATIONS

The role of the nurse in drug therapy with hormones and SERMs involves careful monitoring of the client's condition and providing education as it relates to the prescribed drug regimen. The nurse should carefully evaluate and monitor clients taking this class of medication and obtain a thorough health history. The nurse should also obtain a history of medications and a complete physical examination, including liver function studies and a bone scan to determine the progression of the disease and to establish baseline data. Annual checkups and periodic bone density scans should be repeated throughout therapy to determine the effectiveness of the drug. Raloxifene is a pregnancy category X drug and is therefore contraindicated in pregnant clients.

Clients with a known history of thromboembolism or who are pregnant or lactating, taking HRT, or premenopausal should not take these drugs. SERMs should be used carefully when taking the following drugs: clofibrate, diazepam, diazoxide, ibuprofen, indomethacin, and naproxen.

Client education as it relates to SERMs should include goals, reasons for obtaining baseline data, and possible side effects. Following are important points the nurse should include when teaching clients and caregivers about SERMs:

- Report side effects that may indicate thromboembolic disease, especially sudden chest pain, dyspnea, pain in calves, and swelling in the legs.
- Consume supplements of calcium and vitamin D as directed by the healthcare provider.

- Participate in active weight-bearing exercises such as stair climbing or lifting weights.
- Avoid prolonged periods of immobility.
- Take special safety precautions to prevent falling and fractures.
- Discuss the possibility of using a "hip protector" to prevent hip fractures due to accidental falls.

Bisphosphonates The most common drug class for osteoporosis is the **bisphosphonates**. These drugs are structural analogs of pyrophosphate, a natural substance that inhibits bone resorption. Bisphosphonates inhibit bone resorption by suppressing osteoclast activity, thus increasing bone density and reducing the incidence of fractures by about 50%. Adverse effects include GI problems such as nausea, vomiting, abdominal pain, and esophageal irritation. Because these drugs are poorly absorbed, they should be taken on an empty stomach. Recent studies suggest that once-weekly dosing may give the same bone density benefits as daily dosing, due to the extended duration of drug action.

NURSING CONSIDERATIONS

The role of the nurse in bisphosphonate drug therapy involves careful monitoring of the client's condition and providing education as it relates to the prescribed drug treatment. Obtain a thorough history to determine risk factors (especially a history of fractures), GI conditions, and current medications and dietary supplements. Pre-existing vitamin D deficiency or hypocalcemia should be corrected with supplements before initiating bisphosphonate therapy. A complete physical examination should include CBC, pH, chemistry panel, renal and liver function studies, vital signs, and bone density studies such as a dual x-ray absorptiometry (DXA scan) to establish baseline data. Several months of bisphosphonate therapy are required to obtain desired effects.

Pr **PROTOTYPE DRUG** | Raloxifene (Evista)

ACTIONS AND USES

Raloxifene is a selective estrogen receptor modulator (SERM). It decreases bone resorption and increases bone mass and density by acting through the estrogen receptor. Raloxifene is primarily used for the prevention of osteoporosis in postmenopausal women. This drug also reduces serum total cholesterol and LDL (low-density lipoprotein) without lowering HDL (high-density lipoprotein) or triglycerides.

PHARMACOKINETICS

Because raloxifene undergoes extensive first-pass metabolism in the liver, its bioavailability is about 2%. It is eliminated mainly in feces. Its half-life is 28 to 33 hours.

ADMINISTRATION ALERTS

- Drug may be taken with or without food.
- Raloxifene is pregnancy category X.

ADVERSE EFFECTS AND INTERACTIONS

Common side effects are hot flashes, migraine headache, flu-like symptoms, endometrial disorder, breast pain, and vaginal bleeding. Clients should not take cholesterol-lowering drugs or estrogen replacement therapy concurrently with this medication.

Warfarin use may lead to decreased prothrombin time. Decreased raloxifene absorption will result from concurrent use of ampicillin or cholestyramine. Use of raloxifene with other highly protein-bound drugs (e.g., ibuprofen, indomethacin, diazepam) may interfere with binding sites.

 See the Companion Website for a Nursing Process Focus chart specific to this drug.

These drugs are contraindicated in pregnant or lactating clients and clients with colitis and severe renal disease. Bisphosphonates should be used cautiously in children as safety and efficacy in children have not yet been established.

Client education as it relates to bisphosphonates should include goals, reasons for obtaining baseline data, and possible side effects. Following are important points the nurse should include when teaching clients and caregivers about bisphosphonates:

- Immediately report seizures, muscle spasms, facial twitching, and paresthesias.
- Report difficulty urinating, decreased urination, darkened urine, nausea, vomiting, diarrhea, or bone pain.

- Take medication on an empty stomach 2 hours before eating. Take with a full glass of plain water and sit upright for at least 30 minutes after drug is taken to promote proper absorption.
- Consume calcium-rich foods, such as milk and milk products, dark green vegetables, canned fish with bones (such as salmon), and soy beans.
- Report pain, warmth, inflammation, or decreased movement in joints.
- Participate in light exercise and range of motion exercises, as possible.
- Store medication as recommended by the manufacturer and out of reach of children.

Pr **PROTOTYPE DRUG** | Etidronate Disodium (Didronel)

ACTIONS AND USES

Bisphosphonates are a common treatment for postmenopausal osteoporosis. Etidronate is available in oral and IV forms and has the capability of strengthening bones with continued use by slowing bone resorption. Effects begin 1 to 3 months after therapy starts and may continue for months after therapy is stopped. This drug lowers serum alkaline phosphatase, the enzyme associated with bone turnover, without major adverse effects. Etidronate is also used for Paget's disease and to treat hypercalcemia due to malignancy.

PHARMACOKINETICS

Systemic absorption of oral etidronate is about 3%. Of the absorbed etidronate, about 50% is distributed to bone compartments and slowly eliminated. Etidronate is excreted unchanged in urine and feces. Its half-life is 1 to 6 hours.

ADMINISTRATION ALERTS

- Take drug on an empty stomach 2 hours before a meal.
- Etidronate is pregnancy category B (oral) or C (parenteral).

ADVERSE EFFECTS AND INTERACTIONS

Common side effects of etidronate are diarrhea, nausea, vomiting, esophageal irritation, metallic or altered taste perception, hair loss, bone pain, and leg cramps. Pathological fractures may occur if the drug is taken longer than 3 months.

Calcium supplements may decrease absorption of etidronate; therefore, concomitant use should be avoided. Food-drug interactions are common. Milk and other dairy products and medications such as calcium, iron, antacids, and mineral supplements must be reviewed before beginning bisphosphonate therapy because they have the potential to decrease the effectiveness of bisphosphonates.

 See the Companion Website for a Nursing Process Focus chart specific to this drug.

NURSING PROCESS FOCUS   Clients Receiving Bisphosphonates

Assessment	Potential Nursing Diagnoses/Identified Patterns
Prior to administration: ■ Obtain complete health history including allergies, drug history, and possible drug interactions. ■ Assess for presence/history of pathologic fractures, hypocalcemia, and hypercalcemia. ■ Assess nutritional status. ■ Obtain lab work, including CBC, pH, electrolytes, renal function studies (BUN, creatinine, uric acid), and serum calcium and phosphorous.	■ Need for knowledge regarding to drug therapy ■ Risk for fluid imbalance ■ Risk for fractures ■ Nausea related to side effects of drug ■ Bone pain related to adverse drug reaction ■ Reduced adherence because therapeutic response may take 1–3 months

Planning: Client Goals and Expected Outcomes

The client will:
- Demonstrate decreased progression of osteoporosis or Paget's disease
- Demonstrate decreased risk for pathologic fractures
- Remain free of side effects or adverse reactions
- Demonstrate understanding of dietary needs/modifications
- Maintain adequate fluid volume

Implementation

Interventions (Rationales)	Client Education/Discharge Planning
■ Monitor for pathologic fractures and bone pain. (Drug may cause defective mineralization of newly formed bone.) ■ Monitor for GI side effects. (There may be problems with absorption if client has persistent nausea or diarrhea.) ■ Monitor calcium lab values: serum calcium levels should be 2.05–2.55 mmol/L. (Through inhibition of bone resorption, drug causes blood levels of calcium to fall.)	■ Instruct client to report any sudden bone or joint pain, inability to correctly position self, swelling over bone or joint. ■ Advise client that new-onset nausea or diarrhea may be a symptom of adverse reaction and to report immediately. Advise client to: ■ Have lab studies performed prior to beginning bisphosphonate therapy and periodically during therapy ■ Report symptoms of hypocalcemia (muscle spasms, facial grimacing, convulsions, irritability, depression, psychoses) ■ Report symptoms of hypercalcemia (increased bone pain, anorexia, nausea/vomiting, constipation, thirst, lethargy, fatigue, confusion, depression)
■ Monitor kidney function, especially creatinine level. (Etidronate cannot be used in clients whose creatinine is > 5.) ■ Monitor BUN, vitamin D, urinalysis, and serum phosphate and magnesium levels.	■ Instruct client to report any urinary changes, such as decreased urine production, increased urination.
■ Monitor dietary habits. (Diet must have adequate amounts of vitamin D, calcium, and phosphate.) ■ Monitor adherence with recommended regimen. (Client may discontinue drug due to apparent lack of response.)	■ Advise client to include good food sources of vitamin D, calcium, and phosphate, including dairy products and green leafy vegetables. Advise client: ■ That therapy should continue for 6 months maximum, but full therapeutic response may take 1–3 months ■ That effects continue several months after drug is discontinued ■ To avoid vitamins, mineral supplements, antacids, and high-calcium products within 2 hours of taking bisphosphonates

Evaluation of Outcome Criteria

Evaluate the effectiveness of drug therapy by confirming that client goals and expected outcomes have been met (see "Planning").

See Table 46.2 (page 660), under "Bisphosphonates," for a list of drugs to which these nursing actions apply.

46.5 Pharmacotherapy of Paget's Disease

Paget's disease, or osteitis deformans, is a chronic, progressive condition characterized by enlarged and abnormal bones. With this disorder, the processes of bone resorption and bone formation occur at a high rate. Excessive bone turnover causes the new bone to be weak and brittle; deformity and fractures may result. The client may be asymptomatic or have only vague, non-specific complaints for many years. Symptoms include pain of the hips and femurs, joint inflammation, headaches, facial pain, and hearing loss if bones around the ear cavity are affected. Nerves along the spinal column may be pinched due to compression between the vertebrae.

Paget's disease is sometimes confused with osteoporosis because some of the symptoms are similar. In fact, medical treatments for osteoporosis are similar to those for Paget's disease. The cause of Paget's disease, however, is quite different. The enzyme alkaline phosphatase is elevated in the blood because of the extensive bone turnover, and the disease is usually confirmed by early detection of this enzyme in the blood. Calcium is also liberated because of its close association with phosphate. If diagnosed early enough, symptoms can be treated successfully. If the diagnosis is made late in the progress of the disease, permanent skeletal abnormalities may develop, and other disorders may appear, including arthritis, kidney stones, and heart disease.

Bisphosphonates are drugs of choice for the pharmacotherapy of Paget's disease. Therapy is usually cyclic, with bisphosphonates administered until serum alkaline phosphatase levels return to normal, followed by several months without the drugs. When serum alkaline phosphatase becomes elevated, therapy is begun again. The pharmacological goals are to slow the rate of bone reabsorption and encourage the deposition of strong bone. Calcitonin nasal spray is used as an option for clients who cannot tolerate bisphosphonates. Surgery may be indicated in cases of severe bone deformity, degenerative arthritis, or fracture. Clients with Paget's disease should maintain adequate intake of calcium and vitamin D on a daily basis.

JOINT DISORDERS

Joint conditions such as osteoarthritis, rheumatoid arthritis, and gout are frequent indications for pharmacotherapy. **Osteoarthritis (OA)** is a degenerative, age-onset disease characterized by wearing away of cartilage at articular joint surfaces. **Rheumatoid arthritis (RA)** is a systemic, autoimmune disorder characterized by disfigurement and inflammation of multiple joints that occurs at an earlier age than osteoarthritis. **Gout** is a metabolic disorder that is a form of acute arthritis characterized by joint pain caused by the accumulation of uric acid in the bloodstream or joint cavities. Because joint pain is common to all three disorders, analgesics and anti-inflammatory drugs are important com-

NATURAL THERAPIES

Glucosamine and Chondroitin for Osteoarthritis

Glucosamine sulfate and chondroitin sulfate are available individually or in combination as OTC natural health products used for osteoarthritis. Glucosamine is a natural substance that is an important building block of cartilage. With aging, glucosamine is lost with the natural thinning of cartilage. As cartilage wears down, joints lose their normal cushioning ability, resulting in the pain and inflammation of osteoarthritis. Some studies have shown glucosamine sulfate to be more effective than a placebo in reducing mild arthritis and joint pain. It is purported to promote cartilage repair in the joints. Chondroitin sulfate is also purported to promote cartilage repair. It is a natural substance that forms part of the matrix between cartilage cells. These products are considered relatively safe with few side effects. Recent research suggests that glucosamine combined with chondroitin may be effective only for moderate to severe OA pain (Clegg et al., 2006). More research regarding efficacy is needed.

ponents of pharmacotherapy. A few additional drugs are specific to the particular joint pathology.

46.6 Pharmacotherapy of Arthritis

Arthritis is a general term meaning inflammation of a joint. There are several types of arthritis, each having somewhat different characteristics based on the etiology. Osteoarthritis (OA), the most common type, is due to wear and tear of the cartilage of weight-bearing joints, including knees, hips, and spine. Symptoms of OA include localized pain and stiffness, joint and bone enlargement, and limitations in movement. OA is not accompanied by the degree of inflammation associated with other forms of arthritis. Many consider OA to be a normal part of the aging process. The hand of a client with OA is shown in Figure 46.4.

The goals of pharmacotherapy for OA include reduction of pain and inflammation. Topical medications (capsaicin cream and balms), NSAIDs (including ASA, acetaminophen,

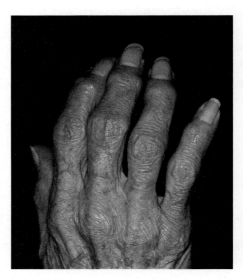

● **Figure 46.4** The hand of a client with osteoarthritis

and COX-2 inhibitors), and tramadol are of value for treatment of pain associated with OA. Celecoxib (Celebrex) is presently the only COX-2 inhibitor approved by Health Canada because of the cardiovascular risk of this drug class. In acute cases, intra-articular glucocorticoids may be used on a temporary basis. Although these drugs help to relieve symptoms, they do not cure the disorder. The actions of NSAIDs are described in Chapter 31.

A newer type of drug therapy for clients with moderate OA who do not respond adequately to analgesics is sodium hyaluronate, a chemical normally found in high amounts within synovial fluid. Sodium hyaluronate is injected directly into the knee joint to replace the body's natural hyaluronic acid that deteriorated due to the inflammation of osteoarthritis. Treatment consists of one injection per week for 3 to 5 weeks. By coating the articulating cartilage surface, sodium hyaluronate helps to provide a barrier, thus preventing friction and further inflammation of the joint. Information given to the client prior to administration should include side effects, such as pain and/or swelling at the injection site, and the advice to avoid any strenuous activity for approximately 48 hours after injection.

Rheumatoid arthritis (RA), the second most common form of arthritis, occurs at an earlier age than OA and has an autoimmune etiology. In RA, **auto-antibodies** called *rheumatoid factors* activate complement and draw leukocytes into the area, where they attack normal cells. This results in persistent injury and the formation of inflammatory fluid within the joints. Joint capsules, tendons, ligaments, and skeletal muscles may also be affected. Unlike OA, which causes local pain in affected joints, clients with RA may develop systemic manifestations that include infections, pulmonary disease, pericarditis, abnormal numbers of blood cells, and symptoms of metabolic dysfunction such as fatigue, anorexia, and weakness. The hands of a client with RA are shown in Figure 46.5.

Pharmacotherapy for relief of RA symptoms includes the same classes of analgesics and anti-inflammatory drugs used for OA. Glucocorticoids may be used for acute RA flare-ups because of their potent anti-inflammatory action.

Disease-modifying antirheumatic drugs (DMARDs) may be used to slow the progression of RA. DMARDs include drugs from several classes. Research has shown that hydroxychloroquine, sulfasalazine, and methotrexate may reduce

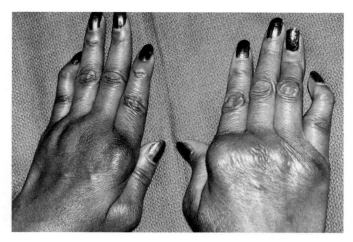

● **Figure 46.5** The hands of a client with rheumatoid arthritis
Source: Courtesy of Dr. Jason L. Smith.

mortality when therapy is started early in the course of the disease. D-penicillamine, gold salts, and immunosuppressants such as leflunomide, azathioprine, cyclosporine, and cyclophosphamide may also be used, although they may produce more toxic effects. Newer agents that inhibit the inflammatory process and produce more tolerable side effects include etanercept, infliximab, and anakinra. Several months may be required before maximum therapeutic effects are achieved. Because many of these drugs can be toxic, clients should be closely monitored. Adverse effects vary depending on the type of drug. These agents are shown in Table 46.3.

Non-pharmacological therapies for relief of arthritic pain are common. The use of non-impact and passive range of motion (ROM) exercises to maintain flexibility along with rest is encouraged. Splinting may help keep joints positioned correctly and relieve pain. Other therapies commonly used to relieve pain and discomfort include thermal therapies, meditation, visualization, distraction techniques, and massage therapy. Knowledge of proper body mechanics and posturing may offer some benefit. Physical and occupational therapists are usually active in helping clients minimize pain through these approaches. Surgical techniques such as joint replacement and reconstructive surgery may become necessary when other methods are ineffective.

TABLE 46.3 Disease-Modifying Drugs for Rheumatoid Arthritis	
Drug	*Route and Adult Dose*
azathioprine (Imuran, Apo-, Gen-, Novo-Azathioprine)	PO; 0.5–1.0 mg/kg/d (max 2.5 mg/kg/d)
gold sodium thiomalate (Myochrysine)	IM; 10 mg wk 1, 25 mg wk 2, then 25–50 mg/wk to a cumulative dose of 1 g
hydroxychloroquine sulfate (Gen-Hydroxychloroquine)	PO; 200–600 mg qd
leflunomide (Apo-, Novo-Leflunomide)	PO; loading dose 100 mg/d for 3 d; maintenance dose 10–20 mg qd
methotrexate (Methotrexate, Apo-, PMS-Methotrexate) (see page 487 for the Prototype Drug box)	PO; 2.5–5 mg q12h for three doses each week or 7.5 mg once/wk
sulfasalazine (Apo-Sulfasalazine)	PO; 1–2 g/d in 4 divided doses (max: 8 g/d)

Pr PROTOTYPE DRUG | Hydroxychloroquine Sulfate (Gen-Hydroxychloroquine)

ACTIONS AND USES

Hydroxychloroquine is prescribed for rheumatoid arthritis and systemic lupus erythematosus in clients who have not responded well to other anti-inflammatory drugs. This agent relieves the severe inflammation characteristic of these disorders. For full effectiveness, hydroxychloroquine is most often prescribed with salicylates and glucocorticoids. This drug is also used for the prophylaxis and treatment of malaria (see Chapter 33).

PHARMACOKINETICS

Hydroxychloroquine is mainly metabolized in the liver. About 25% is excreted unchanged in urine. Its half-life is 32 to 50 days.

ADMINISTRATION ALERTS

- Take drug at the same time every day.
- Administer with milk to decrease GI upset.
- Store drug in a safe place as it is very toxic to children.
- Hydroxychloroquine is pregnancy category C.

ADVERSE EFFECTS AND INTERACTIONS

Adverse symptoms include blurred vision, dizziness, itchiness, GI disturbances, loss of hair, headache, and mood and mental changes. Hydroxychloroquine has possible ocular effects that include blurred vision, photophobia, diminished ability to read, and blacked out areas in the visual field.

Antacids with aluminum and magnesium may prevent absorption. This drug interferes with the client's response to rabies vaccine. Hydroxychloroquine may increase the risk of liver toxicity when administered with hepatotoxic drugs; alcohol use should be eliminated during therapy. It also may lead to increased digoxin levels.

See the Companion Website for a Nursing Process Focus chart specific to this drug.

46.7 Pharmacotherapy of Gout

Gout is due to an accumulation of uric acid crystals that occurs from increased metabolism of DNA or RNA or from the reduced excretion of uric acid by the kidneys. Uric acid is the final breakdown product of DNA and RNA metabolism. One metabolic step that is important to the pharmacotherapy of this disease is the conversion of hypoxanthine to uric acid by the enzyme xanthine oxidase. An elevated blood level of uric acid is called hyperuricemia.

Gout may be classified as primary or secondary. Primary gout, caused by genetic errors in uric acid metabolism, is most commonly observed in Pacific Islanders. Secondary gout is caused by diseases or drugs that increase the metabolic turnover of nucleic acids or that interfere with uric acid excretion. Examples of drugs that may cause gout include thiazide diuretics, ASA, cyclosporine, and alcohol (when ingested on a chronic basis). Conditions that can cause secondary gout include diabetic ketoacidosis, kidney failure, and diseases associated with rapid cell turnover, such as leukemia, hemolytic anemia, and polycythemia.

Acute gouty arthritis occurs when needle-shaped uric acid crystals accumulate in joints, resulting in red, swollen, and inflamed tissue. Attacks have a sudden onset, often occur at night, and may be triggered by diet, injury, or other stresses. Gouty arthritis most often occurs in the big toes, heels, ankles, wrists, fingers, knees, and elbows. Of the clients with gout, 90% are men.

The goals of gout pharmacotherapy are twofold: termination of acute attacks and prevention of future attacks. NSAIDs are the drugs of choice for treating the pain and inflammation of acute attacks. Indomethacin is an NSAID that has been widely used for acute gout, although a COX-2 inhibitor may also be prescribed.

Prophylaxis of gout includes avoidance of foods and drugs that increase uric acid accumulation and worsen gout, and treatment with antigout medications. Clients should avoid high-purine foods such as meat, legumes, alcoholic beverages, mushrooms, and oatmeal because nucleic acids will be formed when they are metabolized. Prophylaxis therapy includes drugs that lower serum uric acid. Sulfinpyrazone is a uricosuric drug that increases the excretion of uric acid by blocking its reabsorption in the

TABLE 46.4 Uric Acid-Inhibiting Drugs for Gout and Gouty Arthritis	
Drug	*Route and Adult Dose*
allopurinol (Apo-Allopurinol)	PO (primary); 100 mg qd; may increase by 100 mg/wk (max 800 mg/day) PO (secondary); 200–800 mg qd for 2–3 d or longer
colchicine	PO; 0.5–1.2 mg followed by 0.5–0.6 mg q1–2h until pain relief (max 4 mg/attack)
probenecid (Benemid, Probalan)	PO; 250 mg bid for 1 wk; then 500 mg bid (max 3 g/d)
sulfinpyrazone (Apo-, Nu-Sulfinpyrazone)	PO; 100–200 mg bid for 1 wk; then increase to 200–400 mg bid

Pr PROTOTYPE DRUG | Colchicine

ACTIONS AND USES

Colchicine is a natural product obtained from the autumn crocus, which is found in Canada and the United States. Colchicine reduces inflammation associated with gouty arthritis by inhibiting the synthesis of microtubules, which are subcellular structures responsible for helping white blood cells infiltrate an area. Although colchicine has no analgesic properties, the reduction in inflammation may lead to pain reduction. Colchicine may be taken to prevent or treat acute gout, sometimes in combination with other uric acid–inhibiting agents.

PHARMACOKINETICS

Colchicine has an unknown onset and peaks in 0.5 to 2 hours. Its half-life is 20 minutes.

ADMINISTRATION ALERTS

- Take drug on an empty stomach, when symptoms first appear.
- Colchicine is pregnancy category C. Parenteral doses must not be given to pregnant women.

ADVERSE EFFECTS AND INTERACTIONS

Side effects such as nausea, vomiting, diarrhea, and GI upset are more likely to occur at the beginning of therapy. These side effects are related to disruption of microtubules responsible for cell proliferation. Colchicine may also directly interfere with the absorption of vitamin B_{12}.

Colchicine interacts with many drugs. For example, NSAIDs may increase GI symptoms, and cyclosporine may increase bone marrow suppression. Erythromycin may increase colchicine levels. Phenylbutazone may increase the risk for blood dyscrasias. Loop diuretics may decrease colchicine effects. Alcohol and products that contain alcohol may cause skin rashes and increase liver damage. Effects of CNS depressants may be increased.

kidney. Allopurinol blocks xanthine oxidase, thus inhibiting the formation of uric acid. Prophylactic therapy is used for clients who suffer frequent and acute gout attacks. Drugs for gout are shown in Table 46.4.

The uric acid inhibitors such as colchicine, sulfinpyrazone, and allopurinol are also used for acute gout. Uric acid inhibitors block the accumulation of uric acid within the blood or of uric acid crystals within the joints. When uric acid accumulation is blocked, symptoms associated with gout diminish. About 80% of the clients using uric acid inhibitors experience GI complaints such as abdominal cramping, nausea, vomiting, and/or diarrhea. These agents are summarized in Table 46.4. Glucocorticoids are useful for the short-term therapy of acute gout, particularly when the symptoms are in a single joint and the medication is delivered intra-articularly.

NURSING CONSIDERATIONS

The role of the nurse in drug therapy with antigout agents involves careful monitoring of the client's condition and providing education as it relates to the prescribed drug regimen. The nurse should carefully evaluate and monitor clients taking this class of drug and obtain a thorough health history. The nurse should obtain a drug history and a complete physical examination, including the following lab studies: CBC, platelets, liver and renal function studies, uric acid levels, and urinalysis. Vital signs should also be taken to establish baseline data. These tests should be repeated

throughout the treatment to assess the effectiveness of the drug.

Clients with known hypersensitivity, pregnancy, or severe GI, renal, hepatic, or cardiac disease should not take antigout agents. These drugs should be used carefully in children and cautiously in clients who have blood dyscrasias or mild liver disease.

Client education as it relates to antigout drugs should include goals, reasons for obtaining baseline data, and possible side effects. Following are important points the nurse should include when teaching clients and caregivers regarding antigout agents:

- Take the medication exactly as ordered.
- Report side effects such as rash, headache, anorexia, lower back pain, pain on urination, hematuria, and decrease in urinary output to the healthcare provider.
- Increase fluid intake to 3 to 4 L/day.
- Decrease or eliminate alcohol consumption; alcohol increases uric acid levels.
- Limit foods that will cause the urine to be more alkaline, such as milk, fruits, carbonated drinks, most vegetables, molasses, and baking soda, in order to decrease the chance of stone formation.
- Avoid taking ASA and large doses of vitamin C; they enhance stone formation.
- Use effective birth control during drug therapy and notify the healthcare provider of any suspicion of pregnancy.

NURSING PROCESS FOCUS Clients Receiving Colchicine

Assessment	Potential Nursing Diagnoses/Identified Patterns
Prior to administration: ■ Obtain complete health history including allergies, drug history, and possible drug interactions. ■ Obtain baseline vital signs. ■ Obtain lab work, including CBC, platelets, uric acid levels, renal and liver function tests, and urinalysis.	■ Need for knowledge regarding drug therapy ■ Activity intolerance related to joint pain ■ Altered body image related to joint swelling

Planning: Client Goals and Expected Outcomes

The client will:
■ Report a decrease in pain and an increase in function of affected joints
■ Demonstrate an understanding of the drug's action by accurately describing drug side effects and precautions and measures to take to decrease any side effects
■ Report side effects and adverse reactions

Implementation

Interventions (Rationales)	Client Education/Discharge Planning
■ Monitor lab results throughout therapy. (Agranulocytosis and thrombocytopenia may occur.) Perform Coombs test for hemolytic anemia. ■ Monitor for signs of toxicity. ■ Monitor for signs of renal impairment such as oliguria. Record intake and output. ■ Ensure that medication is administered correctly. ■ Monitor for pain and mobility. (This is used to assess effectiveness of medication.)	■ Teach client importance of routine lab studies, so deviations from normal can be corrected immediately. ■ Instruct client to report weakness, abdominal pain, nausea, and/or diarrhea. ■ Instruct client to report a decrease in urinary output and to increase fluid intake to 3–4 L/day. ■ Inform client to take medication on an empty stomach. Medication should be taken at first sign of gout attack. ■ Inform client to report an increase or decrease in discomfort and swelling.

Evaluation of Outcome Criteria

Evaluate the effectiveness of drug therapy by confirming that client goals and expected outcomes have been met (see "Planning").

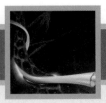

CHAPTER REVIEW

KEY CONCEPTS

The numbered key concepts provide a succinct summary of the important points from the corresponding numbered section within the chapter. If any of these points are not clear, refer to the numbered section within the chapter for review. Expanded versions can be found on the Companion Website.

46.1 Adequate levels of calcium in the body are necessary to properly transmit nerve impulses, to prevent muscle spasms, and to provide stability and movement. Adequate levels of vitamin D, parathyroid hormone, and calcitonin are also necessary for these functions.

46.2 Hypocalcemia is a serious condition that requires immediate therapy with calcium supplements, often concurrently with vitamin D.

46.3 Pharmacotherapy of osteomalacia (softening of bones) includes calcium and vitamin D supplements.

46.4 Pharmacotherapy of osteoporosis includes bisphosphonates, estrogen modulator drugs, and calcitonin.

46.5 Pharmacotherapy of clients with Paget's disease includes bisphosphonates and calcitonin.

46.6 For osteoarthritis, the main drug therapy is pain medication that includes NSAIDs (ASA, acetaminophen, COX-2 inhibitors) or stronger analgesics. Drug therapy for rheumatoid arthritis may include NSAIDs, glucocorticoids, immunosuppressants, and disease-modifying drugs.

46.7 Gout is characterized by a buildup of uric acid in either the blood or the joint cavities. Drug therapy includes agents that inhibit uric acid buildup or enhance its excretion.

REVIEW QUESTIONS

1 Give examples of how unusually low or high levels of blood calcium affect normal body functioning.

2 What are the major drug therapies used for osteoporosis?

3 Identify the two major types of arthritis. What are the differences between the pharmacotherapy of these disorders?

4 What are the differences in pharmacotherapy between gouty arthritis and other arthritic disorders?

CRITICAL THINKING QUESTIONS

1. A young woman calls the triage nurse in her healthcare provider's office with questions concerning her mother's medication. The mother, age 76, has been taking alendronate (Fosamax) after a bone density study revealed a decrease in bone mass. The daughter is worried that her mother may not be taking the drug correctly. She asks for information to make sure that her mother is taking the drug correctly to minimize any chance of side effects. What information should the triage nurse incorporate in a teaching plan regarding the oral administration of alendronate?

2. A community health nurse has decided to discuss the benefits of oral calcium supplements with an 82-year-old female client. The client had a stroke 6 years ago and requires help with most activities of daily living. She rarely leaves home since her husband died 18 months ago and has lost 12 kg because she "just can't get interested" in her meals. She refuses to drink milk. What considerations must the nurse make before recommending calcium supplementation?

3. A 36-year-old man comes to the emergency department complaining of severe pain in the joint of his right big toe. The triage nurse inspects the toe and notes that the joint is red, swollen, and extremely tender. Recognizing this as a typical presentation for acute gouty arthritis, what assessment data should the nurse obtain relevant to this disease process and its pharmacological treatment?

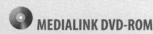

EXPLORE
MediaLink

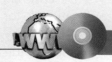 www.pearsoned.ca/adams-king

 MEDIALINK DVD-ROM
- **Audio Glossary**
- **CRNE Review**
- **Videos**
  Arthritis
  Osteoporosis
- **Animation**
  Mechanism of Action: Calcitriol

COMPANION WEBSITE
- **CRNE Review**
- **Case Study:** Drug therapy for rheumatoid arthritis
- **Dosage Calculations**

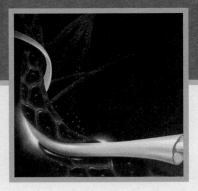

CHAPTER 47

Drugs for Skin Disorders

DRUGS AT A GLANCE

ANTI-INFECTIVES
Antibacterials, antifungals, and antivirals

ANTIPARASITICS
Scabicides
  lindane (Hexit)
Pediculicides

DRUGS FOR SUNBURN AND OTHER MINOR BURNS
Local anesthetics
  lidocaine (Solarcaine, others)

DRUGS FOR ACNE AND ROSACEA
Benzoyl peroxide
Retinoids
  isotretinoin (Accutane)
Antibiotics
Other agents

DRUGS FOR DERMATITIS
Topical glucocorticoids

DRUGS FOR PSORIASIS
Topical glucocorticoids
Topical immunomodulators
Systemic agents

OBJECTIVES

After reading this chapter, the student should be able to do the following:

1. Identify drug classes used for treating skin disorders.
2. Explain the therapeutic action of drug therapies used for bacterial, fungal, or viral infections; mite and lice infestations; sunburn; acne vulgaris; rosacea; dermatitis; and psoriasis in relation to the pathophysiology of the disorders.
3. Describe the nurse's role in the pharmacological management of clients receiving drugs for skin disorders.
4. For each of the drug classes listed in Drugs at a Glance, identify a representative drug and explain its mechanism of action, therapeutic effects, and important adverse effects.
5. Describe and explain, based on pharmacological principles, the rationale for nursing assessment, planning, and interventions for clients receiving drug therapy for skin disorders.
6. Use the nursing process to care for clients receiving drug therapy for skin disorders.

MediaLink

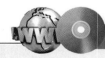

www.pearsoned.ca/adams-king

CRNE review, case studies, and other interactive resources for this chapter can be found on the Companion Website at **www.pearsoned.ca/adams-king**. Click on "Chapter 47" to select the activities for this chapter. For animations, more CRNE review questions, and an audio glossary, access the accompanying DVD-ROM in this textbook.

The integumentary system consists of the skin, hair, nails, sweat glands, and oil glands. The largest and most visible of all organs, the skin normally provides an effective barrier between the outside environment and the body's internal organs. At times, however, external conditions become too extreme or conditions within the body change, resulting in unhealthy skin. When this occurs, pharmacotherapy may be utilized to improve the skin's condition. This chapter examines pharmacotherapy for a broad scope of skin disorders.

47.1 Structure and Function of the Skin

To understand the actions of drugs used for skin disorders, it is necessary to have a thorough understanding of skin structure. The skin is composed of three primary layers: the epidermis, dermis, and subcutaneous layer. The epidermis is the visible, outermost layer that comprises only about 5% of the skin depth. The middle layer is the dermis, or cutis, which comprises about 95% of the entire skin thickness. The subcutaneous layer lies beneath the dermis. The subcutaneous layer is sometimes considered to be separate from the skin and not one of its layers.

Each layer of skin is distinct in form and function. Drugs to treat the skin may be injected or topically applied (see Chapter 8). The epidermis has either four or five sublayers, depending on its location on the body. From the innermost to outermost, the five layers of skin are as follows: stratum basale (also referred to as the stratum germinativum), stratum spinosum, stratum granulosum, stratum lucidum, and the strongest layer, stratum corneum. The stratum corneum is referred to as the horny layer because of the abundance of the protein keratin. Keratin is also found in the hair, hooves, and horns of many mammals. Keratin forms a barrier to repel bacteria and foreign matter, and most substances cannot penetrate it. The largest amount of keratin is found in those areas subject to mechanical stress, for example, the soles of the feet and the palms of the hands.

The innermost sublayer of the epidermis, the stratum basale, continuously supplies the epidermis with new cells as older superficial cells are damaged or lost through normal sloughing. Over their lifetime, these newly created cells migrate from the stratum basale to the outermost layers of the skin. As these cells are pushed to the surface, they are flattened and covered with a water-insoluble material that forms a protective seal. The average time it takes for a cell to move from the stratum basale to the body surface is about 3 weeks. Specialized cells within the deeper layers of the epidermis, called melanocytes, secrete the dark pigment melanin, which offers a degree of protection from the sun's ultraviolet rays. The number and type of melanocytes determine the pigment of the skin. The more melanin, the darker the skin colour. In areas where the melanocytes are destroyed, there are milk-white areas of de-pigmented skin referred to as **vitiligo.**

The second primary layer of skin, the dermis, consists of dense, irregular connective tissue. The dermis provides a foundation for the epidermis and accessory structures such as hair and nails. Most receptor nerve endings, oil glands, sweat glands, and blood vessels are found within the dermis.

Beneath the dermis is the subcutaneous layer, or hypodermis, that consists mainly of adipose tissue that cushions, insulates, and provides a source of energy for the body. The amount of subcutaneous tissue varies in an individual and is determined by nutritional status, age, and heredity.

47.2 Causes of Skin Disorders

Of the various skin disorders, some have vague, generalized signs and symptoms and others have specific and easily identifiable causes. **Pruritus**, or itching, is a general condition associated with dry, scaly skin, or it may be a symptom of mite or lice infestation. Inflammation, a characteristic of burns and other traumatic disorders, occurs when damage to the skin is extensive. Local **erythema**, or redness, accompanies inflammation and many other skin disorders. Trauma to deeper tissues may cause additional symptoms such as bleeding, bruises, and infections.

Skin disorders may be grouped into three general categories: infectious, inflammatory, and neoplastic. A summary of these disorders is given in Table 47.1. Bacterial, fungal, viral, and parasitic infections of the skin are relatively common and are frequent targets of anti-infective pharmacotherapy. Inflammatory disorders encompass a broad range of pathology that includes acne, burns, eczema, dermatitis, and psoriasis. Pharmacotherapy of inflammatory skin disorders includes many of the agents discussed in Chapter 31, such as glucocorticoids. Neoplastic disease includes malignant melanoma and basal cell carcinoma, which are treated with the therapies described in Chapter 35.

Not all skin disorders are localized to the skin. Skin disorders may indicate the presence of underlying systemic conditions associated with other organ systems. If skin conditions are noted, a complete history and physical assessment is needed to identify potential systemic causes such as liver or renal impairment, primary or metastatic tumours, recent injury, or poor nutritional status. During client assessment, the nurse must observe for skin abnormalities, including the colour, size, type, and character of any lesions. Skin turgor and moisture are examined for signs of possible dehydration. The relationship between the integumentary system and other body systems is depicted in Figure 47.1. Common symptoms associated with a range of conditions are shown in Table 47.2.

Although there are many skin disorders, some warrant only localized or short-term pharmacotherapy. Examples include lice infestation, sunburn with minor irritation, and acne. Eczema, dermatitis, and psoriasis are more serious disorders requiring extensive and sometimes prolonged therapy.

SKIN INFECTIONS

Normally, the skin has a diverse population of microorganisms and flora that includes viruses, fungi, and bacteria. Intact skin provides an effective barrier against infection from these organisms. The skin is very dry, and keratin is a poor energy source for microbes. Although perspiration often provides a moist environment, its high salt content discourages microbial growth. Furthermore, the outer layer is continually being sloughed off, and the microorganisms go with it.

47.3 Pharmacotherapy of Bacterial, Fungal, and Viral Skin Infections

Bacterial skin diseases can occur when the skin is punctured or cut or when the outer layer is abraded through trauma or removed through severe burns. Some bacteria also infect hair follicles. The two most common bacterial infections of the skin are caused by *Staphylococcus* and *Streptococcus*, which are normal skin inhabitants. *S. aureus* is responsible for furuncles, carbuncles, and abscesses of the skin. Both *S. aureus* and *S. pyogenes* can cause impetigo, a skin disorder commonly occurring in school-aged children.

Although many skin bacterial infections are self-limiting, others may be serious enough to require pharmacotherapy.

TABLE 47.1	Classification of Skin Disorders	
Type	**Examples**
infectious	bacterial infections such as boils, impetigo, infected hair follicles; fungal infections such as ringworm, athlete's foot, jock itch, nail infection; parasitic infections such as mosquito bites, ticks, mites, lice; viral infections such as cold sores, fever blisters (herpes simplex), chicken pox, warts, shingles (herpes zoster), measles (rubeola), and German measles (rubella)
inflammatory	injury and exposure to the sun such as sunburn and other environmental stresses; disorders marked by a combination of overactive glands, increased hormone production, and/or infection such as acne, blackheads, whiteheads, rosacea; disorders marked by itching, cracking, and discomfort such as eczema (atopic dermatitis), other forms of dermatitis (contact dermatitis, seborrheic dermatitis, stasis dermatitis), and psoriasis
neoplastic	several types of skin cancer: squamous cell carcinoma, basal cell carcinoma, and malignant melanoma; malignant melanoma is the most dangerous; benign neoplasms include keratosis and keratoacanthoma

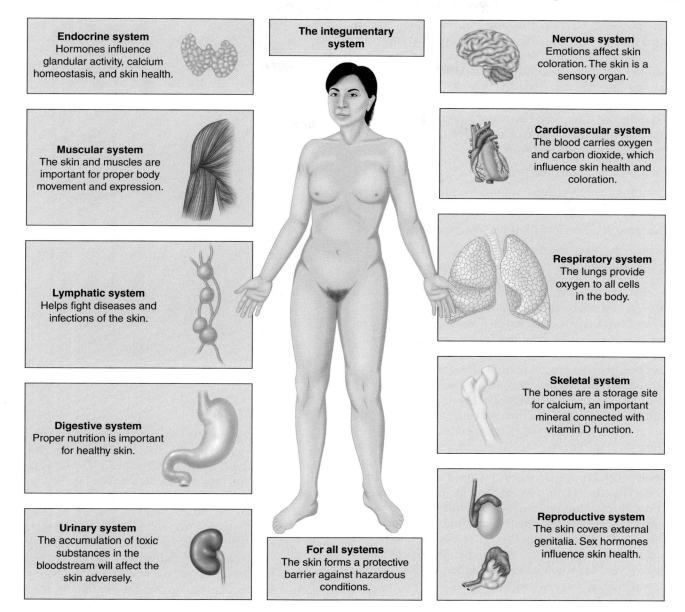

● **Figure 47.1** Interrelationships of the integumentary system with other body systems

TABLE 47.2	Signs and Symptoms Associated with Changing Health, Age, or Weakened Immune System
Sign	**Description**
discoloration of the skin	Discoloration is often a sign of an underlying medical disorder (for example, anemia, cyanoisis, fever, jaundice, and Addison's disease); some medications have photosensitive properties, making the skin sensitive to the sun and causing erythema.
delicate skin, wrinkles, and hair loss	Many degenerative changes occur in the skin; some are found in elderly patients; others are genetically related (fragile epidermis, wrinkles, reduced activity of oil and sweat glands, male pattern baldness, poor blood circulation); hair loss may also be linked to medical procedures, for example, radiation and chemotherapy.
seborrhea/oily skin and bumps	This condition is usually associated with younger patients; examples include cradle cap in infants and an oily face, chest, arms, and back in teenagers and young adults; pustules, cysts, papules, and nodules represent lesions connected with oily skin.
scales, patches, and itchy areas	Some symptoms may be related to a combination of genetics, stress, and immunity; other symptoms are due to a fast turnover of skin cells; some symptoms develop for unknown reasons.
warts, skin marks, and moles	Some skin marks are congenital; others are acquired or may be linked to environmental factors.
tumours	Tumours may be genetic or may occur because of exposure to harmful agents or conditions.

When possible, pharmacotherapy utilizes topical agents applied directly to the site of infection. Topical agents offer the advantage of causing fewer side effects, and many are available OTC for self-treatment. If the infection is deep within the skin, affects large regions of the body, or has the potential to become systemic, then oral or parenteral therapy is indicated. Chapter 32 provides a complete discussion of antibiotic therapy. Some of the more common topical antibiotics include the following:

- Bacitracin ointment (Baciguent)
- Chloramphenicol cream (Chloromycetin)
- Erythromycin ointment (EryDerm, others)
- Gentamicin cream and ointment (Garamycin)
- Neomycin cream and ointment (Myciguent)
- Tetracycline (Topicycline)

Fungal infections of the skin or nails commonly occur in dark areas covered by clothing, such as tinea pedis (athlete's foot) and tinea cruris (jock itch). Tinea capitis (ringworm of the scalp) and tinea unguium (onycholysis of the nails) are also common. These pathogens generally are responsive to therapy with topical antifungal agents. More serious fungal infections of the skin and mucous membranes, such as *Candida albicans* infections that occur in immunocompromised clients, require systemic antifungals (see Chapter 33).

Some viral infections of the skin are considered diseases of childhood and are usually self-limiting. These include varicella (chicken pox), rubeola (measles), and rubella (German measles). Treatment of these infections is directed at controlling symptoms such as pruritus and preventing spread and scarring from skin lesions. Viral infections of the skin in adults include herpes zoster (shingles) and herpes simplex (cold sores and genital lesions). Pharmacotherapy of severe viral skin lesions may include antiviral therapy with acyclovir, as discussed in Chapter 34.

SKIN PARASITES

Common skin parasites include mites and lice. Scabies is an eruption of the skin caused by the female mite *Sarcoptes scabiei,* which burrows into the skin to lay eggs that hatch after about 5 days. Scabies mites are barely visible without magnification and are smaller than lice. Scabies lesions most commonly occur between the fingers, on the extremities, in the axillary and gluteal folds, around the trunk, and in the pubic area, as shown in Figure 47.2. The major symptom is intense itching; vigorous scratching may lead to secondary infections. Scabies is readily spread through contact with upholstery and shared bed and bath linens.

Lice are small parasites ranging from 1 to 4 mm in length. They are readily spread by infected clothing or close personal contact. They require human blood for survival and will die within 24 hours without the blood of a human host. Lice (singular = louse) often infest the pubic area or the

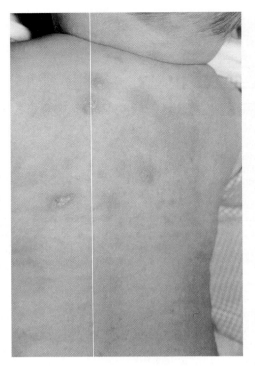

● **Figure 47.2** Scabies
Source: Courtesy of Dr. Jason L. Smith.

scalp and lay eggs, referred to as **nits**, which attach to body hairs. Head lice are *Pediculus capitis*, body lice are *Pediculus corpus*, and pubic lice are *Phthirus pubis. Pediculus capitis*, the most common type in Canada, are shown in Figure 47.3. The pubic louse is referred to as a crab louse because it looks like a tiny crab when viewed under the microscope. Individuals with pubic lice will sometimes say that they have "crabs." Pubic lice may produce sky-blue macules on the inner thighs or lower abdomen. The bite of the louse and the release of saliva into the wound lead to intense itching, followed by vigorous scratching. Secondary infections can result from scratching.

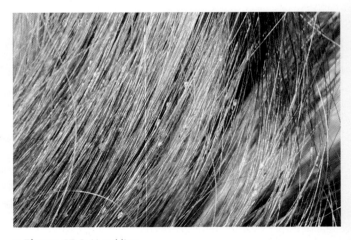

● **Figure 47.3** Head lice
Source: Courtesy of Dr. Jason L. Smith.

47.4 Pharmacotherapy with Scabicides and Pediculicides

Scabicides are drugs that kill mites, and **pediculicides** are drugs that kill lice. Some drugs are effective against both types of parasite. The choice of drug may depend on where the infestation is located, as well as other factors such as age, pregnancy, or breastfeeding.

The traditional drug of choice for both mites and lice is lindane. Lindane is absorbed directly into lice, mites, and their eggs, producing seizures and death of the parasites. Lindane is available as a cream, lotion, and shampoo. Other agents include permethrin, a combination scabicide/pediculicide; crotamiton, a scabicide; and malathion, a pediculicide. All scabicides and pediculicides must be used strictly as directed because their excessive use can cause serious systemic effects and/or skin irritation. Drugs for the treatment of lice or mites must not be applied to the mouth, open skin lesions, or eyes as this will cause severe irritation.

To ensure the effectiveness of pharmacotherapy, clients should inspect hair shafts after treatment, checking for nits by combing with a fine-toothed comb after the hair is dry. This must be conducted daily for at least 1 week after treatment. Some strains of lice and mites have become resistant to common medications, adding to the importance of checking the client several times during the post-application period to be sure all the parasites have been killed. Because nits may be present in bedding, carpets, combs, brushes, seams of clothing, and upholstery, all material coming in close contact with the client must be washed in hot water or treated with medication.

NURSING CONSIDERATIONS

The role of the nurse in scabicide and pediculicide therapy involves careful monitoring of the client's condition and providing education as it relates to the prescribed drug regimen. Before applying a scabicide or pediculicide, the nurse should assess the client's skin and hair, examining for signs of lice, nits, or scabies to verify the need for the medication. Lice may not be obvious on the body but may be found in seams of clothing that contact the axilla, neckline, groin, or beltline. Assess the skin for abrasions, cuts, rashes, and inflammation to determine areas that might be prone to irritation from the medication or increased absorption.

Obtain a complete history, including when the condition began, what treatment, if any, has already been tried (including OTC and home remedies), client allergies, and if anyone in the family has a similar infestation. Assess the client for history of epilepsy as these drugs can lower the seizure threshold in some clients.

Assess females of childbearing age to determine if the client is pregnant or nursing. Scabicides and pediculicides are used with caution in these clients, and precautions should be taken to protect the nursing infant. Lindane is contraindicated in premature infants and should not be applied to

SPECIAL CONSIDERATIONS

Psychosocial and Community Impact of Scabies and Pediculosis

Children and parents, particularly those in relatively affluent areas, may express feeling unclean or that their self-esteem has been lowered when they are diagnosed with scabies or pediculosis. Some clients think that only homeless persons or people of low income get these disorders. The nurse will need to educate the client and family members about the ways in which people contract scabies or pediculosis and how these infestations may be prevented and will need to help those affected to maintain their self-esteem and to adopt a healthy attitude. Persons with scabies or pediculosis may tend to socially isolate themselves, but this is unnecessary if precautions are taken to not share clothing, combs, and other hygiene supplies and to not have bodily contact with others.

Scabies and lice can rapidly spread in a school, nursing home, residential treatment centre, or hospital and become a community health problem. School nurses must assess the potential for students to contact scabies or lice and take preventive measures. These may include frequent assessments of the hair, scalp, and exposed skin and elimination of coat and hat racks and opportunities to share or swap clothing and/or towels. School children and their families need education on prevention and treatment. Clients and their families reporting scabies or pediculosis to the nurse should be treated in an accepting, professional, helpful manner.

children younger than 2 years of age due to increased risk of CNS toxicity. In children ages 2 to 10, lindane is used with caution and sometimes only after other agents such as permethrin and crotamiton have failed to achieve therapeutic goals. Children and older adults may need reduced dosages. Instructions for applying these drugs must be carefully followed. If over-applied, wrongly applied, or accidentally ingested, the client may experience headaches; nausea or vomiting; irritation of the nose, ears, or throat; dizziness; tremors; restlessness; or convulsions.

Wear gloves when applying lindane. Lesions should be cleansed with antibacterial soap and tepid water three times a day to promote healing and reduce chances of secondary infection. The skin should be dried before applying medication.

Client education as it relates to scabicides and pediculicides should include goals, reasons for obtaining baseline data, and possible side effects. Following are important points to include when teaching clients regarding scabicides/pediculicides:

- Keep medication out of the reach of children as it is highly toxic if swallowed or inhaled.
- If breastfeeding, use another source of milk for a minimum of 4 days after using lindane or similar drugs.
- Keep room temperature in the range of 20° to 22.2°C with neither low nor high room humidity in order to reduce itching.
- Prevent re-infestation from household animals by frequently bathing pets and making sure their bedding is washed in hot water or sprayed with a pediculicide or scabicide.

Pr **PROTOTYPE DRUG** | Lindane (Hexit)

ACTIONS AND USES

Lindane is marketed as a cream or lotion for mites and as a shampoo for head lice. Lindane cream or lotion takes longer to produce its effect; therefore, it is usually left on the body for about 8 to 12 hours before rinsing. Lindane shampoo is usually applied and left on for at least 5 minutes before rinsing. Clients should be aware that penetration of the skin with mites causes itching, which lasts up to 2 or 3 weeks even after the parasites have been killed. Lindane kills mites and lice by overstimulating their nervous system.

Treatment may be reapplied in 24 hours when there is evidence of live lice or in 7 days for continued evidence that live mites are present.

PHARMACOKINETICS

Although systemic absorption of lindane is not desired, 10% of the drug (more if skin is damaged from itching) may be absorbed. Lindane is stored in fat. It is metabolized by the liver, excreted in urine, and has a half-life of 17 to 22 hours.

ADMINISTRATION ALERTS

- Do not use for premature infants and children less than 2 years of age.
- Do not use on areas of skin that have abrasions, rash, or inflammation.
- Excessive application may cause dangerous CNS toxicity.
- Lindane is pregnancy category C.

ADVERSE EFFECTS AND INTERACTIONS

CNS adverse effects include restlessness, dizziness, tremors, convulsions (usually after misuse or accidental ingestion), and local irritation. If inhaled, lindane may cause headaches, nausea, vomiting, or irritation of the ears, nose, or throat.

No clinically significant interactions have been established.

- If the child is in daycare, notify caregivers of treatment so that other infected children may be identified.

See "Nursing Process Focus: Clients Receiving Lindane" for specific points the nurse should include when teaching clients regarding this drug.

SUNBURN AND MINOR BURNS

Burns are a unique type of stress that may affect all layers of the skin. Minor, first-degree burns affect only the outer layers of the epidermis, are characterized by redness, and are analogous to sunburn. Sunburn results from overexposure to ultraviolet light, and it is associated with light skin complexions, prolonged exposure to the sun during the more hazardous hours of the day (10 AM until 4 PM), and lack of protective clothing when outdoors. Non-pharmacological approaches to sunburn prevention include the appropriate use of sunscreens and sufficient clothing. Chronic sun exposure can result in serious conditions, including cataracts and skin cancer.

47.5 Pharmacotherapy of Sunburn and Minor Skin Irritation

The best treatment for sunburn is prevention. Clients must be reminded of the acute and chronic hazards of exposure to direct sunlight. Liberal application of a lotion or oil with a very high sun protection factor (SPF) to areas of skin directly exposed to sunlight is strongly recommended.

The symptoms of sunburn include erythema, intense pain, nausea, vomiting, chills, and headache. These symptoms usually resolve within a matter of hours or days, depending on the severity of the exposure. Once sunburn has occurred, medications can only alleviate the symptoms; they do not speed recovery time.

Treatment for sunburn consists of addressing symptoms with soothing lotions, rest, prevention of dehydration, and topical anesthetic agents, if needed. Treatment is usually done on an outpatient basis. Topical anesthetics for minor burns include lidocaine (Solarcaine, Xylocaine), dibucaine (Nupercainal), and tetracaine HCl (Pontocaine). Aloe vera and vitamin E are popular natural therapies for minor skin irritations and burns. These agents may also provide relief from minor pain due to insect bites and pruritus. In more severe cases, oral analgesics such as ASA or ibuprofen may be indicated.

NURSING CONSIDERATIONS

The role of the nurse in drug therapy for sunburn and minor skin irritation involves careful monitoring of the client's condition and providing education as it relates to the prescribed drug regimen. Obtain a drug history, including allergies. When clients present with sunburn, assess the location, body surface area, and extent of injury (erythema, blistering, edema). Assess for weakness, fever, chills, and shock if sunburn is severe. Assess whether any home remedies or OTC medications were used to treat the sunburn. Obtain sunburn and tanning history, including the amount of time the client usually spends in the sun, how easily the client tends to burn, and the SPF rating of sunscreen products if used.

Topical anesthetics are contraindicated in areas of serious burns or infection. Topical lidocaine may cause a hypersensitivity reaction. For clients using the medication for the first time, a trial application on a small area of skin should be conducted to check for allergy. If no adverse reaction has

MediaLink Canadian Dermatology Association

NURSING PROCESS FOCUS   Clients Receiving Lindane (Hexit)

Assessment	Potential Nursing Diagnoses/Identified Patterns
Prior to administration: ■ Obtain complete health history including allergies, drug history, and possible drug interactions. ■ Assess vital signs. ■ Assess skin for presence of lice and/or mite infestation, skin lesions, raw or inflamed skin, and open cuts. ■ Obtain history of seizure disorders. ■ Obtain client's age. ■ Assess pregnancy and lactation status. ■ Obtain social history of close contacts, including household members and sexual partners.	■ Adequate knowledge regarding drug therapy and adverse effects ■ Psychosocial support may be needed to help reduce embarrassment and promote adherence to treatment ■ Risk for impaired skin integrity related to lesions and itching ■ Need for knowledge about ways to reduce risk of re-infestation ■ Need for knowledge of environmental modifications to reduce risk of re-infestation, reduce itch, and promote comfort

Planning: Client Goals and Expected Outcomes

■ Client and significant others will be free of lice or mites and experience no re-infestation.

■ Client will express an understanding of how lice and mites are spread, proper administration of lindane, necessary household hygiene, and the need to notify household members, sexual partners, other close contacts such as classmates of the infestation.

■ Skin will be intact and free of secondary infection and/or irritation.

■ Client will demonstrate an understanding of the drug therapy by accurately describing the drug's intended effects, usage, side effects, and precautions.

Implementation

Interventions (Rationales)	Client Teaching/Discharge Planning
■ Monitor for presence of lice or mites. (This determines the effectiveness of drug therapy.)	Instruct client and caregiver to: ■ Examine for nits on hair shafts and for lice on skin and clothes; inner thigh areas and the seams of clothes that come in contact with axilla, neckline, or beltline may harbour lice ■ Examine for mites between the fingers, on the extremities, in the axillary and gluteal folds, around the trunk, and in the pubic area
■ Apply lindane properly. (Proper application is critical to elimination of infestation.)	Instruct client and caregiver: ■ To wear gloves during application, especially if applying lindane to more than one person, or if pregnant ■ That all skin lotions, creams, and oil-based hair products should be removed completely prior to application by scrubbing the whole body well with soap and water and drying the skin ■ To apply lindane to clean and dry affected body area as directed, using no more than 60 mL per application ■ That eyelashes can be treated with the application of petroleum jelly twice a day for 8 days followed by combing to remove nits ■ To use a fine-tooth comb to comb affected hair following lindane application to the hair and scalp and to treat all household members and sexual contacts simultaneously ■ To re-check affected hair or skin daily for 1 week after treatment
■ Inform client and caregivers about proper care of clothing and equipment. (Contaminated articles can cause re-infestation.)	Instruct client and caregiver to: ■ Wash all bedding and clothing in hot water and dry-clean all non-washable items that came in close contact with client ■ Clean combs and brushes with lindane shampoo and rinse thoroughly

Evaluation of Outcome Criteria

Evaluate the effectiveness of drug therapy by confirming that client goals and expected outcomes have been met (see "Planning").

occurred after 30 to 60 minutes, the medication may be applied to the entire area of mild to moderate sunburn.

Client education as it relates to topical, regional anesthetics should include goals, reasons for obtaining baseline data such as vital signs, and possible side effects. It is important that nurses educate clients about the safe use of topical, regional anesthetic agents, appropriate treatment of sunburn, and prevention of overexposure to the sun. Following are important points to include when teaching clients about topical regional anesthetics:

- Apply topical products as directed.
- Avoid applying medication to open or infected skin.
- Drink plenty of water to avoid dehydration.
- If severe pain persists, notify the healthcare provider.
- Prevent sunburn by wearing a hat and protective clothing and by using sunscreens with an SPF of at least 15.
- Refrigerate topical lotions so that they soothe and cool the skin when applied.

ACNE AND ROSACEA

Acne vulgaris is a common condition affecting 80% of adolescents. Although acne occurs most often in teenagers, it is not unusual to find clients over 30 years of age with acne. This condition in adults is referred to as mature acne or acne tardive. Acne vulgaris is more common in males but tends to persist longer in females.

The etiology of acne vulgaris is unknown, although factors associated with this condition include **seborrhea**, the overproduction of sebum by oil glands, and abnormal formation of keratin that blocks oil glands. The bacterium *Propionibacterium acnes* grows within oil gland openings and changes sebum to an acidic and irritating substance. As a result, small inflamed bumps appear on the surface of the

skin. Other factors associated with acne include androgens, which stimulate sebaceous gland activity, and lower than normal production of linoleic acid in the sebum.

Acne lesions include open and closed **comedones**. Blackheads, or open comedones, occur when sebum has plugged the oil gland, causing it to become black because of the presence of melanin granules. Whiteheads, or closed comedones, develop just beneath the surface of the skin and appear white rather than black.

Rosacea is another skin disorder with lesions affecting mainly the face. Unlike acne, which most commonly affects teenagers, rosacea is a progressive disorder with an onset between 30 and 50 years of age. Rosacea is characterized by small papules or inflammatory bumps without pus that swell, thicken, and become painful, as shown in Figure 47.4. The face takes on a reddened or flushed appearance, particularly around the nose and cheek area. With time, the redness becomes more permanent and lesions resembling acne appear. The soft tissues of the nose may thicken, giving the nose a reddened, bullous, irregular swelling called **rhinophyma.**

Rosacea is exacerbated by factors such as sunlight, stress, increased temperature, and agents that dilate facial blood vessels, including alcohol, spicy foods, skin care products, and warm beverages. It affects more women than men, although men more often develop rhinophyma.

47.6 Pharmacotherapy of Acne and Acne-Related Disorders

Medications used for acne and related disorders are available OTC and by prescription. Because of their increased toxicity, prescription agents are reserved for severe, persistent cases. These drugs are shown in Table 47.3.

Benzoyl peroxide is the most common topical OTC medication for acne. Benzoyl peroxide has a **keratolytic** effect, which helps to dry out and shed the outer layer of the epi-

---

Pr PROTOTYPE DRUG | Lidocaine (Solarcaine, others)

ACTIONS AND USES

Lidocaine is a local anesthetic that provides temporary relief from pain and discomfort in cases of sunburn, pruritus, minor wounds, and insect bites. Its pharmacological action is to cause local anesthesia of skin receptor nerve endings by inhibiting transport of sodium ions across neuronal membranes. Preparations are also available to treat specific areas such as the ear, mouth, throat, and rectal and genital areas.

PHARMACOKINETICS

About 3% of topical lidocaine is absorbed systemically, so it is important to use as directed and not to exceed the maximum dose. Lidocaine is extensively metabolized by the liver, and only 10% is excreted in urine. Its half-life is 1.5 to 2 hours.

ADMINISTRATION ALERTS

- Lidocaine should not be used for treatment of clients with open lesions, traumatized mucosal areas, or a history of sensitivity to local anesthetics.
- Clients should use preparations only in areas of the body for which the medication is intended.
- Lidocaine is pregnancy category C.

ADVERSE EFFECTS AND INTERACTIONS

Topical lidocaine has a low toxicity when used as directed. Lidocaine gel or spray when applied to mucous membranes is rapidly absorbed, and overdose can cause neurological or cardiac toxicity. Allergic reactions and anaphylaxis are rare.

Lidocaine may interfere with the activity of some antibacterial sulfonamides.

 See the Companion Website for a Nursing Process Focus chart specific to this drug.

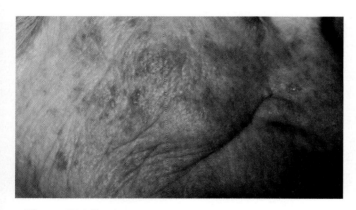

● Figure 47.4 Rosacea
Source: Courtesy of Dr. Jason L. Smith.

dermis. Other effects include possible sebum-suppressing action and antimicrobial activity that lasts up to 48 hours following application. This medication may be dispensed as a topical lotion, cream, or gel and is available in various percent concentrations. Other keratolytic agents used for severe acne include resorcinol, salicylic acid, and sulfur.

Retinoids are newer agents, usually by prescription only, that are effective against severe acne. Tretinoin is a vitamin A derivative with an irritant action that decreases comedone formation and increases extrusion of comedones from the skin. Another use of tretinoin is for wrinkle removal. Topically applied tretinoin is minimally absorbed into the body. Other retinoids include isotretinoin, which is an oral medication and vitamin A metabolite that aids in reducing the size of sebaceous glands, thereby decreasing oil production and the occurrence of clogged pores. Isotretinoin is not recommended during pregnancy because of possible harmful effects to the fetus. A common reaction to retinoids is sensitivity to sunlight. Additional retinoid-like agents and related compounds used to treat

acne include the following prescription medications: adapalene, azelaic acid, and sulfacetamide.

Antibiotics are sometimes used in combination with acne medications to lessen the severe redness and inflammation associated with the disorder. Doxycycline and tetracycline have been the traditional antibiotics used in acne therapy.

Ethinyl estradiol is an estrogen commonly found in oral contraceptives that is also used to help clear the skin of acne. For the actions and contraindications of this and related hormones, see Chapter 41.

Pharmacotherapy for rosacea includes a number of drugs given for acne vulgaris, including isotretinoin, topical azelaic acid 20% cream, sulfacetamide preparations, and systemic antibiotics. In addition, clients with rosacea may be prescribed metronidazole 0.75% to 1% topical preparation, an antibacterial, and an antiprotozoal preparation. Crotamiton 10% cream or lotion may also be prescribed if hair follicle mites are present. In addition to medications, some clients have vascular or carbon dioxide laser surgery for rhinophyma.

NURSING CONSIDERATIONS

The role of the nurse in drug therapy for acne-related disorders includes careful monitoring of the client's condition and providing education as it relates to the prescribed drug regimen. The nurse working with teenagers with acne first needs to establish rapport since many clients may be embarrassed or have an altered body image or self-esteem disturbance because of the acne. Establishing rapport early will help the nurse when obtaining the health history and physical assessment. The nurse should record when the acne began, what treatments have been tried, and with what success. Most acne sufferers will have attempted many OTC therapies before seeing a healthcare provider for a prescription drug, and they may continue to use these preparations

TABLE 47.3 **Drugs for Acne and Acne-Related Disorders**	
Drug	**Remarks**
OTC Agent	
benzoyl peroxide (Benzacin, Benzamyclin, others)	Sometimes combined with tetracycline, erythromycin, or clindamycin in severe cases to fight bacterial infection.
Prescription Agents (Topical)	
adapalene (Differin)	Retinoid-like compound used to treat acne formation.
azelaic acid (Azelex, Finacea, others)	For mild to moderate inflammatory acne.
sulfacetamide sodium (PMS-Sulfacetamide)	For sensitive skin; sometimes combined with sulfur to promote peeling, as in the condition rosacea; also used for conjunctivitis.
tretinoin (Retin-A, others)	To prevent clogging of pore follicles; also used for the treatment of acute promyelocytic leukemia and wrinkles.
Prescription Agents (Oral)	
estradiol (PMS-, Sandoz-Estradiol)	Oral contraceptives are sometimes used for acne; combination drugs may be helpful, for example, ethinyl estradiol plus norgestimate (Ortho Tri-Cyclen-28)
doxycycline (Nu-, PMS-, Ratio-Doxycycline)	Antibiotic; refer to Chapter 32 .
isotretinoin (Accutane)	For acne with cysts or acne formed in small, rounded masses; pregnancy category X.
tetracycline (Tetracycline Cap) (see page 431 for the Prototype Drug box)	Antibiotic; refer to Chapter 32 .

in addition to new prescriptions. Because some medications prescribed for acne are not recommended for the pregnant client, the nurse should ask women of childbearing age their pregnancy status.

The nurse should wear gloves when examining the skin. As with all dermatological conditions, the nurse should have the client undress in order to observe as much of the skin surface as possible. The acne on exposed areas such as the face may present somewhat differently than acne on the back or elsewhere. In some instances, clients are not aware of the extent of their skin disorder.

Isotretinoin is contraindicated in clients with a history of severe depression and suicidal ideation, and clients should sign a consent regarding understanding of suicide risks prior to treatment. Concurrent use of isotretinoin and carbamazepine will decrease blood levels of carbamazepine, which may lead to increased seizure activity. Concurrent use of isotretinoin and hypoglycemic agents may lead to loss of glycemic control as well as increased risk for cardiovascular disease, secondary to elevated triglyceride levels.

A patch test should be done before the acne drug is used for the first time. When applying ointment, lotion, or cream to the skin, cleanse and completely dry the skin and apply the medication to a small area to test for sensitivity. A very small amount of topical medication, about the size of a pea, is enough to cover the face adequately. Topical medication should not be applied to the eyes, mouth, or mucous membranes.

Because isotretinoin may cause severe birth defects or spontaneous abortions, female clients must have a negative pregnancy test result within 2 weeks of beginning treatment. Tetracycline or minocycline use may increase the risk of pseudotumour cerebri, manifested by headache, papilledema, and decreased vision.

Client education as it relates to drugs used to treat acne should include goals, reasons for obtaining baseline data, and possible side effects. Client teaching and understanding is vital to the proper use of acne drugs. Following are the important points the nurse should include when teaching clients about drugs used for the treatment of acne:

- Inform the healthcare provider of all OTC medications used for acne.
- Use acne medications correctly and for the prescribed length of time.
- Avoid foods that seem to make acne worse. Keep a food log to determine which foods tend to worsen the condition.
- Avoid products that will irritate the skin, such as cologne, perfumes, and other alcohol-based products.
- If severe skin irritation or inflammation develops during therapy, discontinue use and call the healthcare provider.

NATURAL THERAPIES

Burdock Root for Acne and Eczema

Burdock root, *Arctium lappa,* comes from a thick, flowering plant sometimes found on the roadsides of Britain and North America. It contains several active substances such as bitter glycosides and flavonoids, and it has a range of potential actions in the body: anti-infective, diuretic, mild laxative, and skin detoxifier. It is sometimes described as an attacker of skin disorders from within because it fights bacterial infections, reduces inflammation, and treats some stages of eczema, particularly the dry and scaling phases. Some claim that it is also effective against boils and sores.

Burdock root is considered safe, having few side effects or drug interactions. It contains 50% inulin, a fibre widely distributed in vegetables and fruits, and it is consumed as a regular part of the daily diet in many Asian countries. In many cases, burdock root is combined with other natural products for a wider range of effectiveness. Such products include sarsaparilla (*Smilax officinalis*), yellow dock (*Rumex crispus*), licorice root (*Glycyrrhiza glabra*), echinacea (*Echinacea purpurea*), and dandelion (*Taraxacum officinale*).

Pr PROTOTYPE DRUG | Isotretinoin (Accutane)

ACTIONS AND USES

The principal action of isotretinoin is regulation of skin growth and turnover. As cells from the stratum germinativum grow toward the skin's surface, skin cells are lost from the stratum pore openings, and their replacement is slowed. Isotretinoin also decreases oil production by reducing the size and number of oil glands. Symptoms take 4 to 8 weeks to improve, and maximum therapeutic benefit may take 5 to 6 months. This drug is most often used in cases of cystic acne or severe keratinization disorders.

PHARMACOKINETICS

Isotretinoin is metabolized by the liver. It is excreted in urine and feces. Its half-life is 21 hours.

ADMINISTRATION ALERTS

- Do not use this drug in clients with a history of severe depression and suicidal ideation.
- Take with meals to minimize GI distress.
- Isotretinoin is pregnancy category X.

ADVERSE EFFECTS AND INTERACTIONS

Isotretinoin is a toxic metabolite of retinol, or vitamin A. Common adverse effects are conjunctivitis, dry mouth, inflammation of the lip, dry nose, nosebleed, increased serum concentrations of triglycerides (by 50% to 70%), bone and joint pain, and photosensitivity. Liver function, serum glucose, and serum triglyceride tests should be performed when taking isotretinoin.

Isotretinoin interacts with vitamin A supplements, which increase toxicity. In addition, tetracycline or minocycline use may increase risk of pseudotumour cerebri. Concurrent use of hypoglycemic agents may lead to loss of glycemic control as well as increased risk for cardiovascular disease, secondary to elevated triglyceride levels. Concurrent use with carbamazepine will decrease blood levels of carbamazepine, which may lead to increased seizure activity.

NURSING PROCESS FOCUS Clients Receiving Isotretinoin (Accutane) Pr

Assessment	Potential Nursing Diagnoses/Identified Patterns
Prior to administration: ■ Obtain complete health history including allergies, drug history, and possible drug interactions. ■ Obtain pregnancy and lactation status. ■ Assess for history of psychiatric disorders. ■ Assess vital signs to obtain baseline information.	■ Need for knowledge regarding drug therapy and adverse effects ■ Psychosocial body image adjustment related to presence of acne and possible worsening of symptoms after treatment begins ■ Risk for impaired skin integrity related to inflammation, redness, and scaling, secondary to treatment ■ Decisional conflict related to desire for pregnancy and necessity of preventing pregnancy during therapy with isotretinoin ■ Difficulty adhering to therapy related to length of treatment time ■ Failure to use effective contraception

Planning: Client Goals and Expected Outcomes

The client will:
■ Experience decreased acne, without side effects or adverse reactions
■ Demonstrate acceptance of body image
■ Demonstrate an understanding of the drug therapy by accurately describing the drug's intended effects, side effects, and precautions

Implementation

Interventions (Rationales)	Client Education/Discharge Planning
■ Monitor lab studies during treatment, including blood glucose.	■ Instruct client on importance of lab studies prior to therapy and periodically during therapy and of doing home blood glucose monitoring if diabetic.
■ Discuss potential adverse reactions to drug therapy. (Understanding of drug effects is important for adherence.)	Instruct client: ■ To use two forms of reliable birth control for 1 month before beginning treatment, during treatment, and for 1 month following completion of treatment ■ Not to donate blood during treatment and for a minimum of 4 weeks after completion of treatment; isotretinoin in donated blood could cause fetal damage if given to a pregnant woman ■ To talk with pediatrician about alternative methods of feeding if breastfeeding ■ To avoid use of vitamin A products
■ Monitor for cardiovascular problems. (Use isotretinoin with caution in clients with heart block, especially if client is also taking a beta-blocker.)	■ Discuss with client importance of complete disclosure regarding medical history and medications.
■ Monitor emotional health. (Client may become depressed secondary to acne itself, length of treatment, possibility of worsening symptoms at beginning of treatment, changed body image, or drug itself.)	Instruct client: ■ To report signs of depression immediately and discontinue isotretinoin ■ Regarding signs and symptoms of depression ■ To report any feelings of suicide ideation
■ Monitor CBC, blood lipid levels, glucose levels, liver function tests, eye exam, GI status, urinalysis.	■ Teach client importance of a complete workup prior to starting isotretinoin therapy and periodically during course of treatment.
■ Monitor for vision changes. (Corneal opacities and/or cataracts may develop as a result of isotretinoin use. Dryness of eyes during treatment is common. Night vision may be diminished during treatment.)	Instruct client: ■ To report any decreased vision and discontinue use of isotretinoin ■ To avoid driving at night if possible ■ That use of artificial tears may relieve dry eyes ■ That use of contact lenses may need to be discontinued during therapy
■ Monitor alcohol use. (Alcohol use with isotretinoin leads to increased triglyceride levels.)	Advise client to: ■ Eliminate or greatly reduce alcohol use, including alcohol-containing preparations such as mouthwashes and OTC medications ■ Read labels for alcohol content
■ Monitor skin problems. (This will determine the effectiveness of drug therapy.)	Advise client: ■ That acne may worsen during beginning of treatment ■ To monitor skin for improvement in 4 to 8 weeks; if no improvement is noted, contact primary healthcare provider

continued

NURSING PROCESS FOCUS Clients Receiving Isotretinoin (Accutane) *(Continued)*

Interventions (Rationales)	Client Education/Discharge Planning
■ Monitor for side effects.	■ Instruct client to be aware of and to report headache (especially if accompanied by nausea and vomiting), fatigue, depression, lethargy, severe diarrhea, rectal bleeding, abdominal pain, dry mouth, hematuria, proteinuria, liver dysfunction (jaundice, pruritus, dark urine).

Evaluation of Outcome Criteria

Evaluate the effectiveness of drug therapy by confirming that client goals and expected outcomes have been met (see "Planning").

DERMATITIS

Dermatitis is an inflammatory skin disorder characterized by local redness, pain, and pruritus. Intense scratching may lead to **excoriation**—scratches that break the skin surface and fill with blood or serous fluid to form crusty scales. Dermatitis may be acute or chronic.

Atopic dermatitis, or **eczema**, is a chronic, inflammatory skin disorder with a genetic predisposition. Clients presenting with eczema will often have a family history of asthma and hay fever as well as allergies to a variety of irritants such as cosmetics, lotions, soaps, pollens, food, and dust. About 75% of clients with atopic dermatitis will have had an initial onset before 1 year of age. In those babies predisposed to eczema, breastfeeding seems to offer protection as it is rare for a breastfed child to develop eczema before the introduction of other foods. In infants and small children, lesions usually begin on the face and scalp, then progress to other parts of the body. A frequent and prominent symptom in infants is the appearance of red cheeks.

Contact dermatitis can be caused by a hypersensitivity response resulting from exposure to specific natural or synthetic allergens, such as plants, chemicals, latex, drugs, metals, or foreign proteins. Accompanying the allergic reaction may be various degrees of cracking, bleeding, or small blisters.

Seborrheic dermatitis is sometimes seen in newborns and in teenagers after puberty. It is characterized by yellowish, oily, crusted patches of skin that appear in areas of the face, scalp, chest, back, or pubic area. Bacterial infection or dandruff may accompany these symptoms.

Stasis dermatitis, a condition found primarily in the lower extremities, results from poor venous circulation. Redness and scaling may be observed in areas where venous circulation is impaired or where deep venous blood clots have formed.

47.7 Pharmacotherapy of Dermatitis

Pharmacotherapy of dermatitis is symptomatic and involves lotions and ointments to control itching and skin flaking. Antihistamines may be used to control inflammation, and analgesics or topical anesthetics may be prescribed for pain relief.

Topical glucocorticoids are the most effective treatment for dermatitis. As shown in Table 47.4, there are many formulations of glucocorticoids available in different potencies. Creams, lotions, solutions, gels, and pads are specially formulated to penetrate deep into the skin layers for relief of local inflammation, burning, and itching. Long-term glucocorticoid use, however, may lead to irritation, redness, and thinning of the skin membranes. If absorption occurs, topical glucocorticoids may produce undesirable systemic effects including adrenal insufficiency, mood changes, serum imbalances, and bone defects, as discussed in Chapter 39.

PSORIASIS

Psoriasis is a chronic, non-infectious, inflammatory disorder characterized by red raised patches of skin covered with flaky, thick, silver scales called plaques, as shown in Figure 47.5. These plaques shed the scales, which are sometimes grayish. The reason for the appearance of plaques is an extremely fast skin cell turnover rate, with skin cells reaching the surface in 4 to 7 days instead of the usual 14 days. Plaques are ultimately shed from the surface, while the underlying skin becomes inflamed and irritated.

The various forms of psoriasis are described in Table 47.5. Lesion size varies, but the shape tends to be round. Lesions are usually discovered on the scalp, elbows, knees, extensor surfaces of the arms and legs, sacrum, and occasionally around the nails. The etiology of psoriasis is unknown, but about 50% of the cases involve a family history of the disorder. One theory of causation is that psoriasis is an autoimmune condition. In psoriasis, certain overactive immune cells release cytokines that cause the increased production of skin cells.

47.8 Pharmacotherapy of Psoriasis

A number of prescription and OTC drugs are available for the treatment of psoriasis, including both topical and systemic agents, as shown in Table 47.6. A primary treatment is topical glucocorticoids, such as betamethasone ointment, lotion, or cream and hydrocortisone acetate cream or oint-

TABLE 47.4   Topical Glucocorticoids for Dermatitis and Related Symptoms

Generic Name	Trade Names
Highest Level of Potency	
betamethasone	Diprosone, Valisone
clobetasol	PMS-, Novo-Clobetasol
Middle Level of Potency	
amcinonide	Ratio-Amcinonide
desoximetasone	Topicort
fluocinonide	Lidex
halcinonide	Halog Cream
mometasone	PMS-, Ratio-Mometasone
triamcinolone	Triamcinolone, Acetonide
Lower Level of Potency	
fluocinolone	Synalar
fluticasone	Flonase
hydrocortisone	Westcort, Dermarest, Vioform
Lowest Level of Potency	
desonide	Tridesilon, Gen-, PMS-Budesonide
dexamethasone	Apo-, Gen-Dexamethasone, Decadron

ment. Topical glucocorticoids reduce the inflammation associated with fast skin turnover.

Another class of preparations is the topical immunomodulators (TIMs), which are agents that suppress the immune system. One example is tacrolimus ointment. Other agents applied topically are retinoid-like compounds such as calcipotriene, a synthetic vitamin D ointment, cream, or scalp solution; and tazarotene, a vitamin A derivative gel or cream. These drugs provide the same benefits as topical glucocorticoids but exhibit a lower incidence of adverse effects. Calcipotriene may produce hypercalcemia if applied over large areas of the body or used in higher doses than recommended. This drug is usually not used on an extended basis.

The most often prescribed systemic drug for severe psoriasis is methotrexate. Methotrexate is used in the treatment of a variety of disorders, including carcinomas and rheumatoid arthritis, in addition to psoriasis. Methotrexate is discussed as a Prototype Drug in Chapter 35 (page 487). Other systemic drugs for psoriasis include acitretin and etretinate. These drugs are taken orally to inhibit excessive skin cell growth.

TABLE 47.5   Types of Psoriasis

Form of Psoriasis	Description of Form	Most Common Location of Lesions	Comments
Guttate (drop-like) or eruptive psoriasis	Lesions smaller than those of psoriasis vulgaris	Upper trunk and extremities	More common in early-onset psoriasis; can appear and resolve spontaneously a few weeks following a streptococcal respiratory infection
Psoriasis annularis	Ring-shaped lesions with clear centres		Rare
Psoriatic arthritis	Resembles rheumatoid arthritis	Fingers and toes at distal interphalangeal joints; can affect skin and nails	About 20% of patients with psoriasis also have arthritis
Psoriasis vulgaris	Lesions are papules that form into erythematous plaques with thick, silver or grey plaques, which bleed when removed; plaques in dark-skinned individuals often appear purple	Skin over scalp, elbows, and knees; lesions possible anywhere on the body	Most common form; requires long-term, specialized management
Psoriatic erythrodema or exfoliative psoriasis	Generalized scaling; erythema without lesions	All body surfaces	
Pustular psoriasis	Eruption of pustules; presence of fever	Trunk and extremities; can appear on palms, soles, and nail beds	

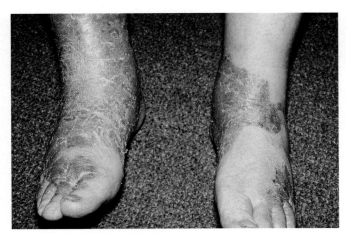

● **Figure 47.5** Psoriasis

Source: Courtesy of Dr. Jason L. Smith.

Other drugs used for different disorders, but which provide relief of severe psoriatic symptoms, are hydroxyurea and cyclosporine. Hydroxyurea is a sickle cell anemia drug. Cyclosporine is an immunosuppressive agent that is presented as a Prototype Drug in Chapter 30 (page 397). In addition, etanercept and infliximab, which are approved for other autoimmune conditions, have been found to improve

symptoms of psoriasis. Etanercept and infliximab are tumour necrosis factor (TNF) blockers.

Other skin therapy techniques may be used with or without additional psoriasis medications. These include various forms of tar treatment (coal tar) and anthralin, which are applied to the skin's surface. Tar and anthralin inhibit DNA synthesis and arrest abnormal cell growth.

Phototherapy with ultraviolet B (UVB) and (ultraviolet A (UVA) are used in cases of severe psoriasis. UVB therapy is less hazardous than UVA therapy. UVB has a wavelength similar to sunlight, and it reduces widespread lesions that normally resist topical treatments. With close supervision, this type of phototherapy can be administered at home. Keratolytic pastes are often applied between treatments. The second type of phototherapy is referred to as PUVA because **psoralens** are often administered in conjunction with the phototherapy. Psoralens are oral or topical agents that, when exposed to UV light, produce a photosensitive reaction. This reaction reduces the number of lesions, but unpleasant side effects such as headache, nausea, and skin sensitivity still occur, limiting the effectiveness of this therapy. Immunosuppressant drugs such as cyclosporine are not used in conjunction with PUVA therapy because they increase the risk of skin cancer.

TABLE 47.6 Drugs for Psoriasis and Related Disorders		
Drug	*Route and Adult Dose*	
Topical Medications		
calcipotriene (Dovonex)	Topically to lesions qd–bid	
tazarotene (Tazorac)	Acne: apply thin film to clean dry area qd Plaque psoriasis: apply thin film qd in the evening	
Systemic Medications		
acitretin (Soriatane)	PO; 10–50 mg qd with the main meal	
cyclosporine (Apo-Cyclosporine)	PO; 1.25 mg/kg bid (max 4 mg/kg/d)	
hydroxyurea (Gen-, Apo-Hydroxyurea)	PO; 80 mg/kg q3d or 20–30 mg/kg qd	
methotrexate (Apo-, Ratio-Methotrexate) (see page 487 for the Prototype Drug box)	PO; 2.5–5 mg bid for three doses each week (max 25–30 mg/wk) IM/IV; 10–30 mg/wk	

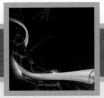

CHAPTER REVIEW

KEY CONCEPTS

The numbered key concepts provide a succinct summary of the important points from the corresponding numbered section within the chapter. If any of these points are not clear, refer to the numbered section within the chapter for review. Expanded versions can be found on the Companion Website.

47.1 Three layers of skin—epidermis, dermis, and subcutaneous layer—provide effective barrier defences for the body.

47.2 Skin disorders that may benefit from pharmacotherapy are acne, sunburns, infections, dermatitis, and psoriasis.

47.3 When the skin integrity is compromised, bacteria, viruses, and fungi can gain entrance and cause infections. Anti-infective therapy may be indicated.

47.4 Scabicides and pediculicides are used to treat parasitic mite and lice infestations, respectively.

47.5 The pharmacotherapy of sunburn includes the symptomatic relief of pain using soothing lotions, topical anesthetics, and analgesics.

47.6 The pharmacotherapy of acne includes treatment with benzoyl peroxide, retinoids, and antibiotics. Therapies for rosacea include retinoids and metronidazole.

47.7 The most effective treatment for dermatitis is topical glucocorticoids.

47.8 Both topical and systemic drugs, including glucocorticoids, immunomodulators, and methotrexate, are used to treat psoriasis.

REVIEW QUESTIONS

1 Name examples of drugs used to treat mite and lice infestations. What precautions should be taken when using these drugs?

2 What is the major purpose of drugs used to treat acne and related skin conditions? Give examples of both topical and systemic drugs.

3 In most cases, which drug category is used to treat symptoms of dermatitis and psoriasis? What other drug therapies and techniques are used to provide a measure of relief for these symptoms?

CRITICAL THINKING QUESTIONS

1. A senior nursing student is participating in well-baby screenings at a public health clinic. While examining a 4-month-old infant, the student notes an extensive, confluent diaper rash. The baby's mother is upset and asks the student nurse about the use of OTC corticosteroid ointment and wonders how she should apply the cream. How should the student nurse respond?

2. A 14-year-old girl has been placed on oral doxycycline (Doxy-Caps) for acne vulgaris because she has not responded to topical antibiotic therapy. After 3 weeks of therapy, the client returns to the dermatologist's office complaining about episodes of nausea and epigastric pain. The nurse learns that the client is "so busy with school activities" that she often forgets a morning dose and

"doubles up" on the drug before bedtime. Devise a teaching plan relevant to drug therapy that takes into consideration the major side effects of this drug and the cognitive abilities of this client.

3. A 37-year-old woman is referred to a dermatologist for increasing redness and painful "acne" lesions. The client is frustrated with her attempts to camouflage her "teenage face" with makeup. She relates to the nurse that she had acne as a teen but had no further problem until the last 11 months. After consultation, the dermatologist suggests a 3-month trial of isotretinoin (Accutane). What are the specific reproductive considerations for this client? What information should this client be provided in relation to reproductive concerns?

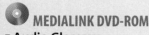

EXPLORE

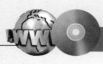 **www.pearsoned.ca/adams-king**

MEDIALINK DVD-ROM
- **Audio Glossary**
- **CRNE Review**

 COMPANION WEBSITE
- **CRNE Review**
- **Dosage Calculations**
- **Case Study:** Acne

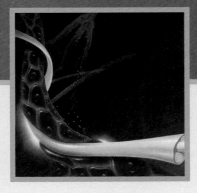

CHAPTER 48

Drugs for Eye and Ear Disorders

DRUGS AT A GLANCE

OBJECTIVES

After reading this chapter, the student should be able to do the following:

1. Identify drug classes used for treating eye and ear disorders.
2. Explain the therapeutic action of drugs therapies used for glaucoma and other eye and ear disorders in relation to the pathophysiology of the disorders.
3. For each of the drug classes listed in Drugs at a Glance, identify a representative drug and explain its mechanism of action, therapeutic effects, and important adverse effects.
4. Explain the two major mechanisms by which drugs reduce intraocular pressure.
5. Describe the nurse's role in the pharmacological management of clients receiving drugs for eye and ear disorders.
6. Describe and explain, based on pharmacological principles, the rationale for nursing assessment, planning, and interventions for clients receiving drug therapy for eye and ear disorders.
7. Use the nursing process to care for clients who are receiving drug therapy for eye and ear disorders.

MediaLink

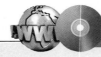

www.pearsoned.ca/adams-king

CRNE review, case studies, and other interactive resources for this chapter can be found on the Companion Website at **www.pearsoned.ca/adams-king**. Click on "Chapter 48" to select the activities for this chapter. For animations, more CRNE review questions, and an audio glossary, access the accompanying DVD-ROM in this textbook.

Eyes and ears are vulnerable to a variety of conditions, many of which can be prevented, controlled, or reversed with proper treatment. The first part of this chapter covers various drugs used for the treatment of glaucoma. Drugs used routinely by ophthalmic healthcare providers are also discussed. The remaining part of the chapter presents drugs used for the treatment of ear disorders, including infections, inflammation, and the buildup of ear wax.

48.1 Anatomy of the Eye

A simple scratch to the eye can cause the client almost unbearable discomfort as well as concern about the effect the damage may have on vision. Some eye disorders may be more bearable, but extremely dangerous—including glaucoma, a leading cause of blindness. A firm knowledge of basic eye anatomy, shown in Figures 48.1 and 48.2, is required to understand eye disorders and their pharmacotherapy. A fluid called **aqueous humour** is found in the anterior cavity of the eye. The anterior cavity has two divisions, the anterior chamber, which extends from the cornea to the iris, and the posterior chamber, which lies between the iris and the lens. The aqueous humour originates in the posterior chamber from a muscular structure called the ciliary body.

Aqueous humour helps to retain the shape of the eye, and it circulates to bring nutrients to the area and remove wastes. From its origin in the ciliary body, the aqueous humour flows through the pupil and into the anterior chamber. Within the anterior chamber and around the periphery is a network of spongy connective tissue, or trabecular meshwork, which contains an opening called the canal of Schlemm. The aqueous humour drains into the canal of Schlemm and out of the anterior chamber into the venous system, thus completing its circulation. Under normal circumstances, the rate of aqueous humour production is equal to its outflow; thus maintaining intraocular pressure (IOP) within a normal range. Interference with either the production or outflow of aqueous humour can lead to an increase in IOP.

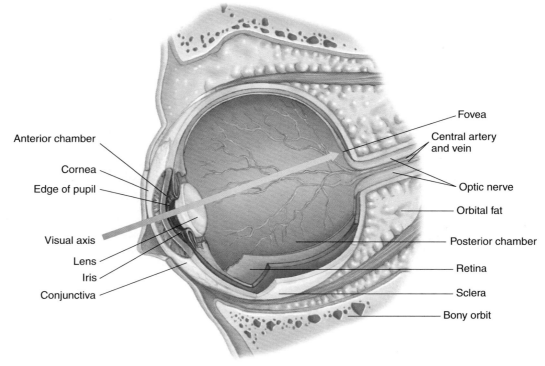

● **Figure 48.1** Internal structures of the eye

Source: Pearson Education/PH College.

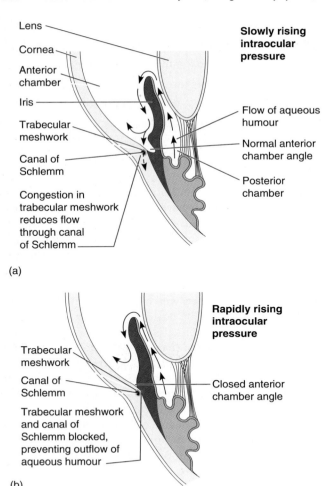

(a)

(b)

● **Figure 48.2** Forms of primary adult glaucoma: (a) in chronic open-angle glaucoma, the anterior chamber angle remains open, but drainage of aqueous humour through the canal of Schlemm is impaired; (b) in acute angle-closure glaucoma, the angle of the iris and anterior chamber narrows, obstructing the outflow of aqueous humour

GLAUCOMA

Glaucoma occurs when the IOP becomes high enough to cause optic nerve damage, leading to visual field loss and possibly advancing to blindness. Although the median IOP in the population is 15 to 16 mm Hg, this pressure varies greatly with age, daily activities, and even time of day. As a rule, IOP consistently above 21 mm Hg is considered abnormal. Many clients, however, tolerate IOP in the mid to high 20s without damage to the optic nerve. IOP above 30 mm Hg requires treatment because it is associated with permanent vision changes. Some clients of Asian descent may experience glaucoma at "normal" IOP values, below 21 mm Hg.

Glaucoma often exists as a primary condition without an identifiable cause. In some cases, glaucoma is associated with genetic factors; it can be congenital in infants and children. Glaucoma can also be secondary to eye trauma, infection, diabetes, inflammation, hemorrhage, tumour, high blood pressure, or cataracts. Some medications may contribute to

the development or progression of glaucoma, including the long-term use of topical or oral glucocorticoids and some antihypertensives, antihistamines, and antidepressants. Glaucoma is the leading cause of *preventable* blindness in Canada.

48.2 Types of Glaucoma

Diagnosis of glaucoma is sometimes difficult because it often occurs without symptoms. **Tonometry** is an ophthalmic technique that tests for glaucoma by measuring IOP. Other routine refractory and visual field tests may uncover signs of glaucoma. One problem with diagnosis is that clients with glaucoma typically do not experience symptoms and therefore do not schedule regular eye exams. In some cases, glaucoma occurs so gradually that clients do not notice a problem until late in the disease process.

As shown in Figure 48.2, the two principal types of glaucoma are **closed-angle glaucoma** and **open-angle glaucoma**. Both disorders result from the same problem: an increase of aqueous humour in the anterior cavity. This increase is caused either by excessive production of aqueous humour or by a blockage of its outflow. In either case, IOP increases, leading to progressive damage to the optic nerve. As degeneration of the optic nerve is occurring, the client will first notice a loss of visual field, then a loss of central visual acuity, and lastly total blindness. Major differences between closed-angle and open-angle glaucoma include how quickly the IOP develops and whether there is narrowing of the anterior chamber angle between the iris and cornea.

Closed-angle glaucoma, also called acute glaucoma or narrow-angle glaucoma, is uncommon. The incidence is higher in older adults and in persons of Asian descent. This acute type of glaucoma is usually unilateral and caused by stress, impact injury, or medications. Pressure inside the anterior chamber increases suddenly, with the iris being pushed over the area where the aqueous humour normally drains. The displacement of the iris is due in part to the dilation of the pupil or accommodation of the lens, causing the narrowed angle to close. Signs and symptoms, caused by acute obstruction of the outflow of aqueous humour from the eye, include intense headaches, difficulty concentrating,

PHARMFACTS

Glaucoma

- More than 250,000 Canadians have glaucoma.
- Glaucoma often has no symptoms until loss of vision occurs.
- Worldwide, over 6 million people have lost their vision as a result of glaucoma.
- People of African and Chinese heritage are at higher risk for glaucoma.
- Glaucoma is most common in clients over 40 years of age.
- Family history of glaucoma, diabetes, previous eye injury, and long-term use of steroids increase the risk of glaucoma.
- Eye drops can control most cases of glaucoma.

Source: Glaucoma Research Society of Canada, "http://www. glaucomaresearch.ca/".

bloodshot eyes, blurred vision, and a bulging iris. Closed-angle glaucoma constitutes an emergency situation.

Open-angle glaucoma, or chronic simple glaucoma, is the most common type, accounting for 90% of the cases. It is usually bilateral, and IOP develops slowly, over a period of years. It is called "open-angle" because the iris does not cover the trabecular meshwork. Clients may be asymptomatic.

48.3 General Treatment of Glaucoma

All of the approaches to glaucoma therapy are directed to the goal of increasing the circulation of aqueous humour that has been reduced (in the case of chronic, open-angle glaucoma) or prevented (in the case of acute, closed-angle glaucoma). In cases of acute, closed-angle glaucoma, surgery such as gonioplasty, laser iridotomy, and peripheral iridectomy may be performed to return the iris back to its original position. In gonioplasty, an argon laser burns the periphery of the iris. When the burn scars heal, tension is created that draws the iris away from the cornea, thus widening the angle. Iridectomy involves the laser creation of a number of small perforations in the iris, which allow the aqueous humour to drain through the normal pathway. Iridectomy involves removal of a small section of the iris to increase the flow of aqueous humour. Although surgery is often performed in acute, closed-angle glaucoma, the majority of cases of open-angle glaucoma are treated with medication.

48.4 Pharmacotherapy of Glaucoma

Pharmacotherapy for glaucoma works by one of two mechanisms: increasing the outflow of aqueous humour at the canal of Schlemm or decreasing the formation of aqueous humour at the ciliary body. Many agents for glaucoma act by affecting the autonomic nervous system (see Chapter 13). Agents for glaucoma, as shown in Table 48.1, include cholinergic agonists, non-selective adrenergics, prostaglandins, beta-adrenergic blockers, alpha$_2$-adrenergic

TABLE 48.1	Selected Drugs for Glaucoma
Drug	*Route and Adult Dose*
Cholinergic Agonists	
carbachol (Carbachol, Isopto, Miostat)	1–2 drops 0.75–3% solution in lower conjunctival sac q4h–tid
demecarium bromide (Humoursol)	1–2 drops 0.125–0.25% solution twice per week
physostigmine sulfate (Eserine Sulfate)	1 drop 0.25–0.5% solution qd–qid
pilocarpine (Miocarpine, Spersacarpine)	Acute glaucoma: 1 drop 1–2% solution every 5–10 minutes for 3–6 doses Chronic glaucoma: 1 drop 0.5–4% solution every 4–12 hours
Non-Selective Adrenergics	
dipivefrin (Apo-Dipivefrin, Propine)	1 drop 0.1% solution bid
epinephrine (Epinal, Eppy/N)	1–2 drops 0.25–2% solution qd–bid
Prostaglandins	
bimatoprost (Lumigan)	1 drop 0.03% solution qd in the evening
⊖ latanoprost (Xalatan)	1 drop (0.005%) solution qd in the evening
Beta-Adrenergic Blockers	
betaxolol (Betaoptic)	1 drop 0.5% solution bid
carteolol (Ocupress)	1 drop 1% solution bid
levobunolol (Betagan)	1–2 drops 0.25–0.5% solution qd–bid
metipranolol (OptiPranolol)	1 drop 0.3% solution bid
⊖ timolol (Apo-Timop, Timoptic, Timoptic XE)	1–2 drops of 0.25–0.5% solution qd–bid; gel (salve); apply qd
Alpha$_2$-Adrenergic Agonists	
apraclonidine (Iopidine)	1 drop 0.5% solution bid
brimonidine tartrate (Alphagan)	1 drop 0.2% solution tid
Carbonic Anhydrase Inhibitors	
acetazolamide (Acetazolam)	PO; 250 mg qd–qid
brinzolamide (Azopt)	1 drop 1% solution tid
methazolamide (Apo-Methazolamide)	PO; 50–100 mg bid or tid
Osmotic Diuretics	
glycerin anhydrous (Ophthalgan)	PO; 1–1.8 g/kg 1–1.5 h before ocular surgery; may repeat q5h
isosorbide (PMS-Isosorbide)	PO; 1–3 g/kg bid–qid
mannitol (Osmitrol)	IV; 1.5–2 mg/kg as a 15–25% solution over 30–60 minutes

agonists, carbonic anhydrase inhibitors, and osmotic diuretics.

Cholinergic Agonists   Drugs that activate cholinergic receptors in the eye produce constriction of the pupil, known as **miosis**, and contraction of the ciliary muscle. These agents are sometimes called **miotics**. These actions change the trabecular meshwork to allow greater outflow of aqueous humour and a lowering of the IOP. Agents such as carbachol and pilocarpine act *directly* on cholinergic receptors. Demecarium, echothiophate, isoflurophate, and physostigmine act *indirectly* by blocking acetylcholinesterase (AchE), the enzyme responsible for breaking down the neurotransmitter acetylcholine. The indirect-acting AchE inhibitors produce essentially the same effects as direct-acting drugs, except they have a longer duration of action. Because of greater toxicity and longer action, these drugs are normally used only in clients with open-angle glaucoma who do not respond to other agents. The cholinergic agonists are applied topically to the eye. The antidote for serious drug toxicity from cholinergic agonists is atropine or pralidoxime chloride.

Non-Selective Adrenergics   Adrenergics (sympathomimetics) activate the sympathetic nervous system. Dipivefrin and epinephryl borate are non-selective adrenergics administered topically for open-angle glaucoma. Epinephrine produces mydriasis (pupil dilation) and increases the outflow of aqueous humour, resulting in a lower IOP. Dipivefrin is converted to epinephrine in the eye. Should epinephrine reach the systemic circulation, it increases blood pressure and heart rate.

Prostaglandins   Latanoprost is a prostaglandin analog available as a 0.005% eye drop solution, which decreases aqueous humour formation and increases outflow in open-angle glaucoma. Latanoprost is presented in this chapter as a Prototype Drug. Another prostaglandin used in the treatment of glaucoma is bimatoprost. The main side effect of these medications is heightened pigmentation, usually a brown colour of the iris in clients with lighter coloured eyes. These drugs cause cycloplegia, local irritation, and stinging of the eyes. Because of these effects, prostaglandins are normally administered just before bedtime.

Beta-Adrenergic Blockers   Beta-adrenergic blockers are drugs of choice for open-angle glaucoma. These include betaxolol, carteolol, levobunolol, metipranolol, and timolol. These drugs act by decreasing the production of aqueous humour, thus reducing IOP. They generally produce fewer ocular adverse effects than cholinergic or adrenergic agonists. The topical administration of beta-blockers for glaucoma treatment does not result in significant systemic absorption. Should absorption occur, however, systemic side effects may include bronchoconstriction, bradycardia, and hypotension.

Alpha$_2$-Adrenergic Agonists   Alpha$_2$-adrenergic agonists are prescribed less frequently than the other antiglaucoma medications. These drugs include apraclonidine, which is used for short-term therapy, and brimonidine, which is approved for long-term therapy. These drugs produce minimal cardiovascular and pulmonary side effects. The most significant side effects are headache, drowsiness, dry mucosal membranes, blurred vision, and irritated eyelids.

Carbonic Anhydrase Inhibitors   Carbonic anhydrase inhibitors may be administered topically or systemically to reduce IOP in cases of open-angle glaucoma. They act by decreasing the production of aqueous humour. Usually these medications are used as a second choice if beta-blockers have not produced therapeutic results. Examples include acetazolamide, brinzolamide, dichlorphenamide, dorzolamide, and methazolamide. Clients must be cautioned when taking these medications because they contain sulfur and may cause an allergic reaction. Because these drugs are diuretics and can reduce IOP quickly, serum electrolytes should be monitored during treatment.

Osmotic Diuretics   Osmotic diuretics are occasionally used in cases of eye surgery or acute, closed-angle glaucoma. Examples include glycerin anhydrous, isosorbide, and mannitol. Because they have the ability to quickly reduce plasma volume (see Chapter 21), they are effective in reducing the formation of aqueous humour. Side effects include headache, tremors, dizziness, dry mouth, fluid and electrolyte imbalances, and thrombophlebitis or venous clot formation near the site of IV administration.

NURSING CONSIDERATIONS

The role of the nurse in drug therapy for glaucoma involves careful monitoring of the client's condition and providing education as it relates to the prescribed drug regimen. The initial assessment of a client with glaucoma includes a general health history to determine past and current medical problems and medications. The nurse should determine if the client has a history of second- or third-degree heart block, bradycardia, heart failure, or COPD. Antiglaucoma agents that affect the autonomic nervous system may be contraindicated for clients with these conditions because of possible drug absorption into the systemic circulation.

Several preparations used in glaucoma have a potential risk of cardiorespiratory side effects that will occur if the medication is systemically absorbed. Prior to starting drug therapy, baseline blood pressure and pulse should be established. When a beta-blocker is used, the client should be taught how to check pulse and blood pressure before medication administration. The nurse should review the parameters of the pulse and blood pressure with the client and family members and establish guidelines when the healthcare provider should be notified. Because the safety of ophthalmic beta-blocker preparations during pregnancy or lactation has not been established, the nurse should obtain information concerning the possibility of pregnancy or breastfeeding.

A key factor in preventing further ocular pathology is client adherence with the medication regimen. The nurse should determine any factors that could decrease adherence, such as insufficient financial resources, lack of knowledge, lack of dexterity or skill in inserting eye drops, or forgetting the dosing schedule. Fear and anxiety about potential blindness and disability may also be evident in the client diagnosed with glaucoma. It is crucial that the nurse allow the client to verbalize feelings and provide emotional support to the client and family. An explanation of the how the disease can be controlled may facilitate adherence as well as alleviate the client's anxiety.

Client education as it relates to drugs to treat glaucoma should include goals, reasons for obtaining baseline data such as vital signs and tests for cardiac and respiratory function, possible side effects, and safe administration of eye medications.

Frequently the person with glaucoma is elderly, so a caregiver will administer the eye drops or gels. The nurse should review the proper method for administering eye medications outlined in Chapter 8. Following are the important points the nurse should include when teaching clients and caregivers regarding ophthalmic solutions used in glaucoma therapy:

- The client is at risk for falls and accidents secondary to decreased vision. Assess for environmental hazards and simple methods to ensure safety.

- Visual difficulty is often worse immediately following instillation of eye drops as vision may be blurred. Remain still until the blurring diminishes.

- Report side effects including eye irritation, conjunctival edema, burning, stinging, redness, blurred vision, pain,

irritation, itching, sensation of foreign body in the eye, photophobia, and visual disturbances.

- Remove contact lenses before instilling drops and wait at least 15 minutes before reinserting them to allow the medication sufficient contact time with the eye.

- Report any reactions to the medication as well as any possibility of pregnancy.

See "Nursing Process Focus: Clients Receiving Ophthalmic Solutions for Glaucoma" for additional client teaching points.

LIFESPAN CONSIDERATIONS

Ophthalmic Drugs in the Home Setting

Older adults may live alone or with family or friends. Ophthalmic drugs often need to be used at home. The ability of the aging individual to safely administer ophthalmic drugs in the home setting should be assessed. Return demonstration by the client may be critical for the nurse to assess the older adult's dexterity and skill in self-administering eye medications. If needed, seek reasonable alternatives, such as help from a neighbour, family member, or caregiver.

Teaching is critical for positive outcomes in this population. The older adult needs to understand that touching or rubbing the eye can result in infection or damage to the eye. Because vision may already be compromised, the older adult may experience blurred vision that should clear in a reasonable time after using ophthalmic drugs. Caution older adults about trying to drive or even ambulate until this unclear vision improves. Additionally, diminished vision puts the older adult at increased risk for falls. The nurse can assess the home and make suggestions to improve safety.

Care should be taken to label eye medicines to indicate which is for the left eye and which is for the right eye. Scheduling medications around a routine, such as meals, also may help the older adult remember to take the ophthalmic medications as prescribed, increasing the adherence necessary for healing.

Medications should be stored safely out of reach of children.

Pr PROTOTYPE DRUG | Latanoprost (Xalatan)

ACTIONS AND USES

Latanoprost is a prostaglandin analog believed to reduce IOP by increasing the outflow of aqueous humour. The recommended dose is one drop in the affected eye(s) in the evening. It is used to treat open-angle glaucoma and elevated IOP.

ADMINISTRATION ALERTS

- Remove contact lens before instilling eye drops. Do not reinsert contact lens for 15 minutes.
- Avoid touching the eye or eyelashes with any part of eyedropper to avoid contamination from one area to another.
- Wait 5 minutes before/after instillation of a different eye prescription to administer eye drops.
- Latanoprost is pregnancy category C.

PHARMACOKINETICS

Latanoprost is absorbed through the cornea. Onset of action is 3 to 4 hours. It is metabolized to its active form in the cornea, reaching its peak effect in about 12 hours. It is excreted by the kidneys.

ADVERSE EFFECTS AND INTERACTIONS

Adverse effects include ocular symptoms such as conjunctival edema, tearing, dryness, burning, pain, irritation, itching, sensation of foreign body in the eye, photophobia, and/or visual disturbances. The eyelashes on the treated eye may grow, thicken, and/or darken. Pigmentation changes may occur in the iris of the treated eye and in the periocular skin. The most common systemic side effect is a flu-like upper respiratory infection. Rash, asthenia, or headache may occur.

Latanoprost interacts with thimerosal: if mixed with eye drops containing thimerosal, precipitation may occur.

 See the Companion Website for a Nursing Process Focus chart specific to this drug.

Pr PROTOTYPE DRUG | Timolol (Apo-Timop, others)

ACTIONS AND USES

Timolol is a non-selective beta-adrenergic blocker available as a 0.25% or 0.5% ophthalmic solution. Timolol reduces elevated IOP in chronic, open-angle glaucoma by reducing the formation of aqueous humour. The usual dose is one drop in the affected eye(s) twice a day. Timoptic XE allows for once-a-day dosing. Treatment may require 2 to 4 weeks for maximum therapeutic effect. It is also available in tablets, which are prescribed to treat mild hypertension.

PHARMACOKINETICS

Onset of action is 30 minutes. It reaches peak effect in about 1 to 2 hours. Duration of action is 24 hours.

ADMINISTRATION ALERTS

- Proper administration lessens the danger of the drug being absorbed systemically, which can mask symptoms of hypoglycemia.
- Timolol is pregnancy category C.

ADVERSE EFFECTS AND INTERACTIONS

The most common side effects are local burning and stinging upon instillation. In most clients, there is no significant systemic absorption to cause adverse effects as long as timolol is applied correctly. If significant systemic absorption occurs, however, drug interactions could occur. Anticholinergics, nitrates, reserpine, methyldopa, and/or verapamil use could lead to increased hypotension and bradycardia. Indomethacin and thyroid hormone use could lead to decreased antihypertensive effects of timolol. Epinephrine use could lead to hypertension followed by severe bradycardia. Theophylline use could lead to decreased bronchodilation.

 See the Companion Website for a Nursing Process Focus chart specific to this drug.

NURSING PROCESS FOCUS   Clients Receiving Ophthalmic Solutions for Glaucoma

Assessment	Potential Nursing Diagnoses/Identified Patterns
Prior to drug administration: ■ Obtain complete health history including allergies, drug history, and possible drug interactions. ■ Obtain complete physical examination focusing on visual acuity and visual field assessments. ■ Assess for the presence/history of ocular pain.	■ Risk for injury if vision is impaired ■ Self-care challenges if vision is impaired ■ Pain related to disease process ■ Need for knowledge regarding drug therapy

Planning: Client Goals and Expected Outcomes

The client will:
- Exhibit no progression of visual impairment
- Demonstrate an understanding of the disease process
- Safely function within own environment without injury
- Report absence of pain
- Demonstrate an understanding of the drug by accurately describing the drug's purpose, action, side effects, and precautions

Implementation

Interventions (Rationales)	Client Education/Discharge Planning
■ Monitor visual acuity, blurred vision, papillary reactions, extraocular movements, and ocular pain.	■ Instruct client to report changes in vision and headache.
■ Monitor the client for specific contraindications to prescribed drug. (There are many physiological conditions in which ophthalmic solutions may be contraindicated.)	■ Instruct client to inform healthcare provider of all health-related problems and prescribed medications.
■ Remove contact lenses before administration of ophthalmic solutions.	■ Instruct client to remove contact lenses prior to administering eye drops and wait 15 minutes before reinsertion.

continued

NURSING PROCESS FOCUS Clients Receiving Ophthalmic Solutions for Glaucoma *(Continued)*	
Interventions (Rationales)	**Client Education/Discharge Planning**
■ Administer ophthalmic solutions using proper technique.	Instruct client in the proper administration of eye drops. ■ Wash hands prior to eye drop administration. ■ Avoid touching the tip of the container to the eye, which may contaminate the solution. ■ Administer the eye drop in the conjunctival sac. ■ Apply pressure over the lacrimal sac for 1 minute. ■ Wait 5 minutes before administering other ophthalmic solutions. ■ Schedule glaucoma medications around daily routines such as waking, mealtimes, and bedtime to lessen the chance of missed doses.
■ Monitor for ocular reaction to the drug such as conjunctivitis and lid reactions.	■ Instruct client to report itching, drainage, ocular pain, or other ocular abnormalities.
■ Assess intraocular pressure readings. (These are used to determine effectiveness of drug therapy.)	■ Instruct client that intraocular pressure readings will be done prior to beginning treatment and periodically during treatment.
■ Monitor colour of iris and periorbital tissue of treated eye.	Instruct client that: ■ More brown colour may appear in the iris and in the periorbital tissue of treated eye ■ Any pigmentation changes develop over months to years
■ Monitor for systemic absorption of ophthalmic preparations. (Ophthalmic drugs for glaucoma can cause serious cardiovascular and respiratory complications if the drug is systemically absorbed.)	■ Instruct client to immediately report palpitations, chest pain, shortness of breath, and irregularities in pulse.
■ Monitor and adjust environmental lighting to aid in client's comfort. (People who have glaucoma are sensitive to excessive light, especially extreme sunlight.)	Instruct client to: ■ Adjust environmental lighting as needed to enhance vision or reduce ocular pain ■ Wear darkened glasses as needed
■ Encourage compliance with treatment regimen.	Instruct client: ■ To adhere to medication schedule for eye drop administration ■ About the importance of regular follow-up care with ophthalmologist

Evaluation of Outcome Criteria

Evaluate the effectiveness of drug therapy by confirming that client goals and expected outcomes have been met (see "Planning").

See Table 48.1 (page 689) for a list of drugs to which these nursing actions apply.

48.5 Pharmacotherapy for Eye Exams and Minor Eye Conditions

Some drugs are specifically designed to enhance eye examinations during ophthalmic procedures. **Cycloplegic drugs** paralyze the ciliary muscles and prevent the lens from moving during assessment. **Mydriatic drugs** dilate the pupils to allow better observation of retinal structures. These agents include anticholinergics, such as atropine and tropicamide, and adrenergics such as phenylephrine. Cycloplegics cause severe blurred vision and a loss of near vision. Mydriatics cause intense photophobia and pain in response to bright light.

Anticholinergic mydriatics can worsen glaucoma by impairing aqueous humour outflow and thereby increasing IOP. In addition, anticholinergics have the potential for producing central side effects such as confusion, unsteadiness, or drowsiness. Examples of cycloplegic, mydriatic, and lubricant drugs are listed in Table 48.2.

Drugs for minor irritation and dryness come from a broad range of classes including antimicrobials, local anesthetics, glucocorticoids, and NSAIDs. In each case, a range of drug preparations may be employed, including drops, salves, optical inserts, and injectable formulations. Some

NATURAL THERAPIES

Bilberry for Eye Health

Bilberry (*Vaccinium myrtillus*), a plant whose leaves and fruit are used medicinally, is found in central and northern Europe, Asia, and North America. It has been shown in clinical studies to increase conjunctival capillary resistance in clients with diabetic retinopathy, thereby providing protection against hemorrhage of the retina. Bilberry contains anthocyanosides, which have a collagen stabilizing effect. Increased synthesis of connective tissue (including collagen) is one of the contributing factors that may lead to blindness caused by diabetic retinopathy. Bilberry has also been used to reduce eye inflammation and improve night vision. It may be taken as a tea to treat non-specific diarrhea and topically to treat inflammation of the mucous membranes of the mouth and throat.

TABLE 48.2 Drugs for Mydriasis, Cycloplegia, and Lubrication of the Eye

Drug	Route and Adult Dose
Mydriatics: Adrenergics	
phenylephrine HCl (Mydfrin, Neo-Synephrine)	1 drop 2.5% or 10% solution before eye exam
Cycloplegics: Anticholinergics	
atropine sulfate (Atropine AK, Dioptic's Atropine, Isopto Atropine)	1 drop 0.5% solution qd
cyclopentolate (Cyclogyl, PMS-Cyclopentolate)	1 drop 0.5–2% solution 40–50 min before eye exam
homatropine (Minims Homatropine)	1–2 drops 2% or 5% solution before eye exam
scopolamine hydrobromide (Isopto Hyoscine)	1–2 drops 0.25% solution 1 h before eye exam
tropicamide (Mydriacyl, Tropicacyl)	1–2 drops 0.5–1% solution before eye exam
Lubricants	
lanolin alcohol (Lacri-lube)	Apply a thin film to the inside of the eyelid
methylcellulose (Methulose, Visculose, others)	1–2 drops prn
naphazoline HCl (Albalon, ClearEyes, others)	1–3 drops 0.1% solution every 3–4 hours prn
oxymetazoline HCl (Visine)	1–2 drops 0.025% solution qid
polyvinyl alcohol (Liquifilm)	1–2 drops prn
tetrahydrozoline HCl (Visine)	1–2 drops 0.05% solution bid–tid

agents only provide lubrication to the eye's surface, whereas others are designed to penetrate and affect a specific area of the eye.

EAR CONDITIONS

The ear has two major sensory functions: hearing and maintenance of equilibrium and balance. As shown in Figure 48.3, three structural areas—the outer ear, middle ear, and inner ear—carry out these functions.

Otitis, inflammation of the ear, most often occurs in the outer and middle ear compartments. **External otitis**, commonly called swimmer's ear, is inflammation of the outer ear that is most often associated with water exposure. **Otitis media**, inflammation of the middle ear, is most often associated with upper respiratory infections, allergies, or auditory tube irritation. Of all ear infections, the most difficult ones to treat are inner ear infections. **Mastoiditis**, or inflammation of the mastoid sinus, can be a serious problem because if left untreated it can result in hearing loss.

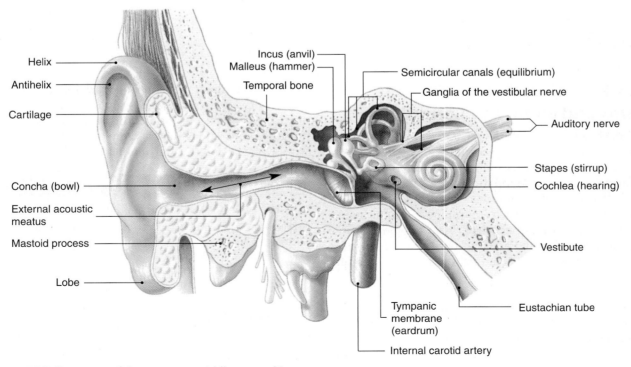

● **Figure 48.3** Structures of the outer ear, middle ear, and inner ear

48.6 Pharmacotherapy with Otic Preparations

The basic treatment for ear infections is topical antibiotics in the form of ear drops. Chloramphenicol is the most commonly used topical otic antibiotic. Systemic antibiotics may be needed in cases when outer ear infections are extensive or in clients with middle or inner ear infections.

In cases of otitis media, drugs for pain, edema, and itching may also be necessary. Glucocorticoids are often combined with antibiotics or other drugs when inflammation is present. Examples of these drugs are listed in Table 48.3.

Mastoiditis is frequently the result of chronic or reoccurring bacterial otitis media. The infection moves into the bone and surrounding structures of the middle ear. Antibiotics are usually given for a trial period. If the antibiotics are not effective and symptoms persist, surgery such as mastoidectomy or meatoplasty may be indicated.

Cerumen (ear wax) softeners are also used for proper ear health. When cerumen accumulates, it narrows the ear canal and may interfere with hearing. This is especially true for older clients and may be part of the changes associated with aging. Healthcare providers working with older adults should be trained to take appropriate measures when removing impacted cerumen. This procedure usually involves instillation of an ear wax softener and then a gentle lavage of the wax-impacted ear with tepid water using an asepto-type syringe to gently insert the water. An instrument called an ear loop may be used to help remove ear wax, but it should be used only by healthcare providers who are skilled in using it. Nurses should advise clients not to perform ear wax removal, especially in children, due to the potential for damage to the eardrum.

NURSING CONSIDERATIONS

The role of the nurse in drug therapy with otic preparations involves careful monitoring of the client's condition and providing education as it relates to the prescribed drug regimen. Before any of the otic preparations are administered, the nurse should assess the client's baseline hearing/auditory status. The nurse should assess the client's symptoms and any current medical conditions. Because the structure of the inner ear changes according to the client's age, the nurse should have a thorough understanding of the anatomy of the ear.

The nurse should obtain information regarding hypersensitivity to hydrocortisone, neomycin sulfate, or polymyxin B. The use of these medications is contraindicated in the presence of perforated eardrum. Chloramphenicol ear drops are contraindicated in hypersensitivity and eardrum perforation. Side effects include burning, redness, rash, swelling, and other signs of topical irritation.

When instilling otic preparations, the ear should be thoroughly cleansed and the cerumen removed through irrigation. The nurse should review the proper method for administering otic medications outlined in Chapter 8. Eardrops should be warmed to body temperature before instillation (but not higher than body temperature). The nurse should administer wax emulsifiers according to the manufacturer's guidelines or healthcare provider's orders.

Client education as it relates to otic preparations should include goals, reasons for obtaining baseline data such as hearing/auditory tests, and possible side effects. Following are important points the nurse should include when teaching clients regarding otic preparations:

- Lie down while instilling chloramphenicol drops since dizziness may occur. Also, do not touch dropper to the ear.
- Administer ear drops at body temperature by running warm water over the bottle.
- With adults and children older than 3 years, the pinna should be held up and back during instillation. With children younger than 3 years of age, the pinna should be gently pulled down and back during instillation.
- Massage the area around the ear gently after instillation to promote thorough administration to the ear canal.
- Lie on the opposite side of the affected ear for 5 minutes after instillation.

TABLE 48.3   Otic Preparations

Drug	Route and Adult Dose
acetic acid and hydrocortisone (Vosol HC)	3 to 5 drops q4h–qid for 24 hours, then 5 drops tid–qid
aluminum sulfate and calcium acetate (Domeboro)	2 drops 2% solution tid–qid
benzocaine and antipyrine (Auralgan)	Fill ear canal with solution tid for 2 or 3 days
carbamide peroxide (Debrox)	1–5 drops 6.5% solution bid for 4 days
ciprofloxacin hydrochloride and hydrocortisone (Cipro)	3 drops of the suspension instilled into ear bid for 7 days
polymixin B, neomycin, and hydrocortisone (Cortisporin)	4 drops in ear tid–qid
triethanolamine polypeptide oleate 10% condensate (Cerumenex)	Fill ear canal with solution; wait 10–20 minutes

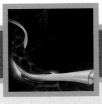

CHAPTER REVIEW

KEY CONCEPTS

The numbered key concepts provide a succinct summary of the important points from the corresponding numbered section within the chapter. If any of these points are not clear, refer to the numbered section within the chapter for review. Expanded versions can be found on the Companion Website.

48.1 Knowledge of basic eye anatomy is fundamental for an understanding of eye disorders and pharmacotherapy.

48.2 Glaucoma develops because the flow of aqueous humour in the anterior eye cavity becomes disrupted, leading to increasing intraocular pressure (IOP). Two principle types of glaucoma are closed-angle glaucoma and open-angle glaucoma.

48.3 General therapy of glaucoma may require laser surgery to correct the underlying pathology.

48.4 Drugs used for glaucoma decrease IOP by increasing the outflow of aqueous humour or by decreasing the formation of aqueous humour.

48.5 Mydriatic (pupil-dilating) drugs and cycloplegic (ciliary muscle–relaxing) drugs are routinely used for eye examinations.

48.6 Otic preparations treat infections, inflammation, and ear wax buildup.

REVIEW QUESTIONS

1 Which components of the eye are specifically affected by glaucoma?

2 Describe two major approaches for controlling intraocular pressure in glaucoma clients. What major drug classes are used in each case?

3 List examples of commonly used drugs for minor eye irritation and injury. What are the major actions of cycloplegic and mydriatic drugs?

4 Identify areas of the ear where microbial infections are most likely. What kind of otic preparations treat infections, inflammation, and ear wax buildup?

CRITICAL THINKING QUESTIONS

1. A 3-year-old girl is playing nurse with her dolls. She picks up her mother's flexible metal necklace and places the tips of the necklace in her ears for her "stethoscope." A few hours later, she cries to her mother that her "ears hurt." The child's mother takes her to see the advanced practice nurse (APN) at an after-hours clinic. An examination reveals abrasions in the outer ear canal and some dried blood. The APN prescribes corticosporin otic drops. What does the healthcare provider need to teach the mother about instillation of this medication?

2. A 64-year-old man has been diagnosed with primary, open-angle glaucoma. He has COPD following a 40-year history of smoking. Is he a candidate for treatment with timolol maleate? Why or why not? Is there a preferred agent?

3. To determine her ability to administer glaucoma medications, the nurse asks the 82-year-old client to instill her own medications prior to discharge. The nurse notes that the client is happy to cooperate and watches as the client quickly drops her head back, opens her eyes, and drops the medication directly onto her cornea. The client blinks several times, smiles at the nurse, and says, "There, no problem at all!" What correction should the nurse make in the client's technique?

EXPLORE
MediaLink

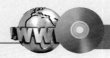

MEDIALINK DVD-ROM
- Audio Glossary
- CRNE Review

COMPANION WEBSITE
- CRNE Review
- Case Study: Client with glaucoma
- Dosage Calculations
- Nursing Process Focus Charts

CHAPTER 6

1 Pyelonephritis is frequently associated with preterm labour in pregnancy. Before initiating antibiotic therapy, the nurse should first determine the client's gestational age. The potential for a drug to be teratogenic is highest during the first trimester. The nurse should also look up the pregnancy classification of the antibiotic. Selected agents, for example, tetracyclines, should not be used during pregnancy. The nurse should address any concerns regarding the drug category with the prescriber.

2 Prior to considering a sedative agent, the client should be assessed for other physical causes of confusion. For example, in the frail elderly, alterations in electrolytes, drug side effects, and rapid environmental changes can contribute to confusion. Attempts at reorientation should be made. Age-related changes that can contribute to altered pharmacotherapeutics include decreases in liver, renal, and cardiovascular function. Thus, the nurse should determine how diazepam (Valium) is distributed and metabolized. Because diazepam is a fat-soluble drug, the drug has a much longer half-life in older adults with increased total body fat. In addition, numerous drugs decrease the metabolism of diazepam and may contribute to an increased half-life and enhanced CNS depression. If sedation is deemed necessary, other drugs should be considered.

3 This question requires the student to go to chapter 8 on drug administration to review techniques for infants (students may wish to address this question after completing chapter 8). The nurse should consult with the prescriber regarding the need to repeat the dose. Many oral elixirs are absorbed, to some degree, in the mucous membranes of the oral cavity. Therefore, the nurse may not need to repeat the dose. The nurse should consider using an oral syringe, which is used to accurately measure and administer medications to infants. The syringe tip should be placed in the side of the mouth, not forced over the tongue. Conditions affecting the GI tract, such as gastroenteritis, can impact drug absorption due to the effect on peristalsis.

CHAPTER 7

1 The purpose of the question is to encourage use of communication skills required for the assessment phase of the nursing process. It is recommended that students consult a nursing diagnosis handbook to support their answers.

The nurse would need to determine that the client's poor eating habits are related to a non-therapeutic environment. One might be tempted to make this initial judgment due to the mother's appearance. Instead, the nurse should determine if other indicators of non-adherence exist; for example, unused medications, missed medical appointments, and other signs of progression of the disease process may suggest non-adherence. The nurse should also determine if the financial cost of therapy is impacting adherence. He or she should also evaluate the type and quality of diabetic education that the client and her mother received.

The nurse should use open-ended questions to encourage the client's mother to verbalize her concerns about her daughter's diagnosis and well-being. He or she should determine if the client's mother has unrealistic expectations about her daughter's ability to manage her disease process (i.e., diet, medications, and exercise).

2 The instructor, depending on what system of nursing diagnosis is being used, could modify this question. The question also assumes that the student has a basic understanding of the pathophysiology of diabetes and the use of the subcutaneous insulin pumps.

Typical client needs would include the following:

* Support in coping with a complex self-care treatment plan
* Sufficient knowledge of condition and medication to manage the treatment plan safely and effectively
* Nutritional information
* Information to reduce risk of infection
* Body image disturbances
* Self-concept disturbances (13 years old)

3 Accountability is the act of being professionally responsible and accountable for one's behaviour. The client has a right to information about drug therapy including the name of the drug, purpose, action, and potential side effects. The nurse is the professional who is responsible for client-family education. Failing to teach can impact the client's ability to safely self-administer medications and may impact adherence to pharmacological therapy. The nurse should routinely integrate teaching as a critical part of drug administration.

CHAPTER 8

1 Medication incidents continue to occur in spite of efforts to prevent errors and increase client safety. The nurse can prevent most errors by following the six rights and three checks of drug administration. However, errors can occur when the client takes drugs or herbal products that are not disclosed to the healthcare provider or an incomplete drug history is obtained. Human errors include misspelling; ordering the wrong drug, dose, and route; entering a drug order in the wrong client's record; and incomplete or inaccurate assessment, such as failing to assess blood pressure before and at peak effect when a drug that lowers blood pressure is being administered. Other factors may include distractions, poor lighting, or other workplace factors.

2 When a client refuses to take a prescribed medication, the nurse should first attempt to discover the reason for the refusal. A common reason for refusal to take a prescribed medication is lack of knowledge regarding the intended effect of a drug, in which case specific information about the drug can be provided at the level the client is able to understand. Sometimes the refusal may be because of intolerable side effects, fear related to previous serious reaction, or allergy to a drug by the client or a family member.

3 IV route has the fastest onset of drug action because the drug is given directly into the bloodstream. Oral, topical, IM, and SC must be absorbed through the capillary wall into the bloodstream and circulated to the site of action. Oral drugs only undergo the hepatic first-pass effect. IM, SC, and IV routes require strict aseptic technique because the skin is penetrated.

CHAPTER 9

1 The nurse should be well organized in preparing for drug administration. The medication administration record must be assessed at the beginning of the shift, and the nurse should develop a systematic time plan (i.e., lists of room numbers and times for scheduled drug administration on the report sheet) that will serve as a reminder of when drugs are due.

In most institutions, regularly scheduled drugs may be administered 30 minutes before and 30 minutes after the assigned time (up to 60 minutes before and after in some institutions), provided this doesn't cause medications to be administered in an unsafely increased time frame. If administered within this time frame, the drugs are considered to have been given "on time." Institutional policies vary and should be consulted.

2 This order as written does not contain an indication for "right dose." Tylenol 3 is a combination drug, acetaminophen and codeine, given orally, and the typical mistake is to assume that the healthcare provider meant for the client to have one tablet by mouth. The nurse should not make this assumption due to the risk of an unintended drug error. Prior to administering the dose, the nurse should consult with the healthcare provider to clarify the intent of the order.

3 A change in prescriptive authority requires an amendment to the act governing nursing practice in the province or territory in which the nurse practises. To learn about this process in your province or territory, visit the website for your professional nursing organization or government.

4 There are numerous persons potentially "at fault" in this scenario. The nurse is ultimately responsible for the dosage error because a quick check of a drug handbook and a simple dosage calculation might have revealed that the dosage was too high. The prescriber was also responsible for writing the wrong dosage; however, the nurse should have notified the healthcare provider to get the dosage corrected. The pharmacist was also responsible for not checking to see that the dosage was correct for the age and weight of the client. There are numerous possibilities for error. Nurses must work within an institution's incident reporting system to ensure that such errors are identified and that mechanisms to prevent subsequent errors are implemented. The nurse is responsible for reporting the error as soon as it is identified to the physician and nurse in charge. It is stressful to make an error, and you could consult the nurse in charge or another respected nurse on your unit to discuss your concerns and get advice about how to manage the situation.

CHAPTER 10

1 The primary concern for this client would be the potential for drug–diet interactions. Warfarin (Coumadin) achieves its anticoagulant effect by interfering with the synthesis of vitamin K-dependent clotting factors. The anticoagulant effect of Coumadin can be decreased by a diet high in vitamin K. Fresh greens and tomatoes from the garden are excellent sources of vitamin K. The nurse must include questions related to the dietary intake of these foods. Consider cultural, seasonal, and socioeconomic factors when assessing diet. It is common for rural people to "eat out of their gardens" during the growing season. The nurse must also determine if other medications have been added to the client's regimen that could interfere with the action of Coumadin.

2 As women age, they experience a 10% decrease in total body water. In general, body weight also decreases in this aging population. Carefully assess the client's current weight and compare it to the previously documented weight. In addition, because body weight has decreased, she may also have a decreased serum protein. Because the dose of furosemide is dependent on the degree of protein binding, less serum protein could make the drug more pharmacologically active. The client may need to have the dosage adjusted.

3 Knowledge of the client's culture and the student's own perceptions and biases can lead to a general discussion about the impact of culture and ethnicity on healthcare. The primary point of any discussion is to emphasize the limited access to care that the culture of poverty creates. This client may be more affected by poverty and a transient living style than either culture or ethnicity in the matter of managing his own healthcare.

CHAPTER 11

1 This question requires information about tamoxifen (Nolvadex). Tamoxifen is a selective estrogen receptor modulator (SERM) that acts by preventing estrogen from binding to the estrogen receptor in breast cells. Therefore, breast cell proliferation is inhibited. Many women assume that because they are taking a SERM, estrogen replacement is indicated. In fact, tamoxifen's effect in tissues other than the breast is similar to estrogen. Tamoxifen does not cause menopause and does not prevent pregnancy. If the client takes a "natural" soy product, this may interfere with the desired action of tamoxifen. Her concern should be acknowledged, but she should be warned not to consume any herbal product without first consulting her healthcare provider.

2 Both garlic and ginseng have a potential drug interaction with the anticoagulant warfarin sodium (Coumadin). It is known that ginseng is capable of inhibiting platelet activity. When taken in combination with an anticoagulant, these herbals are capable of producing increased bleeding potential.

3 The nurse would need to consider the possibility of illicit drug use (and ETOH use, as withdrawal seizures in this age category are not uncommon); however, the nurse should also consider the possibility that the client is using an ephedra product. These herbals are commonly used as dietary supplements for weight loss. Side effects include those seen in this client (i.e., hypertension, rapid heart rate, and seizure). Because these preparations are sold in traditional pharmacies as well as health food stores, many consumers believe them to be safe.

CHAPTER 12

1 The Canadian Centre on Substance Abuse website has information about substances of addiction such as MDMA. MDMA is a neurotoxic agent. When taken in high doses, it can produce malignant hyperthermia, which can lead to muscle damage and renal and cardiovascular system failure. Physical symptoms of MDMA use include hyperthermia, muscle tension, nausea, rapid eye movement, faintness, chills, sweating, increase in heart rate and blood pressure, and involuntary teeth clenching.

2 Aggression is a common psychiatric side effect of anabolic steroid abuse. Research indicates that users may experience paranoid jealousy, extreme irritability, delusions, and impaired judgment. Other symptoms are extreme mood changes and manic-like symptoms even when the user reports feeling "good."

3 The principal danger associated with prolonged use of barbiturates is tolerance and physical addiction. Barbiturates generally lose their effectiveness as hypnotics within 2 weeks of continued usage. This client is demonstrating signs of developing tolerance. He needs to gradually discontinue the drug to decrease the risk of complications associated with sudden withdrawal. These symptoms include severe anxiety, tremors, marked excitement, delirium, and rebound rapid eye movement (REM) sleep. Today, non-barbiturates are usually prescribed as first-line hypnotics.

CHAPTER 13

1 Prazosin is an alpha-adrenergic blocker. The drug's therapeutic action is to dilate peripheral blood vessels and increase blood flow to the client's hands and feet. The pharmacodynamics of prazosin is to prevent norepinephrine from stimulating alpha-adrenergic receptors by blocking the receptors. Because the drug is an alpha-adrenergic blocker, the client should be informed about potential adverse reactions such as drowsiness and orthostatic hypotension. Drowsiness may affect her studies. Evidence that the drug is effective would include warm, normal-coloured hands and feet and increased comfort.

2 Bethanechol is a direct-acting cholinergic agent that works by stimulating the cholinergic receptors of the parasympathetic nervous system. The desired effect, in this case, is an increase in smooth muscle tone in the bladder. Possible side effects would be related to an over-stimulation of the parasympathetic nervous system (such as urgency, nausea, vomiting, and diarrhea) and inhibition of the sympathetic nervous system (such as hypotension, bradycardia, and syncope). Assess vital signs. The drug should be taken on time for increased efficacy and safety.

3 Benztropine is an anticholinergic. Blocking the parasympathetic nerves allows the sympathetic nervous system to dominate. The drug is given as an adjunct in PD to reduce muscular tremor and rigidity. Anticholinergics affect many body systems and produce a wide variety of side effects. The nurse should monitor for increased heart rate, dilated pupils, decreased peristalsis, and decreased salivation in addition to decreased muscular tremor and rigidity. Many of the side effects of anticholinergics are dose dependent. Adverse effects include typical signs of sympathetic nervous system stimulation. Assess vital signs. These drugs are potent and should be taken on time.

4 Isoproterenol is a non-selective beta-adrenergic agonist. Isoproterenol is used as a bronchodilator to treat bronchial asthma and bronchospasm. Stimulation of beta receptors in his heart likely caused his increased heart rate. It is important to assess vital signs and signs of excessive sympathetic nervous system activity. Parasympathetic activity will be decreased. Interventions to enhance the effectiveness and minimize the side effects of this drug include administering the drug on time and providing a calm, supportive environment to minimize anxiety and promote rest.

CHAPTER 14

1 Pain is currently emphasized as being the fifth vital sign. The assessment and appropriate management of pain is a nursing responsibility. A nurse might be tempted to give this client a sleeping medication alone, fearing the side effects that might occur when giving an opioid narcotic in combination. Secobarbital is a short-acting barbiturate. Barbiturates are not effective analgesics and generally do not produce significant hypnosis in clients with severe pain. The barbiturate may intensify the client's reaction to painful stimuli. Administering a barbiturate with a potent analgesic appears to reduce analgesic requirements by about 50%. The nurse may need to consult with the prescriber regarding lowering or titrating the dose of the narcotic.

2 The nurse may immediately recognize lorazepam as an anti-anxiety agent and assume that the purpose of the drug in this case is to control anxiety related to the client's diagnosis and treatment. However, lorazepam also has an unlabelled use as an antiemetic prior to chemotherapy. The treatment modality that will control chemotherapy-related nausea must be individualized.

3 Consider conducting a thorough assessment of the client's sleep patterns. In addition, consider non-pharmacological interventions. In older adults the total amount of sleep does not change; however, the quality of sleep deteriorates. Time spent in REM sleep and stages 3 and 4 NREM sleep shortens. Older adults awaken more often during the night. This can be compounded by the presence of a chronic illness. The alteration in sleep patterns may also be due to changes in the CNS that affect the regulation of sleep. After a thorough assessment, the nurse should discuss age-related issues, health concerns, and environmental factors that may be impacting the quality of sleep.

CHAPTER 15

1 Carbamazepine is a widely prescribed antiepileptic drug. Common side effects are drowsiness, dizziness, nausea, ataxia, and blurred vision. Serious and sometimes fatal blood dyscrasias secondary to bone-marrow suppression have occurred with carbamazepine. The client's hematocrit suggests anemia, and the petechiae and bruising suggest thrombocytopenia. Evaluate the client for complaints of fever and sore throat, which would suggest leukopenia. This client needs immediate evaluation by the healthcare provider who is responsible for monitoring the seizure disorder.

2 This question requires that the student consult a laboratory reference manual. The therapeutic blood level of phenytoin is 10 to 20 mcg/mL. Clients may become drug toxic and demonstrate signs of CNS depression when the serum level is > 20mcg/mL. Exaggerated effects of Dilantin can be seen if the drug has been combined with alcohol or other agents. Dilantin also demonstrates dose-dependent metabolism. When hepatic enzymes necessary for metabolism are saturated, any increase in drug concentration results in a disproportionate increase in plasma concentration level. Priority nursing interventions include alerting the attending physician to the increased serum phenytoin, monitoring vital signs, observing for any change in level of consciousness, and providing for physical safety.

3 Long-term phenytoin therapy can produce an androgenic stimulus. Reported skin manifestations include acne, hirsutism, and an increase in subcutaneous facial tissue—changes that have been characterized as "Dilantin facies." These changes, coupled with the risk for gingival hypertrophy, may be difficult for the adolescent to cope with. In addition, the adolescent with a seizure disorder may be prohibited from operating a motor vehicle at the very age when driving becomes a key to achieving young adult status. Consider the range of possible support groups for this client once she is discharged, and encourage the client to discuss her concerns about the drug regimen with her healthcare provider. The thoughtful nurse will consider the meaning that seizures may have for clients with various ethnic backgrounds and individualize care accordingly.

CHAPTER 16

1 Although many children cope effectively with treatment for ADHD, a 10-year-old Aboriginal boy might be concerned about being "singled out" for therapy. He is old enough at the time of treatment to be aware of his problems in performance. Children who have difficulty in school perceive themselves as being inferior to peers, regardless of cultural group. Aboriginal children may be particularly vulnerable. Children in this age group like to be similar to their peers, and their self-esteem is tied to success in school. This is characteristic of Erikson's developmental stage of industry versus inferiority.

Methylphenidate therapy may be prescribed. It is usually administered twice a day, with one dose before breakfast and one dose before lunch. A child in school may be required to visit a school nurse or a Community Health Nurse in order to receive a dose of Ritalin before lunch. Amphetamine requires once-a-day dosing and may be better accepted by the child and his or her family because treatment can be privately managed at home. Helping the child with ADHD pharmacologically may require the healthcare provider to be sensitive to cultural and social factors.

2 The nurse should teach the client that it might take 2 to 4 weeks before she begins to notice therapeutic benefits. The nurse should help the client identify a support person or network to help assist as she works through her grief. The nurse needs to inform the client that both caffeine and nicotine are CNS stimulants and will decrease the effectiveness of the medication. Also inform the client about the side effects that should be monitored and about the dosage plan. Referral to community resources for bereaved spouses may be helpful. Cultural differences in the time frame considered appropriate for grieving and resumption of activities should be considered when planning care and referrals.

3 The use of any drug during pregnancy must be carefully evaluated. Setraline is a pregnancy category B drug, which means that studies indicate no risk to animal fetuses, although safety in humans has not been established. The prescriber must weigh risks and benefits of any medication during pregnancy. The nurse should recognize this client's risk for ineffective coping as evidenced by her history of depression and help the client to identify support groups in the community. She may be functioning in some degree of isolation from family or other parenting women, which is typical of women who suffer postpartum depression. Identifying culturally appropriate community resources for the client is one intervention designed to provide more holistic care for the client.

CHAPTER 17

1 The client is exhibiting signs of extrapyramidal symptoms (EPS). Initially, the nurse would assess the client to ensure there is no recent neck injury, trauma, and so forth, but if the neck spasms started spontaneously, the nurse would then assess for the possibility that this is due to EPS. The client probably needs to be on a medication such as benztropine to decrease the EPS effects. Teach the client to recognize the symptoms of EPS and to seek medical evaluation when the symptoms occur.

2 The client is elderly, and safety is a priority when taking this medication. Postural hypotension and dizziness are common; therefore, teach the client to move and change position slowly. Constipation is also a concern while on this medication, especially in the elderly.

3 The nurse should initially assess if the client has been taking the medication as ordered or has altered the dose in any way. A client may "cheek" the medication or attempt to cut back on the dose because of the lack of desire to take the medication on a continual basis—especially when the client begins to feel better. It is important that the client understand the importance of adhering to the treatment regime and not adjusting the dose without consulting a healthcare provider.

4 This creates a dilemma for the nurse. The right of the client to refuse treatment must be weighed against whether the client is able to provide informed consent and whether lack of treatment would present a danger to self or others. This requires that the nurse assess the client's condition and whether the client understands the treatment, its risks and benefits, and is capable of making a decision. It is important for the nurse to collaborate with other health team members when uncertain.

CHAPTER 18

1 The client should reassess with a healthcare provider the need for regular Mylanta. This drug contains magnesium, which may cause increased absorption and therefore toxicity. The client needs instruction about decreasing foods that contain vitamin B_6 (e.g., bananas, wheat germ, and green vegetables), as vitamin B_6 may also cause an increase in the absorption of the medication. Teaching should include information about a potential loss of glycemic control (the client is a diabetic) and safety issues related to postural hypotension.

2 A client on benztropine has a decreased ability to tolerate heat. Arizona in July is hot, so the client should be taught to avoid hot climates if at all possible or to increase rest periods, avoid exertion, and notice signs of heat intolerance. When symptoms occur, the client must immediately get out of the heat and rest.

3 The nurse should refer the client and his wife to a healthcare provider regarding the appropriateness of this medication (this is not a nursing function). The couple should be educated about the intended effects of the medication, side effects, when to take it, and safety issues such as postural hypotension and bradycardia that may occur with this medication. Anorexia is also a potential problem—this client is diabetic, and dietary changes may make glucose control more difficult.

CHAPTER 19

1 The nurse does not know how long the client has been hypoxic. The nurse should initially manage the client's ABCs (airway, breathing, and circulation—open airway provide respiratory support) and then stop the PCA pump. Although the nurse will want to go directly to the PCA, it is important to initially manage the patient's airway before stopping the PCA. Stimulating the client (with a sternal rub, etc.) concurrently with managing ABCs and chin lift may rouse the patient and cause him to breathe more effectively. If stimulation and chin lift are unsuccessful, the nurse should call for help. Delegate another nurse to obtain naloxone (Narcan), which is a narcotic antagonist to give the client intravenously in accordance with the agency's protocol for Narcan use. After these initial steps have been completed and the client is stabilized, the nurse must inform the healthcare provider of this adverse effect of the morphine.

2 Sumatriptan is not recommended for clients with CAD, diabetes, or hypertension due to the drug's vasoconstrictive properties. The nurse should refer the client to the prescriber for review of medications and possible adverse reactions related to sumatriptan.

3 The client should be taught to refrain from taking any medication, including OTC medications, without consulting the healthcare provider. This client is on anticoagulant therapy, and aspirin increases bleeding time. The client needs to be taught how to recognize the signs and symptoms of bleeding related to the anticoagulant therapy. The client should review with the prescriber all her medications, with a possible change of aspirin as the anti-inflammatory medication for arthritis.

CHAPTER 20

1 The nurse should question the prescriber regarding this order. Lidocaine is an appropriate choice for local anesthesia, but not if it includes epinephrine. Epinephrine has alpha-adrenergic properties, is a potent vasoconstrictor, and may cause cardiac dysrhythmias in this elderly client. Epinephrine is traditionally not used in the areas of "fingers, nose, penis, toes," as these areas may suffer adverse effects from the vasoconstrictive properties of the drug.

2 The nurse understands that this drug is a depolarizing medication and therefore has the potential to increase potassium release. The nurse is aware that this client is on digoxin and has renal failure, and therefore would not be a good candidate for this drug due to the potential hyperkalemia that may result in life-threatening cardiac dysrhythmias.

3 Digoxin requires careful monitoring, as it may prolong the effects of anesthesia as well as opioids in the client's system, causing depression of the CNS and respiratory system. The client should also be monitored for postoperative bleeding related to the use of ibuprofen. The digoxin concentration should be at a therapeutic level prior to surgery to decrease possible adverse effects of the cardiovascular system postoperatively.

CHAPTER 21

1 Traditionally, anytime a systolic BP is less than 110, blood pressure–reducing medicines should be held unless it has been verified with the healthcare provider that the dose should be given. The client is on a low-sodium, low-protein diet that may contribute to hypotension. Because the client has mild renal failure, the excretion of the drug may be prolonged and may also contribute to the hypotensive effects. If the healthcare provider wants the client to receive the benazepril, then the BP should be rechecked at 30 minutes and 60 minutes after giving the medication. The client should be cautioned about postural hypotension.

2 Atenolol is a beta$_1$-adrenergic blocker medication that works directly on the heart. The nurse and the client need to be aware that the client's heart rate will rarely go above 80 beats per minute (bpm) due to the action of the medication. Tachycardia is one of the adrenergic signs of hypoglycemia that would not be evident with this client. Both the nurse and client need to be aware of the more subtle signs of hypoglycemia (or any other condition that may be recognized by tachycardia) that would not be evident with a client on beta-blocking medications.

3 The nurse must be careful that the client's BP is not lowered too dramatically, or hypotension can occur. This is an example when 120/80 is not necessarily an ideal BP. Typically, the BP is not lowered below 160 systolic—the client is re-evaluated and then (often many hours later) the BP is brought down further. This drip is light sensitive and must remain covered with foil during infusion. Once prepared, the drip is stable only for 24 hours. Nitroprusside is a cyanide by-product; therefore, any client on this drug must be monitored for cyanide toxicity.

CHAPTER 22

1 Atorvastatin may cause muscle damage in some clients. The client taking atorvastatin should be advised to report unexplained leg or muscle pain to her prescriber.

2 This medication has the possibility of causing esophageal irritation, so taking the proper fluids or food with this medication is important. Cholestyramine should be taken before meals with water, milk, fruit juice, or non-carbonated beverages. Fruit juices have a laxative effect and may help prevent the constipation due to the drug.

3 The nurse should advise this client to seek medical advice before self-medicating—especially as this client is a diabetic, and many drugs affect antihyperglycemic medications and blood glucose. Niacin can cause hyperglycemia in this client, and serum glucose should be evaluated. The flushing and hot flashes may be normal side effects of this medication.

CHAPTER 23

1 The nurse should instruct the client to lie down and rest. An expected effect of nitroglycerin is hypotension. The nurse must be cautious in administering NTG to clients whose systolic BP is less than 100 mm Hg. Thus, the nurse should notify the healthcare provider of the client's chest pain and blood pressure prior to administration.

2 Beta-blockers slow the heart rate to a desired 50 to 65 beats per minute (bpm). Many clients suffer from postural hypotension if the heart rate drops below 60 bpm, and therefore the nurse needs to educate the client about the necessity of changing positions slowly. The nurse must be aware that a cardinal sign of decreasing cardiac output is tachycardia—a heart rate >100 bpm for the client not on beta-blockers. If the client is on beta-blocking medication, the heart rate may not go above 80 to 85 bpm and is considered tachycardia for this type of client.

3 Diltiazem has been given to lower the heart rate and to decrease the myocardial oxygen consumption for this client with chest pain. The nurse must monitor closely for hypotension, as this medication lowers the heart rate but also lowers the BP, and this client already has a borderline low BP of 100/60. The client should be on a cardiac monitor with frequent monitoring of BP.

CHAPTER 24

1 The nurse should first note improved signs of perfusion if this medication is effective. The nurse would evaluate the client's skin colour, BP, heart rate, and urinary output. If the medication is effective, all of these will be within normal limits, or at least improved from the client's baseline. The EKG may show improvement by switching to a normal sinus rhythm once the digoxin has reached therapeutic level.

2 The nurse understands that there is a cross-sensitivity between sulfa and furosemide and therefore will inform the healthcare provider of the client's allergy status so a different diuretic can be utilized. Morphine is an appropriate medication for this client not only for its analgesic and sedative effects, but also for the increased venous capacitance that it causes.

3 This diabetic client needs to be educated about the importance of regular glucose checks because this medication may cause the blood sugar to vary sporadically. Typically, hypoglycemia is more of a problem, so the client needs to be especially aware of the symptoms and treatment of hypoglycemia. Safety should be emphasized, especially regarding postural hypotension.

CHAPTER 25

1 Propranolol is a non-selective beta-blocking drug, which means that it not only works on the intended system (cardiac), but also acts on the lungs. This may cause the client to have adverse lung symptoms, such as bronchospasm and shortness of breath; therefore, propranolol is contraindicated for this client, and the nurse should consult the prescriber regarding the order and monitor the client's vital signs.

2 The client should be monitored closely for hypotension, especially in the first few weeks of treatment, and should be taught about postural hypotension. Pulmonary toxicity is a major complication of this drug, so the client should be monitored for cough or shortness of breath. Because digoxin slows the heart rate, as does amiodarone, the client must be monitored closely for bradycardia. Safety and pulmonary symptoms are priorities of care for this client. Amiodarone often increases the effects of digoxin and warfarin and thus must be closely monitored.

3 Bradycardia is a potential problem for a client taking verapamil and digoxin. The client should be assessed for signs of decreased cardiac output, such as pallor, chest pain, shortness of breath, hypotension, and altered level of consciousness. The client needs to be taught to recognize the signs of decreasing cardiac output, as well as how to assess and monitor his or her heart rate.

CHAPTER 26

1 The nurse should question the healthcare provider about this order. No client who appears to be having a CVA (brain attack) should have heparin until a CT scan of the head has been done. Approximately 20% of CVAs are hemorrhagic, and this needs to be ruled out before an anticoagulant is given. The nurse needs to provide supportive care for the client, who may be quite frightened, and his family. This includes information about the diagnostic and treatment plan.

2 The major adverse effect of a fibrinolytic drug is bleeding. All tubes (NG, Foley, ETT), blood draws, arterial lines, and central and peripheral IV insertions need to be done prior to the medication being given, or they may potentiate bleeding in this client.

3 Whether the nurse gives this drug or is teaching the client to self-administer the medication, proper placement in the abdomen is vital. The injection must be given at least 1 to 2 inches away from the umbilicus. There are major blood vessels that run close to the umbilicus, and if the LMWH is given near one of these vessels, there is an increased chance of bleeding into the abdomen or a large (and often occult initially) hematoma forming in the abdomen.

CHAPTER 27

1 A major action of this vasopressor medication is the positive inotropic action that it has on a damaged myocardium that is having difficulty maintaining a good cardiac output (and therefore BP). The drip must be slowly tapered to a point that the BP is well maintained, normally a systolic BP greater than 100. The nurse must never stop the vasopressor drip abruptly, as the client may become acutely hypotensive.

2 This isotonic solution is appropriate for this client. Based on history and assessment, the client is demonstrating signs of being hypovolemic (a heart rate of 122) and requires a solution that will meet the intracellular need. As the client responds to the fluid, the nurse expects to note a corresponding decrease in the heart rate and other symptoms, e.g., weakness, lethargy, and dry mouth.

3 This is not an appropriate IV solution for a head injury client. Once this IV solution is infused into the client, it is considered to be a hypotonic solution that moves fluids into the cells. A client with an increased ICP cannot tolerate an increase of fluid at the cellular level, as this may cause the brain to herniate and lead to death.

CHAPTER 28

1 Chronic renal failure clients often have decreased secretion of endogenous erythropoietin and therefore require a medication such as epoetin alfa to stimulate RBC production and reduce the potential of becoming anemic (or to decrease the effects of anemia).

2 Clients who are receiving filgrastim should have their vital signs assessed every 4 hours (especially pulse and temperature) to monitor for signs of infection related to a low WBC count. The order to obtain vital signs every shift is not appropriate. The nurse should implement q4h assessment of vital signs and notify the healthcare provider of abnormal results.

3 Clients taking this drug need to be educated especially about the GI distress that may occur while on iron supplements. This medication may be taken with food to reduce the potential for GI upset. Constipation is a common complaint of clients on this medication, so preventative measures are required. The client needs to ensure that this medication has a childproof cap and is safely secured, as overdose of iron supplements is a common toxicology emergency for children.

CHAPTER 29

1 The nurse needs to ensure that the client understands the potential side effects related to the anticholinergic effects of this medication. The client (based on age) is at higher risk for urinary retention, glaucoma or visual changes, and constipation. These are common problems for clients who are taking this medication.

2 Although codeine is a more powerful antitussive, it can cause dependence, as well as constipation. Dextromethorphan is a more appropriate choice for this client initially, with codeine syrup as a potential later choice for more severe cough symptoms. Non-pharmacological interventions, such as humidification and increasing p.o. fluids, may be helpful.

3 The client with asthma who is taking a glucocorticoid medication utilizes this as an anti-inflammatory medication to prevent exacerbation of lung problems. As with any steroid, the client's serum glucose must be monitored periodically, as hyperglycemia is a common problem while on this medication. The client should be assessed for other adverse effects such as weight gain, fluid retention, fat redistribution (in the face and upper back), and sleep disturbance (nightmares).

CHAPTER 30

1 The nurse should assess the client for signs of bleeding due to the decreased platelets and for signs of infection due to decreased leukocytes. The client should be taught ways to reduce risk of bleeding (using a soft toothbrush and avoiding falls, etc.) and infection (handwashing and avoiding crowds, etc.).

2 The client needs the protection of this passive form of immunity after an exposure to such an illness. The gamma globulin will act as a protective mechanism for 3 weeks while the client is in the window of opportunity of developing hepatitis A. This drug does not stimulate the client's immune system but will help protect the client from developing the disease. Inform the client of the intended effects of the shot and about the disease.

3 Cyclosporine is a toxic medication with many serious adverse effects. The nurse must understand that this drug cannot be given with grapefruit juice. Clients who take this medication need their kidney function assessed regularly (not because of the kidney transplant, but because cyclosporine reduces urine output). Assess if this client is taking steroids, which are often given concurrently with cyclosporine, as the serum glucose will need to be monitored regularly.

CHAPTER 31

1 This client has many potential problems related to the use of prednisone over a sustained period of time. The primary current concern is the hyperglycemia—an adverse effect of the prednisone that can become serious when the client is diabetic. Blood pressure must be monitored for potential hypertension, which is related to sodium retention and therefore increased water retention caused by the prednisone. The client is also at high risk for infection while on the prednisone due to suppression of the immune system, which is also related to the diabetes. The nurse should explore with the client cultural and socioeconomic factors that may impact diabetes self-care.

2 The nurse should ensure that the client is not allergic to sulfa and then give the client celecoxib for the elbow inflammation and pain. This medication should provide adequate relief of the symptoms. The client should not take acetaminophen due to the related potential liver compromise secondary to the alcohol abuse. The client should not take ibuprofen because of the potential gastric bleeding that may occur (also, the stomach is already at risk because of the alcohol abuse, and the chance of bleeding is elevated due to the potential liver problems secondary to the alcohol abuse).

3 The nurse should advise the client to stop taking the diphenhydramine (Benadryl) and refer him or her to the healthcare provider for advice regarding treatment for allergy symptoms. Diphenhydramine has the potential to increase intraocular pressure in the client with glaucoma and should not be used. This medication also has anticholinergic properties and may cause urinary retention (the client is already at risk related to an enlarged prostate). The client must also be cautioned about the potential for postural hypotension and hypoglycemia while taking diphenhydramine.

CHAPTER 32

1 This client should not be on tetracycline while pregnant because tetracycline is a category D drug that has teratogenic effects on the fetus. Counselling should be provided for alternative sources of care for her acne, as well as the use of drugs when pregnant.

2 The nurse should not give the erythromycin because this medication is metabolized by the liver. An alternative type of antibiotic should be utilized. Otitis externa can also be treated by topical ear drops so that less drug is absorbed. The nurse should explore with the client cultural and socioeconomic factors that may impact healthcare, including beliefs about the meaning of the infection and its treatment. Some aboriginal peoples believe that evil spirits are the underlying cause and employ strategies to remove the spirits.

3 The nurse should monitor the drug levels before and following the third dose. A priority assessment for this client would also be renal function. The nurse should monitor urinary output and urine for protein, the serum BUN, and creatinine on a regular basis. A secondary priority would be hearing assessment, as ototoxicity is not uncommon for clients on gentamycin.

CHAPTER 33

1 As always, the ABCs are a priority for any client and must be considered. The nurse must monitor the client's airway for evidence of bronchospasm and/or decreased gas exchange, such as coughing, poor colour, and decreased oxygen saturation. The nurse must understand that leukopenia is a problem for these clients (related to the amphotericin B and the client's own depressed immune status), and prevention of infection is always a priority. The client's renal status (urinary output, serum BUN, and creatinine) also must be closely monitored, as approximately 30% of clients on this medication suffer renal damage.

2 This client has trichomonas vaginalis, and it must be stressed that her partner should be treated if he is demonstrating symptoms or if unprotected sex is confirmed, otherwise re-infection may occur. Alcohol must be avoided while on this medication, or profound vomiting may occur. It is important to stress that alcohol is found not only in the traditional substances (alcoholic drinks), but also in products such as cough medicine, vanilla, and perfume; at times, even application of perfume that is absorbed via the dermis may cause this vomiting effect.

3 This drug can have profound adverse effects, and the client must be carefully screened as well as educated about this drug prior to taking it. The client must have a baseline physical assessment prior to initiating pharmacotherapy. A priority would be an EKG and blood pressure assessment, liver and renal function tests, and a hearing and visual assessment screening. Because the client may suffer permanent organ damage while taking this medication, baseline information is crucial.

CHAPTER 34

1 Amantadine is an antiviral drug. Explain to the client that he is to receive the drug for prophylaxis of influenza A infection, and about the infection. Because amantadine has anticholinergic side effects such as dry mouth, orthostatic hypotension, dizziness or blurred vision, the client must be taught what signs to watch for and report, and ways to manage the side effects for safety and to increase adherence with treatment. He should be advised to avoid OTC drugs, cold remedies, and herbal products, as many contain ingredients with anticholinergic properties. Plan a method with the client to ensure that the doses are taken as prescribed. Advise the client to immediately report signs of infection.

2 This medication may cause bone marrow suppression. This client is already immune compromised and the potential for leukopenia is high. The client should be taught to watch for any evidence of infection, monitor temperature, and have regular lab tests. The client also needs instruction about the importance of good handwashing and safeguarding against potential sources of infection.

3 The nurse should inform the healthcare provider that the medication needs to be administered over a minimum of 1 hour and the nurse is unable to give the medication as a bolus or "intravenous piggyback" for less than 1 hour. The IV site must be monitored closely while the medication is infusing for potential infiltration. If this occurs, the IV must be stopped immediately.

CHAPTER 35

1 Priorities will include nutrition, safety, comfort, and emotional support. The client needs to be taught strategies for coping with the side effects of the chemotherapy regimen. A major focus would be on the nutritional issues: The client should always take antiemetics 1 hour prior to chemotherapy, eat small, frequent meals, drink high-calorie liquids if unable to eat solid food, and increase fluids if diarrhea occurs, providing the client is not actively vomiting or nauseated.

2 The client and family should be taught about the risk for infection related to immunosuppression. The nurse should stress frequent handwashing, avoiding large crowds, self-assessing temperature accurately at home, and knowing when to call the healthcare provider. Children will be in contact with other children and sources of infection, so hygiene and healthy diet for the children are important. Fatigue is a frequent problem for clients with cancer, and the family with young children will need strategies to assist the mother to obtain rest.

3 The nurse caring for clients receiving vesicant drugs should be familiar with agency protocols for managing incidents that may occur with their use. The nurse should remain with the client and solution and call immediately for someone qualified to bring and use the chemo spill kit. The spill must be cleaned up and waste disposed of per hospital protocols. At no time should the chemo spill be left unattended. The nurse must ensure that any staff who are pregnant do not have contact with the solution or come into the vicinity. Clients and visitors must not come into contact with the spill. While waiting for the spill kit, the nurse may cover the contaminated fluid with paper towels (the nurse must not touch the solution without wearing protective equipment).

CHAPTER 36

1 Regular use of aluminum hydroxide (Amphojel) may cause hypercalcemia—calcium and phosphorus have a reciprocal relationship in that if the calcium goes up, the phosphorus goes down. A client with low serum phosphorus often exhibits signs of increasing weakness. The treatment would be to replace the aluminum hydroxide with a different antacid and take oral phosphorus supplements until serum phosphorus returns to a normal level.

2 The stomach is empty during the sleep cycle, and this is the time when the protective protein peptide (TFF2) is most effective at repairing the mucoprotective lining of the stomach. For the TFF2 protein to reach its maximum effectiveness, the person needs a minimum of 6 hours uninterrupted sleep, which is uncommon in people who sleep during the daytime. Healthy food choices and stress reduction may also enhance healing.

3 This client has a history of peptic ulcer disease and therefore alcohol and smoking are contraindicated, as they will exacerbate the condition. Smoking decreases the effectiveness of ranitidine. Alcohol is a CNS depressant and can cause increased drowsiness in combination with the ranitidine. This client should be advised to stop smoking and drinking alcohol if the PUD is to be resolved.

CHAPTER 37

1 A priority for nursing care is the potential for dehydration. Assess the client for weight loss, hypotension, tachycardia, and fluid/electrolyte imbalance. Administer fluids and electrolytes as ordered. The cause of this ongoing diarrhea needs to be investigated by the physician. Universal precautions are required in case the causative agent is infectious.

2 The client needs to be informed that the prochlorperazine is administered in its own syringe and must not be mixed with any other drug. The nurse could notify the healthcare provider that the client wants a change of antiemetic to one that could be combined with an analgesic and given in the same syringe.

3 This client needs to take a contact laxative to stimulate the nerve endings to facilitate a bowel movement, as opposed to a bulk-forming laxative to promote bowel regularity. The liquid stool may be a result of fecal impaction with only liquid being able to seep out. If this client has ongoing bowel irregularity problems, the bulk-forming laxative may be helpful at a later date. Educate the client to drink plenty of fluids when taking bulk-forming laxatives.

CHAPTER 38

1 The client is experiencing a normal reaction to the niacin but should be instructed to follow up with the healthcare provider for guidance on the appropriate amounts of niacin to take.

2 This client should be advised to see a healthcare provider for guidance on the appropriate doses of vitamins. Vitamin A can cause increased intracranial pressure, which could be the cause of the headaches. Clients need to be instructed on the appropriate amounts of vitamins and about the potential adverse effects—especially when taking megadoses of vitamins.

3 This client needs to be assessed for possible renal calculi. The client is taking 500 mg of vitamin C daily to prevent an upper respiratory infection, but vitamin C is contraindicated in a client with a history of renal calculi, as this may exacerbate the problem.

CHAPTER 39

1 A child with diabetes insipidus will produce large amounts of pale or colourless urine with a low specific gravity of 1.001 to 1.005. A daily volume of urine may be 4 to 10 L or more and may result in excessive thirst and rapid dehydration. Desmopressin is a synthetic analog of ADH. It may be administered intranasally and therefore may be better tolerated by a child. With pharmacotherapy, there should be an immediate decrease in urine production and an increase in urine concentration. The child's mother or caregiver should be taught to use a urine dipstick to check specific gravity during the initiation of therapy. A normal specific gravity would range from 1.005 to 1.030 and would indicate that the kidneys are concentrating urine. The caregiver also should be taught to monitor urine volumes, colour, and odour until a dosing regimen is established.

2 The nurse must be empathetic to the client's father and allow him to express his concerns. He may feel guilty about contributing to his son's current health crisis. Once the client's condition begins to improve, the nurse should assess the father's understanding of the asthma regimen. The father and the client should receive instruction on the side effects of glucocorticoid therapy. Glucocorticoids used for anti-inflammatory purposes can suppress the hypothothalamic-pituitary axis. Abruptly discontinuing a glucocorticoid after long-term therapy (greater than 10 days) can cause a systemic stress response and produce cardiovascular collapse. The father needs to be instructed on the dosage regimen for prednisone, which may include an incremental decrease in the drug dosage when discontinuing the drug. An additional concern the nurse might have is related to the economic needs of this family. Referrals to a resource providing medication financial support would be appropriate.

3 In this situation, the parents need to be instructed as follows:

a. Drug action—stimulates growth on most body tissues, especially epiphyseal plates; also increases cellular size

b. How to reconstitute the medication, site selection, and technique for IM or SC injection

c. Dosing schedule—somatropin injections usually scheduled 48 hours apart

d. Pain and swelling at the injection site

e. Importance of regular follow-up with healthcare provider, including checks on height, weight, and bone age

CHAPTER 40

1 The nurse should first explain that management of gestational diabetes is initiated with diet, exercise, and home blood glucose monitoring. Adherence to prescribed regimens may reduce the client's fasting and post-prandial blood glucose values to acceptable levels. Mothers with gestational diabetes must keep their blood glucose within a very narrow range to prevent the numerous complications that can occur as a result of elevated blood glucose during pregnancy. These complications can range from fetal deformity to fetal macrosomia and its subsequent sequelae. Prepare the client for insulin therapy should diet and exercise fail to maintain control. Oral hypoglycemic agents cross placental membranes and have been implicated as teratogenic agents. Their use is not recommended during pregnancy.

2 There is variation in the absorption rates of subcutaneous insulin among various body areas. It is known that the abdomen has the fastest rate of absorption, followed by the arms, thighs, and buttocks. It is also generally accepted that exercise of a body area can increase the rate of insulin absorption. Rotating from arm to leg to abdomen for each injection will impact glucose control due to the variation in absorption rates. For this reason and also to reduce lipoatrophy, systematic rotation within one area at a time is recommended. The nurse in this situation should review a correct system of rotation for this client.

3 Aboriginal peoples are at increased risk of type 2 DM. Socioeconomic factors (decreased income, education, and living conditions), lifestyle factors (decreased exercise and nutrition), and cultural factors (beliefs about illness and treatment and help-seeking) are among the risk factors. Treatment options may be oral agents or insulin if weight loss and exercise alone are not effective. Seek out and evaluate current resources specifically designed for Aboriginals with diabetes.

CHAPTER 41

1 The student should be able to use this example to help illustrate neuroendocrine control of the female reproductive system. Leuprolide acetate is a synthetic GnRH agonist that acts by stimulating the anterior pituitary to secrete FSH and LH. The pituitary receptors become desensitized, with a resultant decrease in FSH and LH secretion. Consequently, estrogen production, which is dependent on ovarian stimulation, is diminished and the client's menstrual cycle is suppressed. The goal of suppressing the menstrual cycle is to decrease hormonal stimuli to abnormal endometrotic tissue. It is expected that amenorrhea will result, and that there will be a decrease in endometrosis lesions. A decrease in lesions will likely enhance the client's fertility or improve her level of comfort during menstruation. The client will remain on this drug therapy for approximately 6 months. Menstrual periods usually resume 2 months after the completion of therapy.

2 Misoprostol is a prostaglandin that may be prescribed as an antiulcer agent. The drug also has two unlabelled uses, which include cervical ripening prior to induction of labour or termination of pregnancy when used with mifepristone. It is known that prostaglandins have a role in the initiation of labour. This has been demonstrated with the intra-vaginal application of prostaglandin E. Misoprostol is a prostaglandin E analog that has been clearly demonstrated to produce uterine contractions. In this example, the fetus was not tolerating the uterine contractions, and the nurse used correct judgment in quickly acting to remove the drug.

3 Oxytocin exerts an antidiuretic effect when administered in doses of 20 mU/minute or greater. This will result in a decrease in urine output and an increase in fluid retention. Most clients begin a postpartum diuresis and are able to balance fluid volumes relatively quickly. However, the nurse should evaluate the client for signs of water intoxication that include hypertension, drowsiness, listlessness, headache, blurred vision (pappiledema), and oliguria.

CHAPTER 42

1 This client's age puts him at risk for a variety of health problems. Conditions such as renal or hepatic dysfunction may alter the manner in which the drug is metabolized or excreted. Potential impact on clients with coronary artery disease using nitrates has been well documented (e.g., profound hypotension, heart attack, and death). Because the client is requesting a prescription for sildenafil, the nurse should ensure that the history includes the following data:

- Sexual dysfunction
- Cardiovascular disease and use of organic nitrates
- Severe hypotension
- Renal impairment or hepatic impairment, which requires a decrease in the prescribed dose
- Hypertension and use of antihypertensives (concurrent treatment can increase risk of hypotension)

Nurses can be effective in initiating conversations about sexuality. Studies have shown that clients are often forthcoming with concerns about sexual performance when an interviewer is open and professional.

2 According to Erikson's theory of psychosocial development, this young man is in the stage of identity versus isolation. The influence of the family has been replaced, to a large extent, by that of the adolescent's peer group. This young man's desire to be accepted as an athlete and a team member may produce a willingness to "do what it takes" to fit in. In addition, he may aspire to a career in sports and recognizes the need to be in optimum physical condition.

The nurse should inform him about the risks of anabolic steroid use. He may not realize that the use of testosterone in immature males has not been associated with significant increases in muscle mass. This has been documented only in mature males. In addition, testosterone can produce premature epiphyseal closure, potentially impacting this young man's adult height.

3 Finasteride, an androgen inhibitor, is used to shrink the prostate and relieve symptoms associated with hypertrophy. Finasteride inhibits 5-alpha-reductase, an enzyme that converts testosterone to a potent androgen, 5-alpha-dihydrotestosterone (DHT). The prostate gland depends on this androgen for its development, but excessive levels can cause prostate cells to increase in size and divide. A regimen of 6 to 12 months may be necessary to determine client response. Saw palmetto is a herbal preparation derived from a shrublike palm tree. This phytomedicine compares pharmacologically to finasteride in that it is an anti-androgen. The mechanism of action is virtually the same in these two agents. Authorities note no significant adverse effects of saw palmetto extract and no known drug-drug interactions. Just as with finasteride, long-term use is required.

CHAPTER 43

1 Losartan is an angiotensin II receptor antagonist commonly prescribed for hypertension. Because some clients do not respond adequately to monotherapy, Hyzaar combines losartan with hydrochlorothiazide, a diuretic. This combination decreases blood pressure initially by reducing blood volume and arterial resistance. Over time, the diuretic is effective in maintaining the desired change in sodium balance, with a resultant decrease in the sensitivity of vessels to norepinephrine. Angiotensin II receptor antagonists appear to prevent the hypokalemia associated with thiazide therapy.

2 The nurse should carefully monitor fluid status. Because the primary concern is cardiopulmonary, the nurse should assess and document lung sounds, vital signs, and urinary output. A Foley catheter is usually inserted to permit the measurement of hourly outputs. Daily weights should be obtained. Edema should be evaluated and documented as well as status of mucous membranes and skin turgor. Because furosemide is a loop diuretic, the nurse would anticipate a rapid and profound diuresis. Therefore, also observe for signs of hypotension, dehydration, and potassium depletion over the course of therapy.

3 Cerebral edema occurs as a result of the body's response to an initial head trauma. In this case, the client sustained a skull fracture and the trauma of required surgery. The nurse should explain to the mother that mannitol helps to reduce swelling or cerebral edema at the site of her son's injury. The nurse might explain that the drug helps to "pull" water from the site of injury and carry it to the kidneys where it is eliminated. The client's mother should understand that the goal of decreasing swelling is to promote tissue recovery. Nurses must be sensitive to the fact that family members may have severe emotional reactions to a client's injury and need help to focus on short-term goals for recovery when the long-term prognosis is not known.

For additional information on the action or administration of mannitol, consult a drug handbook.

CHAPTER 44

1 Aggressive treatment with loop diuretics is a common cause of hypokalemia. As in this example, hypokalemia can produce many effects including a variety of dyshythmias. KCl is indicated for clients with low potassium levels and is preferred over other potassium salts because chloride is simultaneously replaced.

The nurse administering the KCl must keep in mind several critical concerns to safeguard the client. The primary concern is the risk of potassium intoxication. High plasma concentrations of potassium may cause death through cardiac depression, arrhythmias, or arrest.

The signs and symptoms of potassium overdose include mental confusion, weakness, listlessness, hypotension, and EKG abnormalities. In a client with heart disease, cardiac monitoring may be indicated during potassium infusion.

Consult a drug handbook and institutional policy, and look up the maximum rates for infusing KCl in adults and children.

To prevent potassium intoxication, carefully regulate the infusion of IV fluids. Most institutions require that any solution containing KCl be administered using an infusion pump. Prior to beginning and throughout the infusion, assess the client's renal function (urinary output, BUN, and creatinine levels). A client with diminished renal function is more likely to develop hyperkalemia.

2 This client is dehydrated from an intravascular standpoint, despite her appearance. The client's elevated hemoglobin and hematocrit are one indication of her degree of "dehydration." Most pregnant women present with dilution anemia. This client does not. The midwife recognizes the need to increase the intravascular fluid compartment to promote renal and uterine perfusion.

CHAPTER 45

1 The nurse would anticipate a decrease in the client's spasticity after 1 week of therapy. If there has been no improvement in 45 days, the medication regimen is usually discontinued. In this case, evaluate the client's muscle firmness, pain experience, range of motion, and ability to maintain posture and alignment when in a wheelchair. When spasticity is used to maintain posture, dantrolene should not be used. In this case, the client's spasticity involved only the lower extremities.

2 Leg and foot cramps have anecdotally been associated with tamoxifen, an anti-estrogenic drug. Tamoxifen, which has been shown to reduce the reccurrence of some breast cancers, has been demonstrated to preserve bone density. Tamoxifen has several side effects that impact lifestyle, including the potential for weight gain and leg cramps. Assess several factors before responding to this client's concerns:

- What is the client's activity level? Muscle cramps are associated with muscle fatigue.
- Does she take exogenous calcium?
- Can she tolerate dietary sources of calcium?
- Interventions for leg cramps include the following:
- Stretching exercises before sleep
- Daily calcium and magnesium supplements
- Increasing dietary calcium intake
- Glass of tonic water (containing quinine) at bedtime

This client needs to relate her concerns to the oncologist. A healthcare provider may consider starting the client on quinine (200 to 300 mg) at bedtime. This is an unlabelled use and requires careful client evaluation.

3 Cyclobenzaprine has been demonstrated to produce significant cholinergic activity. Anticholinergics block the action of the neurotransmitter Ach at the muscarinic receptors in the parasympathetic nervous system. This allows the activities of the sympathetic nervous

system to dominate. In this case, the result has been a decrease in oral secretions and relaxation of the smooth muscle of the GI tract. Decreased peristalsis and motility can result in constipation. The anticholinergic effect is also responsible for urinary retention by increasing constriction of the internal sphincter. Discuss non-pharmacological means such as dietary intake of fibre and fluids to manage constipation. Refer the client to his prescriber because the dosage may need to be adjusted or the medication changed.

CHAPTER 46

1 Alendronate is poorly absorbed after oral administration and can produce significant GI irritation. It is important that the client be educated regarding several elements of drug administration.

To promote absorption, the drug should be taken first thing in the morning with 8 ounces of water before ingesting food, beverages, or any other medications. It has been shown that certain beverages, such as orange juice and coffee, interfere with drug absorption. By delaying eating for 30 minutes or more, the client is promoting absorption of the drug. Additionally, the client should be taught to sit upright after taking the drug to reduce the risk of esophageal irritation. Alendronate must be used carefully in clients with esophagitis or gastric ulcer.

If the client misses a dose, she should be told to skip it and not to double up on the next dose. Alendronate has a long half-life and missing an occasional dose will do little to interfere with the therapeutic effect of the drug.

2 Frail elderly clients may be susceptible to hypocalcemia due to dietary deficiencies of calcium and vitamin D or because of decreased physical activity and lack of exposure to sunshine. This client has all of these risk factors. She is uninterested in eating, has physical limitations, and is not able to get out of the house into the sunshine without assistance. Orally administered calcium requires vitamin D for absorption to take place. Because this client does not consume milk, the most recognizable source of vitamin D, she needs to be encouraged to increase her intake of other dietary sources of this vitamin. Vitamin D-rich foods include canned salmon, cereals, lean meats, beans, and potatoes. To promote the effectiveness of calcium supplementation, inform the client about drug–nutrient interactions.

3 The nurse should obtain information about the onset of symptoms, degree of discomfort, and frequency of attacks. A familial history of gout can be predictive due to the fact that primary gout is inherited as an X-linked trait. A past medical history of renal calculi may also be predictive of acute gouty arthritis.

The nurse should ask the client questions about his diet and fluid intake. An attack of gout can be precipitated by alcohol intake (particularly beer and wine), starvation diets, and insufficient fluid intake. In addition, obtain information about prescribed drugs and the use of OTC drugs containing salicylates. Thiazide diuretics and salicylates can precipitate an attack. Also ask about recent lifestyle events. Stress, illness, trauma, or strenuous exercise can precipitate an attack of gouty arthritis.

CHAPTER 47

1 To establish a rapport with the baby's mother, the nurse should first respond to the mother's anxiety. She should validate that the baby's condition is indeed cause for concern and commend the mother for seeking medical guidance. She should consider that the availability of OTC preparations can be a temptation to a young mother who wants only to see her infant more comfortable and relieved of symptoms.

Topical use of corticosteroid ointments can be potentially harmful, especially for young children. Corticosteroids, when absorbed by the skin in large enough quantities over a long period, can result in adrenal suppression and skin atrophy. Children have an increased risk of toxicity from topically applied drugs because of their greater skin surface-area-to-weight ratio compared to that of adults. Ensure that the healthcare provider at the public health clinic sees this client. Once a drug treatment modality is prescribed, ensure that the baby's mother understands the correct method for drug administration. (Severe diaper rash may also be a sign of more serious complications in infants, such as diabetes or neglect; the nurse must consider these as well.)

2 According to Piaget, this 14-year-old client is capable of formal operations, the highest level of cognitive development. A person in this age group is able to think logically and make decisions regarding healthcare problems, as well as being in control of a treatment regimen. To safely self-medicate, the teenager needs information about the medication, its administration, and side effects to anticipate. Teenagers need clear instructions and often respond to a caregiver outside the family as a resource for information.

This client is experiencing GI side effects that are common in doxycycline treatment, as well as with all tetracyclines. Recent studies have demonstrated cases of esophagitis in teenage clients. To develop an effective teaching plan, the nurse will need to assess the client's dosing regimen, as well as current dietary patterns. A teaching plan would include the following:

- Encouraging oral fluids to maintain hydration, even if nausea occurs
- Drinking a full glass of water with the medication to reduce gastric irritation
- Sitting up for 30 minutes after the nighttime dose to reduce gastric irritation and reflux
- Consuming small, frequent meals to ensure adequate nutrition
- Taking the drug 1 hour before or 2 hours after meals to promote its absorption and effectiveness (If nausea persists, however, the client should be encouraged to take the doxycycline with food.)

Taking doxycycline with milk products or antacids decreases the absorption of the drug. Therefore, other remedies for GI irritation will need to be discussed with the healthcare provider.

Birth control should be used if the client is sexually active at this age.

3 This client's presentation is typical of rosacea. To prevent long-term changes in the skin, therapy should be aggressive despite the fact that this client is also of childbearing age. Isotretinoin is a pregnancy category X drug and has a picture of a fetus overlaid by the "No" symbol on the package. Reported teratogenic effects include severe CNS abnormalities such as hydrocephalus, microcephalus, cranial nerve deficits, and compromised intelligence scores.

Teach the client to use contraception while receiving drug therapy and for up to 6 months after therapy is discontinued. She should not begin therapy unless first demonstrating a negative pregnancy test. In addition, teach her to begin therapy on the second or third day of her normal menstrual cycle. Teenagers who are on isotretinoin should anticipate monthly pregnancy tests.

CHAPTER 48

1 Cortisporin Otic is a combination of neomycin, polymyxin B, and 1% hydrocortisone. The technique for instilling this drug applies to most eardrops. Instruct the mother to position her daughter reclining on her side with the affected ear facing up. The mother needs to inspect the ear for the presence of drainage or cerumen and, if present, to gently remove it with a cotton-tipped applicator. Any unusual odour or drainage could be suggestive of a ruptured tympanic membrane and should be reported to the healthcare provider. Next, the mother should be taught to straighten the child's external ear canal by pulling down and back on the auricle to promote distribution of the medication to deeper external ear structures. After the drops are instilled, the mother can further promote medication distribution by gently pressing on the tragus of the ear. The mother should be taught to keep her daughter reclining on her side for 3 to 5 minutes after the drops are instilled. If a cotton ball has been prescribed, the cotton ball should be placed in the ear without applying pressure. The cotton ball can be removed in 15 minutes.

2 Timolol maleate, a beta-adrenergic blocking agent, is contraindicated in individuals with chronic obstructive pulmonary disease, an air-trapping disorder, and may be contraindicated in chronic asthma. This agent has been known to produce bronchospasm by blocking the stimulation of beta$_2$-adrenergic receptors if systemically absorbed. When beta$_2$-receptors are stimulated, relaxation of bronchial smooth muscles is facilitated. In both cases, the beta-adrenergic blocking effect of timolol could be potentially life-threatening. Betaxolol is also a beta-adrenergic blocking agent but is considered safer for use in clients with COPD who require treatment for glaucoma.

3 All ophthalmic agents should be administered in the conjunctival sac. The cornea is highly innervated, and direct application of medication to the cornea can result in excessive burning and stinging. The conjunctival sac normally holds one or two drops of solution.

Following administration of the medication, the client should be reminded to place pressure on the inner canthus of the eye to prevent the medication from flowing into the nasolacrimal duct. This manoeuvre helps to prevent systemic absorption of medication and decreases the risk of side effects commonly associated with antiglaucoma agents.

A-delta fibres nerves that transmit sensations of sharp pain

absence seizure seizure with a loss or reduction of normal activity, including staring and transient loss of responsiveness

absorption the process of moving a drug across body membranes

acetylcholine (Ach) primary neurotransmitter of the parasympathetic nervous system; also present at somatic neuromuscular junctions and at sympathetic preganglionic nerves

acetylcholinesterase (AchE) enzyme that degrades acetylcholine within the synaptic cleft, enhancing effects of the neurotransmitter

acidosis condition of having too much acid in the blood; plasma pH below 7.35

acne vulgaris condition characterized by small inflamed bumps that appear on the surface of the skin

acquired immunodeficiency syndrome (AIDS) infection caused by the human immunodeficiency virus (HIV)

acquired resistance condition in which a microbe is no longer affected by a drug following anti-infective pharmacotherapy

action potential electrical changes in the membrane of a muscle or nerve cell due to changes in membrane permeability

activated partial thromboplastin time (aPTT) blood test used to determine how long it takes clots to form, to regulate heparin dosage

active immunity resistance resulting from a previous exposure to an antigen

active transport the process by which molecules move across the cell membrane against a concentration or electrochemical gradient

acute gouty arthritis condition in which uric acid crystals accumulate in the joints of the big toes, ankles, wrists, fingers, knees, or elbows, resulting in red, swollen, or inflamed tissue

acute radiation syndrome life-threatening symptoms resulting from acute exposure to ionizing radiation, including nausea, vomiting, severe leukopenia, thrombocytopenia, anemia, and alopecia

acute toxicity severe or sudden onset of poisoning

addiction the continued use of a substance despite its negative health and social consequences

Addison's disease hyposecretion of glucocorticoids and aldosterone by the adrenal cortex

adenohypophysis anterior portion of the pituitary gland

adherence taking a medication in the manner prescribed by the healthcare provider, or, in the case of OTC drugs, following the instructions on the label

adolescence period of life from 13 to 18 years of age

adrenergic relating to nerves that release norepinephrine or epinephrine

adrenergics class of antagonist drugs that block the actions of the sympathetic nervous system

adrenergic antagonist drug that blocks the actions of the sympathetic nervous system

adrenocorticotropic hormone (ACTH) hormone secreted by the anterior pituitary that stimulates the release of glucocorticoids by the adrenal cortex

adverse drug reaction (ADR) an undesired response to a drug

aerobic pertaining to an oxygen environment

aerosol suspension of minute liquid droplets or fine solid particles suspended in a gas

affinity chemical attraction that impels certain molecules to unite with others to form complexes

afterload pressure that must be overcome for the ventricles to eject blood from the heart

agonist drug that is capable of binding with receptors to induce a cellular response

akathisia inability to remain still; constantly moving

albumin protein that acts as a carrier molecule in the blood and helps to maintain blood volume and blood pressure

aldosterone hormone secreted by the adrenal cortex that increases sodium reabsorption in the distal tubule of the kidney

alimentary canal hollow tube in the digestive system that starts in the mouth and includes the esophagus, stomach, small intestine, and large intestine

alkalosis condition of having too many basic substances in the blood; plasma pH above 7.45

alkylation process by which certain chemicals attach to DNA and change its structure and function

allergic reaction acquired, hyperresponse of body defences to a foreign substance (allergen)

allergic rhinitis syndrome of sneezing, itchy throat, watery eyes, and nasal congestion resulting from exposure to antigens; also known as hay fever

alopecia hair loss

alpha (α)-receptor type of subreceptor found in the sympathetic nervous system

Alzheimer's disease (AD) most common dementia, characterized by loss of memory, delusions, hallucinations, confusion, and loss of judgment

amide type of chemical linkage found in some local anesthetics involving carbon, nitrogen, and oxygen (-NH-CO-)

amyloid plaque abnormal protein fragments related to neuronal damage; a sign of Alzheimer's disease observed during autopsy

anabolic steroid compound resembling testosterone with hormonal activity; commonly abused by athletes

anaerobic pertaining to an environment without oxygen

analgesic drug used to reduce or eliminate pain

anaphylactic shock type of shock caused by an acute allergic reaction

anaphylaxis acute allergic response to an antigen that results in severe hypotension and may lead to life-threatening shock if untreated

anastomoses natural communication networks among the coronary arteries

androgen steroid sex hormone that promotes the appearance of masculine characteristics

anemia lack of adequate numbers of red blood cells or decreased oxygen-carrying capacity of the blood

angina pectoris acute chest pain upon physical or emotional exertion due to inadequate oxygen supply to the myocardium

angiotensin II chemical released in response to falling blood pressure that causes vasoconstriction and release of aldosterone

angiotensin II receptor blocker (ARB) a drug that lowers blood pressure by selectively blocking angiotensin II from binding to its receptor, which causes vasodilatation

angiotensin-converting enzyme (ACE) enzyme responsible for converting angiotensin I to angiotensin II

anion negatively charged ion

anorexiant drug used to suppress appetite

antacid drug that neutralizes stomach acid

antagonism type of drug interaction in which one drug inhibits the effectiveness of another

antagonist drug that blocks the response of another drug

anthrax a bacterial infection that can cause severe disease and high mortality in humans

antiadrenergic drug used to block adrenergic receptors in the sympathetic nervous system

antibiotic substance produced by a microorganism that inhibits or kills other microorganisms

antibody protein produced by the body in response to an antigen; used interchangeably with the term *immunoglobulin*

anticholinergic drug that blocks the actions of the parasympathetic nervous system

anticoagulant agent that inhibits the formation of blood clots

antidiuretic hormone (ADH) hormone produced by the hypothalamus and secreted by the posterior pituitary that stimulates the kidneys to conserve water

antidote a substance used to block the effects of another substance or drug

antiemetic drug that prevents vomiting

antifibrinolytic drug used to prevent and treat excessive bleeding from surgical sites

antigen foreign organism or substance that induces the formation of antibodies by the immune system

anti-infective general term for any medication that is effective against pathogens

antimicrobial (antibacterial) resistance the development of resistance by microbes to the effects of an antimicrobial drug

antipyretic drug that lowers body temperature

antiretroviral drug that is effective against retroviruses

antithrombin III protein that prevents abnormal clotting by inhibiting thrombin

antitussive drug used to suppress cough

anxiety state of apprehension and autonomic nervous system activation resulting from exposure to a non-specific or unknown cause

anxiolytic drug that relieves anxiety

apoprotein protein component of a lipoprotein

apothecary system of measurement older system of measurement using drams; rarely used

aqueous humour fluid that fills the anterior and posterior chambers of the eye

aromatase inhibitor hormone inhibitor that blocks the enzyme aromatase, which normally converts adrenal androgen to estradiol

ASAP order as soon as possible order, which should be available for administration to the patient within 30 minutes of the written order

assessing appraisal of a client's condition that involves gathering and interpreting data

asthma chronic inflammatory disease of the lungs characterized by airway obstruction

astringent effect shrinkage of swollen mucous membranes or loosening of secretions and facilitation of drainage

atherosclerosis condition characterized by a buildup of fatty plaque and loss of elasticity of the walls of the arteries

atonic seizure very short-lasting seizure during which the client may stumble and fall for no apparent reason

atrial fibrillation rapid irregular heart rhythm originating in the atria of the heart

atrioventricular (AV) node cardiac tissue that receives electrical impulses from the SA node and conveys them to the ventricles

atrioventricular bundle cardiac tissue that receives electrical impulses from the AV node and sends them to the bundle branches; also known as the *bundle of His*

attention deficit disorder (ADD) condition characterized by an inability to focus attention on a task for a sufficient length of time

attention deficit–hyperactivity disorder (ADHD) condition typically diagnosed in childhood and adolescence characterized by hyperactivity as well as attention, organization, and behaviour control issues

atypical antidepressant drug used to treat depression that has a mechanism of action that differs from traditional classes of antidepressants

atypical antipsychotic drug used to treat both the positive and negative symptoms of psychosis or schizophrenia

aura sensory cue such as bright lights, smells, or tastes that precedes a migraine

auto-antibody protein called *rheumatoid factor*, released by B lymphocytes, that tears down the body's own tissue

automaticity ability of certain myocardial cells to spontaneously generate an action potential

autonomic nervous system (ANS) portion of the peripheral nervous system that provides involuntary control over smooth muscle, cardiac muscle, and glands

azoles major class of drugs used to treat mycoses

azoospermia complete absence of sperm in ejaculate

azotemia accumulation of nitrogenous waste products in the kidneys that can result in death if untreated

bacilli bacteria that are oblong in shape; also called *rods*

bactericidal ability to kill bacteria

bacteriostatic ability to inhibit the growth of bacteria

balanced anesthesia use of multiple medications to rapidly induce unconsciousness, cause muscle relaxation, and maintain deep anesthesia

baroreceptor a collection of nerves located in the walls of the atria, aortic arch, vena cava, and carotid sinus that sense changes in blood pressure

basal metabolic rate resting rate of metabolism in the body

baseline data client information that is gathered before pharmacotherapy is implemented

B cell lymphocyte responsible for humoral immunity

beneficence ethical principle of doing good

benign prostatic hyperplasia (BPH) non-malignant enlargement of the prostate gland

benzodiazepines major class of drugs used to treat anxiety disorders

beriberi deficiency of thiamine

beta-lactam ring chemical structure found in most penicillins and some cephalosporins

beta-lactamase (penicillinase) enzyme present in certain bacteria that is able to inactivate many penicillins and some cephalosporins

beta (β)-receptor type of subreceptor found in the sympathetic nervous system

bile acid resin drug that binds bile acids, thus lowering cholesterol

bioavailability ability of a drug to reach the bloodstream and its target tissues

biological response modifier substance that is able to enhance or stimulate the immune system

biologics substances that produce biological responses within the body; synthesized by cells of the human body, animal cells, or microorganisms

bioterrorism intentional use of infectious biological agents, chemical substances, or radiation to cause widespread harm or illness

biotransformation the process by which drug molecules are metabolized and prepared for excretion from the body

bipolar disorder (manic depression) syndrome characterized by extreme and opposite moods, such as euphoria and depression

bisphosphonates class of drugs that block bone resorption by inhibiting osteoclast activity

blood-brain barrier anatomical structure that prevents certain substances from gaining access to the brain

bone deposition the process of depositing mineral components into bone; opposite of bone resorption

bone resorption process of bone demineralization or the breaking down of bone into mineral components

botanical plant extract used to treat or prevent illness

Bowman's capsule portion of the nephron that filters blood and receives the filtrate from the glomerulus

bradykinesia difficulty initiating movement and controlling fine muscle movements

bradykinin chemical released by cells during inflammation that produces pain and side effects similar to those of histamine

broad-spectrum antibiotic anti-infective that is effective against many different gram-positive and gram-negative organisms

bronchospasm rapid constriction of the airways

buccal route administration method in which a tablet or capsule is placed in the oral cavity between the gum and the cheek

buffer chemical that helps maintain normal body pH by neutralizing strong acids or bases

bundle branch electrical conduction pathway in the heart leading from the AV bundle and through the wall between the ventricles

C fibres nerves that transmit dull, poorly localized pain

calcifediol substance formed in the first step of vitamin D formation

calcineurin intracellular messenger molecule to which immunosuppressants bind

calcitonin hormone secreted by the thyroid gland that increases the deposition of calcium in bone

calcitriol substance that is transformed in the kidneys during the second step of the conversion of vitamin D to its active form

calcium channel blocker drug that blocks the flow of calcium ions into myocardial cells

calcium ion channel pathway in a plasma membrane through which calcium ions enter and leave

camptothecins class of antineoplastics that inhibit the enzyme topoisomerase

Canadian Association of Poison Control Centres (CAPCC) an organization that provides a centralized forum for communication, information, and exchange of ideas among Canadian Poison Control Centres

cancer malignant disease characterized by rapidly growing, invasive cells that spread to other regions of the body and eventually kill the host

capsid protein coat that surrounds a virus

carbonic anhydrase enzyme that forms carbonic acid by combining carbon dioxide and water

cardiac output amount of blood pumped by a ventricle in 1 minute

cardiogenic shock type of shock caused when the heart is diseased such that it cannot maintain circulation to the tissues

cardioversion (defibrillation) conversion of fibrillation to a normal heart rhythm

carotenes class of yellow-red pigments that are precursors to vitamin A

catecholamines class of agents secreted in response to stress that include epinephrine, norepinephrine, and dopamine

cathartic substance that causes complete evacuation of the bowel

cation positively charged ion

CD4 receptor protein that accepts HIV and allows entry of the virus into the T4 lymphocyte

cell signalling the transfer of information from one cell to another

central nervous system (CNS) division of the nervous system consisting of the brain and spinal cord

cerebrovascular accident (CVA), also called *stroke* or *brain attack*; acute condition of a blood clot or bleeding in a vessel in the brain

chemical name strict chemical nomenclature used for naming drugs; established by the International Union of Pure and Applied Chemistry (IUPAC)

chemoreceptor collection of nerves located in the aortic arch and carotid sinus that sense changes in oxygen content, pH, or carbon dioxide levels in the blood

chemotherapy drug treatment of cancer

chief cell cell located in the mucosa of the stomach that secretes pepsinogen, an inactive form of the enzyme pepsin that chemically breaks down proteins

cholecalciferol vitamin D_3 formed in the skin by exposure to ultraviolet light

cholesterol a sterol that is synthesized in the liver and is a normal constituent of bile; it is an important precursor in the formation of steroid hormones

cholinergic relating to nerves that release acetylcholine

cholinergics drugs that stimulate cholinergic receptors in the parasympathetic nervous system

chronic bronchitis recurrent disease of the lungs characterized by excess mucus production, inflammation, and coughing

chronic obstructive pulmonary disease (COPD) generic term used to describe several pulmonary conditions characterized by cough, mucus production, and impaired gas exchange

chronic toxicity poisoning that occurs during prolonged exposure to a substance

chyme semifluid, partly digested food that is passed from the stomach to the duodenum

clinical trial testing of a new drug in selected patients

clonic spasm multiple, rapidly repeated muscular contractions

closed-angle glaucoma acute glaucoma that is caused by decreased outflow of aqueous humour from the anterior chamber

clotting factor substance contributing to the process of blood hemostasis

coagulation process of blood clotting

coagulation cascade complex series of steps to stop blood flow

cocci bacteria that are spherical in shape

colloid type of IV fluid consisting of large organic molecules that are unable to cross membranes

colony-stimulating factor (CSF) hormone that regulates the growth and maturation of specific WBC populations

combination drug drug product with more than one active generic ingredient

comedone type of acne lesion that develops just beneath the surface of the skin (whitehead) or as a result of a plugged oil gland (blackhead)

Compendium of Pharmaceuticals and Specialties (CPS) a compilation of drug monographs that are prepared by pharmaceutical manufacturers

complement series of proteins involved in the non-specific defence of the body that promote antigen destruction

complementary and alternative medicine (CAM) system of medicine that considers the health of the whole person and promotes disease prevention

complementary and alternative therapies treatments considered outside the realm of conventional Western medicine

conjugate side chain that, during metabolism, makes drugs more water soluble and more easily excreted by the kidney

constipation infrequent passage of abnormally hard and dry stools

continuing order an order for a drug to be administered at prescribed intervals over a period of days or weeks

contractility the strength by which the myocardial fibres contract

controlled substance in the United States, a drug whose use is restricted by the Comprehensive Drug Abuse Prevention and Control Act; in Canada, a drug subject to guidelines outlined in Part III, Schedule G of the Canadian Food and Drugs Act

conventional (typical) antipsychotic a drug that is used to treat the positive symptoms of schizophrenia

convulsion uncontrolled muscle contractions or spasms that occur in the face, torso, arms, or legs

coronary arterial bypass graft (CABG) surgical procedure performed to restore blood flow to the myocardium by using a section of the saphenous vein or internal mammary artery to go around the obstructed coronary artery

coronary artery disease (CAD) narrowing of the coronary arteries, usually as a result of atherosclerosis

corpora cavernosa tissues in the penis that fill with blood during an erection

corpus luteum ruptured follicle that remains in the ovary after ovulation and secretes progestins

corpus striatum area of the brain responsible for unconscious muscle movement; a point of contact for neurons projecting from the substantia nigra

Crohn's disease chronic inflammatory bowel disease affecting the ileum and sometimes the colon

cross-tolerance situation in which tolerance to one drug makes the client tolerant to another drug

crystalloid type of IV fluid resembling blood plasma minus proteins, which is capable of crossing membranes

culture set of beliefs, values, religious rituals, and customs shared by a group of people

culture and sensitivity testing laboratory exam used to identify bacteria and to determine which antibiotic is most effective

Cushing's syndrome condition of having too much corticosteroid in the blood, caused by excessive secretion by the adrenal glands or by overdosage with corticosteroid medication

cyclooxygenase (COX-1, COX-2) key enzyme in the prostaglandin metabolic pathway that is blocked by ASA and other NSAIDs

cycloplegic drug drug that relaxes or temporarily paralyzes ciliary muscles and causes blurred vision

cytokine chemical produced by white blood cells, such as interleukins, leukotrienes, interferon, and tumour necrosis factor, that guides the immune response

cytotoxic T cell lymphocyte responsible for cell-mediated immunity that kills target cells directly or by secreting cytokines

date rape drug the use of a drug to facilitate forced or involuntary sexual intercourse

deep vein thrombosis (DVT) the formation of a blood clot in a deep vein such as the femoral vein or the popliteal vein

defecation evacuation of the colon; bowel movement

delusion false idea or belief not founded in reality

dementia degenerative disorder characterized by progressive memory loss, confusion, and the inability to think or communicate effectively

dependence strong physiological or psychological need for a substance

depolarization reversal of the plasma membrane charge such that the inside is made less negative

depression disorder characterized by depressed mood, lack of energy, sleep disturbances, abnormal eating patterns, and feelings of despair, guilt, and misery

dermatitis inflammatory condition of the skin characterized by itching and scaling

dermatophytic characteristic of a superficial fungal infection

designer drug substance produced in a laboratory and intended to mimic the effects of other psychoactive controlled substances

diabetes insipidus condition characterized by excessive urination due to lack of secretion of antidiuretic hormone

diabetic ketoacidosis (DKA) type of metabolic acidosis due to an excess of ketone bodies; most often occurring when diabetes mellitus is uncontrolled

diagnosing the process of identifying clients' needs or problems based on analysis of assessment findings

diarrhea abnormal frequency and liquidity of bowel movements

diastolic pressure blood pressure during the relaxation phase of heart activity

dietary fibre ingested substance that is neither digested nor absorbed that contributes to the fecal mass

dietary reference intakes (DRIs) the nutrient values that guide decision-making on nutrition policies and programs to promote the health of Canadians

diffusion the tendency of molecules to move from a region of high concentration to a region of lower concentration

digestion the process by which the body breaks down ingested food into small molecules that can be absorbed

distal tubule portion of the nephron that collects filtrate from the loop of Henle

distribution the process of transporting drugs throughout the body

diuretic substance that increases urine output

dopamine D$_2$-receptor receptor for dopamine in the basal nuclei of the brain that is associated with schizophrenia and antipsychotic drugs

drug general term for any substance capable of producing biological responses in the body

Drug Identification Number (DIN) a unique number located on the label of a prescription or over-the-counter drug product that has been evaluated by the Therapeutic Products Directorate (TPD) and approved for sale in Canada

Drug Product Database a database maintained by Health Canada that contains product and company information on drug products marketed in Canada

drug-protein complex drug bound reversibly to plasma proteins, particularly albumin, that makes the drug unavailable for distribution to body tissues

dry powder inhaler (DPI) device used to convert a solid drug to a fine powder for the purpose of inhalation

duodenum first section of the small intestine

dysentery severe diarrhea that may include bleeding

dysfunctional uterine bleeding hemorrhage that occurs at abnormal times or in excessive quantity during the menstrual cycle

dyslipidemia abnormal (excess or deficient) levels of lipoproteins in the blood

dysrhythmia abnormality in cardiac rhythm

dystonia severe muscle spasms, particularly of the back, neck, tongue, and face; characterized by abnormal tension starting in one area of the body and progressing to other areas

ectopic foci/pacemakers cardiac tissue outside the normal cardiac conduction pathway that generates action potentials

eczema skin disorder with unexplained symptoms of inflammation, itching, and scaling; also called *atopic dermatitis*

efficacy ability of a drug to produce a desired response

electrocardiogram (ECG, EKG) device that records the electrical activity of the heart

electroconvulsive therapy (ECT) treatment used to treat serious and life-threatening mood disorders in patients who are unresponsive to pharmacotherapy

electroencephalogram (EEG) diagnostic test that records brainwaves through electrodes attached to the scalp

electrolytes charged substances in the blood such as sodium, potassium, calcium, chloride, and phosphate

embolus blood clot carried in the bloodstream

emesis vomiting

emetic drug used to induce vomiting

emphysema terminal lung disease characterized by permanent dilation of the alveoli

endogenous opioid chemical produced naturally within the body that decreases or eliminates pain; closely resembles the actions of morphine

endometriosis presence of endometrial tissue in non-uterine locations such as the pelvis and ovaries; common cause of infertility

endothelium inner lining of a blood vessel

enteral nutrition nutrients supplied orally or by feeding tube

enteral route administration method in which drugs are given orally, including through nasogastric or gastrostomy tubes

enteric-coated having a hard, waxy coating designed to dissolve in the alkaline environment of the small intestine

enterohepatic recirculation recycling of drugs and other substances by the circulation of bile through the intestine and liver

enzyme induction process in which a drug changes the function of the hepatic microsomal enzymes and increases metabolic activity in the liver

epilepsy disorder of the CNS characterized by seizures and/or convulsions

ergocalciferol activated form of vitamin D

ergosterol lipid substance in fungal cell membranes

erythema redness associated with skin irritation

erythrocytic stage phase in malaria during which infected red blood cells rupture, releasing merozoites and causing fever and chills

erythropoietin hormone secreted by the kidney that regulates the process of red blood cell formation, or erythropoiesis

esophageal reflux backward flow of stomach contents into the esophagus

ester type of chemical linkage found in some local anesthetics involving carbon and oxygen (-CO-O-)

estrogen class of steroid sex hormone secreted by the ovary

estrogen replacement therapy (ERT) a treatment for women who are post-menopausal or whose ovaries have been damaged or removed that involves taking the hormone estrogen on a regular basis to replace their own

ethics branch of philosophy that deals with distinguishing between right and wrong and the moral consequences of human actions

ethnic having a common history and similar genetic heritage

evaluating systematic, objective assessment of the effectiveness and impact of interventions

excoriation condition in which scratches that break the skin surface fill with blood or serous fluid to form crusty scales

excretion process of removing substances from the body

exocrine glands that excrete hormones to the epithelial surface

expectorant drug used to increase bronchial secretions

exposure contact with an agent that is able to cause disease or injury such as a microbe, a chemical, or the radioactive source

external otitis inflammation of the outer ear; commonly called *swimmer's ear*

extracellular fluid (ECF) compartment body fluid lying outside of cells, which includes plasma and interstitial fluid

extrapyramidal signs (EPS) symptoms of acute dystonia, akathisia, Parkinsonism, and tardive dyskinesia often caused by antipsychotic drugs

febrile seizure tonic-clonic motor activity lasting 1 to 2 minutes with rapid return of consciousness that occurs in conjunction with elevated body temperature

ferritin one of two protein complexes that maintains iron stores inside cells (hemosiderin is the other)

fetal-placental barrier special anatomical structure that inhibits many chemicals and drugs from entering the fetus

fibrin insoluble protein formed from fibrinogen by the action of thrombin in the blood clotting process

fibrinogen blood protein that is converted to fibrin by the action of thrombin in the blood coagulation process

fibrinolysis removal of a blood clot

fight-or-flight response characteristic set of signs and symptoms produced when the sympathetic nervous system is activated

filtrate fluid in the nephron that was filtered by Bowman's capsule

first-pass effect mechanism whereby drugs are absorbed across the intestinal wall and enter the hepatic portal circulation

folic acid (folate) B vitamin that is a coenzyme in protein and nucleic acid metabolism

follicle-stimulating hormone (FSH) hormone secreted by the anterior pituitary gland that regulates sperm or egg production

follicular cell cell in the thyroid gland that secretes thyroid hormone

formulary list of drugs and drug recipes commonly used by pharmacists

Frank-Starling law the greater the degree of stretch on the myocardial fibres, the greater will be the force by which they contract

frequency distribution curve graphical representation that illustrates inter-individual variability in responses to drugs

fungi kingdom of organisms that includes mushrooms, yeasts, and moulds

gamma-aminobutyric acid (GABA) neurotransmitter in the CNS

ganglion collection of neuron cell bodies located outside the CNS

gastroesophageal reflux disease (GERD) condition characterized by regurgitation of stomach contents into the esophagus

general anesthesia medically induced condition of unconsciousness and loss of sensation throughout the entire body

generalized anxiety disorder (GAD) difficult to control, excessive anxiety that lasts 6 months or more, focuses on a variety of life events, and interferes with normal day-to-day functions

generalized seizure seizure that travels throughout the entire brain

generic name non-proprietary name of a drug assigned by the government

genetic polymorphism change in enzyme structure and function due to mutation of the encoding gene

glaucoma a group of eye diseases characterized by increased intraocular pressure, leading to atrophy of the optic nerve and possibly blindness

glucocorticoids class of hormones secreted by the adrenal cortex that help the body respond to stress

glycoprotein IIb/IIIa enzyme that binds fibrinogen and von Willebrand's factor to begin platelet aggregation and blood coagulation

goal any object or objective that the client or nurse seeks to attain or achieve

gonadotropin-releasing hormone (GnRH) a hormone secreted by the hypothalamus that stimulates the secretion of follicle-stimulating hormone (FSH) and luteinizing hormone (LH)

gout metabolic disorder characterized by the accumulation of uric acid in the bloodstream or joint cavities

graded dose-response relationship between the client's response and different doses of a drug

gram negative describes bacteria that do not retain a purple stain because they have an outer envelope

gram positive describes bacteria that stain purple because they have no outer envelope

Graves' disease syndrome caused by hypersecretion of thyroid hormone

growth fraction ratio of the number of replicating cells to resting cells in a tumour

H^+, K^+-ATPase enzyme responsible for pumping acid to the mucosal surface of the stomach

H_1-receptor site located on smooth muscle cells in the bronchial tree and blood vessels that is stimulated by histamine to produce bronchodilation and vasodilation

H_2-receptor site located on cells of the digestive system that is stimulated by histamine to produce gastric acid

H_2-receptor antagonist drug that inhibits the effects of histamine at its receptors in the gastrointestinal tract

hallucination seeing, hearing, or feeling something that is not real

Health Canada federal department responsible for helping the people of Canada maintain and improve their health

heart failure (HF) disease in which the heart muscle cannot contract with sufficient force to meet the body's metabolic needs

Helicobacter pylori bacterium associated with a large percentage of peptic ulcer disease

helminth type of flat, round, or segmented worm

helper T cell lymphocyte that coordinates both the humoral and cell-mediated immune responses and that is the target of the human immunodeficiency virus

hematopoiesis process of blood cell production, which begins with primitive stem cells that reside in bone marrow

hemophilia hereditary lack of a specific blood clotting factor

hemorrhagic stroke type of stroke caused by bleeding from a blood vessel in the brain

hemosiderin one of two protein complexes that maintains iron stores inside cells (ferritin is the other)

hemostasis the slowing or stopping of blood flow

hepatic microsomal enzyme system as it relates to pharmacotherapy, liver enzymes that inactivate drugs and accelerate their excretion; sometimes called the P450 system

hepatitis viral infection of the liver

herb plant with a soft stem that is used for healing or as a seasoning

high-density lipoprotein (HDL) lipid-carrying particle in the blood that contains high amounts of protein and lower amounts of cholesterol; considered to be "good" cholesterol

highly active antiretroviral therapy (HAART) drug therapy for HIV infection which includes high doses of multiple medications that are given concurrently

hippocampus part of the limbic system of the brain that is responsible for learning and memory

histamine chemical released by mast cells in response to an antigen that causes dilation of blood vessels, bronchoconstriction, tissue swelling, and itching

HIV-AIDS acronym for human immunodeficiency virus-acquired immune deficiency syndrome; characterized by profound immunosuppression that leads to opportunistic infections and malignancies not commonly found in clients with functioning immune defences

HMG-CoA reductase primary enzyme in the biochemical pathway for the synthesis of cholesterol

holistic viewing a person as an integrated biological, psychosocial, cultural, communicating whole, existing and functioning within the communal environment

hormone chemical secreted by endocrine glands that acts as a chemical messenger to affect homeostasis

hormone replacement therapy (HRT) drug therapy consisting of estrogen and progestin combinations that is used to treat symptoms associated with menopause

host flora normal microorganisms found in or on a client

household system of measurement older system of measurement using teaspoons, tablespoons, and cups

humoral immunity branch of the immune system that produces antibodies

hypercholesterolemia high levels of cholesterol in the blood

hyperemia increase in blood supply to a body part or tissue space causing swelling, redness, and pain

hyperglycemic effect the tendency of a drug or substance to cause an increase in blood glucose

hyperkalemia high potassium level in the blood

hyperlipidemia excess amount of lipids in the blood

hypernatremia high sodium level in the blood

hyperosmolar non-ketotic coma (HNKC) life-threatening metabolic condition that occurs in people with type 2 diabetes

hypertension high blood pressure

hypervitaminosis excess intake of vitamins

hypnotic drug that causes sleep

hypoglycemic effect the tendency of a drug or substance to cause a decrease in blood glucose

hypogonadism below normal secretion of the steroid sex hormones

hypokalemia low potassium level in the blood

hyponatremia low sodium level in the blood

hypovolemic shock type of shock caused by loss of fluids such as occurs during hemorrhage, extensive burns, or severe vomiting or diarrhea

idiosyncratic response unpredictable and unexplained drug reaction

ileum third portion of the small intestine extending from the jejunum to the ileocecal valve

illusion distorted perception of actual sensory stimuli

immune response specific reaction of the body to foreign agents involving B and/or T lymphocytes

immunosuppressant any drug, chemical, or physical agent that lowers the immune defence mechanisms of the body

implementing the step of the nursing process in which actual client care is provided

impotence inability to obtain or sustain an erection; also called *erectile dysfunction*

infancy period of childhood under the age of 1 year

infertility inability to become pregnant after at least 1 year of frequent, unprotected intercourse

inflammation non-specific body defence that occurs in response to an injury or antigen

influenza common viral infection; often called *flu*

inotropic agent drug or chemical that changes the force of contraction of the heart

insomnia inability to fall asleep or stay asleep

insulin resistance the condition in which normal amounts of insulin are inadequate to produce a normal insulin response from fat, muscle, and liver cells

interferon type of cytokine secreted by T cells in response to antigens to protect uninfected cells

interleukin type of cytokine synthesized by lymphocytes, monocytes, macrophages, and certain other cells that enhances the capabilities of the immune system

intermittent claudication condition caused by insufficient blood flow to skeletal muscles in the lower limbs, resulting in ischemia of skeletal muscles and severe pain on walking, especially in calf muscles

International System of Units (SI) an internationally standardized system of units of measurement

intracellular fluid (ICF) compartment body fluid that is inside cells; accounts for about two-thirds of the total body water

intracellular parasite infectious microbe that lives inside host cells

intradermal (ID) administration method that delivers the drug into the dermis layer of the skin

intramuscular (IM) administration method that delivers the drug into specific muscles

intravenous (IV) administration method that delivers the drugs and fluids directly into the bloodstream

intrinsic factor chemical substance secreted by the parietal cells in the stomach that is essential for the absorption of vitamin B_{12}

ionizing radiation radiation that is highly penetrating and can cause serious biological effects

irritable bowel syndrome (IBS) inflammatory disease of the small or large intestine, characterized by intense abdominal cramping and diarrhea

islets of Langerhans cell clusters in the pancreas responsible for the secretion of insulin and glucagon

jejunum middle portion of small intestine between the duodenum and the ileum

kappa receptor type of opioid receptor

keratolytic action that promotes shedding of old skin

keto acid acidic waste product of lipid metabolism that lowers the pH of the blood

latent phase of HIV infection period during which there are no symptoms

laxative drug that promotes defecation

lecithin phospholipid that is an important component of cell membranes

leukotriene chemical mediator of inflammation stored and released by mast cells with effects similar to those of histamine

libido interest in sexual activity

ligand any chemical that binds to a specific receptor site

limbic system area of the brain responsible for emotion, learning, memory, motivation, and mood

lipoatrophy decrease of subcutaneous fat at an insulin injection site, resulting in an indenture

lipoprotein substance carrying lipids in the bloodstream that is composed of proteins bound to fat

liposome small sac of lipid designed to carry drugs inside it

loading dose comparatively large dose given at the beginning of treatment to rapidly obtain the therapeutic effect of a drug

local anesthesia loss of sensation to a limited part of the body without loss of consciousness

loop of Henle portion of the nephron between the proximal and distal tubules

low-density lipoprotein (LDL) lipid-carrying particle that contains relatively low amounts of protein and high amounts of cholesterol; considered to be "bad" cholesterol

low molecular weight heparin (LMWH) drug closely resembling heparin that inhibits blood clotting

luteinizing hormone (LH) secreted by the pituitary gland, triggers ovulation in the female and stimulates sperm production in the male

macromineral inorganic compound needed by the body in amounts of 100 mg or more daily

maintenance dose dose that keeps the plasma drug concentration continuously in the therapeutic range

major depressive episode a period of pronounced and intense low mood that lasts for more than two weeks

malaria tropical disease characterized by severe fever and chills caused by the protozoan *Plasmodium*

mania condition characterized by an expressive, impulsive, excitable, and overreactive nature

mast cell connective tissue cell located in tissue spaces that releases histamine following injury

mastoiditis inflammation of the mastoid sinus

mechanism of action how a drug exerts its effects

median effective dose (ED_{50}) dose required to produce a specific therapeutic response in 50% of a group of people

median lethal dose (LD_{50}) often determined in preclinical trials, the dose of drug that will be lethal in 50% of a group of animals

median toxicity dose (TD_{50}) dose that will produce a given toxicity in 50% of a group of people

medication drug that is considered medically therapeutic

medication administration record (MAR) documentation of all pharmacotherapies received by the client

medication error any preventable event that may cause or lead to inappropriate medication use or client harm while the medication is in the control of the healthcare provider, client, or consumer

menopause period of time when females stop secreting estrogen and menstrual cycles cease

merozoite a body formed by segmentation and breaking up of a schizont that is capable of invading other corpuscles

metabolism total of all biochemical reactions in the body

metastasis travel of cancer cells from their original site to distant tissue

metered dose inhaler (MDI) device used to deliver a precise amount of drug to the respiratory system

methadone maintenance treatment of opioid dependence by using methadone

methylxanthine chemical derivative of caffeine

metric system of measurement most common system of drug measurement that uses grams and litres

micromineral (trace mineral) inorganic compound needed by the body in amounts of 20 mg or less daily

middle adulthood period of life from 40 to 65 years of age

migraine severe headache often preceded by auras that may include nausea and vomiting

minimum effective concentration amount of drug required to produce a therapeutic effect

miosis constriction of the pupil

miotic drug that causes pupil constriction

monoamine oxidase (MAO) enzyme that destroys norepinephrine in the nerve terminal

monoamine oxidase (MAO) inhibitor drug inhibiting monoamine oxidase, an enzyme that terminates the actions of neurotransmitters such as dopamine, norepinephrine, epinephrine, and serotonin

mood disorder condition characterized by changes in mood such as clinical depression, emotional swings, or manic depression

mood stabilizer drug that moderates mood that is used to treat bipolar disorder and mania

mu receptor type of opioid receptor

mucolytic drug used to loosen thick mucus

mucosa inner lining of the alimentary canal that provides a surface area for the various acids, bases, and enzymes to break down food

muscarinic type of cholinergic receptor found in smooth muscle, cardiac muscle, and glands

muscle spasm involuntary contractions of a muscle or group of muscles that become tightened, develop a fixed pattern of resistance, and result in a diminished level of functioning

mutation permanent, inheritable change to DNA

myasthenia gravis motor disorder caused by a destruction of nicotinic receptors on skeletal muscles and characterized by profound muscular fatigue

mycoses diseases caused by fungi

mydriatic drug that causes pupil dilation

myocardial infarction (MI) ischemia and necrosis of cardiac muscle caused by a blood clot blocking a portion of a coronary artery

myocardial ischemia lack of blood supply to the myocardium due to a constriction or obstruction of a blood vessel

myoclonic seizure seizure characterized by brief, sudden contractions of a group of muscles

myxedema condition caused by insufficient secretion of thyroid hormone

nadir the lowest concentration of blood cells found after taking a drug that suppresses the bone marrow

narcotic natural or synthetic drug related to morphine; may be used as a broader legal term referring to hallucinogens, CNS stimulants, marijuana, and other illegal drugs

narrow-spectrum antibiotic anti-infective that is effective against only one or a small number of organisms

National Emergency Stockpile System (NESS) the program within the Public Health Agency of Canada responsible for maintaining sufficient quantities of supplies to alleviate pain and suffering and to save the lives of Canadians and others affected by natural and human-caused disasters

natural health product (NHP) a product that does not require a prescription and is a vitamin, mineral, herbal remedy, homeopathic medicine, traditional Chinese medicine, or other traditional medicine; a probiotic; or another product such as an amino acid or essential fatty acid

nausea uncomfortable wave-like sensation that precedes vomiting

nebulizer device used to convert liquid drugs into a fine mist for the purpose of inhalation

negative feedback regulatory mechanism in homeostasis in which the first hormone in a pathway is shut off by the last hormone or product in the pathway

negative symptoms in schizophrenia, symptoms that subtract from normal behaviour, including a lack of interest, motivation, responsiveness, or pleasure in daily activities

neoplasm tumour

nephron structural and functional unit of the kidney

nerve agent chemical used in warfare or by bioterrorists that can affect the central nervous system and cause death

neurofibrillary tangle bundle of nerve fibres found in the brain of clients with Alzheimer's disease on autopsy

neurogenic shock type of shock resulting from brain or spinal cord injury

neurohypophysis posterior portion of the pituitary gland

neurolept analgesia type of general anesthesia that combines fentanyl with droperidol to produce a state in which clients are conscious but insensitive to pain and unconnected with surroundings

neuroleptic a drug that is also called antipsychotic and is used to treat psychosis

neuroleptic malignant syndrome (NMS) potentially fatal condition caused by certain antipsychotic medications characterized by an extremely high body temperature, drowsiness, changing blood pressure, irregular heartbeat, and muscle rigidity

neuromuscular blocker drug used to cause total muscle relaxation

neuropathic pain pain caused by injury to nerves and typically described as burning, shooting, or numbness

neurotransmitter a substance that, when released from the axon terminal of a presynaptic neuron, is capable of inhibiting or exciting a target cell

New Drug Submission (NDS) an application made by a drug manufacturer to Health Canada to authorize a safe, efficacious, and high-quality drug

nicotinic type of cholinergic receptor found in ganglia of both the sympathetic and parasympathetic nervous systems

nit egg of the louse parasite

nitrogen mustard alkylating agent used to treat a variety of tumours

nociceptor receptor connected with nerves that receive and transmit pain signals to the spinal cord and brain

nocioceptor pain pain caused by injury to tissues, producing either somatic pain (sharp, localized sensations) or visceral pain (described as generalized dull pain, throbbing, or aching)

non-maleficence ethical obligation to not harm the client

non-specific defences defences such as inflammation that protect the body from invasion by general hazards

non-specific cellular response drug action that is independent of cellular receptors and not associated with other mechanisms, such as changing the permeability of cellular membranes, depressing membrane excitability, or altering the activity of cellular pumps

norepinephrine (NE) primary neurotransmitter in the sympathetic nervous system

nosocomial infection infection acquired in a healthcare setting such as a hospital, physician's office, or nursing home

Notice of Compliance (NOC) certifies that a drug complies with the *Food and Drugs Act* and *Regulations* and may be marketed in Canada

nursing diagnosis clinical-based judgment about the client and his or her response to health and illness

nursing process five-part systematic decision-making method that includes assessment, nursing diagnosis, planning, implementation, and evaluation

objective data information gathered through physical assessment, laboratory tests, and other diagnostic sources

obsessive-compulsive disorder (OCD) recurrent, intrusive thoughts or repetitive behaviours that interfere with normal activities or relationships

older adulthood period of life over age 65

oligospermia presence of less than 20 million sperm in an ejaculate

oncogene gene responsible for the conversion of normal cells into cancer cells

oncotic pressure a form of osmotic pressure exerted by proteins in blood plasma that tends to pull water into the circulatory system

open-angle glaucoma chronic, simple glaucoma caused by hindered outflow of aqueous humour from the anterior chamber of the eye

opiate substance closely related to morphine extracted from the poppy plant

opioid substance obtained from the unripe seeds of the poppy plant; natural or synthetic morphine-like substance

orthostatic hypotension fall in blood pressure that occurs when changing position from recumbent to upright

osmolality number of dissolved particles or solutes in 1 kg (1 L) of water

osmosis process by which water moves from areas of low solute concentration (low osmolality) to areas of high solute concentration (high osmolality)

osteoarthritis (OA) disorder characterized by degeneration of joints, particularly the fingers, spine, hips, and knees

osteomalacia rickets in children; caused by vitamin D deficiency and characterized by softening of the bones without alteration of basic bone structure

osteoporosis condition in which bones lose mass and become brittle and susceptible to fracture

otitis media inflammation of the middle ear

outcome objective measure of goals

ovulation release of an egg by the ovary

oxytocics agents used to stimulate uterine contractions

Paget's disease disorder of bone formation and resorption characterized by weak, enlarged, and deformed bones

palliation form of cancer chemotherapy intended to alleviate symptoms rather than cure the disease

pancreatitis inflammation of the pancreas that may be acute or chronic

panic disorder anxiety disorder characterized by intense feelings of immediate apprehension, fearfulness, terror, or impending doom accompanied by increased autonomic nervous system activity

parafollicular cell cell in the thyroid gland that secretes calcitonin

paranoia having an extreme suspicion and delusion that one is being followed and that others are trying to inflict harm

parasympathetic nervous system portion of the autonomic nervous system that is active during periods of rest and that results in the rest or relaxation response

parenteral nutrition nutrients administered via a route other than ingestion

parenteral route administration method in which the drug is delivered via a needle into the skin layers

parietal cell cell in the stomach mucosa that secretes hydrochloric acid

Parkinson's disease degenerative disorder of the nervous system caused by a deficiency of the brain neurotransmitter dopamine that results in disturbances of muscle movement

Parkinsonism symptoms of tremor, muscle rigidity, stooped posture, and a shuffling gait

partial (focal) seizure seizure that starts on one side of the brain and travels a short distance before stopping

partial agonist medication that produces a weaker, or less efficacious, response than an agonist

passive immunity immune defence that lasts 2 to 3 weeks; obtained by administering antibodies

passive transport the movement of molecules from high to low concentration with no energy input

patent protection a guaranteed period of market exclusivity given to the manufacturer of a new drug

pathogen organism capable of causing disease

pathogenicity ability of an organism to cause disease in humans

pediculicide medication that kills lice

pegylation process that attaches polyethylene glycol (PEG) to an interferon to extend its pharmacological activity

pellagra deficiency of niacin

penicillin-binding protein a protein that binds penicillin

peptic ulcer erosion of the mucosa in the alimentary canal, most commonly in the stomach and duodenum

percutaneous transluminal coronary angioplasty (PTCA) procedure by which a balloon-shaped catheter is used to compress fatty plaque against an arterial wall for the purpose of restoring normal blood flow

perfusion blood flow through a tissue or organ

peripheral edema swelling in the limbs, particularly the feet and ankles, due to an accumulation of interstitial fluid

peripheral nervous system division of the nervous system containing all nervous tissue outside the CNS, including the autonomic nervous system

peripheral resistance amount of friction encountered by blood as it travels through the vessels

peristalsis involuntary wave-like contraction of smooth muscle lining the alimentary canal

pernicious (megaloblastic) anemia type of anemia usually caused by lack of secretion of intrinsic factor

pH measure of the acidity or alkalinity of a solution

pharmacodynamics study of how the body responds to drugs

pharmacogenetics area of pharmacology that examines the role of genetics in drug response

pharmacokinetics study of how drugs are handled by the body

pharmacological classification method for organizing drugs on the basis of their mechanism of action

pharmacology study of medicines; discipline pertaining to how drugs improve or maintain health

pharmacotherapy (pharmacotherapeutics) treatment or prevention of disease by means of drugs

phobia fearful feelings attached to a situation or object such as snakes, spiders, crowds, or heights

phosphodiesterase enzyme in muscle cells that cleaves phosphodiester bonds; its inhibition increases myocardial contractility

phospholipid type of lipid that contains two fatty acids, a phosphate group, and a chemical backbone of glycerol

physical dependence condition of experiencing unpleasant withdrawal symptoms when a substance is discontinued

planning linking strategies, or interventions, to established goals and outcomes

plaque fatty material that builds up in the lining of blood vessels and may lead to hypertension, stroke, myocardial infarction, or angina

plasma cell cell derived from B lymphocytes that produces antibodies

plasma half-life ($t_{1/2}$) length of time required for a drug to decrease its concentration in the plasma by one-half after administration

plasmid small piece of circular DNA found in some bacteria that is able to transfer resistance from one bacterium to another

plasmin enzyme formed from plasminogen that dissolves blood clots

plasminogen protein that prevents fibrin clot formation; precursor of plasmin

polarized condition in which the inside of a cell is more negatively charged than the outside of the cell

polyene antifungal class of drugs containing amphotericin B and nystatin

polypharmacy the taking of multiple drugs concurrently

positive symptoms in schizophrenia, symptoms that add on to normal behaviour, including hallucinations, delusions, and a disorganized thought or speech pattern

postsynaptic neuron in a synapse, the nerve that has receptors for the neurotransmitter

posttraumatic stress disorder (PTSD) type of anxiety that develops in response to re-experiencing a previous life event that was psychologically traumatic

potassium ion channel pathway in a plasma membrane through which potassium ions enter and leave

potency strength of a drug at a specified concentration or dose

preclinical investigation procedure implemented after a drug has been licensed for public use, designed to provide information on use and on occurrence of side effects

preload degree of stretch of the cardiac muscle fibres just before they contract

prenatal preceding birth

preschool child child from 3 to 5 years of age

presynaptic neuron nerve that releases the neurotransmitter into the synaptic cleft when stimulated by an action potential

PRN order (Latin: *pro re nata*) order for medication to be administered as required by the client's condition

prodrug drug that becomes more active after it is metabolized

progesterone hormone secreted by the corpus luteum and placenta that is responsible for building up the uterine lining in the second half of the menstrual cycle and during pregnancy

prostaglandins class of local hormones that promote local inflammation and pain when released by cells in the body

protease viral enzyme that is responsible for the final assembly of the HIV virions

prothrombin blood protein that is converted to thrombin in blood coagulation

prothrombin activator enzyme in the coagulation cascade that converts prothrombin to thrombin; also called *prothrombinase*

prothrombin time (PT) blood test used to determine the time needed for plasma to clot for the regulation of warfarin dosage

proton pump inhibitor drug that inhibits the enzyme H^+, K^+-ATPase

prototype drug well-understood model drug to which other drugs in a pharmacological class may be compared

protozoan single-celled animal

provitamin inactive chemical that is converted to a vitamin in the body

proximal tubule portion of the nephron that collects filtrate from Bowman's capsule

pruritus itching associated with dry, scaly skin

pseudo-Parkinsonism symptoms of Parkinsonism that are drug-induced

psoralen drug used along with phototherapy for the treatment of psoriasis and other severe skin disorders

psychedelic substance that alters perception of reality

psychological dependence intense craving for a drug that drives people to continue drug abuse

psychology science that deals with normal and abnormal mental processes and their impact on behaviour

psychosis a mental disorder in which there is a loss of contact with reality

Purkinje fibres electrical conduction pathway leading from the bundle branches to all portions of the ventricles

rapid eye movement (REM) sleep stage of sleep characterized by quick, scanning movements of the eyes

reabsorption movement of filtered substances from the kidney tubule back into the blood

rebound congestion condition of hypersecretion of mucus following use of intranasal sympathomimetics

rebound insomnia increased sleeplessness that occurs when long-term antianxiety or hypnotic medication is discontinued

receptor structural component of a cell to which a drug binds in a dose-related manner to produce a response

red-man syndrome rash on the upper body caused by certain anti-infectives

reflex tachycardia temporary increase in heart rate that occurs when blood pressure falls

refractory period time during which the myocardial cells rest and are not able to contract

releasing hormone hormone secreted by the hypothalamus that affects secretions in the pituitary gland

renal failure occurs when the kidneys are no longer able to adequately filter and excrete urine and serum creatinine levels increase

renin-angiotensin system series of enzymatic steps by which the body raises blood pressure

respiration exchange of oxygen and carbon dioxide in the lungs; also the process of deriving energy from metabolic reactions

rest-and-digest response signs and symptoms produced when the parasympathetic nervous system is activated

reticular activating system (RAS) part of the brain responsible for sleeping and wakefulness and performing an alerting function for the cerebral cortex; includes the reticular formation, hypothalamus, and part of the thalamus

reticular formation portion of the brain affecting awareness and wakefulness

retinoid compound resembling vitamin A used in the treatment of severe acne and psoriasis

reverse cholesterol transport process by which cholesterol is transported away from body tissues to the liver

reverse transcriptase viral enzyme that converts RNA to DNA

Reye's syndrome potentially fatal complication of infection associated with ASA use in children

rheumatoid arthritis (RA) systemic autoimmune disorder characterized by inflammation of multiple joints

rhinophyma reddened, bulbous, irregular swelling of the nose

rosacea chronic skin disorder characterized by clusters of papules on the face

salicylism poisoning due to ASA and ASA-like drugs

scabicide drug that kills scabies mites

schizo-affective disorder psychosis with symptoms of both schizophrenia and mood disorders

schizophrenia psychosis characterized by abnormal thoughts and thought processes, withdrawal from other people and the outside environment, and apparent preoccupation with one's own mental state

school-aged child child from 6 to 12 years of age

scurvy deficiency of vitamin C

seborrhea skin condition characterized by overactivity of oil glands

second messenger chemical in a cascade of biochemical events that initiates a drug's action by either stimulating or inhibiting a normal activity of the cell

secretion in the kidney, movement of substances from the blood into the tubule after filtration has occurred

sedative substance that depresses the CNS to cause drowsiness or sleep

sedative-hypnotic drug with the ability to produce a calming effect at lower doses while having the ability to induce sleep at higher doses

seizure symptom of epilepsy characterized by abnormal neuronal discharges within the brain

selective estrogen receptor modulator (SERM) drug that produces an action similar to estrogen in body tissues; used for the treatment of osteoporosis in postmenopausal women

selective serotonin reuptake inhibitor (SSRI) drug that selectively inhibits the reuptake of serotonin into nerve terminals; used mostly for depression

septic shock type of shock caused by severe infection in the bloodstream

serotonin syndrome (SES) set of signs and symptoms associated with overmedication with antidepressants that includes altered mental status, fever, sweating, and lack of muscular coordination

seven rights of drug administration principles that offer simple and practical guidance for nurses to use during drug preparation, delivery, and administration

shock condition in which there is inadequate blood flow to meet the body's metabolic needs

single order medication that is to be given only once, and at a specific time, such as a preoperative order

sinoatrial (SA) node pacemaker of the heart located in the wall of the right atrium that controls the basic heart rate

sinus rhythm number of beats per minute normally generated by the SA node

situational anxiety anxiety experienced by people faced with a stressful environment

sleep debt lack of sleep

sociology study of human behaviour within the context of groups and societies

sodium ion channel pathway in a plasma membrane through which sodium ions enter and leave

somatic nervous system division of the nervous system that provides voluntary control over skeletal muscle

somatostatin synonym for growth hormone inhibiting factor that is released from the hypothalamus

somatotropin synonym for growth hormone

Somogyi phenomenon rapid decrease in blood glucose which stimulates the release of hormones (epinephrine, cortisol, glucagon), resulting in an elevated morning blood glucose

spasticity inability of opposing muscle groups to move in a coordinated manner

Special Access Program (SAP) Canadian program that provides for drugs that are not generally available to be used under certain conditions

spirilla bacteria that have a spiral shape

spirituality capacity to love, to convey compassion and empathy, to give and forgive, to enjoy life, and to find peace of mind and fulfillment in living

SSRI discontinuation syndrome symptoms that occur in some individuals when selective serotonin reuptake inhibitor therapy is stopped

stable angina type of angina that occurs in a predictable pattern, usually relieved by rest

standards of care skills and learning commonly possessed by members of a profession

standards of professional practice criteria established by a profession to guide safe and competent actions

standing order order written in advance of a situation that is to be carried out under specific circumstances

STAT order order for a medication that is needed immediately and is to be given only once

status epilepticus condition characterized by repeated seizures or one prolonged seizure attack that continues for at least 30 minutes

steatorrhea stool containing high content of fat as occurs in some malabsorption syndromes

stem cell cell that resides in the bone marrow and is capable of maturing into any type of blood cell

steroid type of lipid that consists of four rings that comprises certain hormones and drugs

sterol nucleus ring structure common to all steroids

stroke volume amount of blood pumped out by a ventricle in a single beat

subcutaneous (SC) administration method in which medication is delivered beneath the skin

subjective data information gathered regarding what a client states or perceives

sublingual (SL) administration method in which medication is placed under the tongue and allowed to dissolve slowly

substance abuse self-administration of a drug that does not conform to the medical or social norms of the client's given culture or society

substance P neurotransmitter within the spinal cord that is involved in the neural transmission of pain

substantia nigra region in the brain where dopamine is synthesized that is responsible for regulation of unconscious muscle movement

superinfection new infection caused by an organism different from the one causing the initial infection; usually a side effect of anti-infective therapy

supraventricular located above the ventricle

surgical anesthesia stage 3 of anesthesia, where most major surgery occurs

sustained-release tablets or capsules designed to dissolve slowly over an extended time

sympathetic nervous system portion of the autonomic system that is active during periods of stress and results in the fight-or-flight response

synapse junction between two neurons consisting of a presynaptic nerve, a synaptic cleft, and a postsynaptic nerve

synaptic transmission process by which a neurotransmitter reaches receptors to regenerate the action potential

systolic pressure blood pressure during the contraction phase of heart activity

tardive dyskinesia unusual tongue and face movements such as lip-smacking and worm-like motions of the tongue that occur during pharmacotherapy with certain antipsychotics

taxoid antineoplastic drug obtained from the Pacific yew tree

T cell type of lymphocyte that is essential for the cell-mediated immune response

tension headache common type of head pain caused by stress and relieved by non-narcotic analgesics

teratogen drug or other agent that causes developmental birth defects

tetrahydrocannabinol (THC) active chemical in marijuana

therapeutic classification method for organizing drugs on the basis of their clinical usefulness

therapeutic index ratio of a drug's LD_{50} to its ED_{50}

therapeutic range dosage range or serum concentration that achieves the desired drug effects

therapeutics branch of medicine concerned with the treatment of disease and suffering

three checks of drug administration in conjunction with the seven rights, these ascertain client safety and drug effectiveness

thrombin enzyme that causes clotting by converting the plasma fibrinogen to fibrin strands

thrombocytopenia reduction in the number of circulating platelets

thromboembolic disorder condition in which the client develops blood clots

thrombolytic drug used to dissolve existing blood clots

thrombopoietin hormone produced by the kidneys that controls megakaryocyte activity

thrombotic stroke type of stroke caused by a blood clot blocking an artery in the brain

thrombus blood clot obstructing a vessel

thyrotoxic crisis (thyroid storm) acute form of hyperthyroidism that is a medical emergency

tissue plasminogen activator (t-PA) natural enzyme and a drug that dissolves blood clots

titre measurement of the amount of a substance in the blood

tocolytic drug used to inhibit uterine contractions

tocopherol generic name for vitamin E

toddlerhood period of childhood from 1 to 3 years of age

tolerance process of adapting to a drug over a period of time and subsequently requiring higher doses to achieve the same effect

tonic spasm single, prolonged muscular contraction

tonic-clonic seizure seizure characterized by intense jerking motions and loss of consciousness

tonicity ability of a solution to cause a change in water movement across a membrane due to osmotic forces

tonometry technique for measuring intraocular tension and pressure

topoisomerase I enzyme that assists in the repair of DNA damage

total parenteral nutrition (TPN) nutrition provided through a peripheral or central vein

toxic concentration level of drug that will result in serious adverse effects

toxicology the study of poisoning

toxoid substance that has been chemically modified to remove its harmful nature but is still able to elicit an immune response in the body

trade (proprietary) name name of a drug assigned by the manufacturer; also called the *brand name* or *product name*

transferrin protein complex that transports iron to the sites in the body where it is needed

transplant rejection reaction of the immune system in which it recognizes a transplanted tissue as being foreign and attacks it

tricyclic antidepressant (TCA) class of drugs used in the pharmacotherapy of depression

triglyceride type of lipid that contains three fatty acids and a chemical backbone of glycerol

tubercle cavity-like lesion in the lung characteristic of infection by *Mycobacterium tuberculosis*

tumour abnormal swelling or mass

type 1 diabetes mellitus (DM) metabolic disease characterized by hyperglycemia and caused by a lack of secretion of insulin by the pancreas

type 2 diabetes mellitus (DM) chronic metabolic disease caused by insufficient secretion of insulin by the pancreas and a lack of sensitivity of insulin receptors

tyramine form of the amino acid tyrosine that is found in foods such as cheese, beer, wine, and yeast products

ulcerative colitis inflammatory bowel disease of the colon

undernutrition lack of adequate nutrition to meet the metabolic demands of the body

unit (U) one of anything

unstable angina severe angina that occurs frequently and is not relieved by rest

urinalysis diagnostic test that examines urine for the presence of blood cells, proteins, pH, specific gravity, ketones, glucose, and microorganisms

vaccination (immunization) using a vaccine or toxoid to prevent disease

vaccine biological material that confers protection against infection; preparation of microorganism particles that is injected into a patient to stimulate the immune system, with the intention of preventing disease

variant angina chest pain that is caused by acute spasm of the coronary arteries rather than by physical or emotional exertion

vasomotor centre area of the medulla that controls baseline blood pressure

ventilation process by which air is moved into and out of the lungs

very low–density lipoprotein (VLDL) lipid-carrying particle that is converted to LDL in the liver

vestibular apparatus portion of the inner ear responsible for the sense of position

vinca alkaloid chemical obtained from the periwinkle plant that has antineoplastic activity

virilization appearance of masculine secondary sex characteristics

virion virus particle capable of causing an infection

virulence severity of disease that a pathogen is able to cause

virus non-living particle containing nucleic acid that is able to cause disease

vitamin organic compound required by the body in small amounts

vitiligo milk-white areas of depigmented skin

vomiting centre area in the medulla that controls the vomiting reflex

von Willebrand's disease (vWD) decrease in quantity or quality of von Willebrand factor (vWF), which acts as a carrier of factor VIII and has a role in platelet aggregation

withdrawal physical signs of discomfort associated with the discontinuation of an abused substance

withdrawal syndrome symptoms that result when a client discontinues taking a substance upon which he or she was dependent

young adulthood period of life from 18 to 40 years of age

Zollinger-Ellison syndrome disorder of excess acid secretion in the stomach, resulting in peptic ulcer disease

BIBLIOGRAPHY AND REFERENCES

General References

Adams, M. P., Holland, L. N., & Bostwick, P. M. (2008). *Pharmacology for nurses: A pathophysiologic approach* (2nd ed.). Upper Saddle River, NJ: Pearson/Prentice-Hall.

Adams, M. P., Josephson, D. L., & Holland, L. N. (2005). *Pharmacology for nurses: A pathophysiologic approach.* Upper Saddle River, NJ: Pearson/Prentice-Hall.

Beers, M .H., & Berkow, R. (Eds.). (2006). *Merck Manual: Diagnoses and Therapy* (18th ed.). Whitehouse Station, NJ: Merck & Co.

Deglin, J. H., & Vallerand, A. H. (2009). *Davis's drug guide for nurses* (11th ed.). Philadelphia: Davis.

Epocrates Online. (2008). https://www.epocrates.com/sessionManager.do?referurl=/online.do&refernext=https://online.epocrates.com/rxmain.jsp

Health Canada. (2008). *Drug Product Database.* http://cpe0013211b4c6d-cm0014e88ee7a4.cpe.net.cable.rogers.com/dpdonline/startup.do?applanguage=en_CA

Health Canada. (2008). *MedEffect,* http://www.hc-sc.gc.ca/dhp-mps/medeff/advisories-avis/prof/2006/index_e.html

Institute for Safe Medication Practices Canada. (2008). ISMP Medication Safety Alert! *Nurse Advise-ERR.*

Krogh, D. (2005). *Biology: A guide to the natural world* (3rd ed.). Upper Saddle River, NJ: Prentice Hall.

Marieb, E. N., & Hoehn, K. (2007). *Human anatomy & physiology* (7th ed). Upper Saddle River, NJ: Prentice Hall.

Mulvihill, M. L., Zelman, P., Holdaway, P., Tompary, E., & Turchany, J. (2006). *Human diseases: A systemic approach* (6th ed.). Upper Saddle River, NJ: Prentice Hall.

Neal, M. J. (2002). *Medical pharmacology at a glance* (4th ed.). Oxford: Blackwell.

Public Health Agency of Canada. *Economic Burden of Illness Database, Custom Tabulation,* Retrieved May 15, 2007, from www.phac-aspc.gc.ca

Silverhorn, D. U. (2006). *Human physiology: An integrated approach* (4th ed.). San Francisco: Benjamin Cummings.

Statistics Canada. (2008). www.statcan.ca

Chapter 1

Canada. Controlled Drug and Substances Act, S.C. 1996, c. 19.

Canada. Government Organization Act, R.S.C. 2000, c. G-10.

Canada. Health Professions Act, R.S.C. 2000, c. H-7.

Canada. Regulations Amending the Marihuana Medical Access Regulations (2003), SOR/2003-387.

Canadian Coordinating Office for Health Technology Assessment. *Common drug review.* URL: https://www.ccohta.ca/CDR/cdr_intro_e.cfm

Carrico, J. M. (2000). Human Genome Project and pharmacogenomics: Implications for pharmacy. *Journal of the American Pharmacists Association, 40*(1), 115–116.

Consumer Healthcare Practices Association (2006). *Healthcare, self-care and self-medication.* Retrieved May 11, 2006, from http://www.chpa-info.org/ChpaPortal/International/WSMI/Health

Health Canada. (2008). *Drug products.* URL: http://www.hc-sc.gc.ca/dhp-mps/prodpharma/index_e.html

Health Canada. (2005). Meeting notes. *Canada's research-based pharmaceutical companies (rx&d) and the therapeutic products directorate (TPD).* Retrieved from http://www.hc-sc.gc.ca/dhpmps/alt_formats/hpfb-dgpsa/pdf/prodpharma/2005-03-21_e.pdf

Marra, C. A., Lynd, L. D., Anis, A. H., & Esdaile, J. M. (2006). Approval process and access to prescription drugs in Canada. *Arthritis Care & Research, 55*(1), 9–11.

Rawson, N. S. (2005). Assessing prescription medications for priority regulatory review. *Regulatory Toxicology and Pharmacology, 42,* 70–6.

Oats, J. A. (2006). The science of drug therapy. In L. L. Brunton, J. S. Lazo, & K. L. Parker (Eds.), *Goodman & Gilman's The pharmacological basis of therapeutics* (11th ed., pp. 117–136). New York: McGraw-Hill.

Rawson, N. S., & Kaitin, K. I. (2003). Canadian and US drug approval times and safety considerations. *Annals of Pharmacotherapy, 37,* 1403–1408.

The Lung Association and the Arthritis Society. *Access to prescription drugs in Canada: A guide.* August 2004. URL: http://www.lung.ca/drugs/2005.02.12.pres.drugs.pdf

Chapter 2

Brass, E. P. (2001). Drug therapy: Changing the status of drugs from prescription to over-the-counter availability. *New England Journal of Medicine, 345,* 810–816.

Canada. Controlled Drug and Substances Act, S.C. 1996, c. 19.

Canada. Regulations Amending the Marihuana Medical Access Regulations (2003), SOR/2003-387.

Gaither, C. A., Kirking, D. M., Ascione, F. J., & Welage, L. S. (2001). Consumers' views on generic medications. *Journal of the American Pharmacists Association, 41*(5), 729–736.

Kacew, S. (1999). Effects of over-the-counter drugs on the unborn child: What is known and how should this influence prescribing? *Paediatric Drugs, 1*(2), 75–80.

World Health Organization. (1997). Guidelines on the Use of International Nonproprietary Names (INNs) for Pharmaceutical Substances, Programme of International Nonproprietary Names, Division of Drug Management and Policies, WHO/Pharm S/NOM 1570.

Chapter 3

Bartlett, J. G., Sifton, D. W., & Kelly, G. L. (Eds.). (2002). *PDR guide to biological and chemical warfare response.* Montvale, NJ: Medical Economics.

Blendon, R. J., Des Roches, C. M., Benson, J. M., Herrmann, M. J., Taylor-Clark, K., & Weldon, K. J. (2003). The public and the smallpox threat. *New England Journal of Medicine, 348*(5), 426–432.

Bozeman, W. P., Dilbero, D., & Schauben, J. L. (2002). Biologic and chemical weapons of mass destruction. *Emergency Medicine Clinics of North America, 20*(4), xii, 975–993.

Canadian Nursing Association. *Standards and best practices: Bioterrorism.* Retrieved May 11, 2006, from http://www.cna-aiic.ca/CNA/practice/standards/bioterrorism/default_e.aspx

Canadian Nurses Association. (2007). *Standards and best practices: Emergencies, disease outbreaks and disasters,* http://cna-nurses.ca/CNA/practice/standards/emergencies/default_e.aspx

Canadian Nurses Association. (2007). *What every nurse should know about bioterrorism and emergency preparedness,* http://cna-nurses.ca/CNA/practice/standards/emergencies/default_e.aspx

Cangemi, C. W. (2002). Occupational response to terrorism. *American Association of Occupational Health Nurses Journal, 50*(4), 190–196.

Chyba, C. F. (2001). Biological security in a changed world. *Science, 293*(5539), 2349.

Committee on Drugs. (2001). Acetaminophen toxicity in children. *Pediatrics, 108*(4), 1020–1024.

Crupi, R. S., Asnis, D. S., Lee, C. C., Santucci, T., Marino, M. J., & Flanz, B. J. (2003). Meeting the challenge of bioterrorism: Lessons learned from West Nile virus and anthrax. *American Journal of Emergency Medicine, 21*(1), 77–79.

International Congress of Nurses. (revised 2006). *ICN Position Statement: Nurses and Disaster Preparedness,* http://www.icn.ch/psdisasterprep01.htm

Kimmel, S. R., Mahoney, M. C., & Zimmerman, R. K. (2003). Vaccines and bioterrorism: Smallpox and anthrax. *Journal of Family Practice, 52*(1 Suppl.), S56–S61.

Lett, D. (2005). Feds to stockpile antivirals as pandemic "speed bump." *Canadian Medical Association Journal, 172*(9), 1167.

McLaughlin, S. (2001). Thinking about the unthinkable: Where to start planning for terrorism incidents. *Health Facilities Management, 14*(7), 26–30, 32.

Mortimer, P. P. (2003). Can postexposure vaccination against smallpox succeed? *Clinical Infectious Diseases, 36*(5), 622–629.

Public Health Agency of Canada. (2008). *Centre for Emergency Preparedness and Response (CEPR),* http://www.phac-aspc.gc.ca/ep-mu/index-eng.php

Public Health Agency of Canada. (2008). *National Emergency Stockpile System (NESS),* http://www.phac-aspc.gc.ca/ep-mu/ness-eng.php

Public Health Agency of Canada. (2008). *Responding to stressful events.* http://www.phac-aspc.gc.ca/publicat/oes-bsu-02/index.html

Rose, M. A., & Larrimore, K. L. (2002). Knowledge and awareness concerning chemical and biological terrorism: Continuing education implications. *Journal of Continuing Education in Nursing, 33*(6), 253–258.

Stephenson, J. (2003). Smallpox vaccine program launched amid concerns raised by expert panel, unions. *Journal of the American Medical Association, 289*(6), 685–686.

Stokes, E., Gilbert-Palmer, D., Skorga, P., Young, C., & Persell, D. (2004). Chemical agents of terrorism: Preparing nurse practitioners. *The Nurse Practitioner Journal, 29*(5), 30–39.

Tasota, F. J., Henker, R. A., & Hoffman, L. A. (2002). Anthrax as a biological weapon: An old disease that poses a new threat. *Critical Care Nurse, 22*(5), 21–32, 34.

World Health Organization. (2007). *Epidemic and Pandemic Alert and Response (EPR),* http://www.who.int/

World Health Organization. (2007). *Health Aspects of Biological and Chemical Weapons,* http://www.who.int/csr/en/

Chapter 4

Brunton, L. L., Lazo, J. S., & Parker, K. L. (Eds.). (2006). *Goodman & Gilman's The pharmacological basis of therapeutics* (11th ed.). New York: McGraw-Hill.

Buxton, I. L. O. (2006). Pharmacokinetics and pharmacodynamics: The dynamics of drug absorption, distribution, action, and elimination. In L. L. Brunton, J. S. Lazo, & K. L. Parker (Eds.), *Goodman & Gilman's The pharmacological basis of therapeutics* (11th ed., pp. 1–40). New York: McGraw-Hill.

Lares-Asseff, I., Flores-Perez, J., Juarez-Olguin, H., Ramirez-Lacayo, M., Loredo-Abdala, A., & Carbajal-Rodriguez, L. (1999). Influence of nutritional status on the pharmacokinetics of acetyl-salicylic acid and its metabolites in children with autoimmune disease. *American Journal of Clinical Nutrition, 69*(2), 318–324.

Marroum, P. J., & Gobburu, J. (2002). The product label: How pharmacokinetics and pharmacodynamics reach the prescriber. *Clinical Pharmacokinetics, 41*(3), 161–169.

Monster, T. B. M., de Jong, P. E., & de Jong-van den Berg, L. T. W. (2003). Drug-induced renal function impairment: A population-based survey. *Pharmacoepidemiology and Drug Safety, 12*(2), 135–143.

Oats, J. A. (2006). The science of drug therapy. In L. L. Brunton, J. S. Lazo, & K. L. Parker (Eds.), *Goodman & Gilman's The pharmacological basis of therapeutics* (11th ed., pp. 117–136). New York: McGraw-Hill.

Thames, G. (2004). Drug forum: Making pharmacokinetics clinically useful. *Gastroenterology Nursing, 27*(2), 74–75.

Chapter 5

Evans, W. E., & McLeod, H. (2003). Pharmacogenomics—Drug disposition, drug targets, and side effects. *New England Journal of Medicine, 348*, 538–549,

Gandhi, M., Aweeka, F., Greenblatt, R. M., & Blaschke, T. F. (2004). Sex differences in pharmacokinetics and pharmacodynamics. *Annual Review of Pharmacology and Toxicology, 44*(1), 499–523.

Neal, M. J. (2002). *Medical pharmacology at a glance* (4th ed.). Oxford: Blackwell.

Chapter 6

Abi Khaled, L., Ahmad, F., Brogan, T., Fearnley, J., Graham, J., MacLeod, S., et al. (2003). Prescription medication use by one million Canadian children. *Journal of Paediatrics and Child Health, 8*(Suppl. A), 6A–56A.

American Academy of Pediatrics, Committee on Drugs. (2001). The transfer of drugs and other chemicals into human breast milk. *Pediatrics, 3*, 776–782.

Auerbach, K. G. (2000). Breastfeeding and maternal medication use. *Journal of Obstetrics, Gynecology and Neonatal Nursing, 28*(5), 554–563.

Bánhidy, F., Lowry, R. B., & Czeize, A. E. (2005). Risk and benefit of drug use during pregnancy. *International Journal of Medical Science, 2*, 100–106.

Bressler, R., & Katz, M. (2003). *Geriatric pharmacology* (2nd ed.). New York: McGraw-Hill Professional.

Briggs, G. G. (2002). Drug effects on the fetus and breast-fed infant. *Clinical Obstetrics and Gynecology, 45*(1), 6–21, 170–171.

Canadian Pediatric Society, Drug therapy and hazardous substances committee. (2003; reaffirmed 2006). Drug investigation for Canadian children: The role of the Canadian Pediatric Society. *Pediatrics & Child Health, 8*(4), 231–234.

Dellasega, C., Klinefelter, J. M., & Halas, C. J. (2000). Psychoactive medications and the elderly patient. *Clinical Review, 10*(6), 53–74.

Friedman, J. M. (2006). ACE inhibitors and congenital anomalies. *New England Journal of Medicine, 354*(23), 2498–2500.

Gibson, P. (2003). Baby safe: Which drugs are safe in pregnancy? *The Canadian Journal of CME,* 67–76.

Hale, T. W. (2004). Maternal medications during breastfeeding. *Clinical Obstetrics and Gynecology, 47*(3), 696–711.

Hattis, D., Russ, A., Banati, P., Kozlak, M., & Goble, R. (2001). Comparative child/adult pharmacokinetic database based upon the therapeutic drug literature. *EPA/State of Connecticut Assistance Agreement #827195-0.*

Health Canada. (2002). *Congenital Anomalies in Canada: A Perinatal Health Report,* p. 1–87. Retrieved March 2006 from http://www.phac-aspc.gc.ca/publicat/cac-acc02/index.html

Health Canada. *Infant Feeding.* Retrieved March 2006 from http://www.hc-sc.gc.ca/fn-an/nutrition/child-enfant/infant-nourisson/index_e.html

Health Canada. (2004). *Canadian perinatal surveillance system.* Retrieved June 15, 2006, from http://www.phac-aspc.gc.ca/rhs-ssg/about_e.htm

Heinrich, J. (2001). Pediatric drug research: Substantial increase in studies of drugs for children but some challenges remain. Testimony before the Committee on Health, Education, Labor and Pensions, U.S. Senate, Washington, DC.

Holmes, L. B., Wyszynski, D. F., & Lieberman, E. (2004). The AED (antiepileptic drug) pregnancy registry: A 6-year experience. *Archives of Neurology, 61*(5), 673–678.

Kwan, C., Steer, E., Rieder, M. J., Matsui, D. (2002). Barriers to drug investigation in children in Canada: Perspectives from academic and community practice. *Journal of Paediatrics and Child Health,* 7(Suppl. A), 44A.

Litalien, C., Théorêt, Y., & Faure, C. (2005). Pharmacokinetics of proton pump inhibitors in children. *Clinical Pharmacokinetics, 44*(5), 441–466.

Leipzig, R. M. (Ed.). (2003). *Drug prescribing for older adults: An evidence-based approach.* Philadelphia: American College of Physicians.

Lo, W. Y., & Friedman, J. M. (2002). Teratogenicity of recently introduced medications in human pregnancy. *Obstetrics and Gynecology, 100*(3), 465–473.

Matsui, D., Kwan, C., Steer, E., & Rieder, M. J. (2003). The trials and tribulations of doing drug research in children. *Canadian Medical Association Journal, 169*(10), 1033–1034.

von Moltke, L. L., Greenblatt, D. J., Harmatz, J. S., & Shader, R. I. (2000). *Psychotropic drug metabolism in old age: Principles and problems of assessment.* Retrieved April 20, 2006, from http://www.acnp.org/g4/GN401000140/CH137.html

Mone, S. M., Gillman, M. W., Miller, T. L., Herman, E. H., & Lipshultz, S. E. (2004). Effects of environmental exposures on the cardiovascular system: Prenatal period through adolescence. *Pediatrics, 113*(4), 1058–1069.

Moore, T. J., Weiss, S.R., Kaplan, S., Blaisdell, C. J. (2002). Reported adverse drug events in infants and children under 2 years of age. *Pediatrics, 110,* e53.

Nice, F. J., Snyder, J. L., & Kotansky, B. C. (2000). Breastfeeding and over-the-counter medications. *Journal of Human Lactation, 16*(4), 319–331.

Pharmacoepidemiology and drug safety. (2000). *Current Awareness, 9*(7), 615–630.

Public Health Agency of Canada. (2002). *Congenital anomalies in Canada: A perinatal health report.* Retrieved June 15, 2007, from http://www.phac-aspc.gc.ca/publicat/cac-acc02/index.html

Spencer, J. P., Gonzalez, L. S., III, & Barnhart, D. J. (2001). Medications in the breast-feeding mother. *American Family Physician, 64,* 19–126.

Spiers, M. V., Kutzik, D. M., & Lamar, M. (2004). Variation in medication understanding among the elderly. *American Journal of Health-System Pharmacy, 61*(4), 373–380.

Steinbrook, R. (2002). Testing medications in children. *New England Journal of Medicine, 347,* 1462–1470.

Wynne, A. L., Woo, T. M., & Millard, M. (2002). *Pharmacotherapeutics for nurse practitioner prescribers.* Philadelphia: F. A. Davis.

Chapter 7

Bakker, D. A., Blais, D., Reed, E., Vaillancourt, C., Gervais, S., & Beaulieu, P. (1999). Descriptive study to compare patient recall of information: Nurse-taught versus video supplement. *Canadian Oncology Nursing Journal, 9*(3), 115–120.

Carpenito, L. J. (2000). *Nursing diagnosis: Application to nursing practice* (8th ed.). Philadelphia: J. B. Lippincott.

College and Association of Registered Nurses of Alberta (2005). *Medication Administration: Guidelines for Registered Nurses.* Edmonton, AB.

Gardner, P. (2003). *Nursing process in action.* New York: Thompson Delmar Learning.

Herdman, T. H. (2008). Nursing diagnosis: Is it time for a new definition? *International Journal of Nursing Terminologies and Classifications, 1,* 1–13.

Hogan, M. A., Bowles, D., & White, J. E. (2003). *Nursing fundamentals: Reviews & rationales.* Upper Saddle River, NJ: Prentice Hall.

Jahraus, D., Sokolosky, S., Thurston, N., & Guo, D. (2002). Evaluation of an education program for patients with breast cancer receiving radiation therapy. *Cancer Nursing, 24*(4), 266–275.

Kozier, B., Erb, G., Berman, A. J., Burke, K., Bouchal, D. S. R., & Hirst, S. P. (2003). *Fundamentals of nursing: The nature of nursing practice in Canada* (1st Canadian ed.). Toronto: Pearson Education Canada.

North American Nursing Diagnosis Association. (2003). *Nursing diagnoses: Definitions and classification 2003–2004.* Philadelphia: Author.

Smith, S., Duell, D., & Martin, B. (2003). *Clinical nursing skills: Basic to advanced skills* (6th ed.). Upper Saddle River, NJ: Prentice Hall Health.

Chapter 8

Armitage, G., & Knapman, H. (2003). Adverse events in drug administration: A literature review. *Journal of Nursing Management, 11*(2), 130–140.

Bankston, J., Deshotels, J. M., Daughtry, L., & Metules, T. J. (Eds). (2001). SJS Same trigger, less deadly. *RN, 64*(10), 39–41.

Berman, A. J., Snyder, S., Kozier, B., & Erb, G. (2008). *Kozier & Erb's fundamentals of nursing concepts, process, and practice* (8th ed.). Upper Saddle River, NJ: Prentice Hall.

Billups, S. J., Malone, D. C., & Carter, B. L. (2000). The relationship between drug therapy noncompliance and patient characteristics, health-related quality of life, and health care costs. *Pharmacotherapy, 20*(8), 941–949.

Blais, K. K., Hayes, J., Kozier, B., & Erb, G. (2002). *Professional nursing practice: Concepts and perspectives* (4th ed.). Upper Saddle River, NJ: Prentice Hall.

College and Association of Registered Nurses of Alberta. (2005). *Medication administration: Guidelines for registered nurses.* Edmonton AB.

Deedwania, P. C. (2002). The changing face of hypertension: Is systolic blood pressure the final answer? *Archives of Internal Medicine, 162*(5), 506–508.

Great Ormond Street Hospital for Children. (2004). *Ear drops: Administration.*

Khaldi, N., Miras, A., & Gromb, S. (2005). Toxic epidermal necrolysis and clarithromycin. *Canadian Journal of Clinical Pharmacology, 12*(3), e264–268.

Koo, M. M., Krass, I., & Aslani, P. (2003). Factors influencing consumer use of written drug information. *Annals of Pharmacotherapy, 37*(2), 259–267.

Kozma, C. M. (2002). Why aren't we doing more to enhance medication compliance? *Managed Care Interface, 15*(1), 59–60.

Lesaffre, E., & de Klerk, E. (2000). Estimating the power of compliance-improving methods. *Controlled Clinical Trials, 21*(6), 540–551.

Madlon, K., Diane, J., & Mosch, F. S. (2000). Liquid medication dosing errors. *Journal of Family Practice, 49*(1), 741–744.

Mitchell, J. F. (2006). Oral dosage forms that should not be crushed. *Institute for Safe Medication Practices.*

Nicholas, P., & Agius, C. (2005). Toward safer IV medication administration: The narrow safety margins of many IV medications make this route particularly dangerous. *American Journal of Nursing, 105*(3), Supplement, 25–30.

Nisbet, A. C. (2006). Intramuscular gluteal injections in the increasingly obese population: Retrospective study. *British Medical Journal, 332,* 637–638.

Olsen, J. L., Giangrasso, A. P., & Shrimpton, D. M. (2004). *Medical dosage calculations* (8th ed.). Upper Saddle River, NJ: Prentice Hall.

Seal. R. (2000). How to promote drug compliance in the elderly. *Community Nurse, 6*(1), 41–42.

Smith, D. I. (2001). *Taking control of your medicines.* Newsletter 1(1). Consumer Health Information Corporation, www.consumer-health.com

Smith, S., Duell, D., & Martin, B. (2003). *Clinical nursing skills: Basic to advanced skills* (6th ed.). Upper Saddle River, NJ: Prentice Hall Health.

Urquhart, J. (2000). Erratic patient compliance with prescribed drug regimens: Target for drug delivery systems. *Clinical Pharmacology and Therapeutics, 67*(4), 331–334.

Ward, D. (2005). Guidelines to good practice administration of medication—nasal/ear drops. *Greater Peterborough Primary Care Partnership.*

Wooten, J. (2001). Toxic epidermal necrolysis. *Nursing 2001, 64*(10), 35–38.

Zaybak, A., Güneş Ü. Y., Tamsel, S., Khorshid, L., & Eşer, İ. (2007). Does obesity prevent the needle from reaching muscle in intramuscular injections? *Journal of Advanced Nursing, 58*(6), 552–556.

Chapter 9

Bates, D. W., Clapp, M., Federico, F., Goldmann, D., Kaushal, R., Landrigan, C., & McKenna, K. J. (2001). Medication errors and adverse drug events in pediatric inpatients. *Journal of the American Medical Association, 285*(16), 2114–2120.

Baker, G. R., & Norton, P. G. (2001). Making patients safer! Reducing error in Canadian health care. *Healthcare Papers, 2*(1), 10–31.

Baker, G. R., Norton, P. G., Flintoft, V., Blais, R., Brown, A., Cox, J., et al. (2004). The Canadian adverse events study: The incidence of adverse events among hospital patients in Canada. *Canadian Medical Association Journal, 170*(11), 1678–1686.

Barnsteiner, J. H. (2005). Medication reconciliation. Transfer of medication information across settings—Keeping it free from error. *American Journal of Nursing.* March, Suppl., 31–36.

Canadian Medication Incident Reporting and Prevention System (CMIRPS). (2006). http://www.hc-sc.gc.ca/dhp-mps/medeff/advers-react-neg/fs-if/cmirps-scdpim_e.html

Canadian Nurses Association. (2004). *CNA position statement on patient safety.* Ottawa: Author.

Canadian Nurses Association. (2008). *Code of ethics for Registered Nurses.* http://www.cna-nurses.ca/CNA/practice/ethics/code/default_e.aspx

Canadian Nurses Protective Society (1996). *Medication errors: A legal information sheet for nurses.* 5(2).

Capital Health. (2007). *Briefing note prohibited abbreviations.* Retrieved September 17, 2006, from http://www.capitalhealth.com

Cohen, M. R. (2000). Preventing medication errors related to prescribing. In M. R. Cohen (Ed.), *Medication errors. Causes, preventions and risk management.* Sudbury, MA: Jones and Bartlett Publishers.

College and Association of Registered Nurses of Alberta. (2003). *Nursing practice standards.* Edmonton, AB: Author

Drug Innovation and Patient Safety—The need for a new paradigm. Proceedings of a Satellite Symposium. (2006). *Canadian Journal of Clinical Pharmacology, 13*(1), Supplement, e1–e49.

Force, M. V., Deering, L., Hubbe, J., Anderson, M., Hagermann, B., Cooper-Hahn, M., et al. (2006). Effective strategies to increase reporting of medication errors in hospitals. *Journal of Nursing Administration, 36*(1), 34–41.

Garg, A. (2004). Review: ordering medications by computer can reduce medication errors. *ACP Journal Club, 140*(2), 52.

Gregory, D. M., Guse, L. W., Davidson, D., & Russell, C. K. (2005). Patient safety: Where is nursing education? *Research Briefs, 46*(2).

Health Canada. (2005). Canadian adverse drug reaction monitoring program (cadrmp) guidelines for the voluntary reporting of suspected adverse reactions to health products by health professionals and consumers: Government of Canada.

Health Canada. (2006). *Canadian medication incident reporting and prevention system (CMIRPS)*. Retrieved May 11, 2006, from http://www.hc-sc.gc.ca/dhp-mps/medeff/advers-react-neg/fs-if/cmirps-scdpim_e.html

Health Canada. (2006). *MedEffect program*, http://www.hc-sc.gc.ca/dhp-mps/medeff/

Hodgkinson, B., Koch, S., Nay, R., & Nichols, K. (2006). Strategies to reduce medication errors with reference to older adults. *International Journal of Evidence-Based Healthcare, 4*(1), 2–41.

Institute for Safe Medication Practices Canada. (2000). *Full and timely disclosure of errors to patients: Honesty is the best policy*. Retrieved May 11, 2006, from http://www.ismp.org/newsletters/acutecare/articles/20000223.as

Institute for Safe Medication Practices Canada. (2005). Lowering the risk of medication errors: Independent double-checks. *ISMP Canada Safety Bulletin, 5*(1).

Institute for Safe Medication Practices Canada. (2006). Medication reconciliation—in the hospital and beyond. *ISMP Canada Safety Bulletin, 6*(3).

Institute for Safe Medication Practices Canada. (2005). Root cause analysis of mediation incidents. *ISMP Canada Safety Bulletin, 5*(10).

Institute for Safe Medication Practices Canada. (1999). *The "five rights."* Retrieved June 17, 2006, from http://www.Ismp.Org/newsletters/acutecare/articles/19990407.Asp?Ptr=y

Kaushal, R., Shojania, K. G., Bates, D. W. (2003). Effects of computerized physician order entry and clinical decision support systems on medication safety: A systematic review. *Archives of Internal Medicine, 163*(12), 1409–1416.

Levy, A., & MacLeod, S. (2005). Drug innovation and patient safety: The need for a new paradigm. *The Canadian Journal of Clinical Pharmacology, 13*(1), e1–e49.

McMorran, M., & Morawiecka, I. (2000). Canadian adverse drug reaction newsletter. *Canadian Medical Association Journal, 162*(7).

Mitchell, A. (2001). Challenges in pediatric pharmacotherapy: Minimizing medication errors. *Medscape Pharmacy, 2*(1), 1–8.

Movement for Canadian Literacy. (2004). *Literacy in Canada: It's time for action*, http://www.literacy.ca

National Steering Committee on Patient Safety. (2002). *Building a safer system: A national integrated strategy for improving safety in Canadian health care*. Ottawa: Author.

Orser, B. (2000). Reducing medication errors. *Canadian Medical Association Journal, 162*(8), 1150–1151.

Pharmacoepidemiology and Drug Safety. (2000). *Current Awareness, 9*(7), 615–630.

Proceedings of a satellite symposium. (2006). Drug innovation and patient safety—the need for a new paradigm. *Canadian Journal of Clinical Pharmacology, 13*(1), Suppl., e1–e49.

Walton, M. (2004). Creating a "no blame" culture: Have we got the balance right? *Quality and Safety in Health Care. 13*(3), 163–134.

Wong, I. C., Ghaleb, M. A., Franklin, B. D., Barber, N. (2004). Incidence and nature of dosing errors in paediatric medications: A systematic review. *Drug Safety, 27*(9), 661–670.

Chapter 10

Andrus, M. R., & Roth, M. T. (2002). Health literacy: A review. *Pharmacotherapy 22*(3), 282–302.

Brody, H., & Hunt, L. M. (2006). Bidil: Assessing a race-based pharmaceutical. *Annals of Family Medicine Inc., 4*(6), 482–483.

Burroughs, V., Maxey, R., Crawley, L., Levy, R. (2002). *Cultural and genetic diversity in America: The need for individualized pharmaceutical treatment*. National Pharmaceutical Council, National Pharmaceutical Association. Available online at: http://www.npcnow.org/issues_productlist/PDF/culturaldiversity. Retrieved November 3, 2003.

Canadian Language and Literacy Research Network. (2006). http://www.cllrnet.ca/

Canadian Nurses Association. (2004). *Promoting culturally competent care*. Ottawa: Author.

Canadian Nurses Association. (2006). *Toward 2020: Visions for nursing*. Ottawa: Author.

Chen, J. (2002, October 20–23). *The role of ethnicity in medication use*. Presented at the American College of Clinical Pharmacy 2002 Annual Meeting, Albuquerque, NM.

Chin, J. L. (2000). Viewpoint: Culturally competent health care. *Public Health Reports 115*(1), 25–33.

Crow, K., & Matheson, L. (2000). Informed consent and truth-telling: Cultural directions for healthcare providers. *Journal of Nursing Administration, 30*(3), 148–152.

Davidhizar, R. (2002). Strategies for providing culturally appropriate pharmaceutical care to the Hispanic patient. *Hospital Pharmacy, 37*(5), 505–510.

Dreher, M., & McNaughton, N. (2002). Cultural competence in nursing: Foundation or fallacy? *Nursing Outlook, 50*, 181–186.

Gallagher, R. M. (2002). *The pain-depression conundrum: Bridging the body and mind*. Medscape clinical update based on session presented at the 21st Annual Scientific Meeting of the American Pain Society. Medscape Clinical Update at http://www.medscape.com/viewprogram/2030

Humma, L. M., & Terra, S. G. (2002). Pharmacogenetics and cardiovascular disease: Impact on drug response and applications to disease management. *American Journal of Health-System Pharmacy, 59*(13), 1241–1252.

Indian & Inuit Nurses of Canada. (2008). http://www.sicc.sk.ca/saskindian/a89mar14.htm

Kral, M. J., Burkhardt, K. J., & Kidd, S. (2002). The new research agenda for a cultural psychology. *Canadian Psychology, 43*(3), 154–162.

Kudzma, E. C. (2001). Cultural competence: Cardiovascular medications. *Progress in Cardiovascular Nursing, 16*(4), 152–160, 169.

Leininger, M. M. (Ed.). (2001). *Culture care diversity and universality: A theory of nursing*. Sudbury, MA: Jones & Bartlett Publishers.

Martin, L., Miracle, A. W., & Bonder, B. R. (2001). *Culture in clinical care*. Thorofare, NJ: Slack, Inc.

Nichols-English, G., & Poirier, S. (2000). Optimizing adherence to pharmaceutical care plans. *Journal of the American Pharmacists Association, 40*(4), 475–485.

Phillips, K. A., Veenstra, D. L., Oren, E., Lee, J. K., & Sardee, W. (2001). Potential role of pharmacogenomics in reducing adverse drug reactions: A systematic review. *Journal of the American Medical Association, 286*, 2270–2279.

Richardson, L. G. (2003). Psychosocial issues in patients with congestive heart failure. *Progress in Cardiovascular Nursing, 18*(1), 19–27.

Sleath, B., & Wallace, J. (2002). Providing pharmaceutical care to Spanish-speaking patients. *Journal of the American Pharmacists Association, 42*, 799–801.

Spector, R. E. (2004). *Cultural diversity in health & illness* (6th ed.). Upper Saddle River, NJ: Prentice Hall.

Statistics Canada. (2006). http://www.statscan.ca

Chapter 11

Blumenthal, M. (Ed.). (2000). *Herbal medicine: Expanded commission E monographs.* Austin, TX: American Botanical Council.

College and Association of Registered Nurses of Alberta. (2005). *Alternative and/or complementary therapy: Standards for registered nurses.* Edmonton, AB.

Consumer Healthcare Practices Association (2006). *Healthcare, self-care and self-medication.* Retrieved May 11, 2006, from http://www.chpa-info.org/ChpaPortal/International/WSMI/Health

Ebadi, M. (2002). *Pharmacodynamic basis of herbal medicine.* Boca Raton, FL: CRC Press.

First Annual Complementary and Alternative Health Care and Paediatrics Forum. (2004). *Canadian Journal of Clinical Pharmacology, 11*(2), e245–e256.

Fontaine, K. L. (2000). *Healing practices: Alternative therapies for nursing.* Upper Saddle River, NJ: Prentice Hall.

Foster, S., & Hobbs, C. (2002). *A field guide to western medicinal plants and herbs.* Boston and New York: Houghton Mifflin Co.

Goldman, P. (2001). Herbal medicines today and the roots of modern pharmacology. *Annals of Internal Medicine, 135*(8), 594–597.

Hardy, M. L. (2000). Herbs of special interest to women. *American Pharmaceutical Association, 40*(2), 234–242.

Health Canada. (2006). *Natural Health Products Directorate,* http://www.hc-sc.gc.ca

Hatcher, T., Dokken, D., & Sydnor-Greenberg, N. (2000). Exploring complementary and alternative medicine in pediatrics: Parents and professionals working together for new understanding. *Pediatric Nursing, 26*(4), 383.

Medical Economics Staff (Ed.). (2000). *Physician's desk reference for herbal medicines* (2nd ed.). Montvale: Medical Economics.

Murch, S. J., KrishnaRaj, S., & Saxena, P. K. (2000). Phytopharmaceuticals: Problems, limitations, and solutions. *Scientific Review of Alternate Medicine, 4*(2), 33–37.

Scott, G. N., & Elmer, G. W. (2002). Update on natural product-drug interactions. *American Journal of Health-System Pharmacy, 59*(4), 339–347.

Statistics Canada. (2006). http://www.statscan.ca

Tyler, V. E. (2000). Product definition deficiencies in clinical studies of herbal medicines. *Scientific Review of Alternate Medicine, 4*(2), 17–21.

White, L. B., & Foster, S. (2000). *The herbal drugstore.* Emmaus, PA: Rodale.

Chapter 12

Ashton, H. (2005). The diagnosis and management of benzodiazepine dependence. *Current Opinion in Psychiatry, 18*(3), 249–255.

Barangan, C. J., & Alderman, E. M. (2002). Management of substance abuse. *Pediatric Review, 23*(4), 123–131.

British Columbia Centre of Excellence for Women's Health. (2005). Girls, women, substance use and addiction. *The Women's Health Contribution Program.*

Brust, J. C. M. (2004). Abused agents: Acute effects, withdrawal, and treatment. *CONTINUUM: Lifelong Learning in Neurology. Neurologic Complications of Substance Abuse, 10*(5), 14–47.

Canadian Centre on Substance Abuse (CCSA). (2006). http://www.ccsa.ca/ccsa/

Chychula, N. M., & Sciamanna, C. (2002). Help substance abusers attain and sustain abstinence. *Nurse Practitioner, 27*(11), 30–47.

Freese, T. E., Miotto, K., & Reback, C. J. (2002). The effects and consequences of selected club drugs. *Journal of Substance Abuse Treatment, 23*(2), 151–156.

Hardie, T. L. (2002). The genetics of substance abuse. *AACN Clinical Issues, 13*(4), 511–522.

Haseltine, E. (2001). The unsatisfied mind: Are reward centers in your brain wired for substance abuse? *Discover, 22*(11), 88.

Health Canada. (2007). *Federal drug legislation,* http://www.hc-sc.gc.ca

Health Canada. (2006). *National Native Alcohol and Drug Abuse Program,* http://www.hc-sc.gc.ca/fnih-spni/substan/ads/nnadap-pnlaada_e.html

Jason, L. A., Davis, M. I., Ferrari, J. R., & Bishop, P. D. (2001). A review of research and implications for substance abuse recovery and community research. *Journal of Drug Education 31*(1), 1–28.

Kandel, D. B. (2003). Does marijuana use cause the use of other drugs? *Journal of the American Medical Association, 289*(4), 482–483.

Manoguerra, A. S. (2001). Methamphetamine abuse. *Journal of Toxicology: Clinic Toxicology, 38*(2), 187.

Naegle, M. A., & D'Avanzo, C. E. (2001). *Addictions and substance abuse: Strategies for advanced practice nursing.* Upper Saddle River, NJ: Prentice Hall.

O'Brien, C. P. (2001). Drug addiction and drug abuse. In J. G. Hardman, L. E. Limbird, & A. G. Goodman (Eds.), *The pharmacological basis of therapeutics* (pp. 621–642). New York: McGraw-Hill.

Peterson, K. (2004/2005). Biomarkers for alcohol use. *Alcohol Research and Health, 28*(1), 1–28.

Sindelar, J. L., & Fiellin, D. A. (2001). Innovations in treatment for drug abuse: Solutions to a public health problem. *Annual Review of Public Health, 22*, 249.

Statistics Canada. (2006). http://www.statscan.ca

Tuttle, J., Melnyk, B. M., & Loveland-Cherry, C. (2002). Adolescent drug and alcohol use. Strategies for assessment, intervention, and prevention. *Nursing Clinics of North America, 37*(3), 443–460, ix.

Wasilow-Mueller, S., & Erickson, C. K. (2001). Drug abuse and dependency: Understanding gender differences in etiology and management. *Journal of the American Pharmacists Association, 41*(1), 78–90.

Chapter 13

Bouchard, R., Weber, A. R., & Geiger, J. D. (2002). Informed decision-making on sympathomimetic use in sport and health. *Clinical Journal of Sports Medicine 12*(4), 209–224.

Chapple, C. R., Yamanishi, T., & Chess-Williams, R. (2002). Muscarinic receptor subtypes and management of the overactive bladder. *Urology, 60*(5 Suppl. 1), 82–88; discussion 88–89.

Cilliers, L., & Retief, F. P. (2003). *Poisons, poisoning and the drug trade in ancient Rome,* http://www.sun.ac.za

Defilippi, J., & Crismon, M. L. (2003). Drug interactions with cholinesterase inhibitors. *Drugs & Aging, 20*(6), 437–444.

Herbison, P., Hay-Smith, J., Ellis, G., & Moore, K. (2003). Effectiveness of anticholinergic drugs compared with placebo in the treatment of overactive bladder: Systematic review. *British Medical Journal, 19,* 326(7394), 841–844.

Hoffman, B. B., & Taylor, P. (2001). Neurotransmission: The autonomic and somatic motor nervous systems. In J. G. Hardman, L. E. Limbird, & A. G. Goodman (Eds.), *The pharmacological basis of therapeutics* (pp. 115–154). New York: McGraw-Hill.

Kolpuru, S. (2003). *Doctor corner: Approach to a case of Down's syndrome. Pediatric OnCall*™, http://www.pediatriconcall.com

Lemstra, A. W., Eikelenboom, P., & van Gool, W. A. (2003). The cholinergic deficiency syndrome and its therapeutic implications. *Gerontology, 49*(1), 55–60.

McCrory, D. C., & Brown, C. D. (2002). Anti-cholinergic broncho-dilators versus beta$_2$-sympathomimetic agents for acute exacerbations of chronic obstructive pulmonary disease. *Cochrane Database of Systematic Reviews, 4,* CD003900.

Medical Economics Staff (Ed.). (2000). *PDR for herbal medicines.* Montvale, NJ: Author.

Miller, C. A. (2002). Anticholinergics: The good and the bad. *Geriatric Nursing 23*(5), 286–287.

MSN Health. (2003). *Drugs & herbs: Phenylephrine ophthalmic,* http://www.content.health.msn.com

Rodrigo, G. J., & Rodrigo, C. (2002). The role of anticholinergics in acute asthma treatment: An evidence-based evaluation. *Chest,121*(6), 1977–1987.

Roe, C. M., Anderson, M. J., & Spivack, B. (2002). Use of anti-cholinergic medications by older adults with dementia. *Journal of the American Geriatrics Society, 50,* 836–842.

ThinkQuest On-line Library. (2003). *Belladonna, deadly nightshade. Poisonous Plants and Animals,* http://www.library.thinkquest.org

Wang, H. E. (2002). Street drug toxicity resulting from opiates combined with anticholinergics. *Prehospital Emergency Care, 6*(3), 351–354.

Chapter 14

AventisPharmaLtd. (2004). *Imovane: Data Sheet for Professionals.* Auckland: Aventis Pharma Ltd.

Baldessarini, R. J. (2001). Drugs and the treatment of psychiatric disorders: Depression and anxiety disorders. In J. G. Hardman, L. E. Limbird, & A. G. Goodman (Eds.), *The pharmacological basis of therapeutics* (pp. 447–484). New York: McGraw-Hill.

Charney, D. S., Mihic, J., & Harris, A. (2001). Hypnotics and sedatives. In J. G. Hardman, L. E. Limbird, & A. G. Goodman (Eds.), *The pharmacological basis of therapeutics* (pp. 399–428). New York: McGraw-Hill.

Gorman, J. N. (2001). Generalized anxiety disorder. *Clinical Cornerstone, 3*(3), 37–46.

Health A to Z. (2003). *Benzodiazepines,* http://www.healthatoz.com

Health Canada. (2006). *Drug Product Database,* http://search.hc-sc.gc.ca/cgi-bin/query?mss=dpd/english/active/

Holcomb, S. S. (2006). Sedative hypnotics in older people with insomnia: Meta-analysis of risks and benefits. Recommendations for assessing insomnia. *Obstetrics & Gynecology, 107*(3), 736–737.

Imovane: Data sheet for professionals. (March 2004). Auckland: Aventis Pharma Ltd.

Lippmann, S., Mazour, I., & Shahab, H. (2001). Insomnia: Therapeutic approach. *Southern Medical Journal, 94*(9), 866–873.

McClung, C. A. (2007). Circadian genes, rhythms and the biology of mood disorders. *Pharmacology & Therapeutics, 114*(2), 222.

Mistraletti, G., Donatelli, F., & Carli, F. Metabolic and endocrine effects of sedative agents. (2005). *Current Opinion in Critical Care, 11*(4), 312–317.

Morgan, K., Dixon, S., Mathers, N., Thompson, J., & Tomeny, M. (2004). Psychological treatment for insomnia in the regulation of long-term hypnotic drug use. *Health Technology Assessment, 8*(8), 1–68.

Pagel, J. F. (2005). Medications and their effects on sleep. *Primary Care Clinics in Office Practice, 32,* 491–509.

Ruyak, P. S., Bilsbury, C. D., & Rajda, M. (2004). A survey of insomnia treatment at Canadian sleep centres: Is there a role for clinical psychologists? *Canadian Psychology, 45*(2),165–173.

Smock, T. K. (2001). *Physiological psychology: A neuroscience approach.* Upper Saddle River, NJ: Prentice Hall.

Vitiello, M. V. (2000). Effective treatment of sleep disturbances in older adults. *Clinical Cornerstone, 2*(5), 16–27.

Yang, C. M., Spielman, A. J., & Glovinsky, P. (2006). Nonpharmacologic strategies in the management of insomnia. *Psychiatric Clinics of North America, 29,* 895–919.

Chapter 15

Burstein, A. H., Horton, R. L., Dunn, T., et al. (2000). Lack of effect of St. John's wort on carbamazepine pharmacokinetics in healthy volunteers. *Clinical Pharmacology and Therapeutics, 68,* 6.

Health Canada. (2006). *Drug Product Database,* http://search.hc-sc.gc.ca/cgi-bin/query?mss=dpd/english/active/

Johnson, K. (2002). Epilepsy and pregnancy. *Medscape Ob/Gyn & Women's Health 7*(2).

Murphy, P. A., & Blaylock, R. L. (2001). *Treating epilepsy naturally: A guide to alternative and adjunct therapies.* New York: McGraw-Hill Contemporary Books.

Pack, A. M., & Morrell, M. J. (2003). Treatment of women with epilepsy. *Seminars in Neurology, 22*(3), 289–298.

Patel, P., & Mageda, M. (2002, April). *Vitamin K deficiency.* E-Medicine: Instant Access to the Minds of Medicine, http://www.emedicine.com

Snelson, C., & Dieckman, B. (2000, June). Recognizing and managing purple glove syndrome. *Critical Care Nurse, 20*(3), 54–61.

Tierney, L. M., McPhee, S. J., and Papadakis, M. A. (Eds.). (2002). The nervous system. In M. J. Minoff (Ed.), *Current medical diagnosis and treatment* (ch. 24). New York: Lange Medical Books/McGraw-Hill Medical Publishing Division.

Trimble, M., & Schmitz, B. (Eds.). (2002). *The neuropsychiatry of epilepsy.* New York: Cambridge University Press.

University of Illinois at Chicago, College of Pharmacy Drug Information Center. (2003). *Is there an interaction between phenytoin and enteral feedings?* http://www.uic.edu

Wyllie, E. (2001). *The treatment of epilepsy: Principles and practice* (3rd ed.). Philadelphia: Lippincott, Williams & Wilkins.

Chapter 16

American Academy of Pediatrics. (2000). Diagnosis and evaluation of the child with attention deficit-hyperactivity disorder. *Pediatrics, 105*(5), 1158–1170.

Baker, G. B., Coutts, R. T., & Greenshaw, A. J. (2000). Neurochemical and metabolic aspects of antidepressants: An overview. *Journal of Psychiatry & Neuroscience, 25*(5), 481–496.

Baldessarini, R. J. (2001). Drugs and the treatment of psychiatric disorders: Depression and anxiety disorders. In J. G. Hardman, L. E. Limbird, & A. G. Goodman (Eds.), *The pharmacological basis of therapeutics* (pp. 447–484). New York: McGraw-Hill.

Black, K., Shea, C., Dursun, S., & Kutcher, S. (2000). Selective serotonin reuptake inhibitor discontinuation syndrome: Proposed diagnostic criteria. *Journal of Psychiatry & Neuroscience, 25*(3), 255–261.

Bodkin J. A., & Amsterdam, J. D. (2002). Transdermal selegiline in major depression: A double-blind, placebo-controlled study in outpatients. *Journal of Psychiatry, 159*(11), 1869–1875.

Brown, C. S., Markowitz, J. S., Moore, T. R., & Parker, N. G. (1999). Atypical antipsychotics: Part II. Adverse effects, drug interactions, and costs. *Annals of Pharmacotherapy, 33*, 210–217.

Burns, M. J. (2001). The pharmacology and toxicology of atypical antipsychotic agents. *Journal of Toxicology: Clinical Toxicology, 39*(1), 1.

Centre for Effective Practice. (2007). *Guidelines Advisory Committee: Management of moderate to severe depression.* Available: http://www.gacguidelines.ca/index.cfm?ACT=topics&Summary_ID=216&Topic_ID=23

DeBattista, C., Solvason, H. B., Poirier, J., Kendrick, E., & Schatzberg, A. F. (2003). A prospective trial of bupropion SR augmentation of partial and non-responders to serotonergic antidepressants. *Journal of Clinical Psychopharmacology, 23*(1), 27–30.

Desai, H. D., & Jann, M. W. (2000). Major depression in women: A review of the literature. *Journal of the American Pharmacists Association, 40*(4), 525–537.

Eli Lilly & Company. (2003). *Strattera: Safety information for health care professionals.* Indianapolis, IN: Author. http://www.strattera.com

Emslie, G. J., & Mayes, T. L. (1999). Depression in children and adolescents: A guide to diagnosis and treatment. *CNS Drugs, 11*(3), 181–189.

Entsuah, R. A., Huang, H., & Thase, M. E. (2001). Response and remission rates in different subpopulations with major depressive disorder administered venlafaxine, selective serotonin reuptake inhibitors, or placebo. *Journal of Clinical Psychiatry, 62*, 869–877.

Furukawa, T. A., McGuire, H., & Barbui, C. (2002). Meta-analysis of effects and side effects of low dosage tricyclic antidepressants in depression: Systematic review. *British Medical Journal, 325*(7371), 991–1000.

Goodwin, F. K., & Goldstein, M. A. (2003). Optimizing lithium treatment in bipolar disorder: A review of the literature and clinical recommendations. *Journal of Psychiatric Practice, 9*(5), 333–343.

Health Products and Food Branch, Health Canada. (2006). *Drug Product Database.* Retrieved April 10, 2006, from http://www.hc-sc.gc.ca/hpfb-dgpsa/tpd-dpt/index_drugs_dpd_e.html

Health Products and Food Branch, Health Canada. (2005). *Important safety information regarding the discontinuation of sales of nefazodone in Canada.* Retrieved April 4, 2005, from http://druginjurylaw.com/serzone-canada.pdf

Hong Ng, C., Norman, T. R., Naing, K. O., Schweitzer, I., Kong Wai Ho, B., Fan, A., et al. (2006). A comparative study of sertraline dosages, plasma concentrations, efficacy and adverse reactions in Chinese versus Caucasian patients. *International Clinical Psychopharmacology, 21*(2), 87–92.

Janicak, P. (2002). *Research report: rTMS vs. ECT in depressed patients.* Chicago: University of Illinois.

Medical Economics Staff (Ed.). (2000). *PDR for herbal medicines.* Montvale, NJ: Author.

Modell, J. G., Katholi, C. R., Modell, J. D., & et al. (1997). Comparative sexual side effects of bupropion, fluoxetine, paroxetine, and sertraline. *Clinical Pharmacology and Therapeutics, 61*, 476–487.

Moses, S. (2003). *Imipramine. Family practice notebook.* Lino Lakes, MN: Family Practice Notebook, LLC, http://www.fpnotebook.com

Nelson, J. C., Mazure, C. M., Jatlow, P. I., & et al. (2004). Combining norepinephrine and serotonin reuptake inhibition mechanisms for treatment of depression: A double-blind, randomized study. *Biological Psychiatry, 55*, 296–300.

Hong Ng, C., Norman, T., Naing, K. O., Schweitzer, I., Kong Wai Ho, B., Fan, A., et al. (2006). A comparative study of sertraline dosages, plasma concentrations, efficacy and adverse reactions in Chinese versus Caucasian patients. *International Clinical Psychopharmacology, 21*(2), 87–92.

Schellenburg, R. (2001). Treatment for the premenstrual syndrome with agnus castus fruit extract: Prospective, randomized placebo-controlled study. *British Medical Journal, 322*(279), 134.

Serretti, A., Artioli, P., & Quartesan, R. (2005). Pharmacogenetics in the treatment of depression: Pharmacodynamic studies. *Pharmacogenetics & Genomics, 15*(2), 61–67.

Sifton, D. (Ed.). (2002). *Health care provider's desk reference (PDR).* Montvale, NJ: Medical Economics Company.

Spector, R. E. (2000). *Cultural diversity in health and illness.* Upper Saddle River, NJ: Prentice Hall Health.

Stahl, S. M. (2005). Antidepressant treatment of psychotic major depression: Potential role of the sigma receptor. *CNS Spectrums, 10*(4), 319–323.

Stahl, S. M., & Grady, M. M. (2003). Differences in mechanism of action between current and future antidepressants. *Journal of Clinical Psychiatry, 64*(Suppl. 13), 13–17.

Stahl, S. M., Pradko, J. F., Haight, B. R., Modell, J. G., Rockett, C. B., & Learned-Coughlin, S. (2004). A review of the neuropharmacology of bupropion, a dual norepinephrine and dopamine reuptake inhibitor. *Primary Care Companion to the Journal of Clinical Psychiatry, 6*, 159–166.

Statistics Canada (2003). Canadian community health survey, 2003. (Catalogue no. 82-401).

Willner, P., Hale, A. S., & Argyropoulos, S. (2005). Dopaminergic mechanism of antidepressant action in depressed patients. *Journal of Affective Disorders, 86*(1), 37–45.

Yatham, L. N., Kennedy, S. H., O'Donovan, C., Parikh, S., MacQueen, G., McIntyre, R., et al. (2005). Canadian network for mood and anxiety treatments (canmat) guidelines for the management of patients with bipolar disorder: Consensus and controversies. *Bipolar Disorders, 7*(s3), 5–69.

Chapter 17

Bailey, K. (2003). Aripiprazole: The newest antipsychotic agent for the treatment of schizophrenia. *Psychosocial Nursing and Mental Health Services, 41*(2), 14–18.

Baldessarini, R. J., & Tarazi, F. I. (2001). Drugs and the treatment of psychiatric disorders: Psychosis and mania. In J. G. Hardman, L. E. Limbird, & A. G. Goodman (Eds.), *The pharmacological basis of therapeutics* (pp. 485–520). New York: McGraw-Hill.

Barclay, L. (2002, July 1). Quetiapine well-tolerated, effective in refractory schizophrenia. *Medscape Medical News,* http://www.medscape.com

Barthel, R. (2002, October 27). Early interventions in psychosis. *Medscape Medical News,* http://www.medscape.com

Brown University Child and Adolescent Psychopharmacology Update. (2002, July 19). Drugs in the pipeline: New drugs and indications for children and adolescents. *Medscape Medical News* http://www.medscape.com

Brown University Geriatric Psychopharmacology Update. (2002, December 9). Treating bipolar disorder in older adults: Gaps in knowledge remain, *Medscape Medical News,* http://www.medscape.com

Burns, M. J. (2001). The pharmacology and toxicology of atypical antipsychotic agents. *Journal of Toxicology: Clinical Toxicology, 39*(1), 1.

Cada, D., Levien, T., & Baker, D. (2003). Aripiprazole. *Hospital Pharmacy 38*(3), 247–254.

Health Canada. (2006). *Drug Product Database,* http://search.hc-sc.gc.ca/cgi-bin/query?mss=dpd/english/active/

Kneisl, C. R., Wilson, H. S., & Trigoboff, E. (2004). *Contemporary psychiatric-mental health nursing.* Upper Saddle River, NJ: Prentice Hall.

Markowitz, J. S., Brown, C. S., & Moore, T. R. (1999). Atypical antipsychotics: Part I. Pharmacology, pharmacokinetics, and efficacy. *Annals of Pharmacotherapy 33,* 73–85.

Medical Economics Staff (Ed.). (2000). *PDR for herbal medicines.* Montvale, NJ: Author.

Medscape Medical News. (2003, February 13). *Dispensing errors reported for serzone and seroquel,* http://www.medscape.com

Vitiello, B. (2001). Psychopharmacology for young children: Clinical needs and research opportunities. *Pediatrics, 108*(4), 983.

Wahlbeck, K., Cheine, M., & Essali, M. A. (2002, April 1). Clozapine versus typical neuroleptic medication for schizophrenia. *Cochrane Review Abstracts, Medscape Medical News,* http://www.medscape.com

Chapter 18

Alzheimer's disease. (2003, April 11). *Unraveling the mystery: The search for new treatments,* http://www.alzheimers.org

Alzheimer's disease fact sheet, http://www.alzheimers.org

Birks, J., Grimley-Evans, J., & Van Dongen, M. (2003). Ginkgo biloba for cognitive impairment and dementia. *Medscape Medical News,* http://www.medscape.com

Brain-cell growth protein shows promise for Parkinson's in early human trial, http://www.parkinsons-foundation.org

Capozza, K. (2003, April 2). *Drug slows progression of Alzheimer's,* http://www.nlm.nih.gov/medlineplus

Cummings, J. L. (2000). Treatment of Alzheimer's disease. *Clinic Corner, 3*(4), 27–39.

Dooley, M., & Lamb, H. M. (2000). Donepezil: A review of its use in Alzheimer's disease. *Drugs and Aging 16*(3), 199–226.

Gruetzner, H. (2001). *Alzheimer's: A caregiver's guide and sourcebook* (3rd ed.). Indianapolis: John Wiley & Sons.

Health Canada. (2006). *Drug Product Database,* http://search.hc-sc.gc.ca/cgi-bin/query?mss=dpd/english/active/

Hristove, A. H., & Koller, W. C. (2000). Early Parkinson's disease: What is the best approach in treatment? *Drugs and Aging, 17*(3), 165–181.

Kahle, P. (2003). *Molecular mechanisms of Parkinson's disease.* Georgetown, TX: Eurekah.com, Inc.

Lambert, D., & Waters, C. H. (2000). Comparative tolerability of the new generation antiparkinson agents. *Drugs and Aging, 16*(1), 55–65.

Olanow, C. W., & Tatton, W. G. (1999). Etiology and pathogenesis of Parkinson's disease. *Annual Review of Neuroscience, 2,* 123–144.

Richter, R. (Ed.). (2003). *Alzheimer's disease: The physicians' guide to practical management.* Totowa, NJ: Human Press.

Sacco, K. A., Bannon, K. L., & George, T. P. (2004). Nicotinic receptor mechanisms and cognition in normal states and neuropsychiatric disorders. *Journal of Psychopharmacology, 18*(4), 457–474.

Standaert, D. G., & Young, A. B. (2001). Treatment of central nervous system degenerative disorders. In J. G. Hardman, L. E. Limbird, & A. G. Goodman (Eds.), *The pharmacological basis of therapeutics* (pp. 549–568). New York: McGraw-Hill.

Warren, S. A., Svenson, L. W., Metz, L. M., Schopflocher, D. P., & Warren, K. G. (2004). Prevalence of multiple sclerosis (MS) among First Nations people in Alberta, Canada: P03.063. *Neurology, 62*(7, Suppl. S5), A215–A216.

Chapter 19

Bannwarth, B. (1999). Risk-benefit assessment of opioids in chronic noncancer pain. *Drug Safety 21*(4), 283–296.

Barkin, R. L., & Barkin, D. (2001). Pharmacologic management of acute and chronic pain: Focus on drug interactions and patient-specific pharmacotherapeutic selection. *Southern Medical Journal, 94*(8), 756–812.

Bloodworth, D. (2005). Issues in opioid management. *American Journal of Physical Medicine & Rehabilitation-Pain Science and Rational Polypharmacy, 84*(3) Suppl., S42–S55.

Botting, R., & Ayoub, S. S. (2005). Cox-3 and the mechanism of action of paracetamol/acetaminophen. *Prostaglandins, Leukotrienes and Essential Fatty Acids, 72*(2), 85.

Broadbent, C. (2000). The pharmacology of acute pain—Part 3. *Nursing Times, 96*(26), 39.

Canadian Pain Society. (2008). *Evidence-based recommendations for medical management of chronic non-malignant pain: Reference guide for clinicians.* Available: http://meds.queensu.ca/cpd/che/assets/cpso-painguidelines.pdf

Canadian Pain Society. (2007). *Pharmacological Management of Chronic Neuropathic Pain—Consensus statement and guidelines from the Canadian Pain Society,* pharmamgmtofcnp.pdf

Committee on Drugs. (2001). Acetaminophen toxicity in children. *Pediatrics, 108*(4), 1020–1024.

Diamond, M. (2003). *Emergency treatment of headache.* Chicago: Internal Medicine Department, Columbus Hospital, http://www.usdoctor.com

Drenth, J. P. H., & Verheugt, F. W. A. (2007). Do cox-2 inhibitors give enough gastrointestinal protection? *Lancet, 369*, 439–440.

Evers, S., & Frese, A. (2005). Recent advances in the treatment of headaches. *Current Opinion in Anaesthesiology, 18*(5), 563–568.

Glajchen, M. (2001). Chronic pain. Treatment barriers and strategies for clinical practice. *Journal of the American Board of Family Practice,14*(3), 178–183.

Guay, D. R. P. (2001). Adjunctive agents in the management of chronic pain. *Pharmacotherapy, 21*(9), 1070–1081.

Gunsteuin, H., & Akil, H. (2001). Opioid analgesics. In J. G. Hardman, L. E. Limbird, & A. G. Goodman (Eds.), *The pharmacological basis of therapeutics* (pp. 569–620). New York: McGraw-Hill.

Health Canada. (2006). *Drug Product Database,* http://search.hc-sc.gc.ca/cgi-bin/query?mss=dpd/english/active/

Health Canada. (2008). *Important Safety Information on Tylenol with Codeine in Nursing Mothers and Ultra-Rapid Metabolizers of Codeine. MedEffect* advisory. Available: http://www.hc-sc.gc.ca/dhp-mps/medeff/advisories-avis/prof/_2008/index-eng.php

Holmer Pettersson, P., Hein, A., Owall, A., Anderson, R. E., & Jakobsson, J. G. (2005). Early bioavailability in day surgery: a comparison between orally, rectally, and intravenously administered paracetamol. *Ambulatory Surgery, 12*(1), 27.

Khouzam, H. R. (2000). Chronic pain and its management in primary care. *Southern Medical Journal, 93*(10), 946–952.

Maharaj, H., Maharaj, D. S., Saravanan, K. S., Mohanakumar, K. P., & Daya, S. (2004). Aspirin curtails the acetaminophen-induced rise in brain norepinephrine levels. *Metabolic Brain Disease, 19*(1–2), 71.

McKeever, T. M., Lewis, S. A., Smit, H. A., Burney, P., Britton, J. R., & Cassano, P. A. (2005). The association of acetaminophen, aspirin, and ibuprofen with respiratory disease and lung function. *American Journal of Respiratory and Critical Care Medicine, 171*(9), 966–971.

Onen, S. H., Onen, F., Courpron, P., & Dubray, C. (2005). How pain and analgesics disturb sleep. *Clinical Journal of Pain Childhood Abuse and Pain in Adulthood, 21*(5), 422–431.

RxList.com. (2003). B*ayer ASA side effects & ASA drug interactions.* http://www.rxlist.com

Tepper, S. J., & Rapoport, A. M. (1999). The triptans: A summary. *CNS Drugs, 12*(5), 403–417.

Tfelt-Hansen, P., DeVries, P., & Sexena, P. R. (2000). Triptans in migraine: A comparative review of pharmacology, pharmacokinetics, and efficacy. *Drugs, 60*(6), 1259–1287.

Vadivelu, N., & Sinatra, R. (2005). Recent advances in elucidating pain mechanisms. *Current Opinion in Anaesthesiology, 18*(5), 540–547.

White, P. F. (2005). The changing role of non-opioid analgesic techniques in the management of postoperative pain. *Anesthesia & Analgesia, November, 101*(5S) Suppl., S5–S22.

Chapter 20

Catterall, W. A., & Mackie, K. (2001). Local anesthetics. In J. G. Hardman, L. E. Limbird, & A. G. Goodman (Eds.), *The pharmacological basis of therapeutics* (pp. 367–384). New York: McGraw-Hill.

Colbert, B. J., & Mason, B. J. (2001). *Integrated cardiopulmonary pharmacology.* New Jersey: Prentice Hall.

DeBalli, P. (2003). The use of propofol as an antiemetic. *International Anesthesiology Clinics Fall, 41*(4), 67–77.

Evers, A., & Crowder, C. M. (2001). General anesthetics. In J. G. Hardman, L. E. Limbird, & A. G. Goodman (Eds.), *The pharmacological basis of therapeutics* (pp. 337–366). New York: McGraw-Hill.

Health Canada. (2006). *Drug Product Database,* http://search.hc-sc.gc.ca/cgi-bin/query?mss=dpd/english/active/

Kanaya, N., Satoh, H., Seki, S., Nakayama, M., & Namiki, A. (2002). Propofol anesthesia enhances the pressor response to intravenous ephedrine. *Anesthesia & Analgesia, 94*(5), 1207–1211.

Kids Health for Parents. (2003). *Your child's anesthesia.* The Nemours Foundation, http://www.kidshealth.org

Nagelhout, J. J., Nagelhout, K., & Zaglaniczny, V. H. (2001). *Handbook of nurse anesthesia* (2nd ed.). Philadelphia: W. B. Saunders.

Omogui, S. (1999). *Sota Omogui's anesthesia drugs handbook* (3rd ed.). Hawthorne, CA: State of the Art Technologies.

Stoelting, R. K. (1999). *Pharmacology and physiology in anesthetic practice* (3rd ed.). Philadelphia: Lippincott, Williams, & Wilkins.

Waugaman, W. R., Foster, S. D., & Rigor, B. M. (1999). *Principles and practice of nurse anesthesia* (3rd ed.). Upper Saddle River, NJ: Prentice Hall.

Chapter 21

Allergy Resources International. (2003). *Angioedema,* http://allallergy.net/articles/index.cfm/edeoc/AO

Asmar, R. (2006). Targeting effective blood pressure control with angiotensin receptor blockers. *International Journal of Clinical Practice, 60*(3), 315–320.

Bolli, P., Hemmelgarn, B., Myers, M. G., McKay, D., Tremblay, & G., Tobe S., for the Canadian Hypertension Education Program. (2007). High Normal blood pressure and prehypertension: The debate continues. *Canadian Journal of Cardiology, 23*(7), 581–583.

Campbell, N., with the assistance of the CHEP executive. (2007). Canadian Hypertension Education Program Guidelines: An annual update. *The Canadian Journal of Diagnosis.* May, 77–81.

Campbell, N.R. (2007, May). The 2007 Canadian Hypertension Education Program Recommendations: The Scientific Summary—an annual update. *Canadian Journal of Cardiology, 23*, 521– 527.

Canadian Hypertension Society. (2006, 2008). *Canadian Hypertension Education Program Recommendations.* Available: http://www.hypertension.ca/chep/recommendations/recommendations-overview/

Cook, N. R., Cutler, J. A., Obarzanek, E., Buring, J. E., Rexrode, K. M., Kumanyika, S. K., et al. (2007). Long term effects of dietary sodium reduction on cardiovascular disease outcomes: observational follow-up of the trials of hypertension prevention (TOHP). *British Medical Journal, 334*(7599), 885.

Kaplan, M. S., Chang, C., Newsom, J. T., & McFarland, B. H. (2002). Acculturation status and hypertension among Asian immigrants in Canada. *Journal of Epidemiology and Community Health, 56*(6), 455–456.

Khan, N.A., Hemmelgarn, B., Padwal, R. et al., (2007, May). The 2007 Canadian Hypertension Education program Recommendations for the management of Hypertension: Part 2—therapy. *Canadian Journal of Cardiology, 23*(7), 539–550.

Klag, M. J., Wang, N. Y., Meoni, L. A., Brancati, F. L., Cooper, L. A., Liang, K. Y., Young, J. H., & Ford, D. E. (2002). Coffee: Intake and risk of hypertension. The Johns Hopkins Precursors Study. *Archives of Internal Medicine, 162*, 657–662.

McLean, D., Kingsbury, K., Costello, J., Cloutier, L., & Matheson, S. (2007). Canadian Hypertension Education Program (CHEP) Recommendations: Management of hypertension by nurses. *Canadian Journal of Cardiovascular Nursing, 17*(2), 10–16.

Nurko, S. (2001). At what level of hyperkalemia or creatinine elevation should ACE inhibitor therapy be stopped or not started? *Cleveland Clinic Journal of Medicine 68*, 9, 754–760.

Oates, J. A., & Brown, N. J. (2001). Antihypertensive agents and the drug therapy of hypertension. In J. G. Hardman, L. E. Limbard, & A. G. Goodman (Eds.), *The pharmacological basis of therapeutics* (pp. 871–900). New York: McGraw-Hill.

Thadhani, R., Camargo, Jr., C. A., Stampfer, M. J., Curhan, G. C., Willett, W. C., & Rimm, E. B. (2002). Prospective study of moderate alcohol consumption and risk of hypertension in young women. *Archives of Internal Medicine, 162*, 569–574.

Touyz, R., & CHEP executive. (2006). Canadian Hypertension Education Program Recommendations: A new key message and some old but still important considerations. *Hypertension Canada,* Bulletin 86.

Woods, A. D. (2001). Improving the odds against hypertension. *Nursing, 31*(8), 36–42.

Chapter 22

Beaird, S. L. (2000). HMG-CoA reductase inhibitors: Assessing differences in drug interactions and safety profiles. *Journal of the American Pharmacists Association, 40*(5), 637–644.

Canadian Cardiovascular Society. (2006). Canadian Cardiovascular Society Position Statement—Recommendations for the diagnosis and treatment of dyslipidemia and prevention of cardiovascular disease.

Canadian Diabetes Association. (2003). Clinical practice guidelines: Management of obesity in diabetes.

Genest, J., Frohlich, J., Fodor, G., & McPherson, R. (2003). Recommendations for the management of dyslipidemia and the prevention of cardiovascular disease: Summary of the 2003 update. *Canadian Medical Association Journal, 169*(9), 921–924.

Go, A. S., Lee, W. Y., Yang, J., Lo, J. C., & Gurwitz, J. H. (2006). Statin therapy and risks for death and hospitalization in chronic heart failure. *Journal of the American Medical Association, 296*(17), 2105–2111.

Illingworth, D. R. (2000). Management of hypercholesterolemia. *Medical Clinics of North America, 84*(1), 23–42.

Law, M. (2000). Plant stanol and sterol margarines. *British Medical Journal, 320*, 861–864.

Meagher, E. A. (2004). Addressing cardiovascular disease in women: Focus on dyslipidemia. *Journal of the American Board of Family Practice, 17*(6), 424–437.

Maltin, L. (2002, April 9). *Statin drugs may fight Alzheimer's, too.* WebMD Medical News, my.webmd.com/content/article/16/1626_50907

Nutrition and Metabolism Advisory Committee, Heart Foundation. (2001) Plant sterols and stanols, a position statement. Melbourne, Australia: Heart Foundation.

Oberman, A. (2000). Role of lipids in the prevention of cardiovascular disease. *Clinical Review,* (Spring), 10–15.

Pilote, L., Dasgupta, K., Guru, V., Humphries, K. H., McGrath, J., Norris, C., et al. (2007). A comprehensive view of sex-specific issues related to cardiovascular disease. *Canadian Medical Association Journal, 176*(6), S1–S44.

Robinson, A. W., Sloan, H. L., & Arnold, G. (2001). Use of niacin in the prevention and management of hyperlipidemia. *Progress in Cardiovascular Nursing, 16*(1), 14–20.

Roche. (2004). *Xenical.* Retrieved January 24, 2006, from http://www.roche.com

Tamargo, J., Caballero, R., Gomez, R., Nunez, L., Vaquero, M., & Delpon, E. (2007). Lipid-lowering therapy with statins, a new approach to antiarrhythmic therapy. *Pharmacology & Therapeutics, 114*(1), 107.

Young, K. L., Allen, J. K., & Kelly, K. M. (2001). HDL cholesterol: Striving for healthier levels. *Clinical Review, 11*(5), 50–61.

Chapter 23

Ambrose, J., & Dangas, G. (2000). Unstable angina: Current concepts of pathogenesis and treatment. *Archives of Internal Medicine, 160*, 25–37.

Deedwania, P. C. (2000). Silent myocardial ischemia in the elderly. *Drugs & Aging, 16*(5), 381–389.

Karp, I., Chen, S. F., & Pilote, L. (2007). Sex differences in the effectiveness of statins after myocardial infarction. *Canadian Medical Association Journal, 176*(3): 333–338.

Kerins, D. M., Robertson, R. M., & Robertson, D. (2001). Drugs used for the treatment of myocardial ischemia. In J. G. Hardman et al. (Eds.), *The pharmacological basis of therapeutics* (10th ed.). New York: McGraw-Hill.

Kreisberg, R. A. (2000). Overview of coronary heart disease and selected risk factors. *Clinical Review,* (Spring), 4–9.

Larsen, J. A., Kadish, A. H., & Schwartz, J. B. (2000). Proper use of antiarrhythmic therapy for reduction of mortality after myocardial infarction. *Drugs & Aging, 16*(5), 341–350.

Levine, G. N., Ali, M. N., & Schafer, A. I. (2001). Antithrombotic therapy in patients with acute coronary syndromes. *Archives of Internal Medicine, 161,* 937–948.

Manuel, D. G., Kwong, K., Tanuseputro, P., Lim, J., Mustard, C. A., Anderson, G. M, Ardal, S., Alter, D. A., & Laupacis, A. (2006). Effectiveness and efficiency of different guidelines on statin treatment for preventing deaths from coronary heart disease: Modelling study. *British Medical Journal, 332*(7555), 1419.

McDonald, M. A., Simpson, S. H., Ezekowitz, J. A., Gyenes, G., & Tsuyuki, R. T. (2005). Angiotensin receptor blockers and risk of myocardial infarction: Systematic review. *British Medical Journal, 331*(7521), 873–879.

O'Rourke, F., Dean, N., Akhtar, N., & Shuaib, A. (2004). Current and future concepts in stroke prevention. *Canadian Medical Association Journal, 170*(7), 1123–1133.

Parchure, N., & Brecker, S. J. (2002). Management of acute coronary syndromes. *Current Opinion in Critical Care, 8*(3), 230–235.

Selim, M., Savitz, S., Linfante, I., Caplan, L., & Schlaug, G. (2005). Effect of pre-stroke use of ACE inhibitors on ischemic stroke severity. *BMC Neurology, 5*(10), 1–7.

Sloan, M. A. (2005). Use of anticoagulant agents for stroke prevention. *Continuum: Lifelong Learning in Neurology Stroke Prevention, 11*(4), 97–127.

Smellie, W. S., & Coleman, J. J. (2007). Pitfalls of testing and summary of guidance on safety monitoring with amiodarone and digoxin. *British Medical Journal, 334*(7588), 312–315.

Staniforth, A. D. (2001). Contemporary management of chronic stable angina. *Drugs & Aging, 18*(2), 109–121.

Zhou, Z., Rahme, E., Abrahamowicz, M., Tu, J. V., Eisenberg, M. J., Humphries, K., Austin, P. C., & Pilote, L. (2005). Effectiveness of statins for secondary prevention in elderly patients after acute myocardial infarction: An evaluation of class effect. *Canadian Medical Association Journal, 172*(9), 1187–1194.

Chapter 24

Ahmed, A., Rich, M. W., Love, T. E., et al. (2006). Digoxin and reduction in mortality and hospitalization in heart failure: A comprehensive post hoc analysis of the DIG trial. *European Heart Journal, 27,*178–186.

Ahmed, A., Young, J. B., & Gheorghiade M. (2007). The underuse of digoxin in heart failure, and approaches to appropriate use. *Canadian Medical Association Journal, 176*(5), 641–643.

Allen, L. A., & O'Connor, C. M. (2007). Management of acute decompensated heart failure. *Canadian Medical Association Journal, 176*(6), 797–805.

Arnold, J. M. O., Howlett, J. G., Dorian, P., Ducharme, A., Giannetti, N., Haddad, H., et al. (2007). Canadian Cardiovascular Society Consensus Conference recommendations on heart failure update 2007: Prevention, management during intercurrent illness or acute decompensation, and use of biomarkers. *Canadian Journal of Cardiology, 23*(1), 21–45.

Arnold, J. M. O., Liu, P., et al. (2006). Canadian Cardiovascular Society consensus conference recommendations on heart failure:

Diagnosis and management. *Canadian Journal of Cardiology, 22*(1), 23–45.

Asmar, R (2006). Targeting effective blood pressure control with angiotensin receptor blockers. *International Journal of Clinical Practice, 60*(3), 315–320.

Bhatia, R. S., Tu, J. V., Lee, D. S., et al. (2006). Outcome of heart failure with preserved ejection fraction in a population-based study. *New England Journal of Medicine, 355,* 260–269.

Bursi, F., Weston, S. A., Redfield, M. M., et al. (2006). Systolic and diastolic heart failure in the community. *Journal of the American Medical Association, 296,* 2209–2216.

Canadian Cardiovascular Society. (2008). *Canadian Cardiovascular Society Consensus Conference Guidelines on Heart Failure 2008.* Available: http://www.hfcc.ca/stage2/guidelines.aspx

Canadian Cardiovascular Society. (2006). *CCS Heart Failure Consensus Recommendations Slide Kit.* Retrieved March 12, 2007, from http://www.hfcc.ca/educational_tools/

Chang , W. T., Dao, J. & Shao, J. H. (2005). Hawthorn: Potential roles in cardiovascular disease. *American Journal of Chinese Medicine, 33*(1), 1–10.

Chow, C. M. et al. (2005). Regional variation in self-reported heart disease prevalence in Canada. *Canadian Journal of Cardiology, 21*(14), 1265–1271.

Dobre, D., van Veldhuisen, D. J., Dejongste, M. J., et al. (2007). Prescription of beta-blockers in patients with advanced heart failure and preserved left ventricular ejection fraction. Clinical implications and survival. *European Journal of Heart Failure, 9*(3), 280–286.

Friedman, J. M. (2006). ACE inhibitors and congenital anomalies. *New England Journal of Medicine, 354*(23), 2498–2500.

Go, A. S., Lee, W. Y., Yang, J., Lo, J. C., & Gurwitz, J. H. (2006). Statin therapy and risks for death and hospitalization in chronic heart failure. *Journal of the American Medical Association, 296*(17), 2105–2111.

Heckman, G. A., & McKelvie, R.S. (2007). Necessary cautions when considering digoxin in heart failure. *Canadian Medical Association Journal, 176*(5), 644–645.

Heart and Stroke Foundation of Canada. (May 2003). The growing burden of heart disease and stroke in Canada 2003.

Jamali, A. H., Tang, A. H. W., Khot, U. N., & Fowler, M. B. (2001). The role of angiotensin receptor blockers in the management of chronic heart failure. *Archives of Internal Medicine, 161,* 667–672.

Johansen, H., et al. (2003). On the rise: The current and projected future burden of congestive heart failure hospitalization in Canada. *Canadian Journal of Cardiology, 19*(4), 430–435.

Lee, D. S., et al. (2004). Regional outcomes of heart failure in Canada. *Canadian Journal of Cardiology, 20*(6), 599–607.

Owan, T. E., Hodge, D. O., Herges, R. M., Jacobsen, S. J., Roger, V. L., & Redfield, M. M. (2006). Trends in prevalence and outcome of heart failure with preserved ejection fraction. *New England Journal of Medicine, 355,* 251–259.

Owan, T. E., & Redfield, M. M. (2005). Epidemiology of diastolic heart failure. *Progress in Cardiovascular Disease, 47*c, 320–332.

Paul, S. (2002). Balancing diuretic therapy in heart failure: Loop diuretics, thiazides, and antagonists. *Congestive Heart Failure, 8*(6), 307–312.

Pittler, M. H., Schmidt, K., & Ernst, E. (2003). Hawthorn extract for treating chronic heart failure: Meta-analysis of randomized trials. *American Journal of Medicine, 114*(8), 665–674.

Richardson, L. G. (2003). Psychosocial issues in patients with congestive heart failure. *Progressive Cardiovascular Nursing, 18*(1), 19–27.

Solomon, S. D. et al. (2005). Influence of ejection fraction on cardiovascular outcomes in a broad spectrum of heart failure patients. *Circulation, 112,* 3738–3744.

Sperelakis, N., Kurachi, Y., Terzic, A., & Cohen, M. (Eds.). (2001). *Heart physiology and pathophysiology* (4th ed.). San Diego: Academic Press.

Tankanow, R., Tamer, H. R., Streetman, D. S., Smith, S. G., Welton, J. L., Annesley, T., et al. (2003). Interaction study between digoxin and a preparation of hawthorn (*Crataegus oxyacantha*). *Journal of Clinical Pharmacology, 43*(6), 637–642.

Young, J. B., et al. (2004). Mortality and morbidity reduction with candesartan in patients with chronic heart failure and left ventricular systolic dysfunction: results of the CHARM low-left ventricular ejection fraction trials. *Circulation, 110,* 2618–2626.

Yusuf, S., Pfeffer, M. A., Swedberg, K., & CHARM Investigators and Committees. (2006). Effects of candesartan in patients with chronic heart failure and preserved left-ventricular ejection fraction: The CHARM-Preserved Trial. *Lancet, 362,* 777–781.

Chapter 25

Antzelevitch, C. & Belardinelli, L. (2006) The role of sodium channel current in modulating transmural dispersion of repolarization and arrhythmogenesis. *Journal of Cardiovascular Electrophysiology, 17*(Suppl. 1), S79–S85.

Beattie, W. S., & Elliot, R. F. (2005). Magnesium supplementation reduces the risk of arrhythmia after cardiac surgery. *Evidence-based Cardiovascular Medicine, 9*(1), 82–5.

Canadian Cardiovascular Society. (2005). *2004 Consensus Conference: Atrial Fibrillation.* Retrieved March 12, 2007, from http://www.ccs.ca/consensus_conferences/2004_AF_chapters_e.aspx

Dayer, M., & Hardman, S. (2002). Special problems with antiarrhythmic drugs in the elderly: Safety, tolerability, and efficacy. *American Journal of Geriatric Cardiology, 11*(6), 370–375.

Diner, B. M., Yiannakoulias, N., Holroyd, B. R., Bullard, M., Spooner, C. H., Rosychuk, R., et al. (2003). Emergency department presentations of atrial fibrillation (AF) in Alberta, Canada. *Academy of Emergency Medicine, 10,* 544.

Dorian, P. & Connors, S. P. (2005). Pharmacological and non-pharmacological methods for rate control. *Canadian Journal of Cardiology, 21*(Suppl. B), 26B–30B.

Everett, T. H. & Olgin, J. E. (2007). Atrial fibrosis and the mechanisms of atrial fibrillation. *Heart Rhythm, 4*(3 Suppl.), S24–S27.

Falk, R. H. (2001). Medical progress: Atrial fibrillation. *New England Journal of Medicine, 344,* 1067–1078.

Fenton, J. M. (2001). The clinician's approach to evaluating patients with dysrhythmias. *AACN Clinical Issues, 12*(1), 72–86.

Haugh, K. H. (2002). Antidysrhythmic agents at the turn of the twenty-first century: A current review. *Critical Care Nursing Clinics of North America, 14*(1), 53–69.

Huikuri, H. V., Castellanos, A., & Myerburg, R. J. (2001). Medical progress: Sudden death due to cardiac arrhythmias. *New England Journal of Medicine, 345,* 1473–1482.

Humphries, K., Jackevicius, C., Gong, Y., Svensen, L., Cox, J., Tu, J., Laupacis, A. (2004). Population rates of hospitalization for atrial fibrillation/flutter in Canada. *Canadian Journal of Cardiology, 20*(9), 869–876.

Kudzma, E. C. (2001). Cultural competence: *Cardiovascular medications. Progress in Cardiovascular Inderal.* Medscape DrugInfo (2003), http://www.medscape.com/druginfo/

Morrill, P. (2000). Pharmacotherapeutics of positive inotropes. *AORN-Journal, 71*(1), 173–178, 181–185.

Podrid, P. J., & Kowey, P. R. (Eds.). (2001). *Cardiac arrhythmia: Mechanisms, diagnosis, and management* (2nd ed.). Philadelphia: Lippincott, Williams, & Wilkins.

Roden, D. M. (2006). Antiarrhythmic drugs. In L. L. Brunton, J. S. Lazo, & K. L. Parker (Eds.), *Goodman & Gilman's The pharmacological basis of therapeutics* (11th ed., pp. 899–932). New York: McGraw-Hill.

Somberg, J. C., Cao, W., Cvetanovic, I., Ranade, V. V., & Molnar, J. (2005). The effect of magnesium sulfate on action potential duration and cardiac arrhythmias. *American Journal of Therapeutics, 12*(3), 218–222.

Tong, G. M., & Rude, R. K. (2005). Magnesium deficiency in critical illness. *Journal of Intensive Care Medicine, 20*(1), 3–17.

Ueshima, K. (2005). Magnesium and ischemic heart disease: A review of epidemiological, experimental, and clinical evidences. *Magnesium Research, 18*(4), 275–284.

Chapter 26

Alligood, K. A., & Iltz, J. L. (2001). Update on antithrombotic use and mechanism of action. *Progress in Cardiovascular Nursing, 16*(2), 81–85.

Allison, G. L., Lowe, G. M., & Rahman, K. (2006). Aged garlic extract and its constituents inhibit platelet aggregation through multiple mechanisms. *Journal of Nutrition, 136*(Suppl. 3), 782S–788S.

Connolly, S. J., & Gillis, A. M. (2005). Therapies for the prevention of stroke and other vascular events in atrial fibrillation and atrial flutter. *Canadian Journal of Cardiology, 21*(Suppl. B), 71B–73B.

Health Canada. (2006). *It's your health: Warfarin and natural products.* Retrieved from http://www.hc-sc.gc.ca/iyh-vsv/med/warfarin_e.html

HealthSquare.com. (2003). *Coumadin: Prescription drug reference,* http://www.healthsquare.com

Hiatt, W. R. (2001). Drug therapy: Medical treatment of peripheral arterial disease and claudication. *New England Journal of Medicine, 344,* 1608–1621.

Hirsh, J., & Raschke, R. (2004). Heparin and low-molecular-weight heparin: The Seventh ACCP Conference on Antithrombotic and Thrombolytic Therapy. *Chest, 126*(3 Suppl.), 188S–203S.

Huyen, T., & Anand, S. S. (2004). Oral antiplatelet therapy in cerebrovascular disease, coronary artery disease, and peripheral arterial disease. *Journal of the American Medical Association, 292,* 1867.

Majerus, P. W., & Tollefson, D. M. (2001). Anticoagulant, thrombolytic, and antiplatelet drugs. In J. G. Hardman, L. E. Limbard,

& A. G. Goodman (Eds.), *The pharmacological basis of therapeutics* (pp. 1519–1538). New York: McGraw-Hill.

Pereira, J. A., Holbrook, A. M., Dolovich, L., Goldsmith, C., Thabane, L., Douketis, J. D., et al. (2005). Are brand-name and generic warfarin interchangeable? A survey of Ontario patients and physicians. *Canadian Journal of Clinical Pharmacology, 12*(3), e240–e245.

Pilote, L., Dasgupta, K., Guru, V., Humphries, K. H., McGrath, J., Norris, C., et al. (2007). A comprehensive view of sex-specific issues related to cardiovascular disease. *Canadian Medical Association Journal, 176*(6), S1–S44.

Rahman, K., & Lowe, G. M. (2006). Garlic and cardiovascular disease: A critical review. *Journal of Nutrition, 136*(3), 736S–740S.

Sifton, D. (Ed.). (2002). *Health care provider's desk reference (PDR).* Montvale, NJ: Medical Economics Company.

Sloan, M. A. (2005). Use of anticoagulant agents for stroke prevention. *CONTINUUM: Lifelong Learning in Neurology Stroke Prevention, 11*(4), 97–127.

Thrombosis Interest Group of Canada. (2008). http://www.tigc.org/

van Walraven, C., Hart, R. G., Singer, D. E., et al. (2002). Oral anticoagulants vs aspirin in non-valvular atrial fibrillation: An individual patient meta-analysis. *Journal of the American Medical Association, 288*, 2441–2448.

Vasant, B. P., & Moliterno, D. J. (2000). Glycoprotein IIb/IIIa antagonist and fibrinolytic agents: New therapeutic regimen for acute myocardial infarction. *Journal of Invasive Cardiology, 12*(B), 8B–15B.

Chapter 27

Dellinger, R. P. (2003). Cardiovascular management of septic shock. *Critical Care Medicine, 31*(3), 946–955.

Hasdai, D., Berger, P. B., Battler, A., & Holmes, D. R. (2002). *Cardiogenic shock: Diagnosis and treatment.* Totowa, NJ: Humana Press.

Kolecki, P., & Menckhoff, C. R. (2001, December 11). Hypovolemic shock. *eMedicine Journal, 2*(12).

Menon, V., & Fincke, R. (2003). Cardiogenic shock: A summary of the randomized SHOCK trial. *Congestive Heart Failure, 9*(1), 35–39.

Moser-Wade, D. M., Bartley, M. K., & Chiari-Allwein, H. L. (2000). Shock: Do you know how to respond? *Nursing, 30*(10), 34–40.

Von Rosenstiel, N., von Rosenstiel, I., & Adam, D. (2001). Management of sepsis and septic shock in infants and children. *Paediatric Drugs, 3*(1), 9–27.

Chapter 28

Bailey, L. B., Rampersaud, G. C., & Kauwell, G. P. (2003). Folic acid supplements and fortification affect the risk for neural tube defects, vascular disease and cancer: Evolving science. *Journal of Nutrition, 133*(6), 1961S–1968S.

Dharmarajan, T. S., Adiga, G. U., & Norkus, E. P. (2003). Vitamin B_{12} deficiency. Recognizing subtle symptoms in older adults. *Geriatrics, 58*(3), 30–34, 37–38.

Dietitians of Canada. (2006). *Vitamin D—many Canadians may not be getting enough.* Retrieved October 11, 2006, from http://www.dietitians.ca/news/mediaPrint.asp?fn=print&id=6542&idstring

Eden, A. N. (2003). Preventing iron deficiency in toddlers: A major public health problem. *Contemporary Pediatrics, 20*(2), 57–67.

Edroso, R. (2003). *Understanding HIV fatigue: What's dragging you down?* WebMDHealth, http://my.webmd.com

Health Canada. (2006). *Dietary reference intakes.* Retrieved October 18, 2006, from http://www.hc-sc.gc.ca/fn-an/nutrition/reference/table/ref_vitam_tbl_e.html

Glanville, T. (2005). Nutrition and health: The role of vitamin and mineral supplements. *Canadian Pharmacists Association.*

Kaushansky, K., & Kipps, T. J. (2006). Hematopoietic agents: Growth factors, minerals, & vitamins. In L. L. Brunton, J. S. Lazo, & K. L. Parker (Eds.), *Goodman & Gilman's The pharmacological basis of therapeutics* (11th ed., pp. 1433–1466). New York: McGraw-Hill.

Marcus, R., & Coulston, A. M. (2001). Water-soluble vitamins: The vitamin B complex and ascorbic acid. In J. G. Hardman, L. E. Limbard, & A. G. Goodman (Eds.), *The pharmacological basis of therapeutics* (pp. 1753–1772). New York: McGraw-Hill.

Oh, R., & Brown, D. L. (2003). Vitamin B_{12} deficiency. *American Family Health Care Provider, 67*(5), 979–986.

Rampersaud, G. C., Kauwell, G. P., & Bailey, L. B. (2003). Folate: A key to optimizing health and reducing disease risk in the elderly. *Journal of the American College of Nutrition, 22*(1), 1–8.

Somer, E. (2003). *Ironing out anemia.* WebMDHealth, http://my.webmd.com

Chapter 29

Canadian Asthma Consensus Conference Guidelines for the Management of Asthma, 2003. Available: http://www.asthmaguidelines.com

Canadian Thoracic Society. (2007). *Canadian Thoracic Society recommendations for management of chronic obstructive pulmonary disease—2007 update.* Available: new2007cts-copdguidelines.pdf

Celli, B. (2003). *Pharmacotherapy in chronic obstructive pulmonary disease.* New York: Marcel Dekker.

Colbert, B. J., & Mason, B. J. (2001). *Integrated cardiopulmonary pharmacology.* Upper Saddle River, NJ: Prentice Hall.

Drazen, J. M., Israel, E., & O'Bryne, P. M. (1999, January 21). Treatment of asthma with drugs modifying the leukotriene pathway. *New England Journal of Medicine, 340*, 197–206.

Fink, J. (2000). Metered dose inhalers, dry powder inhalers and transitions. *Respiratory Care, 45*, 623–635.

Global Initiative for Asthma. (2006). Global Strategy for Asthma Management and Prevention.

Mascitelli, L. & Pezzetta, F. (2007). Treatment of chronic respiratory diseases in obese people. *Canadian Medical Association Journal, 176*, 1130-a.

National Emphysema Foundation. (2003). *Grapefruit juice and drugs,* http://emphysemafoundation.org

Rogers, D. F. (2003). Airway hypersecretion in allergic rhinitis and asthma: New pharmacotherapy. *Current Allergy and Asthma Reports, 3*(3), 238–248.

Rosenwasser, L. J. (2002). Treatment of allergic rhinitis. *American Journal of Medicine, 16*(113, Suppl. 9A), 17S–24S.

Stanbrook, M. B. (2005). Is daily inhaled steroid use necessary in the treatment of mild persistent asthma? *Canadian Medical Association Journal, 172,* 1439.

Stevens, N. (2003). Inhaler devices for asthma and COPD: Choice and technique. *Professional Nurse, 18*(11), 641–645.

Taylor, D. W., & Fowler, E. (2008). Patient-centred care: Does asthma pass the test? *Journal of Medical and Biological Sciences, 2*(1), 1–13.

Undem, B. J., & Lichtenstein, L. M. (2001). Drugs used in the treatment of asthma. In J. G. Hardman, L. E. Limbard, & A. G. Goodman (Eds.), *The pharmacological basis of therapeutics.* New York: McGraw-Hill.

Vega, C. (2005). Budesonide/formoterol may be effective for maintenance and acute relief of asthma. *American Journal of Respiratory Critical Care Medicine, 171,* 129–136.

Wheeler, L. (2003, Mar-April). The last word: Asthma management in schools. *FDA Consumer 37*(2).

Wooltorton, E. (2005). Long-acting ß2-agonists in asthma: Safety concerns. *Canadian Medical Association Journal, 173,* 1030–1031.

Chapter 30

Agnew, L. L., Guffogg, S. P., Matthias, A., Lehmann, R. P., Bone, K. M., & Watson, K. (2005). Echinacea intake induces an immune responses through altered expression of leucocyte hsp70, increased white cell counts, and improved erythrocyte antioxidant defences. *Journal of Clinical Pharmacy and Therapeutics, 30*(4), 363–369.

Canadian Nursing Coalition on Immunization (CNCI). (2004). National Surveys of Provincial and Territorial Immunization Programs. Available: http://www.cps.ca/english/statements/ID/CNCI.pdf

Capriotti, T. (2001). Monoclonal antibodies: Drugs that combine pharmacology and biotechnology. *MedSurg Nursing, 10*(2), 89.

Centers for Disease Control and Prevention. (2004). *Vaccine safety: Misconceptions: About vaccinations and how to respond to them.* Retrieved May 24, 2007, from http://www.cdc.gov/vaccines/vac-gen/6mishome.htm

Fitzgerald, K. A., O'Neill, L. A., & Gearing, A. J. (Eds.). (2001). *The cytokine factsbook* (2nd ed.). Burlington, MA: Elsevier Science & Technology Books.

Health Canada. (2006). *Canadian immunization guide* (7th ed.). Ottawa: Public Health Agency of Canada.

Health Canada. (2006). *Canadian national report on immunization.* Retrieved June 10, 2007, from http://www.phac-aspc.gc.ca/publicat/ccdr-rmtc/06vol32/32s3/4epi_e.html#43

Karam, U. S., & Reddy, K. R. (2003). Pegylated interferons. *Clinical Liver Disease, 7*(1), 139–148.

Krensky, A. M., Strom, T. B., & Bluestone, J. A. (2001). Immunomodulators: Immunosuppressive agents, toleragens, and immunostimulants. In J. G. Hardman, L. E. Limbard, & A. G. Goodman (Eds.), *The pharmacological basis of therapeutics* (pp. 1463–1484). New York: McGraw-Hill.

Public Health Agency of Canada. (2008). *Canadian Adverse Event Following Immunization Surveillance System (CAEFISS),* http://www.phac-aspc.gc.ca/im/aefi-form_e.html

Public Health Agency of Canada. *Canada Communicable Disease Report (CCDR),* http://www.phac-aspc.gc.ca

Public Health Agency of Canada. *Canadian Immunization Awareness Program (CIAP),* http://www.immunize.cpha.ca

Public Health Agency of Canada. (2006). *Canadian national report on immunization. Canada Communicable Disease Report, 32*(S3), 1–44.

Public Health Agency of Canada. (2008). *National Immunization Strategy,* http://www.phac-aspc.gc.ca

Public Health Agency of Canada. (2008). *Vaccine Updates: National Advisory Committee on Immunization (NACI),* http://www.phac-aspc.gc.ca/naci-ccni/

Robinson, J. L. (2007). Vaccine controversies in Canada. *Canadian Pharmacists Journal, 140*(3), S9.

Santamaria, P. (2003). *Cytokines and autoimmune disease.* New York: Kluwer Academic/Plenum Publishers.

Schoop, R., Klein, P., Suter, A., Johnston, S. L. (2006). Echinacea in the prevention of induced rhinovirus cold: meta-analysis. *Clinical Therapeutics, 28*(2), 174–183.

Sharma, M., Arnason, J. T., Burt, A., & Hudson, J. B. (2006). Echinacea extracts modulate the pattern of chemokine and cytokine secretion in rhinovirus-infected and uninfected epithelial cells. *Phytotherapy Research, 20*(2), 147–152.

Sur, D. K., Wallis, D. H., & O'Connell, T. X. (2003). Vaccinations in pregnancy. *American Family Physician, 68,* E299–E309.

The National Advisory Committee on Immunization (2006). Statement on influenza vaccination for the 2006–2007 season. *Canada Communicable Disease Report, 32*(7).

Thomson, A. W., & Lotze, M. T. (2003). *The cytokine handbook* (4th ed., vols. 1–2). Burlington, MA: Elsevier Science & Technology Books.

Chapter 31

Agnew, L. L., Guffogg, S. P., Matthias, A., Lehmann, R. P., Bone, K. M., & Watson, K. (2005). Echinacea intake induces an immune response through altered expression of leucocyte hsp70, increased white cell counts, and improved erythrocyte antioxidant defences. *Journal of Clinical Pharmacy and Therapeutics, 30*(4), 363–369.

Bachert, C., Chuchalin, A. G., Eisebitt, R., Netayzhenko, V. Z., & Voelker, M. (2005). Aspirin compared with acetaminophen in the treatment of fever and other symptoms of upper respiratory tract infection in adults: A multicenter, randomized, double-blind, double-dummy, placebo-controlled, parallel-group, single-dose, 6-hour dose-ranging study. *Clinical Therapeutics, 27*(7), 993.

Baigent, C., & Patrono, C. (2003). Selective cyclooxygenase-2 inhibitors, aspirin, and cardiovascular disease: A reappraisal. *Arthritis & Rheumatism, 48*(1), 12–20.

Berger, W. E. (2003). Overview of allergic rhinitis. *Annals of Allergy and Asthma Immunology, 90*(6, Suppl. 3), 7–12.

Botting, R., & Ayoub, S. S. (2005). COX-3 and the mechanism of action of paracetamol/acetaminophen. *Prostaglandins, Leukotrienes and Essential Fatty Acids, 72*(2), 85.

Braunstahl, G., & Hellings, P. W. (2003). Allergic rhinitis and asthma: The link further unraveled. *Current Opinion in Pulmonary Medicine, 9*(1), 46–51.

Galley, H. F. (2002). *Critical care focus: Vol. 10. Inflammation and immunity.* London: BMJ Books.

Marhsall S. F., et al. (2005). Nonsteroidal anti-inflammatory drug use and breast cancer risk by stage and hormone receptor status. *Journal of the National Cancer Institute, 97*, 805–812.

McKeever, T. M., Lewis, S. A., Smit, H. A., Burney, P., Britton, J. R., & Cassano, P. A. (2005). The association of acetaminophen, aspirin, and ibuprofen with respiratory disease and lung function. *American Journal of Respiratory and Critical Care Medicine, 171*(9), 966–971.

Maharaj, H., Maharaj, D. S., Saravanan, K. S., Mohanakumar, K. P., & Daya, S. (2004). Aspirin curtails the acetaminophen-induced rise in brain norepinephrine levels. *Metabolic Brain Disease, 19*(1–2), 71.

Minghetti, L. P. (2004). Cyclooxygenase-2 (COX-2) in inflammatory and degenerative brain diseases. *Journal of Neuropathology & Experimental Neurology, 63*(9), 901–910.

Nathan, R. A. (2003). Pharmacotherapy for allergic rhinitis: A critical review of leukotriene receptor antagonists compared with other treatments. *Annals of Allergy and Asthma Immunology, 90*(2), 182–190.

Oh, R. (2005). Practical applications of fish oil (omega-3 fatty acids) in primary care. *Journal of American Board of Family Practice, 18*(1), 28–36.

Raffa, R. B., Walker, E. A., & Sterious, S. N. (2004). Opioid receptors and acetaminophen (paracetamol). *European Journal of Pharmacology, 503*(1–3), 209.

Sklar, G. E. (2002). Hemolysis as a potential complication of acetaminophen overdose in a patient with glucose-6-phosphate dehydrogenase deficiency. *Pharmacotherapy, 22*(5), 656–658.

White, P. F. (2005). The changing role of non-opioid analgesic techniques in the management of postoperative pain. *Anesthesia & Analgesia, 101*(Suppl.), S5–S22.

Woo, W., Man, S.-Y., Lam, P., & Rainer, T. H. (2005). Randomized double-blind trial comparing oral paracetamol and oral nonsteroidal antiinflammatory drugs for treating pain after musculoskeletal injury. *Annals of Emergency Medicine, 46*(4), 352.

Chapter 32

Andresen, M. (2007). Macrolides resistance rising. *Canadian Medical Association Journal, 176*, 159.

Beyer, D., Kroll, H. P., Endermann, R., Schiffer, G., Siegel, S., Bauser, M., Pohlmann, J., Brands, M., Ziegelbauer, K., Haebich, D., Eymann, C., & Brötz-Oesterhelt. H. (2004). New class of bacterial phenylalanyl-tRNA synthetase inhibitors with high potency and broad-spectrum activity. *Antimicrobial Agents and Chemotherapy, 48*, 525–532

Canadian Integrated Program for Antimicrobial Resistance Surveillance. *Recovery rate and final number of isolates submitted for antimicrobial resistance (AMR) testing across the bacterial species, the active surveillance components and the animal species, 2002–2005.* Ottawa: Public Health Agency of Canada. Available: http://www.phac-aspc.gc.ca/cipars-picra/pdf/cipars-picra-2005_pr-t1_e.pdf (Retrieved May 8, 2007).

Chambers, H. F. (2006). General considerations of antimicrobial therapy. In L. L. Brunton, J. S. Lazo, & K. L. Parker (Eds.), *Goodman & Gilman's The pharmacological basis of therapeutics* (11th ed., pp. 1095–1110). New York: McGraw-Hill.

Conly, J. (2002). Antimicrobial resistance in Canada. *Canadian Medical Association Journal 167*(8)

Dancer, S. J. (2007). Attention prescribers: Be careful with antibiotics. *Lancet, 369*(9560), 442.

Drew, R. H. (2007). Emerging options for treatment of invasive, multidrug-resistant Staphylococcus Aureus infections. *Pharmacotherapy, 27*(2), 227–249.

Erlendsdottir, H., Dahl-Knudsén, J., Odenholt, I., et al. (2001). Penicillin pharmacodynamics in four different experimental pneumococcal infection models. *Antimicrobial Agents and Chemotherapy, 45*, 1078–1085.

Freiberg, C., Fischer, H. P., & Brunner, N. A. (2005). Discovering the mechanism of action of novel antibacterial agents through transcriptional profiling of conditional mutants. *Antimicrobial Agents and Chemotherapy, 49*(2), 749–759.

Hibbard, J. (2005). Analysis comparing the antimicrobial activity and safety of current antiseptic agents. *Journal of Infusion Nursing, 28*(3), 194–207.

Hutter, B., Schaab, C. Albrecht, S. Borgmann, M. Brunner, N. A. Freiberg, C. Ziegelbauer, K. Rock, C. O. Ivanov, I., & Loferer, H. (2004). Prediction of mechanisms of action of antibacterial compounds by gene expression profiling. *Antimicrobial Agents and Chemotherapy, 48*, 2838–2844.

Krensky, A. M., Strom, T. B., & Bluestone, J. A. (2006). Immunomodulators: Immunosuppressive agents, toleragens, and immunostimulants. In L. L. Brunton, J. S. Lazo, & K. L. Parker (Eds.), *Goodman & Gilman's The pharmacological basis of therapeutics* (11th ed., pp. 1463–1484). New York: McGraw-Hill.

LeBlanc, L., Pépin, J., Toulouse, K., Ouellette, M.-F., Coulombe, M.-A., Corriveau, M.-P., et al. (2006). Fluoroquinolones and risk for methicillin-resistant staphylococcus aureus. *Emerging Infectious Diseases, 12*(9), 1398–1405.

Malhotra-Kumar, S., Lammens, C., Coenen, S., Van Herck, K., & Goossens, H. (2007). Effect of azithromycin and clarithromycin therapy on pharyngeal carriage of macrolide-resistant streptococci in healthy volunteers: a randomised, double-blind, placebo-controlled study. *Lancet, 369*, 482.

Nielsen, E., Viberg, A., Lowdin, E., Cars, O., Karlsson, M, O., & Sandstrom, M. (2007). Semimechanistic pharmacokinetic/pharmacodynamic model for assessment of activity of antibacterial agents from time-kill curve experiments. *Antimicrobial Agents and Chemotherapy, 51*(1), 128–136.

Norén, T., Wullt, M., Åkerlund, T., Bäck, E., Odenholt, I., & Burman, L. G. (2006). Frequent emergence of resistance in Clostridium difficile during treatment of C. difficile-associated diarrhea with fusidic acid. *Antimicrobial Agents and Chemotherapy, 50*, 3028–3032.

Nyhlén, A., Ljungberg, B., Nilsson-Ehle, I., & Odenholt, I. (2002). Bactericidal effect of combinations of antibiotic and antineoplastic agents against Staphylococcus aureus and Escherichia coli. *Chemotherapy, 48*, 71–77.

Ofner-Agostini, M., Simor, A. E., Mulvey, M., Bryce, E., Loeb, M., McGeer, A., et al. (2006). Methicillin-resistant staphylococcus aureus in Canadian Aboriginal people. [Canadian Nosocomial Infection Surveillance Program, Health Canada]. *Infection Control & Hospital Epidemiology, 27*(2), 204–207.

Odenholt, I., Cars, O. & Löwdin, E. (2004). Pharmacodynamic studies of amoxicillin against Streptococcus pneumoniae: Comparison of a new pharmacokinetically enhanced formulation (2000 mg twice daily) with standard dosage regimens. *Journal of Antimicrobial Chemotherapy, 54*, 1062–1066.

Petri, W. A. (2006). Chemotherapy of tuberculosis, *Mycobacterium avium* complex disease, and leprosy. In L. L. Brunton, J. S. Lazo, & K. L. Parker (Eds.), *Goodman & Gilman's The pharmacological basis of therapeutics* (11th ed., pp. 1203–1224). New York: McGraw-Hill.

Petri, W. A. (2006). Penicillins, cephalosporins, and other beta-lactam antibiotics. In L. L. Brunton, J. S. Lazo, & K. L. Parker (Eds.), *Goodman & Gilman's The pharmacological basis of therapeutics* (11th ed., pp. 1127–1154). New York: McGraw-Hill.

Petri, W. A. (2006). Sulfonamides, trimethoprim-sulfamethoxazole, quinolones, and agents for urinary tract infections. In L. L. Brunton, J. S. Lazo, & K. L. Parker (Eds.), *Goodman & Gilman's The pharmacological basis of therapeutics* (11th ed., pp. 1111–1126). New York: McGraw-Hill.

Sheff, B. (2001). Taking aim at antibiotic-resistant bacteria. *Nursing, 31*(11), 62–68.

Wooten, J., & Sakind, A. (2003). Superbugs: Unmasking the threat. *RN, 66*(3), 37–43.

Chapter 33

Bennet, J. E. (2006). Antifungal agents. In L. L. Brunton, J. S. Lazo, & K. L. Parker (Eds.), *Goodman & Gilman's The pharmacological basis of therapeutics* (11th ed., pp. 1225–1242). New York: McGraw-Hill.

Dickson, R., Awasthi, S., Dimellweek, C., & Williamson, P. (2003). Antihelminthic drugs for treating worms in children: Effects on growth and cognitive performance. *Cochrane Review*, http://www.medscape.com

Dodds, E. S., Drew, R. H., & Perfect, J. R. (2000). Antifungal pharmacodynamics: Review of the literature and clinical applications. *Pharmacotherapy, 20*(11), 1335–1355.

Health Canada. (2003). Medical Access to Quinine for Malaria Treatment Streamlined in Canada through the Canadian Malaria Network.

Kontoyiannis, D. P., Mantadakis, E., & Samonis, G. (2003). Systemic mycoses in the immunocompromised host: An update in antifungal therapy. *Journal of Hospital Infection, 53*(4), 243–258.

Oh, R. (2005). Practical applications of fish oil (omega-3 fatty acids) in primary care. *Journal of American Board of Family Practice, 18*(1), 28–36.

Pray, W. S. (2001). Treatment of vaginal fungal infections. *U.S. Pharmacist 26*(9).

Shapiro, A. C., & Goldberg, D. E. (2006). Chemotherapy of protozoal infections: Malaria. In L. L. Brunton, J. S. Lazo, & K. L. Parker (Eds.), *Goodman & Gilman's The pharmacological basis of therapeutics* (11th ed., pp. 869–898). New York: McGraw-Hill.

Steile, R. W. (2002). Focus on infection, prevention detection and treatment. *Medscape Medical News*, http://www.medscape.com

Re, V. L., & Gluckman, S. J. (2003). Prevention of malaria in travelers. *American Family Physician, 68*, 509–514, 515–516.

Suh, K. N., Kain, K. C., & Keystone, J. S. (2004). Malaria. *Canadian Medical Association Journal, 170*(11), 1693–1702.

Tracy, J. W., & Webster, L. T. (2001). Drugs used in the chemotherapy of protozoal infections: Malaria. In J. G. Hardman et al. (Eds.), *The pharmacological basis of therapeutics* (10th ed.). New York: McGraw-Hill.

Turness, B. W., Beach, M. J., & Roberts, J. M. (2000). Giardiasis surveillance. *Morbidity and Mortality Weekly Report*, Centers for Disease Control.

Wilson, C. (2005). Recurrent vulvovaginitis candidiasis: An overview of traditional and alternative therapies. *Advance for Nurse Practitioners, 13*(5), 24–29.

Chapter 34

Almuente, V. (2002). Herbal therapy in patients with HIV. *Medscape Pharmacists, 3*(2), 1–4.

American Academy of Pediatrics. (1997). Use of codeine- and dextromethorphan-containing cough remedies in children. *Pediatrics, 99*(6), 918–920.

Brenner, B. G., Roger, M., Routy, J. P., Moisi, D., Ntemgwa, M., Matte, C., et al. (2007). High rates of forward transmission events after acute/early HIV-1 infection. *Journal of Infectious Diseases, 195*, 951–959.

Burdge, D., Money, D., Forbes, J., Walmsley, S., Smaill, F., Boucher, M., et al. (2003). Canadian consensus guidelines for the care of HIV-positive pregnant women: Putting recommendations into practice. *Canadian Medical Association Journal, 168*(13), 1683–1688.

Canada. (2004). *Federal initiative to address HIV/AIDS in Canada.* Available: http://www.hawaii.edu/hivandaids/Federal_Initiative_ to_Address_HIVAIDS_in_Canada.pdf

Canadian Association for Study of the Liver. *Canadian Consensus Conference on the Management of Viral Hepatitis.* CASL and Health Canada. Available: http://www.lhsc.on.ca/casl/cont.htm.

Center for Infectious Disease Prevention and Control, Public Health Agency of Canada. (2007). HIV and AIDS in Canada Surveillance Report to December 31, 2005.

Duggan, J., Peterson, W. S., Schutz, M., Khuder, S., & Chakraborty, J. (2001). Use of complementary and alternative therapies in HIV-infected patients. *AIDS Patient Care and STDs, 15*, 159–167.

Goldschmidt, R. H., & Dong, B. J. (2001). Treatment of AIDS and HIV-related conditions. *Journal of the American board of Family Practice, 14*(4), 283–309.

Hayden, F. G. (2001). Antimicrobial agents: Antiviral agents (nonretroviral). In J. G. Hardman, L. E. Limbard, & A. G. Goodman (Eds.), *The pharmacological basis of therapeutics* (pp. 1313–1348). New York: McGraw-Hill.

Idemyor, V. (2003). Twenty years since human immunodeficiency virus discovery: Considerations for the next decade. *Pharmacotherapy, 23*, 384–387.

Kirkbride, H. A., & Watson, J. (2003). Review of the use of neuraminidase inhibitors for prophylaxis of influenza. *Communicable Diseases and Public Health, 6*(2), 123–127.

Kuritzkes, D. R., Boyle, B. A., Gallant, J. E., Squires, K. E., & Zolopa, A. (2003). Current management challenges in HIV: Antiretroviral resistance. *AIDS Reader, 13*(3), 133–135, 138–142.

Lesho, E. P., & Gey, D. C. (2003). Managing issues related to anti-retroviral therapy. *American Family Physician, 68*, 675–686, 689–690.

Miller, C. L, Spittal, P. M., Wood, E., Chan, K., Schechter, M. T., Montaner, J. S., et al. (2006). Inadequacies in antiretroviral therapy use among aboriginal and other Canadian populations. *AIDS Care, 18,* 968–976.

Mills, E., Montori, V., Perri, D., Phillips, E., & Koren, G. (2005). Natural health product-HIV drug interactions: A systematic review. *International Journal of STDs and AIDS, 16*(3), 181–186.

Ofotokun, I., & Pomeroy, C. (2003). Sex differences in adverse reactions to antiretroviral drugs. *Topics in HIV Medicine, 11*(2), 55–59.

Paul, I. M. (2005). Effect of dextromethorphan, diphenhydramine, and placebo on nocturnal cough and sleep quality for coughing children and their parents: In reply. *Pediatrics, 115*(2), 512–b-513.

Public Health Agency of Canada. (2007). *HIV/AIDS epidemiology reports and updates.* Available: http://www.phac-aspc.gc.ca/aids-sida/publication/epi/epi2007-eng.php

Public Health Agency of Canada. (2007). *Influenza updates.* Available: http://www.phac-aspc.gc.ca/im/influenza-eng.php

Public Health Agency of Canada. (2007). *Notifiable diseases online.* Available: http://dsol-smed.phac-aspc.gc.ca/dsol-smed/ndis/index_e.html (retrieved May 3, 2007).

Public Health Agency of Canada. (2008). *Severe Respiratory Illness (SRI) in the SARS "Post-outbreak" period.* Available: http://www.phac-aspc.gc.ca/sars-sras/sri-eng.php

Public Health Agency of Canada. (2008). *Current Avian influenza (H5N1).* Available: http://www.phac-aspc.gc.ca/h5n1/index-eng.php

Raffanti, S. P., & Haas, D. W. (2001). Antimicrobial agents: Antiretroviral agents. In J. G. Hardman, L. E. Limbard, & A. G. Goodman (Eds.), *The pharmacological basis of therapeutics* (pp. 1349–1380). New York: McGraw-Hill.

Schoop, R., Klein, P., Suter, A., Johnston, S. L. (2006). Echinacea in the prevention of induced rhinovirus cold: meta-analysis. *Clinical Therapeutics, 28*(2), 174–183.

Sharma, M., Arnason, J. T., Burt, A., & Hudson, J. B. (2006). Echinacea extracts modulate the pattern of chemokine and cytokine secretion in rhinovirus-infected and uninfected epithelial cells. *Phytotherapy Research, 20*(2), 147–152.

Walker, B. D. (2002). *Immune reconstitution and immunotherapy in HIV infection.* Medscape Clinical Update, http://www.medscape.com/viewprogram/2435

Chapter 35

Birner, A. (2003). Safe administration of oral chemotherapy. *Clinical Journal of Oncological Nursing, 2,* 158–162.

Breed, C. D. (2003). Diagnosis, treatment, and nursing care of patients with chronic leukemia. *Seminars in Oncology Nursing, 19*(2), 109–117.

Buzdar, A. U. (2000). Tamoxifen's clinical applications: Old and new. *Archives of Family Medicine, 9,* 906–912.

Chabner, B. A., Ryan, D. P., Paz-Ares, L., Garcia-Carbonero, R., & Calabresi, P. (2001). Antineoplastic agents. In J. G. Hardman, L. E. Limbard, & A. G. Goodman (Eds.), *The pharmacological basis of therapeutics* (10th ed.). New York: McGraw-Hill.

Chemoprevention of Breast Cancer: Recommendations and Rationale, U.S. Preventive Services Task Force. (2003). *American Family Physician, 67*(6), 1309–1314.

Dalton, R. R., & Kallab, A. M. (2001). Chemoprevention of breast cancer. *Southern Medical Journal, 94*(1), 7–1.

Health Canada. (2005). *Lung cancer.* Retrieved August 8, 2007, from http://www.hc-sc.gc.ca/hl-vs/tobac-tabac/body-corps/disease-maladie/lung-poumon/lung-poumon_e.html

Hood, L. E. (2003). Chemotherapy in the elderly: Supportive measures for chemotherapy-induced myelotoxicity. *Clinical Journal of Oncological Nursing, 7*(2), 185–190.

Lee, S. O., Yeon Chun, J., Nadiminty, N., Trump, D. L., Ip, C., Dong, T., et al. (2006). Monomethylated selenium inhibits growth of LNCaP human prostate cancer xenograft accompanied by a decrease in the expression of androgen receptor and prostate-specific antigen (PSA). *The Prostate, 66*(10), 1070–1075.

Levine, M. N., & Whelan, T. (2006). Adjuvant chemotherapy for breast cancer—30 years later. *New England Journal of Medicine, 355*(18), 1920–1922.

Moran, P. (2000). Cellular effects of cancer chemotherapy administration. *Journal of Infusion Nursing, 23*(1), 44.

Peters, U., Chatterjee, N., Church, T. R., Mayo, C., Sturup, S., Foster, C. B., et al. (2006). High serum selenium and reduced risk of advanced colorectal adenoma in a colorectal cancer early detection program. *Cancer Epidemiology, Biomarkers, and Prevention, 15*(2), 315–320.

Reid, M. E., Duffield-Lillico, A. J., Sunga, A., Fakih, M., Alberts, D. S., & Marshall, J. R. (2006). Selenium supplementation and colorectal adenomas: An analysis of the nutritional prevention of cancer trail. *International Journal of Cancer, 118*(7), 1777–1781.

Rieger, P. (2001). *Biotherapy: A comprehensive overview* (2nd ed.). Sudbury, MA: Jones and Bartlett.

Rugo, H. (2001, October 15). *How to succeed with breast cancer adjuvant therapy,* http://healthology.com

Smith, B., Waltzman, R., & Rugo, H. (2002, December 10). *Living longer with cancer: Preserving quality of life,* http://healthology.com

Seitz, S., Hohla, F., Schally, A. V., Moder, A., Engel, J. B., Horn, F., et al. (2008). Inhibition of estrogen receptor positive and negative breast cancer cell lines with a growth hormone-releasing hormone antagonist. *Oncology Reports, 20,* 1289–94.

Wood, L. (2001). Antineoplastic agents. *Journal of Infusion Nursing, 24*(1), 48.

Chapter 36

Hoogerwerf, W. A., & Pasricha, P. J. (2001). Agents used for the control of gastric acidity and treatment of peptic ulcers and gastroesophageal reflux disease. In J. G. Hardman, L. E. Limbard, & A. G. Goodman (Eds.), *The pharmacological basis of therapeutics* (10th ed.). New York: McGraw-Hill.

Huggins, R. M., Scates, A. C., & Latour, J. K. (2003). Intravenous proton-pump inhibitors versus H_2-antagonists for treatment of GI bleeding. *Annals of Pharmacotherapy, 37*(3), 433–437.

Litalien, C., Théorêt, Y., & Faure, C. (2005). Pharmacokinetics of proton pump inhibitors in children. *Clinical Pharmacokinetics, 44*(5), 441–466.

Louw, J. A., & Marks, I. N. S. (2003). *The management of peptic ulcer disease.* Retrieved September 29, 2006, from http://www.medscape.com/viewarticle/463485_print

Meurer, L. N., & Bower, D. J. (2002). Management of Helicobacter pylori infection. *American Family Physician, 65,* 1327–1336, 1339.

Patel, A. S., Pohl, J. F., & Easley, D. J. (2003). What's new: Proton pump inhibitors and pediatrics. *Pediatric Review, 24*(1), 12–5.

Paterson, W. (1998). Canadian association of gastroenterology practice guidelines: Management of noncardiac chest pain. *Canadian Journal of Gastroenterology, 12*(6), 401–408.

Petersen, A. M. (2003). *Helicobacter pylori*: An invading microorganism? A review. *FEMS Immunology and Medical Microbiology, 36*(3), 117–126.

Sharma, P., & Vakil, N. (2003). Review article: *Helicobacter pylori* and reflux disease. *Aliment Pharmacological Therapy, 17*(3), 297–305.

Stanghellini, V. (2003). Management of gastroesophageal reflux disease. *Drugs Today, 39*(Suppl. A), 15–20.

Vanderhoff, B. T., & Tahboub, R. M. (2002). Proton pump inhibitors: An update. *American Family Physician, 66,* 273–280.

Chapter 37

Apotex. (2005). *Prescribing information: Lactulose solution usp.* Retrieved March 22, 2007, from http://www.apotexcorp.com

Crohn's and Colitis Foundation of Canada, http://www.ccfc.ca

Glazer, G. (2001). Long-term pharmacotherapy of obesity: A review of efficacy and safety. *Archives of Internal Medicine, 161,* 1814–1824.

Golembiewski, J., Chernin, E., & Chopra, T. (2005). Prevention and treatment of postoperative nausea and vomiting. *American Society of Health-System Pharmacists.*

Guglietta, A. (2003). *Pharmacotherapy of gastrointestinal inflammation.* Basel, Switzerland: Birkhauser Verlag.

International Foundation for Functional Gastrointestinal Disorders, http://www.IFFGD.org

Jafri, S., & Pasricha, P. J. (2001). Agents used for diarrhea, constipation and inflammatory bowel disease: Agents used for biliary and pancreatic disease. In J. G. Hardman, L. E. Limbard, & A. G. Goodman (Eds.), *The pharmacological basis of therapeutics* (10th ed.). New York: McGraw-Hill.

Knutson, D., Greenberg, G., & Cronau, H. (2003). Management of Crohn's disease—A practical approach. *American Family Physician, 68,* 707–714, 717–718.

Pasricha, P. J. (2001). Prokinetic agents, antiemetics and agents used in irritable bowel syndrome. In J. G. Hardman, L. E. Limbard, & A. G. Goodman (Eds.), *The pharmacological basis of therapeutics* (10th ed.). New York: McGraw-Hill.

Recommendations of the Canadian Paediatric Society's Nutrition Committee, February 2006, http://www.cps.ca/

Recommendations of the World Health Organization for home management of diarrhea, 2006, http://www.who.int

Spanier, J. A., Howden, C. W., & Jones, M. P. (2003). A systematic review of alternative therapies in the irritable bowel syndrome. *Archives of Internal Medicine, 163*(3), 265–274.

University of Alberta. (2006). *Canada high in ulcerative colitis and Crohn's cases: Is Canada too clean?* Retrieved September 29, 2006, from http://www.sciencedaily.com/releases/2006/08/060823184850.htm

Wald, A. (2003). Is chronic use of stimulant laxatives harmful to the colon? *Journal of Clinical Gastroenterology, 36*(5), 386–389.

Weigle, D. S. (2003). Pharmacological therapy of obesity: Past, present, and future. *Journal of Clinical Endocrinology and Metabolism, 88*(6), 2462–2469.

Chapter 38

Bhagavan, N. V. (2002). *Medical biochemistry.* Burlington, MA: Harcourt/Academic Press.

Campbell, S. M. (2006). An anthology of advances in enteral tube feeding formulations. *Nutrition in Clinical Practice, 21*(4), 411–415.

Canadian Parenteral-Enteral Nutrition Association (CPENA), http://www.cpena.ca/home.html

Dieticians of Canada. (2006). Vitamin D—Many Canadians may not be getting enough. *Dietitians of Canada—News Room Print Resource,* May 25, 2006, http://www.dietitians.ca/news/media

Glanville, T. (2005). Nutrition and health: The role of vitamin and mineral supplements. *Canadian Pharmacists Association.*

Health Canada (2006). *Dietary Reference Intakes tables.* Retrieved October 11, 2006, from http://www.hc-sc.gc.ca/fn-an/nutrition/reference/table/ref_vitam_tbl_e.html

Hise, M. E., Kattelmann, K. & Parkhurst, M. (2005). Evidence-Based Clinical Practice: Dispelling the Myths. *Nutrition in Clinical Practice, 20*(3), 294–302.

Indian and Northern Affairs Canada. (2006). *Inuit macronutrient intake.* Retrieved October 11, 2006, from http://www.ainc-inac.gc.ca/index_e.html

Marcus, R., & Coulston, A. M. (2001). Fat-soluble vitamins: Vitamins A, K and E. In J. G. Hardman, L. E. Limbard, & A. G. Goodman (Eds.), *The pharmacological basis of therapeutics* (10th ed.). New York: McGraw-Hill.

Marcus, R., & Coulston, A. M. (2001). Water-soluble vitamins: The vitamin B complex and ascorbic acid. In J. G. Hardman, L. E. Limbard, & A. G. Goodman (Eds.), *The pharmacological basis of therapeutics* (10th ed.). New York: McGraw-Hill.

McDermott, J. H. (2000). Antioxidant nutrients: Current dietary recommendations and research update. *Journal of the American Pharmacists Association, 40*(6), 785–799.

Oh, R. C., & Brown, D. L. (2003). Vitamin B_{12} deficiency. *American Family Physician 67,* 979–986, 993–994.

Padayatty, S. J., Katz, A., Wang, Y., Eck, P., Kwon, O., Lee, J. H., Chen, S., Corpe, C., Dutta, A., Dutta, S. K., & Levine, M. (2003). Vitamin C as an antioxidant: Evaluation of its role in disease prevention. *Journal of the American College of Nutrition, 22*(1), 18–35.

Perrotta, S., Nobili, B., Rossi, F., Di Pinto, D., Cucciolla, V., Borriello, A., Oliva, A., Della Powers, H. J. (2003). Riboflavin (vitamin B_2) and health. *American Journal of Clinical Nutrition, 77*(6), 1352–1360.

Ragione, F. (2003). Vitamin A and infancy. Biochemical, functional, and clinical aspects. *Vitamins and Hormones, 66,* 457–591.

Rampersaud, G. C., Kauwell, G. P., & Bailey, L. B. (2003). Folate: A key to optimizing health and reducing disease risk in the elderly. *Journal of the American College of Nutrition, 22*(1), 1–8.

Chapter 39

Coureau, B., Bussières , J. F., & Tremblay, S. (2008). Cushing's syndrome induced by misuse of moderate- to high-potency topical corticosteroids. *Annals of Pharmacotherapy.*

Dehdashti, A. R., & Gentili, F. (2007). Current state of the art in the diagnosis and surgical treatment of Cushing disease: Early experience with a purely endoscopic endonasal technique. *Neurosurgery Focus, 23*(3), E9.

Demester, N. (2001). Diseases of the thyroid: A broad spectrum. *Clinical Review, 11*(7), 58–64.

Farwell, A. P., & Braverman, L. E. (2006). Thyroid and antithyroid drugs. In L. L. Brunton, J. S. Lazo, & K. L. Parker (Eds.), *Goodman & Gilman's The pharmacological basis of therapeutics* (11th ed., pp. 1511–1540). New York: McGraw-Hill.

Griffiths, H., & Jordan, S. (2002). Corticosteroids: Implications for nursing practice. *Nursing Standard, 17*(12), 43–53.

Holcomb, S. S. (2002). Thyroid diseases: A primer for the critical care nurse. *Dimensions of Critical Care Nursing, 21*(4), 127–133.

Joffe, R. T., Brimacombe, M., Levitt, A. J., & Stagnaro-Green, A. (2007). Treatment of clinical hypothyroidism with thyroxine and triiodothyronine: A literature review and metaanalysis. *Psychosomatics, 48,* 379–384.

Margioris, A. N., & Chrousos, G. P. (Eds). (2001). *Adrenal disorders.* Totowa, NJ: Humana Press.

Parker, K. L., & Schimmer, B. P. (2006). Pituitary hormones and their hypothalamic releasing factors. In L. L. Brunton, J. S. Lazo, & K. L. Parker (Eds.), *Goodman & Gilman's The pharmacological basis of therapeutics* (11th ed., pp. 1489–1510). New York: McGraw-Hill.

Pimentel, L., & Hansen, K. N. (2005). Thyroid disease in the emergency department: A clinical and laboratory review. *Journal of Emergency Medicine, 28(2),* 201–209.

Schori-Ahmed, D. (2003). Defenses gone awry. Thyroid disease. *RN, 66*(6), 38–43.

Winqvist, O., Rorsman, F., & Kämpe, O. (2000). Autoimmune adrenal insufficiency: Recognition and management. *BioDrugs, 13*(2), 107–114.

Chapter 40

Bates, N. (2002). Overdose of insulin and other diabetic medication. *Emergency Nurse, 10*(7), 22–26.

Bloomgarden, Z. T. (2006). Aspects of type 2 diabetes and related insulin-resistant states. *Diabetes Care, 29*(3), 732–740.

Bohannon, N. J. V. (2002). Treating dual defects in diabetes: Insulin resistance and insulin secretion. *American Journal of Health-System Pharmacists, 59,* 59.

Bell, D. S. H., & Ovalle, F. (2000). Management of type 2 diabetes. *Clinical Review,* (Spring), 93–96.

Boctor, M. A. (2003). Diabetes mellitus. In J. Gray (Ed.), *Therapeutic choices* (4th ed., p. 805). Ottawa: Canadian Pharmacists Association.

Buchanan, T. A., & Xiang, A. H. (2005). Gestational diabetes mellitus. *Journal of Clinical Investigations, 115,* 485–491.

Canadian Diabetes Association. (2008). *Carbohydrate counting.* Available: http://www.diabetes.ca/about-diabetes/nutrition/carbohydrate-counting/

Canadian Diabetes Association. (2003). Clinical practice guidelines for the prevention and management of diabetes in Canada. *Canadian Journal of Diabetes, 27,* 1–163.

Canadian Diabetes Association. (2008). *Clinical practice guidelines for the prevention and management of diabetes in Canada.* Available: http://www.diabetes.ca/files/cpg2008/cpg-2008.pdf.

Canadian Institute for Health Information. (2006). *Treatment of end-stage organ failure in Canada, 1995 to 2004* [2006 annual report].

Chehade, J. M., & Mooradian, A. D. (2000). A rational approach to drug therapy of type 2 diabetes mellitus. *Drugs, 60*(1), 95–113.

Chen, S. W. (2002). Editorial: Insulin glargine: Basal insulin of choice? *American Journal of Health-System Pharmacists, 59,* 609, 643.

Chiasson, J. L., Aris-Jilwan, N., Belanger, R., et al. (2003). Diagnosis and treatment of diabetic ketoacidosis and the hyperglycemic hyperosmolar state. *Canadian Medical Association Journal, 168,* 859–866.

Cole, L. (2002). Unraveling the mystery of acute pancreatitis. *Dimensions of Critical Care Nursing, 21,* 86–91.

Danne, T., Becker, R. H. A., Heise, T., Bittner, C., Frick, A. D., & Rave, K. (2005). Pharmacokinetics, prandial glucose control, and safety of insulin glulisine in children and adolescents with type 1 diabetes. *Diabetes Care, 28*(9), 2100–2105.

Davis, S. N. (2006). Insulin, oral hypoglycemic agents, and the pharmacology of the endocrine pancreas. In L. L. Brunton, J. S. Lazo, & K. L. Parker (Eds.), *Goodman & Gilman's The pharmacological basis of therapeutics* (11th ed., pp. 1613–1646). New York: McGraw-Hill.

Gottlieb, S. W. (2003). Just the facts: The importance of diabetic research. *Diabetes Forecast 56,* 39–42.

Goulet, S., Trepman, E., Mmath, M. C., Koulack, J., Fong, H., Duerksen, F., et al. (2006). Revascularization for peripheral vascular disease in Aboriginal and non-Aboriginal patients. *Journal of Vascular Surgery, 43,* 735–741.

Harrigan, R. A., Nathan, M. S., & Beattie, P. (2001). Oral agents for the treatment of type 2 diabetes mellitus: Pharmacology, toxicity, and treatment. *Annals of Emergency Medicine, 38*(1), 68.

Health Canada. (2002). *Canada's Physical Activity Guide.* Retrieved October 15, 2007, from http://www.phac-aspc.gc.ca

Health Canada. (2007). *Eating Well with Canada's Food Guide.* Retrieved October 15, 2007, from http://www.hc-sc.gc.ca

Hjelm, K., Mufunda, E., Nambozi, G., & Kemp, J. (2003). Preparing nurses to face the pandemic of diabetes mellitus: A literature review. *Journal of Advanced Nursing, 41,* 424–435.

Hovens, M. M., Tamsam, J. t., Beishuzien, E. D., & Huisman, M. V. (2005). Pharmacological strategies to reduce cardiovascular risk in type 2 diabetes mellitus: An update. *Drugs, 65*(4), 433–445.

Inzucchi, S. E. (2006). Management of hyperglycemia in the hospital setting. *New England Journal of Medicine, 355*(18), 1903–1911.

Leiter, L. A., et al. (2001). Diabetes Screening in Canada (DIASCAN) Study: Prevalence of undiagnosed diabetes and glucose intolerance in family physician offices. *Diabetes Care, 24*(6), 1038–1043.

Mantis, A. K. et al. (2001). Continuous subcutaneous insulin infusion therapy for children and adolescents: An option for routine diabetes care. *Pediatrics, 107,* 351–357.

McKnight-Menci, H., Sababu, S., & Kelly, S. D. (2005). The care of children and adolescents with type 2 diabetes. *Journal of Pediatric Nursing, 20*(2), 96–106.

Mitchell, R. M. S., Byrne, M. F., & Baillie, J. (2003). Pancreatitis. *Lancet, 361,* 1447–1456.

Mokdad, A. H., Bowman, B. A., & Ford, E. S. (2001). The continuing epidemics of obesity and diabetes in the United States. *Journal of the American Medical Association, 286,* 1195–1200.

Nissen, S. E., & Wolski, K. (2007). Effect of rosiglitazone on the risk of myocardial infarction and death from cardiovascular causes. *New England Journal of Medicine, 356,* 2457–2471.

Norris, S. L., et al. (2005). Long-term effectiveness of weight-loss interventions in adults with pre-diabetes: A review. *American Journal of Preventive Medicine, 28*(1), 126–139.

Public Health Agency of Canada. *Economic Burden of Illness Database, Custom Tabulation,* Retrieved May 15, 2007, from http://www.phac-aspc.gc.ca

Public Health Agency of Canada, Using National Diabetes Surveillance System (NDSS) data files contributed by all provinces and territories, as of October 31, 2007.

Rao, S. S., et al. (2004). Impaired glucose intolerance and impaired fasting glucose. *American Family Physician, 15,* 69(8), 1961–1968.

Rosenstock, J., Zinman, B., Murphy, L. J., Clement, S. C., Moore, P., Bowering, C. K., et al. (2005). Inhaled insulin improves glycemic control when substituted for or added to oral combination therapy in type 2 diabetes: A randomized, controlled trial. *Annals of Internal Medicine,* 549–558.

Statistics Canada. (2003). Canadian Community Health Survey (CCHS) *The Daily* (self-reported data). Retrieved October 15, 2007, from http://www.statcan.ca

Statistics Canada. (2004). Canadian Community Health Survey (CCHS) Cycle 2.2, Nutrition. *The Daily.* Retrieved October 15, 2007, from http://www.statcan.ca

Chapter 41

Brown, J., & Fortier, M. (2006). Canadian consensus conference on osteoporosis, 2006 update. *Society of Obstetricians and Gynaecologists of Canada, 172,* S95–S112.

Conley, C. (2003). *Hormonal therapy for breast cancer: Current issues,* http://healthology.com

Frackiewicz, E. J., & Shiovitz, T. M. (2001). Evaluation and management of premenstrual syndrome and premenstrual dysphoric disorder. *Journal of the American Pharmacists Association, 41*(3), 437–447.

Kusiak, V. (2002). *FDA approves prescribing information for postmenopausal hormone therapies,* http://www.premarin.com/hep/html

Leeman, L., Fontaine, P., King, V., Klein, M. C., & Ratcliffe, S. (2003). The nature and management of labor pain: Part II. Pharmacologic pain relief. *American Family Physician, 68,* 1115–1120, 1121–1122.

Loose, D. S., & Stancel, G. M. (2006). Estrogens. In L. L. Brunton, J. S. Lazo, & K. L. Parker (Eds.), *Goodman & Gilman's The pharmacological basis of therapeutics* (11th ed., pp. 1541–1572). New York: McGraw-Hill.

Ludwig, M., Westergaard, L. G., Diedrich, K., & Andersen, C. Y. (2003). Developments in drugs for ovarian stimulation. *Best Practice and Research. Clinical Obstetrics and Gynecology, 17*(2), 231–247.

Nelson, A. (2000). Contraceptive update Y2K: Need for contraception and new contraceptive options. *Clinic Corner 3*(1), 48–62.

Olds, S. B., London, M. L., Ladewig, P. A., & Davidson, M. R. (2004). *Maternal-newborn nursing and women's health care* (7th ed.). Upper Saddle River, NJ: Prentice Hall Health.

Osmers, R., Friede, M., Liske, E., Schnitker, J., Freudenstein, J., & Henneicke-von Zeplin, H. H. (2005). Efficacy and safety of isopropanolic black cohosh extract for climacteric symptoms. *Obstetrics and Gynecology, 105*(5 pt 1), 1074–1083.

Shepherd, J. E. (2001). Effects of estrogen on cognition, mood, and degenerative brain diseases. *Journal of the American Pharmacists Association, 41*(2), 221–228.

Snyder, P. J. (2001). Androgens. In J. G. Hardman, L. E. Limbard, & A. G. Goodman (Eds.), *The pharmacological basis of therapeutics* (10th ed.). New York: McGraw-Hill.

Understanding the WHI study: Assessing the results. (2003). Available: http://www.premarin.com/pdf/Risk.Tearsheet.pdf

Chapter 42

Bent, S., Kane, C., Shinohara, K., Neuhaus, J., Hudes, E. S., Goldberg, H., et al. (2006). Saw palmetto for benign prostatic hyperplasia. *New England Journal of Medicine, 354*(6), 557–566.

Brock, G. B. (2003). Tadalafil: A new agent for erectile dysfunction. *Canadian Journal of Urology, 10*(Suppl. 1), 17–22.

Bullock, T. L., & Andriole, G. L. (2006). Emerging drug therapies for benign prostatic hyperplasia. *Expert Opinion on Emergency Drugs, 11*(1), 111–123.

Canadian Urological Society, http://www.cua.org.

Carrier, S. (2003). Pharmacology of phosphodiesterase 5 inhibitors. *Canadian Journal of Urology, 10*(Suppl. 1), 12–6.

Gordon, A. E., & Shaughnessy, A. F. (2003). Saw palmetto for prostate disorders. *American Family Physician, 67*(6), 1281–1283.

Grover, S. A., Lowensteyn, I., Kaouache, M., Marchand, S., Coupal, L., DeCarolis, E., et al. (2006). The prevalence of erectile dysfunction in the primary care setting: Importance of risk factors for diabetes and vascular disease. *Archives of Internal Medicine, 166,* 213–219.

Padma-Nathan, H., Saenz de Tejada, I., Rosen, R. C., & Goldstein, I. (Eds.). (2001). *Pharmacotherapy for erectile dysfunction.* London: Taylor & Francis Books Ltd.

Kassabian, V. S. (2003). Sexual function in patients treated for benign prostatic hyperplasia. *Lancet, 361*(9351), 60–62.

Khastgir, J., Arya, M., Shergill, I. S., Kalsi, J. S., Minhas, S., & Mundy, A. R. (2002). Current concepts in the pharmacotherapy of benign prostatic hyperplasia. *Expert Opinion on Pharmacotherapy, 3*(12), 1727–1737.

Mcleod, D. G. (2003). Hormonal therapy: Historical perspective to future directions. *Urology, 61*(2, Suppl. 1), 3–7.

Steiner, B. S. (2002). Hypogonadism in men. A review of diagnosis and treatment. *Advanced Nursing Practice, 10*(4), 22–27, 29.

Susman, E. (2003). *ACC: Investigative anti-impotence drug appears with antihypertensive medications,* http://www.docguide.com/news/content.nsf/PatientResAllCateg/Erectile%20Dysfunction?OpenDocument#News

Suzuki, T., Nakamura, Y., Moriya, T., & Sasano, H. (2003). Effects of steroid hormones on vascular functions. *Microscopy Research and Technique, 60*(1), 76–84.

The Canadian Prostate Health Council, http://www.canadian-prostate.com

Thiyagarajan, M. (2002). Alpha-adrenoceptor antagonists in the treatment of benign prostate hyperplasia. *Pharmacology, 65*(3), 119–128.

Chapter 43

Armstrong, L. E., Casa, D. J., Maresh, C. M., & Ganio, M. S. (2007). Caffeine, fluid-electrolyte balance, temperature regulation, and exercise-heat tolerance. *Exercise and Sport Sciences Reviews.* Available: http://www.medscape.com/viewarticle/559762_1

Bard, R. L., Barry, M. A., Bleske, E. & Nicklas, J. M. (2004). Food: An unrecognized source of loop diuretic resistance. *Pharmacotherapy, 24,* 630–637.

Costello-Boerrigter, L. C., Boerrigter, G., & Burnett, J. C. (2003). Revisiting salt and water retention: New diuretics, aquaretics, and natriuretics. *Medical Clinics of North America 87*(2), 475–491.

Hawkins, R. G., & Houston, M. C. (2005). Is population-wide diuretic use directly associated with the incidence of end-stage renal disease in the United States? A hypothesis. *American Journal of Hypertension, 18,* 744–749.

Kidney Foundation of Canada. (2006). *Winter 2006 statistics.* Retrieved August 8, 2007, from http://www.kidney.sk.ca/prevention/statistics/canada.html

Klarenbach, S. W., Moist, L. M., Foley, R. N., Barrett, B. J., Madore, F., White, C. T., et al. (2008). Clinical practice guidelines for supplemental therapies and issues. *Canadian Society of Nephrology. Kidney International, 110,* S19–24.

Moist, L. M., Foley, R. N., Barrett, B. J., Madore, F., White, C. T., Klarenbach, S. W., et al. (2008). Clinical practice guidelines for evidence-based use of erythropoietic-stimulating agents. *Canadian Society of Nephrology. Kidney International, 110,* S12–18.

Verbalis, J. G., Goldsmith, S. R., Greenberg, A., Schrier, R. W., & Sterns, R. H. (2007). Hyponatremia treatment guidelines 2007: Expert panel recommendations. *American Journal of Medicine, 120*(11 Suppl. 1), S1–21.

Wassertheil-Smoller, S., Psaty, B., Greenland, P., et al. (2004). Association between cardiovascular outcomes and antihypertensive drug treatment in older women. *Journal of the American Medical Association, 292,* 2849–2859.

Chapter 44

Adrogue, H. J. (2006). Metabolic acidosis: Pathophysiology, diagnosis and management. *Journal of Nephrology, 19*(Suppl. 9), S62–9.

Bhananker, S. M., Paek, R., & Vavilala, M. S. (2004). Water intoxication and symptomatic hyponatremia after outpatient surgery. *Anesthesia & Analgesia, 98*(5), 1294–1296.

Chio, P. T. L., Gordon, Y., Quinonez, L. G., et al. (1999). Crystalloids vs. colloids in fluid resuscitation: A systemic review. *Critical Care Medicine, 27*(1), 200–203.

Kamel, K. S., & Halperin, M. L. (2006). An improved approach to the patient with metabolic acidosis: A need for four amendments. *Journal of Nephrology,19*(Suppl. 9), S76–85.

Moviat, M., van Haren, F.,& van der Hoeven, J. G. (2003). Conventional or physicochemical approach in intensive care unit patients with metabolic acidosis. *Critical Care, 7*(3), R41–R45.

Pham, P. C., Pham, P. M., & Pham, P. T. (2000). Vasopressin excess and hyponatremia. *American Journal of Kidney Disease, 47,* 727–737.

Rose, B. D. (2000). *Clinical physiology of acid-base and electrolyte disorders* (5th ed.). New York: McGraw-Hill.

Rosenthal, K. (2006). The whys and wherefores of I.V. fluids. *Nursing Made Incredibly Easy, 4*(3), 8–11.

Takil, A., Eti, Z., Irmak, P., et al. (2002). Early postoperative respiratory acidosis after large intravascular volume infusion of lactated ringer's solution during major spine surgery. *Anesthesia & Analgesia, 95,* 294–298.

Wilmore, D. (2000). Nutrition and metabolic support in the 21st century. *Journal of Parenteral & Enteral Nutrition, 4*(1), 1–4.

Chapter 45

Dystonia. (2003). *Botulism toxin injections.* Dystonia Medical Research Foundation, http://www.dystonia-foundation.org/treatment/botox.asp

Dystonia. (2003). *Complementary therapy.* Dystonia Medical Research Foundation, http://www.dystonia-foundation.org/treatment/comp.asp

Dystonia. (2003). *Dystonia defined.* Dystonia Medical Research Foundation, http://www.dystonia-foundation.org/defined/

Health Canada. (2008). *Health Canada reviewing issue of distant toxin spread potentially associated with Botox and Botox Cosmetic.* Available: http://www.hc-sc.gc.ca/ahc-asc/media/advisories-avis/_2008/2008_32-eng.php

Medlineplus. (2003). *Spasticity.* National Institute of Health, http://www.nlm.nih.gov/medlineplus/ency/article/003297.htm

National Institute of Neurological Disorders and Stroke. (2003). *NINDS spasticity information page.* National Institute of Health, http://nindsupdate.ninds.nih.gov/health_and_medical/disorders/spasticity_doc.htm

Nelson, A., Ragan, B. J., Bell, G. W., Ichiyama, R. M., & Iwamoto, G. A. (2004). Capsaic in-based analgesic balm decreases pressor responses evoked by muscle afferents. *Medicine & Science in Sports & Exercise, 36*(3): 444–450.

Van Beek A.L., Lim P.K., Gear A.J., & Pritzker M. R. (2007). Management of vasospastic disorders with botulinum toxin A. *Plastic and Reconstructive Surgery, 119,* 217–26.

Ward, A. B., Molenaers, G., Colosimo, C., & Berardelli, A. (2006). Clinical value of botulinum toxin in neurological indications. *European Journal of Neurology, 13*(Suppl. 4), 20–26.

Chapter 46

Brown, J. P., & Josse, R. G. (2002). Clinical practice guidelines for the diagnosis and management of osteoporosis in Canada. *Canadian Medical Association Journal, 167,* S1–34.

Brown, J., & Fortier, M. (2006). Canadian Consensus Conference on Osteoporosis, 2006 Update. *Society of Obstetricians and Gynaecologists of Canada, 172,* S95–S112.

Canadian Arthritis Society publications and guidelines for management. (2008). Available: http://www.arthritis.ca/local%20programs/ontario/publications%20and%20resources/publications/default.asp?s=1

Canadian Institutes of Health Research. (2007). *Bone research—a structural support—an important mineral depot.* Retrieved March 19, 2007, from http://www.cihr-irsc.gc.ca/cgi-bin/print-imprimer.pl

Centre for Effective Practice. (2008). http://www.effectivepractice.org/

Clegg, D. O., Reda, D. J., Harris, C. L., Klein, M. A., O'Dell, J. R., Hooper, M. M., et al. (2006). Glucosamine, chondroitin sulfate, and the two in combination for painful knee osteoarthritis. *New England Journal of Medicine, 354*(8), 795–808.

Clemett, D., & Goa, K. L. (2000). Celecoxib. A review of its use in osteoarthritis, rheumatoid arthritis and acute pain. *Drugs, 59*(4), 957–980.

Curry, L. C., & Hogstel, M. O. (2002). Osteoporosis. *American Journal of Nursing, 102,* 26–32.

Drenth, J. P. H., & Verheugt, F. W. A. (2007). Do cox-2 inhibitors give enough gastrointestinal protection? *Lancet, 369,* 439–440.

Health & Welfare Canada, Health Protection Branch: Mandatory Addition of Vitamins A and D to Milk—Background Paper. Ottawa: Nutrition Evaluation Division, Food Directorate, 1990.

Jelley, M. J., & Wortmann, R. (2000). Practical steps in the diagnosis and management of gout. *BioDrugs, 14*(2), 99–107.

Lacki, J. K. (2000). Management of the patient with severe refractory rheumatoid arthritis. Are the newer treatment options worth considering? *BioDrugs, 13*(6), 425–435.

Laine, L., Curtis, S. P., Cryer, B., Kaur, A., & Cannon, C. P. (2007). Assessment of upper gastrointestinal safety of etoricoxib and diclofenac in patients with osteoarthritis and rheumatoid arthritis in the Multinational Etoricoxib and Diclofenac Arthritis Long-term (MEDAL) programme: A randomised comparison. *Lancet, 369*(9560), 465.

Love, C. (2003). Dietary needs for bone health and the prevention of osteoporosis. *British Journal of Nursing, 12*(1), 12–21.

Manek, N., & Lane, N. (2000). Osteoarthritis: Current concepts in diagnosis and management. *American Academy of Family Physicians, 61*(6).

Marcus, R. (2001). Agents affecting calcification and bone turnover: Calcium, phosphate, parathyroid hormone, vitamin D, calcitonin and other compounds. In J. G. Hardman, L. E. Limbard, & A. G. Goodman (Eds.), *The pharmacological basis of therapeutics* (10th ed.). New York: McGraw-Hill.

Orwoll, E. S. (1999). Osteoporosis in men. *New Dimensions in Osteoporosis, 1*(5), 2–8, 12.

Prestwood, K. M. (2000). Prevention and treatment of osteoporosis. *Clinical Cornerstone, 2*(6), 34–44.

Roberts, L. J., Morrow, J. D. (2001). Analgesic-antipyretic and anti-inflammatory agents employed in the treatment of gout. In J. G. Hardman, L. E. Limbard, & A. G. Goodman (Eds.), *The pharmacological basis of therapeutics* (10th ed.). New York: McGraw-Hill.

Rucker, D., Allan, J. A., Fick, G.H., & Hanley, D. A. (2002). Vitamin D insufficiency in a population of healthy Western Canadians. *Canadian Medical Association Journal,166,* 1517–1524.

Sanofi-synthelabs. (2003). *Hyalgan-sodium hyaluraonte solutions,* http://www.sanofi-synthelabous.com

Siminoski, K., Leslie, W. D., Frame, H., Hodsman, A., Josse, R. G., Khan, A., et al. (2005). Recommendations for bone mineral density reporting in Canada. *CAR Clinical Practice Guidelines, 56*(3), 178–188.

Vieth, R., Cole, D. E., Hawker, G. A., Trang, H. M., & Rubin, L. A. (2001). Wintertime vitamin D insufficiency is common in young Canadian women, and their vitamin D intake does not prevent it. *European Journal of Clinical Nutrition, 55,* 1091–1097.

Chapter 47

Canadian Dermatology Association, http://www.dermatology.ca

Feldman, S. (2000). Advances in psoriasis treatment. *Dermatology Online, 6*(1), 4.

Fox, L. P., Merk, H. F., & Bickers, D. R. (2006). Dermatological pharmacology. In L. L. Brunton, J. S. Lazo, & K. L. Parker (Eds.), *Goodman & Gilman's The pharmacological basis of therapeutics* (11th ed., pp. 1679–1706). New York: McGraw-Hill.

Hooper, B. J. (1999). *Primary dermatologic care.* St. Louis: Mosby, Inc.

Leung, D. Y., & Boguniewicz, M. (2003). Advances in allergic skin diseases. *Journal of Allergy and Clinical Immunology, 111*(3, Suppl.), S805–S812.

Lindow, K. B., & Warren, C. (2001). Understanding rosacea: A guide to facilitating care. *American Journal of Nursing, 101,* 44–51.

Murphy, K. D., Lee, J. O., & Herndon, D. N. (2003). Current pharmacotherapy for the treatment of severe burns. *Expert Opinion in Pharmacotherapy, 4*(3), 369–384.

Oprica, C., Emtestam, L., & Nord, C. E. (2001). Overview of treatments for acne. *Dermatology Nursing, 14,* 242–246.

Psoriasis Society of Canada, http://www.psoriasissociety.org

Roos, T. C., & Merk, H. F. (2000). Important drug interactions in dermatology. *Drugs 59*(2), 181–192.

Smith, G. (2003). Cutaneous expression of cytochrome P-450 CYP25: Individuality in regulation by therapeutic agents for psoriasis and other skin diseases. *Lancet, 361,* 1336–1344.

Wyatt, E. L., Sutter, S. H., & Drake, L. A. (2001). Dermatological pharmacology. In J. G. Hardman, L. E. Limbard, & A. G. Goodman (Eds.), *The pharmacological basis of therapeutics* (pp. 1795–1818). New York: McGraw-Hill.

Chapter 48

Academy of Family Physicians. (2004). Diagnosis and management of acute otitis media. *Pediatrics, 113,* 1451–1465.

Clinical Practice Committee (2004). *Clinical procedure guideline—Ear drops: Administration.* London: Great Ormond Street Hospital.

De, M., McDonald, P., & Vaughan-Jones, R. (2007). Variability of ear drops in normal population: An accurate delivery device required. *The Internet Journal of Otorhinolaryngology, 6*(1), 143–147.

Eskola J, Kilpi T, Palmu A, et al. (2001). Efficacy of a pneumococcal conjugate vaccine against acute otitis media. *New England Journal of Medicine, 344,* 403–409.

Fireman, B., Black, S. B., Shinefield, H. R., et al. (2003). Impact of the pneumococcal conjugate vaccine on otitis media. *Pediatric Infectious Diseases, 22,* 10–16.

Henderer, J. D., & Rapuano, C. J. (2006). Ocular Pharmacology. In L. L. Brunton, J. S. Lazo, & K. L. Parker (Eds.), *Goodman & Gilman's The pharmacological basis of therapeutics* (11th ed., pp. 1707–1737). New York: McGraw-Hill.

Johnson, D. L., Swank, P. R., Owen, M. J., et al. (2000). The effects of early middle ear effusion on child intelligence at 3, 5 and 7 years of age. *Journal of Pediatric Psychology, 25,* 5–13.

Leibovitz, E., & Dagan, R. (2001). Pediatric infection: Otitis media therapy and drug resistance. Part 2: Current concepts and new directions. *Infections in Medicine, 18*(5), 263–270.

Little, P., Gould, C., Williamson, I., et al. (2001). Pragmatic randomized controlled trial of two prescribing strategies for childhood acute otitis media. *British Medical Journal, 322,* 336–342.

McCaig, L. F., Besser, R. E., & Hughes, J. M. (2002). Trends in antimicrobial prescribing rates for children and adolescents. *Journal of the American Medical Association, 287,* 3096–3102.

McCormick, D. P., Baldwin, C. D., Friedman, N., et al. (2003). Bullous myringitis: A case-control study. *Pediatrics, 112,* 982–986.

Pappas, S., Nikolopoulos, T. P., Korres, S., Papacharalampous, G., Tzangarulakis, A., & Ferekidis, E. (2006). Topical antibiotic ear drops: Are they safe? *International Journal of Clinical Practice, 60,* 1115–1119.

Siegel, R. M., Kiely, M., Bien, J., et al. (2003). Treatment of otitis media with observation and a safety-net prescription. *Pediatrics, 112,* 527–531.

INDEX

Page numbers followed by *f* indicate figures and those followed by *t* indicate tables, boxes, or special features. The titles of special features (e.g. PharmFacts) are also capitalized.

Prototype drugs appear in **boldface**, drug classifications are in SMALL CAPS, and trade names are capitalized and cross-referenced to their generic name. Diseases, disorders, and conditions are in red type.

A

abacavir 466*t*
Abbokinase. *See* urokinase
abciximab
    for angina pectoris 291*t*
    for anticoagulant therapy 336*t*
    for myocardial infarction 299
Abelcet. *See* **amphotericin B**
abortion
    pharmacological agents for
        carboprost tromethamine 589*t*, 590–591
        dinoprostone 589*t*, 590–591
        mechanism of action 590–591
        methotrexate with misoprostol 589*t*, 590–591
        mifepristone with misoprostol 589*t*, 590–591
Abreva. *See* docosanol
abscesses 422*t*
absence (petit mal) seizures 157, 162, 163, 164–166
absorption
    definition 27
    factors affecting 28–28*f*
    mechanisms 26*f*–27*f*, 27
acarbose 576*t*, 578
Accolate. *See* zafirlukast
Accupril. *See* quinapril
Accutane. *See* **isotretinoin**
acebutolol 138*t*, 322*t*
ACE inhibitors. *See* ANGIOTENSIN-CONVERTING ENZYME INHIBITORS
acetaminophen
    actions and uses 408*t*
    administration alerts 408*t*
    adverse effects 17*t*, 50, 408*t*
    for allergic rhinitis 411*t*
    as an antipyretic 408
    ethnic considerations 408*t*
    as an non-opioid analgesic 220, 225, 225*t*
    pharmacokinetics 408*t*
Acetazolam. *See* acetazolamide
acetazolamide 623, 624*t*, 689*t*–690*t*, 690
acetic acid and hydrocortisone 695*t*
acetohexamide 576*t*
Acetonide. *See* **prednisone**
acetylcholine (Ach)
    physiology 21–22
    receptors 126–128, 127*t*
acetylcholinesterase (AchE) 127–128, 129

ACETYLCHOLINESTERASE INHIBITORS. *See* CHOLINERGICS, indirect-acting
acetylcysteine 17*t*, 380*t*, 381
acetylsalicylic acid
    actions and uses 28, 28*f*, 227*t*
    administration alerts 227*t*
    adverse effects 227*t*
    for inflammation 403*t*
    pharmacokinetics 227*t*
    pharmacotherapy with 225
    route and dosage 225*t*
    trade names 12*t*
AchE. *See* acetylcholinesterase
acid-base balance. *See also* acidosis; alkalosis 636–637, 637*f*
acidophilus 107*t*, 451*t*, 522*t*
acidosis
    causes 637*f*, 637*t*
    natural therapy with sea vegetables 639*t*
    nursing considerations 637–639
    pharmacotherapy 637
acid production 502, 502*f*–503*f*
acitretin 683, 683*t*
acne vulgaris
    characteristics 678
    natural therapy with burdock root 680*t*
    pharmacotherapy 678–679
        adapalene 679*t*
        azelaic acid 679*t*
        benzoyl peroxide 678–679, 679*t*
        doxycycline 679, 679*t*
        estradiol 679, 679*t*
        isotretinoin. *See* **isotretinoin**
        nursing considerations 679–680
        sulfacetamide sodium 679*t*
        tetracycline. *See* **tetracycline**
        tretinoin 679, 679*t*
Acova. *See* argatroban
acquired antimicrobial resistance 424, 425*f*
acquired immunodeficiency syndrome. *See also* HIV-AIDS 464
ACTH. *See* adrenocorticotropic hormone; corticotropin
Actifed. *See* pseudoephedrine; triprolidine
Actifed Cold and Allergy tablets 411*t*
Actifed Cold and sinus caplets 411*t*
action potentials 319
Activa C. *See* vitamin C
Activase. *See* **alteplase**
activated partial thromboplastin time (aPTT) 333

active immunity 389–390*f*
active transport 26–27
Actonel. *See* risedronate sodium
Actos. *See* pioglitazone
acute gouty arthritis 666, 667*t*
acute insulin response 576
acute radiation syndrome 23
acute toxicity 16
acyclovir
    actions and uses 472*t*
    administration alerts 472*t*
    adverse effects 472*t*
    for herpes viruses 471*t*, 472
    pharmacokinetics 472*t*
AD. *See* Alzheimer's disease
Adalat. *See* nifedipine
Adamsite 22*t*
adapalene 679, 679*t*
ADD. *See* attention deficit disorder
addiction. *See also* substance addiction 113
Addison's disease 562
adefovir 474, 474*t*
A-delta fibres 218
Adenocard. *See* adenosine
adenohypophysis 550
adenosine 130, 326
ADHD. *See* attention deficit-hyperactivity disorder
adolescence
    definition 51
    pharmacotherapy for 51–52
    psychosocial impacts of diabetes 575*t*
ADR. *See* adverse drug reaction
adrenal cortex. *See also* adrenal glands
    disorders 550*t*
    feedback control 561–561*f*
adrenal glands
    diseases
        Addison's disease 562
        Cushing's syndrome 563, 564–566*t*
        pharmacotherapy
        glucocorticoids. *See* GLUCOCORTICOIDS
    glucocorticoid secretion control 561
    normal function 561
Adrenalin. *See* epinephrine
ADRENERGIC AGONISTS (SYMPATHOMIMETICS)
    ALPHA. *See* ALPHA-ADRENERGIC AGONISTS (SYMPATHOMIMETICS)
    BETA. *See* BETA-ADRENERGIC AGONISTS (SYMPATHOMIMETICS)

Credits

All photographs not listed below are acknowledged on page.

Interior Art and Photographs: Unit 1: Shirley L. King (Figures 1.1, 1.2, 4.3). Units 2 and 3: Shirley L. King (Figures 8.5, 11.1, 11.2); Jim Dowdalls/Photo Researchers, Inc.; © Jan Hurd/Phototake. Unit 4: Custom Medical Stock. Unit 5: Figures 21.4, 24.2, and 24.4 adapted with the permission of the Canadian Cardio-vascular Society; David Mack/Photo Researchers, Inc. Unit 6: © Steve Oh, M.S./Phototake. Unit 7: Shirley L. King (Figure 38.1); © Steve Oh, M.S./Phototake. Unit 8: Michael Freeman/Phototake; Unit 9: Custom Medical Stock.

Interior Illustrations: Precision Graphics, Imagineering

"AS IS" LICENSE AGREEMENT AND LIMITED WARRANTY